OXFORD MEDICAL PUBLICATIONS

Effective Care in
Pregnancy and Childbirth

EDITORS

Iain Chalmers MB BS, MSc, DCH, FFCM, FRCOG
Director, National Perinatal Epidemiology Unit,
Oxford

Murray Enkin MD, FRCS(C), FACOG
Professor Emeritus,
Departments of Obstetrics and Gynaecology, and
Clinical Epidemiology and Biostatistics,
McMaster University

Marc J. N. C. Keirse MD, DPhil, DPH
Professor of Obstetrics,
Leiden University and
Visiting Professor of Obstetrics,
University of Leuven

Effective Care in Pregnancy and Childbirth

VOLUME 2: CHILDBIRTH

PARTS VI–X AND INDEX

Edited by

IAIN CHALMERS   MURRAY ENKIN

MARC J. N. C. KEIRSE

Foreword by

ARCHIE COCHRANE

Oxford · New York · Toronto
OXFORD UNIVERSITY PRESS

Oxford University Press, Walton Street, Oxford OX2 6DP

Oxford New York Toronto
Delhi Bombay Calcutta Madras Karachi
Petaling Jaya Singapore Hong Kong Tokyo
Nairobi Dar es Salaam Cape Town
Melbourne Auckland
and associated companies in
Berlin Ibadan

Oxford is a trade mark of Oxford University Press

Published in the United States
by Oxford University Press, New York

First published 1989
Reprinted (with corrections) 1991

British Library Cataloguing in Publication Data
Effective care in pregnancy and childbirth.
1. Pregnant women. Medical care.
I. Chalmers, Iain.   II. Enkin, Murray.   III. Keirse
Marc J. N. C.
618.2'4
ISBN 0–19–261558–0 v.1.
ISBN 0–19–261880–6 v.2.

Library of Congress Cataloging in Publication Data
(Data available)

Set by Latimer Trend & Company Limited, Plymouth
Printed and bound by Bookcraft (Bath) Ltd.

Contents

Contributors

Sophie Alexander MD. Obstetrician, École de Santé Publique, Université Libre de Bruxelles, Campus Erasme CP 590/5, 808 route de Lennik, 1070 Brussels, Belgium.

Douglas Altman BSc. Head, Medical Statistics Laboratory, Imperial Cancer Research Fund, P O Box 123, Lincoln's Inn Fields, London WC2A 3PX, UK.

Jill Astbury BA, MEd, PhD. Lecturer, Key Centre for Women's Health in Society, Department of Community Medicine, University of Melbourne, Parkville 3052, Australia.

Cornelia J. Baines MD, MSc. Associate Professor, Dept Preventive Medicine & Biostatistics, University of Toronto, Toronto, Ontario, Canada M5S 1A8.

Leiv S. Bakketeig MD. Head, Department of Epidemiology, National Institute of Public Health, Geitmyrsveien, N-0462 Oslo 4, Norway.

David Banta MD, MPH, MS. Professor of Technology Assessment, Department of Health Economics, University of Limburg, P O Box 616, 6200 MD Maastricht, The Netherlands.

Jack Bennebroek Gravenhorst MD. Professor of Obstetrics and Gynaecology, Leiden University, University Hospital, Rijnsburgerweg 10, 2333 AA Leiden, The Netherlands.

Howard M. Berger MD, MRCP, BSc. Senior Lecturer, Department of Neonatology, University of Leiden, University Hospital, Rijnsburgerweg 10, 2333 AA Leiden, The Netherlands.

Per Bergsjø MD, PhD. Professor and Head of Department of Obstetrics and Gynaecology, University of Bergen, Kvinneklinikken, Haukeland Sykehus, N-5021, Bergen, Norway.

Eve Blair PhD. Research Officer, NH and MRC Research Unit in Epidemiology and Preventive Medicine, University Department of Medicine, The Queen Elizabeth II Medical Centre, University of Western Australia, Nedlands, Perth, Western Australia 6009, Australia.

Béatrice Blondel BA, MA, PhD. Chargée de Recherches, Groupe de Recherches Épidémiologiques sur la Mère et l'Enfant, INSERM Unité 149, 16 Avenue Paul-Vaillant-Couturier, 94807 Villejuif, France.

Martin Bobrow DSc, MB BCh, FRCP, MRCPath. Prince Philip Professor of Paediatric Research, University of London, Paediatric Research Unit, Division of Medical and Molecular Biology, United Medical and Dental Schools of Guy's and St Thomas' Hospitals, 8th Floor, Guy's Tower, Guy's Hospital, London Bridge, London SE1 9RT, UK.

Michael Bracken PhD, MPH, MPhil, BSc, FACE. Professor of Epidemiology, and Obstetrics and Gynaecology, Department of Epidemiology and Public Health, Yale University Medical School, 60 College Street, New Haven, Connecticut 06510, USA.

Ian Brown MB BS, FRCOG. Honorary Lecturer, Department of Obstetrics and Gynaecology, University of Zimbabwe, Harare Maternity Hospital, P O Box ST14, Southerton, Harare, Zimbabwe.

Robert Bryce MB BS, MSc, MRCOG, FRACOG. Senior Research Officer, NH and MRC Unit in Epidemiology and Preventive Medicine, University Department of Medicine, The Queen Elizabeth II Medical Centre, University of Western Australia, Nedlands, Perth, Western Australia 6009, Australia.

Pierre Buekens MD. Obstetrician, Université Libre de Bruxelles, École de Santé Publique, Campus Erasme CP 590/5, 808 route de Lennik, 1070 Bruxelles, Belgium.

Hubert Campbell MA, MB BS, FRCP, FFCM, FSS. Emeritus Professor of Medical Statistics, University of Wales College of Medicine, Pwll Coch Uchaf, Druidstone Road, Cardiff CF3 9XE, UK.

Iain Chalmers MB BS, MSc, DCH, FFCM, FRCOG. Director, National Perinatal Epidemiology Unit, Radcliffe Infirmary, Oxford OX2 6HE, UK.

Thomas Chalmers MD. Distinguished Physician, Veterans Administration; Lecturer, Harvard School of Public Health; President and Dean Emeritus, Mt Sinai Medical Center, New York. Technology Assessment Group, Harvard University School of Public Health, 677 Huntington Avenue, Boston, Massachusetts 02115, USA.

Rory Collins MB BS, MSc. British Heart Foundation Senior Research Fellow, University of Oxford, Clinical Trials Service Unit, Radcliffe Infirmary, Oxford OX2 6HE, UK.

Patricia Crowley MB BCh, DCH, MRCOG, MRCPI. Senior Lecturer, Department of Obstetrics and Gynaecology, University College Dublin, Coombe Lying-in Hospital, Dolphins Barn, Dublin 8, Republic of Ireland.

Caroline Crowther MB ChB, DCH, MRCOG. Senior Lecturer in Obstetrics and Gynaecology, University of Adelaide, Department of Obstetrics, Queen Elizabeth Hospital, Woodville Road, Woodville, South Australia 5011, Australia.

Michael Daker PhD. Senior Lecturer in Cytogenetics, University of London, Paediatric Research Unit, Division of Medical and Molecular Biology, United Medical and Dental Schools of Guy's and St Thomas' Hospitals, 8th Floor, Guy's Tower, Guy's Hospital, London Bridge, London SE1 9RT, UK.

Kay Dickersin MA PhD. Assistant Professor, Department of Ophthalmology, University of Maryland School of Medicine, 22 South Greene St, Baltimore, Maryland 21201, USA.

Michael Drummond BSc, MCom, DPhil. Director, Health Services Management Centre, University of Birmingham, Park House, 40 Edgbaston Park Road, Birmingham B15 2RT, UK.

Diana Elbourne BSc, MSc, PhD. Social Statistician, National Perinatal Epidemiology Unit, Radcliffe Infirmary, Oxford OX2 6HE, UK.

Eleanor Enkin BHSc. Honorary Research Assistant, National Perinatal Epidemiology Unit, 47 Bowman Street, Hamilton, Ontario, Canada L8S 2T5.

Murray Enkin MD, FRCS(C), FACOG. Professor Emeritus, Departments of Obstetrics and Gynaecology, and Clinical Epidemiology and Biostatistics, McMaster University, 1200 Main Street West, Hamilton, Ontario, Canada L8N 3Z5.

Gillian C. Forrest MB BS, MRCPsych, MRCGP. Consultant Child Psychiatrist, The Park Hospital for Children, Old Road, Headington, Oxford OX3 7LQ, UK.

Robert Fraser MD, MRCOG, DCH. Senior Lecturer/Honorary Consultant, Department of Obstetrics and Gynaecology, University of Sheffield, Clinical Sciences Centre, Northern General Hospital, Herries Road, Sheffield S5 7AU, UK.

Jo Garcia BA, MSc. Social Scientist, National Perinatal Epidemiology Unit, Radcliffe Infirmary, Oxford OX2 6HE, UK.

Sally Garforth BNurs, SCM. Formerly Research Midwife, National Perinatal Epidemiology Unit, 15 Clifton Park Road, Caversham, Reading PG4 7PD, UK.

Peter A. Goldstein BA. Medical Student, Mt Sinai School of Medicine of the City University of New York (CUNY), Clinical Trials Unit, Mt Sinai Medical Center, One Gustave Levy Place, New York, NY 10029, USA.

Adrian Grant DM, MSc, MRCOG. Epidemiologist, National Perinatal Epidemiology Unit, Radcliffe Infirmary, Oxford OX2 6HE, UK.

John Grant MB ChB, MRCP, MRCOG. Consultant Obstetrician and Gynaecologist, Bellshill Maternity Hospital, North Road, Bellshill NL4 3JN, UK.

Jane Green BA, BM BCh, DPhil. Honorary Research Associate, National Perinatal Epidemiology Unit, Radcliffe Infirmary, Oxford OX2 6HE, UK.

Elina Hemminki MD. Assistant Professor, Department of Public Health, University of Helsinki, Haartmaninkatu 3, 00290 Helsinki, Finland.

Jini Hetherington. Unit Administrator, National Perinatal Epidemiology Unit, Radcliffe Infirmary, Oxford OX2 6HE, UK.

G. Justus Hofmeyr MB BCh, MRCOG. Professor and Head, Department of Obstetrics and Gynaecology, Coronation Hospital and University of the Witwatersrand Medical School, York Road, Parktown 2193, South Africa.

David J. S. Hunter MB ChB, FRCOG, FRCS(C). Professor, Department of Obstetetrics and Gynaecology, McMaster University, 1200 Main Street West, Hamilton, Ontario, Canada L8N 3Z5.

Frank Hytten MD, PhD, FRCOG. Editor Emeritus, British Journal of Obstetrics and Gynaecology, 27 Sussex Place, Regent's Park, London NW1 4RG, UK.

Sally Inch SRN, SCM. Midwife, Oxfordshire Health Authority, 3 Willow Close, Garsington, Oxford OX9 9AN, UK.

Claire Johnson. Medical Student, University of Oxford, Green College, 43 Woodstock Road, Oxford OX2 6HG, UK.

Humphrey H. H. Kanhai MD. Senior Lecturer, Leiden University, Department of Obstetrics, University Hospital, Rijnsburgerweg 10, 2333 AA Leiden, The Netherlands.

Marc J. N. C. Keirse MD, DPhil, DPH. Professor of Obstetrics, Leiden University and Visiting Professor University of Leuven, Belgium; Leiden University Hospital, Rijnsburgerweg 10, 2333 AA Leiden, The Netherlands.

James King MB BS, FRCS, FRCOG, FRACOG. Medical Superintendent, Mater Mothers' Hospital, South Brisbane, Queensland 4101, Australia.

Sheila Kitzinger MLitt. Standlake Manor, Standlake, nr Witney, Oxon OX8 7RH, UK.

Michael Klein MD, CCFP, FCFP, ABFP, FCPS, FAAP. Professor Family Medicine, Chief and Director, The Herzl Family Practice Centre, McGill University School of Medicine, 5750 Côte de Neiges, Montreal PQ, Canada H3S 1Y7.

Alessandro Liberati MD. Chief, Clinical Epidemiology Unit, Mario Negri Institute, Istituto Mario Negri, Via Eritrea 62, 20157 Milano, Italy.

Jonathan Lomas MA. Associate Professor; Associate Coordinator, Centre for Health Economics and Policy Analysis, Department of Clinical Epidemiology and Biostatistics, McMaster University, 1200 Main Street West, Hamilton, Ontario, Canada L8N 3Z5.

Judith Lumley MA, MB BS, PhD. Senior Lecturer, Monash University, Department of Paediatrics, Queen Victoria Children's Hospital, Monash Medical Centre, 246 Clayton Road, Clayton, Victoria 3168, Australia.

Sally MacIntyre BA, MSc, PhD. Director, Medical Research Council Medical Sociology Unit, University of Glasgow, 6 Lilybank Gardens, Glasgow G12 8QQ, UK.

Kassam Mahomed MB ChB, MRCOG. Lecturer, Department of Obstetrics and Gynaecology, University of Zimbabwe, Harare Maternity Hospital, P O Box ST14, Southerton, Harare, Zimbabwe.

Patrick Mohide MD, FRCS(C), MSc. Associate Professor, Department of Obstetrics and Gynaecology, McMaster University, 1200 Main Street West, Hamilton, Ontario, Canada L8N 3Z5.

Miranda Mugford BA. Economist, National Perinatal Epidemiology Unit, Radcliffe Infirmary, Oxford OX2 6HE, UK.

Cornelis Naaktgeboren PhD. Former leader, Research Group for Comparative Obstetrics, University of Amsterdam, Dorpsweg K157, 1676 GK Twisk, The Netherlands.

James Neilson BSc, MD, MRCOG. Senior Lecturer, Department of Obstetrics and Gynaecology, University of Edinburgh, Centre for Reproductive Biology, 37 Chalmers Street, Edinburgh EH3 9EW, UK.

Ann Oakley MA PhD. Deputy Director, Thomas Coram Research Unit, 41 Brunswick Square, London WC1N 1AZ, UK.

Arne Ohlsson MD, FRCP(C). Staff Neonatologist, Regional Perinatal Unit, University of Toronto, Women's College Hospital, 76 Grenville Street, Toronto, Ontario, Canada M5S 1B2.

A. Carla C. van Oppen. Staff Obstetrician, Department of Obstetrics, Leiden University Hospital, Rijnsburgerweg 10, 2333 AA Leiden, The Netherlands.

Fabio Parazzini MD. Researcher, Epidemiology Unit, Mario Negri Institute, Istituto Mario Negri, Via Eritrea 62, 20157 Milano, Italy.

John Parboosingh MB ChB, BSc, FRCOG, FRCP(C). Professor, Department of Obstetrics and Gynaecology, University of Calgary, Foothills Hospital, 1403 – 29th Street NW, Calgary, Alberta, Canada T2N 2T9.

James F. Pearson MD, FRCOG. Reader in Obstetrics and Gynaecology, University of Wales College of Medicine, Department of Obstetrics and Gynaecology, University Hospital of Wales, Heath Park, Cardiff CF4 4XN, UK.

Maureen Porter BSc, MSc, PhD. Honorary Research Fellow, Department of Sociology, Edward Wright Building, University of Aberdeen, Old Aberdeen AB9 2ZE, UK.

Shirley Post MHA. Formerly Executive Director, Canadian Institute of Child Health, Suite 105, 17 York Street, Ottawa, Ontario, Canada K1N 5S7.

Walter J. Prendiville MRCOG, MAO, FRACOG. Senior Lecturer, Department of Obstetrics and Gynaecology, University of Western Australia, King Edward Memorial Hospital, Subiaco, Western Australia 6008, Australia.

Gareth Rees MB BCh, FFARCS. Consultant Anaesthetist, Department of Anaesthetics, University Hospital of Wales, Heath Park, Cardiff CF4 4XN, UK.

Margaret Reid MA, PhD. Lecturer, Department of Community Medicine and Social and Economic Research, University of Glasgow, 2 Lilybank Gardens, Glasgow G12 8QQ, UK.

Joan Reisch PhD. Associate Professor of Family Practice and Community Medicine, Department of Paediatrics, University of Texas, Southwestern Medical Center, 5323 Harry Hines Blvd, Dallas, Texas 75235-9063, USA.

Mary J. Renfrew BSc, RGN, SCM, PhD. Midwife Researcher, National Perinatal Epidemiology Unit, Radcliffe Infirmary, Oxford OX2 6HE, UK.

Joyce Roberts CNM, PhD. Director, Graduate Nurse-Midwifery Program; Professor, School of Nursing; Associate Professor, School of Medicine. Department of Obstetrics and Gynaecology, School of Nursing C-288, University of Colorado Health Sciences Center, 4200 East Ninth Avenue, Denver, Colorado 80262, USA.

Jane Robinson MA, PhD, AIPM, RGN, ONC, RHV, HVT, Cert Ed. Director, Nursing Policy Studies Centre, University of Warwick, Coventry, Warwickshire CV4 7AL, UK.

Sarah Robinson BSc. Senior Research Fellow, Nursing Research Unit, Department of Nursing Studies,

King's College, University of London, Coleridge Building, 552 King's Road, London SW10 0UA, UK.

Patrizia Romito PhD. Researcher, Istituto di Puericultura, Ospedale Burlo Garofalo, Via dell' Istria 65/1, I-34100 Trieste, Italy.

Janet Rush RN, BScN, MHSc. Assistant Clinical Professor, Department of Nursing, McMaster University and Patient Care Coordinator, Chedoke McMaster Hospitals, Department of Nursing, 1200 Main Street West, Hamilton, Ontario, Canada L8N 3Z5.

David Rush MD. Head of Epidemiology Program, Human Nutrition Research Center on Aging, Tufts University, 711 Washington Street, Boston, Massachusetts 02111, USA.

Henry S. Sacks PhD, MD. Director, Clinical Trials Unit/Associate Professor, Department of Medicine and Biomathematics, Mt Sinai Medical Center, One Gustave Levy Place, New York, NY 10029, USA.

Marie-Josèphe Saurel-Cubizolles BA, MA, PhD. Chargée de Recherches, Groupe de Recherches Epidémiologiqes sur la Mère et l'Enfant (INSERM Unité 149), 16 Avenue Paul-Vaillant-Couturier, 94807 Villejuif, France.

Madeleine Shearer Editor, *Birth*, 110 El Camino Real, Berkeley, California 94705, USA.

William Silverman MD. 90 La Cuesta Drive, Greenbrae, California 94904, USA.

Penny Simkin BA, PT. Childbirth Educator, Consultant in Family Centred Maternity Care, 1100 23rd Avenue East, Seattle, Washington 98112, USA.

Jennifer Sleep BA. District Research Co-ordinator, West Berkshire Health Authority, Department of Midwifery, Royal Berkshire Hospital, Craven Road, Reading RG1 5AN, UK.

Fiona Smaill MB ChB, FRACP, FRCP(C). Assistant Professor, Infectious Disease and Microbiology, Department of Microbiology, McMaster University, 1200 Main Street West, Hamilton, Ontario, Canada L8N 3Z5.

Fiona Stanley MD, MSc, MFCM. Director, Western Australian Research Institute for Child Health, Princess Margaret Hospital, Subiaco, Perth 6008, Western Australia.

Rosalind Stanwell-Smith MB BCh, MRCOG, MFCM. Specialist in Community Medicine, Bristol and Weston Health Authority, 10 Marlborough Street, Bristol BS1 3NP, UK.

Michel Thiery MD, PhD, FRCOG. Professor and Chairman, Department of Obstetrics, University Hospital, De Pintelaan 135, B-900 Gent, Belgium.

Mary Ellen Thomson PhD, MSc, BSc. Manager of Research Projects, Research and Evaluation, Ministry of Health, 1515 Blanchard Street, Victoria, British Columbia, Canada V8W 3C8.

Gianni Tognoni MD. Chief, Laboratory of Clinical Pharmacology, Istituto Mario Negri, Via Eritrea 62, 20157 Milano, Italy.

Pieter Treffers MD. Professor of Obstetrics and Gynaecology, University of Amsterdam, Meibergdreet 9, 1105 Amsterdam Zuidoost, The Netherlands.

Jon E. Tyson MD. Associate Professor of Pediatrics and Obstetrics/Gynecology, University of Texas, Southwestern Medical Center, 5323 Harry Hines Blvd, Dallas, Texas 75235-9063, USA.

Aldo Vacca MB BS, DGO, MRCOG, FRACOG. Director of Obstetrics and Gynaecology, Mater Mothers' Hospital, South Brisbane, Queensland 4101, Australia.

Raymond G. De Vries BA, MA, PhD. Associate Professor, Department of Sociology, St Olaf College, Northfield, Minnesota 55057, USA.

Henk C. S. Wallenburg MD, PhD. Director of Obstetrics, Department of Obstetrics and Gynaecology, Erasmus University Medical School EE 2283, P O Box 1738, 3000 DR Rotterdam, The Netherlands.

Elaine Wang MD, CM, MSc, FRCP(C). Assistant Professor, Pediatrics, University of Toronto, Department of Infectious Diseases, Hospital for Sick Children, 555 University Avenue, Toronto, Canada M5G 1X8.

Robert Watson MB ChB, MRCOG. Consultant Obstetrician and Gynaecologist, Department of Obstetrics and Gynaecology, Barnsley District General Hospital, Gawber Road, Barnsley, S Yorks S75 2EP, UK.

Ruta Westreich MA. Staff Psychologist, Institute of Community and Family Psychiatry, Jewish General Hospital, 5750 Côte de Neiges, Montreal PQ, Canada H3T 1E2.

Flavia Zanaboni MD. Resident, Third Obstetric Gynecology Clinic, University of Milan, Istituto Provinciale Maternita Infanzio, Via M Melloni, 20188 Milano, Italy.

Luke Zander MB BChir, DCH, DObstRCOG, FRCGP. Senior Lecturer, Department of General Practice, United Medical and Dental Schools of Guy's and St Thomas', Lambeth Road Group Practice, 80 Kennington Road, London SE11 6SP, UK.

Part VI

Care during labour

48 The biology of childbirth

Cornelis Naaktgeboren

1 Introduction

Parturition is not an isolated event, but a part of the total reproductive process; all aspects of reproductive biology are interrelated. The physiology and behaviour of all mammals at the time of birth are closely regulated and integrated. From the biological point of view, the purpose of reproduction is the maintenance of the species in the struggle for life. Many adaptations have evolved to serve this purpose, and it is amazing to see the ways in which different solutions in different species effectively achieve the same end.

The differences in reproduction among different species can best be understood as adaptations to the ecology of the species. Since the aim of childbirth is to help the species to survive, it is necessary for maternal behaviour to commence immediately after birth. In many species this behaviour is mediated by the same endocrine factors that regulate the onset of parturition. From a biological as well as social point of view, bonding is a part of giving birth.

Comparative studies have contributed substantially to our knowledge and our understanding of reproductive processes. The differences that have evolved among species all developed from adaptive mutations in homologous structures in the embryo. General conclusions can, however, only be drawn when many species are studied: specific adaptations may not be extrapolated from one species to another.

All aspects of human parturition can be compared with those seen in other mammalian species. The only unique characteristic of human birth, not found in any other species is an anatomical one: the internal and external rotation of the fetal head as an adaption to the sigmoid birth tract that resulted from our upright posture. Even apes have a more or less straight birth tract, and this rotation does not occur.

All mammals try to find a safe place before they deliver their young. It is clear that this pattern of behaviour, common to all mammalian species including humans, favours the chance of survival for the off-spring. If a labouring animal is disturbed, uterine contractions are inhibited and the female is able to leave the spot and to find another safe place before she actually gives birth. This adaptive mechanism clearly shows the importance of a perception of safety and avoidance of disturbance during parturition (Naaktgeboren and Slijper 1970; Naaktgeboren and Bontekoe 1976).

In nest-building animals, the mother builds a nest well before the onset of the expulsion phase. The rabbit doe furnishes the nest with wool plucked from her fur (Fig. 48.1). The wild sow makes a nest of twigs (Martys 1982); the domestic sow does the same with straw if this

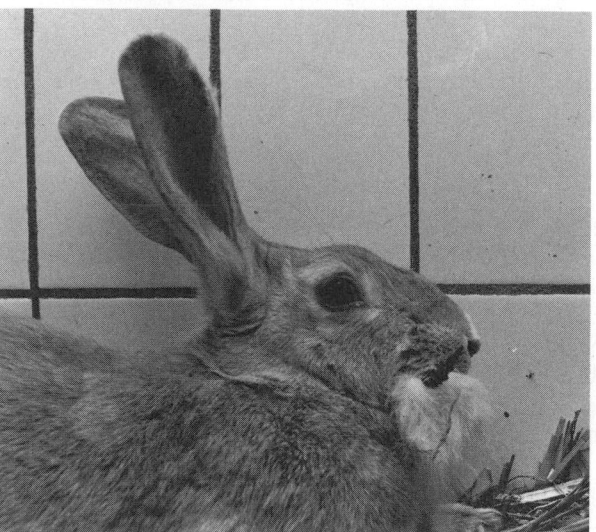

Fig. 48.1 The rabbit doe furnishes the nest with wool plucked from her fur.

is available in adequate quantity. Rats make nests of leaves or of pieces of paper. In these species it has been shown that nest-building behaviour is associated with the hormonal changes that lead to the onset of parturition or lactation (Terkel and Rosenblatt 1971). Preparation for delivery and retrieval of pups thus seem to be patterns of behaviour regulated by endocrine mechanisms. Pseudopregnant rats also build nests.

In popular scientific books and films concerned with animals and their young, the anthropomorphic term 'maternal love' is too often used. Maternal love and maternal behaviour may occur at the same time, but they are not synonymous. This was proven beyond doubt by cross-circulation experiments (Terkel and Rosenblatt 1971) which showed that maternal behaviour could be induced in virgin female rats by infusing them with blood from newly delivered rats. The changing progesterone/oestrogen ratio in the pre-parturient rabbit (Ross *et al.* 1963), or the increasing levels of prolactin in the blood of sows shortly before delivery are considered to be necessary factors for the induction of nest building.

The regulation of maternal behaviour and of the physiology of parturition and lactation are controlled by the same endocrine stimuli. It must be clear, however, that an animal is not a hormone-triggered computer. Cross-transfusions do not always induce the donor's behaviour in the recipient (Terkel and Rosenblatt 1971). To understand and appreciate an animal's maternal behaviour towards her offspring one must keep in mind the complex and strong interactions that exist between the animal's endocrine system, its physiology, and its behaviour. Overestimating or underestimating any of these aspects may lead to serious misunderstanding.

Humans are not exceptions in this respect. Lind *et al.* (1972) and Wasz-Höckert *et al.* (1972) showed that the milk ejection reflex and a rise in deep body temperature within the female breasts often takes place as soon as the mother hears or sees her baby. These physiologic responses thus occur before suckling and are not initiated by it.

It would serve little purpose to describe more examples from the vast literature of comparative research in reproduction. Two main points have been made: different species have made specific adaptations to the ecology of which they form a part; and common mechanisms, which have a fundamental value, are observed in all mammals. This is just as true for the behavioural as for the physiological, endocrinological, anatomical (and many other) aspects of parturition.

The lessons of comparative biology can only be understood when these principles of species-specific adaptation to ecology, and fundamental mechanisms applicable to all, are appreciated; otherwise, comparisons of human reproduction with that of other animals will inevitably lead to false interpretations.

Our culture, ways of living, judicial systems, and religions are parts of the ecological niche in which human beings live. These factors, which are typically human, make comparisons between humans and animals even more complicated, especially when birth in different cultures is considered (see Chapter 6). Comparative ethno-obstetrics, however, can be of great value to help us distinguish uniquely human behaviour in the biologic sense from that due to cultural influences (Schiefenhövel and Sich 1983; Naaktgeboren 1988a,b).

2 History of comparative obstetrics

The study of comparative obstetrics dates back to antiquity. Scenes depicted on Egyptian graves dating back to the third millennium BC show the birth of a calf with human assistance to the labouring cow, and of copulation, delivery, and suckling of cattle and other animals. The hieroglyph, which clearly used the bicornuate uterus of the cow for its model, was the *symbol for fertility*. This demonstrates that knowledge of reproduction and of the reproductive organs was already available in the old Egyptian kingdom.

The modern study of comparative obstetrics began in the nineteenth century, shortly after publications on veterinary obstetrics appeared at the end of the eighteenth century. In 1819, Stein delivered his professorial inaugural address on 'the differences between man and animals for clarifying the need for obstetric help in humans'. From his work it is clear that he had observed animal deliveries, and his conclusions benefited human obstetrical care. The works of Kehrer (1864, 1867), who first described the operation of lower segment caesarean section, dealt with all major problems of comparative obstetrics, including the onset of labour, parturient behaviour, duration of labour, morphology of the birth tract, size of the developed fetus, presentation of the fetus, first breathing, and severing of the umbilical cord.

Birth has been observed in many mammals, and the many scattered observations were collected by Slijper in 1960. The birth of a giraffe was first described in 1849; that of monkeys in 1906; and that of a great ape in 1915 (Slijper 1960). The first major textbook on comparative obstetrics (Naaktgeboren and Slijper 1970) is still a useful reference source.

Comparative fetal and neonatal physiology had also become a field of investigation on its own by this time (Dawes 1968; Perry 1972), and the importance of comparative reproductive biology was firmly established.

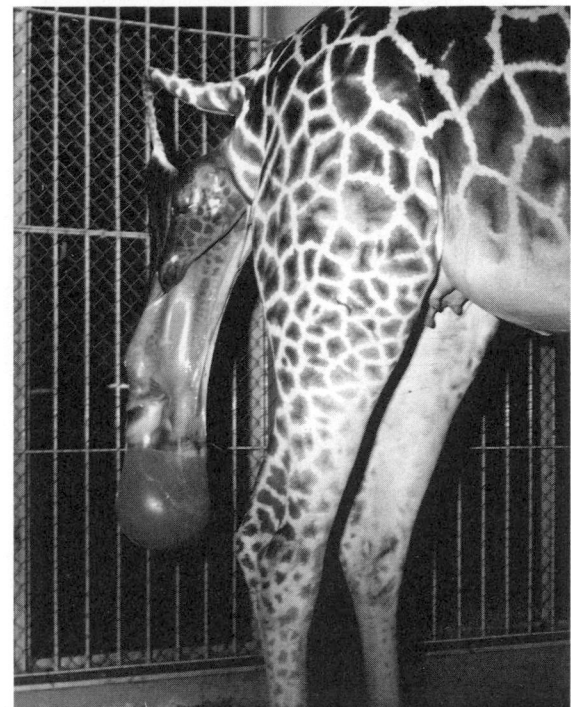

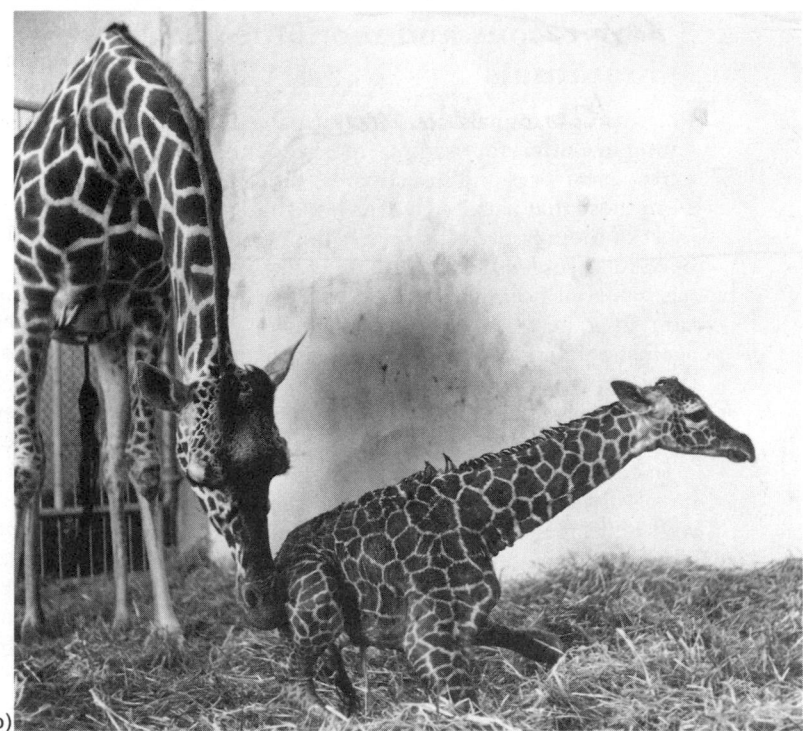

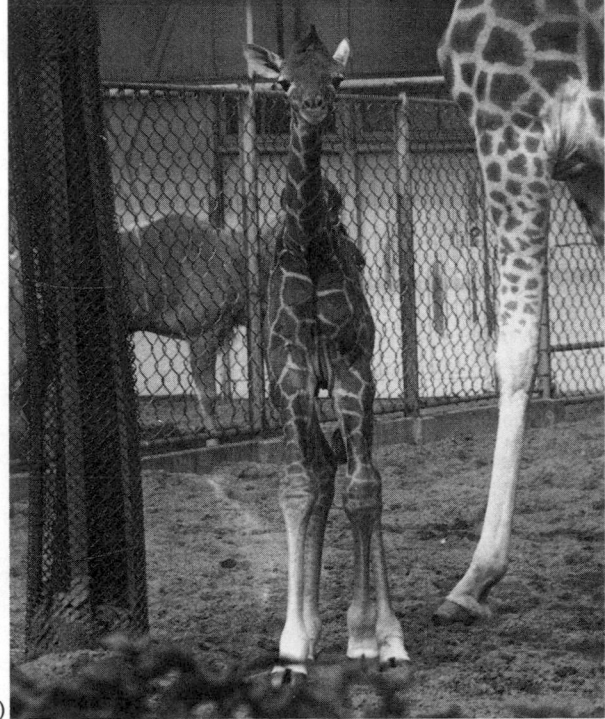

Fig. 48.2 (a) Birth of a giraffe, still in amniotic sac.
(b) Nuzzling of newborn.
(c) Newborn standing shortly after birth.

3 Polytocous and monotocous mammals

Polytocous mammals (those that usually deliver several young in a litter; for example, most rodents, rabbits and hares, carnivores and insectivores) differ in many ways from those that usually give birth to single offspring. In most of these polytocous species the newborn animal is born relatively undeveloped, blind and deaf, and either has a coat of nest hair, or lacks hair entirely. Intensive care in a nest is necessary to protect the newborn against cold and predators. During this nesting period their sense organs and coat develop. After some time they can leave the nest from time to time, although they still need parental care.

In contrast, monotocous mammals (those that usually have only a single offspring) usually give birth to very well developed young, which can follow their mother almost immediately after birth (such as giraffes, horses or whales), or which can clamp themselves to their mother's breast (such as bats or monkeys). Nevertheless, these offspring also need parental care to survive.

4 How animals behave at birth

4.1 Introduction

Pregnant females in many species show components of maternal behaviour shortly before giving birth. Ewes have a changed vocalization, and may utter lamb-calling sounds, sometimes several days before labour begins. Kitten-calling in cats may also occur some days before delivery. Self-licking behaviour is modified in rats. For most species, however, little is known about preparation for delivery and for maternal care, apart from the fact that most nest-building animals look for a nesting place and begin nest-building.

This lack of knowledge about preparturitional behavioural changes does not imply that these changes do not occur. Such changes can be very subtle (Rosenblatt and Lehrman 1963; Naaktgeboren 1987), and would not be detected except by special investigations. They are much less dramatic than the behavioural changes that take place during and after birth.

4.2 Polytocous animals

As soon as parturition begins, genital licking becomes frequent in most polytocous species. By licking, the labouring animal removes protruding fetal membranes, mucus and blood from her genital region (Fig. 48.3(a)). Labouring females in many species show signs of discomfort, perhaps of severe pain. Trembling movements in the abdomen can be observed in rats, cats and dogs. After some time straining is seen, the fetal membranes appear at the vulva, and the young are expelled by several straining movements (Fig. 48.3(b),(c)). Of the animals that give birth to several offspring, only the rabbit gives birth easily and quickly. Most animals deliver their young with great effort, with intervals of 5 to 45 minutes between each delivery. The whole sequence is repeated for every birth.

The close correlation between the physiology of birth and maternal behaviour is well illustrated in the classic work of Rosenblatt and Lehrman (1963) on the laboratory rat. Maternal behaviour in the rat is observed immediately after birth. If the young are removed, maternal behaviour diminishes rapidly and disappears. Even if young rats are later given to a female rat whose own pups were removed she will not display maternal behaviour. If the litter is replaced by younger pups, maternal behaviour will continue for a longer period than it does normally. At parturition the mother is responsive to newborn animals and her behaviour is adapted to the needs of the growing young. Immediately after parturition female rats also retrieve alien pups, even if they are much older and do not resemble newborns. A few days later, however, the mother no longer behaves in this way, but will usually attack or ignore alien young rats. She has by now learned to recognize her own pups.

The following quotation from Rosenblatt and Lehrman (1963) describes this concisely: 'The shift from self-licking to licking of the young, the increase in nest-building behaviour and the change in its character, the appearance of retrieving responses, and the occurrence of the first nursing responses, all coming when the helpless and practically immobile young appear on the scene, encourage the establishment of a nursing–suckling relationship between mother and young. If this relationship becomes established, the maternal responsiveness of the female increases and is maintained throughout the litter period. If the young do not stimulate the mother just after parturition, her readiness to perform maternal responses declines rapidly and completely. The special nature of the condition of the female immediately postpartum is emphasized by the fact that reintroduction of young after several days of such isolation does not restore the maternal condition to anything like the level which it would have reached if the young have been present continuously since birth. By contrast, when the young animals are removed for equivalent periods later during the litter period, the decline in maternal responsiveness is not nearly so drastic, and recovery readily follows the reintroduction of the young. Parturition therefore represents a crucial point of change, or point of inflection, in the relationship between the mother and her (litter) environment'.

The environment also plays an important role in the establishment and maintenance of maternal behaviour. A female rat may abandon her nest due to crowded social conditions, or due to changes in lighting or in temperature. She makes a new nest and brings the

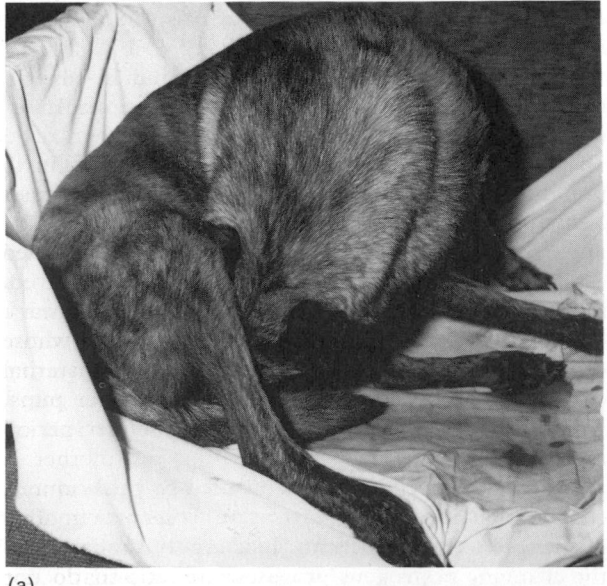

(a)

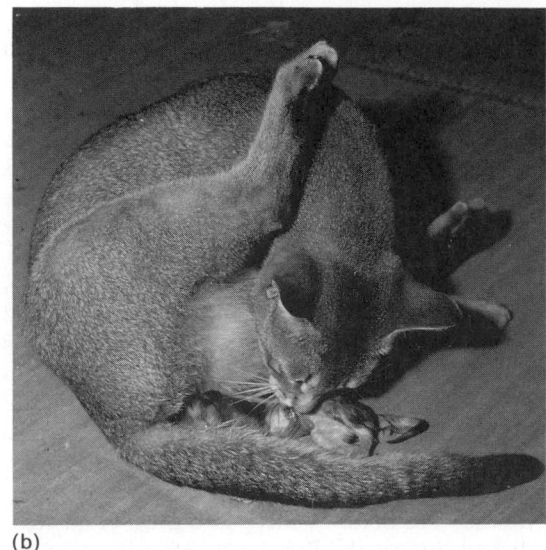

(b)

(c)

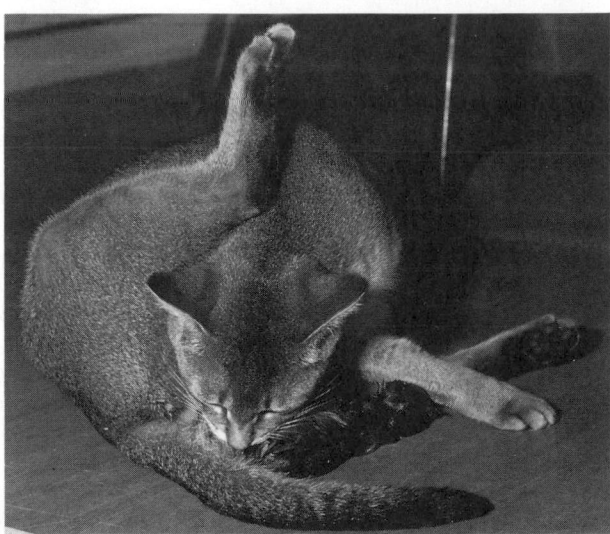

Fig. 48.3 Parturition in polytocous animals
    (a) genital licking in the dog at the onset of birth
    (b) a mother cat licks her newborn kitten
    (c) a mother cat severs the umbilical cord by biting through it.

young to the new nest. If the environmental disturbance is too stressful, she continues carrying pups and depositing them in different places. The young get exhausted and finally they die.

4.3 Monotocous animals

Unlike the polytocous mammals that characteristically build nests, the birth environment for monotocous animals varies widely. Whales and dolphins deliver their young while swimming: the young is expelled tail first, and must swim to the surface for its first breath. Seals give birth on the seashore. The hippopotamus, which gives birth in shallow water, is the only land mammal for which it is natural to have an underwater confinement. Bats deliver their young while hanging,

and the umbilical cord functions as a safety belt if the newborn fails to grasp the mother's fur at the right moment. Many monkeys give birth in a tree, watched with vivid interest by other members of the group. Detailed descriptions of parturition in many species have been reported (see Naaktgeboren and Slijper 1970). In this chapter, birth in ungulates and primates will be described as representative of the monotocous mammals.

4.3.1 Ungulates

In many ungulates (such as cows, sheep, and horses) the udder becomes harder and warmer, and the vulva becomes reddened and swollen one or two days before parturition. Somewhat later a mucous discharge from the vulva may be observed. The exact time of birth cannot be predicted, however, from either external appearance or behaviour. Cows, horses, and sheep make no nest, and the only behavioural change is perhaps an increasing restlessness. The mare often shows no behavioural changes at all. If someone is observing her, the labour may be suppressed, and the foal will be born just as soon as the unwanted observer has left.

A spontaneous delivery in monotocous ungulates is only possible if the fetus presents with the head first and back dorsally directed. The slightest variation from this position will lead to severe difficulties, which in wild animals would cause the death of both fetus and mother. The only obstetric help in nature is that offered by predators who will shorten the period of pain by killing the 'patient' and eating her.

The mother–kid bond in sheep and goats (Fig. 48.4) is established during the first hours after birth of the kid, often even before the afterbirth is expelled. If the bond is not established during this short phase of sensitivity, the mother rejects the newborn, whose chance of survival then becomes extremely small. During delivery the mother licks fetal fluids, and as soon as the young is expelled she starts licking the newborn intensively (Naaktgeboren 1966). If maternal licking of the newborn lamb is prevented, and the dry kid is offered to the ewe some hours afterwards, the mother is not capable of accepting her own young. If the young is removed (even no more than five minutes) after brief contact between mother and newborn, however, the ewe has no difficulties in recognizing her young after

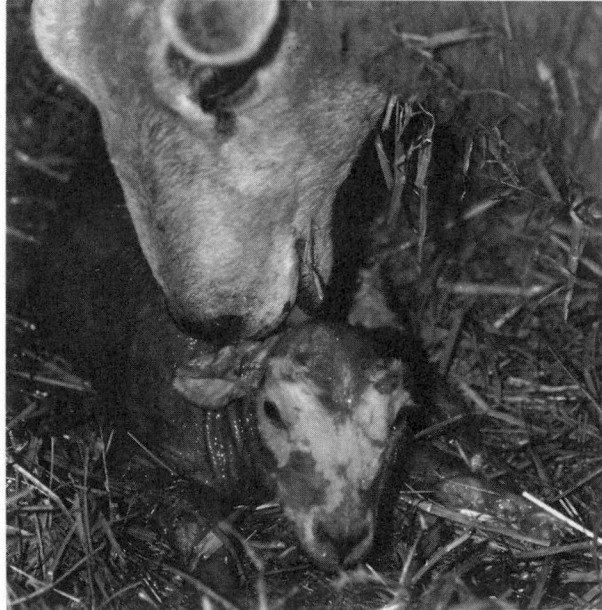

Fig. 48.4 Mother-lamb bonding in the sheep.

one to three hours separation (Collias 1956; Klopfer and Gamble 1966; Hersher *et al.* 1963).

Shortly before giving birth, ewes tend to separate themselves from the flock and thus deliver alone. Bonding starts by licking, and the ewe learns to recognize her offspring. If an alien lamb, wet with fetal fluids is presented to her, she will also accept it at this moment. Sometimes, just prior to giving birth, ewes have the opportunity to meet another parturient ewe. In these cases it is regularly observed that both ewes lick the first newborn lamb to be born, and sometimes the lamb is bonded to the other ewe instead of its mother. Bonding occurs in these ruminants by a process of imprinting, during a short sensitive phase. The ewe or the goat is willing to lick a wet newborn only just before and just after delivery.

Leaving the flock or herd is induced by the hormonal changes that also lead to parturition. It secures bonding of the ewe to her own lamb. It is highly probable that the changing oestrogens/progesterone ratio that occurs prior to parturition makes the ewe sensitive to the smell of fetal fluids. Anosmic females are unable to distinguish between their own and alien kids or lambs, but maternal behaviour is not eliminated by ablation of olfaction (Bouissou 1968; Poindron 1976). In contrast to the situation of the rat, the period of imprinting in the sheep and goat results in a well-developed recognition of their own newborn. Alien young are butted away.

It must be kept in mind that vision and acoustic signals also play a role in the maintenance of the mother–child bond. The development of the interaction is also dependent on the kid's behaviour. The following description by Klopfer and Gamble (1966) offers a clear illustration of behavioural interactions in the goat: 'We were able to show that immediate separation of the kids from their mothers for a period as brief as one hour led to a rejection of the young by the mother, or, at the very least a permanent impairment in the development of the normal relationship. Even where the impairment seemed initially to be very slight, it led to progressively greater disturbances whose final effect was of large magnitude. An example will illustrate this last point: a particular mother, on being presented her kid subsequent to a two-hour separation, showed herself somewhat ambivalent toward it. The mother sniffed and licked the kid, but then repulsed it (by lowering the head and gently pushing it away) when the kid attempted to crawl beneath her abdomen toward the udder. After the first few pushes by the mother, the kid withdrew even when the mother merely feinted. The withdrawal appeared to trigger a stronger rejection response by the mother. This, in turn, intensified the withdrawal response of the kid, which, in its turn, finally culminated in the doe's rejection activities totally overriding or replacing licking and grooming. Thus this animal, initially ambivalent, after a period of an hour showed active and intense rejection of its kid, butting it vigorously and biting it even as it sought to retreat. In contrast, mothers of the control group were first allowed a few minutes contact with their young. During this period they assiduously licked and nuzzled their offspring. Subsequent isolation of even several hours duration did not, in these animals, in any way interfere with the re-acceptance of the young, nor the care lavished upon them, nor, indeed, any other phase of the maternal–young relationship.'

4.3.2 Primates

Maternal behaviour in primates is much different from, and more complex than, that seen in ungulates. The behaviour of the young is important, as it is in other mammals, but in the primates the role played by vision is particularly important. In the *Macaca fuscata* monkey, it has been observed that crippled young received special attention. The mother can learn to give more care if the young animal asks for it (Carpenter 1972). Eye-to-eye contact seems to be of great importance, both in non-human primates and in the human. In the human, the possible role of a 'critical phase' or time period after birth that determines parent–infant attachment has not been clearly defined. Human mother–infant attachment results from a complex interaction between genetic endowment, sociocultural environment, and the infant's responses.

In summary, it can be said that in all species, including humans, the establishment of maternal behaviour is the result of interactions between mother and newborn. The different forms in which this behaviour develops and manifests itself can be regarded as specific adaptations to different ecologies, but in all mammals for which data are available, the behaviour of the young plays an integral role in triggering and maintaining maternal behaviour. Abnormal newborn behaviour may lead to either abandonment or special care. The human falls well within the range of mammalian parent–young interactions (Gubernick and Klopfer 1981; Naaktgeboren 1988b). The young in all species ask in a specific way for the care that they need. Usually they receive a positive response which favours the survival of the species. Cases of failure demonstrate the complexity of the interactions and the adaptations that are necessary to ensure the future of the next generation.

5 Biological effects of stress

Severe stress can cause miscarriage in several species of mammals. This has been described in detail for both rabbits and primates. The intensity of the response is determined by other characteristics of the species. Stress induced miscarriages are hardly ever seen, for example, in cattle or sheep.

In the rabbit, fetal death and reabsorption of embryos, miscarriage, or preterm birth of non-viable young occur if population density increases beyond tolerance. This causes psychological stress in the animals, leading to high levels of circulating adrenaline which in turn affect placental function. Myers (1971) described differences in the colour and lobulation of placentae between free-ranging and caged rhesus monkeys, as well as a significant difference in mean birthweight (613 g in free ranging and 519 g in caged monkeys). Myers' findings have been replicated by the work of other investigators in other primates (Naaktgeboren and Bontekoe 1976). Thus, stress can influence fetal growth, placental morphology, and structure and cause miscarriage, preterm delivery, or fetal death in several mammalian species. High levels of catecholamines in the pregnant rhesus monkey can cause fetal asphyxia (Adamsons *et al.* 1971). It seems to be clear that the effects of stress are mediated directly by the output of adrenaline. The myometrial reaction to stress can either be an increase or a decrease in activity and both effects are due to the extra output of adrenaline (Bontekoe 1978; Bontekoe *et al.* 1977). The effects of stress on the pattern of myometrial activity during parturition and during the postpartum period can also be mimicked by exogenous adrenaline.

In all mammalian species the course of delivery can be influenced by environmental disturbances (Naaktgeboren and Bontekoe 1976; Naaktgeboren 1979). Anxiety and fright invariably lead to prolongation of the duration of labour, or, in polytocous species, to excessively long intervals between the births of successive young. As soon as the cause of anxiety has disappeared, the labouring animal recommences its discontinued activity. Suppression of uterine activity is a life-saving adaptation for the labouring animal, because in cases of danger the animal is able either to fight or to flee. Afterwards the animal can give birth to the young in peace and safety.

For many animals the mere presence of an observer during parturition acts as a stress-stimulus. This often results in fruitless waiting. If the observer leaves the animal alone, the mother delivers the newborn in his absence. We started recording uterine activity in a ewe which had already begun to strain but in whom the uterus was completely quiescent. We then stopped recording and left the ewe alone. Within one hour the lamb was born (Naaktgeboren 1979).

Increasing uterine activity leading to miscarriage, preterm delivery or fetal death, and decreasing uterine activity stopping the progress of labour, are of great adaptive value. These stress responses help in the struggle for life. In times of severe stress, such as overpopulation or extremely cold winters, the loss of a pregnancy increases the chances that the female will survive and reproduce during the next breeding season.

Likewise, suppression of labour is of importance for the protection of the mother and the newborn. These mechanisms are of fundamental importance and human beings have not lost them during the process of civilization. The disappearance of uterine contractions that is seen in some women after arrival in the hospital is not pathology, but a normal and readily understandable response in a healthy woman.

Patterns of uterine contractility and their endocrine regulation vary greatly among species. Some of the interspecies differences found in experimental studies can be explained in the context of other characteristics of the species. Extrapolation of findings from one species to another is unwise, however. Women are neither rats nor ewes.

6 Time of delivery

All mammals can deliver their young at any time of the day or night, but in all species most deliveries take place at whatever time of day or night the animals usually rest. Thus, night-active species deliver preferentially during the day, and day-active animals during the night. In ruminants an extra peak in the frequency of delivery sometimes occurs at the time they chew the cud. The onset of labour is easiest during parasympathetic dominance, whereas sympathetic stimuli inhibit labour. In the mare it has been observed that the preferred time for delivery changed by one hour from winter to summer. This has to do with the changed working rhythms of people in the stable, and the mares delivered their foals during the new phase of rest. It is evident that a close correlation exists between the time of delivery and the mechanisms mediating psychogenic suppression of labour.

7 Place of birth, parturient behaviour, and the role of other animals

All mammals look for a safe and quiet place to give birth, which may be their nest, a tree, or on the seashore. Sometimes an animal delivers in complete solitude, leaving the herd before parturition, as we have described for the ewe, whereas in other species, such as the elephant, the labouring female prefers to be surrounded by members of the group. In still other species, such as mice, the young are born in a family nest (Fig. 48.5).

Assistance at parturition by other members of the group is characteristic of many species, and not a uniquely human activity. In many mammalian species that live in groups, the labouring female is assisted by members of the group. Mice prefer to give birth in a family nest. Elder females assist at the birth, by helping

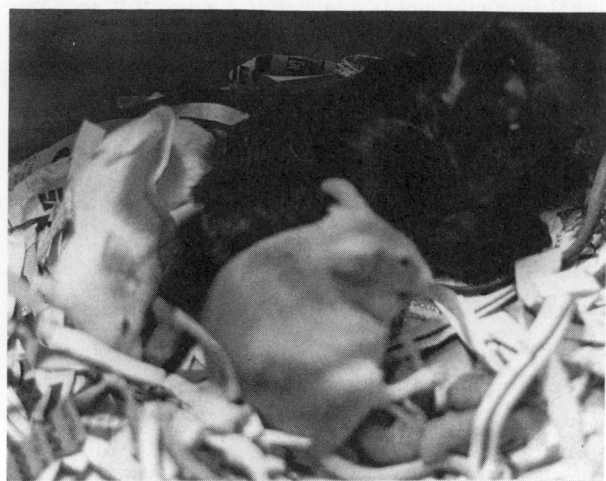

Fig. 48.5 Mice in a family nest.

the labouring female, by cleaning the newborn animals, by biting the umbilical cord, and even by eating the placenta (Fig. 48.5).

A comparable kind of behaviour is seen in dolphins. If a young dolphin, born within the group, fails to swim to the surface immediately after being born, two or three members of the group join together to push it towards the surface, where it can take its first breath. In an orang-utan, assistance at parturition is given by the father, who acts as a midwife, skilfully gripping the emerging newborn with large fleshy lips and drawing it out of the birth canal—a primitive form of vacuum extraction. The mother shows no interest in her baby before it cries (Gensch 1965). In wolves, the father also shows a vivid interest in his offspring and cares for the labouring female. This can also be observed in the domestic dog (Naaktgeboren 1987).

The behaviour of other members of the species is not always helpful to the parturient. In rats, for example, other females sometimes try to steal newborn animals, which leads to fighting and inhibition of labour (Naaktgeboren 1979).

My own observations do not leave me with the impression that other animals are urged to help primarily by the mother. It seems highly probable that this behaviour is triggered mainly by signals from the newborn animal itself. The 'midwifery-behaviour' thus proves that in many species the mere presence of conspecific young can influence behaviour, even in males, so that the young are cared for. I have described these phenomena in detail and discussed their relevance for the adoption of alien young (Naaktgeboren 1988a,b).

Adoptive behaviour is normal in species living in small social groups, such as certain monkeys, wolves, elephants, and humans at the beginning of their existence. In these species, care of the young is less dependent on the endocrine changes leading to delivery, which in turn enables also males to care for children, and makes it less difficult for a dog, or a human mother, to accept a child after a caesarean than for a ewe. Comparative obstetrics reveals not only similarities but also essential differences between species.

8 Conclusions

Although the place of birth, parturient behaviour, and the role of other members of the species varies considerably among mammals, they all have one fundamental feature in common: the need for a feeling of being safe. Removal of the labouring animal from her safe environment invariably results in inhibition of uterine contractions. Our own species is not an exception. Even in countries where hospital birth is the norm, for some women, leaving home and going to the hospital is the greatest stress of the whole process of parturition (Friedman 1975).

Human biology and the basic patterning of the human mind cannot change as quickly as can patterns of civilization. In the light of what has been said, it is not surprising that, from the viewpoint of the biologist, human birth as carried out in the industrialized world does not fit well into the range of mammalian parturient behaviour. The environment of the modern hospital, with its unfamiliar surroundings and strange personnel is not the home environment with family and friends to which the woman is accustomed. Practices such as daylight obstetrics, restrictions of spontaneous activity during labour, the supine position for delivery, and the separation of the newborn infant from its mother are not in accord with our biological heritage. The lessons of comparative biology remain to be learned.

The safest way to help labouring women is to respect nature and not to interfere with spontaneous events unless there is clear evidence that to do so would be beneficial. It is a dangerous practice to overestimate the ability of obstetric technology and to underestimate the spontaneous reactions and the innate biological behaviour of the parturient woman.

References

Adamsons K, Mueller-Heubach E, Myers RE (1971). Production of fetal asphyxia in the rhesus monkey by administration of catecholamines to the mother. Am J Obstet Gynecol, 109: 248–262.

Bontekoe EHM (1978). The influence of sex steroid hormones on the uterine response to epinephrine and to stress in the laboratory rabbit. Z Säugetierkd, 43: 357–369.

Bontekoe EHM, Blacquière JF, Naaktgeboren C, Dieleman SJ, Willems PPM (1977). Influence of environmental disturbances on uterine motility during pregnancy and parturition in rabbit and sheep. Behavioural Processes, 2: 41–73.

Bouissou MF (1968). Effet de l'ablation des bulbes olfacifs sur la reconnaissance du juene par sa mere chez les ovins. Rev du Comportement Animal, 3: 77–83.

Carpenter CR (1972). *Macaca fuscata* (cercopithecidae): maternal behavior. Film E 1468 of Enclycopaedia Cinematographica (1971). Accompanying publication 7 pages, 1972.

Collias NE (1956). The analysis of socialization in sheep and goats. Ecology, 37: 228–239.

Dawes GS (1968). Foetal and Neonatal Physiology. A Comparative Study of the Changes at Birth. Chicago: Year Book Medical Publications.

Friedman DD (1975). Conflict behavior in the parturient. In: The Family. Hirsch H (ed). Proceedings of the 4th International Congress of Psychosomatic Obstetrics and Gynaecology. Basel: Karger Verlag, pp 373–376.

Gensch W (1965). Die geburt eines orang-utans im Zoo Dresden. Freunde des Kölner Zoo, 4: 133.

Gubernick DJ, Klopfer PH (eds) (1981). Parental Care in Mammals. New York: Plenum Press.

Hersher L, Richmond JB, Moore A (1963). Maternal behavior in sheep and goats. In: Maternal Behavior in Mammals. Rheingold HL (ed). New York: John Wiley, Chapter 6.

Kehrer FA (1864). Über die zusammenziehungen des weiblichen genitalkanals. Beitr zur vergleichenden und experimentellen Geburtskunde I Giessen.

Kehrer FA (1867). Vergleichende physiologie der geburt. Beitr zur vergleichenden und experimentellen Geburtskunde II Giessen.

Klopfer PH, Gamble J (1966). Maternal 'imprinting' in goats: the role of chemical senses. Z Tierpsychol, 23: 588–592.

Lind J, Vuorenkoski V, Wasz-Höckert D (1972). The effect of crystimulus on the temperature of the lactating breast in primipara. A thermographic study. Proceedings of the 3rd International Congress of Psychosomatic Obstetrics and Gynaecology. Basel: Karger-Verlag, pp 293–295.

Martys M (1982). Gehegebeobachtungen zur geburts- und reproduktions-biologie des Europäischen wildschweines (Sus Scrofa L). Thesis, Utrecht University.

Myers RE (1971). The pathology of the rhesus monkey placenta. In: The Use of Non-human Primates in Research on Human Reproduction. Diczfalusy E, Standly CC (eds). World Health Organization Symposion-Sukhumi.

Naaktgeboren (1966). Cervus elaphus (Cervidae) Geburt. Film E1114 from Encyclopaedia cinematographica.

Naaktgeboren C (1979). Behavioural aspects of parturition. Animal Reprod Science, 2: 155–166.

Naaktgeboren (1987). De geboorte bij de hond (3rd ed). Naarden: Strengholt.

Naaktgeboren C (1988a). Ouders en kinderen. Vruchtbaarheid, zwangerschap en geboorte in verschillende culturen. Deventer: Ankh-Hermes.

Naaktgeboren C (1988b). Het aangenomen kind. Biologische en culturele aspecten van de ouder-kind relatie. Deventer: Ankh-Hermes.

Naaktgeboren C, Bontekoe EHM (1976). Vergleichendgeburtskundliche betrachtungen und experimentelle untersuchunger über psychosomatische störungen der schwangerschaft und des geburtsablaufes. Z Tierzüchtung Züchtungsbiol, 93: 264–320.

Naaktgeboren C, Slijper EJ (1970). Biologie der geburt. Hamburg: Paul Parey Verlag.

Perry JS (1972). Control of parturition. J Reprod Fertil, Supplement 16.

Poindron P (1976). Mother-young relationships in intact or anosmic ewes at the time of sucking. Biology of Behaviour, 2: 161–177.

Rosenblatt JS, Lehrman DS (1963). Maternal behavior of the laboratory rat. In: Maternal behavior in mammals. Rheingold HL (ed). New York: John Wiley, Chapter 1.

Ross S, Sawin PB, Zarrow MX, Denenberg VH (1963). Maternal behavior in the rabbit. In: Maternal Behavior in Mammals. Rheingold HL (ed). New York: John Wiley, Chapter 3.

Schiefenhövel W, Sich D (1983). Die Geburt aus ethnomedizinischer Sicht Curare—Sonderband. Vieweg: Braunschweig.

Slijper EJ (1960). Die Geburt der Säugetiere. Handbuch der Zoologie 9(9), 1–108. Berlin: de Gruyter.

Stein GW (1819). Der Unterschied zwischen Mensch und Thier im Gebären; zur Aufklärung über das Bedürfnis der Geburtshilfe für den Menschen. Bonn, 1–100.

Terkel J, Rosenblatt JS (1971). Aspects of nonhormonal maternal behavior in the rat. Hormones and Behavior, 2: 161–171.

Wasz-Höckert O, Seitamo L, Vuorenkoski V, Partanen T, Lind J (1972). Emotional attitudes toward the child and child rearing and the effect of crystimulus on the skin temperature of the lactating breasts in primiparas. Proceedings of the 3rd International Congress of Psychosomatic Obstetrics and Gynaecology. Basel: Karger Verlag, p 284–286.

49 Social and professional support during childbirth

Marc J. N. C. Keirse, Murray Enkin, and Judith Lumley

1 Introduction

One of the factors that is believed to be important as a cause of the high intervention rates during labour that are seen in many industrialized societies is the hospital environment, with its separation of family members, rigid procedures, lack of choice over positions for labour, and so on. Yet the opening up of labour wards in industrialized societies, first to fathers and then to other support people, has been associated in time with a staggering increase in caesarean birth and other interventions. How can these facts be reconciled? The unanswered questions are legion.

Support during childbirth can be provided by the professionals who are also responsible for the clinical care of the woman in labour; by professionals specifically designated to provide support rather than clinical care; or by the woman's partner, family, or friends.

Experimental studies thus far have only examined the contribution of the second group, i.e. a 'doula' as a person specifically designated to provide social but not clinical support in labour. Only three such studies are available and they all emanate from the same group, although they have been conducted in two different countries, Guatemala and the United States (Sosa *et al.* 1980; Klaus *et al.* 1986; Kennell *et al.* 1988). In the first of these experimental studies support was defined as 'physical contact (e.g. rubbing the mother's back and holding her hands), conversation, and the presence of a friendly companion whom the mother has not met before' (Sosa *et al.* 1980). In the report of the second study it was made clear that support has both emotional and physical components, with the provision of explanation and encouragement an explicit factor (Klaus *et*

al. 1986). A central feature of support in these studies is the promise that the labouring woman will not, at any time, be left alone.

Another setting where support and not being left alone in labour form part of the management protocol is the National Maternity Hospital, Dublin. Here there is a 'prior guarantee of continuous personal attention during labour' (O'Driscoll and Meagher 1980). Describing the policy, O'Driscoll and Meagher stress the point that mere physical presence is not enough. Labouring women's companions, who are usually student midwives but sometimes medical students, have a primary duty of providing emotional support to the mother. This includes walking with her in the early part of labour, holding her hands, maintaining eye contact, 'consciously striving to establish a strong sense of rapport . . . to ensure the patient understands clearly the purpose of every medical procedure and the result of every examination performed, and that she is kept informed of progress, with regular updating of the time at which her baby is expected to be born' (O'Driscoll and Meagher 1980). This description includes the emotional, the tangible and the informational components which typically make up social support.

Other descriptions of the support role mention advocacy as well as explanation, physical comfort and encouragement. Advocacy, which is particularly associated with plans and expectations before labour, is a common component of partners' and labour coaches' supportive activities.

Many of the people involved in pregnancy and childbirth may, as a part of their role, provide some or all the components of the support described above.

The separation of support from other functions of

caregiving is slightly artificial. The caregivers often combine support with assessment and diagnosis. Autonomous midwives, for example, would be involved with physical comforting, explanation and encouragement, information and feedback. Traditionally and at least in theory, they would 'be there' all the time. The advocacy part of support would apply whenever complications developed and a doctor was called in. Throughout labour and birth the autonomous midwife would also assess progress, diagnose any complications and assist the parents in deciding what action should be taken.

In hospital settings the separation of support from management may be far greater (see for example Sosa *et al.* 1980; Klaus *et al.* 1986), with doctors and nurses carrying out tasks of a technical nature. Among the professionals there is even more splitting of functions, with control and decision-making vested in the obstetrician, while the midwife is either restricted to monitoring and assessment, or loses this role to fetal heart rate and uterine activity monitors. The loss of diagnostic and decision-making roles seems not to free the midwife for providing emotional and psychological support, since her time is then taken up with caring for the equipment and assisting the physician.

In a Canadian study of matched women planning home and hospital births, women in the two groups had very different expectations about support. 'In the home group, more than half expected their midwife to be with them all or most of the time during labour, while in the hospital group only 15 per cent expected to have a nurse with them throughout all or most of labour' (Hodnett 1983; Hodnett and Abel 1986). These expectations were in line with what actually happened: 89 per cent of the women in the home group had a midwife with them throughout all or most of labour; less than a third of the women in the hospital group had a nurse with them for that length of time.

When caregivers do not or cannot provide consistent support during labour, then support develops into a separate issue. Either it becomes the province of family and friends, or it becomes a problem to be dealt with by the institution.

2 The birth environment: implications for support

Klaus *et al.* (1986) refer to developments in obstetrical care over the past 75 years which have resulted in the mother's isolation during labour. For perhaps a third of that time, this distressing feature of the birth environment was not apparent. The subjective experiences of labour and birth were submerged by twilight sleep and general anaesthesia. While women were unconscious, questions of support were irrelevant. Birth was in some

places (particularly but not exclusively in North America) a forceful and violent event, met and overcome by equally violent forces (Arney and Neill 1982). When the natural childbirth movement made labouring women visible and redefined the experience of giving birth as potentially positive, aspects of the birth environment took on a new significance (see Chapter 7).

There are many features of the contemporary birth environment that may increase its stressfulness: the unfamiliarity of the place and most of the people; the variable use of procedures such as routine insertion of intravenous lines; restriction of fluids and foods; shaving the perineum; enemas; regular vaginal examinations; restriction of movement; fetal monitoring; augmentation of labour; epidural anaesthesia; and, increasingly, the high probability of an operative outcome (World Health Organization 1985; Hewson *et al.* 1985; Lumley 1987) and (see Chapter 5, this volume).

Many people believe that fear, pain and anxiety are increased by the mechanized, clinical environment and the unknown attendants, with adverse effects on the progress of labour; and that being in hospital exposes one to all the hazards of the intervention cascade, one unwanted manoeuvre leading to another. Four observational studies suggest that more intensive care may have adverse effects on low risk mothers and infants (Neutra *et al.* 1978; Klein *et al.* 1983; Shear *et al.* 1983; de Regt *et al.* 1986).

If it is true that a stress-inducing environment during labour can have adverse effects, then the perinatal outcomes of the control groups in the three experimental studies previously mentioned (Sosa *et al.* 1980; Klaus *et al.* 1986; Kennell *et al.* 1988) may have a major iatrogenic component. The setting in the Guatemalan studies, with 56 to 60 deliveries a day, an open observation ward for early labour, and 'hospital policies (which) did not permit any family member, friend or a continuous nurse caretaker to be present' (Sosa *et al.* 1980) sounds as if it might indeed be conducive to fear, pain, and anxiety. In Dublin, too, the presence of a constant companion is part of a management package that includes active management of labour, aggressive use of oxytocin, and a lack of enthusiasm about the presence in the labour ward of family members or friends (O'Driscoll and Meagher 1980). O'Driscoll and Meagher describe 'labour that is not properly supervised' as characterized by a woman showing 'steady emotional disintegration ... withdrawn from contact ... contorted features and restless movements interrupted by outbursts of terror until finally a state of panic is reached and self-control is lost completely.'

The assumption that rigid policies in the birth environment lead to an increased resort to major interventions is not necessarily correct, however. A comparison of hospital policies and practices in a large Australian city was analysed with reference to features of family

Table 49.1 Rate (per cent) of intrapartum interventions, by maternity hospital flexibility (Lumley and Davey 1987).

Intervention	Hospital flexibility score	
	Low (< 60/120)	High (> 90/120)
Oxytocin use	23.7–42.5 (median 33.8)	21.2–53.3 (median 37.6)
Forceps delivery	8.6–21.1 (median 16.0)	9.7–23.0 (median 18.0)
Caesarean delivery	9.1–23.7 (median 19.0)	11.0–24.8 (median 16.0)

centred maternity care, leading to the construction of a 'flexibility' score for each hospital. The lowest and highest quartiles on the flexibility scale were then compared, using data from the state birth forms. Table 49.1 shows that the range and median values for caesarean delivery did not differ between low and high flexibility hospitals.

A survey in the National Maternity Hospital in Dublin showed that 65 per cent (102/157) of women had a companion constantly throughout labour. Most of the remaining 35 per cent, who were left alone for less than five minutes, were distressed by this (Garcia *et al.* 1985). The perception of isolation and the reality of being left alone, even momentarily, is often compounded by the intermittent appearance and disappearance of large numbers of unknown people: physicians, midwives, nurses, and medical, nursing, or midwifery students. One commentator has dubbed them 'masked intruders' (Odent 1984). A Canadian study found that women giving birth in hospital encountered an average of 6.4 unfamiliar professionals during labour (range 3–14) (Hodnett 1983). Chard and Richards reported in 1977 that one low risk mother having her first child in a teaching hospital was attended by 16 people during six hours of labour. Despite this bevy of caregivers, most of the time she was alone, including long periods at crucial points such as the end of the first stage of labour.

The obstetric practices described above extend throughout the industrialized world. However, within that world, or in its ambit, live women who are not part of the dominant culture. They may speak a different language, particularly with regard to private, personal, or family happenings. They may retain strong ties to other ways of life, ties which for them have the status of laws. Such laws often prescribe who should be present during the labour and birth, often exclude men from any role at all, may require the placenta or the cord to be treated in a particular way, or the mother to be given special foods after delivery (see Chapter 6). Contravention of the 'laws' creates extreme shame and guilt, and the foreknowledge that the 'laws' will be broken creates

fear, discourages early attendance for antenatal care, and contributes to unattended birth and 'absconding' from hospital care (Central Australian Aboriginal Congress 1985). In Australia, for example, aboriginal women giving birth in such hospitals have very high rates of fetal distress, failure to progress in labour and caesarean delivery (Mukerjee and McNicol 1985).

Support is clearly one of the missing elements of birth in settings similar to the one just described. There are immediate needs for full-time interpreters, and for access and facilities for family members to be constant, culturally appropriate companions, but it is also necessary to modify the other culturally inappropriate aspects of care at the same time (Central Australian Aboriginal Congress 1985).

3 Men during labour and at birth

The entry of men as accoucheurs into what had always and everywhere been considered women's business is discussed elsewhere in this book (see Chapter 9). The arrival of men as husbands and partners into labour and birth was a later phenomenon. A questionnaire survey conducted in the European Region of the World Health Organization found that fathers may be present during labour in some hospitals in 13 out of 23 countries, and be present during an uncomplicated birth in some hospitals in 12 out of 23 countries (World Health Organization 1985).

Husbands have entered the labour ward for two reasons. The first is the reclaiming of birth by women as a positive experience. This has meant that the exclusion of a woman's sexual partner and father of the newborn, while another man is allowed to preside over the event, is widely seen as incongruous. The presence of fathers has fitted in well with other recent changes. In the decades when natural childbirth and psychoprophylaxis were not well understood or accepted, partners were expected to reinforce what had been taught in childbirth education and if necessary to act as advocates.

The second reason for partners' presence in labour wards has been to fill the gaps. The women planning a hospital birth in the Canadian study cited earlier (Hodnett 1983) rarely expected to have a nurse with them throughout labour. They felt the nurses would be too busy, or saw them as unwelcome strangers, or viewed the nurse's role as purely technical in nature. They intended to rely on their partners for support, assistance with breathing techniques and comfort measures. Hodnett (1983) comments: 'Recognizing that labouring women require psychological support, and realizing that nurses have little time to give it, hospitals have increasingly permitted and encouraged husbands to assume active roles in the care of their wives during labor.'

There are countries in North America and Europe, as well as most of Australia and New Zealand, where the presence of women's partners during labour has, within twenty years, gone from being occasionally permitted to very assertive couples, to being normative and virtually universal. The report of a recent Australian opinion poll was headed 'Father in the delivery ward: most say yes' (The Age, 29 August 1985).

Unfortunately studies of the impact of the father's presence on labour and birth have been impaired by small sample sizes and self-selection. Research in the 1970s, carried out when the presence of fathers was relatively unusual, studied a group where there was almost total confounding of the variable of interest (fathers in labour or at birth) with social class, attendance at childbirth education classes and preference for non-medicated birth (see, for example, Henneborn and Cogan 1975).

Some doubts have been expressed about handing over the supportive role to fathers. One concern relates to whether they are equipped for tasks that were formerly the responsibility of an experienced and professionally trained person. In Dublin there is, or was, little doubt on the point: 'Women, in general, have more to gain from the presence of a female companion who is not just sympathetic but is informed as well, and therefore in a much better position to provide the sense of firm reassurance which is so sorely needed at this time' (O'Driscoll and Meagher 1980).

Other questions relate to the way in which the father's presence might influence either the labouring woman or the male obstetrician. Odent (1984) writes:

'It may not always be best, however, for a woman to have her partner there. Certain men have a beneficial presence, while others only slow labor down. Sometimes an over-anxious man will get worried and will then try to hide it by talking too much; his chatter can keep the woman from concentrating on her labor.

I think of one incident when a woman couldn't seem to get beyond eight centimetres dilation; when her husband left the room for a short time to rest, their baby was born. Though this woman had told us that she wanted her husband present, her body was saying the reverse. A particularly overprotective and possessive man can also have a negative effect on labor. He continually massages, caresses, and holds *his* woman, who belongs to *him*. He anticipates her demands rather than responds to them. The woman in labor requires calm, but he can provide only stimulation. Men sometimes find it hard to observe, accept, and understand a woman's instinctive behaviour during childbirth. Instead they often try to keep her from slipping out of a rational, self-controlled state' (Odent 1984).

Odent suggests that some support people, the woman's partner being no exception, can interfere with the normal progress of labour by their effects on the woman. In addition, when there are major tensions in the couple's relationship, practical and emotional support in labour may be difficult to provide or to accept.

It is certainly true that the general entry of partners into labour wards has not been associated with fewer perinatal interventions. To give just one example, a recent paper from a London teaching hospital reported that 44 per cent of women had epidural anaesthesia, 47 per cent a forceps delivery, and 47 per cent an augmented labour, despite the presence throughout labour of a supportive (male) companion (Copstick et al. 1986). Moreover, failure to progress/dystocia is being diagnosed much more often than it was 20 years ago, with a concomitant increase in caesarean delivery rates (National Institutes of Health 1981).

However, since the interventions in labour are much more related to caregiver differences than to differences between labouring women—as variations in practice demonstrate (Garcia et al. 1987, Garforth and Garcia 1987, Lumley 1987, World Health Organization 1985) (see Chapter 70)—a more important mechanism for any influence of the partner's presence on the outcome of labour is likely to be a change in the behaviour of the physician. Cartoonists have often portrayed the males in labour rooms either talking to each other and ignoring the woman, or jointly engrossed in the output from a machine. Perhaps the identification of the physician with the partner in some way promotes a different pattern of care, including more intervention? We do not know.

There has been almost no research on the support actually provided by husbands and partners. An attempt to define and classify the supportive behaviours which might be provided by a partner, midwife, or other companion was described by Standley and Nicholson (1980). These behaviours were systematically sampled by the same group in a later study in which the activities of partners and nurses in early labour were compared (Klein et al. 1981). More extensive studies using random assignment to different supportive companions and using systematic assessment of support behaviour are in progress (E Hodnett, personal communication).

Also unresearched are the expectations that women bring to labour concerning the support that they will have and what they will need. Hodnett (1983) compared such expectations in two matched groups of women planning home and hospital birth. Women in the home group expected their partners to be more helpful during labour than did those in the hospital group. Ironically, the latter had much lower expectations of support from professional caregivers than the former. Interviews after birth found that in relation to support, what had happened matched the expectations.

Table 49.2 Retrospective ratings of support in labour

Study	Rating	*n*
Hodnett (1983)		
Support from significant others	6.72 (home birth)	40
	6.08 (hospital)	40
Support from significant others	6.77 (home birth)	40
and professionals	5.99 (hospital)	40
Lumley, unpublished data		
Support from husband/partner	4.82 (birth centre)	81
Support from midwife	4.93 (birth centre)	81
Klein *et al.* (1981)		
Helpfulness of partner	4.97 (hospital)	29
Helpfulness of nurse	4.07 (hospital)	29
Bennet *et al.* (1985)		
Support of partner or friend	5.4 (hospital)	398
Support of main midwife	4.8 (hospital)	398
Support of other midwife	3.5 (hospital)	398
Support of doctor	3.5 (hospital)	398

All studies used forced choice rating scales with higher scores denoting more perceived support.

Several surveys using retrospective interviews have asked women to rate the quality of the support provided during labour and birth. These are summarized in Table 49.2. The results are remarkably similar in very different settings with partners almost uniformly rated very highly and in most cases more highly than midwives.

Other types of study have had less positive findings. A recent study of pain in labour found that all primiparae had someone with them throughout labour (98 per cent had the baby's father). The presence of a labour partner who provided specific encouragement in pain control techniques—*not* just a reassuring presence and emotional support—was associated with much lower epidural rates and with fewer women describing panic, exhaustion or overwhelming pain, although pain ratings in the two groups were not different (Copstick *et al.* 1986). Similar results were described among Lamaze-trained women a decade earlier (Block *et al.* 1975), although an attempt at systematic training of fathers in these skills could detect little impact (Cambell and Worthington 1981). Self-selection presents a problem in the interpretation and generalizibility of the results of both studies: couples were recruited only from women attending childbirth preparation classes.

A recent exploratory study in Scotland found husbands unable to provide effective support in the conventional labour ward (Barbour 1986). Occasionally a husband was co-opted by the midwife to confirm her statements or to add his encouragement to hers, but in general, husbands were marginal figures. They were treated as children might be; given a 'pretend' role in the birth (e.g. allowed to cut the cord) and referred to as if they were spoilt babies unaware of the real world of women's lives. These dismissive attitudes coexisted uneasily with ideas of father involvement and family togetherness (Barbour 1986).

Another puzzling fact is that virtually all research has been on primiparae. One of the few exceptions found that multiparae were much less likely to have husband support or presence in labour, and their easier obstetric experience was not associated with any improvement compared with their first birth in terms of enjoyment, or pain (Norr *et al.* 1980).

In Dublin, where the presence of husbands throughout labour and birth is not yet normative, more women found the nurses (74/177) and other staff (35/177) to be reassuring than they found their husbands to be (10/120). This was quite a different dimension from feeling positive about the husband's presence, since 89 per cent of women whose husbands were there for at least part of the labour had positive feelings about this (Garcia *et al.* 1985).

4 Other support people

Apart from institutionally employed doulas, midwives, and partners, two other categories of people are currently providing support in labour: other family members and friends, and professional coaches or monitrices. There is a great deal of variation between hospitals in whether or not they permit other support people in labour wards. A recent survey in one Australian city found that nearly 40 per cent of units now allowed this (Davey 1984) but it seems to be less usual in most European countries (World Health Organization 1985). Hodnett's Canadian study (1983) reported that 18 per cent of women in the hospital group had more than one person with them during labour (up to six) and a few women would have liked more supporters than they had. In alternative birth settings it is customary for several people to be present for at least some of the time. The freedom to choose who will be present, and when, is often a factor in choosing to give birth outside hospital. It would be unwise to assume, though, that the mere presence of several people will provide additional support: 90 per cent of Hodnett's (1983) study group would have preferred to have fewer people present than the three to six who were there.

Family and friends, like husbands and partners, may be there to share in the experience rather than to provide support. An anecdotal account which presents this view comes from Odent (1984):

'Other women prefer to have several people with them at the clinic. We have noticed that many of these women have long and difficult labors. One night while the midwives and I were watching television we saw a big car pull up outside. A pregnant woman, apparently in labor, stepped out of the car, followed by a man, a woman, a very young girl, and another man with a camera. The first reaction from the midwives was, "Well, looks like we're in for a long night". They were right: the labor was long and drawn-out. Perhaps certain women want to be surrounded by people at this time because of some fear or insecurity about labor. Yet these anxious feelings may become even stronger if the woman in labor senses she is being watched or feels she must play some specific role in relation to those present. On the other hand, women from tight-knit families or communities are often comforted during labor by the presence of the people they are used to seeing every day' (Odent 1984).

The Australian hospitals which allow other support people in labour do not differ in caesarean delivery rates from those that do not permit people other than the father to be present (both 16 per cent) (Lumley and Davey 1987) (Table 49.1).

To some extent, the move to have additional family support arose from disillusionment with what the husband could provide, especially when the labour was a long one. (Doulas and student midwives, after all, work shifts rather than 24 hours a day.) Family and friend support is particularly appropriate where support is seen in terms of physical comfort, being there, maintaining eye contact, and encouragement. When coping with labour and normal progress are seen more in terms of utilizing learned skills, such as controlled breathing patterns and relaxation, then the chosen additional support person is likely to be a monitrice, a labour coach or childbirth educator. Her role has been defined as a continuous presence, tailored to the couple's needs and wishes, but focused on physical and emotional support and advocacy, assisting the couple in the interpretation of their wishes to the hospital staff.

Just as the role of support person, typified by the doula, arose because of the splitting of care into management and support, so the role of the labour coach comes from the splitting of education from care.

Once education becomes a separate activity, those responsible for care and management in labour may not know what antenatal education consists of and may be unwilling or unable to support labouring women in the use of their learned skills. Belittling the usefulness of the education programme may also occur, along with complaining about the unreal expectations it has created. When a labour coach is recruited as an advocate for the labouring woman, territorial rivalries with other staff, especially with midwives, are almost inevitable and the intended support may end up as a casualty of the conflict. A study of the impact of monitrice support on physiological and psychological childbirth outcomes and on the role of the husband/partner during labour is being carried out in Canada (E Hodnett, personal communication).

5 Randomized trials of social support

The three trials that are relevant to these issues were carried out by the same researchers in two settings (Sosa *et al.* 1980; Klaus *et al.* 1986; Kennell *et al.* 1988). The three doulas employed in the Guatemalan studies were single and childless, highly trained research workers who had worked at the Institute of Nutrition of Central America and Panama for several years and had obtained more advanced training and degrees before joining the support project. All three were similar to the patients in ethnicity, culture, and language but they were better educated (J Kennell, personal communication).

The findings in these trials are consistent, though certain comparisons in the smaller trial are not statistically significant. The presence of a supportive companion during labour was associated with a striking reduction in the length of labour, with a consequent reduced resort to augmentation of labour with oxytocics (Table 49.3). Fetal passage of meconium during labour was reduced (Table 49.4), and this, together with the effect of the supportive companions on uterine action, resulted in fewer instrumental deliveries (Table 49.5) and caesarean sections (Table 49.6). Low Apgar

Table 49.3 Effect of social support in labour on oxytocin augmentation

Study	EXPT		CTRL		Odds ratio	Graph of odds ratios and confidence intervals						
	n	(%)	*n*	(%)	(95% CI)	0.01	0.1	0.5	1	2	10	100
Sosa *et al.* (1980)	2/32	(6.25)	16/95	(16.84)	0.42 (0.13–1.32)							
Klaus *et al.* (1986)	4/168	(2.38)	33/249	(13.25)	0.26 (0.13–0.52)							
Typical odds ratio (95% confidence interval)					0.30 (0.16–0.53)							

Table 49.4 Effect of social support in labour on meconium-stained liquor

Study	EXPT		CTRL		Odds ratio	Graph of odds ratios and confidence intervals						
	n	(%)	n	(%)	(95% CI)	0.01	0.1	0.5	1	2	10	100
Sosa *et al.* (1980)	3/32	(9.38)	24/95	(25.26)	0.39 (0.15–1.03)							
Klaus *et al.* (1986)	21/168	(12.50)	44/249	(17.67)	0.68 (0.39–1.16)							
Typical odds ratio (95% confidence interval)					0.59 (0.37–0.95)							

Table 49.5 Effect of social support in labour on forceps delivery

Study	EXPT		CTRL		Odds ratio	Graph of odds ratios and confidence intervals						
	n	(%)	n	(%)	(95% CI)	0.01	0.1	0.5	1	2	10	100
Sosa *et al.* (1980)	1/32	(3.13)	4/95	(4.21)	0.75 (0.10–5.85)							
Klaus *et al.* (1986)	2/168	(1.19)	7/249	(2.81)	0.47 (0.12–1.78)							
Typical odds ratio (95% confidence interval)					0.54 (0.17–1.65)							

Table 49.6 Effect of social support in labour on caesarean delivery

Study	EXPT		CTRL		Odds ratio	Graph of odds ratios and confidence intervals						
	n	(%)	n	(%)	(95% CI)	0.01	0.1	0.5	1	2	10	100
Sosa *et al.* (1980)	6/32	(18.75)	26/95	(27.37)	0.64 (0.25–1.59)							
Klaus *et al.* (1986)	11/168	(6.55)	43/249	(17.27)	0.39 (0.22–0.69)							
Typical odds ratio (95% confidence interval)					0.45 (0.27–0.73)							

Table 49.7 Effect of social support in labour on Apgar score <8 at 5 minutes

Study	EXPT		CTRL		Odds ratio	Graph of odds ratios and confidence intervals						
	n	(%)	n	(%)	(95% CI)	0.01	0.1	0.5	1	2	10	100
Sosa *et al.* (1980)	0/32	(0.00)	3/95	(3.16)	0.26 (0.02–3.56)							
Klaus *et al.* (1986)	4/168	(2.38)	8/249	(3.21)	0.74 (0.23–2.39)							
Typical odds ratio (95% confidence interval)					0.62 (0.21–1.81)							

Table 49.8 Possible mechanisms for the findings in the randomized controlled trials of social support during labour

---

1. A reduction in fear, pain, and anxiety in the intervention group
      > shorter labour
      less need for pain relief or oxytocin
      fewer caesarean deliveries

2. An increase in fear, pain anxiety in the control group
      > longer labour
      more analgesics, more anaesthetics
      oxytocin
      fetal distress
      caesarean delivery for fetal distress and/or failure to
         progress

3. More attention from the staff to the control group
      > more intervention
      more problems

4. No change in fear, pain, or anxiety but a change in the behaviour of the women in the intervention group: less overt disress or contained distress
      > less intervention

5. Culturally appropriate care in the intervention group which partly or completely counterbalances the stressful effects of the hospital setting

---

scores were less common among the babies born to mothers who had had companions, but this difference could easily be a reflection of chance (Table 49.7). The main questions about these randomized controlled trials are the mechanisms of action and the generalizability of the results (Table 49.8). Since these are pragmatic trials, it might be thought that the mechanisms are irrelevant, but discussions of the possible reasons for better outcomes in the intervention group may have important implications for generalizing to other settings.

Sosa *et al.* (1980) and Klaus *et al.* (1986) believe that the most important factor is a reduction in fear, pain, and anxiety when women have a supportive companion, and they link these possible changes with effects of catecholamines on uterine contractility and uterine and placental blood flow as hypothesized by Myers (1975).

Two other randomized trials have shown a shortening of labour in women assigned to an obviously different form of care from the standard one: Leboyer delivery (Nelson *et al.* 1980) and a birth room (Chapman *et al.* 1986). These suggest that the length of labour may be readily influenced by a variety of factors. Whether it is the nature of the change or its novelty that is most important is not clear.

Since assignment to the intervention programme in these trials was always apparent to all the staff, it is possible that it affected staff patient interaction and decision-making. The relative importance of staff judgements compared with patient differences is shown by

the dramatic fall in caesarean delivery rates between the two Guatemalan studies: 23 per cent overall in the 1980 paper, 12 per cent overall in the 1986 paper, though the patients and the setting are described identically. Another example of the importance of caregiver factors is that while the control group in Guatemala were three to five times more likely to get oxytocin for augmentation of labour than were the doula group, in Dublin, 30 per cent of primigravidae receive oxytocin despite the provision of continuous personal care from a student midwife (O'Driscoll and Meagher 1980).

Another suggested mechanism may relate to an adverse birth environment. The routines at the Guatemalan hospital where the trial was carried out were established in the 1950s and based on North American practices of that era. By contrast, birth in Guatemala had been until that time something which occurred at home, with women assisted by the mother's mother, the father's mother, and a village midwife. Thus women in the study would have been the first generation to labour alone and to give birth among strangers and in the presence of men. However, the women, the nurses and the doulas were similar in background, ethnicity and language (J Kennell, personal communication). Given this information and the accounts of the overcrowded and hectic labour and delivery wards by the research team in the two papers, it seems possible that the environment might well have been particularly stressful.

The generalizability of the results of these trials must be seriously questioned, in part because of the special features of the environments in which they were carried out, and in part because of the special characteristics of the doulas, which are unlikely to be reflected in other categories of support persons such as partners, midwives, and others.

6 Conclusions

6.1 Implications for current practice

The paucity of good research evidence on the nature and effects of social and professional support in labour does not leave us without direction for policy and future research. Where there are extremes of isolation, overcrowding, use of painful procedures, a rapidly changing cast of professional staff and no familiar person, particularly for primigravidae, it is not too fanciful to compare their state with that of the absolutely terrified pregnant monkeys so often cited in relation to psychological stress and fetal asphyxia (Myers 1975). Where, in addition, aspects of birth care are culturally inappropriate, an additional component of shame and fear will be present (Central Australian Aboriginal Congress 1985). How common these extreme situations are we do not know, but wherever they exist, the provision of a friendly companion chosen by the labouring woman to be with her is likely to improve her well-being. As a matter of public policy also, such extreme situations should not be permitted to continue unchanged.

The potential for territorial rivalries over the provision of support is very great indeed. 'One can legitimately ask if, given the constraints posed by institutional norms and policies, an employee of the hospital (e.g. a nurse or midwife) can provide the same quality of support and advocacy that a professional "outsider" can. On the other hand, the presence of an outsider can pose a threat to the institution, which may have a negative influence on the quality of care received by the labouring woman' (E Hodnett; personal communication).

In a review of social support in pregnancy, Oakley (1985) drew attention to the very real possibility that an interaction which is beneficial to most people may have the reverse effect on some. Sensitivity to the possible negative effects of any support policy for a minority of those exposed to it is essential. The presence of husbands during labour, once grudgingly permitted, is now normative; yet, observations of father-attendance suggest that in some settings neither active support nor supportive companionship is manifested (Barbour 1986).

Given the difficulties of generalizing from the few available randomized trials and the present state of collective ignorance, an interim conclusion might be that it is inappropriate for hospitals to take it upon themselves to exclude any category of support person from labour and birth. Where women have strong preferences for who should be with them at this time, these should be respected.

6.2 Implications for future research

A change in support may be an important variable in any experimental intervention, and one with unforeseen and often unresearched consequences. In a recent comparison of universal with selective electronic fetal monitoring it was found that universal monitoring was inadvertently associated with less nursing support. The researchers commented: 'we cannot preclude the possibility that the potential advantages of universal monitoring may have been diminished by this change in obstetrical management' (Leveno *et al.* 1986).

In clinical trials it is essential for researchers to consider the implications that an intervention may have on the support provided or accessible to the woman in labour. Even when strenuous attempts to control for this factor have been made in the design, differences tend to creep in. Garcia *et al.* (1985) found that, even in Dublin with its policy of never leaving women alone, women allocated to electronic fetal monitoring were more often left alone for brief periods than were those assigned to intermittent auscultation. It is essential to look for differences in what did happen as opposed to what was supposed to happen.

There is also a need for detailed, perhaps anthropological, non-experimental research on what actually happens in labour (see Chapter 4). Such studies would provide better specification of support activities and descriptions of the interaction between professional and non-professional support people, as well as more consistent and reliable ways of rating the environment (Standley and Nicholson 1980).

In settings where there is currently no continuous support or caregiving, there is an opportunity to implement changes within the context of randomized trials that might answer some of the vexing questions raised at the beginning of this chapter: What is important in providing effective support? Is it enough to be there, or is it necessary to provide encouragement or physical comfort? What is the relationship between supporters and caregivers? Is it better for the support person to be a stranger than to be familiar, to be a peer or a professional? The results of the available studies provide important evidence but to date, the main lesson from them is that we have a lot to learn.

References

The Age (1985). Melbourne. 29 August.

Arney WR, Neill J (1982). The location of pain in childbirth: natural childbirth and the transformation of obstetrics. Sociol Health Illness, 4: 1–24.

Barbour R (1986). Being there: fathers on the labour ward. Paper presented at the BSA Medical Sociology Conference, York, 26–28 September.

Bennett A, Hewson D, Booker E, Holliday S (1985). Antenatal preparation and labor support in relation to birth outcomes. Birth, 12: 9–16.

Block CR, Block R, Shrock P (1975). The effect of support of the husband and obstetrician on pain perception and control in childbirth. Birth Family J, 2: 43–50.

Cambell A, Worthington EL (1981). A comparison of two methods of training husbands to assist their wives with labour and delivery. J Psychosom Res, 25: 557–563.

Central Australian Aboriginal Congress (1985). Borning. Ampe Mbareke Pmere Alaltye. The Congress Alukura by the Grandmother's Law. Report to the Policy and Planning Division, Commonwealth Department of Health, Canberra.

Chapman MG, Jones M, Spings JE, de Swiet M, Chamberlain GVP (1986). The use of a birth-room—a randomized controlled trial comparing delivery with that in a labour ward. Br J Obstet Gynaecol, 93: 182–187.

Chard T, Richards M (1977). Lesson for the future. In: Benefits and Hazards of the New Obstetrics. Clinics in

Developmental Medicine No 64. Chard T, Richards M (eds). London: Heinemann, p 157–163.

Copstick SM, Taylor KE, Hayes R, Morris N (1986). Partner support and the use of coping techniques in labour. J Psychosom Res, 30: 497–503.

Davey BA (1984). Leboyer, family-centred birth in Melbourne. Survey: March 1984. Published by the author.

de Regt RH, Minkoff HL, Feldman J, Schwarz RH (1986). Relation of private or clinic care to the cesarean birth rate. New Engl J Med, 315: 619–624.

Garcia J, Corry M, MacDonald D, Elbourne D, Grant A (1985). Mothers' views of continuous electronic fetal monitoring and intermittent auscultation in a randomized controlled trial. Birth, 12: 79–86.

Garcia J, Garforth S, Ayers S (1987). The policy and practice of midwifery study: introduction and methods. Midwifery, 3: 2–9.

Garforth S, Garcia J (1987). Admitting—a weakness or a strength? Routine admission of a woman in labour. Midwifery, 3: 10–24.

Henneborn WJ, Cogan R (1975). The effect of husband participation on reported pain and probability of medication during labour and birth. J Psychosom Res, 19: 215–222.

Hewson D, Bennett A, Holliday S, Booker E (1985). Childbirth in Sydney teaching hospitals : a study of low-risk primiparous women. Community Health Studies, 9: 195–202.

Hodnett ED (1983). The Effects of Person-Environment Interaction on Selected Childbirth Outcomes of Women having Home and Hospital births. Ph D thesis, University of Toronto.

Hodnett ED, Abel SM (1986). Person–environment interaction as a determinant of labor length variables. Health Care For Women International, 7: 341–356.

Kennel J, Klaus M, McDrath S, Robertson S, Hinkley C (1988). Medical intervention: the effect of social support. Pediatric Research, 23: 211A.

Klaus MH, Kennell JH, Robertson SS, Sosa R (1986). Effects of social support during parturition on maternal and infant morbidity. Br Med J, 2930: 585–587.

Klein RP, Gist NF, Nicholson J, Standley K (1981). A study of father and nurse support during labor. Birth Family J, 8: 161–164.

Klein M, Lloyd I, Redmam C, Bull M, Turnbull AC (1983). A comparison of low-risk pregnant women booked for delivery in two systems of care: shared care (consultant) and integrated general practice unit. Br J Obstet Gynaecol, 90: 118–128.

Leveno KJ, Cunningham FG, Nelson S, Roark M, Williams ML, Guzick D, Dowling S, Rosenfeld CR, Buckley A (1986). A prospective comparison of selective and universalla electronic fetal monitoring in 34,995 pregnancies. New Engl J Med, 3150: 615–619.

Lumley J (1987). Trends in birth style in Australia. Perinatal Medicine. Proceedings of the 4th conference of the Australian Perinatal Society.

Lumley J, Davey BA (1987). Do hospitals with family-centred maternity care policies have lower intervention rates? Birth, 14: 132–134.

Mukerjee B, McNicol J (1985). Alice Springs Hospital Maternity Report 1981–1983. Alice Springs: Northern Territory Department of Health.

Myers RE (1975). Maternal psychological stress and fetal asphyxia: a study in the monkey. Am J Obstet Gynecol, 122: 47–59.

National Institutes of Health (1981). Cesarean Childbirth. Report of a Consensus Development Conference, pp 8–9. US Department of Health and Human Services. Public Health Service. National Institutes of Health. Bethesda : NIH Publication No. 82–2067.

Nelson NM, Enkin MW, Saigal S, Bennett KJ, Milner R, Sackett DL (1980). A randomized clinical trial of the Leboyer approach to childbirth. New Engl J Med, 302: 655–660.

Neutra RR, Fienberg SE, Greenland S (1978). Effect of fetal monitoring on neonatal death rates. New Engl J Med, 299: 324–326.

Norr KL, Block CR, Charles AG, Meyering S (1980). The second time around: parity and birth experience. J Obstet Gynecol Neonatal Nurs, January–February, 30–36.

Oakley A (1985). Social support in pregnancy: the 'soft' way to improve birth-weight? Soc Sci Med, 21: 1259–1268.

Odent M (1984). Birth Reborn. London: Souvenir Press.

O'Driscoll K, Meagher D (1980). Active Management of Labour. London: W B Saunders.

Shear GL, Gipe BT, Matheis JK, Levy MR (1983). Provider continuity and quality of medical care. Medical Care, 21: 1204–1210.

Sosa R, Kennell JH, Klaus M, Robertson S, Urrutia J (1980). The effect of a supportive companion on perinatal problems, length of labor and mother-infant interaction. New Engl J Med, 303: 597–600.

Standley K, Nicholson J (1980). Observing the childbirth environment: a research model. Birth Family J, 7: 15–20.

World Health Organization (1985). Having a Baby in Europe. Public Health in Europe 26. Copenhagen: WHO Regional Office for Europe.

50 Hospital policies for labour and delivery

Iain Chalmers, Jo Garcia, and Shirley Post

Because of the importance of the birth event for individuals, for the continuity of families, the existence of communities and indeed the species, no society known to us has left the management of birth up to the individual. Rather, people everywhere have regulated the event'

Jordan 1985

1 Introduction

There may have been a time, not too long ago, when one might have been excused for believing that women were reasonably content with the way that care during childbirth was regulated by society in Europe and North America. As earlier chapters in this book have made clear (see Chapters 7 and 8), if this conclusion was ever justified, it would certainly have been difficult to sustain it during the last decade. In many countries the maternity services have been the subject of unprecedented public criticism. A recurrent target in these attacks has been the type of care women receive during labour and delivery.

Most births now take place in hospitals. Like other large institutions, hospitals (and the professionals working within them) depend on rules and routines for efficient functioning—and it is probably essential that they continue to do so. What is often at issue, however, is the extent to which rules and routines are based on sound evidence that they do more good than harm, and the extent to which professionals use discretion in applying them. The routines surrounding birth in hospital have come under attack, not only because they have been applied inflexibly, but also because there is often no evidence that they serve the best interests of childbearing women and their babies.

Detailed evaluations of the various routines and procedures that have come to characterize modern intrapartum care are presented in later chapters in this book.

In this chapter we want to set the scene for some of these evaluations by documenting the marked variations that exist in the type of care women receive, variations that depend more on which maternity unit a woman happens to attend and which particular professional she consults than on her individual needs or preferences. These differences in practice are often so dramatic that they cannot conceivably be explained by differences in either medical indications, or the expressed preferences of the women attending the different hospitals concerned. Rather, they constitute persuasive evidence that there is collective professional uncertainty about the value of many of the rules and routines in which women are often required to acquiesce during labour and delivery.

Most of the data we shall use to illustrate these variations were obtained in two, fairly detailed, national surveys of maternity hospitals which were conducted in the mid-1980s. One of these was conducted in England in 1984 (Garcia *et al.* 1986). A set of questionnaires was sent to each of the 193 Directors of Midwifery Services in the Health Districts of England. One hundred and eighty (93 per cent) responded, providing information about the maternity units for which they were responsible. A similar survey was conducted in Canada in 1985 (Post and Hanvey 1986; Hanvey and Post 1986). In this survey, a questionnaire was sent to the Director of Nursing at each of the 636 hospitals in Canada with more than twenty births a year. Responses were received for 69 per cent of the hospitals. When the definitions used in the two surveys were sufficiently similar, comparative data have been tabulated.

To make it clear that the variations in labour routines and rules which characterize the situation in English and Canadian maternity units is not unique, however, we have also drawn on the results of a survey conducted in ten of the countries within the European Region of the World Health Organization (Phaff 1986; World Health Organization 1986). In most of these ten countries, a questionnaire was sent by a local co-ordinator to a sample of between eight and sixteen hospitals selected to ensure representation of different sizes and types of maternity units (Maratos 1986). It is obviously necessary to be cautious about the extent to which these samples are representative of practice in each of the countries concerned, but the survey results nevertheless provided some interesting contrasts.

2 Controlling the environment of labour and delivery

2.1 Birth plans

The maternity hospital is home territory for professionals. This reality will always tend to put individual 'visitors' to this territory at a disadvantage when it comes to influencing the institution's rules and routines about aspects of care. In particular, early or advanced labour is not a time at which women can begin effective negotiations about aspects of their care on what is often strange and daunting foreign territory (see Chapter 51). Evidence emerged in both the English and Canadian surveys that this problem was appreciated in some maternity units. In addition to the antenatal classes organized by many hospitals, just over half the units in Canada were giving parents written information about care during labour. Nearly half of the maternity units in England said that women's expressed preferences were recorded. In 30 per cent of units this was achieved by recording women's views in the clinical record; in 14 per cent of units the device of a 'birth plan' had been formally adopted.

2.2 Companions

A woman's ability to cope in unfamiliar territory controlled by people who will often be strangers to her may be enhanced if she is accompanied by supportive relations or friends (see Chapter 16). The vast majority of the Canadian hospitals surveyed allowed the father and another friend of the woman to be with her, without restrictions, during labour. Only one Canadian hospital still did not allow this; in six others, fathers were allowed in the labour room only if they had attended prenatal classes. Virtually all of the Canadian hospitals also allowed fathers to attend vaginal births, and almost half allowed them to attend caesarean sections. Just over a quarter of the hospitals allowed a woman's other children in the labour room as well, but a majority did not allow children to attend the birth.

The survey of English maternity units revealed a rather more restrictive situation. More than half of the units said that there were circumstances in which the father would be required to leave the labour and delivery room. Some units specified particular circumstances (general anaesthesia, instrumental deliveries and, more rarely, vaginal examinations); others simply stated that he would be asked to leave on occasions 'at the discretion of the medical staff'. A few units indicated that a father would only be excluded at the woman's request. Only a third of English maternity units permitted a woman to be accompanied by a companion in addition to the father, although two-thirds of the units were happy for the woman to have such a companion with her if the father was not available or if the woman did not want him to be with her. The attitude of English maternity units to the presence of children during labour and delivery was very similar to that of Canadian units.

The report of the survey in other European countries states that, in Czechoslovakia and Greece, nobody apart from professional staff may be present with the woman during labour and delivery. Only the father is admitted to labour rooms in the Federal Republic of Germany, Finland, and Italy. The father and other relatives, chosen by the mother, may attend in Denmark, France, The Netherlands, and Norway. If accompanied by their father, children may be with their mother during the first stage of labour in The Netherlands and Norway, and throughout labour in Denmark (Maratos 1986).

2.3 Clothing

One of the ways in which the strangeness of institutions to outsiders is reinforced is by the special clothes sometimes worn by both visitors and staff. In almost half of the English maternity units surveyed a woman's companion had to wear a gown or apron, and in 8 per cent a face mask as well. A wide variation was found in the extent to which midwives working in English maternity units wore masks, hats and special shoes (Table 50.1). In some units these garments were never worn, in others they were worn all the time; sometimes all individuals will be masked, sometimes only the doctor or midwife and not others in the room.

Table 50.1 Policies with respect to midwives wearing masks, caps, and special shoes in the labour wards of English consultant maternity units, 1984

	Proportion (%) of maternity units		
	Masks	Hats	Shoes
Never	43	81	90
Always	2	3	6
For specified procedures only	44	14	1
Other	11	2	3

3 Routines during labour and delivery

3.1 Enemas and perineal shaving

Table 50.2 shows the extent to which, on admitting women in labour, maternity units in England and Canada prepared them by shaving the perineum and emptying the lower bowel with either an enema or a suppository (see Chapter 51). Although both interventions were used more frequently in Canada than in England, in both countries some hospitals hardly used them at all, while others used them routinely. At the time that the European survey was done in the early 1980s, both perineal shaving and bowel preparation were reported to have been obligatory in Czechoslovakia, Finland, Greece, Italy, and Norway (Maratos 1986).

Table 50.2 Estimated proportion of women having a perineal shave and bowel preparation on admission in labour, English and Canadian maternity units, 1984 and 1985

| Estimated proportion of women | Proportion (%) of maternity units | | | |
| | Perineal shave | | Bowel preparation | |
	England	Canada	England	Canada
Almost all	24	45	15	38
More than half	17	18	20	30
Less than half	10	8	31	16
Hardly any	49	29	35	16

3.2 Food and drink

Concern about the possibility that a women might inhale stomach contents during emergency induction of general anaesthesia is the factor which prompts maternity units to have rules about food and drink during labour (see Chapter 52). But as Table 50.3 shows, opinions clearly differed in English maternity units about the importance of this risk and the ways in which it may be contained. A substantial minority of units had

Table 50.3 Policies in respect of food, drinks other than water, and water alone during labour, English consultant maternity units, 1984

| | % Consultant units | | |
	Food	Drinks other than water	Water
Never	39	26	2
In early labour only	50	33	0
Throughout labour	7	34	86
Other	4	8	12

Table 50.4 Estimated proportion of women receiving intravenous infusion during labour, Canadian maternity units, 1985

Estimated proportion of women	Proportion (%) of maternity units
Almost all	22
More than half	14
Less than half	27
Hardly any	37

a policy forbidding women to eat at any stage during labour; just over a quarter denied women any drink other than water; and some of the units surveyed actually denied even water to women in labour. By contrast, 7 per cent of units permitted women to take food throughout labour if they so wished, and over a third allowed drinks other than water. The Canadian survey did not obtain information about policies concerning food and drink explicitly. What it did show (Table 50.4) was that setting up an intravenous infusion is a common practice in many units and that it is routine in nearly a quarter of them. Here again, however, there were contrasts: in over a third of Canadian maternity units very few women received fluids by intravenous drip.

3.3 Monitoring

It appeared that English maternity units were somewhat more likely than those in Canada to use continuous electronic fetal heart-rate monitoring (see Chapter 54). In a third of English units, compared to a fifth of Canadian units, continuous electronic monitoring was used routinely. Very few English units, but one in five units in Canada used the method only very rarely. (Table 50.5).

Policies for monitoring the progress of labour using vaginal examinations (see Chapter 53) varied among English maternity units. While almost two-thirds of the units surveyed had either no policy at all, or one which they described as flexible, in over a third of the units the progress of labour was assessed by vaginal examinations conducted according to a fixed schedule, usually 4-hourly, but as frequently as 2-hourly in some units

Table 50.5 Estimated proportions of women receiving continuous electronic fetal heart monitoring, English obstetric consultant units, 1984, and Canadian maternity units, 1985

| Estimated proportion of women | Proportion (%) of maternity units | |
	England	Canada
Almost all	32	21
More than half	38	17
Less than half	27	41
Hardly any	3	21

Table 50.6 Policies for vaginal examination to assess progress of labour, English consultant maternity units, 1984

Vaginal examination	Proportion (%) of maternity units
No policy	30
Flexible policy	34
Fixed schedule	36
4-hourly	27
3-hourly	2
2-hourly	3
Other	4

(Table 50.6). Although partograms were being used to record the progress of labour graphically in nine out of ten maternity units in England, in only a quarter was a specific rate of cervical dilatation used to make a diagnosis of abnormally slow progress.

3.4 Position for delivery

Most maternity units in England (87 per cent), but only 43 per cent of those surveyed in Canada, reported that they respected women's choices of position for delivery (see Chapter 55). This difference was reflected in differences in the most usual positions adopted by women during delivery (Table 50.7). Maternity units in Canada were substantially more likely than English units to report that women were usually supine or in lithotomy position during delivery. The fact that over a quarter of English maternity units had a birth chair compared with less than 5 per cent of Canadian units may be either a reflection of, or a cause of, the more flexible policies in England. One in ten English maternity units reported having mattresses on the floor for women who wished to use them, 6 per cent had a birth stool, and 2 per cent a birth bar.

This evidence of a preparedness to be flexible within many English maternity units contrasts strikingly with the conclusion reached after surveying hospitals in other European countries. Mothers were said to have had virtually no choice of position for delivery in Italy, Greece, France, Finland, and Czechoslovakia (Maratos 1986). The situation in some of these countries is

Table 50.7 Most usual position during delivery, English consultant maternity units, 1984, and Canadian maternity units, 1985

Position	England	Canada
Sitting upright	11	3
Semi-recumbent	74	52
Left-lateral	3	0
Supine	3	27
Lithotomy	—	18
Other	10	—

unlikely to be quite as restrictive as implied by this statement, however. At least one hospital in France, for example, not only encourages women to adopt whatever position they find comfortable (Odent 1981), but also has an international reputation (Gillett 1979) as a result of promoting this more flexible attitude.

3.5 Length of second stage

Four out of five maternity units in England had policies restricting the length of the second stage of labour to one hour or less for women having their first baby (Table 50.8). The remainder used more discretionary approaches which were guided by assessments of fetal and maternal well-being (see Chapter 67). A relatively long second stage of labour was less likely to be accepted in multiparae, with 66 per cent of the units surveyed restricting the length to 30 minutes and a further 23 per cent proceeding to assisted delivery an hour after full dilatation of the cervix (Table 50.8). The estimated ranges of episiotomy rates across maternity hospitals within nine European countries stretch from less than 5 per cent to nearly 100 per cent (World Health Organization 1986).

Table 50.8 Policies for limiting the length of the second stage of labour, English obstetric consultant units, 1984

	% Consultant units	
	Primiparae	Multiparae
½ hour	5	66
¾ hour	8	9
1 hour	69	14
Other	18	11

4 Conclusions

The variation in intrapartum practices and routines which we have documented is *a priori* evidence of a collective professional uncertainty concerning the value of the rules which have come to govern the care of women during labour and delivery. As a general working rule we would suggest that professionals are not justified in maintaining and introducing routines into care unless good evidence exists that these are more likely to do good than harm to women using the maternity services. This is not the case for many of the elements of care during labour which we have mentioned.

Implementing change in these matters can be painfully slow. Canadian maternity units have made considerable progress in terms of opening their doors to companions for women during labour and childbirth. Comparison of the results of the 1985 survey with a similar enquiry mounted in 1980 (Post 1981), however, reveals little change in the extent to which women undergo the rituals of shaving and bowel preparation, or in the extent to which they are encouraged to choose the position for delivery which they find most comfortable and effective.

Professionals need a structure within which to do their work, and this structure must necessarily involve working rules and at least some routines; this applies whether the professional is working independently or within an institution. Those who work in institutions, however, are more likely to have to work within a framework of rules intended to serve the interests of other people working in and using the institution. Change can be slow because familiar rules and routines are comforting, and also simply because it takes time to develop and agree new policies—time that may be seen

as better spent providing clinical care. The challenge faced by professionals working in maternity units is firstly to maintain and introduce only those routines and rules which have been shown, on balance, to do more good than harm; and secondly, to apply such routines flexibly and in a way which takes the needs of individual childbearing women into account. A prerequisite for moving in the right direction is that both professionals working in the maternity services and women using those services should be aware of the relevant evidence. This is necessary, not only to enable them make informed choices concerning which routines to accept, but also to assess when these should be applied flexibly to take into account the special needs of individual women.

References

Garcia J, Garforth S, Ayers, A (1986). Midwives confined? Labour ward policies and routines. Proceedings of the 1985 Conference on Research and the Midwife, University of Manchester, pp 2–30.

Gillett J (1979). Childbirth in Pithiviers, France. Lancet, 2: 894–896.

Hanvey L, Post SE (1986). Changing patterns in maternity care. Canadian Nurse, September: 28–34.

Jordan B (1985). Sistemi natali ed etno-ostetrica: frammenti di una ricerca transculturale. In: Culture del parto. Milano: Feltrinelli, pp 73–84.

Maratos O (1986). Rooming-in and other psychosocial aspects of routine perinatal practices in the European Region: consumers' choice and promotion of mother–newborn bonding. In: Perinatal Health Services in Europe. Phaff JML (ed). London: Croom Helm, pp 10–16.

Odent M (1981). The evolution of obstetrics at Pithiviers. Birth Family J, 8: 7–16.

Phaff JML (ed) (1986). Perinatal Health Services in Europe. London: Croom Helm.

Post SE (1981). Family-centred maternity care: the Canadian picture. Dimensions in Health Service, 58: 26–31.

Post SE, Hanvey L (1986). Family-centred maternity care—what has happened in five years. Dimensions in Health Service, 63:14–16.

World Health Organization (1986). Having a baby in Europe. Copenhagen: WHO Regional Office for Europe.

51 Hospital admission practices

Sally Garforth and Jo Garcia

1 Introduction

A woman entering a hospital in labour may have experienced months or even years of anticipation, fear, and uncertainty about childbirth, all focused on the moment when she will walk past the 'point of no return' through the doors into the labour ward. This is the time when she feels, and is, at her most vulnerable. She may be in hospital for the first time. Strange things over which she has limited control are beginning to happen to her body. She may be in considerable physical distress, and at the same time excited at the beginning of a major event in her life. She may have a great deal of anxiety associated with factors that are totally irrelevant to the admission, but are still of utmost importance to her; concern about a child at home with a neighbour sitting in; worry about the puddle on the new mattress, or whether she remembered all the items on the list the hospital gave her; anxiety perhaps about how her partner will react. Above all she is wondering how much it will hurt, and whether she will be able to cope. It is a woman preoccupied with both trivia and life-shattering realizations, in physical and emotional turmoil, who needs to be welcomed into a strange environment and given comfort and care.

The midwife or labour room nurse may have an entirely different set of priorities. Her main concerns are probably to discover what stage of labour the woman is in, and to reassure herself that the mother and baby are well. She will also have record keeping tasks, and sometimes may be responsible for other women in labour. Providing appropriate care for each individual woman, with her individual and idiosyncratic needs, is a daunting task.

This chapter will examine English midwifery practice at admission to hospital of a woman in labour, and set it within the context of research evidence about effective and appropriate care. The data presented in this chapter come from a survey of the directors of midwifery services in all the English Health Districts and an in-depth study of aspects of policy and practice in eight Health Districts selected to provide a range of circumstances and policies (Garcia *et al.* 1987). The in-depth study included observation of care in the labour ward, and interviews with the women and midwives observed. In the course of this field-work 62 admissions of women in normal labour at term were observed with the consent of couples and their midwives.

2 First impression

Various recommendations for changes in admission practices have been made because of a recognition that women are probably anxious, if not actually frightened when they come in labour. The Maternity Services Advisory Committee, in its report on intrapartum care (1984) includes a check-list about admission in labour. This emphasizes the need to welcome and support mothers and their companions and suggests that care-givers should introduce themselves and give information about shift arrangements. Respect for a woman's individual needs, her involvement in decisions about her care, and efforts to preserve her dignity are all crucial, especially at admission.

Women in the present study were asked how confident they had felt when they first arrived in hospital. The majority stated that they were 'very confident' or 'fairly confident' and only 7 out of the 51 who answered this question said that they were 'not very confident'. Forty-one women said, in answer to a second question, that they felt 'very welcome', 8 'fairly welcome', and only one 'not very welcome'.

2.1 Information

Although there is little data available about information and decision-making specifically in regard to admission in labour, there is a large body of general literature about these aspects of maternity care. Cartwright (1979), in the conclusions relating to her study of induction of labour, writes: 'There is clear evidence from the study that many women were not given information they would have liked about various aspects of childbearing. It is also apparent that the large majority, four-fifths, wanted to be involved in making decisions about their care.' Macintyre (1982) describes four 'unproductive stereotypes' which get in the way of communication in maternity care: 'lower class women do not want information or explanation'; 'women do not understand technical terms'; 'the best reply to questions is reassurance'; 'no news is good news'. Kirkham (1983a) suggests that the efforts of midwives to meet women's needs for information are sometimes unsuccessful because women are often reluctant to ask the 'busy' people for information, and so direct questions at staff who are less likely to be decision-makers. Women in her study also gained some of their information from 'eavesdropping', a mechanism which is bound to increase the possibility for misunderstanding.

Kirkham (1983b) makes detailed suggestions about ways to improve the interactions between women and midwives at admission. She describes some of the possible barriers to good communications, and suggests that the admission, which has the potential to be a source of reassurance, may instead become a place where the woman is 'stripped' both literally and metaphorically.

Admission in labour provides an important opportunity for discussion of women's requests, plans, and worries for labour and delivery. One District had a questionnaire built into the system of care at admission so that women's preferences about aspects of labour care would be raised automatically In other areas it was left to individual midwives or women.

Women whose care had been observed made some relevant comments about this aspect of care in the interviews carried out after delivery. One said: 'You feel they would be happy to listen if you wanted things done in a particular way.' And another: 'Not when I came in. But they did ask me a few weeks ago at clinic. When she thinks you're nearly there they ask you what you want so when you come in you've already been asked.' But one respondent was rather disillusioned and said: 'The questionnaire—when they said what sort of a labour do you want?—it's very nice them asking you, then they strap you on a monitor and you're there. Anything you ask for, you can't have.'

In addition to providing an opportunity for the general discussion of a women's needs, the time of admission provides an opportunity for midwives to inform and reassure women, as they explain the various examinations and procedures that are being carried out. Of the admissions observed in this study, a large majority of women (88 per cent) were considered to have received adequate information, only 12 per cent to have received 'minimal, scant or negligible' explanation. There was a tendency, however, for midwives to concentrate on a description of *what* was happening, rather than explaining *why* certain procedures were carried out. Explanations of the results of tests and examinations varied from 'That's fine' to a detailed description of the woman's progress in labour illustrated with diagrams. Individual midwives, as one would expect, varied in their skill in communication and sensitivity, from those who offered unlimited explanation ('Ask any questions you like; what I am doing is routine to me but not to you!') to those whose brisk competence did not invite enquiry or offer information. Occasionally, when there were two caregivers present, there was a tendency to 'talk over' the woman (for example: 'She's about 3 cm'). Complete lack of communication was sometimes observed, especially when obstetric jargon was used. One woman was told by a junior doctor that her cervix was effaced and she later sought clarification from the observer as to what the doctor had meant about its face!

2.2 Forms of address

In less than one in five of the encounters we observed did midwives ask women how they wished to be addressed. Some assumed that she did not mind being called by her first name; some remained on a formal basis using 'Mrs', while others adopted some more familiar term such as 'lovey' or 'pet' depending on the locality. Although some women found this friendly, one woman remarked: 'I don't like being called "lovey" and things like that. I think I could have been treated a bit more as an adult. It made me feel as if I was a child.' Midwives frequently used the phrase 'Good girl' when addressing women. Just over half the midwives introduced themselves by name to the woman. 'I'm Jill and I'll be looking after you while you are here.' This practice of a midwife introducing herself, using whatever title and name she feels appropriate, represents common courtesy and we feel that it should be universal.

2.3 Accompanying persons

The support of a partner or some other companion may be particularly important to a woman in labour at the time of admission to hospital. Considerable variation was found between the eight Health Districts where observation was carried out. In four of the eight Health Districts visited, it was routine practice for the partner to be present at admission, whereas he was usually excluded in the other four Districts. Of the 62 admissions observed, eight of the women (13 per cent) arrived alone, 28 (45 per cent) arrived with a companion or partner who was allowed to stay with them, and 25 (40 per cent) arrived with a partner or companion who was asked to wait elsewhere.

This aspect of care appears to be influenced by the policy or custom in a particular place, although a minority of midwives made individual decisions. In one of the Districts every midwife, when interviewed about this, indicated that companions were encouraged, with comments such as: 'Yes for admission they are encouraged. There are no restrictions now. They can have parents or other relatives.' 'It's the Mum's choice. There are no exceptions.' In another District, the only midwife who allowed a partner to stay during admission (at the woman's request) intimated that she was 'not supposed to'. When interviewed about this, midwives gave a variety of reasons for excluding the partner, including the small size of rooms; that women preferred it; that they were excluded for a vaginal examination or shave or enema; or simply that it was the usual practice. One midwife said: 'I don't know why—probably because of getting them changed and examining them. I suppose it's largely for our convenience. It's what usually happens here.'

In some of the cases where partners had been excluded, the midwives said that partners could have stayed if they had wished. In many of these cases it was observed that they had been asked to wait as a matter of course without being given any real choice. Occasionally couples were met by a ward clerk or auxiliary nurse who automatically asked partners to wait elsewhere. It may seem that this is a minor detail of care, and it may not directly affect the obstetric outcome; but interviews carried out with these women the following day indicated that the presence of a companion at admission was often central to their concerns, and those of their partners. Only two women from our sample (3 per cent) preferred not to have anyone with them at admission. The vast majority of women expressed pleasure and relief when their partner could stay, or disappointment when he was unable to do so, whether because he was at work or looking after other children, or excluded as the result of hospital routine. These particular comments are typical and speak for themselves. 'I was upset. I think you need someone who knows you.' 'I would have liked him to be with me but they told him to wait. He wanted to come in but did not say anything although we had talked about it at home.' 'I thought it was very good. I think it all depends on your choice.'

2.4 Privacy and dignity

In a recent paper about privacy in the labour ward, Flint (1984) drew attention to the contrast between the sort of privacy one can expect at home and that likely to be experienced in a typical maternity hospital: '. . . (I) realised that if I transferred my bedroom to the labour ward I'd want to be able to bolt or lock the door to stop strangers from walking in, especially if I were undressing, having a vaginal examination, having my abdomen palpated, using a bedpan or being emotional. . . .'

From our observation provision for privacy in admission rooms sometimes seemed to be unsatisfactory, often involving curtains and screens of various designs, rather than a door which could be closed. One woman's comment indicates that perceptions of privacy and dignity can vary. 'I felt walking through from the first room to the other room I would have liked to put my dressing gown on. I don't suppose anyone takes any notice, but it's you—how you feel.' Another women felt humiliated by being treated as if she was sick. 'I would have preferred to walk but the man (a porter) insisted that I go in a wheelchair because of the slippy floors.' Perhaps the porter was obeying one of a myriad of written and unwritten hospital rules familiar to maternity unit staff.

One of the first procedures undertaken when women arrive is to ask them to undress. If this is done insensitively it can be quite a humiliating experience, especially because the woman is often already feeling anxious and vulnerable. One midwife said: 'Just take all your clothes off and pop up on the bed. What buttons there are, go down the front and you'll find there's a slit up the back.' Hospital gowns are not usually an aid to confidence and dignity.

Six of the Districts provided a hospital gown, while two asked women to bring an old, comfortable nightshirt from home. This appeared popular with women, as it gave them a little more dignity and individuality. The economic advantage to the health service budget in these stringent times also warrants consideration, in that only a few gowns would have to be provided for women who arrived in an emergency or forgot to bring one.

3 Clinical assessment

The main clinical tasks at admission are to assess a woman's progress in labour, her condition, and that of her baby, and to make decisions about their care. In carrying out these tasks caregivers have various means at their disposal, including a discussion with the woman about her history and symptoms, and obstetric records; observation of her temperature, blood pressure, and general condition; abdominal palpation and vaginal examination; and some form of monitoring of the fetal heart (see Chapters 53 and 54).

The 'diagnosis' of labour has received relatively little research attention, and some important practical questions remain unanswered. For example, the advice given to a woman antenatally, and over the telephone, about the onset of labour will have an influence on her decision to come into hospital. Her experiences in labour may well be affected by the timing of admission in relation to her progress in labour. As Klein and his co-workers (1985) found, different patterns of care can influence the timing of admission. In their study, women booked for delivery in a general practitioner maternity unit, who had often been seen by a community midwife at home, came into hospital further advanced in labour than a matched group of women booked for consultant unit care in the same hospital. Once a woman comes into hospital her experience will vary depending on hospital policies and on the decisions made by her caregivers. If she is judged not to be in labour she may be sent home or to another hospital ward. There is very little evidence about the effects of this process or the consequences of differing policies (see Chapter 53).

3.1 Clinical procedures

Certain clinical procedures appear to be more or less universal when a woman arrives at hospital in labour. In our study 58 (94 per cent) of the women had their temperature taken and blood pressure measured, 54 (87 per cent) had their pulse counted, and 37 (60 per cent) had their urine tested. An explanation of why this was necessary was given to 11 (18 per cent) of the women. Only 21 (34 per cent) were given any indication of whether all was well following these observations. One midwife said jokingly 'You can't but come into a hospital without having a thermometer stuck in your mouth.'

All of the women had abdominal palpation on admission and all the midwives listened to the fetal heart with a Pinard stethoscope, except in one hospital where a period of electronic fetal monitoring was part of the routine admission. The use of electronic fetal monitoring at admission ranged from routine use, through selective use, to units where it was never seen at admission. In units where it was routine, women were occasionally asked if they minded, but often monitoring in this way was accepted as a matter of course. 'I think I'll just put you on this machine for a little while to see how you are doing.'

The majority of women in our study had a vaginal examination at admission, the exception to this being in one hospital where there was a policy for the doctor to carry out a speculum examination if the membranes had ruptured. Overall the membranes were ruptured artificially on admission in 7 cases (11 per cent) and a fetal scalp electrode was attached in 3 of these. In an additional 4 women, with spontaneous rupture of membranes, a fetal scalp electrode was attached at admission. The amount of discussion and explanation about this varied. Some of the women were given a choice while in other cases agreement was assumed. 'I'm just going to do an internal and see how you are doing. If I can I will break your waters and put a clip on baby's head. O.K.?'

3.2 Midwives' priorities

When we asked midwives about their priorities when admitting women to hospital in labour, about two-thirds either mentioned or gave priority to welcoming the woman, making her feel at ease or discussing her needs; the remainder gave clinical priorities only. Some contrasting approaches are shown in the following answers: 'First impressions are important. Win them over. Establish a rapport . . .' 'Onto the bed, palpate and listen-in . . .' 'Make sure they are clean . . .'

Midwives seemed to vary in the extent to which they could adjust their admission routine to allow for women's individual needs. Less experienced midwives may find it harder to be flexible because the clinical and record keeping tasks are less familiar to them. On the other hand, some of the experienced midwives who we observed found it difficult to abandon familiar practices such as bowel preparation. Admission is particularly challenging because neither the clinical tasks nor the personal contact and reassurance can be put to one side. Good midwifery care involves an impressive and seemingly effortless balancing of the two.

4 Preparation procedures

Admission to hospital in labour has often involved the routine use of bowel preparation with enemas or suppositories, and the shaving of some or all of the pubic and perineal area. A bath or shower is often part of the process as well. In their review of preparation for labour, Mahan and McKay (1983) begin with a description of care at the Sloane Maternity Hospital in New York in the early part of this century. Women admitted for labour care '. . . were given an enema followed by a vaginal douche with bichloride of mercury. Their heads were cleansed with kerosene, ether, or ammonia and their nipples and navels doused with ether. Charity patients, who were assumed to harbour an abundance of germs, had their pubic hair shaved, whereas that of private patients was merely clipped.'

This zealous preparation for labour was part of the aggressive onslaught on infective organisms which typified the approach in the early 1900s. Even today, some aspects of admission convey the suggestion that a woman needs to be cleaned-up before she can be 'admitted' to the labour ward. A bath, for example, can be offered as comfort or relaxation, or can be part of the 'cleaning' routine.

4.1 Enemas

The routine use of bowel preparation has been recommended to allow the fetal head to descend; to stimulate contractions and thereby shorten labour; to reduce contamination at delivery and so to minimize infection rates for the mother and the baby. Myles (1981) recommends routine use of an enema principally to allow more room for the fetus. She also asserts that an enema will disperse the contractions of 'false labour'. Mahan and McKay (1983), on the other hand, have drawn attention to the potential risks involved in the use of enemas, particularly those with soapsuds. They cite documented cases of rectal irritation, colitis, gangrene, and anaphylactic shock.

There are two reports of randomized controlled trials mounted to evaluate the effects of routinely giving women enemas on admission to hospital in labour (Romney and Gordon 1981; Drayton and Rees 1984). The available evidence suggests that the rate of faecal soiling is unaffected during the first stage of labour (Table 51.1), but reduced during the second stage (Table 51.2). However, in both studies the investigators noted that the soiling in the control group was mainly slight and easier to remove than soiling in the enema group. No effects on the duration of labour or on neonatal or perineal wound infection have been detected (Drayton and Rees 1984).

Of the 19 women who had an enema or suppositories whom we questioned in our in-depth study, 3 were pleased or had requested this, 6 did not mind or were prepared to have whatever was necessary, and 6 expressed negative feelings about it such as embarrassment, discomfort, or reluctance. The majority of women who did not have an enema were pleased or relieved not to, but some did not have strong views.

The reasons offered by midwives for giving an enema included hospital policy, policies of individual consultants, a belief that most women would be more comfortable with an empty bowel, or a belief that this particular woman had a need for an enema. Reasons for not giving an enema included 'no fixed policy', 'no time', and an assessment of 'no need'.

4.2 Pubic shaving

The stated purpose of routine predelivery shaving has been to lessen the risk of infection and, presumably, to make suturing easier and safer. As early as 1922, Johnston and Sidall provided evidence which challenged these assumptions. Their controlled trial, and the only other controlled trial (Kantor 1965), were unable to detect any protective effect of perineal shaving in respect of puerperal febrile morbidity (Table 51.3), a finding which was supported by the results of a non-randomized cohort comparison reported by Romney (1980). Bond (1980) and Mahan and McKay (1983) have drawn attention to the disadvantages in terms of discomfort as the hair grows back, and this problem (as well as the minor abrasions caused by shaving), was noted by Romney (1980) in her non-randomized cohort comparison of women receiving no shave, a partial shave, or a complete shave because of their consultants' preferences. She found no statistically significant difference in infection rates between the groups.

Of the admissions we observed, 10 per cent involved

Table 51.1 The effect of enema on admission in labour on faecal soiling in first stage of labour

Study	EXPT		CTRL		Odds ratio	Graph of odds ratios and confidence intervals						
	n	(%)	n	(%)	(95% CI)	0.01	0.1	0.5	1	2	10	100
Romney and Gordon (1981)	1/25	(4.00)	4/25	(16.00)	0.27 (0.04–1.69)							
Drayton and Rees (1984)	15/109	(13.76)	14/113	(12.39)	1.13 (0.52–2.46)							
Typical odds ratio (95% confidence interval)					0.91 (0.44–1.86)							

Table 51.2 The effect of enema on admission in labour on faecal soiling during delivery

Study	EXPT		CTRL		Odds ratio	Graph of odds ratios and confidence intervals						
	n	(%)	n	(%)	(95% CI)	0.01	0.1	0.5	1	2	10	100
Romney and Gordon (1981)	6/25	(24.00)	4/25	(16.00)	1.63 (0.41–6.44)							
Drayton and Rees (1984)	24/109	(22.02)	63/113	(55.75)	0.24 (0.14–0.42)							
Typical odds ratio (95% confidence interval)					0.31 (0.19–0.52)							

Table 51.3 The effect of perineal shaving on admission in labour on postpartum febrile morbidity

Study	EXPT		CTRL		Odds ratio	Graph of odds ratios and confidence intervals						
	n	(%)	*n*	(%)	(95% CI)	0.01	0.1	0.5	1	2	10	100
Kantor *et al.* (1965)	4/75	(5.33)	5/75	(6.67)	0.79 (0.21–3.03)							
Johnston and Sidall (1922)	32/196	(16.33)	22/193	(11.40)	1.51 (0.85–2.68)							
Typical odds ratio (95% confidence interval)					1.37 (0.81–2.31)							

a complete shave, 26 per cent a partial shave, and the majority involved no shave. Of the 22 women who had a shave of some sort, 1 felt it better to be shaved, 3 expected to be shaved, 8 did not mind, and 6 women did not want a shave or did not feel that they had any real choice. The majority of women who did not have a shave were pleased or relieved not to, but some did not mind.

4.3 Providing information about routines

Our data on shaving and bowel preparation showed that midwives' decisions and actions are affected by the policies in the hospitals in which they work, but within this framework there are more subtle ways in which caregivers communicate with women and which can enlarge or inhibit the options that women actually have. The following examples are from direct observation of midwives and women at admission. The first example is an open question: 'How do you feel about a shave?' The midwife then goes on to present the woman with the opportunity to refuse without being difficult. 'Would you rather not?' The second is a statement: 'We usually give a small shave'. This statement does not insist that the woman has a shave, but it does make it obvious that she would be breaking the norm if she were to say that she does not want one. In the third example the midwife gives the woman a nominal choice by the use of the word 'All right?': I'm going to give you an enema. All right?' When the question is presented in this way it affords little choice unless the woman is prepared to be quite assertive, as she then would have to indicate that it is *not* 'all right'. The fourth example shows a case where a woman is given warning but not really *any* choice. A student midwife asks the midwife 'Can I have a razor please? I'll give her a quick shave while I've got her in this position.' She then tells the mother: 'It's only so I've got a good view when the baby is coming.' In the last case: 'The next thing I'm going to do is give you a shave and an enema.' The midwife realizes that she needs to give information, but again she presents no real choice.

These examples of the way in which midwives com-municate with the women in their care are not a representative sample from the field-work. They have been selected to illustrate how choices can be given or restricted. In many of the admissions observed, the subject of a shave or enema was fully discussed and in many units the woman was told that these procedures would not be carried out if she objected. Individual midwives certainly differ in the way that they allow or inhibit choice and implement policies.

5 Conclusions

The presence of a companion is now a generally accep-ted part of labour care, and important to many women during admission when they may be in most need of support. The presence of the companion or companions that they choose should be encouraged and facilitated.

Because admission is a time when women may be particularly vulnerable, caregivers should pay attention to ways of maintaining women's dignity. Maternity units should consider possible ways of providing more privacy and of treating women more as adults, for example, in styles of address and introductions by staff. Abandoning the traditional hospital gown could be one other step towards this goal.

Women appreciate the efforts that midwives make to inform and consult them about their progress in labour and the care they are to receive. When choices about care are offered to women, caregivers should present those choices in a manner that allows women to ask for what they want, and discuss their uncertainties.

There is no justification for continuing to administer enemas routinely or for perineal shaving. The midwife admitting a woman to the labour ward is faced with a challenging task as she seeks to give appropriate and individual care and to balance the clinical and personal aspects of care. The effects of what she says and does to a woman at such a crucial time may be far reaching and long remembered. She has it in her power to make admission a weakness or a strength.

References

Bond S (1980). Shave it . . . or save it? Nursing Times, Feb. 28: 362–363.

Cartwright A (1979). The Dignity of Labour? London: Tavistock.

Drayton S, Rees C (1984). They know what they're doing. Nursing Mirror, 159: 4–8.

Flint C (1984). Coziness in the delivery suite. Nursing Times, 13 June: 28–30.

Garcia J, Garforth S, Ayers S (1987). The policy and practice in midwifery study: Introduction and methods. Midwifery, 3: 2–9.

Garforth S, Garcia J (1987). Admitting—a weakness or a strength? Routine admission of a woman in labour. Midwifery, 3: 10–24.

Johnston RA, Sidall RS (1922). Is the usual method of preparing patients for delivery beneficial or necessary? Am J Obstet Gynecol, 4: 645–650.

Kantor HI, Rember R, Tabio P, Buchanon R (1965). Value of shaving the pudendal-perineal area in delivery preparation. Obstet Gynaecol, 25: 509–512.

Kirkham M (1983a). Labouring in the dark: Limitations on the giving of information to enable patients to orient themselves to the likely events and timescale of labour. In: Nursing Research—Ten Studies in Patient Care. Wilson-Barnet J (ed). Chichester: John Wiley, pp 81–89.

Kirkham M (1983b). Admission in labour: Teaching the patient to be patient? Midwives' Chron, Feb: 44–45.

Klein M, Elbourne D, Lloyd I (1985). A prospective study comparing the experiences of low risk women booked for delivery in two systems of maternity care. Occasional Paper No. 31, April. London: Royal College of General Practitioners.

Macintyre S (1982). Communications between pregnant women and their medical and midwifery attendants, Midwives' Chron, Nov: 387–394.

Mahan CS, McKay S (1983). Preps and enemas—keep or discard? Contemporary Obstet Gynaecol, Nov: 241–248.

Maternity Services Advisory Committee (1984). Maternity care in action, Part II—care during childbirth. London: Her Majesty's Stationery Office.

Myles M (1981). Textbook for Midwives (9th edn). Edinburgh: Churchill Livingstone.

Romney ML, (1980). Predelivery shaving: an unjustified assault? J Obstet Gynaecol, 1: 33–35.

Romney ML, Gordon H (1981). Is your enema really necessary? Br Med J, 282: 1269–1271.

52 Nutrition and hydration in labour

Claire Johnson, Marc J. N. C. Keirse, Murray Enkin, and Iain Chalmers

1 Introduction

Many aspects of care during labour and childbirth are debatable; few of these debates, however, are fought with so much heat and so little light as those concerning whether or not women in labour should have free access to food and drink. The opinion that food and drink should be withheld once labour has commenced is most widely held. A small minority, however, hold equally strongly that, except for women at high risk of needing general anaesthesia, the benefits of allowing women nourishment as they wish far outweigh the minuscule benefits of more restrictive policies.

These contrasting opinions are expressed in practice. A survey of labour ward policies in England revealed that over a third of consultant maternity units allowed no fluid and drink whatsoever during labour (Garcia et al. 1986). In only 7 per cent of the units surveyed was the stated policy to allow women food as desired. The remaining maternity units had intermediate policies, but most prohibited all solid foods. A recent survey in the United States showed a similar picture (McKay and Mahan 1988). Almost 50 per cent of the responding units in their survey allowed no oral intake except ice chips; most of the remainder allowed only sips of clear fluids; only about one in ten units allowed women to drink as much fluid as they desired. None permitted the woman to eat and drink as she wished.

For many women these restrictions would not present a problem. A substantial proportion of women do not want to eat during labour, particularly during its later phases. For those who do, however, enforced hunger during the first stage of labour can be a highly unpleasant experience (Simkin 1986). More than thirty years ago Crawford (1956b), commenting on a policy of no oral intake during labour for women at above average risk of requiring general anaesthesia in the unit in which he was the obstetric anaesthetist, noted that 'even those who eventually came to forceps delivery commented that their only unpleasant memory of their stay in hospital was of their hunger during the first stage of labour'. Why then are such restrictive policies with regard to food and drink employed when some women so obviously find them distressing? The explanation lies in the widespread concern that eating and drinking during labour will put women at an increased and unacceptable risk of regurgitation and aspiration of gastric contents.

This concern is real, and serious. The risk of aspiration is, however, almost entirely associated with the use of general anaesthesia. The degree of risk will therefore relate directly to the frequency with which general anaesthesia accompanies childbirth, and to the care and skill with which the anaesthetic is administered (see Chapter 72).

Policies that restrict oral intake during labour have the laudable objective of reducing the risk of regurgitation and inhalation of gastric contents. In this chapter we will examine the magnitude of the risk; the degree to which these policies are effective in achieving their objective; the efficacy of other policies with the same aim; and the untoward effects that may be associated with them. Examination of the effects of these policies is seriously hampered by the lack of research evidence. The inadequacy of this evidence is disturbing in view of the importance of the problem, and surprising in view of the vehemence with which the arguments supporting these policies are expressed.

2 Risks of aspiration

There are two quite separate risks associated with the regurgitation and aspiration of gastric contents. First, aspiration of food particles of sufficient size to obstruct a main stem or segmental bronchus may result in atelectasis distal to the obstruction, possibly with severe hypoxaemia as a consequence. Second, even in the absence of particulate matter, gastric aspirate, if sufficiently acidic, will cause chemical burns in the airways, resulting in disruption and necrosis of the bronchial, bronchiolar, and alveolar lining. It is this syndrome of acid aspiration in particular, described by Mendelson (1946) over 40 years ago, that constitutes the greatest risk in pregnant women who undergo general anaesthesia (see Chapter 72).

The absolute level of the risk of aspiration has always been low, and now is very low. Mendelson's (1946) classic paper, in which he first described the syndrome of acid aspiration that bears his name, reported no deaths, despite aspiration and the subsequent development of aspiration pneumonia. Scott (1986) pointed out that '. . . the rarity of this condition must be noted. The prevention of even one death by increasing gastric pH would not be apparent until 200,000 women in labour had been treated.' In the United States, between 1974 and 1978, 408 of the 2475 maternal deaths (16 per cent) were related to complications of analgesia and anaesthesia, but only a quarter of these (4 per cent of maternal deaths) were due to aspiration of gastric contents (Kaunitz *et al.* 1985). Between 1979 and 1981, of a total of 176 direct obstetric maternal deaths in England and Wales, 29 (16.5 per cent) were associated with anaesthesia, and 8 (4.5 per cent of the total) of these were due to inhalation of gastric contents (Department of Health and Social Security 1986). A Massachusetts maternal mortality report showed that the leading causes of maternal death from 1982 to 1985 were trauma, pulmonary embolus, and pregnancy induced hypertension, followed by intracranial haemorrhage, infection, and amniotic fluid embolus. Anaesthesia ranked tenth as a cause of maternal death, with an anaesthesia-related maternal mortality rate of 0.3 per 100,000 births from 1982 to 1985 (Sachs *et al.* 1987).

Even one avoidable maternal death is a terrible tragedy. It is clear, however, that aspiration of gastric contents now plays a very small role, in both absolute and relative terms, as a cause of maternal death. Nevertheless, it remains a cause of unquantified mater-

nal morbidity in women who aspirate gastric contents but do not die.

Over the years a number of specific measures have been introduced in attempts to avoid aspiration. Before considering these, however, it is important to remember that the competence of those administering general anaesthetics to pregnant women has been a matter of concern for over a generation. In 1956 Parker stated 'it is probable that the skilled anaesthetist can invariably avoid disaster . . . but by the nature of obstetric work it is unlikely that a skilled anaesthetist can be always and everywhere available.' Thirty years later Morgan (1986), commenting on the most recent report on confidential enquiries into maternal deaths in England and Wales stated: 'A factor which is repeatedly noted is the frequency with which inexperienced anaesthetists are involved with these disasters.' A detailed discussion of anaesthetic techniques is beyond the scope of this chapter, but it has been repeatedly pointed out that failure to apply proper anaesthetic technique is the major reason that deaths from aspiration of gastric contents still occurs (Moir 1978; Levinson and Shnider 1986; Gibbs *et al.* 1986; Morgan 1986; Crawford 1986). Of the various elements of good technique, the most important is undoubtedly the use of cricoid pressure (Sellick 1961) to stop regurgitation of gastric contents during the critical time period between induction of anaesthesia and intubation (see Chapter 72).

Whether or not aspiration problems could be completely abolished if proper anaesthetic technique were always to be employed remains uncertain. It is clear, however, that most of these problems could be prevented by a combination of the avoidance of unnecessary procedures that require anaesthesia, particularly caesarean section (see Chapter 70), the use of regional anaesthesia whenever feasible, and meticulous attention to safe anaesthetic technique (see Chapter 72). Measures to reduce the volume and to increase the pH of gastric contents cannot compensate for inadequate anaesthetic technique; such measures are, however, widely used. The following sections will review the evidence concerning their efficacy.

3 Measures to reduce gastric volume and acidity

3.1 Restriction of oral intake

Fasting, with the aim of ensuring an empty stomach, is the most commonly used measure aimed at reducing the volume of the gastric contents. There is, however, no guarantee that withholding food and drink during labour will ensure that the stomach will be empty in the event that general anaesthesia should become necessary. Roberts and Shirley (1976), who obtained information about gastric volume in 146 women during labour by tube aspiration of gastric contents at the time of anaesthesia, found that although the volume diminished with time since the last meal, reaching a minimum average of about 20 ml after 20 hours, the volume then began to rise again due to gastric secretions. Women who had not eaten for more than eight hours before labour started had the lowest average volume of gastric aspirate, but the authors noted that no time interval between the last meal and the onset of labour guaranteed a stomach volume of less than 100 ml.

Howard and Sharp (1973), in the course of a double blind randomized controlled trial of the effect of metoclopramide on gastric emptying during labour in nulliparous women, found that, even in women who had had no solid food for at least 18 hours previously, the mean volume of the gastric contents was 567 ml in the placebo-treated group and still as much as 363 ml in the women who had received metoclopramide.

It should be noted that in the study reported by Howard and Sharp (1973), pethidine had been administered to women in both groups for analgesia when needed. Nimmo and colleagues (1975), among others (Crawford 1956a,b; Holdsworth 1978; Wilson 1978), showed that pethidine, diamorphine, and pentazocine given to labouring women greatly delayed gastric emptying compared to those women not given narcotics in labour. Advanced labour may result in a modest reduction in gastric emptying time, but the evidence supporting this belief is very weak (Crawford 1987). Indeed, in one of the very few studies to use a reliable technique for measuring gastric emptying (Crawford 1956b), ten of the twelve women studied showed normal gastric emptying of semi-solid material during active labour. Whatever the magnitude of any real effect of pregnancy or labour that may exist, it is likely to be small compared to the effect of narcotics (Wilson 1978).

In addition, as pointed out by Crawford as early as 1956, 'starving women in labour is obviously impracticable'. He suggested, instituted in its place, and maintained (Crawford 1978) the use of a low residue, low fat diet with the aim of providing palatable, attractive, small meals at frequent intervals, avoiding foods with long fibres and foods which form a large clot or ball in the stomach, e.g. milk, soft bread, and foods which remain in the stomach for long periods or which delay the emptying of the stomach, e.g. fats. The diet consisted of tea, fruit juice, lightly cooked eggs, crisp toast and butter, plain biscuits, clear broth, and tinned fruits. Crawford (1978) maintained that 'Those women—and they form the great majority of the patient population— who are unlikely to require general anaesthesia, are classified as "low risk", and may be offered the prepared diet at any appropriate time during labour'. Fasting, he believed, should be reserved for women who are at high risk of requiring general anaesthesia, who should receive no food or drink except sips of

water or sweets to suck. 'The diet has proved acceptable to the many thousands of patients who have taken it during labour in our hospital. It has never been a source of concern to patients or staff.'

From the above it is clear that fasting during labour does not have the desired effect of ensuring an empty stomach, and, to quote Roberts and Shirley (1974), 'the myth of considering the time interval between the last meal and either delivery or the onset of labour as a guide to gastric content volume should now be laid firmly to rest.'

Nor can fasting during labour be relied on to lower the acidity of the gastric contents. Roberts and Shirley (1976) reported that 50 per cent of women whose last meal was within 12 hours, and 33 per cent who had eaten more than 12 hours before, had gastric contents with a pH of below 2.5 if no antacid had been given. Four of six women whose last meal was more than 20 hours before delivery and who did not take antacids, had a gastric pH below 1.8. Crawford (1986) commented provocatively 'Is it not intriguing that, in England and Wales, the number of maternal deaths from acid-aspiration apparently rose only after the appearance of Parker's (1956) paper led to severe dietary restriction in labour, amounting in most units almost to starvation?'

3.2 Pharmacologic approaches

The frequency of unpredictably large volumes and equally unpredictable low pH values of the gastric contents, whether women fast or do not fast during labour, has led to the deployment of a number of agents in an attempt both to lower the gastric volume and to decrease the gastric acidity of labouring women.

3.2.1 Pharmacologic measures to decrease gastric volume

An increase in the rate of gastric emptying can be achieved with both cimetidine (Qvist and Storm 1983) and metoclopramide (Howard and Sharp 1973; Bylsma-Howell *et al.* 1983; Murphy *et al.* 1984), and this results in quite striking decreases in gastric volume, as shown in controlled comparisons of cimetidine and antacids (Table 52.1).

The stomach contents can be emptied mechanically with a stomach tube, or vomiting induced with apomorphine pre-operatively. Holdsworth *et al.* (1980) compared these two methods by using them in alternate women in labour who required a general anaesthetic. There was no statistically significant difference in the mean gastric aspirate during operation (24 ± 6.91 ml for the apomorphine, 30 ± 7 ml for the stomach tube). The majority of the women having the stomach tube passed found it 'very unpleasant', whereas the majority of those receiving apomorphine found the procedure only 'slightly unpleasant'. It should be noted that neither

Table 52.1 The effect of hydrogen ion antagonists versus antacids on mean (SD) gastric volume (ml) prior to delivery

Study	N	H+antagonist		Antacid		Diff.
Husemeyer and Davenport (1980)	62	7.6	(8.8)	18.4	(25.3)	−10.8
Pickering et al. (1980)	16	72.0	(9.0)	104.0	(43.0)	−32.0
Ostheimer et al. (1982)	24	21.1	(12.9)	46.6	(28.3)	−25.5
Tettambel (1983)	20	23.5	(18.4)	29.6	(21.2)	−6.1
Hodgkinson et al. (1983)	89	11.0	(2.0)	33.4	(5.2)	−22.4
Frank et al. (1984)	25	11.5	(9.1)	51.9	(27.9)	−40.4

Table 52.2 The effect of hydrogen ion antagonists versus antacids on mean (SD) gastric pH prior to delivery

Study	N	H+antagonist	Antacid	Diff
Husemeyer and Davenport (1980)	62	4.3 (2.1)	7.8 (1.0)	−3.5
Pickering et al. (1980)	16	5.0 (NA)	4.6 (NA)	+0.4
Ostheimer et al. (1982)	24	5.5 (2.3)	4.2 (2.0)	+1.3
Tettambel (1983)	20	4.0 (2.0)	3.7 (1.8)	+0.3
Hodgkinson et al. (1983)	89	6.3 (0.2)	5.5 (0.3)	+0.8
Frank et al. (1984)	25	5.2 (2.2)	7.6 (1.3)	−2.4

method guarantees that the stomach will be empty; maximum residual gastric volumes were 300 ml for the apomorphine treated women and 120 ml for women for whom gastric 'emptying' with a stomach tube was employed.

3.2.2 Pharmacologic measures to increase gastric pH

A survey of 317 departments of anaesthesia in the United Kingdom (Sweeney and Wright 1986) showed a remarkable diversity of practices aimed at lowering gastric acidity. No prophylaxis at all was used in 18.5 per cent of the units surveyed; 53.5 per cent used magnesium trisilicate (in 46.7 per cent, it was the only prophylactic used); 23 per cent used sodium citrate (in 12 per cent, as the sole agent); 3.4 per cent used cimetidine (in 0.7 per cent, as the sole agent); and 11.3 per cent used ranitidine (in 5.5 per cent, as the sole agent).

In view of the rarity of the acid aspiration syndrome, it is hardly surprising that none of these has been adequately tested in terms of their ability to reduce the incidence of this fearful complication. Evaluation of their efficacy has been limited to examining whether or not they are capable of raising gastric pH above an arbitrarily defined cut-off point of 2.5.

The results of controlled trials have shown that gastric pH can be raised prior to delivery by the use of aluminium hydroxide (Taylor and Pryse-Davies 1966), magnesium trisilicate (Taylor and Pryse-Davies 1966), sodium citrate (Dewan et al. 1984; Abboud et al. 1984), metoclopramide (Cohen et al. 1984), and the hydrogen ion antagonist cimetidine (McCaughey et al. 1981; Qvist and Storm 1983). Randomized comparisons between different agents have provided no evidence that any particular agent or class of agents influences gastric pH prior to delivery any more effectively than others agents or classes of agents (Taylor and Pryse-Davies 1966; Tettambel 1983; and Table 52.2).

The effectiveness of these agents in raising gastric pH, however, does not necessarily mean that they will have an effect on the incidence or severity of Mendel-son's syndrome. Although from 1966 onward there has been a movement towards the routine administration of alkalis to all women in labour, Scott (1978) noted that cases of Mendelson's syndrome occurred in women who had had a full regimen of antacid treatment, and so the efficacy of this prophylaxis is still in doubt. Scott (1978) also questioned the safety of repeated administration of alkalis, and pointed out that their use 'has certainly led to a false sense of security'.

4 Intravenous hydration and nourishment

Restricting food and drink during labour may result in dehydration and ketosis. Whether the degree of ketosis that occurs in some women during labour is a harmless physiological state or a pathological condition that interferes with uterine action is uncertain (Dumoulin and Foulkes 1984). There has been no research published about the nutritional needs of the labouring woman. For some women, these are likely to be similar to those of an individual engaged in strenuous athletic activity (Hazle 1986).

The most common response to the problem of ketosis in maternity units where eating during labour is prohibited is the use of intravenous infusion of glucose and fluid. The effects of this practice should be carefully weighed against those of the alternative course of allowing women to eat and drink as they desire.

The maternal effects of intravenous infusion of carbohydrate-containing solutions during labour have been evaluated in a number of controlled trials. The rise in mean serum glucose levels (Inman 1971; Ames et al. 1975; Lawrence et al. 1982; Morton et al. 1985; Evans et al. 1986) appears to be accompanied by a rise in maternal insulin levels (Morton et al. 1985), and a reduction in mean levels of 3-hydroxybutyrate (Ames et al. 1975; Morton et al. 1985; Evans et al. 1986). The available data show no consistent direction of effect on either maternal pH or lactate levels (Inman 1971; Ames

Table 52.3 Effect of maternal dextrose infusions during labour on plasma glucose levels in the newborn (mmol/litre; mean ± SD)

Study	N	Dilution	Dextrose	Control	Diff.
Evans *et al.* (1986)	50	2.5%	4.0 (1.7)	2.9 (0.6)	+3.1
Inman (1971)	20	5%	4.2 (NA)	3.4 (NA)	+0.8
	20	10%	4.9 (NA)	3.4 (NA)	+1.6
Lawrence *et al.* (1982)	19	10%	14.3 (2.3)	2.5 (0.6)	+11.9

Table 52.4 Effect of maternal dextrose infusions during labour on mean (SD) umbilical arterial blood pH

Study	N	Dilution	Dextrose	Control	Diff.
Inman (1971)	20	5%	7.19 (NA)	7.25 (NA)	−0.06
	20	10%	7.28 (NA)	7.25 (NA)	+0.03
Lawrence *et al.* (1982)	19	10%	7.26 (0.07)	7.33 (0.03)	−0.07

et al. 1975; Lawrence *et al.* 1982; Morton *et al.* 1985; Evans *et al.* 1986).

As far as the baby is concerned, however, infusion of carbohydrate-containing solutions to the mother results not only in an increase in plasma glucose levels (Table 52.3) but may also result in a decrease in umbilical arterial blood pH (Table 52.4). Iatrogenic hyperinsulinism in the fetus can occur when women receive more than 25 g glucose intravenously during labour (Rutter *et al.* 1980; Lucas *et al.* 1980). This can result in neonatal hypoglycemia and raised levels of blood lactate (Aynsley-Green and Saltesz 1986). Furthermore, the excessive use of salt-free intravenous solutions can result in serious hyponatraemia in both the mother and the fetus (Tarnow-Mordi et al. 1981).

The use of intravenous infusion of glucose and fluids to combat ketosis and dehydration in the mother may thus have potentially serious unwanted effects on the baby. These potential hazards might be obviated by the more physiologic approach of using the oral route for supplying calories and fluids during labour.

5 Conclusions

No presently known measures can ensure that a labouring woman's stomach is empty, or that her gastric juices will have a pH greater than 2.5. Enforced fasting in labour, the use of antacids, or pre-anaesthetic mechanical or chemical emptying of the stomach are only partially effective. All of these have unpleasant consequences, and are potentially hazardous to the mother and possibly her baby.

The syndrome of aspiration of gastric contents under general anaesthesia is rare but serious. It is wise whenever feasible to avoid general anaesthesia for delivery whenever possible, and to use a proper anaesthetic technique with meticulous attention to the known safeguards, especially cricoid pressure.

References

Abboud TK, Curtis J, Earl S, Henriksen EH, Hughes SC, Levinson G, Shnider SM (1984). Efficacy of clear antacid prophylaxis in obstetrics. Acta Anaesthesiol Scand, 28: 301–304.

Ames AC, Cobbold S, Maddock J (1975). Lactic acidosis complicating treatment of ketosis of labour. Br Med J, 4: 611–613.

Aynsley-Green A, Soltesz G (1986). Metabolic and endocrine disorder. Part I. Disorder of blood glucose homeostasis in the neonate. In: Textbook of Neonatology. Roberton NRC (ed). Edinburgh: Churchill Livingstone.

Bylsma-Howell M, Riggs KW, McMorland GH, Rurak DW, Ongley R, McErlane B, Price JDE, Axelson JE (1983). Placental transport of metoclopramide: assessment of maternal and neonatal effects. Can Anaesth Soc J, 30: 487–492.

Cohen SE, Jasson J, Talafre M-L, Chauvelot-Moachon L, Barrier G (1984). Does metoclopramide decrease the volume of gastric contents in patients undergoing cesarean section? Anesthesiology, 61: 604–607.

Crawford JS (1956a). Some aspects of obstetric anaesthesia. Br J Anaesth, 28: 146–158

Crawford JS (1956b). Some aspects of obstetric anaesthesia: Part III. Br J Anaesth, 28: 201–208.

Crawford JS (1978) Principles and practice of obstetric anaesthesia (4th edn). Oxford: Blackwell Scientific Publications.

Crawford JS (1986). Maternal mortality from Mendelson's syndrome. Lancet, 1: 920–921.

Crawford JS (1987) Preoperative oral fluids. Anesth Analg, 66: 914–915.

Crawford JS, Potter SR (1984). Magnesium trisilicate mixture BP: its physical characteristics and effectiveness as a prophylactic. Anaesthesia, 39: 535–539.

Department of Health and Social Security (1986). Report on confidential enquiries into maternal deaths in England and Wales 1979–1981. Report on Health and Social Subjects 29. London: Her Majesty's Stationery Office.

Dewan DM, Floyd HM, Thistlewood JM, Bogard TD (1984). Sodium citrate premedication for elective cesarean section (abstract). Anesth Analg, 63: 205.

Dumoulin JG, Foulkes JEB (1984). Ketonuria during labour. Br J Obstet Gynaecol, 91: 97–98.

Evans SE, Crawford JS, Stevens ID, Durbin GM, Daya H (1986). Fluid therapy for induced labour under epidural analgesia: biochemical consequences for mother and infant. Br J Obstet Gynaecol, 93: 329–333.

Frank M, Evans M, Flynn P, Aun C (1984). Comparison of the prophylactic use of magnesium trisilicate mixture BPC, sodium citrate mixture or cimetidine in obstetrics. Br J Anaesth, 56: 355–361.

Garcia J, Garforth S, Ayers S (1986). Midwives confined? Labour ward policies and routines. Research and the Midwife Conference, Manchester 1985. Proceedings, pp 2–30.

Gibbs CP, Krischer J, Peckham BM, Sharp H, Kirschbaum TH (1986). Obstetric anesthesia; a national survey. Anesthesiology, 65: 298–306.

Hazle NR (1986). Hydration in labor: is routine intravenous hydration necessary? J Nurs Midwifery, 31: 171.

Hodgkinson R, Glassenberg R, Joyce TH, Coombs DW, Ostheimer GW, Gibbs CP (1983). Comparison of cimetidine (Tagamet) with antacid for safety and effectiveness in reducing gastric acidity before elective caesarean section. Anesthesiology, 59: 86–90.

Holdsworth JD (1978). The place of apomorphine prior to obstetric analgesia. J Int Med Res, 6: 26–32.

Holdsworth JD, Johnson K, Mascall G, Roulston RG, Tomlinson PA (1980). Mixing of antacids with stomach contents. Another approach to the prevention of the acid aspiration (Mendelson's) syndrome. Anaesthesia, 35: 641–650.

Howard FA, Sharp DS (1973). Effect of metoclopramide on gastric emptying during labour. Br Med J, 1: 446–448.

Husemeyer RP, Davenport HT (1980). Prophylaxis for Mendelson's syndrome before elective caesarean section. A comparison of cimetidine and magnesium trisilicate mixture regimens. Br J Obstet Gynaecol, 87: 565–570.

Inman SE (1971).The treatment of ketosis in labour. J Obstet Gynaecol Br Cmmnwlth, 78: 624–627.

Kaunitz AM, Hughes JM, Grimes DA, Smith JC, Rochat RW, Kafrissen ME (1985). Causes of maternal mortality in the United States. Obstet Gynecol, 65: 605–621.

Lawrence GF, Brown VA, Parsons RJ, Cooke ID (1982). Feto-maternal consequences of high-dose glucose infusion during labour. Br J Obstet Gynaecol, 89: 27–32.

Levinson G, Shnider SM (1986). Obstetric anesthesia coverage—a continuing problem. Anesthesiology, 65: 245–246.

Lucas A, Adrian TE, Aynsley-Green A, Bloom SR (1980). Iatrogenic hyperinsulinism at birth. Lancet, 1: 144–145.

McCaughey W, Howe JP, Moore J, Dundee JW (1981). Cimetidine in elective caesarean section. Effect on gastric acidity. Anaesthesia, 36: 167–172.

McKay S, Mahan C (1988). I. Modifying the stomach contents of labouring women: why, how, with what success, and at what risks? II. How can aspiration of vomitus in obstetrics best be prevented? Birth, 15: in press.

Mendelson CL (1946). The aspiration of stomach contents into the lungs during obstetric anesthesia. Am J Obstet Gynecol, 52: 191–205.

Moir DD (1978). The contribution of anaesthesia to maternal mortality. J Int Med Res, 6: 40–44.

Morgan M (1986). The confidential enquiry into maternal deaths. Anaesthesia, 41: 689–691.

Morton KE, Jackson MC, Gillmer MDG (1985). A comparison of the effects of four intravenous solutions for the treatment of ketonuria during labour. Br J Obstet Gynaecol, 92: 473–479.

Murphy DF, Nally B, Gardiner J, Unwin A (1984). Effect of metoclopramide on gastric emptying before elective and emergency caesarean section. Br J Anaesth, 56: 1113–1116.

Nimmo WS, Wilson J, Prescott LF (1975). Narcotic analgesics and delayed gastric emptying during labour. Lancet, 1: 890–893.

Ostheimer GW, Morrison JA, Lavoie C, Sepkoski C, Hoffman J, Datta S (1982). The effect of cimetidine on the mother, newborn and neonatal behavior. Anesthesiology, 57: A405.

Parker RB (1956). Maternal death from aspiration asphyxia. Br Med J, 2: 16–19.

Pickering BG, Palahniuk RJ, Cumming M (1980). Cimetidine premedication in elective caesarean section. Can Anaesth Soc J, 27: 33–35.

Qvist N, Storm K (1983). Cimetidine pre-anesthetic. A prophylactic method against Mendelson's syndrome in cesarean section. Acta Obstet Gynecol Scand, 62: 157–159.

Roberts RB, Shirley MA (1974). Reducing the risk of acid aspiration during caesarean section. Anesth Analg, 53: 859–868.

Roberts RB, Shirley MA (1976). The obstetrician's role in reducing the risk of aspiration pneumonitis. With particular reference to the use of oral antacids. Am J Obstet Gynecol, 124: 611–617.

Rutter N, Spencer A, Mann N, Smith M (1980). Glucose during labour. Lancet, 2: 155.

Sachs BP, Brown DAJ, Driscoll SG, Schulman E, Acker D, Ransil BJ, Jewitt JF (1987). Maternal mortality in Massachusetts. Trends and prevention. New Engl J Med, 316: 667–672.

Scott DB (1978). History of Mendelson's syndrome. J Int Med Res, 6: 47–51.

Scott DB (1986). Endotracheal intubation: friend or foe. Br Med J, 292: 157–158.

Sellick BA (1961). Cricoid pressure to control regurgitation of stomach contents during induction of anaesthesia: preliminary communication. Lancet, 2: 404–406.

Simkin P (1986). Stress, pain, and catecholamines in labour. Part 2. Stress associated with childbirth events: a pilot survey of new mothers. Birth, 13: 234–240.

Sweeney B, Wright I (1986). The use of antacids as a prophylaxis against Mendelson's syndrome in the United Kingdom. A survey. Anaesthesia, 41: 419–422.

Tarnow-Mordi WO, Shaw JCL, Liu D, Gardner DA, Flynn FV (1981). Iatrogenic hyponatraemia of the newborn due to maternal fluid overload: a prospective study. Br Med J, 283: 639–642.

Taylor G, Pryse-Davies J (1966). The prophylactic use of antacids in the prevention of the acid-pulmonary-aspiration syndrome (Mendelson's syndrome). Lancet, 1: 288–291.

Tettambel MA (1983). Preoperative use of antacids to prevent Mendelson's syndrome in cesarean section: a pilot study. J Am Osteopath Assoc, 82: 858–860.

Wilson J (1978) Gastric emptying in labour: some recent findings and their clinical significance. J Int Med Res, 6: Suppl (1) 54–60.

53 Monitoring the progress of labour

Caroline Crowther, Murray Enkin, Marc J. N. C. Keirse, and Ian Brown

1 Introduction

Labour, the culmination of pregnancy, is a special time both emotionally and physically for each woman. It is a time of intense physical activity, stress, and pain, and it may prove to be a time of overt or hidden dangers. As well as minimizing or removing the dangers, the care that a woman receives during labour must not only help her to cope with the effort, stress, and pain of labour.

The purpose of monitoring progress in labour is to recognize incipient problems, so that their progression to serious problems may be prevented. Prolonged labour is strongly associated with several adverse outcomes. It can lead to maternal exhaustion, perinatal asphyxia, and even death. Thus the anticipation of prolonged labour cannot be considered a trivial issue, as inefficient uterine action can be corrected and some adverse outcomes can be prevented. This monitoring must, however, be carried out with thought and consideration, rather than as an unthinking routine or a procrustean attempt to make all women fit predetermined criteria of so called 'normal'.

2 Recognition of the onset of labour

The diagnosis of labour is usually a self-diagnosis made by the woman. She will most commonly recognize that she is in labour by the onset of painful, regular contractions. Sometimes she will make the diagnosis after a show of mucus or blood, or after rupture of the membranes. On admission to hospital the diagnosis of labour may, or may not, be confirmed by the professional staff.

Labour is, by definition, the presence of regular uterine contractions, leading to progressive effacement and dilatation of the cervix, and ultimately to the delivery of the baby. While there is no difficulty in confirming the diagnosis of labour when it is strong and well established, the diagnosis is not always as clear-cut as the above definition would suggest. The time of onset of the contractions is sometimes difficult to determine; at least two assessments are required to establish whether or not progressive effacement and dilatation of the cervix is occurring; and delivery of the baby, although a clear criterion, can only be established retrospectively.

Cervical dilatation often begins several weeks before the end of pregnancy, and may progress slowly to the time of labour (Anderson and Turnbull 1969; Hendricks *et al.* 1970). If plotted on a graph, the degree of cervical dilatation of late pregnancy, like the degree of cervical dilatation during labour, would show gradual progression. In the last three days prior to labour Hendricks *et al.* (1970) found the mean cervical dilatation to be 1.8 cm in primigravidae, and 2.2 cm in multiparae. He considered the onset of active labour to start where the pre-labour cervical dilatation curve intersected the cervical dilatation curve of active labour, a point made by extrapolation of both curves. Although this may define the onset of labour in retrospect, it is of no use in clinical care.

A semi-objective surrogate index of the time of onset of labour, and a practical starting point from which subsequent progress can be monitored would be the time of admission of the woman to hospital. (For women not hospitalized for delivery this point could be taken as the time when she initially requests care for her labour.) This starting point for measuring the progress of labour (Hendricks *et al.* 1970; Philpott and Castle 1972a; O'Driscoll *et al.* 1973) is commonly used in clinical practice.

2.1 Time of admission

The point in labour at which a woman presents herself for admission to hospital will vary from woman to woman. Several factors may influence her decision about when to go to the hospital. These will include the way she feels, her expectations of labour, her anxiety about arriving too early or too late, and any complications that may have arisen. It will also depend on the advice that she has been given as to how and when she should recognize herself to be in labour and when to come to the hospital, which in turn will depend on the admission criteria of each maternity unit.

External factors such as the distance from her home to the hospital, and the help and support she has available will also influence her, as will her previous experience and parity. Hendricks *et al.* (1970) found the mean cervical dilatation at admission to be 2.5 cm in primiparae and 3.5 cm in multiparae. Studies in other settings have also shown that the mean dilatation at admission in labour is less in primiparae than that in multiparae (Duignan *et al.* 1975; Gibb *et al.* 1982).

All of these factors will affect when a woman is admitted to hospital and hence, the apparent length of her labour. In a group of low risk women who were admitted when they thought they were in labour, the mean dilatation on admission was significantly greater in women booked for general practice unit care than in women booked for care in the consultant unit (Klein *et al.* 1983). This may have been because domiciliary midwives often assessed women at home before recommending admission to the general practitioner unit, whereas women booked for delivery in the consultant unit were not similarly assessed. Not surprisingly, these women were subsequently reported to have shorter labours, illustrating the arbitrary nature of length of labour defined by time of admission to hospital.

The timing of hospital admission may have important consequences on the progress of labour. Hemminki and Sumukka (1986), in a retrospective study of 436 healthy primigravid women with a normal pregnancy anticipating a normal delivery, found that although the women who came to hospital early (regular contractions for 4 hours or less before admission) had a shorter total length of labour than those who were admitted in more advanced labour, they had more diagnoses of difficult labour recorded. More intrapartum interventions were carried out on them, more caesarean sections were performed, and they had a longer postpartum hospital stay than did the women who were admitted later in labour.

It is unlikely that any universal 'best' time for hospital admission in labour will be determined. For most women, the best time would be when they feel that they would be happier or more comfortable in hospital.

2.2 Confirming the diagnosis of labour

One of the most important decisions in care in labour is to recognize that labour has started (O'Driscoll *et al.* 1973). 'True' labour must be differentiated from 'false labour'. The clinical diagnosis of active labour is easy when 'pains' plus progress in cervical dilatation are present. To confirm or deny the diagnosis of labour in a woman self-admitted as 'in labour' is not so easy when the cervix is uneffaced and closed.

O'Driscoll *et al.* (1973) reported that over 10 per cent of women self-admitted in labour to the National Maternity Hospital, Dublin were considered not to be in labour by the staff. Somewhat less than half of these women went into active labour within 24 hours of admission. Almost all the women initially thought not to be in labour by staff, but who subsequently laboured within 24 hours, had a show or rupture of the membranes to support their contention of being in labour. This study shows first, that the professional staff do not always agree with a woman's self-diagnosis that labour has begun, and second, that the professional staff are not always right.

The frequency, duration, and strength of contractions, the state of the membranes, the presence or absence of a show, and the state of effacement and dilatation of the cervix are all important criteria to be considered in making or confirming the diagnosis of labour. The individual or combined sensitivities, specificities, and predictive values for each of these criteria have not been well studied or reported. Such studies could well point the way toward clearer delineation of which criteria are useful for the diagnosis of labour and which are not.

In spite of the difficulties in reliably establishing that labour has started, the most convenient and most used marker of the onset of labour (although recognized as an arbitrary starting point and not a biologically correct one), remains the time when the woman is admitted in labour.

3 Assessing the progress of labour

3.1 Maternal condition

The physical and mental state, the comfort and well-being of the woman must be just as carefully monitored during labour as the progress of contractions or the state of the cervix. Symptoms she experiences such as nausea, dyspnoea, or dizziness should be fully assessed as to their cause, and treatment provided if necessary. Fear can be allayed and stress alleviated by the presence of companions and competent, caring staff (see Chapter 49). The intensity of pain she experiences will determine her need for and the timing of pain relief (see Chapters 56 and 57).

3.2 General observations

Adequate attention must be paid to the general condition of the woman and in most circumstances this will include at least blood pressure, pulse, and temperature. It is questionable whether any useful purpose is served by routine repeated observations of these parameters in healthy women in apparently normal labour. Although these observations are of value in some clinical situations, there has been no evaluation of their routine use in normal labour.

Although such assessments have become traditional, there is little agreement as to how frequently they should be performed. Pulse and blood pressure observations have been recommended from half-hourly to every 2 hours (O'Driscoll *et al.* 1969; Philpott 1972; Studd 1973; Melmed and Evans 1976). The value, if any, of such frequent assessments of pulse and blood pressure in normal labour to screen for problems such as intrapartum pre-eclampsia is unknown. It is likely to be small. In the presence of known or suspected abnormality (e.g. antepartum or intrapartum haemorrhage, pre-eclampsia), such assessments should be made as frequently as necessary, or even continuously, rather than being dictated by the regulations of a rigid scheme that is applied to all women.

In many units temperature is commonly taken every four hours throughout normal labour. As with pulse and blood pressure assessments, this is probably unnecessary in normal labour, but not frequent enough when problems are suspected. The first sign of intra-uterine infection may be a rise in the mother's temperature, although fetal tachycardia is sometimes an earlier recognized alerting sign.

In many centres all urine passed in labour is measured and tested for protein, acetone, and glucose. An adequate record of fluid output and input may be needed when there is a risk of fluid retention, for instance in women with pre-eclampsia or when large doses of oxytocin are used (see Chapter 58). Similarly, when epidural analgesia is instituted it is useful to record whether and when urine was passed in order to avoid an overfilled bladder. When instrumental delivery is undertaken it is again useful to know whether and when the bladder was emptied. It is difficult to believe, however, that the collection and measurement of all urine passed as a routine procedure can serve any useful purpose.

3.3 Uterine contractions

Labour is initiated, and progress maintained, by the contractions of the uterus. Almost always the woman herself is aware of the contractions, their frequency, their duration and their strength. These parameters can be confirmed by abdominal palpation. The self-report by the woman, supplemented by abdominal examination when required, is quite sufficient to monitor the contractions adequately in most situations.

Abdominal palpation cannot, however, accurately quantitate the changes in uterine pressure resulting from the contraction, and this constraint also applies to the record of uterine contractions made by an external tocodynamometer (Miller 1983). It may provide an accurate record of the frequency and, to a lesser extent, of the duration of contractions but not of their intensity. The latter information can be important when progress in labour is slow and augmentation of the strength of contractions is considered (see Chapter 58).

Several methods of quantifying uterine activity have been described (Figure 53.1). Caldeyro-Barcia *et al.* (1957) introduced the 'Montevideo Unit' (strength of contractions times frequency per 10 minutes). El Sahwi *et al.* (1967) added the duration of the contraction and defined the 'Alexandria Unit'. Advances in computer technology can now provide rapid on-line quantification of uterine activity. Hon and Paul (1973) showed that the total area under the contraction curve was a good indicator of uterine activity, and introduced the 'Uterine Activity Unit'. Steer (1977) measured active contraction area as the area under the pressure curve, excluding basal tone. This was measured over a period of time and termed the 'uterine activity integral', expressed in kiloPascals per 15 minutes. Phillips and Calder (1987) suggested assessment of uterine activity on a continuous basis rather than over a defined period of time. In the active phase of labour the rate of cervical dilatation was found to correlate better with uterine contractility expressed in terms of active contraction area than in terms of Montevideo Units, frequency, or active pressure (Steer *et al.* 1984).

The clinical utility of all these suggested units remains unclear, and for the moment they must be considered of research interest only. No study has demonstrated improvements in the outcome of labour by the use of more sophisticated measurements of uterine activity. If labour progress is considered abnormal because the cervix does not adequately efface or dilate, the precise information on uterine activity that can be obtained from intrauterine pressure recording may enable better evaluation of the problem, and may provide a means of monitoring changes in uterine activity in response to treatment. Although theoretically reasonable, these postulated benefits have not been demonstrated by prospective controlled trials.

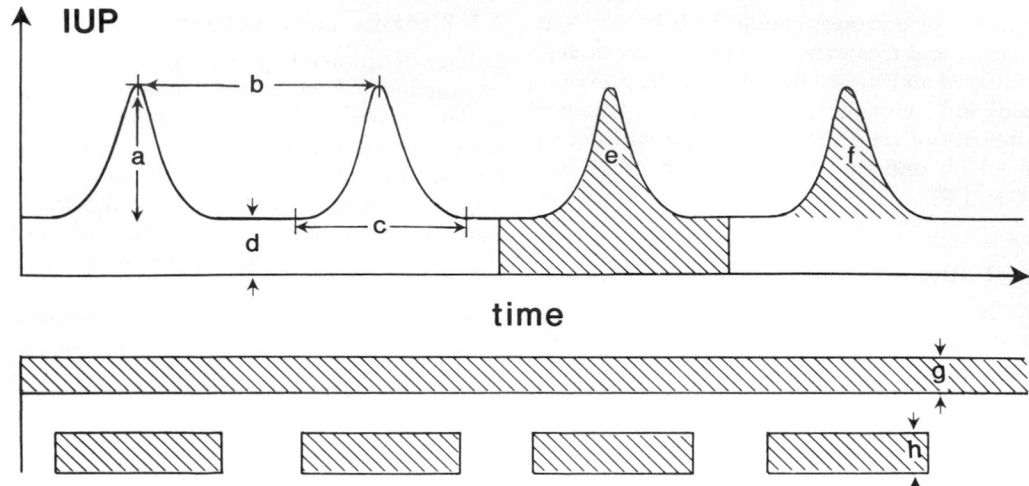

Fig. 53.1 Record of uterine contractions showing measures that are used for quantifying uterine activity.

Legend

a = active pressure; height of contraction
b = contraction interval
c = duration of contraction
d = baseline pressure or tone

e = total area under the (contraction) curve
f = active contraction area
g = mean active pressure
h = mean contraction active pressure

4 Progress of labour

4.1 Cervical dilatation and effacement

Cervical dilatation in the past was often expressed in terms of coinage such as dimes, quarters, and silver dollars in North America, or in terms of finger-breadths. Such units of measure are now obsolete and today cervical dilatation is usually estimated in centimetres, from 0 cm when closed to 10 cm at full dilatation. Friedman (1954) considered the rate of dilatation of the cervix to be the most exact measure of the progress of labour. Assessment of cervical dilatation is not, however, as precise as one would like to believe. To our knowledge, no studies of either inter-observer or intra-observer reproducibility have been reported. Personal experience has shown substantial variations in estimates by different observers in the same situation, and even by the same observer on repeat examination. (At times this may explain the embarrassing phenomenon of the 'shrinking cervix'.)

From the standpoint of the woman's comfort, cervical dilatation is best assessed between contractions. Friedman (1954), however, measured dilatation at the peak of a contraction, and Richardson *et al.* (1978) reported that the cervix was maximally dilated 15 seconds after the peak of each contraction. There is no clear guidance from the literature as to the most accurate time to assess the dilatation in relation to a contraction, and consistency of the time of observation is

probably only important when assessing progress in difficult situations.

Effacement or thinning of the cervix is usually measured by estimating the length of the cervix in centimetres, but is sometimes expressed in percentage effaced. Once again, there is likely to be considerable variation in estimations by different examiners.

Cervical dilatation and effacement can be assessed directly by vaginal examination or indirectly by rectal examination. Rectal examinations were advocated by Kroening and Reis (cited in Peterson *et al.* 1965) toward the end of the nineteenth century in the belief that, unlike vaginal examinations, they did not cause contamination of the genital tract. Their use was prompted by Semmelweis's observation in 1847 that puerperal infection was caused by the introduction of septic material into the vagina by the examining hand of the obstetrical attendant (Manning 1961).

Several studies comparing vaginal and rectal examinations were made in the United States in the mid 1950s–1960s. All showed a similar incidence of puerperal infection whether rectal or vaginal examinations were employed during labour (Prystowsky 1954; Fara *et al.* 1956; Manning 1961; Bertelsen and Johnson 1963; Peterson *et al.* 1965). On the basis of these studies vaginal examinations became standard practice for the assessment of cervical dilatation during labour, although some units (O'Driscoll and Meagher 1980) continued to recommend the use of rectal examination for assessment.

Women's preference for vaginal over rectal examinations was clearly demonstrated in a randomized clinical trial (Murphy *et al.* 1986). In this trial, 307 women were randomly allocated to either vaginal or rectal examinations for assessments in labour. The women, regardless of their parity, expressed a preference for vaginal assessments. The examination was described as 'very uncomfortable' by 28 per cent in the rectal examination group compared to only 11 per cent in the vaginal group (which might lead one to conclude that they would have preferred neither examination if not necessary). No difference in maternal or neonatal morbidity was found between the two groups, although the authors recognized that a far larger trial would be required to exclude the possibility of a difference. Overall, the available evidence would suggest that there is no place whatsoever for rectal examinations in monitoring the progress of labour.

Vaginal examination in labour is usually conducted under aseptic conditions, to minimize the risk of infection. Antiseptic creams and lotions are usually used, and sterile gloves worn. In 44 per cent of units in England masks are worn when vaginal examinations are performed (Garcia *et al.* 1986), although there is no evidence that they are of any benefit. In view of the fact that masks have not been shown to be of value during vaginal surgery (Chamberlain and Houang 1984) or in the delivery room (Turner *et al.* 1984) it is highly unlikely that any infections are prevented by this practice. Units in which it still takes place could save resources by phasing it out, and might consider doing so in the context of a randomized trial to settle the question for others as well.

The recommended frequency of internal examinations to assess the progress of cervical dilatation varies tremendously among units and in the literature. Philpott and Castle (1972b) advised four-hourly assessment, and if delay was detected, two-hourly. O'Driscoll and Meagher (1980) recommended rectal assessment on admission followed by an examination at one hour, then two-hourly examinations unless slow progress prompted more frequent examinations. Studd *et al.* (1982) advised three-hourly assessment; Duignan (1985) suggested assessment every one to two hours; and Cardozo and Studd (1985) recommended three- to four-hourly examinations. In her survey of English labour ward policies and routines, Garcia *et al.* (1985) found that 30 per cent of the units surveyed had no policy on the timing of cervical assessments, 36 per cent had a fixed schedule for assessment, and 34 per cent had a flexible policy (see Chapter 50). In the units where there was a fixed policy, 77 per cent used four-hourly assessment, 5 per cent three-hourly assessment, and 8 per cent two-hourly assessment. In the units with a flexible policy, over half had a four-hourly policy, 15 per cent an 'at least four-hourly' policy, and 5 per cent a 'not greater than 4 hourly' policy. This variation amply illustrates the lack of consensus for the optimal timing of vaginal examinations in labour.

Like all assessments in labour, it would seem most sensible that the number and timing of vaginal examinations should be frequent enough to permit adequate assessment of progress and to promptly detect any problems, but no more frequent than necessary to accomplish this end.

4.2 Descent of the presenting part

If the head is presenting, its relationship to the brim of the pelvis can be determined by abdominal or vaginal examination. On vaginal examination the level of the presenting part can be related to the ischial spines. Moulding of the fetal head, an important observation in following the progress of labour, particularly if cephalopelvic disproportion is suspected (see Chapter 31), can also be determined by vaginal examination. Stewart (Stewart 1977; Stewart and Philpott 1980) described a method of grading moulding between the two parietal bones, and between the occipital bone and the parietal bones. His method of recording is shown in Table 53.1 (see Chapter 71). Formation of a caput succedaneum is also related to the progress of labour, but Stewart (1977) showed that this assessment is subjective and of little clinical value.

Descent can be estimated abdominally by determining the amount of the baby's head that is still above the pelvic brim. Crichton (1974) introduced the 'fifths' terminology for this, in which the amount of head above the pelvis is related to the pelvic brim in fifths (Fig. 53.2). Abdominal assessment avoids the need for vaginal examination, and is not influenced by the presence of a caput succedaneum or moulding.

No studies comparing the relative accuracy of these two approaches in relation to the outcome of labour have been reported. Given the additional information that can be obtained, it would seem reasonable that both methods of examination be carried out before operative delivery is undertaken (see Chapter 71).

Table 53.1 Assessment of moulding (after Stewart 1977)

Degree of moulding	Clinical findings
−	Bones normally separated.
+	Bones just touching. No overlap.
+ +	Overlap of suture lines. Reducible on gentle digital pressure.
+ + +	Overlap of suture lines. Reducible on gentle digital pressure.

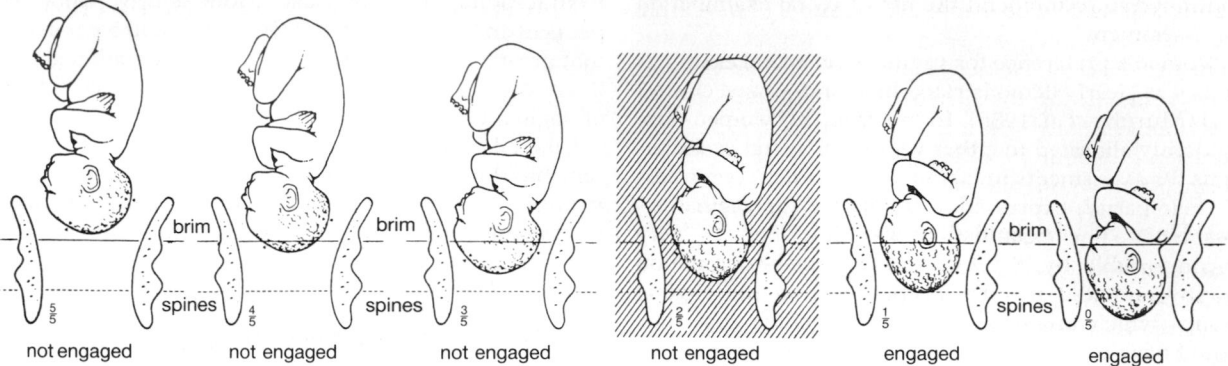

Fig. 53.2 Abdominal method for determining descent of the fetal head into the pelvis (after Crichton 1974).

5 Normal labour

Labour has been defined as normal 'when a baby is born within a period of 12 hours, via the natural passage, through the efforts of the mother, and when no harm befalls either party as a result of the experience' (O'Driscoll and Meagher 1980). This simple definition, while useful for retrospective classification, is of no value whatsoever for assessing the normality of an ongoing labour. Normal labour can more usefully be defined in terms of the rate of progress of cervical dilatation (usually expressed in centimetres per hour).

Several surveys have described the duration and velocity of labour in different groups of women (Friedman 1955; Hendricks *et al.* 1970; O'Driscoll *et al.* 1970; Philpott and Castle 1972a; Beazley and Kurjak 1972; Studd 1973; Duignan *et al.* 1975; Melmed and Evans 1976; Sokol *et al.* 1977; Bergsjo *et al.* 1979; Cardozo *et al.* 1982; Gibb *et al.* 1982; Hunter *et al.* 1983; Klein *et al.* 1983; Tuck *et al.* 1983). From such descriptive data, statistical ranges for 'normality' can be drawn, although it should be realized that these are statistical ranges only, and they are not necessarily clinically relevant. Direct comparisons among studies are difficult because of differences in inclusion and exclusion criteria.

The definition of the range of 'normal', in terms of both length of labour and rate of cervical dilatation, obviously depends on the inclusion and exclusion criteria and on the proportion of women who are considered to be 'normal' (see Chapter 3). With too narrow a definition of 'normality' an increased number of labours would be defined as 'abnormal', and the women concerned may be subjected to unnecessary 'therapeutic' interventions to treat non-existent dystocia.

5.1 Duration of labour

Baird (1952) defined a normal labour as 'one in which the vertex presents and which is completed in 24 hours or less by spontaneous delivery without injury or undue discomfort to the mother'. O'Driscoll *et al.* (1969) also considered 24 hours as the upper limit of normal, but more recently suggested 12 hours as the upper limit of normal labour (O'Driscoll *et al.* 1984). Current obstetrical opinion tends towards acceptance of the shorter time period.

Studies on the duration of labour have mainly involved primiparae, and the available data are summarized in Table 53.2. These data suggest that normal

Table 53.2 Studies on the duration of labour: mean values and 90th–95th centiles

Intervals studied	Duration in hours		Centiles	
	Primi-gravidae	Multi-gravidae	90th	95th
Onset of regular contractions to delivery				
Friedman 1955*	13.3	—		< 32
Sokol *et al.* 1977*	11.4	8.0		< 25
Bergsjo *et al.* 1979*	8.3	—	< 17	
Admission to delivery				
Philpott and Castle 1972b	—	—		< 12
O'Driscoll and Meagher 1980*	—	—		< 10
Admission to 2nd stage				
Studd 1973	6.3	4.6		
Duignan *et al.* 1975	5.6	3.7	88% < 10	
Cardozo *et al.* 1982*	6.3	—	< 12	
Gibb *et al.* 1982*	—	3.4	88%	< 10
Klein *et al.* 1983 (GPU)	10.6	6.0		
(Consultant)	8.3	5.4		
Tuck *et al.* 1983* (White)	5.9	3.1		
(Asian)	7.2	3.2		
(Black)	6.9	3.3		
Active phase				
Friedman 1955*	—	—		< 12
Hendricks *et al.* 1970	—	—	< 8	

*Studies involving a wide cross-section of a childbearing population in spontaneous labour.

labour will usually be completed within 24 hours from the onset of regular contractions, or within 12 hours from the onset of the active phase of labour. As previously stated, the total length of labour can only be determined in retrospect, and definitions based on the duration of labour are of limited value in assessing the normality of an ongoing labour.

5.2 Rate of cervical dilatation

Statistical analysis of labour parameters was first described by Friedman (1955), based on the now classic 'Friedman curve' of cervical dilatation in labour (Friedman 1954; Fig. 3). Friedman initially described the graph as 'a realistic tool for the study of individual labours in progress, by obstetricians outside of university hospitals'.

Friedman's curve of cervical dilatation in centimetres plotted against time in hours, was derived from 100 primigravid women in spontaneous labour ('with few exceptions'). No exclusions were made for malpresentations, malposition, or multiple pregnancy, nor for the use of oxytocin, caudal analgesia, or operative delivery. The onset of labour was taken as the time when regular contractions were established and dilatation of the cervix was measured by hourly rectal examinations. The sigmoid curve so obtained was divided into four phases:

1. Phase 1—the latent phase—from the onset of regular contractions to the acceleration period. During this period the rate of dilatation was slow, with a mean duration of 7.3 hours from the onset of contractions to a cervical dilatation of 2 to 2.5 cm.

2. Phase 2—the acceleration phase—continuous changing and increasing rate of cervical dilatation.

3. Phase 3—the phase of maximum slope—where there was linear progress in cervical dilatation. This phase

corresponded to a mean cervical dilatation from 3.5 to 8.5–9.0 cm.

4. Phase 4—the deceleration phase—where the slope of dilatation decreased until full dilatation at 10 cm was reached.

Following the early work by Friedman, graphs of cervical dilatation for different obstetric populations have been produced by others.

Philpott and Castle (1972a) established cervicographic parameters of normality for an African population. The 624 primigravidae in their study constituted a more selected group than that described by Friedman, since women with malpresentation, malposition, and multiple pregnancy were excluded, and since the women had a cervical dilatation of 3 cm or more at entry into the study. The mean rate of cervical dilatation found by Philpott and Castle (1972a) in the active phase was 1.6 cm per hour, considerably slower than the mean rate of 3.5 cm per hour found by Friedman (1955). The higher prevalence of mild cephalopelvic disproportion in the African 'normals' studied by Philpott and Castle was suggested as an explanation for the difference.

On their cervicograph Philpott and Castle (1972a) constructed a straight line, joining the point of 1 cm dilatation at 0 time and the point of 10 cm dilatation 9 hours later and called this the alert line. This corresponded to a rate of dilatation of 1 cm per hour (Fig. 53.4). The alert line corresponded roughly to the mean rate of cervical dilatation in the slowest 10 per cent of the primigravidae studied, similar to the 95th percentile rate of 1.2 cm per hour in the primigravidae studied by Friedman (1955). They hoped that by the use of this population-derived cervical dilatation rate (less than 1 cm per hour) the women destined to have prolonged labour would be identified.

Although the purpose of the 'alert line' was to differentiate normal labour (progress to the left of the alert line) from abnormal labour (deviation across the alert line), in use Philpott and Castle (1972a,b) found that it was crossed by 22 per cent of the women. Nevertheless, they considered it to be useful in differentiating women in normal labour from those with cephalopelvic dispro-

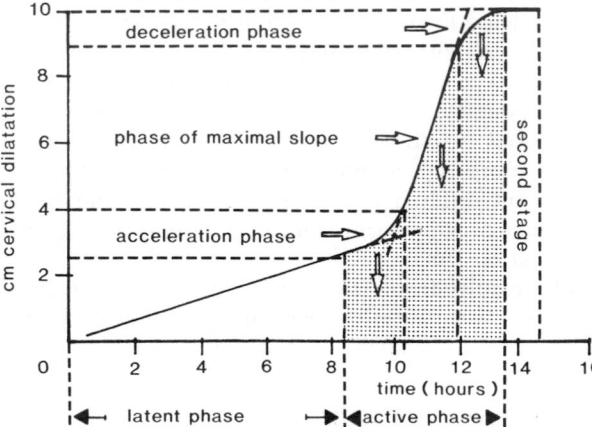

Fig. 53.3 Friedman's curve of cervical dilatation versus time in labour (after Friedman 1954).

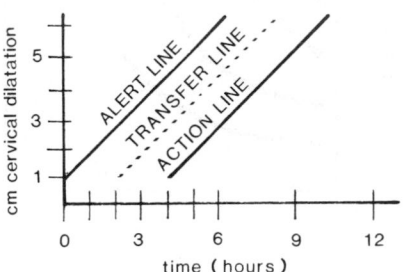

Fig. 53.4 Cervicograph showing alert and action lines (after Philpott and Castle 1972a).

portion or inefficient uterine action (Philpott and Castle 1972a,b).

The value of the alert line as a screening procedure for abnormal labour has received only limited investigation (Philpott and Castle 1972b; Melmed and Evans 1976; Hunter *et al.* 1983). The rate of 1 cm per hour in the active phase of labour as the cut-off between normal and abnormal labour (Philpott and Castle 1972a) was also accepted by Beazley and Kurjak (1972), O'Driscoll *et al.* (1973), Cowan *et al.* (1982a,b) and Gibb *et al.* (1984). A Canadian national consensus conference suggested 0.5 cm per hour as the cut-off point for normality (National Consensus Conference on Aspects of Caesarean Section Planning Committee 1985).

The same principle was used by Studd (1973) to derive 5 slopes of standard cervical dilatation in primigravid labour for each of 5 different values of cervical dilatation on admission. These slopes or curves were termed nomograms (Fig. 53.5). As with the alert line of Philpott and Castle (1972a) the nomograms also aimed to distinguish normal from abnormal progress in labour.

Studd (1973) retrospectively evaluated the nomogram in 292 consecutive primigravidae in spontaneous labour. He found that in 44 per cent of labours the cervical dilatation curve crossed to the right of the nomogram curve. These women had longer first and second stages of labour, and more instrumental deliveries than did women whose cervical dilatation pattern remained to the left of the nomogram, and their babies had lower Apgar scores.

When tested prospectively in 741 women in spontaneous labour, 156 of 349 primigravidae (44.7 per cent) and 46 of 392 multigravidae (11.7 per cent) had a cervical dilatation pattern that crossed to the right of the nomogram (Studd *et al.* 1975). Studd (1973) judged cervimetric progress greater than 2 hours to the right of the nomogram to be abnormal and suggested this should be the cut-off for the use of oxytocin stimulation.

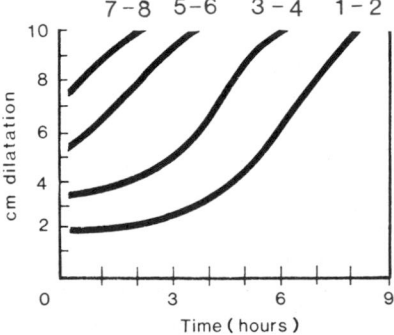

Fig. 53.5 Nomograms of cervimetric progress during labour; progress in dilatation is shown in relation to the dilatation at the onset of the measurement (after Studd 1973).

Table 53.3 Studies on the rate of cervical dilatation in the active phase of labour in primiparae: mean/or median cervical dilatation rates and 90th–95th centiles

Authors, year		Mean dilatation cm/hour	Centiles 90th	95th
Friedman (1955)*		3.00		1.2
Hendrick *et al.* (1970)		2.00		—
Philpott and Castle (1972a)		1.75	1.0	
Melmed and Evans (1976)	(spontaneous labour)	1.84		—
	(forceps delivery)	0.93		
	(caesarean section)	0.42		
Bergsjo *et al.* (1979)*		—	1.2	
Cowan *et al.* (1982a)		2.50†		< 1.0
Hunter *et al.* (1983)	(spontaneous labour)	2.00		—
	(forceps delivery)	1.20		
	(caesarean section)	< 0.90		

*Studies involving a wide cross-section of obstetric population in spontaneous labour.
†Median

Although initial cervimetric studies concentrated on labour in primiparae, the rate of cervical dilatation in the active phase of spontaneous labour is similar in primigravidae and in multigravidae (Hendricks *et al.* 1970; Duignan *et al.* 1975).

It appears that within a stringent definition of statistical normality the cervical dilatation pattern is unaffected by parity or racial differences (Duignan *et al.* 1975; Melmed and Evans 1976). If this is indeed so, concepts of statistical normality (and therefore abnormality) can be applied to any woman regardless of parity or race. Nevertheless, further studies to support this hypothesis are needed. Studies of unselected groups of women that give a more representative picture, show statistically significant differences in length of labour and in the incidence of abnormal labour in different racial groups (Tuck *et al.* 1983).

The results from studies that list rates of cervical dilatation with mean/median rates and 90th/95th percentiles, where available, are shown in Table 53.3.

6 Abnormal labour

Slow progress in labour does not necessarily mean abnormal labour or the presence of a problem. It should however, alert the caregiver to the potential or the possibility of a problem. Slow progress in the first stage of labour can occur in either the latent or the active phase. These appear to be clinically different and should probably be considered separately.

6.1 Prolonged latent phase

The latent phase of labour is poorly understood. Some consider it to be the end of pre-labour (Hendricks *et al.* 1970). Others, however, believe it to be a true entity (Koontz and Bishop 1982). There is limited understanding of the aetiology of a prolonged latent phase, little information about its significance, and no controlled studies of its management.

As this phase usually starts before the women is admitted to hospital, the precise time of onset is often difficult to determine. Although the mean length of the latent phase was found by Friedman to be 6.4 hours in primigravidae (Friedman 1955) and 4.8 hours in multigravidae (Friedman and Sachtleben 1961), means are of little clinical value. The duration of the latent phase varies so greatly from woman to woman that a normal range is virtually impossible to define. Friedman (1955) considered greater than 20 hours in a primigravida and greater than 14 hours in a multigravida to be prolonged, but not of clinical importance. These figures correspond to the 95th centile for the duration of the latent phase in the women studied. Cardozo *et al.* (1982), using time from admission to the onset of the active phase, considered an interval greater than 6 hours to indicate prolongation of the latent phase in primiparae, and Gibb *et al.* (1982) suggested an interval of greater than 4 hours in a multigravidae.

According to Friedman (1955, 1973) a prolonged latent phase is not associated with increased perinatal morbidity, mortality, or other adverse outcome. This opinion was not shared by all other workers. Cardozo *et al.* (1982), who used admission to hospital as the time of commencement, found a significantly higher incidence of caesarean section, and of lower 5 minute Apgar scores in the 3.5 per cent of primigravidae with a prolonged latent phase than in women who had a normal pattern of labour. In multigravidae Gibb *et al.* (1982) found 1.4 per cent of women to have a prolonged latent phase; these women had a higher caesarean section rate and their babies had lower Apgar scores. Whether these adverse effects were due to the underlying condition or to the management policy of amniotomy and oxytocin stimulation is uncertain, however (Cardozo *et al.* 1982).

One of the major problems in care is differentiating between a prolonged latent phase and false labour. Unfortunately, this distinction can only be made retrospectively. Philpott (1982) suggested that, if no progress in effacement or cervical dilatation occurs within 4 hours after admission, the woman should be given 100 mg pethidine for analgesia and sedation. If at 8 hours she is still in the latent phase with no progress, amniotomy and oxytocin is advised. No trials of this approach have been carried out. There is an urgent need for controlled studies about this common, distressing, and poorly understood phase of labour, its aetiology, its significance, and the best policy of care (see Chapter 58).

6.2 Prolonged active phase

Slow progress or failure to progress in the active phase of labour has been defined either as an overall measurement (e.g. longer than x hours), or as a rate related measurement (e.g. a rate of cervical dilatation of less than y cm per hour). It should be noted that the commonly cited 12-hour duration of the active phase is roughly equivalent to a rate of 0.5 cm per hour, half as fast as the 1 cm per hour that is also commonly used.

Deviation from this arbitrarily defined 'normal' rate of dilatation is, however, an indication for consideration rather than for intervention. Philpott and Castle (1972b) found that graphs of over a fifth of the labours in primigravid women studied crossed their 'alert line', and would, by their definition, be considered abnormal. They did not, however, recommend intervention in the form of oxytocin therapy until a line drawn 4 hours to the right of the 'alert line' had been crossed. This line, known as the 'action line', represents a cervical dilatation rate of 0.6 cm per hour or less. In their population, partograms of 11 per cent of the women crossed it (Fig. 53.4). For rural areas a 'transfer line' drawn 2 hours to the right of the 'alert line', was incorporated. If the cervicographic pattern crossed the 'transfer line', this was taken as an indication for transfer to a hospital where further assessment and treatment could be carried out, and where operative delivery facilities were available if needed.

Philpott and Castle (1972b) suggested a policy of active management of labour if the action line was crossed, to distinguish between primary inefficient uterine action on the one hand, and cephalopelvic disproportion on the other. This involved a pelvic assessment to exclude gross cephalopelvic disproportion, monitoring the mother and the fetus, intravenous fluids, epidural anaesthesia, and a trial of oxytocin.

If satisfactory progress (>1 cm per hour) with improved uterine action was made, vaginal delivery was allowed. A caesarean section was performed if fetal distress developed prior to full dilatation, or if progress was unsatisfactory in the face of increased uterine activity. In their unit, the incidence of prolonged labour, the percentage of women given oxytocin, the caesarean section rate, and the perinatal mortality were lower after that policy was instituted than before, but no concurrent control group was used for comparison.

O'Driscoll and his colleagues (1970) at the National

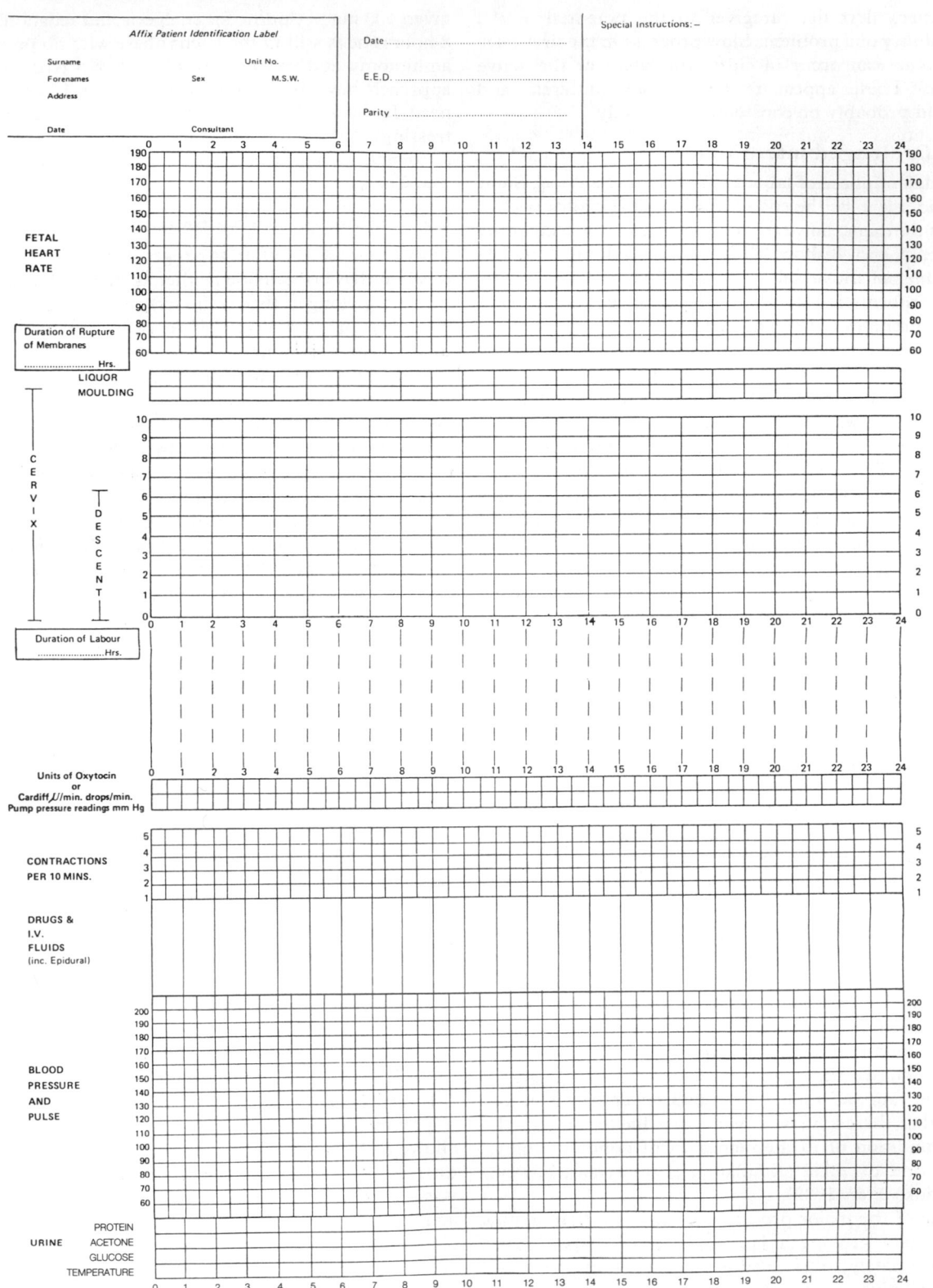

Fig. 53.6 Example of a partogram.

Maternity Hospital in Dublin, on the other hand, pursue a policy of more active management of labour from the moment of admission. They advocate augmentation with oxytocin whenever cervical dilatation is less than 1 cm per hour. Some 30 per cent of primigravid labours are augmented with oxytocin (O'Driscoll and Meagher 1980). They claim that this policy has virtually eliminated prolonged labour, as 98 per cent of women were delivered within 12 hours of admission, while the caesarean section rate remained low, at 4.8 per cent (O'Driscoll *et al.* 1984), but, once again, control data are not available.

Cephalopelvic disproportion must be considered when progress in labour is slow. If gross cephalopelvic disproportion or marked moulding of the fetal skull is present, the diagnosis may be clear enough to warrant caesarean section. In suspected mild cases efficient uterine action must be assured, as otherwise cephalopelvic disproportion cannot be excluded.

7 Recording the progress of labour

When monitoring the progress of labour, recording the findings is almost as important as making the assessments. The primary reasons for doing so are to make that progress readily apparent, so that problems will be recognized early, and to facilitate transfer of information to other caregivers. Several methods of recording measures of progress are in current use.

A time-based diary of events permits a detailed documentation of all important maternal and fetal assessments, but the recording and inspection of such a record can be tedious. It is often difficult to follow, particularly when labour is prolonged or when there is a change of staff. A more structured representation of events and progress can facilitate early recognition of potentially correctable problems.

The partogram (Fig. 53.6), a structured graphical representation of the progress of labour, has been adopted in many units throughout the world. Graphic analysis of cervical dilatation during labour was first described by Friedman (1954), whereas Philpott (1972) suggested using a 'partogram' for recording all pertinent observations during labour. Garcia *et al.* (1986) found that 89 per cent of consultant maternity units in England recorded labour progress on partograms.

With the use of a partogram the progress of labour can be seen at a glance on one sheet of paper, failure to progress can be readily recognized, and the writing of lengthy descriptions in elaborate prose can be avoided. It is simple to use by all grades of staff, is a practical teaching aid, and is an efficient means of exchange of technical information about labour progress between teams of caregivers.

8 Conclusions

The well-being of the mother as well as that of the fetus must be carefully monitored during labour. This monitoring does not necessarily require the use of special equipment, but it always requires careful and individualized observation.

Although this chapter has dealt mainly with uterine contractions and cervical dilatation, monitoring the progress of labour requires more than the assessment of these physiological variables. The rate of progress must be considered in the context of the woman's total well-being, rather than as simply a physical phenomenon. A dilatation rate of 1 cm per hour in a woman who is having strong contractions and is in severe distress is far more worrying than a rate of 0.3 cm per hour in a woman who is comfortable, walking around, drinking cups of tea and chatting with the midwife.

Vaginal rather than rectal examination should be used to assess the progress of labour, but no more often than deemed necessary. Slow progress should alert one to the possibility of abnormal labour, but should not automatically result in intervention.

In view of the importance of labour progress and the amount of discomfort that slow progress can provoke in the woman, the fetus, and the caregivers, it is rather surprising that so few of the many guidelines to care that have been suggested have been substantiated by solid research evidence.

Important research questions relate to the relative effectiveness of expectant and supportive care versus augmentation of labour for delay in both the latent and active phases of labour. Such questions can never be answered by uncontrolled observational data, but should be readily resolved by properly conducted controlled trials.

References

Anderson ABM, Turnbull AC (1969). Relationship between length of gestation and cervical dilatation, uterine contractility, and other factors during pregnancy. Am J Obstet Gynecol, 105: 1207–1214.

Baird D (1952). The cause and prevention of difficult labour. Am J Obstet Gynecol, 63: 1200–1212.

Beazley JM, Kurjak A (1972). Influence of a partograph on the active management of labour. Lancet, ii: 348–351.

Bergsjo P, Bakketeig L, Eikhom SN (1979). Duration of labour with spontaneous onset. Acta Obstet Gynecol Scand, 58: 129–134.

Bertelsen H, Johnson B (1963). Routine vaginal examinations during labour. A comparative study. Am J Obstet Gynecol, 85: 527–531.

Caldeyro-Barcia R, Sica-Blanco Y, Poseiro JJ, Gonzalen-Panizza V, Mendez-Bauer C, Fielitz C, Alvarez H, Pose SV, Hendricks CH (1957). A quantitative study of the action of synthetic oxytocin on the pregnant human uterus. J Pharmacol Exp Ther, 121: 18–31.

Cardozo LD, Gibb DMF, Studd JW, Vasant RV, Cooper D (1982). Predictive value of cervimetric labour patterns in primigravidae. Br J Obstet Gynaecol, 89: 33–38.

Cardozo L, Studd J (1985). Abnormal labour patterns. In: The Management of Labour. Studd J. (ed). London: Blackwell Scientific Publications, pp 171–187.

Chamberlain GV, Houang E (1984). Trial of the use of masks in the gynaecological operating theatre. Ann R Coll Surg Eng, 66: 432–433.

Cowan DB, Van Middelkoop A, Philpott RH (1982a). Intra-uterine pressure studies in African nulliparae: normal labour progress. Br J Obstet Gynaecol, 89: 364–369.

Cowan DB, Van Middelkoop A, Philpott RH (1982b). Intra-uterine pressure studies on African nulliparae: delay, delivery, and disproportion. Br J Obstet Gynaecol, 89: 370–380.

Crichton D (1974). A reliable method of establishing the level of the fetal head in obstetrics. S Afr Med J, 48: 784–787.

Duignan NM, Studd JWW, Hughes AO (1975). Characteristics of normal labour in different racial groups. Br J Obstet Gynaecol, 82: 593–601.

Duignan N (1985). Active management of labour. In: The Management of Labour. Studd J (ed). Oxford: Blackwell Scientific Publications, pp 146–158.

El-Sahwi S, Gaafar AA, Toppozada HK (1967). A new unit for evaluation of uterine activity. Am J Obstet Gynecol, 98: 900–903.

Fara FJ, Steward M, Standard J (1956). The use of unlimited non-sterile vaginal examinations on the conduct of labour. Am J Obstet Gynecol, 72: 1–11.

Friedman EA (1954). The graphic analysis of labour. Am J Obstet Gynecol, 68: 1568–1575.

Friedman EA (1955). Primigravid labour—a graphicostatistical analysis. Am J Obstet Gynecol, 6: 567–589.

Friedman EA, Sachtleben MR (1961). Dysfunctional labour. I Prolonged latent phase in nullipara. Am J Obstet Gynecol, 17: 135–148.

Friedman EA (1973). Patterns of labour as indicators of risk. Clin Obstet Gynecol, 16: 172–183.

Garcia J, Garforth S, Ayers S (1986). Midwives confined? Labour ward policies and routines. Research and the Midwife Conference. Manchester. Proceedings. 1986: pp 2–30.

Gibb DMF, Cardozo LD, Studd JWW, Magos AL, Cooper DJ (1982). Outcome of spontaneous labour in multigravidae. Br J Obstet Gynaecol, 89: 708–711.

Gibb DMF, Arulkumaran S, Lun KC, Ratnam SS (1984). Characteristics of uterine activity in nulliparous labour. Br J Obstet Gynaecol, 91: 220–227.

Hemminki E, Simukka R (1986). The timing of hospital admission and progress of labour. Eur J Obstet Gynecol Reprod Biol, 22: 85–94.

Hendricks CH, Brenner WE, Kraus G (1970). Normal cervical dilatation pattern in late pregnancy and labour. Am J Obstet Gynecol, 106: 1065–1082.

Hon EH, Paul RH (1973). Quantitation of uterine activity. Obstet Gynecol, 42: 368–370.

Hunter DJS, Enkin MW, Sargeant EJ, Wilkinson J, Tugwell P (1983). The outcome of prolonged labour as defined by partography and the use of oxytocin. A descriptive study. Am J Obstet Gynecol, 145: 189–192.

Klein M, Lloyd I, Redman C, Bull M, Turnbull A (1983). A comparison of low-risk pregnant women booked for delivery in 2 systems of care:- shared care (consultant) and integrated general practice unit. II Labour and delivery management and neonatal outcome. Br J Obstet Gynaecol, 90: 123–128.

Koontz WL, Bishop EH (1982). Management of the latent phase of labour. Clin Obstet Gynecol, 25: 111–114.

Manning R (1961). To do or not to do—a critical review of vaginal examination during labour. Am J Obstet Gynecol, 82: 1356–1358.

Melmed H, Evans MI (1976). Predictive value of cervical dilatation rate. 1. Primipara labour. Am J Obstet Gynecol, 47: 511–515.

Miller FC (1983). Uterine motility in spontaneous labour. Clin Obstet Gynecol, 26: 78–86.

Murphy K, Grieg V, Garcia J, Grant A (1986). Maternal considerations in the use of pelvic examinations in labour. Midwifery, 2: 93–97.

National Consensus Conference on Aspects of Caesarean Section Planning Committee (1985). Criteria used for the diagnosis of dystocia. Hamilton, Canada: McMaster University.

O'Driscoll K, Jackson RJA, Gallagher JT (1969). Prevention of prolonged labour. Br Med J, ii: 477–480.

O'Driscoll K, Jackson RT, Gallagher JT (1970). Active management of labour and cephalo-pelvic disproportion. J Obstet Gynaecol Br Commnwlth, 77: 385–389.

O'Driscoll K, Stronge JM, Minogue M (1973). Active management of labour. Br Med J, 3: 135–137.

O'Driscoll K, Meagher D (1980). Active Management of Labour. London: W B Saunders.

O'Driscoll K, Foley M, MacDonald D (1984). Active management of labour as an alternative to caesarean section for dystocia. Obstet Gynecol, 63: 485–490.

Peterson W, Stauch J, Toth B, Robinson L (1965). Routine vaginal examinations during labour. A comparative study with bacteriological analysis. Am J Obstet Gynecol, 92: 310–318.

Phillips GF, Calder AA (1987). Units for the evaluation of uterine contractility. Br J Obstet Gynaecol, 94: 236–241.

Philpott RH (1972). Graphic records in labour. Br Med J, 4: 163–167.

Philpott RH, Castle WM (1972a). Cervicographs in the management of labour on primigravidae. I. The alert line for detecting abnormal labour. J Obstet Gynaecol Br Commnwlth, 79: 592–298.

Philpott RH, Castle WM (1972b). Cervicographs in the management of labour in primigravidae. II. The action line and treatment of abnormal labour. J Obstet Gynaecol Br Commnwlth, 79: 599–602.

Philpott RH (1982). The recognition of cephalo-pelvic disproportion. In: Obstetric Problems in the Developing World. Philpott RH (ed). London: W B Saunders, p 617.

Prystowsky H (1954). Is the danger of vaginal examination overestimated? Am J Obstet Gynecol, 68: 639–644.

Richardson JA, Sutherland IA, Allen DW (1978). A cervimeter for continuous measurement of cervical dilatation in labour. Preliminary results. Br J Obstet Gynaecol, 85: 178–184.

Sokol RJ, Stojkov J, Chik, L, Rosen M (1977). Normal and abnormal progress. I. A quantitative assessment and survey of the literature. J Reprod Med, 18: 47–53.

Steer P J (1977). The measurement of uterine contractions. In: The current state of fetal heart rate monitoring and ultrasound in obstetrics. Beard RW, Campbell S (eds). London: Royal College of Obstetricians and Gynaecologists, pp 48–70.

Steer PJ, Carter MC, Beard RW (1984). Normal levels of active contraction area in spontaneous labour. Br J Obstet Gynaecol, 91: 211–219.

Stewart KS (1977). MD thesis, University of Edinburgh.

Stewart KS, Philpott RH (1980). Fetal responses to cephalopelvic disproportion. Br J Obstet Gynaecol, 87: 641–649.

Studd J (1973). Partograms and nomograms of cervical dilatation in management of primigravid labour. Br Med J, 4: 451–455.

Studd J, Clegg DR, Saunders RR, Hughes AO (1975). Identification of high risk labours by labour nomogram. Br Med J, ii: 545–547.

Studd JW, Cardozo LD, Gibb DMF (1982). The management of spontaneous labour. In: Progress in Obstetrics and Gynaecology. Studd J (ed). London: Churchill Livingstone, p. 66.

Tuck SM, Cardozo LD, Studd JW, Gibb DMF (1983). Obstetric characteristics in different racial groups. Br J Obstet Gynaecol, 90: 892–897.

Turner MJ, Crowley P, MacDonald D (1984). The unmasking of delivery room routines. J Obstet Gynaecol, 4: 188–190.

World Health Organization (1986). Appropriate Technology for Maternal and Newborn Care. Progress report on activities of WHO and WHO collaborating institutions. Maternal and Child Health Unit, Division of Family Health, Geneva: World Health Organization.

54 Monitoring the fetus during labour

Adrian Grant

1 Introduction

The aim of monitoring the fetus during labour is straightforward: it is to identify fetal problems which, if uncorrected, will cause death, short-term morbidity, or possibly long-term morbidity (but see Chapter 77). Evaluation of the various approaches to intrapartum fetal monitoring, by contrast, is fraught with difficulties. First, as will be discussed in detail in Section 2 of this chapter, the methods of monitoring during labour have evolved over 170 years, whereas modern methods for evaluating such tests have only been in use for the last 30 years. Second, like other tests of fetal 'well-being', it is impossible to assess reliably the 'predictive properties' of methods of intrapartum monitoring. This is discussed in Section 3, but the reader is also referred to Chapter 3 in Volume 1 of this book for a full description of the theoretical bases of these difficulties. For these reasons,

the alternative approaches to fetal monitoring during labour have to be evaluated in conjunction with the interventions which they prompt, ideally in the context of randomized controlled trials. These interventions may be conservative management (see Section 4) or, more usually, operative delivery (see Section 5).

Randomized trials of 'tests', such as those performed to monitor the fetus during labour, do not just evaluate the treatment prompted by the test. Let us assume, for the moment, that intrapartum monitoring can identify a reversible condition which, if left uncorrected, would result in poor fetal outcome. For the monitoring to be effective, the test must be performed correctly; its results must then be interpreted satisfactorily; and finally, this interpretation must provoke an appropriate response. Randomized controlled trials of alternative approaches to intrapartum fetal monitoring evaluate all three of these components as one 'package' of intervention. As discussed at various times during this chapter, there is controversy about how the tests of monitoring should be performed, about how the test results should be interpreted, and about what response an 'abnormal' result should prompt. Failure of any one of these components could negate the usefulness of that particular method of monitoring. This should be taken into account when considering the randomized trials of intrapartum fetal monitoring. Nevertheless, it is reassuring that the randomized trials which have been conducted, have generated consistent evidence about the effects of the alternative methods of monitoring on fetal and maternal outcome (see Section 5).

The focus of the chapter is a discussion of alternative methods of fetal heart rate monitoring. Several other methods of intrapartum surveillance will be mentioned more briefly, however.

2 Evolution of fetal monitoring during labour

2.1 Intermittent auscultation of the fetal heart

Although fetal heart sounds were probably first heard in the middle of the eighteenth century (Pinkerton 1969), it was not until 1821 that Lejumeau de Kergeradec, a French nobleman, suggested that auscultation of the fetal heart might be useful clinically. Kergeradec suggested that the ability to distinguish between fetal and maternal pulse rates could be used to diagnose both fetal life and multiple pregnancy (cited in Pinkerton 1969; and Goodlin 1979). He described fetal bradycardia as a sign of distress, and wondered 'whether it will be possible to judge the state of health or disease of the fetus from the variations that occur in the beat of the fetal heart' (cited in Schifrin and Suzuki 1973).

One of the obstetricians who adopted the technique of stethoscopic auscultation of the fetal heart was Evory Kennedy, Assistant Master at the Rotunda Hospital, Dublin in the late 1820s and early 1830s. Kennedy developed the use of auscultation to assess fetal wellbeing, and in 1833 he published an important book entitled *Observations on Obstetric Auscultation.* Although not all the clinical criteria which Kennedy suggested for 'fetal distress' have stood the test of time, he did conjecture on the nature of meconium-staining of the liquor amnii (see Section 2.2), and many of his impressions about various changes in fetal heart rate are still plausible today.

During the 1840s and 1850s, fetal auscultation slowly became established throughout Europe as the most satisfactory way of ascertaining fetal viability both during pregnancy and during labour. Some obstetricians (for instance, Fleetwood Churchill in Dublin and James Young Simpson in Edinburgh) began to consider

methods such as forceps delivery for earlier intervention in attempts to deliver a baby alive who would otherwise die *in utero*, and interest shifted from the diagnosis of fetal death to the recognition of fetal heart rate changes which might presage intrapartum fetal death.

In 1849, for example, Kilian proposed 'stethoscopic indications for forceps operation': 'The forceps must be applied under favorable conditions without delay when the fetal heart tones diminish in frequency to less than 100 beats per minute or when they increase to 180 beats per minute, when they lose their purity of tone, and when only one tone can be clearly heard' (cited by Goodlin 1979). In 1876, McClintock in Dublin noted that intrapartum death was sometimes signalled by a fetal bradycardia which immediately followed each contraction. Slowness to return to a normal rate following a contraction was documented in greater detail by two French obstetricians, Cazeaux and Tarnier, in 1884. These observations were largely ignored; Evory Kennedy had recommended auscultation between contractions because the fetal heart rate became difficult to measure during contractions. Auscultation between contractions had thus become standard practice and was to remain so for the next 75 years.

In 1893 Von Winkel proposed specific criteria for abnormalities of the fetal heart: a fetal heart rate of more than 160 or less than 120 (cited in Schifrin and Suzuki 1973). These criteria still form the basis for identifying 'fetal distress' using intermittent auscultation. Cazeaux and Tarnier had described a 'state of suffering' of the fetus on the basis of fetal heart rate changes, but it appears that the term 'fetal distress' was first used by Tweedie and Wrench in Dublin in 1908 (cited in Pinkerton 1976).

By the start of the twentieth century the stethoscopic approach had become the predominant method of fetal heart auscultation, commonly using a particular modification of fetal stethoscope ascribed to a French obstetrician, Alphonse Pinard (1844–1934). Although some authorities, such as Seitz in 1903, felt that changes in fetal heart rate during contractions might give an earlier warning sign (Gultekin-Zootzmann 1975), auscultation was used intermittently, usually between contractions. Until the mid-1950s the criteria for 'fetal distress' remained almost unchanged: a fetal heart rate which was above 160 or below 100–120 or irregular, or the passage of fresh meconium.

2.2 Liquor assessment

As mentioned in the previous section, Evory Kennedy conjectured on the significance of meconium-staining of the liquor amnii more than 150 years ago. Passage of meconium is associated with an increased risk of intrapartum stillbirth (Matthews and Martin 1974), neonatal death (Fujikura and Klionsky 1975), and various measures of neonatal morbidity, such as lowered acid–base status (Hobel 1971). Meconium in the liquor carries the risk of the meconium aspiration syndrome (Gregory *et al.* 1974), which explains some but not all of the observed association between meconium staining of the liquor and neonatal mortality and morbidity.

The degree of meconium, and the timing of its evacuation, are related to the strength of the association with poor fetal outcome. Thick meconium recognized at the onset of labour carries the worst prognosis, and is associated with a five-sevenfold increased risk of peri-natal death (Meis *et al.* 1978; MacDonald *et al.* 1985). Thick, undiluted meconium also reflects reduced liquor volume at the onset of labour, and the latter is a risk factor in its own right (see Chapter 30). Thick undi-luted meconium is less likely to be seen at rupture of the membranes, and this is the basis for the recommenda-tion that 'no visible liquor at the time of rupture of membranes' should be treated as if there is thick meconium unless clear liquor subsequently drains (O'Driscoll and Meagher 1980). Slight staining of the liquor at the onset of labour probably carries a small increase in risk (Hobel 1971), but this has been dis-puted (Meis *et al.* 1978; Starks 1980). Like reduced liquor volume, meconium-staining of the liquor at the onset of labour reflects events prior to the onset of labour. O'Driscoll and his colleagues (1977) believe that significant meconium-staining is a sign of impaired placental function that antedates labour and 'which exposes the fetus to the risk of hypoxia during labour'.

Passage of meconium for the first time after the onset of labour is less common, and it seems to carry an associated risk intermediate between heavy and light early passage of meconium (Meis *et al.* 1978).

Whatever the degree or time of passage of meconium, the risks associated are increased importantly if fetal heart rate abnormalities are also present (Miller *et al.* 1975; Starks 1980).

Because of these associations between liquor status and adverse outcomes, routine assessment of the liquor in early labour, if necessary by amnioscopy or artificial rupture of the membranes (O'Driscoll and Meagher 1980), has been recommended as a screening test for identifying fetuses at increased risk. Unfortunately, no controlled evaluation of such a policy has been reported.

2.3 Continuous fetal electrocardiography

The fetal electrocardiogram was first recorded by Cremer in 1906 (Goodlin 1979). An abdominal elec-trode was placed over the uterine fundus and a second electrode lodged in the vagina. The fetal complexes were just visible in Cremer's electrocardiograph (ECG) but were almost completely overshadowed by maternal complexes. The separation of maternal and fetal ECG complexes has remained the outstanding problem of

this technique. Until the 1950s, the fetal signal obtained in this way was so small compared to that of the mother that it was impossible to drive a tachometer to record a fetal heart rate. In the 1950s Hon and Hess (1957) in the USA developed a way of cancelling the maternal ECG by using a second ECG recording of the mother's complexes and subtracting this from the abdominal recording. The technique was laborious and never entirely satisfactory, but despite this Hon was able to document profound bradycardia in a dying fetus and also noticed that manipulation of a prolapsed cord caused fetal heart irregularities and bradycardia (Hon 1959).

The clear need to obtain distinct and large fetal ECG signals was realized in the late 1950s by Caldeyro-Barcia and his colleagues in Uruguay. They implanted an electrode directly into the fetus transabdominally (Caldeyro-Barcia 1958). It was then possible to obtain continuous fetal heart rate and intrauterine pressure tracings simultaneously. This method of obtaining a fetal ECG was clearly unacceptable for normal clinical practice and the breakthrough came in 1960 when Hon (1960) successfully introduced an electrode through the cervix and clipped it onto the fetal head.

The development of the internal scalp electrode led to a rapid growth in research into the relationship between fetal heart rate changes and events during labour. Hon and his co-workers in the USA and, independently, Caldeyro-Barcia in Uruguay and Ham-macher (1967) in Germany, reported various fetal heart rate changes which they related to 'fetal distress'. Although tachycardia and bradycardia were classical signs of 'fetal distress', Hon distinguished between constant or 'baseline' bradycardias, which were almost invariably associated with good fetal outcome, and bradycardias which represented a change in rate from a previously higher level (Hon 1959). He also described late fetal heart rate decelerations, which he thought were due to uteroplacental insufficiency, and variable decelerations, which he ascribed to umbilical cord compression. Caldeyro-Barcia described similar changes (though he called them type II and type III decelerations respectively), and Hammacher related loss of fetal heart rate variability to fetal distress. A common nomenclature was agreed following meetings between the various groups of investigators in 1971 and 1972.

2.4 Fetal heart monitoring with Doppler ultrasound

Callagan and his colleagues first described the applica-tion of the Doppler principle to detect the fetal heart beat in 1964. (The principle is that there is a change in frequency when a waveform is reflected from a moving surface.) Two years later Bishop (1966) and Bernstine and Callagan (1966) used the same technique to measure fetal heart rate. The machinery was relatively simple and inexpensive and gave a strong enough signal to allow reliable fetal heart rate recording. By 1969 this technique was already in use in a number of clinical obstetric units in Britain (Huntingford and Pendleton 1969) and North America (Paul and Hon 1971). Diffusion was accelerated by the consensus opinion of four experts (Hellman *et al.* 1970) that ultrasound did not adversely affect the rate of miscarriage or congenital malformation.

Doppler ultrasound provides the most reliable method for monitoring the fetal heart rate during late pregnancy and for external monitoring of the fetal heart rate during labour. All moving parts of the fetal heart generate an ultrasound pulse. The strongest of these pulses originates from the ventricles during systole; a pulse is also produced by the atria during diastole. Detailed ultrasound examination may therefore provide evidence of fetal heart function, but as currently used to measure the fetal heart rate, the ultrasound beam may wander between the atria and ventricles thus picking up signals at different stages of the cardiac cycle. This has little effect on the estimation of fetal heart rate but gives a misleading impression of the time interval between beats and hence the variability in the fetal heart rate over time. For this reason the raw Doppler signal is usually smoothed, averaged, or filtered. All modern monitors use autocorrelation. Despite this, ultrasound fetal heart rate monitors give a poorer impression of fetal heart rate variability than those which use electro-cardiographic and phonocardiographic recording (Carter 1986). Additional problems are, first, that a maternal heart rate may occasionally be counted in error and this may lead to an inappropriate diagnosis of fetal distress (Amato 1983), and second, that when the fetus or mother moves the signal may be lost or artefactual (Visser *et al.* 1980), necessitating frequent repositioning of the transducer.

2.5 Fetal scalp blood acid–base assessment

The technique of sampling blood from the fetal scalp during labour was first described by Saling in Berlin in the early 1960s (Saling 1961, 1962). A scalpel or stylette is passed through the cervix to make a small incision in the fetal scalp. A sample of blood is then collected in a capillary tube and analysed to determine its acid–base status. Saling (1964) and others (Beard *et al.* 1967; Coltart *et al.* 1969) found that about half the cases with slowing of the fetal heart rate had normal fetal scalp blood pH values and they recommended the introduction of fetal scalp blood sampling into clinical practice as a means of making continuous fetal heart rate monitoring more specific. Modern automated blood microprocessors are much easier to use, require very small quantities of blood, and give a more reliable measurement of acid-base status than the meters used in the

1960s and 1970s (Stewart *et al.* 1983). In other respects, the technique has changed little since Saling's first description and remains somewhat cumbersome and time-consuming.

2.6 Current patterns of fetal monitoring during labour

The use of continuous fetal heart rate monitoring in obstetric practice, using either fetal scalp electrodes or an external Doppler ultrasound transducers, increased rapidly during the 1970s. A survey of all deliveries in Britain during a single week in 1970 revealed that only one fetus in 279 was monitored electronically, one in 333 had a scalp blood sample taken, and one in a thousand had both continuous electronic heart rate monitoring and fetal scalp blood sampling (Chamberlain *et al.* 1975). A national survey in France conducted in 1972 showed that 93.8 per cent of labours were then monitored by intermittent auscultation, 5.5 per cent by continuous electronic monitoring alone, and 0.7 per cent with a combination of continuous electronic monitoring and fetal scalp blood pH estimation. By 1975 the use of continuous electronic monitoring had more than doubled in the one region resurveyed (Rumeau-Roquette and Bréart 1978). In the USA an estimated 1000 electronic fetal monitoring systems were in use by 1972. A 1976 survey of teaching hospitals in North America revealed that, of the 279 for which information was available, all but one used electronic fetal monitoring (Dilts 1976).

In 1978, Gillmer and Combe (1979) conducted a postal survey of specialist obstetric units in the United Kingdom. Of 264 such units only one (in which only 800 babies were delivered each year) did not have an electronic fetal heart rate monitor. Among the units with monitors, the numbers of deliveries per monitor varied widely (172–2702; median 600). Two broad groups of hospitals were identifiable—those in which electronic monitoring was used in as high a proportion of women as possible, and those in which its use was restricted to women whose pregnancies were deemed to be at high risk. Fetal blood pH estimation was used in conjunction with fetal heart rate measurement in 98 hospitals (40 per cent) and a further 38 (16 per cent) had a pH meter in, or adjacent to, the labour ward but did not use it for fetal blood pH estimation.

By 1985, a survey of all British maternity units revealed that 96 per cent of all deliveries took place in units with a continuous fetal heart rate monitor and that all units with 2000 or more deliveries each year had at least one monitor (Grant 1987a). The median annual deliveries per monitor was near 400 (most larger units had between 300 and 750 deliveries per monitor each year). In contrast, only 33 per cent of women were delivered in a unit with a fetal scalp pH meter.

Despite this trend during the 1970s and early 1980s

to replace intermittent auscultation by continuous electronic monitoring, the fetus continues to be monitored using intermittent auscultation very widely. The recently published findings of the 1980 National Natality Survey—a sample survey of ten thousand births in USA hospitals in that year—revealed that an estimated 48 per cent had been monitored with continuous electronic fetal monitoring: 27 per cent by Doppler ultrasound alone, 10 per cent by scalp electrode alone, 6 per cent by a combination of Doppler ultrasound and scalp electrode, and 4 per cent by other methods and combinations (Placek *et al.* 1984).

As this survey suggests, continuous electronic fetal heartrate monitoring during labour is now most commonly achieved either 'externally' by Doppler ultrasound, or 'internally' by electrocardiography. If continuous fetal heart rate monitoring is being used, external monitoring is usually employed during early labour, particularly before the membranes have ruptured. Internal monitoring is the method of choice later in labour because it provides a more reliable trace and allows the mother greater freedom of movement. For this reason it is common practice in Britain to change to internal monitoring as soon as labour is established and when it is possible to attach a fetal scalp electrode. There is no uniformity in the use of fetal scalp blood pH measurement as an adjunct to fetal heart rate monitoring. Some obstetricians feel that fetal heart rate monitoring alone is a reliable means of assessing fetal well-being, whereas others feel that fetal blood pH measurement is a necessary adjunct to fetal heart rate monitoring (Beard 1974; Gillmer and Combe 1979; Beard and Rivers 1979; Perkins 1984).

3 Test characteristics of fetal monitoring tests

There is no question that continuous electronic fetal heart rate monitoring provides more information than intermittent auscultation with a fetal stethoscope: this is the basis for the use of electronic fetal monitoring in clinical practice. Listening for a minute every fifteen minutes between contractions, as is commonly employed with intermittent auscultation in the first stage of labour, samples the fetal heart rate for only about 7 per cent of the time and provides relatively little information about the relationship between changes in the fetal heart rate and uterine contractions and fetal heart rate variability. The question is whether this greater sophistication improves the effectiveness of fetal monitoring during labour in terms of outcome.

The development of new tests for use in clinical practice can be characterized as having three phases, each of which requires a particular form of evaluation (Grant 1984). The first phase is that of technical development; evaluation of this phase requires an assessment of whether the test measures what it is supposed to measure (for example, in this context, fetal heart rate). The second stage of development is the definition of abnormal test results for use in clinical practice; evaluation in this phase is by assessment of whether the test defined in this way actually identifies the clinical condition(s) it is supposed to identify. It is these first two stages of evaluation of methods of intrapartum fetal heart monitoring in 'isolation' from the intervention that they may prompt, which will be discussed in this section. (The principles and terms used have been described in Chapter 3.) The third stage of development is the choice of clinical action to be taken on the basis of abnormal and normal test results. Sections 4 and 5 review the evidence that fetal and maternal problems are more successfully prevented by clinical action taken on the basis of more intensive fetal heart monitoring.

3.1 Accuracy and reproducibility

3.1.1 Intermittent auscultation

Studies in which real or simulated 'intermittent auscultation' has been compared with an audio recording of a heart rate have shown wide margins of error in the rate estimate, particularly when these fall outside the normal range (Hon 1958, Day *et al.* 1968); and in the identification of periodic changes in the rate (Miller *et al.* 1984). The very simple criteria used in clinical practice to define normal and abnormal fetal heart rates recorded by intermittent auscultation, however, circumvent much of this inaccuracy: 'clinical accuracy' (the extent to which individuals are correctly assigned to normal or abnormal test groups) using the conventional cut-offs of 120 and 160 beats per minute appears to be good (Hon 1958). Of course, this begs the question of whether these simple criteria are useful in clinical practice and this will be discussed later.

3.1.2 Continuous electronic fetal heart rate monitoring

Modern electronic fetal heart rate monitors, when functioning correctly, give an accurate measurement of the heart rate (to within 1.5 per cent (Department of Health and Social Security 1984)). Accuracy is greatest using 'internal', continuous ECG methods. These allow accurate measurement of the time interval between heart beats, and hence fetal heart rate variability. As discussed earlier, external ultrasound methods are generally less satisfactory for measuring variability, although when the intervals between impulses are summed and averaged these methods do give an accurate measurement of fetal heart rate.

Interpretation of fetal heart rate changes requires simultaneous recording of uterine contractions. This is accomplished most accurately by direct measurement of the intrauterine pressure by means of a catheter inserted into the uterine cavity. This method is sometimes associated with complications (National Institutes of Health 1979; Ledger 1978), both maternal (Chan *et al.* 1973; Haverkamp and Bowes 1971) and fetal (Trudinger and Pryce-Davies 1978; Cave *et al.* 1979; Stokes 1984). For this reason uterine contractions are also commonly recorded by means of an external pressure transducer. Though safer, this is a less satisfactory method of tocographic recording because it gives a less precise description of the relationship between changes in fetal heart rate and uterine contractions and does not provide a measurement of intrauterine pressure.

The criteria used to interpret continuous recordings of the fetal heart rate are far more complex than those of intermittent auscultation. Thus, despite the fact that electronic fetal monitoring gives a substantially more accurate measurement of the fetal heart rate, the clinical interpretation of fetal heart rate traces is more complicated and open to greater variation in interpretation.

Few studies have been mounted to assess the 'reproducibility' (intra- and inter-observer variation) of trace interpretation. Trimbos and Keirse (1978), Peck (1980), and Flynn *et al.* (1982), have shown variation in the assessment of antepartum cardiotocographic traces. The European Community Project on Perinatal Monitoring (Van Geijn 1987) demonstrated that the widest disagreement was on the classification of heart rate variability and the type of deceleration, the additional elements which are *not* considered during intermittent auscultation. Cohen *et al.* (1982) examined the extent of agreement and disagreement in interpretation and clinical response to intrapartum traces. Twelve obstetricians, recognized in the USA for their scientific and clinical contributions to electronic fetal monitoring, were interviewed. A description of 14 patterns (different combinations of periodic changes and baseline variabilities) was supplied, each of which is generally considered to be 'abnormal', although there was known to be disagreement 'in the literature' over their perceived severity. The obstetricians were asked to classify the traces into three levels of severity: 'ominous', 'non-reassuring' and 'innocuous'. They were then asked what clinical action they would take if conservative treatment failed, firstly if fetal blood acid–base was not available, and secondly, if it was available. In the initial assessment of the 14 traces there was near perfect agreement over five, fair agreement over a further five, but marked disagreement over the remaining four. Faced with the choice of continuous monitoring or immediate delivery, the obstetricians agreed closely in four cases, agreed moderately in eight, and disagreed markedly in two. Where there was a consensus, this reflected the initial assessment of the traces. As might be expected, preference for continued monitoring was greatest in those patterns which had been graded as 'innocuous' or 'non-reassuring', whereas immediate delivery was most commonly preferred in traces which were judged to be 'ominous'.

When the choice was expanded to include fetal scalp blood sampling, this proved a popular option. In some situations, obstetricians chose it to improve 'specificity' (cases in which they would otherwise have expedited delivery) and in others to improve 'sensitivity' (cases in which they would otherwise have continued monitoring). (See Chapter 3 for an explanation of these terms.) There was perfect agreement over two patterns (when all of the obstetricians would have performed fetal blood sampling). Disagreement was marked for five of the other patterns.

This variation for individual patterns reflected marked differences between the obstetricians. The number of traces initially classified as 'ominous' varied from 1 to 6. When the choice of action lay between continued monitoring or immediate delivery, anything between 0 and 8 of the patterns were judged to merit immediate delivery. When the option of fetal scalp blood sampling was available, the number of cases in which its use was recommended ranged from 2 to 14. As the authors themselves note, these observers are unlikely to be representative of all obstetricians in the USA. They were all conversant with electronic fetal monitoring and worked in academic centres where facilities for fetal blood sampling are likely to exist. Nevertheless, this study does demonstrate that variation exists not only in trace interpretation but also in the clinical action which it may prompt.

In this study by Cohen and his colleagues (1982), descriptions of trace patterns were supplied to the 14 obstetricians; they were not asked to interpret and categorize actual electronic fetal monitoring traces. More recently, Nielsen and colleagues (1987) compared the assessment of 50 thirty-minute intrapartum cardiotocographs by four experienced obstetricians, in terms of 'need for immediate delivery'. Only 11 (22 per cent) of the traces were assessed in the same way by all four obstetricians. Furthermore, on average, 21 per cent of the traces were interpreted differently by individual obstetricians when reassessed two months later.

Individually, many clinicians believe that they know how to interpret and respond to intrapartum fetal heart rate patterns (even if they think that others can not) (see, for example, Parer 1986). Such feelings underlie strongly held opinions about specific aspects of intrapartum monitoring such as the importance of variability and the choice of paper speed (Keirse 1986). These studies showing wide intra- and inter-observer variation in trace interpretation demonstrate the subjectivity of current methods of visual assessment of fetal heart rate patterns, and suggest that such confidence is misplaced. Training of observers in standardized systems of visual interpretation is likely to reduce variation, but interpretation will always remain subjective to some extent. Objective computerized assessment is therefore a rational development. Nevertheless, the sophisticated assessment of many parameters which constitutes current visual interpretation is not easily simulated by computer. Computerized assessment will undoubtedly reduce observer variation but will not necessarily increase the test's validity if some elements of current visual systems are not considered by the computer. Computerized systems for intrapartum fetal heart rate interpretation should be rigorously evaluated before introduction into clinical practice.

3.2 Predictive properties of fetal monitoring tests

The extent to which the measurement problems discussed above are clinically important will be reflected in the ability of the methods of monitoring to separate 'normal' from 'abnormal' fetuses satisfactorily—the second phase of evaluation mentioned at the beginning of this section.

The rationale for continuous monitoring of the fetal heart rate during labour is that it identifies fetal problems earlier and more efficiently than intermittent auscultation. Continuous monitoring should therefore be more 'sensitive'. The concept of comparing the two approaches in this way is therefore attractive. There are, however, unavoidable reasons why the evaluation of fetal heart rate monitoring in these terms is inexact and unreliable (see below). These problems have been discussed in detail by Grant (1986) and in Chapter 3.

3.2.1 Intermittent auscultation

Formal attempts to 'validate' intermittent auscultation have all taken place at a time when clinical intervention for 'fetal distress' was based on abnormalities of intermittently auscultated fetal heart tones. It is thus impossible to exclude the confounding effects of clinical intervention on outcome. Furthermore, in many studies, the diagnosis of 'fetal distress' was not based solely on fetal heart rate abnormalities, but included meconium-staining of the liquor.

In most studies the predictive properties of intermittent auscultation are expressed in terms of positive predictive values without presentation of the data in a form which allows calculation of sensitivity or specificity (see, for example, Lund 1943). Wood and Pinkerton (1961) reported that, over a two-year period (1957–59) at Queen Charlotte's Hospital, London, 18 out of 30 intrapartum stillbirths (sensitivity 60 per cent) had signs of 'fetal distress', but there is no information about false positive diagnoses of fetal distress. Other studies (McCall and Fulshaw 1953; Hellman *et al.* 1958; Walker J 1959; Fenton and Steer 1962) showed that a variety of auscultated fetal heart rate changes

were predictive of perinatal death, particularly if associated with the passage of meconium, but that only a minority of cases with abnormalities subsequently ended in perinatal death. Later, Benson and his colleagues (1968) using extensive data from the US Collaborative Perinatal Project (Niswander and Gordon 1972) searched for a more sophisticated index of fetal distress based on intermittent auscultation of the fetal heart rate, but concluded that 'no reliable single auscultatory indicator of fetal distress exists in terms of fetal heart rate, save in an extreme degree'.

In summary, evaluation of intermittent auscultation in terms of its ability to predict poor fetal outcome is fraught with methodological and other problems. Taken at face value, intermittent auscultation appears to perform badly, and indeed, this prompted the development of continuous electronic fetal heart rate monitoring.

3.2.2 Continuous electronic fetal heart rate monitoring

Many of the same constraints apply to the evaluation of the predictive properties of continuous electronic fetal monitoring. Most validation studies of electronic fetal monitoring have used the Apgar score as the 'Gold Standard' against which the test was compared. These studies are summarized elsewhere (Grant 1986). The problems of using the Apgar score in this way are discussed in Chapter 3. Abnormal trace patterns are clearly predictive of low Apgar scores, although, with sensitivities around 70 per cent and specificities around 80 per cent, apparently not strongly so. Some cases of low Apgar score do not reflect fetal compromise during labour (such as low Apgar scores due to congenital abnormalities, or opiates administered for pain relief) and in all but one of these studies intervention was based on the trace patterns. Furthermore, variable definitions of abnormal traces have been used. These factors might lead to an underestimate of the true predictive properties of abnormal fetal heart rate traces.

Positive predictive values are, however, generally low (about 30 per cent), whereas negative predictive values are generally high, with many estimates over 90 per cent. This is the reason for the clinical impression that a normal test result (normal trace) indicates that the baby is all right, whereas a positive test result (abnormal trace) is associated with a large number of false positives. This impression is stronger the lower the prevalence of adverse outcome (in this context, low Apgar scores are relatively common when compared, for example, with deaths) (see Chapter 3 for theoretical discussion of this). Schifrin and Dame's study (1972) illustrates this. They found that abnormal fetal heart rate traces seemed to be better predictors of low five-minute Apgar score (sensitivity 83 per cent) than the one-minute score (sensitivity 54 per cent); yet, because low five-minute scores were so infrequent, the positive predictive value appears much less good for this index. This was the only study in which the traces were kept 'blind' from the clinicians responsible for care, and which thus truly estimated the extent to which abnormal traces could predict low Apgar scores in the context of current practice based on intermittent auscultation. It is noteworthy that if two cases of congenital abnormalities had been excluded from this analysis all the cases with low Apgar scores at five minutes would have been correctly predicted (sensitivity 100 per cent).

The ability of electronic fetal monitoring to predict low fetal scalp pH has also been investigated (see Grant 1986). Again, a clear relationship exists, with an estimated sensitivity of 90 per cent. But the large numbers of false positives which are a consequence of relatively low specificity result in a low positive predictive value.

Murphy and his colleagues (1981) examined the relationship between electronic fetal monitoring and a variety of measures of neonatal outcome. There was a statistically significant relationship with Apgar score, but the strength of the relationship with other measures of later outcome was weaker. Painter and his colleagues (1978) examined the relationship of abnormal electronic fetal monitoring traces to Apgar scores, abnormal neonatal neurology, and status at one year of age. They chose to follow up 38 babies who had had the 'most ominous' patterns during the period of case recruitment, together with 12 babies who had had normal fetal heart rate patterns during labour. Two-thirds of the babies with severe, variable or late decelerations in labour had low Apgar scores and abnormal neonatal neurological signs. Of the seven babies who were assessed as abnormal at one year of age the degree of abnormality was 'minor' in five. Borgstedt and colleagues (as described in the National Institutes of Health report 1979) also claimed that fetal heart rate decelerations during labour were correlated with (undefined) 'overt brain damage' at one year of age. Decelerations identified more than 50 per cent of these cases but there was a 'high false positive rate'. The fact that intrapartum traces may predict childhood morbidity (albeit weakly) does not, however, necessarily mean that the problem originated in labour. It has long been recognized that signs during labour, such as abnormal traces, may be the first indication of an underlying problem that predated the onset of labour (Freud 1897).

Saling's rationale for recommending fetal scalp blood pH estimation as a secondary test for those cases with abnormal trace patterns was to reduce the number of false positives. The relationship between scalp pH and Apgar score has also been summarized elsewhere (Grant 1986). Because electronic fetal heart monitoring and scalp blood pH are related, the implications of using scalp blood pH as a 'diagnostic' test when there is a trace abnormality cannot easily be assessed from their performance 'in isolation' (see Chapter 3).

The study by Beard *et al.* (1971) allows an assessment of the effect of using fetal scalp blood pH in this way when the definition of abnormal traces remains fixed. The specificity rose from 43 per cent to 93 per cent—a large reduction in false positives—and this was reflected in an improvement in the positive predictive value from 28 per cent to 60 per cent. But fetal blood pH is not perfectly sensitive, and in this context of a fixed definition of trace abnormality sensitivity fell from 69 per cent to 31 per cent, with a corresponding increase in false negatives. This implies that the use of fetal scalp blood pH measurement may reduce greatly the number of unnecessary caesarean sections performed because of falsely abnormal fetal heart rate traces, but a few babies with abnormal traces who are truly compromised may be falsely deemed to be normal.

In fact, it is likely that the *definition* of an abnormal trace pattern may change when the option to perform fetal scalp sampling is available. As Cohen's study (Cohen *et al.* 1982) suggested (see Section 3.1.2 above), fetal blood sampling may be performed for a trace pattern which on its own would not be considered to warrant caesarean section. In this way the sensitivity may actually be increased by the availability of scalp sampling. Furthermore, as will be discussed in Section 5, there is experimental evidence which suggests that the addition of scalp sampling does indeed improve both the sensitivity and the specificity of electronic fetal heart rate monitoring.

It should be recognized that these studies of the predictive properties of intrapartum fetal heart rate traces are all based on retrospective assessment of a trace pattern after delivery. As the parent of a child whose heart rate was monitored electronically during labour has pointed out (Royston 1982), however, fetal heart rate monitors not uncommonly malfunction during labour and this influences the way in which those providing care react to trace 'abnormalities'. The more often an alarm is false due to malfunctioning, the more likely it is that a true alarm will be ignored. In other words, the interpreter/machine combination is likely to be less sensitive and less specific than when a trace pattern is considered on its own. This 'systems' view (Royston 1982) has received surprisingly little attention in the debate about intrapartum monitoring.

In summary, electronic fetal rate monitoring undoubtedly gives a much more detailed measurement of fetal heart rate than intermittent auscultation; this is reflected in a far more complex method for defining normal and abnormal test results. The problem with electronic fetal heart rate monitoring is in its interpretation rather than with its ability to measure. A variety of methodological and other problems make it impossible to assess whether electronic fetal monitoring is better at identifying intrapartum fetal problems than intermittent auscultation, as has often been claimed. These difficulties can only be circumvented by comparing the extent to which the clinical actions prompted by the alternative monitoring methods successfully prevent poor fetal (and maternal) outcome. This third phase of evaluation is the subject of the next two sections.

4 Conservative management of fetal distress

The most radical and common treatment for intrapartum fetal distress diagnosed by persistent fetal heart rate abnormalities or depressed fetal scalp blood pH is prompt delivery. Many fetal heart rate abnormalities, however, will resolve with simple conservative measures, such as a change in maternal position (to relieve aorto-caval compression) (see Chapter 55); discontinuation of oxytocin administration to maximize utero-placental blood flow; head down tilt to relieve

pressure on the umbilical cord; and maternal oxygen administration to maximize oxygen transport to the placenta.

4.1 Conservative measures versus operative delivery for 'fetal distress'

The effects of conservative measures versus operative delivery for auscultated fetal heart abnormalities (using the criteria discussed earlier), or meconium staining of the liquor amnii, in otherwise uncomplicated pregnancies and labours were assessed in a controlled trial conducted in Natal, South Africa, in the late 1950s (Walker N 1959). The choice of policy 'was determined by drawing a sealed envelope from a drum'. No data are available with which to assess the comparability of the two groups generated. Operative delivery rates were, however, strikingly different: 61 per cent versus 20 per cent overall; 28 per cent versus 7 per cent for caesarean delivery; and 33 per cent versus 13 per cent for operative vaginal delivery (Table 54.1). Operative deliveries in the conservatively managed group were for reasons other than fetal distress alone, such as cephalopelvic

Table 54.1 Effect of operative versus conservative management of intrapartum 'fetal distress' (diagnosed by intermittent auscultation) on operative delivery

Study	EXPT		CTRL		Odds ratio	Graph of odds ratios and confidence intervals						
	n	(%)	n	(%)	(95% CI)	0.01	0.1	0.5	1	2	10	100
Walker (1959)	106/174	(60.92)	35/176	(19.89)	5.48 (3.58–8.39)					⟶		
Typical odds ratio (95% confidence interval)					5.48 (3.58–8.39)					⟶		

Effect of operative versus conservative management of intrapartum 'fetal distress' (diagnosed by intermittent auscultation) on caesarean section

Walker (1959)	48/174	(27.59)	12/176	(6.82)	4.30 (2.47–7.49)					⟶		
Typical odds ratio (95% confidence interval)					4.30 (2.47–7.49)					⟶		

Effect of operative versus conservative management of intrapartum 'fetal distress' (diagnosed by intermittent auscultation) on operative vaginal delivery

Walker (1959)	58/174	(33.33)	23/176	(13.07)	3.11 (1.90–5.12)					⟶		
Typical odds ratio (95% confidence interval)					3.11 (1.90–5.12)					⟶		

Effect of operative versus conservative management of intrapartum 'fetal distress' (diagnosed by intermittent auscultation) on perinatal mortality

Walker (1959)	14/174	(8.05)	12/176	(6.82)	1.19 (0.54–2.65)				⟶			
Typical odds ratio (95% confidence interval)					1.19 (0.54–2.65)				⟶			

disproportion, intrauterine infection and pre-eclampsia. These problems, which carried a much worse prognosis, were therefore acted on in both of the experimental groups and the contrast in management was largely a manifestation of intervention for 'uncomplicated' fetal distress. Thirty-nine per cent of the women allocated to operative delivery had spontaneous vaginal deliveries because 'delivery was imminent' at trial entry.

The rate of perinatal mortality was similar in the two groups (Table 54.1). Unfortunately no details are available for maternal or neonatal morbidity. Nor are details given about the causes of the perinatal deaths; it is therefore impossible to assess whether the similarity in the overall death rates reflected fewer deaths ascribed to 'asphyxia' balanced by more deaths ascribed to trauma in the intervention group. Given that 24 per cent of the deliveries in the intervention group were achieved with the help of symphysiotomy or mid-cavity forceps, such a reciprocity is plausible and there is a hint of such a relationship in one of the more recently conducted trials (MacDonald *et al.* 1985).

4.2 Intravenous preloading before epidural anaesthesia

Maternal hypotension due to vasodilatation often follows the induction of epidural anaesthesia, with consequent fetal heart rate abnormalities. Preloading with intravenous fluids has been shown in a well-conducted trial (Collins *et al.* 1978) to counteract the relative hypovolaemia that follows epidural block, and to reduce the frequency of fetal heart rate abnormalities by a substantial amount (Table 54.2).

4.3 Intravenous betamimetics

Intravenous betamimetics appear to be a useful treatment for 'buying time' when persistent fetal heart rate abnormalities indicate elective delivery. In a randomized controlled trial involving 20 labours characterized by both ominous fetal heart rate changes and a fetal scalp blood pH of less than 7.25 (Table 54.3), 10 of the 11 treated with intravenous terbutaline showed improvement in the heart rate pattern, compared with none in the control group (Patriarco *et al.* 1987). At birth, terbutaline-treated babies were less likely to be acidotic and to have low Apgar scores. There were no perinatal deaths in either group. Terbutaline was reported to have no adverse effects, other than transient maternal tachycardia. This short-term improvement could be very useful in places where facilities for emergency caesarean section are not immediately available, or to 'buy' time to set up regional anaesthesia. Also, the improvement in the trace pattern is sometimes sustained so labour can continue without further intervention.

4.4 Amnioinfusion

Another temporizing manoeuvre, amnioinfusion, has been described for variable deceleration patterns. This fetal heart rate abnormality is often considered to be due to cord compression, particularly when there is oligohydramnios. Correction of 'oligohydramnios' is the basis of amnioinfusion. Saline is infused through an intrauterine catheter into the uterine cavity, either until the variable decelerations have resolved, or until 800 mls have been infused.

In a randomized controlled trial involving 96 women (Miyazaki and Nevarez 1985; Table 54.4), variable decelerations persisted in 49 per cent in the amnioinfusion group compared with 96 per cent in the control group. The difference in the caesarean section rates (7 per cent; 3 women), however, was much less clear-cut, although primigravidae appeared to benefit differentially in this respect. The only complication reported was a case of cord prolapse two hours after amnioinfusion in which the baby was born in very poor condition.

Table 54.2 Effect of intravenous preloading before epidural anaesthesia in labour on maternal hypotension

Study	EXPT		CTRL		Odds ratio	Graph of odds ratios and confidence intervals						
	n	(%)	*n*	(%)	(95% CI)	0.01	0.1	0.5	1	2	10	100
Collins *et al.* (1978)	1/49	(2.04)	15/53	(28.30)	0.14 (0.05–0.41)							
Typical odds ratio (95% confidence interval)					0.14 (0.05–0.41)							

Effect of intravenous preloading before epidural anaesthesia in labour on fetal heart rate abnormality

Collins *et al.* (1978)	6/49	(12.24)	18/53	(33.96)	0.30 (0.12–0.75)							
Typical odds ratio (95% confidence interval)					0.30 (0.12–0.75)							

Table 54.3 Effect of intravenous betamimetics in intrapartum fetal distress (diagnosed by electronic fetal heart rate monitoring) on no improvement in fetal heart rate abnormality

Study	EXPT		CTRL		Odds ratio	Graph of odds ratios and confidence intervals						
	n	(%)	*n*	(%)	(95% CI)	0.01	0.1	0.5	1	2	10	100
Patriarco *et al.* (1987)	1/11	(9.09)	9/9	(100.0)	0.03 (0.01–0.18)							
Typical odds ratio (95% confidence interval)					0.03 (0.01–0.18)							

Effect of intravenous betamimetics in intrapartum fetal distress (diagnosed by electronic fetal heart rate monitoring) on Apgar score <7 at 1 minute

Patriarco *et al.* (1987)	1/11	(9.09)	4/9	(44.44)	0.17 (0.02–1.21)							
Typical odds ratio (95% confidence interval)					0.17 (0.02–1.21)							

Effect of intravenous betamimetics in intrapartum fetal distress (diagnosed by electronic fetal heart rate monitoring) on perinatal mortality

Patriarco *et al.* (1987)	0/11	(0.00)	0/9	(0.00)	1.00 (1.00–1.00)							
Typical odds ratio (95% confidence interval)					1.00 (1.00–1.00)							

Table 54.4 Effect of amnioinfusion in intrapartum fetal distress (diagnosed by electronic fetal heart rate monitoring) on persistent fetal heart rate abnormality

Study	EXPT		CTRL		Odds ratio	Graph of odds ratios and confidence intervals						
	n	(%)	*n*	(%)	(95% CI)	0.01	0.1	0.5	1	2	10	100
Miyazaki and Nevarez (1985)	24/49	(48.98)	45/47	(95.74)	0.10 (0.04–0.25)							
Typical odds ratio (95% confidence interval)					0.10 (0.04–0.25)							

Effect of amnioinfusion in intrapartum fetal distress (diagnosed by electronic fetal heart rate monitoring) on caesarean section for fetal distress

Miyazaki and Nevarez. (1985)	9/49	(18.37)	12/47	(25.53)	0.66 (0.25–1.73)							
Typical odds ratio (95% confidence interval)					0.66 (0.25–1.73)							

Table 54.4—*continued* Effect of amnioinfusion in intrapartum fetal distress (diagnosed by electronic fetal heart rate monitoring) on Apgar score <7 at 1 minute

Miyazaki and Nevarez (1985)	11/47	(22.45)	9/47	(19.15)	1.22 (0.46–3.25)	
Typical odds ratio (95% confidence interval)					1.22 (0.46–3.25)	

Table 54.5 Effect of piracetam for fetal distress in labour on caesarean section

Study	EXPT		CTRL		Odds ratio	Graph of odds ratios and confidence intervals						
	n	(%)	*n*	(%)	(95% CI)	0.01	0.1	0.5	1	2	10	100
Huaman *et al.* (1983)	12/48	(25.00)	21/48	(43.75)	0.44 (0.19–1.02)							
Typical odds ratio (95% confidence interval)					0.44 (0.19–1.02)							

Effect of piracetam for fetal distress in labour on Apgar score <7 at 1 minute

Huaman *et al.* (1983)	2/48	(4.17)	5/48	(10.42)	0.40 (0.09–1.85)	
Typical odds ratio (95% confidence interval)					0.40 (0.09–1.85)	

Effect of piracetam for fetal distress in labour on 'neonatal morbidity'[*]

Huaman *et al.* (1983)	0/48	(0.00)	5/48	(10.42)	0.12 (0.02–0.74)	
Typical odds ratio (95% confidence interval)					0.12 (0.02–0.74)	

*See text for definition

Table 54.6 Description of the randomized comparisons of different methods of intrapartum fetal heart rate monitoring, with operative delivery for 'fetal distress'

Trial	No. women (no. fetuses where different)	Entry characteristics	Method of allocation	Comparability of groups at entry	Study regimens Continuous FHR	pH
1st Denver (Haverkamp *et al.* 1976) 1973–75	242:241	High risk	Seated, opaque envelopes	Similar, though concern about mismatch of abnormal traces in early labour (see comment)	EFM via scalp electrode	No
1st Melbourne (Renou *et al.* 1976) 1974–1975	175:175	High risk: in fetal intensive care unit	Sealed envelopes	Similar, though difference in numbers of proteinurias and antepartum haemorrhages	EFM	Yes: FBS 'when FHR abnormal' in 31 (18%) cases
2nd Denver (Haverkamp *et al.* 1979) 1975–77	230:229:231 [230:232:233] (see comment)	High risk	Sealed envelopes	Similar	(a) EFM via scalp electrode (b) EFM via scalp electrode	No Yes: in 44 (19%) cases
Sheffield (Kelso *et al.* 1978) 1976–77	253:251	Low risk	Sealed, opaque envelopes	Similar	EFM via scalp electrode (use of 'dip area' (Shelley & Tipton, 1971) criticized)	No
2nd Melbourne (Wood *et al.* 1981) 1978–79	445:482	Low risk	Randomized cards *not* in sealed envelopes (see comment)	Important differences especially in gravidity (see comment)	EFM	Yes: FBS 'when trace abnormal' number not stated
Copenhagen (Neldam 1986) 1981–82	482:498	All women except diabetics	Random allocation to one of two policies for whole *week* (see comment)	Similar	EFM from time 'women no longer felt like walking'; 66 (14%) delivered before 10 min strip	Yes but only performed 3 times (0.6%); all in 2nd stage
Dublin (Macdonald *et al.* 1985) 1981–83	6474:6490 [6530:6554]	(a) Live fetus of 28 + weeks (b) no evidence of fetal anomaly (c) in labour (d) liquor without significant meconium-staining	Sealed, opaque envelopes	Similar	EFM; if persistent abnormal pattern: FBS in 1st stage, delivery in 2nd stage. 10% delivered too quickly and a further 9% did not have EFM throughout labour	Yes: 286 (4.4%); 173 for abnormal FHR (see comment)

Intermittent		Co-intervention	Withdrawals after entry	Measurement of outcome	Analysis	Comment
FHR	**pH**					
IA after contractions every 15 min in 1st stage, every 5 min in 2nd stage (EFM trace hidden)	No	Suggested more intensive nursing care to intermittent group – no evidence	No	Paediatricians 'blind' to allocation		All women had continuous monitoring but concealed for intermittent group. More abnormal traces in revealed group early in labour led to accusation that allocation not truly random; but no other evidence for this.
IA regimen not clearly stated (no EFM)	No	Staff may have favoured continuous group because fetal intensive care unit 'on trial'; but no evidence	All cases of one specialist from *both* groups	No 'blinding'	Early termination of trial after 7 'interim' analyses (see comment)	Multiple, repeated analyses with data dependent stopping rule carries risk of type 1 error or exaggeration of true size of treatment effect.
IA after contractions every 15 min in 1st stage, every 5 min in 2nd stage	No	No evidence; all women had study nurse throughout labour	No	No 'blinding'		Random allocation to *3* groups; (a) EFM alone; (b) EFM plus option of FBS and (c) IA alone.
IA every 15 min	No	No evidence	No	No 'blinding'		
IA regimen not clearly stated; 49 women subsequently had EFM	No	No evidence	Yes, in an attempt to adjust for imbalances in original trial groups (see comment)	No 'blinding'	Attempt to adjust for imbalances in 'allocated' groups not successful, 'non-compliers' retained in original group (see comment)	Randomization cards in largest hospital *not* in sealed envelopes. Randomization almost certainly corrupted: 10% more primigravidae in continuous group. Attempt to adjust by 'random withdrawal'; nevertheless, likely to be important selection bias.
IA every 30 min (at least) up to 5 cm cervical dilatation; every 15 min up to full dilatation; every 5 min in 2nd stage	Yes, performed 2 times (0.4%)	Allocation by *week* was chosen to avoid co-intervention bias	No	No 'blinding'		Allocation by week chosen to avoid co-intervention bias but allocation predictable so possibly prone to selection bias-no evidence.
IA after contractions every 15 min in 1st stage; between every contraction in 2nd stage. If abnormality persisted: FBS+EFM in 1st stage; delivery in 2nd stage. 2% had EFM	Yes: 232 (3.5%); 49 for abnormal FHR (see comment)	Staff experienced with both methods of monitoring; nurse/ midwife with women throughout labour	No	Paediatric neurologist 'blind' to allocation	Main analyses based on 12,964 women. Other analyses based on subgroups	Hospital policy to perform FBS after 8 hours in labour; twice as many (139:77) performed for this indication in the intermittent group.

Table 54.6—*continued* Description of the randomized comparisons of different methods of intrapartum fetal heart rate monitoring, with operative delivery for 'fetal distress'

Trial	No. women (no. fetuses where different)	Entry characteristics	Method of allocation	Comparability of groups at entry	Study regimens Continuous FHR	pH
Dallas (Leveno *et al.* (1986) 1982–85	(a) 17,586:17,409 [17,759:17,571]	All deliveries during 36-month trial period	Alternate months over 36-month period	Similar, except imbalance in fetuses 'dead when mother arrived at delivery suite' (see comment)	19 EFM monitors available for 20-bed suite; 79% EFM – about ¾ of those not EFM either dead on arrival or delivered within 60 min. Assessment at least half-hourly	No
	(b) NS:NS [17,641:17,410]	All deliveries excluding fetuses dead when mother first assessed in delivery suite	Alternate months; post-hoc exclusion of fetuses judged to have died before mother arrived	Similar, though concern about possible differential exclusion based on 'dead when mother arrived' (see comment)	As above, but 'dead on arrival' excluded	No
	(c) 7,288:7,330	The 42% of pregnancies with single fetus with cephalic presentation; spontaneous, uncomplicated labour; birthweight > 2500 g	Alternate months; excluding 58% with 'high risk' pregnancies categorized after delivery (see comment)	Few data to check but similar numbers. Concern that decision about selection might be affected by allocation (see comment)	EFM – 94% cases	No
Seattle/Vancouver (Luthy *et al.* 1987) 1981–85	122:124	Women in labour at *26–32* weeks singleton with cephalic presentation; estimated weight 700–1751 g; no recognized malformation, placenta praevia or severe APH (see comment)	Sealed, opaque envelopes stratified by centre and estimated birthweight	Similar	EFM; if persistent abnormal pattern: FBS or delivery	Yes: in 6 (5%) cases

Intermittent		Co-intervention	Withdrawals after entry	Measurement of outcome	Analysis	Comment
FHR	**pH**					
7 EFM monitors available for 20-bed suite; 37% had EFM because 'high risk' (see comment). Assessment at least half-hourly	No	Monthly allocation chosen to avoid co-intervention bias; similar patient:nurse ratio in two trial groups: 2.16:1 and 2.12:1	No	No 'blinding'	Unbiased, but compared liberal EFM (79%) with restricted EFM (37%) and includes many outcomes which could not have been prevented by EFM	Compares liberal (79%) with restricted (37%) use of EFM – high risk had EFM in both groups which were responsible for most bad outcomes. Comparison (a) includes *all* deliveries during the trial including some that could not plausibly be altered by EFM (e.g. antepartum late fetal deaths).
As above, but 'dead on arrival' excluded	No	See above	Fetuses judged to be dead when mother arrived	See above	As above; concern about post-allocation withdrawals of stillbirths (see comment)	Comparison (b) excludes fetuses judged to be 'dead before arrival at labour and delivery unit'. More such deaths in restrictive months (161:118); could be chance but $p < 0.01$, or could be biased ascertainment (and hence biased withdrawal) perhaps because viability was checked later in this group or because assessor knew allocation.
Percentage EFM not stated but likely to be small	No	See above	58% of pregnancies considered at any increased risk. Unclear whether decision made blind to allocation but probably not	See above	Clearer separation of policies but worries about post-allocation selection of groups for comparison (see comment)	Comparison (c) based on labours considered 'low risk'; could be prone to selection bias because allocation known but similar proportion in each met criteria.
IA with stethoscope or amplified Doppler; every 15 min in 1st stage; at least every 5 min in 2nd stage. If persistent ominous rate:delivery	No	All participants had 1:1 nursing from study nurses	Total of 376 women were randomized but 130 were incorrectly judged to be in early labour and had birthweight > 1750 g (see comment)	Not stated	Analyses based on 246 women who delivered babies weighing < 1,751 g (see comment)	130 of total 376 randomized subsequently delivered baby weighing > 1,750 g and so excluded from analysis. No evidence that chances of delivery of baby > 1,750 g related to allocation so selection bias unlikely.

Otherwise, neonatal outcome was similar in the two groups (Table 54.4).

4.5 Piracetam

A third approach to the conservative treatment of persistent fetal distress has been to 'treat' the fetus to prevent any adverse effects. Piracetam, a derivative of gamma-aminobenzoic acid, is thought to promote the metabolism of the brain cells when they are hypoxic. It has been evaluated in a single placebo-controlled trial (Huaman *et al.* 1983; Table 54.5). The results suggest that piracetam treatment reduces the need for caesarean section, and improves neonatal outcome as judged by the Apgar score and neonatal 'respiratory problems, and signs of hypoxia'.

5 Randomized comparisons of different methods for intrapartum fetal heart rate monitoring, with operative delivery for 'fetal distress'

5.1 Description of the trials

Between 1973 and 1987 nine randomized controlled trials of different methods of intrapartum fetal monitoring, with operative delivery for 'fetal distress', were completed and reported (Haverkamp *et al.* 1976; Renou *et al.* 1976; Haverkamp *et al.* 1979 Langendoerfer *et al.* 1980; Kelso *et al.* 1978; Wood *et al.* 1981; MacDonald *et al.* 1985; Neldam *et al.* 1986; Leveno *et al.* 1986; Luthy *et al.* 1987). These are summarized in Table 54.6. This Table presents the numbers of subjects; the entry criteria (some trials involved women at high risk, some women at low risk, and others all women, irrespective of risk); the method of allocation (to assess the possibility of selection bias at entry); the actual monitoring regimens compared (particularly whether or not there was an option to perform fetal scalp blood pH estimation); the possibility of 'co-intervention' (such as

extra nursing attention in one group); withdrawals after entry (to assess selection bias after entry); the 'blinding' of outcome assessment (to assess the likelihood of biased measurement of outcome); unusual aspects of the analysis; and, lastly, comments on special features of each study.

In the following review of the outcomes observed in these trials, a distinction has been drawn between trials in which electronic fetal monitoring was used without fetal pH estimation, trials in which electronic fetal monitoring was backed by fetal scalp blood sampling, and the Dallas trial (Leveno *et al.* 1986) in which liberal use of electronic fetal monitoring was compared with restricted use, in both instances, without the option of scalp blood sampling. For some outcomes, however, such as use of intramuscular and epidural anaesthesia, and maternal or neonatal infection, the first two categories of trial have been reviewed together; that is to say, the policy of electronic fetal monitoring, with or without fetal blood sampling, has been compared with the policy of intermittent auscultation.

5.2 Effects on obstetric intervention

The randomized comparisons of different methods of intrapartum fetal monitoring (with policies of operative delivery for 'fetal distress') are very consistent in the suggested effect of electronic fetal monitoring on operative delivery rates. As might be expected, rates are higher in all the intensively monitored groups, with a typical increase of about one-third, regardless of whether fetal blood pH estimate was available (Table 54.7). However, the use of fetal pH assessment has an important modifying effect on the *types* of operative delivery, tending to limit the increased use of caesarean delivery and promote the use of operative vaginal delivery (see below).

In all 10 comparisons the caesarean section rate is higher in the electronic fetal monitoring group (Tables 54.8 and 54.11). The 3 trials in which electronic fetal monitoring was used without the option of fetal scalp blood pH estimation have the highest odds ratios (all

Table 54.7 Effect of electronic fetal monitoring (no scalp sampling) versus intermittent auscultation in labour on all operative deliveries

Study	EXPT		CTRL		Odds ratio	Graph of odds ratios and confidence intervals						
	n	(%)	*n*	(%)	(95% CI)	0.01	0.1	0.5	1	2	10	100
Haverkamp *et al.* (1979)	105/233	(45.06)	67/232	(28.88)	2.00 (1.37–2.91)							
Kelso *et al.* (1978)	95/253	(37.55)	89/251	(35.46)	1.09 (0.76–1.57)							
Haverkamp *et al.* (1976)	100/242	(41.32)	94/241	(39.00)	1.10 (0.77–1.58)							
Typical odds ratio (95% confidence interval)					1.33 (1.07–1.64)							

Table 54.7—*continued* Effect of electronic fetal monitoring and scalp sampling versus intermittent auscultation in labour on all operative deliveries

Study	EXPT n	(%)	CTRL n	(%)	Odds ratio (95% CI)	Graph of odds ratios and confidence intervals
MacDonald et al. (1985)	686/6530	(10.51)	551/6554	(8.41)	1.28 (1.14–1.44)	
Renou et al. (1976)	109/175	(62.29)	91/175	(52.00)	1.52 (1.00–2.32)	
Haverkamp et al. (1979)	80/230	(34.78)	67/232	(28.88)	1.31 (0.89–1.94)	
Neldam et al. (1986)	113/482	(23.44)	82/487	(16.84)	1.51 (1.10–2.06)	
Luthy et al. (1987)	34/122	(27.87)	28/124	(22.58)	1.32 (0.74–2.35)	
Wood et al. (1981)	138/445	(31.01)	111/482	(23.03)	1.50 (1.12–2.01)	
Typical odds ratio (95% confidence interval)					1.34 (1.21–1.47)	

Table 54.8 Effect of electronic fetal monitoring (no scalp sampling) versus intermittent auscultation in labour on all caesarean sections

Study	EXPT n	(%)	CTRL n	(%)	Odds ratio (95% CI)	Graph of odds ratios and confidence intervals
Haverkamp et al. (1979)	41/233	(17.60)	13/232	(5.60)	3.21 (1.82–5.66)	
Kelso et al. (1978)	24/253	(9.49)	11/251	(4.38)	2.20 (1.11–4.37)	
Haverkamp et al. (1976)	40/242	(16.53)	16/241	(6.64)	2.62 (1.50–4.57)	
Typical odds ratio (95% confidence interval)					2.70 (1.92–3.81)	

Effect of electronic fetal monitoring and scalp sampling versus intermittent auscultation in labour on all caesarean sections

Study	EXPT n	(%)	CTRL n	(%)	Odds ratio (95% CI)	
MacDonald et al. (1985)	158/6474	(2.44)	144/6490	(2.22)	1.10 (0.88–1.38)	
Renou et al. (1976)	39/175	(22.29)	24/175	(13.71)	1.78 (1.04–3.08)	
Haverkamp et al. (1979)	26/230	(11.30)	13/232	(5.60)	2.09 (1.08–4.02)	
Neldam et al. (1986)	28/482	(5.81)	18/487	(3.70)	1.59 (0.88–2.88)	
Luthy et al. (1987)	19/122	(15.57)	19/124	(15.32)	1.02 (0.51–2.03)	
Wood et al. (1981)	18/445	(4.04)	10/482	(2.07)	1.96 (0.92–4.16)	
Typical odds ratio (95% confidence interval)					1.29 (1.08–1.54)	

statistically significant at the 5 per cent level), and this is reflected in a typical odds ratio as high as 2.70 for electronic fetal monitoring used on its own. Electronic fetal monitoring used in conjunction with fetal pH estimation was also associated with a statistically significant increase in the caesarean rate, but to a much smaller extent than electronic fetal monitoring alone (typical odds ratio 1.29; Table 54.8). The increased risk of caesarean section associated with electronic fetal monitoring is most striking when the indication was 'fetal distress' (Table 54.9): again, the odds ratios are twice as high in the trials which did not use fetal pH estimates as those in which fetal acid–base status was assessed. The risk was also increased, however, when the primary indication was 'failure to advance in labour' (Table 54.10). These rates were higher in all the continuously monitored groups but were especially raised in the three trials in which electronic fetal monitoring was used on its own. Universal (as opposed to selective) use of electronic fetal monitoring (Leveno *et al.* 1986) was also associated with a significantly higher caesarean rate (Table 54.11), but this was limited to caesarean delivery

Table 54.9 Effect of electronic fetal monitoring (no scalp sampling) versus intermittent auscultation in labour on caesareans for fetal distress

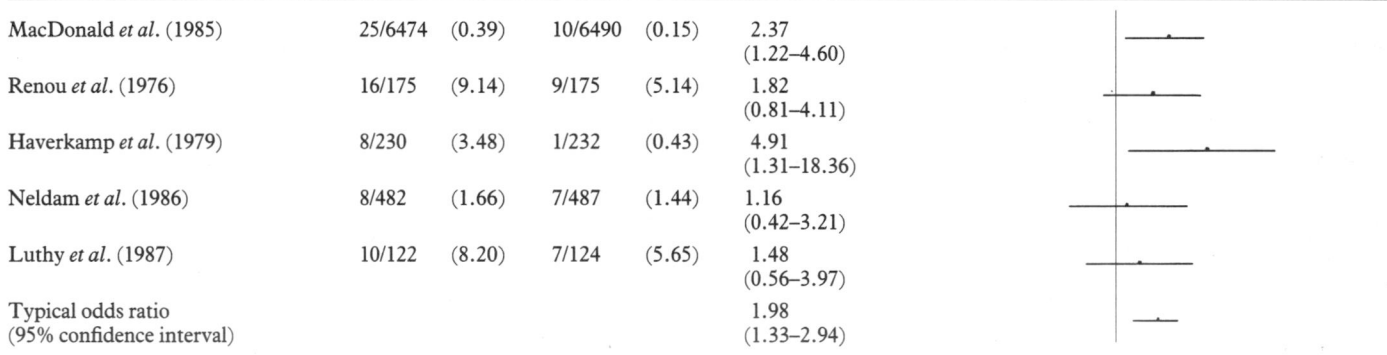

Study	EXPT		CTRL		Odds ratio	Graph of odds ratios and confidence intervals
	n	(%)	*n*	(%)	(95% CI)	0.01 0.1 0.5 1 2 10 100
Haverkamp *et al.* (1979)	16/233	(6.87)	1/232	(0.43)	6.19 (2.35–16.29)	
Kelso *et al.* (1978)	4/253	(1.58)	3/251	(1.20)	1.32 (0.30–5.88)	
Haverkamp *et al.* (1976)	18/242	(7.44)	3/241	(1.24)	4.42 (1.84–10.59)	
Typical odds ratio (95% confidence interval)					4.14 (2.29–7.51)	

Effect of electronic fetal monitoring and scalp sampling versus intermittent auscultation in labour on caesareans for fetal distress

MacDonald *et al.* (1985)	25/6474	(0.39)	10/6490	(0.15)	2.37 (1.22–4.60)	
Renou *et al.* (1976)	16/175	(9.14)	9/175	(5.14)	1.82 (0.81–4.11)	
Haverkamp *et al.* (1979)	8/230	(3.48)	1/232	(0.43)	4.91 (1.31–18.36)	
Neldam *et al.* (1986)	8/482	(1.66)	7/487	(1.44)	1.16 (0.42–3.21)	
Luthy *et al.* (1987)	10/122	(8.20)	7/124	(5.65)	1.48 (0.56–3.97)	
Typical odds ratio (95% confidence interval)					1.98 (1.33–2.94)	

Table 54.10 Effect of electronical fetal monitoring (no scalp sampling) vs. intermittent auscultation in labour on caesareans for failure to progress

Study	EXPT		CTRL		Odds ratio	Graph of odds ratios and confidence intervals
	n	(%)	*n*	(%)	(95% CI)	0.01 0.1 0.5 1 2 10 100
Haverkamp *et al.* (1979)	25/233	(10.73)	12/232	(5.17)	2.13 (1.09–4.17)	
Kelso I *et al.* (1978)	16/253	(6.32)	7/251	(2.79)	2.25 (0.97–5.19)	
Haverkamp *et al.* (1976)	22/242	(9.09)	13/241	(5.39)	1.73 (0.87–3.44)	
Typical odds ratio (95% confidence interval)					2.00 (1.32–3.03)	

Table 54.10—*continued* Effect of electronical fetal monitoring and scalp sampling versus intermittent auscultation in labour on all caesareans for failure to progress

Study	EXPT n	(%)	CTRL n	(%)	Odds ratio (95% CI)	Graph of odds ratios and confidence intervals
MacDonald *et al.* (1985)	88/6474	(1.36)	84/6490	(1.29)	1.05 (0.78–1.42)	
Renou *et al.* (1976)	10/175	(5.71)	7/175	(4.00)	1.45 (0.55–3.83)	
Haverkamp *et al.* (1979)	18/230	(7.83)	12/232	(5.17)	1.55 (0.74–3.24)	
Neldam *et al.* (1986)	18/482	(3.73)	11/487	(2.26)	1.66 (0.79–3.48)	
Luthy *et al.* (1987)	4/122	(3.28)	3/124	(2.42)	1.36 (0.30–6.11)	
Typical odds ratio (95% confidence interval)					1.19 (0.93–1.52)	

Table 54.11 Effect of liberal versus restrictive use of electronic fetal monitoring (all labours) on all caesareans

Study	EXPT n	(%)	CTRL n	(%)	Odds ratio (95% CI)	Graph of odds ratios and confidence intervals
Leveno *et al.* (1986)	1933/17586	(10.99)	1777/17409	(10.21)	1.09 (1.01–1.16)	
Typical odds ratio (95% confidence interval)					1.09 (1.01–1.16)	

Effect of liberal versus restrictive use of electronic fetal monitoring (all labours) on caesareans for fetal distress

Study	EXPT	CTRL	Odds ratio (95% CI)	
Leveno *et al.* (1986)	454/17586 (2.58)	369/17409 (2.12)	1.22 (1.06–1.40)	
Typical odds ratio (95% confidence interval)			1.22 (1.06–1.40)	

Effect of liberal versus restrictive use of electronic fetal monitoring (all labours) on caesareans for failure to advance

Study	EXPT	CTRL	Odds ratio (95% CI)	
Leveno *et al.* (1986)	848/17586 (4.82)	854/17409 (4.91)	0.98 (0.89–1.08)	
Typical odds ratio (95% confidence interval)			0.98 (0.89–1.08)	

Effect of liberal versus restrictive use of electronic fetal monitoring (low-risk labours) on caesareans for fetal distress

Study	EXPT	CTRL	Odds ratio (95% CI)	
Leveno J *et al.* (1986)	64/7288 (0.88)	28/7330 (0.38)	2.21 (1.47–3.33)	
Typical odds ratio (95% confidence interval)			2.21 (1.47–3.33)	

performed for 'fetal distress' rather than for 'failure to advance'; for those women at no apparent increased risk of problems during labour, the odds of a caesarean for 'fetal distress' increased 2.3-fold.

In contrast to these findings in respect of caesarean section, operative vaginal delivery rates (Table 54.12) were no higher in the labours monitored with electronic fetal monitoring alone, but were consistently higher in the groups monitored with electronic fetal monitoring with the option of fetal blood pH estimation; typically, the odds were 30 per cent higher in these trials. Generally speaking, there is therefore an inverse relationship between the effect of intensive monitoring on caesarean delivery on the one hand, and on operative vaginal delivery on the other. Fetal pH estimation, when used in conjunction with electronic fetal monitor-

ing, appears to postpone the decision to deliver from the first to the second stage of labour.

The higher operative delivery rates in the more intensively monitored groups are reflected in higher rates of maternal infection postpartum (Table 54.13; Koszalka *et al.* 1982).

The randomized comparisons of different methods of intrapartum fetal monitoring, with operative delivery for 'fetal distress', have also generated data on aspects of obstetric intervention other than operative delivery. As far as labour is concerned, one concern about the use of continuous electronic monitoring (without telemetry) has been the possibility that it prolongs labour by restricting women's movement during labour (see Chapter 55). In those trials for which data are available, the results are generally reassuring in this respect.

Table 54.12 Effect of electronic fetal monitoring (no scalp sampling) versus intermittent auscultation in labour on operative vaginal deliveries

Study	EXPT		CTRL		Odds ratio	Graph of odds ratios and confidence intervals						
	n	(%)	*n*	(%)	(95% CI)	0.01	0.1	0.5	1	2	10	100
Haverkamp *et al.* (1979)	64/233	(27.47)	54/232	(23.28)	1.25 (0.82–1.89)							
Kelso *et al.* (1978)	71/253	(28.06)	78/251	(31.08)	0.87 (0.59–1.27)							
Haverkamp *et al.* (1976)	60/242	(24.79)	78/241	(32.37)	0.69 (0.47–1.02)							
Typical odds ratio (95% confidence interval)					0.90 (0.71–1.13)							

Effect of electronic fetal monitoring and scalp sampling versus intermittent auscultation in labour on operative vaginal deliveries

Study	EXPT		CTRL		Odds ratio	Graph
MacDonald *et al.* (1985)	528/6530	(8.09)	407/6554	(6.21)	1.33 (1.16–1.52)	
Renou *et al.* (1976)	70/175	(40.00)	67/175	(38.29)	1.07 (0.70–1.65)	
Haverkamp *et al.* (1979)	54/230	(23.48)	54/232	(23.28)	1.01 (0.66–1.56)	
Neldam *et al.* (1986)	85/485	(17.53)	64/493	(12.98)	1.42 (1.00–2.01)	
Luthy *et al.* (1987)	15/122	(12.30)	9/124	(7.26)	1.77 (0.76–4.10)	
Wood *et al.* (1981)	120/445	(26.97)	101/482	(20.95)	1.39 (1.03–1.88)	
Typical odds ratio (95% confidence interval)					1.31 (1.18–1.46)	

Effect of liberal versus restrictive use of electronic fetal monitoring (all labours) on operative vaginal delivery

Study	EXPT	CTRL	Odds ratio	Graph
Leveno *et al.* (1986)	656/15231 (4.31)	742/16121 (4.60)	0.93 (0.84–1.04)	
Typical odds ratio (95% confidence interval)			0.93 (0.84–1.04)	

There is also no clear effect of the fetal monitoring method on the use of analgesia. (The most striking differences in the overall use of systemic analgesics are between the studies rather than within-trial differences associated with different fetal monitoring policies.) In the large Dublin trial fewer women in the electronic fetal monitoring group were given intramuscular analgesia. This difference tends to dominate the overview of the trials in this respect, although in two of the five other trials with available data the pattern is reversed (Table 54.14). There is no clear difference in the use of epidural anaesthesia (Table 54.15). Despite the dif-

ferences in the use of intramuscular analgesia between the two trial groups in Dublin, a survey of a subsample of 200 women in the trial (Garcia *et al.* 1985) did not detect any differences in mothers' perception of pain or in their ratings of adequacy of pain relief (Table 54.16).

Data about the use of general anaesthesia are available for only four trials (Table 54.17). All show an increased use of general anaesthesia associated with electronic fetal monitoring. This reflects the higher rate of caesarean section in these groups; this is why the increase in the 'use of' general anaesthesia is greater in the trials in which electronic fetal monitoring was used

Table 54.13 Effect of electronic fetal monitoring versus intermittent auscultation on maternal infection

Study	EXPT		CTRL		Odds ratio	Graph of odds ratios and confidence intervals
	n	(%)	*n*	(%)	(95% CI)	0.01 0.1 0.5 1 2 10 100
MacDonald *et al.* (1985)	97/4987	(1.95)	83/4999	(1.66)	1.17 (0.87–1.58)	
Renou *et al.* (1976)	64/175	(36.57)	53/175	(30.29)	1.33 (0.85–2.07)	
Haverkamp *et al.* (1979)	27/463	(5.83)	8/232	(3.45)	1.64 (0.80–3.38)	
Kelso *et al.* (1978)	8/253	(3.16)	7/251	(2.79)	1.14 (0.41–3.18)	
Neldam *et al.* (1986)	0/482	(0.00)	0/487	(0.00)	1.00 (1.00–1.00)	
Luthy *et al.* (1987)	13/122	(10.66)	11/124	(8.87)	1.22 (0.53–2.84)	
Haverkamp *et al.* (1976)	31/234	(13.25)	11/237	(4.64)	2.88 (1.53–5.42)	
Typical odds ratio (95% confidence interval)					1.37 (1.11–1.68)	

Table 54.14 Effect of electronic fetal monitoring versus intermittent auscultation on intramuscular analgesia

Study	EXPT		CTRL		Odds ratio	Graph of odds ratios and confidence intervals
	n	(%)	*n*	(%)	(95% CI)	0.01 0.1 0.5 1 2 10 100
MacDonald *et al.* (1985)	2217/4965	(44.65)	2388/4977	(47.98)	0.87 (0.81–0.95)	
Renou *et al.* (1976)	154/175	(88.00)	159/175	(90.86)	0.74 (0.37–1.46)	
Kelso *et al.* (1978)	71/253	(28.06)	79/251	(31.47)	0.85 (0.58–1.24)	
Neldam *et al.* (1986)	258/482	(53.53)	266/487	(54.62)	0.96 (0.74–1.23)	
Haverkamp *et al.* (1976)	49/242	(20.25)	40/241	(16.60)	1.27 (0.80–2.02)	
Wood *et al.* (1981)	394/445	(88.54)	416/482	(86.31)	1.22 (0.83–1.80)	
Typical odds ratio (95% confidence interval)					0.90 (0.83–0.96)	

Table 54.15 Effect of electronic fetal monitoring versus intermittent auscultation on epidural anaesthesia

Study	EXPT		CTRL		Odds ratio	Graph of odds ratios and confidence intervals						
	n	(%)	*n*	(%)	(95% CI)	0.01	0.1	0.5	1	2	10	100
MacDonald *et al.* (1985)	143/4965	(2.88)	167/4977	(3.36)	0.85 (0.68–1.07)							
Haverkamp *et al.* (1979)	93/463	(20.09)	48/232	(20.69)	0.96 (0.65–1.43)							
Kelso *et al.* (1978)	71/253	(28.06)	73/251	(29.08)	0.95 (0.65–1.40)							
Neldam *et al.* (1986)	51/482	(10.58)	34/487	(6.98)	1.57 (1.00–2.45)							
Haverkamp *et al.* (1976)	51/242	(21.07)	69/241	(28.63)	0.67 (0.44–1.01)							
Typical odds ratio (95% confidence interval)					0.92 (0.79–1.07)							

Table 54.16 Effect of electronic fetal monitoring versus intermittent auscultation on women's feelings of a 'lot of pain'

Study	EXPT		CTRL		Odds ratio	Graph of odds ratios and confidence intervals						
	n	(%)	*n*	(%)	(95% CI)	0.01	0.1	0.5	1	2	10	100
Garcia *et al.* (1985)	60/100	(60.00)	58/100	(58.00)	1.09 (0.62–1.90)							
Typical odds ratio (95% confidence interval)					1.09 (0.62–1.90)							

Effect of electronic fetal monitoring versus intermittent auscultation on women's feelings of too little analgesia

| Garcia *et al.* (1985) | 31/100 | (31.00) | 35/100 | (35.00) | 0.84 (0.46–1.50) | | | | | | | |
| Typical odds ratio (95% confidence interval) | | | | | 0.84 (0.46–1.50) | | | | | | | |

Table 54.17 Effect of electronic fetal monitoring (no scalp sampling) versus intermittent auscultation in labour on general anaesthesia

Study	EXPT		CTRL		Odds ratio	Graph of odds ratios and confidence intervals						
	n	(%)	*n*	(%)	(95% CI)	0.01	0.1	0.5	1	2	10	100
Haverkamp *et al.* (1979)	38/233	(16.31)	11/232	(4.76)	3.39 (1.87–6.12)							
Haverkamp *et al.* (1976)	31/242	(12.81)	12/241	(4.98)	2.62 (1.40–4.90)							
Typical odds ratio (95% confidence interval)					3.00 (1.95–4.61)							

Effect of electronic fetal monitoring and scalp sampling versus intermittent auscultation in labour on general anaesthesia

Haverkamp *et al.* (1979)	22/230	(9.57)	11/232	(4.74)	2.07 (1.02–4.19)							
Neldam *et al.* (1986)	27/482	(5.60)	18/487	(3.70)	1.54 (0.85–2.80)							
Typical odds ratio (95% confidence interval)					1.74 (1.10–2.75)							

on its own, than in the trials in which there was an option to use fetal pH estimation.

5.3 Effects on fetal and neonatal outcomes

Only three deaths occurred in the three trials which evaluated electronic fetal monitoring on its own (Table 54.18), and none of these occurred during labour. The 61 perinatal deaths in the trials of electronic fetal monitoring plus fetal pH estimation were evenly distributed between the electronically monitored and control groups (Table 54.19), but because of the small number this distinction is still compatible with a 40 per cent reduction or 60 per cent increase in the risk of perinatal death. Only nine deaths occurred during labour. There is a suggestion in the Dublin trial that continuous monitoring was associated with fewer deaths due to 'asphyxia' and more due to 'trauma'. This observation

Table 54.18 Effect of electronic fetal monitoring (no scalp sampling) versus intermittent auscultation in labour on all perinatal deaths (normally formed)

Study	EXPT		CTRL		Odds ratio	Graph of odds ratios and confidence intervals
	n	(%)	n	(%)	(95% CI)	0.01 0.1 0.5 1 2 10 100
Haverkamp et al. (1979)	1/233	(0.43)	0/232	(0.00)	7.36 (0.15–99.99)	
Kelso et al. (1978)	0/253	(0.00)	1/251	(0.40)	0.13 (0.00–6.77)	
Haverkamp et al. (1976)	1/242	(0.41)	0/241	(0.00)	7.36 (0.15–99.99)	
Typical odds ratio (95% confidence interval)					1.94 (0.20–18.62)	

Effect of electronic fetal monitoring (no scalp sampling) versus intermittent auscultation in labour on intrapartum deaths

Study	EXPT		CTRL		Odds ratio	Graph
Haverkamp et al. (1979)	0/233	(0.00)	0/232	(0.00)	1.00 (1.00–1.00)	
Kelso et al. (1978)	0/253	(0.00)	0/251	(0.00)	1.00 (1.00–1.00)	
Haverkamp et al. (1976)	0/242	(0.00)	0/241	(0.00)	1.00 (1.00–1.00)	
Typical odds ratio (95% confidence interval)					1.00 (1.00–1.00)	

Table 54.19 Effect of electronic fetal monitoring and scalp sampling versus intermittent auscultation in labour on all perinatal deaths

Study	EXPT		CTRL		Odds ratio	Graph of odds ratios and confidence intervals
	n	(%)	n	(%)	(95% CI)	0.01 0.1 0.5 1 2 10 100
MacDonald et al. (1985)	12/6530	(0.18)	12/6554	(0.18)	1.00 (0.45–2.24)	
Renou et al. (1976)	1/175	(0.57)	1/175	(0.57)	1.00 (0.06–16.05)	
Haverkamp et al. (1979)	1/230	(0.43)	0/232	(0.00)	7.45 (0.15–99.99)	
Neldam et al. (1986)	0/485	(0.00)	1/493	(0.20)	0.14 (0.00–6.93)	
Luthy et al. (1987)	15/122	(12.30)	17/124	(13.71)	0.88 (0.42–1.85)	
Wood et al. (1981)	1/445	(0.22)	0/482	(0.00)	8.03 (0.16–99.99)	
Typical odds ratio (95% confidence interval)					0.98 (0.58–1.64)	

Table 54.19—*continued* Effect of electronic fetal monitoring and scalp sampling versus intermittent auscultation in labour on intrapartum deaths

Study	EXPT		CTRL		Odds ratio	Graph of odds ratios and confidence intervals						
	n	(%)	n	(%)	(95% CI)	0.01	0.1	0.5	1	2	10	100
MacDonald *et al.* (1985)	3/6530	(0.05)	2/6554	(0.03)	1.50 (0.26–8.65)							
Renou *et al.* (1976)	0/175	(0.00)	1/175	(0.57)	0.14 (0.00–6.82)							
Haverkamp *et al.* (1979)	0/230	(0.00)	0/232	(0.00)	1.00 (1.00–1.00)							
Neldam *et al.* (1986)	0/485	(0.00)	1/493	(0.20)	0.14 (0.00–6.93)							
Luthy *et al.* (1987)	1/122	(0.82)	1/124	(0.81)	1.02 (0.06–16.35)							
Wood *et al.* (1981)	0/445	(0.00)	0/482	(0.00)	1.00 (1.00–1.00)							
Typical odds ratio (95% confidence interval)					0.81 (0.22–2.98)							

Table 54.20 Effect of liberal versus restrictive use of electronic fetal monitoring (all labours) on all perinatal deaths

Study	EXPT		CTRL		Odds ratio	Graph of odds ratios and confidence intervals						
	n	(%)	n	(%)	(95% CI)	0.01	0.1	0.5	1	2	10	100
Leveno *et al.* (1986)	262/17759	(1.48)	299/17571	(1.70)	0.87 (0.73–1.02)							
Typical odds ratio (95% confidence interval)					0.87 (0.73–1.02)							

Effect of liberal versus restrictive use of electronic fetal monitoring (all labours) on all perinatal deaths (alive on admission)

Study	EXPT		CTRL		Odds ratio							
Leveno *et al.* (1986)	144/17641	(0.82)	138/17410	(0.79)	1.03 (0.81–1.30)							
Typical odds ratio (95% confidence interval)					1.03 (0.81–1.30)							

Effect of liberal versus restrictive use of electronic fetal monitoring (all labours) on normally-formed intrapartum death > 900 g

Study	EXPT		CTRL		Odds ratio							
Leveno *et al.* (1986)	6/17641	(0.03)	7/17410	(0.04)	0.85 (0.29–2.51)							
Typical odds ratio (95% confidence interval)					0.85 (0.29–2.51)							

is based on small numbers, but it is plausible given the extra forceps deliveries in the electronically monitored group (MacDonald *et al.* 1985) and the association between forceps delivery and intracranial trauma (O'Driscoll *et al.* 1981). Interpretation of the perinatal mortality data (Table 54.20) in the trial reported by Leveno *et al.* (1986) is problematic (see also comment on Table 54.6). If all deaths are considered, irrespective of the timing of death, liberal use of continuous monitoring appears to reduce the risk of perinatal mortality.

This protective effect disappears, however, when the imbalance in the number of babies 'judged to be dead before arrival at labour and delivery unit' is taken into account. Furthermore, most deaths occurred amongst very preterm babies and there were only 13 intrapartum deaths of normally-formed babies with birthweights of more than 900 g, 6 among babies monitored during periods when the liberal policy was in use, and 7 among those born during the months when the 'restricted' policy was in operation.

Table 54.21 Effect of electronic fetal monitoring (no scalp sampling) versus intermittent auscultation in labour on Apgar score <7 at one minute

Study	EXPT		CTRL		Odds ratio	Graph of odds ratios and confidence intervals
	n	(%)	n	(%)	(95% CI)	0.01 0.1 0.5 1 2 10 100
Haverkamp et al. (1979)	41/233	(17.60)	33/232	(14.22)	1.29 (0.78–2.11)	
Kelso et al. (1978)	24/253	(9.49)	24/251	(9.56)	0.99 (0.55–1.80)	
Haverkamp et al. (1976)	31/242	(12.81)	29/241	(12.03)	1.07 (0.63–1.84)	
Typical odds ratio (95% confidence interval)					1.13 (0.83–1.54)	

Effect of electronic fetal monitoring and scalp sampling versus intermittent auscultation in labour on Apgar score <7 at one minute

Study	EXPT		CTRL		Odds ratio	
MacDonald et al. (1985)	216/5035	(4.29)	227/5058	(4.49)	0.95 (0.79–1.15)	
Renou et al. (1976)	28/175	(16.00)	25/175	(14.29)	1.14 (0.64–2.05)	
Haverkamp et al. (1979)	35/230	(15.22)	33/232	(14.22)	1.08 (0.65–1.81)	
Neldam et al. (1986)	28/485	(5.77)	32/493	(6.49)	0.88 (0.52–1.49)	
Wood et al. (1981)	39/445	(8.76)	40/482	(8.30)	1.06 (0.67–1.68)	
Typical odds ratio (95% confidence interval)					0.98 (0.84–1.14)	

Effect of electronic fetal monitoring (no scalp sampling) versus intermittent auscultation in labour on Apgar score <4 at one minute

Study	EXPT		CTRL		Odds ratio	
Haverkamp et al. (1979)	14/233	(6.01)	11/232	(4.74)	1.28 (0.57–2.87)	
Kelso et al. (1978)	4/253	(1.58)	7/251	(2.79)	0.57 (0.17–1.88)	
Typical odds ratio (95% confidence interval)					0.99 (0.51–1.94)	

Effect of electronic fetal monitoring and scalp sampling versus intermittent auscultation in labour on Apgar score <4 at one minute

Study	EXPT		CTRL		Odds ratio	
MacDonald et al. (1985)	62/6530	(0.95)	57/6554	(0.87)	1.09 (0.76–1.57)	
Renou et al. (1976)	4/175	(2.29)	6/175	(3.43)	0.66 (0.19–2.33)	
Haverkamp et al. (1979)	10/230	(4.35)	11/232	(4.74)	0.91 (0.38–2.19)	
Neldam et al. (1986)	5/485	(1.03)	7/493	(1.42)	0.73 (0.23–2.26)	
Luthy et al. (1987)	9/122	(7.38)	4/124	(3.23)	2.28 (0.75–6.96)	
Wood et al. (1981)	4/445	(0.90)	6/482	(1.24)	0.72 (0.21–2.52)	
Typical odds ratio (95% confidence interval)					1.04 (0.78–1.40)	

There is no evidence from the ten trial comparisons that intensive fetal heart rate monitoring, with or without fetal pH estimation, reduces the risk of low Apgar score (Table 54.21), even when only the most depressed scores are considered. Overall, the rates of admission to special care nurseries are very similar when the trial groups are compared (Table 54.22). This is reflected in typical odds ratios of 1.00 for the trials in which electronic fetal monitoring was used alone, and 1.03 for the trials in which fetal pH was used as a basis for diagnosing 'fetal distress'.

The one measure of neonatal outcome which does seem to be improved by more intensive intrapartum monitoring is neonatal seizures (Table 54.23). This effect seems to be restricted to electronic fetal monitoring backed by fetal pH estimation, and the odds of neonatal seizures appears to be reduced by about one half. This effect was suggested by an overview of the earlier trials (Chalmers 1979) and subsequently tested and confirmed in the Dublin trial (MacDonald et al. 1985). Secondary analysis of the Dublin trial suggested that the reduced risk of neonatal seizures was limited to labours that were induced or augmented with oxytocin and, or that were prolonged. No effect was seen in preterm babies (Luthy et al. 1987) and so the estimated protective effect is even greater in the term babies. This effect is not seen when electronic fetal monitoring is used on its own, although the total number of cases (nine) is too small to provide a reliable estimate. No difference was observed in the Dallas trial in respect of neonatal seizures and this is consistent with the other trials in which an option to assess fetal acid–base status was not included. The finding of a reduction in the risk of neonatal seizures by 50 per cent associated with continuous monitoring of the fetal heart and fetal acid–base estimation is potentially a very important effect: between a quarter and a third of babies who suffer neonatal seizures die, and a further quarter to a third are seriously impaired in childhood (Dennis 1978; Dennis and Chalmers 1982). However, the neonatal seizures prevented by intensive monitoring do not appear to be those associated with long term impairment (MacDonald et al. 1985; Grant 1987b).

Neonatal infection was uncommon in all the trials but there is no evidence to suggest that intensive monitoring increased this risk (Table 54.24). The data are insufficient to explore differences between types of electrode in this respect. In a small trial comparing the Surgicraft-Copeland (Ghosh and Tipton 1976) with two types of spiral electrode, Calvert and Newcombe

Table 54.22 Effect of electronic fetal monitoring (no scalp sampling) versus intermittent auscultation in labour on admission to special care nursery

Study	EXPT n	(%)	CTRL n	(%)	Odds ratio (95% CI)
Haverkamp et al. (1979)	23/233	(9.87)	29/232	(12.50)	0.77 (0.43–1.37)
Kelso et al. (1978)	45/253	(17.79)	43/251	(17.13)	1.05 (0.66–1.66)
Haverkamp et al. (1976)	35/242	(14.46)	28/241	(11.62)	1.28 (0.76–2.18)
Typical odds ratio (95% confidence interval)					1.03 (0.76–1.38)

Effect of electronic fetal monitoring and scalp sampling versus intermittent auscultation in labour on admission to special care nursery

Study	EXPT n	(%)	CTRL n	(%)	Odds ratio (95% CI)
MacDonald D et al. (1985)	545/6530	(8.35)	547/6554	(8.35)	1.00 (0.88–1.13)
Renou et al. (1976)	11/175	(6.29)	30/175	(17.14)	0.35 (0.18–0.67)
Haverkamp et al. (1979)	29/230	(12.61)	29/232	(12.50)	1.01 (0.58–1.75)
Neldam et al. (1986)	51/485	(10.52)	49/493	(9.94)	1.06 (0.70–1.61)
Wood et al. (1981)	59/445	(13.26)	48/482	(9.96)	1.38 (0.92–2.07)
Typical odds ratio (95% confidence interval)					1.00 (0.90–1.12)

Table 54.23 Effect of electronic fetal monitoring (no scalp sampling) versus intermittent auscultation in labour on neonatal seizures

Study	EXPT n	(%)	CTRL n	(%)	Odds ratio (95% CI)	Graph of odds ratios and confidence intervals
Haverkamp *et al.* (1979)	2/233	(0.86)	2/232	(0.86)	1.00 (0.14–7.11)	
Kelso *et al.* (1978)	0/253	(0.00)	1/251	(0.40)	0.13 (0.00–6.77)	
Haverkamp *et al.* (1976)	2/242	(0.83)	2/241	(0.83)	1.00 (0.14–7.11)	
Typical odds ratio (95% confidence interval)					0.80 (0.21–2.95)	

Effect of electronic fetal monitoring and scalp sampling versus intermittent auscultation in labour on neonatal seizures

Study	EXPT n	(%)	CTRL n	(%)	Odds ratio (95% CI)	
MacDonald *et al.* (1985)	12/6530	(0.18)	27/6554	(0.41)	0.46 (0.25–0.87)	
Renou *et al.* (1976)	0/175	(0.00)	4/175	(2.29)	0.13 (0.02–0.95)	
Haverkamp *et al.* (1979)	0/230	(0.00)	2/232	(0.86)	0.14 (0.01–2.18)	
Neldam *et al.* (1986)	0/485	(0.00)	0/493	(0.00)	1.00 (1.00–1.00)	
Luthy *et al.* (1987)	7/122	(5.74)	7/124	(5.65)	1.02 (0.35–2.99)	
Wood *et al.* (1981)	0/445	(0.00)	0/482	(0.00)	1.00 (1.00–1.00)	
Typical odds ratio 95% confidence interval)					0.49 (0.29–0.82)	

Effect of liberal versus restrictive use of electronic fetal monitoring (all labours) on neonatal seizures

Study	EXPT n	(%)	CTRL n	(%)	Odds ratio (95% CI)	
Leveno *et al.* (1986)	53/17641	(0.30)	45/17410	(0.26)	1.16 (0.78–1.73)	
Typical odds ratio 95% confidence interval)					1.16 (0.78–1.73)	

Table 54.24 Effect of electronic fetal monitoring versus intermittent auscultation on neonatal infection

Study	EXPT n	(%)	CTRL n	(%)	Odds ratio (95% CI)	Graph of odds ratios and confidence intervals
MacDonald *et al.* (1985)	43/5035	(0.85)	43/5058	(0.85)	1.00 (0.66–1.54)	
Renou *et al.* (1976)	4/175	(2.29)	8/175	(4.57)	0.50 (0.16–1.59)	
Haverkamp *et al.* (1979)	6/463	(1.30)	0/232	(0.00)	4.54 (0.83–24.90)	
Kelso *et al.* (1978)	12/253	(4.74)	13/251	(5.18)	0.91 (0.41–2.04)	
Neldam *et al.* (1986)	3/482	(0.62)	3/487	(0.62)	1.01 (0.20–5.03)	
Haverkamp *et al.* (1976)	6/242	(2.48)	3/241	(1.24)	1.96 (0.53–7.33)	
Typical odds ratio 95% confidence interval)					1.03 (0.74–1.43)	

(1980) reported no difference in scalp infection rates. Data on scalp trauma are only available for the Dublin trial. These show an overall rate of 0.3 per cent and no differences between the two trial groups. Much higher rates were reported in a trial which compared two spiral electrodes (Okada *et al* 1977) but Calvert and Newcombe (1980) reported similar rates in their small trial comparing two types of spiral electrode with the Surgicraft-Copeland electrode.

5.4 Maternal opinions

Most studies of women's opinions of intrapartum fetal monitoring have been uncontrolled surveys of their views about continuous electronic monitoring (for example, Starkman 1976; Shields 1978; Molfese *et al.* 1982; Jackson *et al.* 1983; Kruse 1984). These suggest that continuous monitoring is acceptable to most women, but that it can also have important adverse consequences for some women.

Many women interviewed in these surveys reported that continuous monitoring and recording of the fetal heart rate was reassuring because it demonstrated that the baby was alive and provided the information that caregivers need during labour (Youngs and Starkman 1976). These feelings seem to be enhanced if women are given a clear view of the monitor during labour (Jackson *et al.* 1983). Women at relatively high risk of problems during labour and those most knowledgeable about continuous monitoring seem most likely to be reassured. Detailed information given just prior to the start of labour, however, appears to have little positive effect on women's perceptions of intrapartum monitoring (Jackson *et al.* 1983).

Continuous electronic monitoring of the fetal heart rate can generate anxiety in a number of ways which cannot be predicted in advance for individual women. The trace itself may become worrying and this may be particularly disquieting if there is uncertainty about the significance of the 'abnormality' amongst those giving care. The trace may be of poor quality or even artefactual, or the monitor itself may malfunction, sometimes repeatedly (Royston 1982). An external abdominal transducer may become displaced or a scalp electrode detached. Although these problems only apply to a minority of women, they are not uncommon events in a labour ward, particularly if there is a policy of universal electronic monitoring.

Some women interviewed in the surveys reported discomfort and restriction of movement, or worries that an electrode would damage the baby's scalp. Others found the monitor a distraction which interfered with their relationships with caregivers and, or companion in labour.

How much weight should be given to the various maternal views of electronic fetal heart rate monitoring revealed in these uncontrolled surveys? Two of the randomized controlled studies (MacDonald *et al.* 1985; Neldam *et al.* 1986) included an assessment of the mothers' views of the alternative approaches to fetal monitoring during labour (Garcia *et al.* 1985; Hansen *et al.* 1985). Only the former, however, has been reported as a comparison of the two randomized groups.

A subsample of 200 women who took part in the large trial conducted in Dublin were interviewed after delivery (Table 54.25). No difference between the trial groups was detected in respect of the proportions of women who reported 'worries or anxieties' during labour, or that labour had been 'unpleasant'. Nearly all women interviewed reported that they were able to get in touch with a nurse or doctor at any time. The type of monitoring did, however, alter the women's source of reassurance: those in the electronically monitored group were more likely to mention a member of the medical staff as being reassuring, whereas those in the intermittent auscultation group tended to mention a nurse or nurses. In contrast, there was no evidence of a differential effect on the women's relationship with their companions in labour. Hospital staff, in particular, and people in general, were much the most common source of reassurance. Eight per cent in the electronically monitored group did mention the monitor in this respect, however. 'Not being left alone' was a source of reassurance for 20 per cent of women in both groups. It is significant that electronic monitoring appeared to increase the chances of a woman being left alone during labour. As discussed in Section 5.2, more intensive monitoring did not seem to alter the pain of labour (Table 54.16). Some women in the group monitored by intermittent auscultation reported discomfort from the Pinard stethoscope, however. In line with the observational studies, more women in the continuously monitored group felt 'too restricted' during labour (Table 54.25).

6 Other methods of fetal monitoring and diagnosis in labour

6.1 Intrapartum fetal stimulation tests

Fetal heart rate acceleration is commonly accepted as an indicator of fetal well-being in antepartum non-stress testing (see Chapter 30). These accelerations in a non-stress test are commonly associated with fetal movements or uterine contractions but may be evoked by other stimuli such as sound (Smith *et al.* 1986a). Clark and his colleagues (1982) observed that fetal heart rate acceleration sometimes coincided with fetal scalp blood sampling and that scalp blood pH tended to be normal if an acceleration occurred. A further prospective study using 'firm digital pressure on the head followed by a

Table 54.25 Effect of electronic fetal monitoring versus intermittent auscultation on women's reported 'worries and anxieties'

Study	EXPT		CTRL		Odds ratio	Graph of odds ratios and confidence intervals
	n	(%)	n	(%)	(95% CI)	0.01 0.1 0.5 1 2 10 100
Garcia et al. (1985)	41/100	(41.00)	44/100	(44.00)	0.89 (0.51–1.55)	
Typical odds ratio (95% confidence interval)					0.89 (0.51–1.55)	

Effect of electronic fetal monitoring versus intermittent auscultation on women's feelings of unpleasant labour

Garcia et al. (1985)	30/100	(30.00)	31/100	(31.00)	0.95 (0.52–1.74)	
Typical odds ratio (95% confidence interval)					0.95 (0.52–1.74)	

Effect of electronic fetal monitoring versus intermittent auscultation on women's feelings of being left alone

Garcia et al. (1985)	33/100	(33.00)	22/100	(22.00)	1.73 (0.93–3.22)	
Typical odds ratio (95% confidence interval)					1.73 (0.93–3.22)	

Effect of electronic fetal monitoring versus intermittent auscultation on women's feelings of being 'restricted'

Garcia et al. (1985)	17/100	(17.00)	6/100	(6.00)	2.93 (1.23–6.97)	
Typical odds ratio (95% confidence interval)					2.93 (1.23–6.97)	

gentle pinch of the scalp with an atraumatic clamp' seems to confirm these findings (Clark *et al.* 1984). Response (by fetal heart rate acceleration) to either of these stimuli was associated with a scalp blood pH of greater than or equal to 7.19. Of the fetuses which showed no response, about 40 per cent had pH estimations below 7.19.

A study using sound stimulation by an 'electronic artificial larynx' placed over the fetal head had broadly similar results (Smith *et al.* 1986b). Fetal heart rate acceleration in response to sound stimulation was associated with fetal pH values greater than 7.25. Of the 34 fetuses who did not react with an acceleration, 18 had pH values of less than 7.25. In 25 cases who had both sound stimulation and fetal scalp blood sampling, all 12 fetuses who reacted to sound stimulation also reacted to scalp blood sampling. Of the 13 fetuses who failed to react to sound, 5 subsequently showed a fetal heart rate acceleration in response to scalp sampling and all of these had pH values of 7.24 or more. Scalp stimulation may therefore be more specific than sound stimulation, but it is more invasive.

These studies require replication. If their results are confirmed, fetal stimulation tests could be very useful. They could reduce the need for scalp blood sampling or

be used as an alternative when scalp sampling is either technically impossible, or not available. Ideally, on the basis of currently available evidence, a non-reactive stimulation test should, however, be followed by fetal scalp blood acid–base estimation.

6.2 The admission test—short electronic fetal heart rate recording on admission in labour

Intrapartum fetal distress commonly reflects problems which predate the onset of labour (Modanlou *et al.* 1974; Steer 1982). For this reason there is a strong case for careful risk assessment at the beginning of labour (see Section 2.2, above), particularly as risk assessment systems based on the mother are not very satisfactory in this respect (see Chapter 22).

A short (15–20 minute) period of external electronic fetal heart monitoring on admission in labour has been recommended as a screening test for women who otherwise are deemed to be at low risk (Ingemarsson *et al.* 1986). This practice is becoming common. The rationale is that it identifies a subgroup of fetuses who would benefit from more intensive monitoring and might identify major fetal problems which would be missed by intermittent auscultation.

In a study of just over 1000 low risk women conducted in Singapore (Ingemarsson *et al.* 1986), 22 of the fetuses were considered to have suffered fetal distress either because they had a scalp blood pH of less than 7.20, or because they had an Apgar score of less than 7 five minutes after birth. Ten of the total study group had 'ominous' admission tests. One of these fetuses died during labour and a second suffered severe meconium aspiration syndrome. Both were 'missed' by intermittent auscultation, although the latter case could have been identified as high risk because of the passage of meconium. On the debit side, a baby with lethal malformations also had an ominous trace, and in another, 'ominous' case, the maternal pulse rate was probably measured by mistake. Forty-nine women (5 per cent) had 'equivocal' admission tests and 5 of these subsequently met the criteria for fetal distress (see above). The remaining l3 (59 per cent) babies with fetal distress all had normal admission tests. Only 3 of these were delivered within 6 hours, however, suggesting that most cases of fetal distress after a normal admission test reflect problems which developed after the admission test.

The same investigators have since investigated the usefulness of the acoustic stimulation test (see above) as an adjunct to the admission test (Ingemarsson *et al.* 1988). The acoustic stimulation test does appear useful as a basis for further categorizing the group with equivocal admission tests: the minority with an abnormal acoustic stimulation test were at high risk of developing fetal distress.

A screening test on admission in labour used as a basis for deciding on selective intensive monitoring is attractive in principle because it should identify the 'prevalent' cases of fetal distress in fetuses which embark on labour in an already compromised state. The results of the Singapore study (Ingemarsson *et al.* 1986) suggest that the admission test would improve the predictive properties of monitoring in this way. This study does not, however, evaluate the other two components of monitoring that must be fulfilled if the policy is to be effective; that is, whether the test is interpreted accurately and then acted on appropriately, when it is used in clinical practice. These questions can only be addressed satisfactorily in randomized controlled trials. Indeed, as has been pointed out (Goodlin 1987), the randomized trials of continuous electronic monitoring which have already been reviewed in this chapter all included early continuous monitoring in the more intensively managed group, yet failed to provide strong evidence that this had any beneficial effects in practice.

6.3 Fetal electrocardiography

Until recently the problems of electrical background noise and signal distortion have made the study of the components of the fetal electrocardiogram very difficult

(Symonds 1986). Recent technical developments have made this possible (Jenkins 1986) and early clinical research suggests that changes in the ST segment and height of the T wave, which have been observed in studies of hypoxic animal fetuses (Rosen 1986), are also seen in compromised human fetuses (Jenkins *et al.* 1986). The interpretation of electrocardiographic changes during labour is not straightforward and no single index is clearly optimal (Murray 1986). Combinations of changes in the time intervals of the electrocardiographic signal and in the ST and T segments seem the most promising possibilities for electrocardiographic intrapartum monitoring. Shortened QRS complexes at the end of pregnancy or early in labour may be an indication of intrauterine growth retardation (Pardi *et al.* 1986). This approach to intrapartum monitoring is promising, but much further development and evaluation will be required before its clinical usefulness can be assessed reliably.

6.4 Fetal cardiac electromechanical time intervals

Hopes have not been realized concerning the measurement of the time interval between the onset of ventricular depolarization (the electrocardiographic Q wave) and the beginning of the ejection of blood from the ventricles (the pre-ejection period) as a measure of fetal well-being. The pre-ejection time interval tends to be shortened or prolonged when there is other evidence to suggest 'fetal distress', but these changes are not consistent (Martin *et al.* 1984).

6.5 Fetal electroencephalography

Study of brain function during labour is logical given that a primary aim of intrapartum fetal monitoring is to prevent neurological impairment. Continuous recording of the fetal electroencephalogram during labour is now technically possible (Maynard *et al.* 1979). Interpretation is difficult, however, and the technique appears to require considerable development before it could be considered other than a research tool.

6.6 Continuous biochemical monitoring

Methods for continuous measurement of pH, pO_2 and pCO_2 (sometimes simultaneously) have been under development for more than 10 years. None is yet sufficiently reliable or practical for use in routine practice. A general issue is the representativeness of scalp measurements, given that blood flow through the scalp is reduced during labour (O'Connor *et al.* 1979). The formation of caput succedaneum and compression of the electrode also influence the reliability of measurements.

The Roche electrodes commonly used for continuous tissue pH measurements have been unsatisfactory for a number of reasons. They are large and fragile, with a tendency to become detached (Weber and Nickelson 1984). Continuous transcutaneous pO_2 monitoring also remains unsatisfactory. These electrodes, too, have been large and difficult to attach. To maintain capillary blood supply, the electrode has to be heated. Transcutaneous pO_2 measurement using a small needle electrode overcomes some of these problems (Aarnoudse *et al.* 1981) but there are still practical problems to solve (Aarnoudse *et al.* 1985). There are also theoretical reasons for thinking that pO_2 is not the most appropriate biochemical measurement in this context (Steer 1982). Transcutaneous pCO_2 monitoring looks the most promising from a theoretical and technical point of view (Lofgren 1987; Nickelson *et al.* 1986), but the problems common to all methods of continuous biochemical monitoring still have to be solved (Schmidt *et al.* 1985). None of these new techniques has been tried in more than a small series of fetuses.

7 Conclusions

7.1 Implications for current practice

Liquor amnii which is sparse or contains meconium is associated with an increased risk of perinatal mortality and morbidity. The status of the liquor when the membranes have ruptured spontaneously should be assessed early in labour and the presence of meconium or low liquor volume should prompt more intensive fetal surveillance. Whether or not routine amnioscopy or artificial rupture of the membranes to assess the liquor is justified is not clear from the available evidence.

Evidence from the randomized comparisons of different methods of fetal heart rate monitoring, particularly the large trial conducted in Dublin, suggests that intrapartum death is equally preventable by any of the methods of fetal heart rate monitoring currently employed, provided that importance is attached to the prompt recognition of intrapartum fetal heart rate abnormalities, whatever the particular monitoring policy adopted. (During the two years of the Dublin trial, for example, the intrapartum death rate was lower than in the preceding and following years (National Maternity Hospital 1986).)

The reliability of intermittent auscultation may be increased by the use of hand-held ultrasound monitors when heart sounds are difficult to hear with a conventional stethoscope. There are arguments for always using these devices (Crawford 1986), partly because they may cause less maternal discomfort than a Pinard stethoscope (Garcia *et al.* 1985). Compliance with intermittent auscultation should be straightforward if a caregiver has responsibility for only one woman during labour. Such individualized attention is likely to have other benefits for a woman (see Chapter 49), and it is to

be deplored that current staffing and other policies for intrapartum care in many delivery wards make this ideal impossible to meet. The implication is that auscultation may not be performed as frequently or regularly as it should be to provide safe fetal monitoring.

The complexity of continuous electronic monitoring makes it susceptible to technical and mechanical failures. Machine maintenance and replacement and in-service training of personnel are therefore important, particularly as both may fall victim to 'economy' savings. Electronic fetal monitoring may also provide suboptimal surveillance if it reduces the frequency with which the caregiver formally checks the fetal heart rate. A fetal heart monitor should be an adjunct to personal care not a substitute for it.

The wide inter- and intra-observer variation in the interpretation of continuous fetal heart rate records, even amongst 'experts', demonstrates that this is a major problem with current methods of continuous monitoring. Developments to standardize interpretation seem sensible even if it is impossible to judge whether such standard approaches are better or worse than alternative, more individualistic systems of interpretation.

The evidence suggests that not only false positives (false alarms) but also false negatives are reduced by the use of fetal blood sampling as an adjunct to fetal heart rate monitoring. Despite its practical problems, fetal acid–base assessment is, on the basis of current evidence, an essential adjunct to fetal heart rate monitoring and should be much more widely used, during the second stage as well as the first stage of labour.

The policy implications of the review of the randomized comparisons of continuous electronic monitoring and intermittent auscultation will depend on the importance that the reader attaches to the observed reduction in the risk of neonatal seizures (MacDonald *et al.* 1985). Limited follow-up of the children in the Dublin trial who suffered neonatal seizures suggests that the neonatal seizures which are potentially preventable by more intensive monitoring, are *not* associated with long-term problems (Grant 1987b). Nevertheless, some people will consider that neonatal seizures are sufficiently important in their own right for their prevention to form the basis for current policy. On this basis, there is a good case for using more intensive monitoring when labour ceases to be 'physiological': for example, during induction or augmentation of labour; if labour is prolonged; if there is meconium-staining of the liquor; or during the unusual physiological circumstances of multiple pregnancy. For the majority of labours for which no such indications apply, the current evidence suggests that more intensive monitoring increases obstetric intervention with no clear benefit for the fetus. Regular auscultation by a personal attendant, as used in the randomized trials, therefore seems to be the policy of choice in these labours. Such a policy will be difficult to reimplement in the many hospitals whose current policy is universal electronic monitoring. Firstly, individualized care during labour is often perceived as not possible; and secondly, midwives and others have lost the ability and confidence to monitor labour in this way.

The choice of technique for fetal heart monitoring has much wider ramifications than the direct effects on the physical health of fetus and mother. Depending on the prevailing system of care for women during childbirth it may influence the roles and relationships of those involved. With intermittent auscultation the midwife is the centre of caregiving, with the doctor playing a consultative role when the midwife is worried that there may be problems. In contrast, use of continuous electronic monitoring changes the delivery room into an intensive care unit. The midwife takes on a more technical role with doctors becoming more centrally involved in routine care. The presence of a monitor may also change the relationships between the woman and her partner on the one hand, and the woman, midwife, and doctor, on the other. These wider implications must be recognized by policy makers.

7.2 Implications for future research

The evaluation of methods of monitoring the fetus during labour, in common with all tests of fetal well-being, is difficult. Claims to the contrary are likely to be misleading. It will be extremely difficult to demonstrate that new techniques affect fetal and neonatal morbidity, although a demonstration that they offer improvements in terms such as women's satisfaction, staff preference and staff-time saved would be worthwhile.

Selective use of continuous electronic monitoring implies the identification of a subgroup of fetuses at high risk of developing problems during labour. This process needs refinement. Improvement could come from advances in antenatal testing or from fetal assessment at the onset of labour. The place of the admission test is unclear in this respect and this warrants further evaluation, ideally in the context of large randomized trials.

The message from the trials of continuous fetal heart rate monitoring, that 'more information' may lead to harmful as well as beneficial effects should not be forgotten when new techniques are developed. Computerized assessment of intrapartum fetal heart rate patterns is a promising method for reducing inter- and intra-observer variation in trace interpretation. These systems still require extensive evaluation, however, before they can be introduced into clinical practice, other than on an experimental basis.

It is surprising that so few formal randomized comparisons of the alternative electrodes have been conducted. Worries about transmission of the human immunodeficiency virus from an infected mother to her baby give new impetus to the search for non-invasive techniques of monitoring.

Current methods of fetal acid–base assessment by fetal scalp blood sampling are cumbersome and time-consuming. There is an urgent need for a simplified technique for rapid intermittent fetal acid–base assessment. It is surprising that such technology is not already available. Intrapartum fetal stimulation tests are promising complementary tests and warrant further evaluation.

New methods for measuring the short-term effects of intrapartum 'asphyxia' in the newborn nursery (Fitzhardinge *et al.* 1981; Cady *et al.* 1983; Levene and Trounce 1986; Eyre *et al.* 1983; Aziz *et al.* 1986) may provide useful surrogate measures for assessing the predictive properties and effectiveness of new methods of intrapartum monitoring. Those designing studies to evaluate intrapartum monitoring should take these developments into account.

There is unlikely to be any satisfactory alternative to trying to evaluate new methods of monitoring, together with the interventions which they prompt, in the context of randomized trials. The overviews in this chapter have demonstrated that relatively small trials may provide useful information, provided that a sufficiently large number of such trials are conducted. Nevertheless, adverse outcome as a consequence of labour and delivery is now so uncommon that more pragmatic research designs must be pursued if sufficiently large studies are to be mounted. 'Cluster' randomization of different clinics or hospitals, for example, would not only allow large samples to be studied relatively easily, but would also circumvent first, the problems of 'contamination' and 'co-intervention' which may blunt the comparison, and secondly, the need for the investigators to be proficient in using each of the techniques being compared.

References

Aarnoudse JG, Huisjes HJ, Oeseburg B, Zijlstra WG (1981). Subcutaneous oxygen tension in the fetal scalp during labour—continuous monitoring with a needle electrode. Br J Obstet Gynaecol, 88: 517–524

Aarnoudse JG, Huisjes HJ, Gordon H, Oeseburg B, Zijlstra WG (1985). Fetal subcutaneous scalp pO$_2$ and abnormal heart rate during labour. Am J Obstet Gynecol, 153: 565–566.

Amato JC (1983). Fetal heart rate monitoring. Am J Obstet Gynecol, 147: 967–969.

Aziz SS, Wallace SJ, Murphy JF, Sainsbury CPQ, Gray OP (1986). Cotside EEG monitoring using compressed spectral analysis. Arch Dis Child, 61: 242–246.

Beard RW (1974). Detection of fetal asphyxia in labor. Pediatrics, 53: 157–168.

Beard RW, Rivers RPA (1979). Fetal asphyxia in labour. Lancet, ii: 1117–1119.

Beard RW, Morris ED, Clayton SG (1967). pH of foetal capillary blood as an indicator of the condition of the foetus. J Obstet Gynaecol Br Commnwlth, 74: 812–822.

Beard RW, Filshie GM, Knight CA, Roberts GM (1971). The significance of the changes in the continuous fetal heart rate in the first stage of labour. J Obstet Gynaecol Br Commnwlth, 78: 865–881.

Benson RC, Shubeck F, Deutschberger J, Weiss W, Berendes H (1968). Fetal heart rate as a predictor of fetal distress. Obstet Gynecol, 32: 259–266.

Bestine RL, Callagan DA (1966). Ultrasonic Doppler inspection of the fetal heart. Am J Obstet Gynecol, 95: 1001–1004.

Bishop EH (1966). The obstetric uses of ultrasound. Int J Fed Gynecol Obstet, 4: 190–196.

Cady EB, Costello AM de L, Dawson MJ, Delphy DT, Hope PL, Reynolds EOR, Tofts PS, Wilkie DR (1983). Non-invasive investigation of cerebral metabolism in newborn infants by phosphorous nuclear magnetic resonance spectroscopy. Lancet, i: 1059–1062.

Caldeyro-Barcia R (1958). Estudio de la anoxia fetal intrauterina mediante el ECG fetal y el registro continuo de la frecuencia cardiaca fetal. III Cong Lat-Am Obstet Ginecol (Mexico). Reported in: Cibils LA. Electronic Fetal–Maternal Monitoring, Chapter 1, Monitoring of the mother.

Callagan DA, Rowland TC, Goldman DE (1964). Ultrasonic Doppler observation of the fetal heart. Obstet Gynecol, 23: 637.

Calvert JP, Newcombe RG (1980). Which fetal scalp electrode? Lancet, i: 371.

Carter MC (1986). Advances in electronic fetal monitors—real or imaginary? J Perinat Med, 14: 405–410.

Cave DG, Swingler GR, Skew PG (1979). Hypoxic stillbirth due to entangled intrauterine catheter. Br Med J, i: 233.

Chalmers I (1979). Randomised controlled trials of intrapartum monitoring. In: Perinatal Medicine, 6th European Congress, Vienna. Thalhammer O, Baumgarten K, Pollak A (eds), pp 260–265.

Chamberlain R, Chamberlain G, Howlett B, Claireaux A (1975). Care of the Baby. In: British Births 1970, Vol. 1. Heinemann: London, pp 196–234.

Chan WA, Paul RH, Toews J (1973). Intrapartum fetal monitoring—maternal and fetal morbidity and perinatal mortality. Obstet Gynecol, 41: 7–13.

Clark SL, Gimovsky ML, Miller FC (1982). Fetal heart rate response to scalp blood sampling. Am J Obstet Gynecol, 144: 706–708.

Clark SL, Gimovsky ML, Miller FC (1984). The scalp stimulation test: A clinical alternative to fetal blood sampling. Am J Obstet Gynecol, 148: 274–277.

Cohen AR, Klapholz H, Thompson MS (1982). Electronic fetal monitoring and clinical practice—a survey of obstetric opinion. Med Decision Making, 2: 79–95.

Collins KH, Bevan DR, Beard RW (1978). Fluid loading to reduce abnormalities of fetal heart rate and maternal hypotension during epidural analgesia in labour. Br Med J, 2: 1460–1461.

Coltart TM, Trickey NRA, Beard RW (1969). Foetal blood sampling: practical approach to management of foetal distress. Br Med J, 1: 342–346.

Crawford JW (1986). Limitations of current fetal monitoring techniques. J Perinat Med, 14: 379–383.

Day E, Maddern L, Wood C (1968). Auscultation of foetal heart rate: an assessment of its error and significance. Br Med J, 4: 422–424.

Dennis J (1978). Neonatal convulsions: aetiology, late neonatal status and long-term outcome. Dev Med Child Neurol, 20: 143–148.

Dennis J, Chalmers I (1982) Very early neonatal seizure rate: a possible epidemiological indicator of the quality of perinatal care. Br J Obstet Gynaecol, 89: 418–426.

Department of Health and Social Security (1984). Evaluation of Cardiotocographs. Health Equipment Information 133.

Dilts PV (1976). Current practice in antepartum and intrapartum fetal monitoring. Am J Obstet Gynecol, 126: 491–494.

Eyre JA, Oozeer RC, Wilkinson AR (1983). Continuous elecroencephalographic recording to detect seizures in paralysed newborn babies. Br Med J, 286: 1017–1018.

Fenton AN, Steer CM (1962). Fetal distress. Am J Obstet Gynecol, 83: 354–362.

Fitzhardinge MD, Flodmark O, Fitz CR, Ashby S (1981). The prognostic value of computed tomography as an adjunct to assessment of the term infant with postasphyxial encephalopathy. J Pediatr, 99: 777–781.

Flynn AM, Kelly J, Matthews K, O'Connor M, Viegas O (1982). Predictive value of, and observer variability in, several ways of reporting antepartum cardiotocographs. Br J Obstet Gynaecol, 89: 434–440.

Freud S (1897). Infantile cerebral paralysis. Republished 1968, translated by Ruffin LA. Coral Gables, Florida: University of Miami Press.

Fujikura T, Klionsky B (1975). The significance of meconium staining. Am J Obstet Gynecol, 121: 45–50.

Garcia J, Corry M, MacDonald D, Elbourne D, Grant A (1985). Mothers' views of continuous electronic fetal heart monitoring and intermittent auscultation in a randomised controlled trial. Birth, 12: 79–85.

Ghosh AK, Tipton RH (1976). Fetal scalp electrodes. Lancet, i: 1075.

Gillmer MDG, Combe D (1979). Intrapartum fetal monitoring practice in the United Kingdom. Br J Obstet Gynaecol, 86: 753–758.

Goodlin RC (1979). History of fetal monitoring. Am J Obstet Gynecol, 133: 323–352.

Goodlin RC (1987). Admission test: A screening test for fetal distess in labor. Obstet Gynecol, 70: 143.

Grant A (1984). Principles for clinical evaluation of methods of perinatal monitoring. J Perinat Med, 12: 227–233.

Grant A (1986). The Dublin Randomised Controlled Trial of Intrapartum Fetal Heart Rate Monitoring. Thesis, University of Oxford.

Grant A (1987a). Equipment and services. In: Birthplace. Chamberlain GVP, Gunn P (eds). Chichester: John Wiley, pp 50–100.

Grant A (1987b). The relationship between obstetrically preventable intrapartum asphyxia, abnormal neonatal neurological signs and subsequent motor impairment in babies born at or after term. In: Perinatal Events and Brain Damage in Surviving Children. Kubli F, Patel N, Schmidt

880 *Adrian Grant*

W, Linderkamp O (eds). Berlin: Springer Verlag.

Gregory GA, Gooding CA, Phibbs RH, Tooley WH (1974). Meconium aspiration in infants—a prospective study. J Pediatr, 85: 848–852.

Gultekin-Zootzmann B (1975). The history of monitoring the human fetus. J Perinat Med, 3: 135–144.

Hammacher K (1967). Electronische Krontrolle des fetalen Lebens vor und wahrend des gerburt. Arch Gynäkol, 204: 270–271.

Hansen PK, Smith SF, Nim J, Neldam S, Osler M (1985). Maternal attitudes to fetal monitoring. Eur J Obstet Gynec Reprod Biol, 20: 43–51.

Haverkamp AD, Bowes WA (1971). Uterine perforation: a complication of continuous fetal monitoring. Am J Obstet Gynecol, 110: 667–669.

Haverkamp AD, Thompson HE, McFee JG, Cetrulo C (1976). The evaluation of continuous fetal heart rate monitoring in high-risk pregnancy. Am J Obstet Gynecol, 125: 310–320.

Haverkamp AD, Orleans M, Langendoerfer S, McFee J, Murphy J, Thompson HE (1979). A controlled trial of the differential effects of intrapartum fetal monitoring. Am J Obstet Gynecol, 134: 399–408.

Hellman LM, Schiffer MA, Kohl SG, Tolles WE (1958). Studies in fetal well-being: variations in fetal heart rate. Am J Obstet Gynecol, 76: 998–1010.

Hellman L, Donald I, Sunden E, Duffus GM (1970). Safety of diagnostic ultrasound in obstetrics. Lancet, i: 1133–1135.

Hobel CJ (1971). Intrapartum clinical assessment of fetal distress. Am J Obstet Gynecol, 110: 336–342.

Hon EH (1958). The electronic evaluation of the fetal heart rate; preliminary report. Am J Obstet Gynecol, 75: 1215–1230.

Hon EH (1959). Observations on pathologic fetal bradycardia. Am J Obstet Gynecol, 77: 1084–1091.

Hon EH (1960). Apparatus for continuous monitoring of the fetal heart rate. Yale J Biol Med, 32: 397–399.

Hon EH, Hess OW (1957). Instrumentation of fetal electrocardiography. Science, 125: 553–554.

Huaman EJ, Hassoun R, Itahashi CM, Pereda GJ, Mejia MA (1983). Results obtained with piracetam in foetal distress during labour. J Int Med Res, 11: 129–136.

Huntingford PJ, Pendleton HJ (1969). The clinical application of cardiotocography. J Obstet Gynaecol Br Commnwlth, 76: 586–595.

Ingemarsson I, Arulkumaran S, Ingemarsson E, Tambayraja RL, Ratnam SS (1986). Admission test: A screening test for fetal distess in labor. Obstet Gynecol, 68: 800–806.

Ingemarsson I, Arulkumaran S, Paul RH, Ingemarsson E, Tambayraja RL, Ratnam SS (1988). Fetal acoustic stimulation in early labor in patients screened with the admission test. Am J Obstet Gynecol, 158: 70–74.

Jackson JE, Vaughan M, Black P, D'Souza S (1983). Psychological aspects of fetal monitoring: maternal reaction to the position of the monitor and staff behaviour. J Psychosom Obstet Gynaecol, 2: 97–102.

Jenkins HLM (1986). Technical progress in fetal electrocardiography—a review. J Perinat Med, 14: 365–370.

Jenkins HML, Symonds EM, Kirk DL, Smith PR (1986). Can fetal electrocardiography improve the prediction of intrapartum fetal acidosis? Br J Obstet Gynecol, 93: 6–12.

Keirse MJNC (1986). Electronic monitoring in labor: Too good to be put to the test? Birth, 13: 256–258.

Kelso IM, Parsons RJ, Lawrence GF, Arora SS, Edmonds DK, Cooke ID (1978). An assessment of continuous fetal heart rate monitoring in labor—a randomised trial. Am J Obstet Gynecol, 131: 526–532.

Koszalka MF, Haverkamp AD, Orleans M, Murphy J (1982). The effects of internal electronic fetal heart rate monitoring on maternal and infant infections in high-risk pregnancies. J Reprod Med, 27: 661–665.

Kruse J (1984). Long-term reactions of women to electronic fetal monitoring during labor. J Family Practice, 18: 543–548.

Langendoerfer S, Haverkamp AD, Murphy J, Nuwick KD, Orleans M, Pacosa F, van Doornick W (1980). Pediatric follow-up of a randomised controlled trial of intrapartum fetal monitoring techniques. J Pediatr, 97: 103–107.

Ledger WJ (1978). Complications associated with invasive monitoring. Seminars Perinatol, 2: 187–194.

Levene MI, Trounce JQ (1986). Cause of neonatal convulsions: towards more precise diagnosis. Arch Dis Child, 61: 78–87.

Leveno KJ, Cunningham FG, Nelson S, Roark M, Williams ML, Guzick D, Dowling S, Rosenfeld CR, Buckley A (1986). A prospective comparison of selective and universal electronic fetal monitoring in 34,995 pregnancies. New Engl J Med, 315: 615–619.

Lofgren O (1987). Continuous transcutaneous carbon dioxide measurement from the fetal scalp during labor and during the first minutes of extra uterine life. J Perinat Med, 15: 37–44.

Lund CJ (1943). Fetal tachycardia during labor—a fallible sign of fetal distress. Am J Obstet Gynecol, 45: 636–645.

Luthy DA, Shy KK, van Belle G, Larson EB, Hughes JP, Benedetti TJ, Brown ZA, Effer S, King JF, Stenchever MA (1987). A randomised trial of electronic fetal monitoring in preterm labor. Obstet Gynecol, 69: 687–695.

MacDonald D, Grant A, Sheridan-Pereira M, Boylan P, Chalmers I (1985). The Dublin randomised trial of intrapartum fetal heart monitoring. Am J Obstet Gynecol, 152: 524–539.

Martin C-B, van Dis P, Jongsma HW (1984). Clinical applications of fetal cardiac electromechanical intervals. J Perinat Med, 12: 277–278.

Matthews CD, Martin MR (1974). Early detection of meconium-stained liquor during labor: A contribution to fetal care. Am J Obstet Gynecol, 120: 808–811.

Maynard DE, Cohen RJ, Viniker DA (1979). Intrapartum fetal monitoring with the cerebral function monitor. Br J Obstet Gynaecol, 86: 941–947.

McCall JO, Fulshaw RW (1953). A study of fetal distress, its interpretation and significance. Am J Obstet Gynecol, 65: 1006–1019.

Meis PJ, Hall M, Marshall JR, Hobel CJ (1978). Meconium passage: A new classification for risk assessment during labor. Am J Obstet Gynecol, 131: 509–513.

Miller FC, Sacks DA, Yeh S, Paul RH, Schifrin BS, Martin CB, Hon EH (1975). Significance of meconium during labor. Am J Obstet Gynecol, 122: 573–580.

Miller FC, Pearce KE, Paul RH (1984). Fetal heart rate

pattern recognition by the method of auscultation. Obstet Gynecol, 64: 332–336.

Miyazaki FS, Nevarez F (1985). Saline amnioinfusion for relief of repetitive variable decelerations: a prospective randomized study. Am J Obstet Gynecol, 153: 301–306.

Modanlou H, Yeh S, Hon EH (1974). Fetal and neonatal acid-base balance in normal and high-risk pregnancies. Obstet Gynecol, 43: 347–353.

Molfese V, Sunshine P, Bennett A (1982). Reactions of women to intrapartum fetal monitoring. Obstet Gynecol, 59: 705–709.

Murphy JR, Haverkamp AD, Langendoerfer S, Orleans M (1981). The relation of electronic fetal monitoring patterns to infant outcome measures in a random sample of term size infants born to high risk mothers. Am J Epidemiol, 114: 539–547.

Murray HG (1986). The fetal electrocardiogram: current clinical developments in Nottingham. J Perinat Med, 14: 399–404.

National Institutes of Health (1979). Report of a task force on predictors of fetal distress. In: Antenatal Diagnosis. Washington DC: US Department of Health, Education and Welfare.

National Maternity Hospital (1986) Annual Report for 1986, Dublin.

Nielsen PV, Stigsby B, Nickelson C, Nim J (1987). Intra- and inter-observer variability in the assessment of intrapartum cardiotocograms. Acta Obstet Gynecol Scand, 66: 421–424.

Neldam S, Osler M, Hansen PK, Nim J, Smith SF, Hertel J (1986). Intrapartum fetal heart rate monitoring in a combined low- and high-risk population: a controlled clinical trial. Eur J Obstet Gynecol Reprod Biol. 23: 1–11.

Nickelson C, Thomsen SG, Weber T (1986). Fetal carbon dioxide tension during human labour. Eur J Obstet Gynecol Reprod Biol, 22: 205–206.

Niswander KR, Gordon M (1972). The women and their pregnancies. National Institutes of Health Publication 73–379. Washington DC: US Department of Health, Education and Welfare.

O'Connor MC, Hytten FE, Zanelli GD (1979). Is the fetus 'scalped' in labour? Lancet, ii: 947–948.

O'Driscoll K, Meagher D (1980). Active Management of Labour. London: W B Saunders.

O'Driscoll K. Coughlan M, Fenton V, Skelly M (1977). Active management of labour: care of the fetus. Br Med J, 2: 1451–1453.

O'Driscoll K, Meagher D, MacDonald D, Geoghegan F (1981). Traumatic intracranial haemorrhage in first born infants and delivery with obstetric forceps. Br J Obstet Gynaecol, 88: 577–581.

Okada DM, Chow AW, Bruce VT (1977). Neonatal scalp abscess and fetal monitoring: factors associated with infection. Am J Obstet Gynecol, 129: 185–189.

Painter MJ, Depp R, O'Donoghue PD (1978). Fetal heart rate patterns and development in the first year of life. Am J Obstet Gynecol, 132: 271–277.

Pardi G, Ferrazzi I, Cetin I, Rampello S, Baselli G, Cerutti S, Civardi S (1986). The clinical relevence of the abdominal fetal electrocardiogram. J Perinat Med, 14: 371–377.

Parer JT (1986). The Dublin trial of fetal heart rate monitoring: the final word? Birth, 13: 119–121.

Patriarco MS, Viechnicki BM, Hutchinson TA, Klasko SK, Yeh S-Y (1987). A study of intrauterine fetal resuscitation with terbutaline. Am J Obstet Gynecol, 157: 384–387.

Paul RH, Hon EH (1971). Clinical fetal monitoring, a survey of current usage. Obstet Gynecol, 37: 779–784.

Peck TM (1980). Physicians' subjectivity in evaluating oxytocin challenge tests. Obstet Gynecol, 60: 13–16.

Perkins RP (1984). Perinatal observations in a high-risk population managed without intrapartum fetal pH studies. Am J Obstet Gynecol, 149: 327–334.

Pinkerton JHM (1969). Kergaradec, friend of Laennec and pioneer of foetal auscultation. Proc R Soc Med, 62: 477–483.

Pinkerton JHM (1976). Fetal auscultation—Some aspects of its history and evolution. J Irish Med Assoc, 69: 363–368.

Placek PJ, Keppel KG, Taffel SM, Liss TL (1984). Electronic fetal monitoring in relation to cesarean section delivery for live births and stillbirths in the US 1980. Public Health Reports, 99: 173–183.

Renou P, Chang A, Anderson I, Wood C (1976). Controlled trial of fetal intensive care. Am J Obstet Gynecol, 126: 470–476.

Rosen KG (1986). Alterations in the fetal electrocardiogram as a sign of fetal asphyxia—experimental data with a clinical implementation. J Perinat Med, 14: 355–363.

Royston GHD (1982). Fetal heart rate monitoring: a system view. Lancet, 1: 861.

Rumeau-Roquette C, Bréart G (1978). Surveillance électronique de l'accouchement et risque périnatal dans l'enquête nationale de 1972. In: Symposium sur la surveillance foetale, Vol 1. Kontron (ed). Zurich.

Saling E (1961). Neue Untersuchungsmoglichkeiten des Kindes unter Geburt (Einfuhrung and Grundlagen). Zbl Gynäkol, 83: 1906–1908.

Saling E (1962). Neues Vorgehen zur Untersuchung des Kindes unter der gebert. Arch Gynäkol, 197: 108–122.

Saling E (1964). Mikroblutuntersuchungen am Feten: Klinischer Einsatz und erste Ergebausse. Z Geburtsh Gynäkol, 152: 56–75.

Schifrin BS, Dame L (1972). Fetal heart rate patterns—prediction of Apgar score. J Am Med Assoc, 219: 1322–1325.

Schifrin BS, Suzuki K (1973). Fetal surveillance during labour. Int Anesthesiol Clinics, 11: 17–44.

Schmidt S, Langner K, Gesche J, Dudenhausen JW, Saling E (1985). The influence of progress of labor on the reliability of the transcutaneous pCO_2 of the fetus. J Perinat Med, 13: 195–200.

Shelley T, Tipton RH (1971). Dip area: A quantitive measure of fetal heart rate patterns. J Obstet Gynaecol Br Commnwlth, 78: 694–701.

Shields D (1978). Maternal reactions to fetal monitoring. Am J Nursing, 3: 2110–2112.

Smith CV, Nguyen HN, Phelan JP, Paul RH (1986a). Intrapartum assessment of fetal well-being: A comparison of fetal acoustic stimulation with acid-base determinations. Am J Obstet Gynecol, 155: 726–728.

Smith CV, Phelan JP, Platt LD, Broussard P, Paul RH (1986b). Fetal acoustic stimulation testing. II A randomized clinical comparison with the non-stress test. Am J Obstet Gynecol, 155: 131–134

Starkman MN (1976). Psychological responses to the use of the fetal monitor during labor. Psychosom Med, 38: 269–277.

Starks GC (1980). Correlation of meconium-stained amniotic fluid, intrapartum fetal pH, and Apgar scores as predictors of perinatal outcome. Obstet Gynecol, 56: 604–609.

Steer PJ (1982). Has the expression 'fetal distress' outlived its usefulness. Br J Obstet Gynaecol, 89: 690–693.

Stewart P, Hillan E, Calder AA, Nicol SM (1983). A comparative assessment of an automated blood microprocessor for fetal blood pH measurements in the labour ward. Br J Obstet Gynaecol, 90: 522–524.

Stokes IM (1984). Fetal distress associated with malposition of an intra-uterine catheter. J Obstet Gynaecol, 4: 196–197.

Symonds EM (1986). Fetal electrocardiographic monitoring: past, present and future—a historical perspective. J Perinat Med, 14: 385–390.

Trimbos JB, Keirse MJNC (1978). Observer variability in assessment of antepartum cardiotocograms. Br J Obstet Gynaecol, 85: 900–906.

Trudinger BJ, Pryce-Davies J (1978). Fetal hazards of the intrauterine pressure catheter: five case reports. Br J Obstet Gynaecol, 85: 567–572.

van Geijn HP (1987). Fetal monitoring—present and future: the evaluation of fetal heart rate patterns. Eur J Obstet Gynecol Reprod Biol, 24: 117–119.

Visser GHA, Goodman JDS, Dawes GS (1980). Problems with ultrasonic fetal heart rate monitor. Lancet, i: 707–708.

Walker N (1959). The case of conservatism in management of foetal distress. Br Med J, 2: 1221–1226.

Walker J (1959). Fetal distress. Am J Obstet Gynecol, 77: 94–107.

Weber T, Nickelson C (1984). Continuous measurement of pH with a glass electrode. J Perinat Med, 12: 238–239.

Wood C, Pinkerton JHM (1961). Clinical aspects of anoxic stillbirths. J Obstet Gynaecol Br Empire, 68: 552–556.

Wood C, Renou P, Oats J, Farrell E, Beischer N, Anderson I (1981). A controlled trial of fetal heart rate monitoring in a low-risk obstetric population. Am J Obstet Gynecol, 141: 527–534.

Youngs DD, Starkman MN (1976). Psychological and physiological aspects of electronic fetal monitoring. Primary Care, 3: 691–700.

55 Maternal position during the first stage of labour

Joyce Roberts

1 Introduction

Interest in maternal position during the first stage of labour has existed throughout the twentieth century. In 1909, King suggested that 'the recumbent posture during labour is much overdone' and noted, 'it is often persisted in—either by custom or by direct order of the obstetrician—when it does positive harm, by prolonging labour, by exhausting the woman, and sometimes leading to the persistence of faulty presentations, as well as increasing the duration and intensity of the woman's suffering.' Early publications mainly suggested the use of upright positions for labour and delivery in preference to the recumbency that was becoming more common as an increasing proportion of births began to occur in institutions (Markoe 1917; Howard 1951, 1954, 1958; Newton 1956; Newton and Newton 1960). Papers published more recently have promoted the use of the lateral position (Irwin 1978) and have stressed the importance of accepting whatever position the labouring woman chooses for herself (Carlson et al. 1986; Rossi and Lindell 1986).

Until recently there has been relatively little well-controlled research to assess the validity of the various strongly held opinions which exist about position during labour and delivery (Roberts 1980; Roberts and Mendez-Bauer 1980). In these circumstances a reasonable policy might seem to be to encourage women to choose whatever positions they wish to adopt during labour until or unless good evidence can be produced to cast doubt on the wisdom of such an approach. If the results of recent surveys had suggested that a liberal approach of this kind was universal in the institutions in which women give birth, the relevance of a review of the available evidence about the effects of recumbency might justifiably be questioned. As it is, recumbency continues to be required by many of the professionals who provide care during labour (see Chapter 50), so it is important to assess what the consequences of this policy may be.

In this, the first of two chapters on this subject, evidence relating to the effects of adopting different positions during the first stage of labour will be reviewed; in a related chapter (see Chapter 66), position during the second stage of labour and delivery will be considered.

2 Effects of different positions on haemodynamics and uterine contractility

Of the published clinical trials studying the effects of maternal position during the first stage of labour, ten have concentrated on the effects of different positions on haemodynamics and uterine contractility. In these investigations women have been asked to serve as their own controls, with periods of time spent in different positions being either formally randomized or alternated.

Four of these ten studies focused on variables related to haemodynamics (Ueland and Hansen 1969; Eckstein and Marx 1974; Galbert and Marx 1974; Abitol 1985). They have shown not only that cardiac output is significantly reduced in the supine and sitting positions (Ueland and Hansen 1969), but also that even when the compression of the inferior vena cava is partially relieved by the contracting uterus and by engagement and descent of the fetus into the pelvis, the compression of the lower aorta is not relieved. The fact that the supine position is associated with a greater decline in femoral than brachial arterial pressure, and in an increase in extradural pressure, and that this association is not observed in the lateral position or when the uterus is tilted to the left (Galbert and Marx 1974; Eckstein and Marx 1974), suggests that the supine recumbent position can compromise uterine blood flow during labour. In Abitol's (1985) trial, in which women were asked to alternate between the lateral recumbent and supine positions, the supine position was associated with a reduction in both pulse pressure in the big toe and femoral arterial pressure, as well as a statistically significant increase in late decelerations of the fetal heart rate.

A similar research design has been used to study the effects of maternal posture on uterine activity (Caldeyro-Barcia *et al.* 1960; Miller *et al.* 1982; Mendez-Bauer *et al.* 1975, 1976a,b, and 1980; Roberts *et al.* 1981, 1983, 1984). These studies have revealed that contraction intensity is consistently reduced and contraction frequency often increased when the labouring woman sits or lies supine after being upright. Standing and lateral recumbency are thus associated with greater contraction intensity and efficiency—that is, the ability of the contractions to accomplish cervical dilatation (Miller *et al.* 1982; Roberts *et al.* 1983), and this effect has been used in the management of dystocia (Read *et al.* 1981; see Chapter 53).

The results of these studies suggest that the supine position can adversely affect both the condition of the fetus and the progression of labour by interference with uterine haemodynamics and compromising the efficiency of uterine contractions. The fact that these effects were not detected in a comparison of lateral recumbency with the supine position (Roberts *et al.* 1984) probably means that frequent changes of maternal position (at least every half-hour) may be a way of avoiding the adverse effects of supine recumbency. None of the evidence derived from these studies, however, suggests that the supine position should be encouraged.

3 The effects of upright versus recumbent positions on the mother, progress of labour, and the baby

Are the effects of recumbency on haemodynamics and uterine contractility which have been described above reflected in more substantial effects on either the mother or her baby? It is worth noting that there are inevitable difficulties in designing randomized trials to address this question. It is impossible to blind partici-

pants and caregivers to the group to which women have been assigned, and very difficult to blind those assessing outcomes. This reality results in both the possibility of cointerventions (additional measures applied more often to women in one group than in the other) and bias in the assessment of some outcome measures. Furthermore, the primary objective of these studies must be seen as evaluating intended rather than actual positions during labour. Women not infrequently have difficulty in maintaining the position to which they had been assigned: Chan (1963), for example, reported that women assigned to maintain an upright position during labour 'complained bitterly' about remaining erect throughout labour and wanted to rest in bed during the latter part.

In addition to the ten trials cited above in which women served as their own controls, eleven controlled trials have been reported in which women were assigned either to an upright group who were asked to stand, walk or sit during the entire first stage of labour, or to a group asked to remain recumbent in bed in a supine or lateral recumbent position (Chan 1963; Mitre 1974; Liu 1974; McManus and Calder 1978; Diaz *et al.* 1978 [same trial also reported in Caldeyro-Barcia 1978 and 1979, and Diaz *et al.* 1980]; Flynn *et al.* 1978; Williams *et al.* 1980; Read *et al.* 1981; Calvert *et al.* 1982; Hemminki and Saarikoski 1983; Roberts *et al.* 1983 [same trial also reported in Roberts *et al.* 1984]). The trials are summarized in Table 55.1.

Table 55.2 presents data showing the effect of position on the length of labour. These are consistent with the effects of position on uterine activity demonstrated in the crossover trials described above. In the five trials in which women were allocated to either remain upright or supine, women who maintained upright positions had shorter labours (Caldeyro-Barcia 1978, 1979; Diaz *et al.* 1978, 1980; Flynn *et al.* 1978; Liu 1974; Mitre 1974). In the four trials in which upright position was compared with lateral recumbency there were no striking differences in the length of labour (Calvert *et al.* 1982; Chan 1963; McManus and Calder 1978; Williams *et al.* 1980). In one other trial (Hemminki and Saarikoski 1983), labour was actually longer in the ambulant than in the non-ambulant group. This may be explained by the fact that women in the recumbent group were permitted to get up if they desired and women in the ambulant group were allowed to rest in bed 'whenever they wanted'.

In the reports of four trials (Chan 1963; Williams *et al.* 1980; Calvert *et al.* 1982; Hemminki and Saarikoski 1983) it was noted that women in the upright group preferred to recline in bed as labour progressed, often at about 5–6 cm dilatation. These impressions of women's preference to recline as labour progresses are consistent with the findings from a trial in which women were asked to alternate between sitting up in a chair and lying

Table 55.1 Summary of clinical trials of maternal positions during the first stage of labour

Study	Research design	Sample size	Positions compared	Entry criteria	Exclusion criteria	Subject characteristics	Phase of labour studied	Outcomes compared	Results reported
Cadeyro-Barcia *et al* (1960)	Subjects served as own control	84	Supine vs. Side	Prelabour or 1st stage half oxytocin-induced, half spontaneous	Amniotomy, altered oxytocin infusion rate, any medication	Term pregnancies Mixed parity	Early and active labour	Uterine contractions Intensity Frequency Tonus Uterine activity	Greater on side Greater on back Greater on back No difference
Chan (1963)	Alternate assignment	100 100 ⎯⎯ 200	Erect: Standing or Sitting In bed: Lateral or Supine	Primigravida in spontaneous labour	Elective caesarean section	Preterm and term Mixed complications in labour Mixed dilatation entry to study	1st through 2nd stage	Mode of delivery Duration of 1st, 2nd, and 3rd stages Complaints of discomfort Amount of analgesia	No difference No significant differences More complaints in propped position More given in erect group
Ueland and Hansen (1969)	Subjects served as own control	23	Supine vs. Lateral	Term pregnancy-induced labour	Sedation	Mixed parity	Active labour	Cardiac output / Heart rate / Stroke volume	Greater inc. in supine position with contraction. Greater inc. in lateral position without a contraction. Greater dec. in supine position with contraction. Lower in lateral position without a contraction. Greater inc. in supine position with a contraction. Greater in lateral position without a contraction.
Eckstein and Marx (1974)	Subjects served as own control	45	Lateral Supine Supine w/wedge or mechanical displacement	Latent labour or active labour	None indicated	Gravid in labour Healthy Term pregnancy	Latent and active labour	Blood pressure brachial femoral / Maternal heart rate	Incidence of hypotension lower in active labour. Lower in supine position. BP increases when either device used to displace uterus. Greatest in supine position.
Galbert and Marx (1974)	Subjects served as own control	12	Lateral Supine Supine with wedge on mechanical displacement	Various stages of labour	None indicated		Active labour	Lumber extradural pressure Arterial blood pressure	Extradural pressure was significantly higher in the supine position. Maximal epidural pressure was in supine position without lateral displacement and with bearing down effort. Mean arterial pressure was lowest in the supine position.
Mitre (1974)	Assignment alternate	50 50 ⎯⎯ 100	Sitting vs. Supine	Admission in early active labour 1–3 cm dilatation	Need for stimulation of labour Evidence of CPD surgery or trauma to presentation	Normal nulliparae Cephalic presentation	Active phase of labour	Fetal results Time in active labour (hours) Apgar scores	No difference Sitting $\bar{x}5.47 \pm 1.71$ $t = 4.12$ Supine $\bar{x} = 7.25 \pm 1.64$ $p < 0.05$ Sitting 7–10. $\bar{x} = 9$

Table 55.1 Summary of clinical trials of maternal positions during the first stage of labour

Study	Research design	Sample size	Positions compared	Entry criteria	Exclusion criteria	Subject characteristics	Phase of labour studied	Outcomes compared	Results reported
Cadeyro-Barcia et al (1960)	Subjects served as own control	84	Supine vs. Side	Prelabour or 1st stage half oxytocin-induced, half spontaneous	Amniotomy, altered oxytocin infusion rate, any medication	Term pregnancies Mixed parity	Early and active labour	Uterine contractions Intensity Frequency Tonus Uterine activity	Greater on side Greater on back Greater on back No difference
Chan (1963)	Alternate assignment	100 100 ⎯ 200	Erect: Standing or Sitting In bed: Lateral or Supine	Primigravida in spontaneous labour	Elective caesarean section	Preterm and term Mixed complications in labour Mixed dilatation entry to study	1st through 2nd stage	Mode of delivery Duration of 1st, 2nd, and 3rd stages Complaints of discomfort Amount of analgesia	No difference No significant differences More complaints in propped position More given in erect group
Ueland and Hansen (1969)	Subjects served as own control	23	Supine vs. Lateral	Term pregnancy-induced labour	Sedation	Mixed parity	Active labour	Cardiac output Heart rate Stroke volume	Greater inc. in supine position with contraction. Greater inc. in lateral position without a contraction. Greater dec. in supine position with contraction. Lower in lateral position without a contraction. Greater inc. in supine position with a contraction. Greater in lateral position without a contraction.
Eckstein and Marx (1974)	Subjects served as own control	45	Lateral Supine Supine w/wedge or mechanical displacement	Latent labour or active labour	None indicated	Gravid in labour Healthy Term pregnancy	Latent and active labour	Blood pressure brachial femoral Maternal heart rate	Incidence of hypotension lower in active labour. Lower in supine position. BP increases when either device used to displace uterus. Greatest in supine position.
Galbert and Marx (1974)	Subjects served as own control	12	Lateral Supine Supine with wedge on mechanical displacement	Various stages of labour	None indicated		Active labour	Lumber extradural pressure Arterial blood pressure	Extradural pressure was significantly higher in the supine position. Maximal epidural pressure was in supine position without lateral displacement and with bearing down effort. Mean arterial pressure was lowest in the supine position.
Mitre (1974)	Assignment alternate	50 50 ⎯ 100	Sitting vs. Supine	Admission in early active labour 1–3 cm dilatation	Need for stimulation of labour Evidence of CPD surgery or trauma to	Normal nulliparae Cephalic presentation	Active phase of labour	Fetal results Time in active labour (hours) Apgar scores	No difference Sitting $\bar{x}5.47 \pm 1.71$ $t = 4.12$ Supine $\bar{x} = 7.25 \pm 1.64$ $p < 0.05$ Range 7–10. $\bar{x} = 9$ both groups

Study	Assignment	n	Positions	Criteria / risk factors	Stage	Population	Variables	Results (group 1)	Results (group 2)	p	Comments
		— 40	Recumbent: Lateral	≥6 Term pregnancy Amniotomy		primigravidas ea. in upright vs. recumbent groups	required Length of labour induction–delivery interval Mode of delivery Amount of analgesia Fetal condition	No difference No difference No difference No difference No difference			of positions used. Uncontrolled obstetrical variables that influence labour outcome.
Diaz et al. (1978) Caldeyro-Barcia (1979) Diaz et al. (1980)	Random assignment	225 145 — 370	Horizontal movement Vertical	Low risk Normal pelvis Spontaneous 3–5 cm cervical dilatation Cephalic presentation Anterior position CPD Breech	1st stage	Mixed parity (matched in each group) Term pregnancy	Spontaneous rupture of fetal membranes Length of labour Median duration active phase Incidence of caput succedaneum Incidence of forceps Apgar score 48-h neurological examination	No difference Horizontal n 181 180 min No difference 6.7% No difference No difference	Vertical n 143 135 min 0.7%	$p<0.001$ $p<0.05$	
Flynn et al. (1978)	Random assignment	34 34 — 68	Ambulation Lateral recumbency	Amniotomy internal monitoring established	1st stage	Mixed parity (matched in each group) Term pregnancy	Duration of active labour from 2 cm – mean Need for augmentation Need for analgesia Contractions: Frequency per 30 min Intensity – mmHg Basal tone FHR: accelerations decelerations Beat-to-beat variations Apgar – 1 min 5 min	Ambulant 4.1 hr 6 pt 14 needed 8.5 55.53 11.0 10 4 >8 bpm 8.8 9.9	Bed 6.7 hr 12 pt 34 needed 10.1 46.54 11.4 1 17 <8 bpm 7.5 9.4	$p<0.001$ $p<0.001$ $p<0.001$ $p<0.05$ $p<0.05$ NS $p<0.001$ $p<0.005$ $p<0.001$ $p<0.001$ $p<0.05$	
Williams, Thom and Studd (1980)	Assignment by use of hospital number – from 300 consecutive deliveries	55 48 — 103	Recumbency Ambulation	Admission to labour Any 'risk' factors	1st and 2nd stages	Mixed parity in both groups Term pregnancy	Length of labour Mode of delivery Incidence of fetal distress	No difference No difference No difference			87.5% of ambulant patients asked to return to bed in active labour. Poor control of position used.
Read, Miller and Paul (1981)	Random assignment after failure to progress in labour	8 6 — 14	Oxytocin recumbent Ambulation	Failure to progress in labour for ≥1 hr	Changes in labour progress and uterine contractility Uterine activity Units and Montevideo Units	Mixed parity Term pregnancy		Both approaches effective Initially a greater increase in UAU for ambulant group.			

Table 55.1 Summary of clinical trials of maternal positions during the first stage of labour – *continued*

Study	Research design	Sample size	Positions compared	Entry criteria	Exclusion criteria	Subject characteristics	Phase of labour studied	Outcomes compared	Results reported
Calvert, Newcombe, and Hibbard (1982)	Assignment based on hospital number	100 45 55 — 200	Conventional cardiotocography (recumbent-lateral) Telemetry: option to ambulate chose to remain in bed	Admission to delivery unit Term pregnancy Cephalic presentation Cervix ≥2.5 cm dilated Amniotomy	Previous stillbirth Contraindications for vaginal delivery	Mixed parity	1st stage	Use of telemetry to ambulate; Pain, Anxiety, Comfort, Mobility, Uterine Activity – Alexandria Units Apgar scores Length of labour Analgesia	45% elected to ambulate – 75% returned to bed. Ambulatory group reported more pain and less restriction in mobility No difference No difference More patients who ambulated received analgesia $p < 0.04$
Hemminki and Saarikoski (1983)	Random assignment	315 312 — 627	Ambulation ad lib Control lateral recumbency	Spontaneous labour Intact membranes	SGA infants Breech Twins Concomitant disease Induction of labour Spontaneous rupture of membranes or amniotomy	Term pregnancies Mixed parity (unequal in groups more multipara in control group)	1st stage	Proportion of sample who ambulated Time of rupture of membranes Pain Length of labour FHR Apgar score and other neonatal outcomes	Some women in each group ambulated. More women in the ambulatory group ambulated in early labour. 80–94% of the women in both groups remained in bed in late labour after 5 cm. More women in ambulatory group did not experience amniotomy until ≥8 cm (41% vs. 22% control). More pain in control group (52% vs. 62% reported painful or very painful labour). No difference No difference No difference
Roberts et al. (1983, 1984)	Subjects served as own control with random assignment of initial position	18 11 — 29	Side vs. Sitting Side vs. Supine	Spontaneous labour 2–3 cm dilatation	Any medication	Term nullipara	1st stage	Uterine contractions Intensity Frequency Uterine activity Uterine efficiency Maternal comfort FHR Duration of labour $*p < 0.05$	Side vs. Sitting / Side vs. Supine $\bar{x}=$: Side vs. 39* / Sitting 32 / Side vs. 47* / Supine 38 Intensity: 2.9* 3.4 / 3.6* 4.2 Frequency: 108* 98 / 160 153 Uterine activity / efficiency: 311* 175 / 234 309 Maternal comfort: +late labour / +early labour / No difference FHR No difference Duration: 7 hr 21 min / 5 hr 24 min
Abitol (1985)	Systematic selection and alteration of position	902	Supine vs. Lateral recumbency	Admission to labour vertex presentation	Prematurity Postmaturity medical complications CPC or previous caesarean section	Mixed parity and individualised labour care		FHR Blood pressure in brachial artery, popliteal artery, pulse pressure in big toe	14% (126) of patients/fetuses had late decelerations, and in 24% of the 126, these only occurred in the supine position. No change with position. Both dropped significantly in supine position. Conclusion: Aortic compression in the supine position contributes to 20% of late decelerations (fetal distress).

Table 55.2 Influence of maternal position on the average duration (in hours) of the first stage of labour in primiparae

Study	Upright Mean (SD)	Recumbent Mean (SD)	Diff.	p-value
Chan (1963)	8.6 (NA)	7.2 (NA)	+1.4	NS
Mitre (1974)	5.5 (1.7)	7.3 (1.6)	−1.8	<0.05
Liu (1974)	2.7 (NA)	4.2 (NA)	−1.6	<0.05
Caldeyro-Barcia et al. (1978, 1979) Diaz et al. (1978, 1980)	2.5 (NA)	4.3 (NA)	−1.8	<0.05
Flynn et al. (1978)	4.1 (NA)	6.7 (NA)	−2.6	<0.001
Williams et al. (1980)	7.9 (4.9)	6.3 (3.2)	+0.5	NS
Hemminki and Sharikoski (1983)	9.9 (NA)	8.8 (NA)	+1.1	<0.05

on their sides in bed (Roberts *et al.* 1981, 1984). These women were asked about their comfort, contractions, and location of pain as they alternated between these two positions for as long as they were able to do so.

Their responses revealed a statistically significant shift from a preference to sit up prior to about 5 or 6 cm dilatation to a preference to recline on their sides in bed as labour progressed beyond this stage.

Maternal comfort has been considered explicitly in six trials (Liu 1974; McManus and Calder 1978; Flynn *et al.* 1978; Calvert *et al.* 1982; Hemminki and Saarikoski 1983; Williams *et al.* 1980). Its assessment was varied and included need for pain medication; the mean dosage of analgesia administered to each group; pain, anxiety, and comfort assessed using analogue scales (Calvert *et al.* 1982); and the midwives' assessment of the severity of women's pain (Hemminki and Saarikoski 1983). The available data do show, however, that upright posture is associated with a reduced use of narcotic analgesics or epidural anaesthesia (Table 55.3).

The effect of upright posture on the efficiency of uterine contractions and the length of labour is reflected in less frequent use of drugs to augment labour in women who adopt this position (Table 55.4). In part, this may reflect the fact that it is easier to administer

Table 55.3 The effect of upright versus recumbent position in first stage of labour on use of oxytocin/PGs for augmentation

Study	EXPT n	(%)	CTRL n	(%)	Odds ratio (95% CI)	Graph of odds ratios and confidence intervals
Hemminki and Saarikoski (1983)	88/315	(27.94)	98/312	(31.41)	0.85 (0.60–1.19)	
Flynn et al. (1978)	6/34	(17.65)	12/34	(35.29)	0.41 (0.14–1.19)	
McManus and Calder (1978)	2/20	(10.00)	4/20	(20.00)	0.47 (0.08–2.58)	
Williams et al. (1980)	13/48	(27.08)	15/55	(27.27)	0.99 (0.42–2.35)	
Typical odds ratio (95% confidence interval)					0.80 (0.59–1.08)	

Table 55.4 The effect of upright versus recumbent position in first stage of labour on use of pethidine/epidural

Study	EXPT n	(%)	CTRL n	(%)	Odds ratio (95% CI)	Graph of odds ratios and confidence intervals
Hemminki and Saarikoski (1983)	72/200	(36.00)	75/200	(37.50)	0.94 (0.62–1.41)	
Flynn et al. (1978)	14/34	(41.18)	34/34	(100.0)	0.06 (0.02–0.17)	
Liu (1974)	0/30	(0.00)	0/30	(0.00)	1.00 (1.00–1.00)	
Calvert et al. (1982)	43/45	(95.56)	54/55	(98.18)	0.41 (0.04–4.07)	
McManus and Calder (1978)	95/144	(65.97)	88/115	(76.52)	0.60 (0.35–1.03)	
Typical odds ratio (95% confidence interval)					0.63 (0.46–0.86)	

Table 55.5 The effect of upright versus recumbent position in first stage of labour on instrumental vaginal delivery

Study	EXPT n	(%)	CTRL n	(%)	Odds ratio (95% CI)	Graph of odds ratios and confidence intervals
Hemminki and Saarikoski (1983)	16/315	(5.08)	12/312	(3.85)	1.33 (0.63–2.85)	
Flynn *et al.* (1978)	2/34	(5.88)	10/34	(29.41)	0.20 (0.06–0.70)	
Chan (1963)	23/93	(24.73)	25/95	(26.32)	0.92 (0.48–1.77)	
Caldeyro-Barcia (1979)	1/143	(0.70)	12/181	(6.63)	0.22 (0.07–0.66)	
Read *et al.* (1981)	3/8	(37.50)	2/6	(33.33)	1.18 (0.14–9.95)	
Calvert *et al.* (1982)	17/100	(17.00)	13/100	(13.00)	1.37 (0.63–2.96)	
McManus and Calder (1978)	4/19	(21.05)	5/19	(26.32)	0.75 (0.17–3.30)	
Williams *et al.* (1980)	7/48	(14.58)	8/55	(14.55)	1.00 (0.34–2.99)	
Typical odds ratio (95% confidence interval)					0.84 (0.60–1.18)	

Graph scale: 0.01 0.1 0.5 1 2 10 100

Table 55.6 The effect of upright versus recumbent position in first stage of labour on Apgar score <7 at 1 minute

Study	EXPT n	(%)	CTRL n	(%)	Odds ratio (95% CI)	Graph of odds ratios and confidence intervals
Calvert *et al.* (1982)	7/100	(7.00)	11/100	(11.00)	0.62 (0.23–1.62)	
Williams *et al.* (1980)	5/48	(10.42)	4/55	(7.27)	1.48 (0.38–5.78)	
Typical odds ratio (95% confidence interval)					0.82 (0.37–1.81)	

Graph scale: 0.01 0.1 0.5 1 2 10 100

such drugs to women who are lying in bed. The available data (Table 55.5) provide no evidence of a consistent effect of position during the first stage of labour on the likelihood of instrumental delivery, however. Similarly, there is no consistency of the findings with respect to the condition of the baby. Flynn and her colleagues (1978) are the only investigators to have reported significantly lower incidences of fetal heart rate abnormalities and depressed Apgar scores associated with upright position. Other investigators, some of whom used telemetry in conjunction with ambulation (Calvert *et al.* 1982), did not detect differences in fetal heart rate patterns or Apgar scores (Table 55.6). No information is available about the effect of position during the first stage of labour on more substantive indicators of the babies' well-being.

4 Conclusions

Professional requirements that women remain supine during the first stage of labour are less widespread than they used to be, but they still exist. The available evidence suggests that this policy compromises effective uterine activity, prolongs labour and leads to an increased use of drugs to augment contractions. Women should be encouraged to adopt whatever position they find comfortable during the first stage of labour. Many will choose upright positions to begin with and then adopt lateral recumbent positions as labour becomes more advanced.

An area that merits further investigation is that of factors in the birth setting or environment that influence women's choice or options of positions they use during labour. As Rigby (1857) observed more than a century ago, women in labour '... will, in great measure be guided by the arrangements which are made for her confinement and will assume the posture for which they are specially adapted'. These 'arrange-ments', as well as the attitudes and beliefs of birth attendants, might be explored through ethnographic methods to learn how these factors influence the conduct of labour in various settings.

References

Abitol MM (1985). Supine position in labor and associated fetal heart rate changes. Obstet Gynecol, 65: 481–486.

Broadhurst A, Flynn AM, Kelly J, Lynch PF (1979). The effect of ambulation in labour on maternal satisfaction, analgesia and lactation. In: Psychosomatic Medicine in Obstetrics and Gynaecology. Zichella (ed). Rome: 5th International Congress, pp 943–946.

Caldeyro-Barcia R (1978). The influence of maternal position during the first stage of labor. In: Kaleidoscope of Childbearing: Preparation, Birth and Nurturing. Highlights of the 10th Biennial Convention of the International Childbirth Education Association, Inc. Simkin P, Reinke C (eds). Seattle, WA: Pennypress, pp 31–42.

Caldeyro-Barcia R (1979). The influence of maternal position on time of spontaneous rupture of membranes, progress of labor and fetal head compression. Birth Family J, 6: 10–18.

Caldeyro-Barcia R, Noriega-Guerra L, Cibils LA, Alvarez H, Poseiro JJ, Pose SV, Sica-Blanco Y, Mendez-Bauer C, Fielitz C, Gonzalez-Panizza VH (1960). Effect of position changes on the intensity and frequency of uterine contractions during labor. Am J Obstet Gynecol, 80: 284–290.

Calvert JP, Newcombe RG, Hibbard BM (1982). An assessment of radiotelemetry in the monitoring of labour. Br J Obstet Gynaecol, 89: 285–291.

Carlson JM, Diehl JA, Sachtleben-Murray M, McRae M, Fenwick L, Friedman EA (1986). Maternal position during parturition in normal labor. Obstet Gynecol, 68: 443–447.

Chan DP (1963). Positions during labour. Br Med J, 1: 100–102.

Diaz AG, Schwarcz RF, Fescina YR, Caldeyro-Barcia R (1978). Separata de la Revista Clinica e Investigacion en Ginecologia y Obstetricia. Barcelona, Espana: Mayo–Junio, 5:3.

Diaz AG, Schwarcz RF, Caldeyro-Barcia R (1980). Vertical position during the first stage of the course of labor, and neonatal outcome. Eur J Obstet Gynecol Reprod Biol, 11: 1–7.

Eckstein K-L, Marx GF (1974). Aortocaval compression and uterine displacement. Anesthesiology, 40: 92–96.

Flynn AM, Kelly J, Hollins G, Lynch PF (1978). Ambulation in labour. Br Med J, 2: 591–593.

Galbert MW, Marx GF (1974). Extradural pressure in the parturient patient. Anesthesiology, 40: 499–502.

Hemminki E, Saarikoski S (1983). Ambulation and delayed amniotomy in the first stage of labor. Eur J Obstet Gynec Reprod Biol, 15: 129–139.

Howard FH (1951). The physiologic position for delivery. Northwest Med, 50: 98–100.

Howard FH (1954). The application of certain principles of physics to the physiology of delivery. West J Sci Obstet Gynecol, 62: 607–609.

Howard FH (1958). Delivery in the physiologic position. Obstet Gynecol, 11: 318–322.

Irwin HW (1978). Practical considerations for the routine application of left lateral Sims' position for vaginal delivery. Am J Obstet Gynecol, 131: 129–133.

King FA (1909). The significance of posture in obstetrics. New York Med J, 90: 1054–1058.

Liu YC (1974). Effects of an upright position during labor. Am J Nurs, 74: 2202–2205.

Markoe JW (1917). Posture in obstetrics. New York: Bulletin-Lying-In Hospital, 11–26.

McManus TJ, Calder AA (1978). Upright posture and the efficiency of labour. Lancet, 1: 72–74.

Mendez-Bauer C, Arroyo J, Garcia-Ramos C, Mendendez A, Lavilla M, Izquierdo F, Elizaga IV, Zammarriego J (1975). Effects of standing position on spontaneous uterine contractility and other aspects of labor. J Perinat Med, 3: 89–100.

Mendez-Bauer C, Arroya J, Zammarriego (1976a) Maternal standing position in first stage of labor. In: Reviews in Perinatal Medicine, Vol. 1. Scarpelli EM, Cosmi EV (eds). Baltimore: University Park Press.

Mendez-Bauer C, Arroyo J, Menendez A, Salmean J, Manas J, Lavilla M, Martinez San Martin S, Elizaga IV, Zammarriego J (1976b). Effects of different maternal positions during labour. 5th Eur Congr Perinatal Med, Uppsala, Sweden, June 9–12.

Mendez-Bauer C, Arroyo J, Freese U, Garcia-Ramos C, Hundsdorfer P, Izquierdo F, Lavilla M, Manas J, Menendez A, Reina L, Roberts J, Ruiz-Canseco A, Steiner H, Zammarriego-Crespo J (1980). The dynamics of labor in different positions. Paper presented at the 7th Eur Congr Perinatal Med, Barcelona, Spain.

Miller FC, McCart D, Mueller E (1982). Effects of position change during labor on intrauterine resting pressure. J Calif Perinat Assn, 2: 50–52.

Mitre IN (1974). The influence of maternal position on duration of the active phase of labor. Int J Gynaecol Obstet, 12: 181–183.

Newton M (1956). The effect of position on the course of the second stage of labor. Obstet Gynecol, 7: 517–520.

Newton M, Newton N (1960). The propped position for the second stage of labor. Obstet Gynecol, 15: 28–34.

Read JA, Miller FC, Paul RH (1981). Randomized trial of ambulation versus oxytocin for labor enhancement: A preliminary report. Am J Obstet Gynecol, 139: 669–672.

Rigby E (1857). What is the natural position of a woman during labour? Medical Times and Gazette, 15: 345–346.

Roberts J (1980). Alternative positions for childbirth —Part I: First stage of labor. J Nurs Midwifery, 25: 11–18.

Roberts J, Mendez-Bauer C (1980). A perspective of maternal position during labor. J Perinat Med, 8: 255–264.

Roberts J, Malasanos L, Mendez-Bauer C (1981). Maternal

positions in labor: Analysis in relation to comfort and efficiency. March of Dimes Birth Defects Foundation: Original Article Series XVIII: 97–128.

Roberts J, Mendez-Bauer C, Wodell DA (1983). The effects of maternal position on uterine contractility and efficiency. Birth, 10: 243–249.

Roberts J, Mendez-Bauer C, Blackwell J, Carpenter ME, Marchese T (1984). Effects of lateral recumbency and sitting on the first stage of labor. J Reprod Med, 29: 477–482.

Rossi MA, Liddell SG (1986). Maternal positions and pushing techniques in a nonprescriptive environment. J Obstet Gynecol Neonatal Nurs, 15: 203–208.

Ueland K, Hansen JM (1969). Maternal cardiovascular dynamics. II. Posture and uterine contractions. Am J Obstet Gynecol, 103: 1–8.

Williams RM, Thom MH, Studd JWW (1980). A study of the benefits and acceptability of ambulation in spontaneous labour. Br J Obstet Gynaecol, 87: 122–126.

56 Non-pharmacological methods of pain relief during labour

Penny Simkin

1 Beliefs about pain and its relief

Western attitudes toward pain, including childbirth pain, have undergone considerable change over the past several centuries. During the Middle Ages, disease and pain were perceived as punishment for wickedness and sin. Priests officiated at times of sickness, pain, and death, as they did at other major events in peoples' lives: birth, baptism, confirmation, communion, and marriage. They could do little to ease pain or control disease, but they gave comfort (Caton 1985).

Priests also inflicted pain and suffering, in the form of torture and brutal public executions in administering 'justice' or extracting confessions from wrongdoers, witches, and heretics. Pain was perceived as a means of spiritual purification. It was widely accepted that God (and His agents, the priests) controlled sin by inflicting suffering on sinners. Furthermore, if a person, family, or community experienced adversity, such as illness, drought, or epidemic, it was assumed that God was displeased with them and was punishing them. Harshly blaming the sufferer, however, gave way to other interpretations based more on direct observation; many perceived that natural phenomena contributed to, and therefore, could also relieve suffering. They discovered and utilized folk remedies in addition to prayer and reliance upon priests.

Midwives, the traditional birth attendants, drew heavily on their practical knowledge of plants, foods, drugs, poultices, rituals and good luck charms, as well as their wisdom and experience to help women during childbirth (Wertz and Wertz 1977). Such departure from religious doctrine did not go unheeded. Some midwives, even some pious Christians, were condemned as witches and heretics for ignoring or defying the religious customs prevailing during the period (Ehrenreich and English 1973).

With the Renaissance, new attitudes prevailed; thinkers in the Age of Reason questioned accepted dogma, and mastery over Nature became an explicit goal during the Enlightenment. Pain and suffering were no longer passively accepted as the result of sin; they were now perceived as natural phenomena which could be studied, controlled, altered, or wiped out. Pain was now seen to be destructive and unrelated to the deeds or thoughts of the sufferers. The pursuit of pleasure and absence of pain became desirable and both morally and medically acceptable (Caton 1985).

The profession of medicine emerged by separating itself from the Church on the one hand, and from the barber's trade on the other. Until then, surgery was considered a menial and lowly practice, performed by uneducated barbers, who were called in for bloodletting, treating of wounds, tooth extractions, and destruction and removal of fetuses in obstructed labours. Eventually, surgery became a respected and vital part of the repertoire of medicine.

By the mid-nineteenth century, with the introduction of inhalation anaesthesia (chloroform and ether), the means for reducing or obliterating pain became available to contemporary medicine. Although initially there was considerable medical opposition to its use (Wertz and Wertz 1977), this opposition faded when it became obvious that better and more extensive surgery could be performed with anaesthesia.

Chloroform was introduced into childbirth in the mid-nineteenth century, and given a huge boost in acceptance when Queen Victoria used and enjoyed it for the birth of her eighth child in 1853. Twilight sleep, a combination of morphine and scopolamine originating in Germany and well publicized abroad, became a popular method of pain relief for childbirth in the early twentieth century. Women of means and influence travelled to Germany from other European countries and North America in order to give birth with twilight sleep. With their social status, they were able to exert considerable pressure in their home countries to make twilight sleep available to all childbearing women (Sandelowski 1984; Wertz and Wertz 1977).

The steadily increasing use of anaesthesia and pain medication in childbirth from its introduction in the mid-nineteenth century until today has always been accompanied by protests from professional and lay people of varying persuasions, who held the common belief that anaesthesia in childbirth was objectionable. Some based their objections on their belief that the use of anaesthesia was too complex or unsafe. Others felt anaesthesia was morally undesirable because it robbed a woman of the pain considered necessary to ensure that she loved her baby. Some feminists and health advocates believed that a suitable diet and lifestyle were sufficient to ensure painless childbirth. Others retained the earlier church doctrine; they believed the Bible taught that birth pain was a punishment for woman's fall from Grace. Any effort to obliterate the pain of childbirth was perceived as defying God's will. Lastly, some believed that birth, as a natural and normal process, was not inherently painful, and that a woman's beliefs and emotional state were the underlying factors which led to painful perceptions of labour (see Chapter 7).

The use of medications for pain relief spread, however, and some disadvantages of their use began to emerge. Undesirable side-effects and risks occurred even with the proper administration of medications. Scepticism and doubt arose, especially among some segments of the public, giving impetus to the search for alternative methods of pain relief. By the mid-twentieth century the authority to treat pain began to shift from the provider to the woman, or 'client', the person most affected by the pain and its treatment. Over-the-counter drugs which can be self-selected and self-administered have placed relief of pain more in the hands of the sufferer than ever before.

Further evidence of the trend toward non-professional self-treatment of pain can be found in the popularity of alternative, non-pharmacologic methods of pain relief. In no area of medicine has such a trend been more apparent than in the area of childbirth pain. The study of pain transmission and its modulation have produced many exciting new findings in the past twenty-five years which are today being applied in new techniques for relieving pain. In addition, the mechanism of older techniques is now better understood. This chapter contains a discussion of labour pain, a description of many alternative non-pharmacologic methods to relieve it, a theoretical explanation for how these methods might work, and the scientific evidence available about their effectiveness (see also Chapter 57).

2 The complex nature of labour pain

The first step in labour pain perception occurs with activation of sensory receptors in the uterus, cervix and surrounding soft tissue and pelvic joints. Bonica (1984) states that the pain of the first stage of labour is related to the dilatation, distention, and stretching of the cervix and lower uterine segment during contractions, along with stretch and tension and pressure within the bony pelvis. Other writers (Moir 1939; Dick-Read 1953) believed labour pain was caused by ischaemia in the myometrium during contractions, which could be exacerbated by sympathetic hyperactivity secondary to fear and tension. In the second stage, stretching within the pelvis and distention of the perineum and vagina are additional sources of pain. Bonica (1984) also describes referred pain to the dermatomes supplied by the spinal cord segments (T10 to L1 and S2 to S4) that receive input from the uterus, cervix, perineum, and vagina. Thus, a wide area including the low abdomen, low back, perineum, and upper legs represents the area of referred pain.

2.1 Transmission of painful sensation

Painful (noxious) stimuli excite activity in the small, thinly myelinated (A-delta) or unmyelinated (C) afferent nerve fibres, which carry impulses from the site of the painful stimulus to the dorsal horn of the spinal cord. These same fibres transmit innocuous (non-painful) sensations of temperature and pressure as well as pain. Transmission over these fibres is slower than over other more thickly myelinated fibres, a fact which underlies the theoretical explanation for the mechanism of several non-pharmacologic methods of pain relief.

The dorsal horn is a segment of the dorsal column, which extends the entire length of the spinal cord, and receives impulses from all over the body, including the brain. The neurones entering the dorsal horn synapse with other neurones with a variety of functions: some cause reflex motor activity such as 'jumping', muscle tension, or withdrawal; some cause autonomic nervous system activity (the fight or flight response); others ascend through vertical tracts to the reticular formation and limbic system in the brainstem and to the cortex, where conscious recognition, discrimination and interpretation of the stimulus takes place and a response is triggered. Therefore, 'Pain is composed of a distinctive sensation, and the individual's reaction to this sensation, with accompanying emotional overtones, activity in both somatic and autonomic systems, and volitional efforts of avoidance or escape' (Gilman and Winans 1984).

Efforts to modulate pain may be directed toward any one or combination of the components contributing to the perception of pain: (1) avoiding, removing, or diminishing the stimulus causing the pain; (2) providing innocuous sensory stimulation to compete with and inhibit pain awareness; (3) modifying the individual's reaction to the pain; (4) diminishing or replacing the accompanying negative emotional overtones; (5) controlling somatic and autonomic activity. Because of the numerous variables influencing pain sensations and the numerous approaches to pain relief, evaluation of pain-relieving measures is extremely complex and dependent on psychological as well as physical variables. The 'gate control' theory for modulation of pain sensation provides a helpful model for conceptualizing the numerous methods for reducing pain awareness.

2.2 Modification of pain: the gate control theory

The pain message received by the brain is modified in numerous ways between the site of the stimulus (in our example, the contracting uterus or dilating cervix) and the cerebral cortex. The gate control theory of Wall and Melzack (Melzack 1973; Wall 1978) postulates that the dorsal horn in the spinal cord is the site where impulses converge—some excitatory to noxious impulse transmission, and others inhibitory. Depending on the balance of impulses, the conscious perception will be of greater or lesser pain.

While small afferent fibres transmit pain impulses relatively slowly, the large myelinated A fibres which run adjacent to them rapidly transmit innocuous stimuli, such as touch and pressure. These 'fast' fibres activate cells in the substantia gelatinosa of the dorsal horn that inhibit transmission of noxious impulses, thus dampening pain perception at the level of the spinal cord. The faster transmission over these fibres helps to 'close' the gate to pain sensations.

In addition, descending fibres from centres in the brain stem and cortex to the dorsal horn can modulate (increase or decrease) the excitability of the cells which transmit pain information. Therefore, the brain receives messages about injury by way of a gate controlled system which is influenced by (1) injury signals, (2) other types of afferent impulses, and (3) descending control.

Recent findings indicate that synthesis and release of endorphins in the dorsal horn and in higher centres of the brain stem are part of the pain modulation system (Fields and Levine 1984). Endorphins bind to receptor sites at the synapse and are thought to inhibit the transmission of noxious impulses. Thus, according to the gate control theory, one's perception represents the net effect of influences which augment or diminish pain awareness.

Stimuli which are usually interpreted as painful are not perceived as pain under certain conditions. Familiar examples abound: the sportsman or soldier who is injured, but does not even notice the pain when involved in the heat of competition or battle; the headache of which one is unaware when engrossed in a movie or play, but which 'comes back' when it is over; the massage or bath which soothes the aching back or feet. These well-known observations do not lend themselves to easy interpretation and explanation. People respond to pain stimuli in different ways; they even respond differently to the same stimuli at different times and under different circumstances.

Many of the non-pharmacologic methods of pain relief utilized in childbirth take advantage of these varying responses. The methods vary widely in how they affect the nervous system and in how effective they are. They may be classified by the way they alter the transmission of pain impulses or by the way they modify the pain sensation. The general classification is as follows:

1. Techniques which aim to reduce the painful stimuli.
2. Techniques which aim to excite sensory receptors in the skin, bombarding the 'gate' in the dorsal column with competing innocuous stimuli.
3. Techniques which aim to enhance the descending inhibitory pathways from the brain to the synapses in the dorsal horn.

The techniques for alleviating pain to be described in this chapter include: movement and maternal positioning, counterpressure and abdominal decompression, application of heat and cold, hydrotherapy, various kinds of massage, acupuncture and acupressure, transcutaneous electrical nerve stimulation, education, stress reduction, patterned breathing, relaxation, distraction, visualization, attention focusing, audioanalgesia, and hypnosis.

Each of these techniques is claimed to benefit the labouring woman by reducing pain. What is the evidence of their effectiveness? How good is the evidence? How might they alter transmission of pain stimuli?

3 Techniques which reduce painful stimuli

The most obvious solution to the problem of pain is to remove or avoid the stimuli which cause it. If one cannot avoid these stimuli (and few pregnant women can avoid the contractions which cause labour pain), one can use techniques which reduce the painful stimuli elicited by uterine contractions or a particular position of the presenting part. This is the designated purpose of various maternal body positions, movement, counterpressure, and abdominal decompression.

3.1 Maternal movement and position changes

Labouring women find that they experience less pain in some positions than others and if left to their own devices, will select those body positions which are more comfortable. Engelmann (1882) studied labour among primitive peoples by direct observation, library research, and by collecting observations from obstetricians and travellers in foreign countries. He found that women 'whose parturition is governed by instinct and not by modern obstetric custom' tend to labour in more upright or 'inclined' postures as opposed to recumbent or horizontal postures. Atwood's (1976) more recent review confirmed Engelmann's earlier findings (see Chapter 55).

Today's labouring women tend to be restricted to bed because of cultural expectations and obstetric cus-

toms such as electronic fetal monitoring, intravenous hydration, and medications, each of which render movement out of bed difficult or unsafe. Despite these restraints, modern women seem to prefer freedom of movement when it is allowed. Carlson *et al.* (1986) found that when 'given freedom to assume any position in or out of bed during the course of their labour without interference or instruction by attendant personnel', labouring women in their observational study assumed an average of seven to eight positions during labour. They changed positions more frequently in late first stage and second stage than they did earlier in labour. Caldeyro-Barcia (1979) has reported that women spontaneously utilize several upright postures: sitting, standing, and walking. Although women's reasons for changing positions were not sought, it can be assumed that they were far more likely to seek greater comfort than greater discomfort.

Through trial and error and through their instinctive tendency to seek comfort, labouring women learn that some positions (sitting, walking, standing or kneeling and leaning forward) are more comfortable than others, and they naturally prefer those. Certain positions tend to be more comfortable to more women than others. There is, however, no universal acceptance of a particular position or positions by all labouring women. When the mother changes positions, she alters relationships between gravity, the uterine contractions, the fetus, and her pelvis, which may be advantageous in enhancing labour progress and reducing pain (Fenwick and Simkin 1987). For example, pressure of the fetal head against the sacroiliac joint may be relieved if the mother moves from a semi-recumbent to a hands and knees posture. Pain from an occiput posterior position of the fetus may be relieved by rotation of the fetal head which is sometimes accomplished by the same posture, combined with pelvic rocking and abdominal stroking (Andrews 1981).

The effects of maternal position on perceived pain are influenced by a number of factors including fetal size, position, head size and shape, size and shape of the maternal pelvis, quality of uterine contractions. Knowing this, experienced caregivers place trust in the mother's ability to find pain reducing positions. They try not to restrict women, and encourage them to seek comfort, suggesting possible positions and trusting the women's judgement.

Beyond the potential mechanical advantages of alleviating the source of pain, position changes and ambulation also offer distraction and activation of joint receptors as stimuli to compete with pain stimuli for recognition at the level of the cortex (Hilbers and Gennaro 1986).

3.2 Counterpressure

Counterpressure consists of steady strong force applied

to a spot on the low back during contractions, using one's fist, 'heel' of hand, or a firm object. While there are no controlled trials of its effectiveness, it certainly appears to alleviate back pain in the labouring woman. The technique is widely taught in antenatal classes, and testimonials abound from users as to its benefits. It appears to be most effective when a woman suffers extreme back pain which is thought to be related to an occiput posterior position. The steady pressure probably counteracts strain against the sacroiliac ligaments caused by the fetal occiput.

Reasonable speculation suggests that counterpressure probably moves the sacrum slightly, helping to restore a more normal and less painful alignment of the sacrum and ilium.

3.3 Abdominal decompression

Abdominal decompression was introduced in the mid-1950s by the South African obstetrician, O. S. Heyns (1959), as a non-pharmacologic method for shortening labour and reducing labour pain (see Chapter 41). Women were placed in an air-tight plastic bag that enclosed their bodies from the chest down. The bag was connected to a vacuum device which, when activated by the woman, created a negative pressure within the bag; she would increase the negative pressure during, and release it between contractions. Heyns believed that abdominal decompression enhances the efficiency of the uterus by lifting the abdominal wall off the contracting and forward-tilting uterus, thus removing resistance to the contractions. Furthermore, with decompression, the shape of the uterus is altered from ellipsoid to spherical, thus, theoretically, allowing the myometrial fibres in the upper uterine segment to shorten quickly.

Abdominal decompression might reduce pain, partly by altering the uterine contractions and partly by eliminating the source of the pain. Heyns (1959) reported remarkable results, which gained a great deal of attention throughout the British Commonwealth, Europe, and North America. His uncontrolled study comprised 100 primigravidae who used abdominal decompression throughout labour, beginning at one to two centimeters' dilatation. Length of labour was less than 5 hours in half the women, more than 10 hours in only 16. Women's subjective assessments of pain indicated that only 9 had poor pain relief. Pain relief when compared to contractions experienced without decompression was reported by the remainder as complete (2); very good (8); good (42); satisfactory (34); or fair (5).

Similar findings were reported by Scott and Loudon (1960) and Quinn and McKeown (1962), but Shulman and Birnbaum (1966), using 25 labouring women as their own controls, found no benefit in reducing either pain or labour duration. The assessments of pain were made by each woman and her obstetrician; abdominal decompression was used on every other contraction,

and turned off for the contractions between. Furthermore, seven women found the apparatus uncomfortable. They suspended their study after 25 cases, because of the poor initial results they obtained.

Abdominal decompression has now largely disappeared from use, partly because of the lack of good evidence that it is beneficial, but also because the decompression apparatus is cumbersome, constrictive, noisy, uncomfortable, and messy (Editorial 1974).

It was suggested by Dolezal and Hlavaty (1970) that any benefits from abdominal decompression probably stemmed from the relief it brought for the problems it caused. In order to utilize the equipment, women were forced to maintain a supine or semi-recumbent position, which caused supine hypotension, decreased circulation to the uterus and decreased placental perfusion. Abdominal decompression, by lifting the uterus off the aorta and inferior vena cava simply restored the circulation it had impaired. The same explanation may be applied to the decrease in pain. Abdominal decompression probably simply alleviated the pain which had been worsened by the supine position (Roberts *et al.* 1983) and by ischaemia of the uterine muscle secondary to impaired circulation.

4 Techniques which activate peripheral sensory receptors

4.1 Superficial heat and cold

The use of hot compresses applied to the low abdomen, groin, or perineum, a warm blanket over the entire body, or icepacks on the low back, anus, or perineum, relieve pain in labour. The therapeutic use of heat and cold, because of their widespread empirical acceptance and low incidence of harmful side-effects when used reasonably (that is, at safe temperatures that cause neither burns nor frost damage), have not been evaluated in randomized controlled trials.

Superficial heat is generated from hot or warm objects, such as hot water bottles, hot moist towels, electric heating pads, heated silica gel packs, warm blankets, baths, and showers. Superficial cold is generated from ice bags, blocks of ice, frozen silica gel packs, and towels soaked in cool or ice water.

4.1.1 *Mechanism of pain relief achieved with heat or cold*

It is difficult to explain the pain relief achieved by either heat or cold in terms of the gate control theory, because transmission of temperature sensations takes place over the same small neurones that transmit pain stimuli (the A-delta and C fibres) (Gilman and Winans 1984). It is not clear why increasing stimulation of the pain pathways does not result in increased perception of pain. Perhaps by occupying the pain pathways with innocuous or pleasant stimuli along with painful stimuli, the higher brain centres may activate the central biasing mechanism, which, in effect, selects the stimuli which will pass through the pain gate. As hypothesized by Melzack (1973), the higher brain centres discriminate between peripheral heat or cold stimuli and visceral pain stimuli, perceiving heat as a pleasant 'counter-stimulant' or cold as 'counter-irritant'. These counter-stimuli then compete for recognition at the conscious level.

In addition to possible direct effects on pain perception, several well-known physiological responses elicited by heat and cold indirectly result in pain relief. Indirect pain relieving effects may be achieved through reduction of painful muscle spasms or cramps, changes in circulation to an area, a decreased inflammatory response, and relaxation of tiny muscles in the capillaries and hair follicles in the skin. In other words, the application of heat or cold may reverse some conditions that create pain or are associated with it.

Table 56.1 summarizes the physiological effects of heat and cold. As can be seen, heat and cold have the capacity for altering autonomic responses which may be associated with pain or injury, or with anxiety.

As comfort measures, heat and cold are widely accepted, if not fully understood. Because they provide only partial relief from labour pain, they might at best be considered only as adjunct therapy.

4.2 Hydrotherapy: baths and showers

The healing and pain-relieving properties of water— hot or cold, flowing or still, sprayed or poured—have been hailed over the centuries. Although they are a common household remedy for numerous ailments such as aches and pains, sores and burns, fatigue and tension, baths and showers are not available to most women labouring in hospitals. Most obstetric units have few such facilities because they were designed and built when women were routinely confined to bed and

Table 56.1. Physiological effects of heat and cold

Heat	Cold
1. Increased local blood flow	1. Decreased local blood flow
2. Increased local skin and muscle temperature	2. Decreased local skin and muscle temperature
3. Increased tissue metabolism	3. Decreased tissue metabolism
4. Decreased muscle spasm	4. Decreased muscle spasm (longer lasting than heat)
5. Relaxation of tiny muscles in skin (capillaries, hair follicles)	5. Slow transmission of impulses over afferent neurones, leading to decreased sensation
6. Raises pain threshold	

sufficiently drugged to make bathing impossible. While that remains the case to a large extent today, some new birthing facilities provide bath tubs and showers (even whirlpool baths) for labouring women.

4.2.1 Potential benefits of hydrotherapy in labour

Odent (1983), writing about extensive use of the bath by labouring women in his obstetric unit, said, '... Immersion during the second half of the first stage of labour is helpful, particularly for women having painful and inefficient contractions. ... We hope that other experiences would confirm that immersion in warm water is an efficient, easy, and economical way to reduce the use of drugs and the rate of intervention in parturition.'

Brucker (1984) and Brown (1982) advocated hydrotherapy to relieve pain, promote relaxation, reduce psychological tension, and 'decrease the pressure on abdominal muscles, allowing the uterus to contract more efficiently and with better oxygenation' (Brown 1982). This last claimed benefit is similar to one of the benefits attributed to abdominal decompression (see previous section of this chapter).

Smith (1987) described the effects of warm tub baths on 31 low risk women in labour. The women used standard residential tubs with inflatable pillows. Their abdomens were not immersed. They had cold cloths for their foreheads, and water was poured over their abdomens. They left the tub in time for the second stage. She measured 9 variables at 3 times: before the women entered the tub, and 15 and 60 minutes after entering the tub. The time spent in the tub ranged from 12 to 202 minutes (mean 60 minutes). Women left the tub usually either to change position or to deliver.

Mean arterial blood pressure and anxiety level was statistically significantly decreased after 15 minutes in the tub, and remained at the lower level. Maternal pulse and estimated uterine activity decreased after one hour in the tub. Maternal temperature and fetal heart rate did not change with bathing. Pain and distress decreased significantly after 15 minutes, but returned close to the pre-tub level by one hour. Nine primigravidae in active labour dilated at an average rate of 2.7 cm per hour. Smith concluded that warm tub baths in labour are a 'useful and safe practice for low-risk women'. A warm bath, shower or whirlpool bath exerts a soothing action on cutaneous nerve endings, causing vasodilation in the skin, relaxation of tiny muscles in the hair follicles and, generally a reversal of the sympathetic nervous system response (stress or 'fight or flight' response), which frequently arises in labour (Lederman *et al.* 1978). By reducing stress in labour, the bath enhances the woman's sense of well-being and reduces her pain perception (Simkin 1986). The higher brain centres (thalamus and cortex) send inhibitory impulses to the dorsal column to inhibit transmission of pain signals.

Thermal receptors and tactile receptors are activated by immersion in water, and more so by the spray of a shower or the swirling water of the whirlpool bath. Thus, the dorsal column receives stimuli from all over the periphery, and the gate to pain is closed, inhibiting transmission of those impulses to the cortex.

The efficacy of hydrotherapy in reducing labour pain has not been evaluated scientifically. The degree to which hydrotherapy can reduce pain awareness in labour is unknown, although the published empirical observations of Odent (1983) and Brown (1982), and the positive reactions of labouring women to hydrotherapy informally observed by everyone who attends them will ensure continuation of its use.

Controlled trials would be highly desirable, comparing morbidity, length of labour, analgesic use, numbers and types of interventions, and patient satisfaction in groups using and not using hydrotherapy.

4.2.2 Potential adverse effects

Resistance to the idea of immersion in water in prompted by concerns about its safety. If the membranes are ruptured, the possibility exists that bacteria in bath water will enter the vagina and uterus, increasing the likelihood of infection. Odent (1983) reported no infectious complications even when membranes were ruptured. A further concern arises over the comparative inconvenience of monitoring maternal vital signs, contractions, and fetal heart tones with a woman immersed in water or a shower. Although such monitoring is possible (Odent 1983), it is probably less convenient for the staff. The possibility exists that the mother will be unable or unwilling to leave the bath at the time of birth. Odent (1983) has described how this has happened on one hundred occasions in his hospital, with no detectable untoward effects on mother or baby.

Hyperthermia, another potential risk, can be prevented by periodic checking of maternal vital signs and taking appropriate action.

4.3 Touch and massage

The use of touch in various forms conveys pain-reducing messages, depending on the quality and circumstances of the touch. A hand placed on a painful spot, a pat of reassurance, stroking one's hair or cheek in an affectionate gesture, a tight embrace, or more formal purposeful massage techniques—all communicate to the receiver a message of caring, of wanting to be with and help her. While massage is used for numerous purposes other than pain relief, the object of most massage is to make people feel better, or to relieve pain and facilitate relaxation.

Hedstrom and Newton (1986) reported that touch and physical contact during labour are widely practised

in numerous cultures today as they have been in the past. Whereas much of the physical contact in the past and in non-Western cultures is for purposes of position support, massage, and compression of the abdomen to promote descent, in the West today the major purpose is to convey caring and reassurance. Antenatal educators today also teach various forms of touch and massage as pain-relieving measures.

Massage in labour takes numerous forms. Hilbers and Gennaro (1986) describe how various types of massage stimulate different receptors in the skin, increasing neural activity in the larger myelinated fibres. Stimuli are transmitted more rapidly over these pathways than over the pain pathways. The effect of 'bombarding' the central nervous system with innocuous or pleasing stimuli is to bias cortical perceptions away from the awareness of pain. Such competitive large-fibre stimulation probably provides relief for only as long as it is being administered. When discontinued, the woman's awareness of her pain increases. In addition, the phenomenon of adaptation may diminish the pain-relieving effects of massage over a period of time. Therefore, use of intermittent massage, or variation in the type of stroke and location of the touch probably prolongs the pain-reducing effects of massage.

Massage takes the form of light or firm stroking, vibration, kneading, deep circular pressure, continual steady pressure, and joint manipulation. It can be carried out by using fingertips, entire hands, or various devices which roll, vibrate, or apply pressure. In theory, the various forms of massage stimulate different sensory receptors, thus occupying numerous pathways to inhibit pain stimuli at the level of the dorsal horn.

The sense of well-being afforded by soothing touch also reduces pain perception by enhancing the descending inhibitory pathways from the limbic system in the midbrain, where the motivational–affective component of response to pain originates. The autonomic nervous system is controlled by the limbic system; thus, if a woman interprets her sensations as dangerous, painful, or fearful, the limbic system activates a sympathetic response, which facilitates transmission of pain impulses and increases pain perception. In labour, it is easier to prevent than to relieve the effects of a stress response.

How effective are touch and massage in controlling or relieving pain? Are women less likely to require pain medications if they receive touch and massage during labour than if they do not? These questions have not been pursued in a systematic way, although experience strongly suggests that touch and massage relieve many types of pain. Penny (1979) interviewed 150 women and Birch (1986) interviewed 30 nurse midwifery clients within two days after they gave birth, asking them about their perceptions of touch received during labour. The results of the two surveys were very similar. All subjects felt the touch they had received was positive (except for abdominal palpation and vaginal exams); most stated that touch helped them cope with labour. Rubbing, holding, pressure, and patting were the types of touch most often described as helpful. Most said they felt less or somewhat less pain when they were touched. Nearly half stated their husbands or relatives were the people providing the therapeutic touch; the midwife and nurse were also identified by a significant minority. In Penny's survey, the doctor who did vaginal exams was identified most often as one providing 'negative touch'. When asked to describe the meaning of positive touch, more than 80 per cent reported the following: being supported, comforted, cared for, reassured, safe, accepted, encouraged, understood, closer to the person touching them, and able to rely on that person.

As for negative effects of touch, besides those mentioned above, many women in Birch's study reported that their perception of the therapeutic value of touch changed as labour progressed. Most reported that touch was perceived as less helpful with the passage of time. Rubbing and massaging were the types of touch most likely to diminish in benefit.

Both these authors emphasized that touch is a powerful means of non-verbal communication and encouraged caregivers to use touch as a means of providing reassurance and caring, and not only as a method for accomplishing procedures.

In their review, Hedstrom and Newton (1986) described two unpublished theses (Sommer 1979; Saltenis 1962) in which the effects of reassuring touch during labour contractions were compared with no use of touch. Sommer (1979) randomly assigned 90 women to either an experimental group who, during a 30-minute period in late first stage, received the routine care plus a reassuring light touch on the hand for 5 to 10 seconds each time they expressed anxiety, or to a control group who received routine nursing care. She found statistically significantly less anxiety in the experimental group, as expressed in blood pressure readings, verbal expressions of anxiety stated during the late first stage of labour, and women's self reports completed within four hours of delivery.

Saltenis (1962) compared women's ability to work with their contractions in an experimental group receiving touch and a control group not receiving touch from the nurse. The experimental group fared better.

Another form of 'touch', referred to somewhat deceptively as 'therapeutic touch', does not necessarily include physical contact between healer and patient. As described by Krieger (1975), it is the 'simple placing of the hands for about 10 to 15 minutes on or close to the body of an ill person by someone who intends to help or heal that person'.

The technique is based on the premise that each person is surrounded by an energy field which can be assessed and altered by the hands of the healer. The field of a person in pain can theoretically be 'unruffled' and pain reduced if the healer moves her hands in stroking motions a few inches away from the body. This approach, as strange as it seems to those who embrace the Western approach to pain and illness, is arousing interest, not only among alternative health care providers, but in university medical settings as well (Krieger *et al.* 1979).

None of the touch or massage techniques has been subjected to careful scientific investigation. The apparently harmless intervention is well received by labouring women and easily discontinued if she wishes; therefore, it seems unlikely to occupy a high priority in anyone's list of research questions.

4.4 Acupuncture and acupressure

Acupuncture, as practised in China for over 2500 years, consists of the insertion of strategically placed needles in any of more than 365 points along the twelve meridians of the body. It treats disease and pain by correcting 'blockages, excesses, or imbalances in the flow of the vital life force' (Bonica 1974). Acupuncture therapy derives from ancient Chinese philosophy, in which man is perceived as a microcosmic image of the universe, subject to the same tensions and disruptions of Yin and Yang as nature itself. Beginning in 1958, under Mao Tse-tung's direction, the application of acupuncture was broadened to include analgesia for surgery and childbirth. Today it is combined with electrical current, which is stated to augment the pain-relieving effect. It is only since the Cultural Revolution that Western physicians have taken acupuncture seriously as a therapy. Renewed contact between Westerners and the Chinese has brought efforts to understand and evaluate Chinese medical customs in the context of the Western scientific approach.

The precise technique of obstetric acupuncture varies among practitioners in selection of points, size of needle, and method of insertion. Some operators stimulate traditional acupuncture points and others use points in the dermatomes supplied by the same spinal cord segments that supply the cervix and pelvis (Bonica 1974). Abouleish and Depp (1975) utilized electroacupuncture at eight points for first stage: four on the abdomen, one on the hand, and three on the leg below the knee. For the second stage, points were located in the perineal body and behind the anus, with two 'accessory' points beside the vagina. The authors complained that the needles placed in these points were in the way, restricted maternal movement, and tended to become dislodged. They called for further studies to find fewer and more effective points further away from the uterus and perineum.

4.4.1 *Mechanism for pain relief with acupuncture*

Acupuncture appears to block both sensory and emotional components of pain, but the mechanism at work is complex and poorly understood. There are several hypotheses offered by Westerners trying to apply their mode of thinking to this mysterious technique.

Chapman (1984) described acupuncture as having a strong psychological component, which he feels is largely responsible for the analgesic effects. The technique is not used routinely for all women. After patients are carefully selected, they are thoroughly prepared physically, mentally, and emotionally for the procedure. In fact, Chapman draws a parallel between preparation for acupuncture and preparation for childbirth. He cites the following features shared by the two: provision of information about the forthcoming procedures and expected sensations; social support and moment-by-moment coaching; accounts of successful pain control and testimonials from others who have utilized the procedures; and relaxation techniques.

Those receiving acupuncture analgesia, then, may have considerable prior faith in the effectiveness of the technique (Melzack 1975). Put in the terms of the gate control theory, the higher brain centres transmit strong inhibitory impulses to the dorsal horn, serving to close the gate to pain. Melzack (1973) suggested that acupuncture activates a central biasing mechanism in the brainstem, which stimulates descending inhibitory impulses to block synaptic transmission in the pain pathways. This hypothesis is consistent with another, which proposes that endogenous opioid production (known to occur either in the pituitary or the periaqueductal grey matter located in the brainstem) is enhanced with acupuncture and blocked by the narcotic antagonist, naloxone (Pomeranz and Chiu 1976; and Yang and Kok 1979).

Another hypothesis suggests that acupuncture causes presynaptic inhibition of sensory fibres at the level of the dorsal horn, by activating large diameter afferent fibres, thus closing the gate to pain. Since many acupuncture points lie in dermatomal relationship with the site of pain, this hypothesis makes theoretical sense.

In an attempt to further clarify the mechanism by which acupuncture reduces pain, Yang, Cai, and Wu (1984) compared the inhibitory effects of acupuncture on separate sensory and emotional components of pain. Using nine volunteers, they established the intensity of electrical stimulation of the sural nerve required to achieve each of seven sensory levels for each person: touch, the sensory threshold; slight numbness; severe numbness; slight pain (pain threshold); medium pain; intense pain (threshold of unbearable pain); extreme unbearable pain. Emotional components were evaluated as well through subjects' reports of what they felt and observation of their overt behaviour (language,

actions, and facial expression). In addition, the character and extent of sweating were noted.

Electroacupuncture was then applied for thirty minutes to the sural nerve proximal to the pain source, while repeating the electrical stimulation. The pain stimulus was continued for another thirty minutes after electroacupuncture was discontinued.

Both the sensory and emotional components of pain were markedly inhibited during acupuncture, and although sensory components reverted to the original when acupuncture was stopped, the emotional component (or degree of emotional upset with the pain) remained as low as it had been with acupuncture. According to the authors, 'The subjects could bear the stimulus of intense pain mainly because electroacupuncture had improved the emotional experience of pain and reduced the reactions associated with negative emotion: nervousness, dread, ill-ease, anxiety. Accordingly, the endurance of pain rose.'

4.4.2 *Effectiveness of acupuncture for relief of labour pain*

Acupuncture during labour has not been well or frequently studied, and no controlled trials have been published, despite indications that it might provide good analgesia. A recently published well-designed trial of acupuncture for management of primary dysmenorrhea (Helms 1987) indicated considerable improvement in a group of eleven women receiving real acupuncture for three months when compared with a placebo acupuncture group of women (where needles were placed on points other than acupuncture points), a standard control group of women, and a visitation control group of women (who saw their doctor frequently, but had no acupuncture treatment). The real acupuncture group reduced their medication use by an average of 41 per cent at the end of the study period. No other group changed their medication use. The relevance of these findings to childbirth pain is unclear. Long-term use of acupuncture, as done in this study, differs from the acute use in labour, and may produce better results.

Descriptive studies of acupuncture for relief of pain in labour have given little useful information. Of 15 women to whom he administered electroacupuncture during labour, Ledergerber (1976) reported that six had total relief of pain in labour and birth, and three had total relief in labour but required a small amount of novocaine around the rectum during delivery. In the six remaining women, acupuncture was unsuccessful. Abouleish and Depp (1975) utilized electroacupuncture during childbirth with twelve women and produced an 'average of sixty per cent analgesia' in active labour in seven women. In the other five, four received no pain relief and one discontinued very early because of her dislike of the needles. Ten of the eleven received regional anaesthesia. Nine were 'delighted' with the experiment and wanted acupuncture for future deliveries, because they received no drugs and were alert and free from after effects. This degree of satisfaction seems surprising because each woman had eight needles inserted in her abdomen, hand, and leg. Although the authors of the study found acupuncture impractical, time-consuming, restrictive of the woman, and interfering with electronic fetal monitoring, nine of twelve women were pleased with it.

The techniques involved in the use of acupuncture are complex and time-consuming, and the use of multiple needles attached to electrical stimulators is inconvenient and immobilizing to the woman. Its use in labour has not garnered a great deal of interest, and it is doubtful that interest will grow significantly in Western nations.

4.4.3 Acupressure

Acupressure has been called 'acupuncture without needles' (McCaffery 1979). The technique, also called shiatsu, involves the application of pressure or deep massage to the traditional acupuncture points, with thumb, fingertip, fingernail, or palm of hand. Practitioners who use acupressure assume that it works by raising local endorphin levels in the treated area, or possibly by activating the central biasing mechanism in the brain to inhibit painful stimuli. This has never been substantiated. In fact, the only references to acupressure for obstetrical application seem to exist in the lay literature (Jungman 1982; Jiminez 1983; Ohashi and Hoover 1983; Lieberman 1987). Only the barest mention can be found in medical and nursing literature.

The 'New Lamaze method', an adaptation of the Lamaze method, now includes the teaching of acupressure for discomforts of pregnancy and for control of anxiety, back pain in labour and ineffective contractions (Jungman 1982; Jimenez 1983). Specific pain-relieving shiatsu techniques for labour described by Ohashi and Hoover (1983) include thumb pressure at strategic points of the sacrum, occiput, and medial surface of the tibia. Sometimes combined with vibratory massage, shiatsu is applied for five to ten seconds at a time and repeated several times.

Reports of effectiveness, either anecdotal or scientific, are lacking in the literature at this time. Acupressure is easy to learn and can be applied by a non-professional companion of the labouring woman. Formal evaluation of its effectiveness would be worthwhile to establish its place (if any) as a comfort measure for labour.

4.5 Transcutaneous electrical nerve stimulation (TENS)

Transcutaneous electrical nerve stimulation (TENS) is a method of pain management which is non-invasive, portable, easy to use, and quickly discontinued if necessary. Utilized originally for the relief of chronic pain, trauma, and postsurgical pain, transcutaneous electrical nerve stimulation has recently been introduced on a small scale for pain relief in labour.

The transcutaneous electrical nerve stimulation unit consists of a hand-held box containing the battery-powered generator of electrical impulses, some characteristics of which (pulse width, frequency, and amplitude or intensity) may be varied. A low-voltage electric current is transmitted to the skin via surface electrodes, which results in a 'buzzing' or tingling sensation. The therapist may preset certain characteristics; the labouring woman may vary some, such as the intensity, pulse frequency, and patterns of stimulation, so that she can increase, decrease, or pulse the sensations as she wishes.

Most transcutaneous electrical nerve stimulation units used in obstetrics contain two channels, each of which is connected to an independently controlled pair of electrodes. Thus the woman may experience different sensations from the two pairs of electrodes. Quality of sensation is also varied by the placement and the size of the electrodes. When the intensity of electrical stimulation increases, the sensation of buzzing or tingling intensifies and the muscles beneath the electrodes may contract involuntarily. Intensity can reach painful levels, especially if the electrodes are small in area.

Usually, the transcutaneous electrical nerve stimulation unit is set just below the pain threshold intensity of the woman. This level remains continuous between contractions. During contractions, the woman or her partner may increase the intensity to a level which competes successfully with the pain of her contraction.

In all reported investigations of transcutaneous electrical nerve stimulation for labour, one pair of electrodes was placed paravertebrally at the level of T10 to L1, to correspond to the spinal segments where the afferents, carrying painful stimuli from the uterus, enter the spinal cord. The second pair of electrodes was placed either paravertebrally at S2 to S4 (Augustinsson *et al.* 1977; Erkkola *et al.* 1980; Bundsen *et al.* 1981; Miller Jones 1980; Nesheim 1981; Harrison *et al.* 1986) or at either the sacral or suprapubic sites (Robson 1979; Bundsen *et al.* 1982a; Grim and Morey 1985).

Safety concerns have focused on theoretically possible effects of high intensity transcutaneous electrical nerve stimulation on the fetus's heart function, especially when electrodes are placed on the low abdomen close to the fetus. Further concerns arose when interference with electronic fetal monitor tracings were reported by Augustinsson *et al.* (1977); Erkkola *et al.* (1980); Robson (1979); Grim and Morey (1985); and Bundsen *et al.* (1981).

Though no untoward effects on the fetus have been reported, there has been only one investigation of the safety aspects of transcutaneous electrical nerve stimulation, especially as applied to the fetus. Bundsen and Ericson (1982) proposed and studied a preliminary safety norm for transcutaneous electrical nerve stimulation. In 15 supervised births, they established a limit or maximum current density level at 0.5 microampere per square millimetre when transcutaneous electrical nerve stimulation is used in the suprapubic region, and there were no adverse fetal effects. In addition, they tested a filter to suppress the electrical disturbances of the electronic fetal monitor, which had previously occurred.

Less concern has been raised when electrodes are placed only on the back, which is where they have been placed in most studies.

4.5.1 Pain-relieving mechanisms of TENS

Transcutaneous electrical nerve stimulation is thought to work by bombarding the large-diameter afferent fibres with innocuous stimuli, thus closing the gate to pain. Furthermore, evidence suggests that levels of endorphins are increased in cerebrospinal fluid after low frequency and high intensity transcutaneous electrical nerve stimulation (Sjolund *et al.* 1977; Sjolund and Eriksson 1979).

4.5.2 Effectiveness of TENS

Transcutaneous electrical nerve stimulation for childbirth pain, although hardly ever used clinically, has been subjected to more controlled trials than any of the other modalities discussed in this chapter. This somewhat surprising situation can perhaps be explained by the fact that transcutaneous electrical nerve stimulation was conceptualized in the laboratory by scientists whose vocations centre on understanding pain mechanisms. Most other non-pharmacologic methods of pain relief are based on age-old beliefs, discovered through trial and error and handed down through the generations. Scientific validation of their effectiveness has yet to be established. Transcutaneous electrical nerve

stimulation, however, is one modality that has been extensively tested before being widely adopted. Ironically the results of the trials still remain inconclusive as to the value of transcutaneous electrical nerve stimulation for labour pain.

To date there have been at least four randomized controlled trials of transcutaneous electrical nerve stimulation in labour (Erkkola *et al.* 1980; Nesheim 1981; Bundsen *et al.* 1982a; Harrison *et al.* 1986). In summary, the pooled overviews suggest paradoxical conclusions: that the effect of transcutaneous nerve stimulation is to increase the incidence of reported intense pain (Table 56.2), yet to decrease the likelihood of use of epidural anaesthesia (Table 56.3), and to be favourably assessed by the women who use it (Table 56.4). It has no obvious effect on the use of other forms of analgesia (Table 56.5).

Harrison *et al.* (1986) carried out the only randomized double-blind placebo-controlled trial of transcutaneous electrical nerve stimulation reported to date. They studied 100 primigravidae (49 in transcutaneous electrical nerve stimulation group; 51 in transcutaneous electrical nerve stimulation placebo group) and 50 para 2, gravida 3 women (27 in transcutaneous electrical nerve stimulation group; 23 in transcutaneous electrical nerve stimulation placebo group). The results of this, the methodologically best trial, coincided with those of the pooled overviews.

Although the difference in frequency of the most intense pain scores between the groups was not statistically significant, there was a strong trend towards increased pain in the women who had the transcutaneous electrical nerve stimulation, and this also agreed with independent assessments made by the midwives. (The increased pain observed did become statistically significant when the results of all trials were pooled— see Table 56.2.) They found no statistically significant differences in the proportion of women who used no other analgesia besides transcutaneous electrical nerve stimulation or placebo. Among the primigravidae, 6/49

Table 56.2 Effect of transcutaneous electrical nerve stimulus (TENS) in labour on incidence of 'intense pain'

Study	EXPT		CTRL		Odds ratio	Graph of odds ratios and confidence intervals						
	n	(%)	*n*	(%)	(95% CI)	0.01	0.1	0.5	1	2	10	100
Harrison *et al.* (1986)	63/64	(98.44)	55/59	(93.22)	3.77 (0.63–22.44)							
Erkkola *et al.* (1980)	43/100	(43.00)	17/100	(17.00)	3.43 (1.87–6.27)							
Nesheim (1981)	10/35	(28.57)	18/35	(51.43)	0.39 (0.15–1.01)							
Bundsen *et al.* (1982a)	8/15	(53.33)	5/9	(55.56)	0.92 (0.18–4.65)							
Typical odds ratio (95% confidence interval)					1.82 (1.14–2.91)							

Table 56.2 Effect of transcutaneous electric nerve stimulation (TENS) in labour on use of epidural anaesthesia

Study	EXPT		CTRL		Odds ratio	Graph of odds ratios and confidence intervals						
	n	(%)	*n*	(%)	(95% CI)	0.01	0.1	0.5	1	2	10	100
Harrison *et al.* (1986)	15/76	(19.74)	26/76	(34.21)	0.48 (0.24–0.98)							
Erkkola *et al.* (1980)	0/100	(0.00)	0/100	(0.00)	1.00 (1.00–1.00)							
Nesheim (1981)	1/35	(2.86)	2/35	(5.71)	0.50 (0.05–5.00)							
Bundsen *et al.* (1982a)	0/15	(0.00)	0/9 (0.00)	1.00	(1.00–1.00)							
Typical odds ratio (95% confidence interval)					0.48 (0.24–0.96)							

Table 56.4 Effect of transcutaneous electric nerve stimulation (TENS) in labour on unfavourable assessment of procedure

Study	EXPT		CTRL		Odds ratio	Graph of odds ratios and confidence intervals						
	n	(%)	*n*	(%)	(95% CI)	0.01	0.1	0.5	1	2	10	100
Harrison *et al.* (1986)	16/76	(21.05)	52/74	(70.27)	0.14 (0.07–0.26)							
Nesheim (1981)	10/35	(28.57)	16/35	(45.71)	0.48 (0.19–1.27)							
Typical odds ratio (95% confidence interval)					0.20 (0.12–0.35)							

Table 56.5 Effect of transcutaneous electric nerve stimulation (TENS) in labour on use of analgesia in labour

Study	EXPT		CTRL		Odds ratio	Graph of odds ratios and confidence intervals						
	n	(%)	*n*	(%)	(95% CI)	0.01	0.1	0.5	1	2	10	100
Harrison *et al.* (1986)	57/76	(75.00)	58/74	(78.38)	0.83 (0.39–1.76)							
Erkkola *et al.* (1980)	23/100	(23.00)	14/100	(14.00)	1.81 (0.89–3.69)							
Nesheim (1981)	35/35	(100.0)	35/35	(100.0)	1.00 (1.00–1.00)							
Bundsen *et al.* (1982a)	13/15	(86.67)	9/9	(100.0)	0.19 (0.01–3.51)							
Typical odds ratio (95% confidence interval)					1.18 (0.71–1.97)							

(12 per cent) of the women in the transcutaneous electrical nerve stimulation group and 7/51 (14 per cent) of the placebo group used no other analgesia. In the multigravidae, 13/27 (48 per cent) of the transcutaneous electrical nerve stimulation and 9/23 (39 per cent) of the placebo group took no other analgesia. The authors explained that at their hospital self-administered nitrous oxide (Entonox) was readily available and routinely accepted by many women. If use of Entonox is disregarded, the proportion of primigravidae not using other analgesia rises to 20/49 (41 per cent) and 12/51 (24 per cent) in the transcutaneous electrical nerve stimulation and placebo group respectively. For multigravidae the proportions were 22/27 (81 per cent) and 15/23 (65 per cent) respectively.

Use of epidural analgesia was lower in the transcutaneous electrical nerve stimulation group than the control (Table 56.3); all but 3 epidurals were used by primigravida. The women's postpartum assessments of transcutaneous electrical nerve stimulation were more favourable in the transcutaneous electrical nerve stimulation groups compared to the placebo groups (Table 56.4). 38/49 (78 per cent) of the transcutaneous electrical nerve stimulation primigravidae and 25/35 (81 per cent) of the transcutaneous electrical nerve stimulation multigravidae had favourable assessments of transcutaneous electrical nerve stimulation, compared with 15/51 (29 per cent) and 7/23 (30 per cent) of the women in the placebo groups.

In Nesheim's (1981) placebo-controlled, but unblinded, study a wide variety of analgesics was available and extensively used by all the women in both groups, but the women's assessments of pain relief and of transcutaneous electrical nerve stimulation's value were more positive in the transcutaneous electrical nerve stimulation group than the placebo group. Although paracervical block was used for more (20/35) women in the placebo group than in the active treatment group (10/35), the author believed that this was primarily due to observer bias, 'the midwives tending to pity the patients receiving mock stimulation'. She concluded '. . . no clinically significant beneficial effects of transcutaneous nerve stimulation during labour could be demonstrated in this study.'

A smaller randomized trial by Bundsen *et al.* (1982a) compared the effects of transcutaneous electrical nerve stimulation on 15 induced labours with 9 induced controls, finding a trend towards less analgesia use in the former.

Erkkola *et al.* (1980) studied 100 labouring women with transcutaneous electrical nerve stimulation, comparing them to a randomly selected group of 100 without transcutaneous electrical nerve stimulation. At all phases of labour, the transcutaneous electrical nerve stimulation group rated their pain higher than the control group, and they used more analgesia. Despite this, 86 of the transcutaneous electrical nerve stimulation group judged transcutaneous electrical nerve stimulation to have provided good or moderate pain relief!

In addition to the randomized trials, a number of uncontrolled studies (Shealy and Maurer 1974; Andersson *et al.* 1976; Robson 1979; Stewart 1979; Grim and Morey 1985) and non-randomized cohort studies (Miller Jones 1980; Bundsen *et al.* 1981) have also yielded conflicting results, no doubt reflecting the characteristics of the women who chose the modality as much as its effectiveness *per se.*

These trials suggest that some women tend to find transcutaneous electrical nerve stimulation helpful in labour, but that it does not stand alone as an adequate method of pain relief. The question remains as to whether transcutaneous electrical nerve stimulation's effectiveness might be improved if it were used differ-ently, with different physical parameters, and different electrode size and placement, or if it were used more in conjunction with antenatal preparation and other non-pharmaceutical pain-relieving measures.

5 Techniques which enhance descending inhibitory pathways

These techniques include education about the birth process and what to expect, along with re-education or indoctrination to a perception of birth as a normal healthy process. The pain of birth is presented as 'different from ordinary pain . . . "positive" or "functional" pain, "pain with a purpose" or "creative pain" ' (Kitzinger 1978). Goals of childbirth education include imparting knowledge and helping women achieve a sense of confidence and optimism in their abilities to give birth, along with competence in the use of specific comfort measures. Their partners are trained to help and to use specific pain relieving measures. Thus, the cognitive and evaluative abilities of the woman are enlisted in the effort to reduce pain perception.

If one is fearful or anxious, the descending afferent pathways facilitate transmission of pain impulses to the cortex, thus opening the gate to pain. Measures to inhibit autonomic arousal, which takes place at the midbrain level—the relaxation response to pain—are incorporated to combat pain perception.

Emotional support (see Chapter 49), a comfortable environment, presence of loved ones, relaxation techniques, hypnosis, and visualization all contribute to a woman's sense of wellbeing, and help close the gate to pain.

The subcortical levels of the brain—the limbic system and reticular formation where autonomic arousal and primitive responses to pain originate—contain heavy concentrations of endogenous opioid receptors, which suggests that the mechanism of pain inhibition at this level involves release of endorphins or similar substances.

The effectiveness of the cognitive techniques taught in conventional antenatal classes are discussed elsewhere in this book (see Chapter 20). Here, other specific techniques which enhance the descending inhibitory pathways and thus reduce pain—attention-focusing, hypnosis, audioanalgesia and music—will be discussed.

5.1 Attention-focusing and distraction
Numerous methods exist for coping with pain by involving the conscious participation of the individual in attention-focusing or mind-diverting activities designed to 'take one's mind off the pain'. Utilizing the principles of the gate control theory, such strategies close the gate to pain by bombarding the synapses at the

dorsal horn with impulses from the cortex that inhibit transmission of pain stimuli.

Attention-focusing may be accomplished by deliberate intentional activities on the part of the labouring woman. Examples include patterned breathing, attention to verbal coaching, visualization and self-hypnosis, performing familiar tasks such as grooming and eating, and concentration on a visual, auditory, tactile, or other stimulus.

Distraction may be a more passive form of attention-focusing, with stimuli from the environment or from other people drawing a woman's attention from her pain. Television, a walk out of doors, background music, or soothing tones of voice stimulate receptors in the brain which also send inhibitory messages to the dorsal horn. Distraction does not require as much mental concentration as deliberate attention-focusing measures and is probably ineffective when pain is severe.

Attention-focusing and distraction are usually used in combination with other strategies. Discussion of the effectiveness of attention-focusing is included in the chapter on antenatal classes (Chapter 20).

5.2 Hypnosis

Hypnosis was introduced into obstetrics in the early nineteenth century and has been used on a limited scale and in various ways ever since. While the popularity and acceptability of hypnosis in childbirth have fluctuated, it seems to have been most widely accepted by the medical profession in the 1950s and 60s, as indicated by the number of papers appearing in the medical literature during that period.

Hypnosis is defined as 'a temporarily altered state of consciousness, in which the individual has increased suggestibility' (Vardurro and Butts 1982). Under hypnosis a person demonstrates the following characteristics: physical and mental relaxation (deeper than can be achieved without hypnosis); increased focus of concentration; ability to modify perception; ability to modify (increase or decrease) memory; ability to control normally uncontrollable physiological responses (such as blood pressure, blood flow, heart rate, and the healing process; and trance logic (tolerance of logical inconsistencies) (Olson 1984).

Hypnosis is used in two ways to control pain perception in childbirth: self-hypnosis and post-hypnotic suggestion. Most hypnotherapists teach self-hypnosis, so that women may enter a trance during labour and reduce awareness of painful sensations. Among the techniques used are: relaxation; visualization (helping the woman imagine a pleasant, safe scene and placing herself there, symbolizing her pain as an object that can be discarded, or picturing herself as in control or free of pain); distraction (focusing on something other than the pain); glove anaesthesia (through suggestion, creating a

feeling of numbness in one of her hands, and then spreading that numbness wherever she wishes by placing her numb hand on the desired places of her body). The woman is taught to induce these techniques herself; only rarely do hypnotherapists accompany their clients in labour.

Other therapists rely almost completely on post-hypnotic suggestion. They use 'hypnoreflexogenous techniques', which combine hypnosis and Lamaze training, giving the women post-hypnotic suggestions that will allay their fears about the pain and difficulty of labour, and modify their interpretation of and reaction to contractions. The labouring woman will be 'relaxed, fearless, happily expectant' (Werner *et al.* 1982). These hypnotherapists do not teach their clients to enter a hypnotic state routinely during labour, because they will not need to. Most, they claim, will be comfortable as a result of the effectiveness of the post-hypnotic suggestions. Exceptions to this are extraordinary circumstances such as forceps delivery or episiotomy and repair, under which it would be necessary to go into a trance.

The mechanism by which hypnosis alters the labouring woman's perceptions of pain during contractions and descent of the presenting part continues to puzzle both its advocates and its critics. According to the gate control theory, hypnosis works at the level of the cortex and brainstem. By reinterpreting painful stimuli as benign sensations, the brain centres send impulses that keep the gate from opening. Hypnosis influences the cortex and lower brain centres to replace the usual pain messages (which can increase pain perception by opening the gate to pain impulses) with messages of calm and well-being (which close the gate). The autonomic nervous system response is also dampened, and stress hormones (adrenalin, dopamine, and cortisol) which increase pain perception are not produced as they usually are in labour. Therefore, through hypnosis, deep relaxation can be achieved, along with inhibition of the stress response and alteration of the perception of contractions from being painful or frightening to being a 'pleasant hardening' (Werner *et al.* 1982) of the uterine muscle. The 'gate' to pain is thus closed by the bombardment from above by innocuous impulses.

5.2.1 *Effectiveness of hypnosis*

Just how effective is hypnosis in reducing pain in childbirth? To date, only one prospective randomized trial of hypnosis in labour (Freeman *et al.* 1986) has been reported. This trial evaluated the effect of self-hypnosis on pain relief, satisfaction, and analgesic requirements for women in their first labour. Eighty-two primigravidae were randomly allocated to either a hypnosis group or a control group. Both groups received routine antenatal classes; the 42 women in the hypnosis group were also seen individually each week for hypnosis training in relaxation and pain relief.

Thirteen women were ultimately excluded for obstetrical reasons (9 in the hypnosis group and 4 in the control), and an additional 4 women were excluded from the hypnosis group for failure to attend for hypnosis training, leaving 29 women in the hypnosis group and 36 in the control group for the subsequent analysis. Hypnotic depth was assessed in the experimental group: 5 women were good hypnotic subjects; 19 moderate; and 5 poor.

There was no difference in analgesia use between the two groups; 15/29 (52 per cent) of the hypnosis group were 'very satisfied' with labour, compared to 8/36 (23 per cent) of the control group ($p = 0.08$), but of course the women were aware of the group to which they had been allocated.

The mean duration of pregnancy (39.9 weeks versus 39.3 weeks) and mean duration of labour (12.4 hours versus 9.7 hours) were both statistically significantly longer in the hypnosis group ($p < 0.05$), although in neither case did the longer times reach levels of clinical concern. Similar findings have been reported elsewhere; in fact, hypnosis has been utilized in an attempt to stop preterm labour in the belief that one cause of preterm labour is psychosocial stress (see Chapter 15), which Omer *et al.* (1986) claim can be reduced through hypnosis. Werner *et al.* (1982) also reported longer labours among their patients, and asked, 'Why should labour be hurried and intense?'. Since the time factor alone is not of clinical concern as long as mother and fetus are in good condition, it is possible that a longer labour may be better paced for the mother, providing more rest between contractions without raising her levels of anxiety or pain.

In their 1982 review article on hypnosis in obstetrics, Werner *et al.* cited eight studies which found striking reductions in the amount of chemical analgesia used in labour by women who used hypnosis when compared with various norms; ten reports of lower perceived pain in women using hypnosis; and five reports of reduced anxiety before and during labour in women using hypnosis. Although the findings are impressive, these uncontrolled studies are subject to bias in subject selection, analysis, and observation.

Hypnosis appears to have lost its popularity among obstetricians by the early 1970s, probably due to a combination of factors that had little to do with demonstrated safety or effectiveness: the development of better methods of anaesthesia (see Chapter 57) and the amount of time required for adequate hypnosis preparation. In addition, the Council on Mental Health of the American Medical Association (1958) and the American Psychiatric Association (1961) issued warnings that hypnosis is a powerful and potentially harmful technique, which should be used only by physicians with extensive postgraduate psychiatric training. Even

though there were few cited examples of harm done by hypnosis (e.g. dangers to patients' mental health, alleged sexual improprieties), these statements acted as a further deterrent. Since few obstetricians had psychiatric training, many withdrew their use of hypnosis in favour of other less controversial or less 'dangerous' methods.

5.3 Music and audioanalgesia

Music and audioanalgesia are used to control pain in numerous situations, including dental work, post-operative pain, treatment of burns, and occasionally in childbirth. Many childbirth educators use music in antenatal classes to create a peaceful and relaxing environment, and also advocate it for use during labour as an aid to relaxation. They suggest that expectant parents select music that the mother finds soothing, rehearse relaxation to tape recordings of that music, and then play them in labour, as one way to reinforce their ability to relax under the duress of labour.

Music therapists have advocated that music in labour be used for more than achieving a calm environment. They suggest that properly chosen music (pleasing to the mother and containing appropriate rhythms) reinforces the mother's efforts at patterned breathing, assists with relaxation, and provides distraction from discomfort and disturbing hospital sounds (Hanser *et al.* 1983). Other pain specialists advocate the use of audioanalgesia in various pain situations, including childbirth. This involves the use of white noise (sound consisting of all frequencies, suggesting the noise of a waterfall or the ocean) the volume of which can be controlled by the person in pain. Theoretically, the white noise dampens other incoming stimuli from the environment and from other parts of the body, thus decreasing pain perception.

5.3.1 The pain control mechanism of music and audioanalgesia

The gate control theory, when applied in the case of auditory stimulation, would explain the pain-relieving mechanism in terms of enhancement of descending inhibitory pathways. Probably a variety of factors are at play: distraction, if the music or sound is loud enough or compelling enough for the subject to be consciously aware of it; endorphin production, if the music is well liked, pleasing or familiar to the subject; relaxing, if the sound or music is soothing and is associated with pleasant memories; and reinforcing of other behaviours, such as rhythmic breathing.

Both music and white noise, alone or in combination, have been studied for their effectiveness in reducing childbirth pain. Obstetrical applications were inspired by the success in controlling dental pain reported during the 1950s, before the use of local anaesthesia or nitrous oxide for dental procedures became routine.

5.3.2 Audioanalgesia

Audioanalgesia for pain relief in obstetrics consists of the use of soothing music between contractions combined with white sound, the volume of which is controlled by the labouring woman, during contractions. The volume of the white sound drowns out the music during contractions.

Moore *et al.* (1965), in the only published randomized placebo-controlled trial of audioanalgesia, provided each of the 25 study participants with earphones and audioanalgesia. The experimental group (13 women) received background music between contractions and self-controlled 'sea noise' that could be turned up to 120 decibels (the point of 'auditory discomfort') during contractions. The control group (12 women) had a similar arrangement, except that their 'sea noise' could be turned up to only 90 decibels (louder than heavy traffic and almost as loud as subway noise (Jensen 1980)). In other words, the only difference between the two groups was that the experimental group could attain a higher level of white noise. The authors assumed that the music and relatively low noise level would have only placebo effects and no physiologic benefit. Pain-relieving medications were available 'if the midwife considered the pain relief was inadequate'.

Results were obtained from two questionnaires, one answered by the midwife in attendance, the other administered to each woman on the third postpartum day by another midwife who had not been present during labour. There was a trend towards better pain relief in the audioanalgesia group, but the effect was confined to primigravidae, and was not statistically significant. Both the experimental and the control groups were overwhelmingly in favour of having sea noise again in future labours; 11 of the 13 multiparae and 7 of the 11 primiparae wanted to have sea noise again. This might suggest either the ineffectiveness of audioanalgesia, or that the somewhat lower levels of white noise, intended as placebo, offered almost comparable pain relief, with only a trend in favour of the experimental group. One wonders if the manoeuvres in the experimental and control groups were too similar, thus preventing a true test of the value of audioanalgesia.

A number of other investigators (Gardner *et al.* 1960; McDowell 1966; Burt and Korn 1964; Glass 1964; Moore *et al.* 1965) found decreased use of analgesic medication and reports of decreased pain from the use of audioanalgesia in non-randomized cohort studies.

Moore *et al.* discontinued their study of audioanalgesia partly because it was time-consuming for the physicians (the equipment was complicated and technical problems arose frequently), the earphones were cumbersome and uncomfortable for the women, who would need to rest from them periodically, and because they felt that their interim results did not warrant continuing the trial. With today's improvements in tape recorders, earphones, and sound reproduction, the technical difficulties would be minimal. Their findings, though somewhat equivocal, merit further trials with study designs modified to provide a clearer difference between the experimental and control manoeuvre.

5.3.3 Music

Judging from the absence of recently published papers on the subject, the interest in audioanalgesia or white noise for labour pain has faded, while the use of music has elicited a modest degree of interest, especially among the childbearing women, childbirth educators, and a few care-providers. The pleasing qualities of music may offer an added dimension beyond the distraction brought about by white noise. Music from a tape recorder or phonograph creates a pleasant and relaxing ambience; or if the mother uses earphones, music blocks out disturbing, distracting, or unpleasant sounds. Many birthing rooms today are furnished with tape recorders and tapes for use by labouring women. When carefully chosen, music may be used to reinforce rhythmic breathing patterns and massage strokes, or to facilitate visualizations and induction of hypnosis. Thus, music may have the potential to reduce stress and to enhance other pain-relieving measures. Music may also elicit more relaxed and positive behaviour from the staff and from the woman's chosen companions.

Music also increases endorphin production in a sizable minority of people. Goldstein (1980) found that music, primarily that with 'special emotional meaning for a person', elicits 'thrills' in the majority of people responding to his questionnaire. A 'thrill' was described as a usually pleasurable chill, shudder, tingling, or tickling, invariably associated with sudden changes in mood or emotion. In a controlled trial comparing the effects of injectable saline and naloxone (a narcotic antagonist) on music-induced thrills, Goldstein found that naloxone significantly attenuated thrills repeatedly in 3 of 10 subjects. Since naloxone is known to block the effects of endorphins, his findings imply that in some people, music causes increased production of endorphins (Goldstein 1980), endogenous pain relieving substances.

The few small studies of the pain-relieving effects of music in labour have found positive effects (Hanser *et al.* 1983; Clark *et al.* 1981; Sammons 1984; Durham and Collins 1985). Having selected seven women who would act as their own controls, Hanser *et al.* (1983) provided them with two individual music therapy training sessions in addition to their Lamaze training. The women were taught the purposes of background music during labour: to cue rhythmic breathing; to assist relaxation; and to use the music as an auditory focal point, diverting attention from discomfort and anxiety-raising hospital sounds. The music therapist selected music which would fulfil those purposes and match the individual tastes of each woman. She also instructed each woman and her labour partner to use the music to help them carry out the Lamaze breathing and relaxation techniques. The music therapist was present in labour for at least 35 contractions. She played music appropriate to the circumstances for ten contractions, alternating with silence for five contractions. She recorded negative and positive pain-related behaviours (for example, tension or relaxation in specific body parts; irregular, broken breathing patterns or rhythmic Lamaze breathing; negative or positive verbalizations, or vocalizations expressing doubt, pain, or tension) on an observation form during each contraction and the interval following. An independent observer was present for at least five contractions of each labour to determine observer reliability. The resulting inter-observer reliability was 97 per cent. Within one week following delivery, each mother completed an open-ended questionnaire inquiring about her perceptions and preferences for music or no music.

All seven women demonstrated fewer negative pain responses during the music periods ($p < 0.05$). Six of the seven women stated on the questionnaire that they believed the music fulfilled the purposes of helping them relax, cueing breathing, or distracted them from the pain. The other respondent stated she was not always aware of the music, but when she 'thought about it' the music helped her relax.

Clark *et al.* (1981) compared a group of women who had received prepared childbirth training with a group who had received the training plus music relaxation techniques and who were also assisted during labour by a music therapist. The latter were more positive in their responses to a questionnaire about their labours than the former.

Sammons (1984) investigated the likelihood that women from Lamaze classes would use music in labour if they had a single labour rehearsal with musical accompaniment than if they did not. Fifty-four women attending Lamaze classes were randomly assigned to either a music-rehearsal or nonmusic-rehearsal group. Both groups received Lamaze training, were told that music during labour was an option, and answered a postpartum questionnaire asking about their feelings on the use of music in labour. In addition, the experimental group had musical accompaniment during one labour rehearsal in class. There was 'scant elaboration on the potential benefits of music in labour', even in the experimental group. Although the 24 women in the experimental group were more likely than women in the control group to intend to or use music in labour (40 per cent versus 20 per cent), the difference was not statistically significant.

The questionnaire responses indicated that all eight women who used music in labour would do so again, and 61 per cent of the total sample would consider it. If the instructor were to 'make a more definitive statement about the efficacy of music for analgesia and relaxation, greater use might be seen' (Sammons 1984).

In a study of 30 women randomly allocated to either prenatal classes with music played during the exercise sessions and the opportunity to play music during their labours, or to control prenatal classes with a standard curriculum and no music during labour, Durham and Collins (1985) found a decrease in the use of pharmaceutical analgesia in the music group.

These small studies of childbirth pain, when combined with findings of the effects of music or auditory stimulation on other types of pain (for example, postoperative pain, dental pain, pain associated with burn therapy (Maslar 1986)), suggest that music has the capacity to reduce pain, at least in selected women. Its efficacy, however, seems to depend on the degree of prior education, preparation, and accommodation to the personal musical tastes of each woman.

6 Conclusions

Studies of the effectiveness of techniques to enhance descending inhibitory pathways indicate highly variable results. Well designed trials are rare and the subjective assessments by patients tend to be far more positive than objective measures of pain relief, such as reduction in use of pharmacologic methods of pain relief.

All methods of labour pain relief must be measured against the current 'Gold Standard' of pain relief, the epidural block, which boasts a high rate of success (from 67 per cent to 90 per cent) (Melzack *et al.* 1984; Morgan *et al.* 1982; Bundsen *et al.* 1982b; Bonica 1980) (see Chapter 57). Disadvantages to epidural block exist, however, and these, along with the desire among many women to experience labour, mandate continuing development of non-pharmacological labour pain relief measures.

Techniques like the ones described in this chapter cannot match epidural analgesia for effectiveness, but they are likely to have fewer harmful side-effects, and are well liked by some women. All that need be said about them is that they seem to help some women. Many of them require time and effort to learn and master, and their effectiveness is unpredictable, partly because of the complexities of the pain system and the human personality.

Satisfaction in childbirth is not necessarily contingent upon the absence of pain (Morgan *et al.* 1982; Norr *et al.* 1977). Many women are willing to experience pain in childbirth, but do not want the pain to overwhelm them. For those women whose goals for childbirth include the use of self-help measures to manage pain with minimal drug use, and for those who have little or no access to pharmacologic methods of pain relief, many of the methods described here are available and useful alternatives.

References

Abouleish E, Depp R (1975). Acupuncture in obstetrics. Anesth Analg, 54: 83–8.

American Psychiatric Association (1961). Training in medical hypnosis: a statement of position by the APA. Document available from the Central Office Washington DC 3.

Andersson SA, Block E, Holmgren E (1976). English summary of: Logfrekvent transkutan elektrisk stimulering for smartlindring vid farlossning. Lakartidningen, 73: 2421–2423.

Andrews CM (1981). Nursing intervention to change a malpositioned fetus. Adv Nurs Sci, 3: 53.

Atwood RJ (1976). Parturitional posture and related birth behaviour. Acta Obstet Gynecol Scand, 57: 5–25.

Augustinsson L, Bohlin P, Bundsen P, Carlsson C, Forssman L, Sjoberg P, Tyreman NO (1977). Pain relief during delivery by transcutaneous electrical nerve stimulation. Pain, 4: 59–65.

Birch ER (1986). The experience of touch received during labor: postpartum perceptions of therapeutic value. J Nurse Midwifery, 31: 270–276.

Bonica JJ (1974). Acupuncture anesthesia in the People's Republic of China: implications for British medicine. Acupuncture Anesth, 229: 1317–1325.

Bonica JJ (1980). Obstetric Analgesia and Anesthesia. World Federation of Societies of Anaesthesiologists, Amsterdam.

Bonica JJ (1984). Labour pain. In: Textbook of Pain. Melzack R, Wall P D (eds). Edinburgh: Churchill Livingstone, pp 377–392.

Brown C (1982). Therapeutic effects of bathing during labor. J Nurse Midwifery, 27: 13–16.

Brucker MC (1984). Nonpharmaceutical methods for relieving pain and discomfort during pregnancy. Matern Child Nurs J, 9: 390–394.

Bundsen P, Peterson L, Selstam U (1981). Pain relief in labor by transcutaneous electrical nerve stimulation: a prospective matched study. Acta Obstet Gynecol Scand, 60: 459–468.

Bundsen P, Ericson K (1982). Pain relief in labor by transcutaneous electrical nerve stimulation: safety aspects. Acta Obstet Gynecol Scand, 61: 1–5.

Bundsen P, Ericson K, Peterson L, Thiringer K (1982). Pain relief in labor by transcutaneous electrical nerve stimulation. Testing of a modified technique and evaluation of the neurological and biochemical condition of the newborn infant. Acta Obstet Gynecol Scand, 61: 129–136.

Bundsen P, Peterson L, Selstam U (1982b). Pain relief during delivery: an evaluation of conventional methods. Acta Obstet Gynecol Scand, 61: 289.

Burt RK, Korn GW (1964). Audioanalgesia in obstetrics: 'white sound' analgesia during labor. Am J Obstet Gynecol, 88: 361–365.

Caldeyro-Barcia R (1979). Physiological and psychological bases for the modern and humanised management of normal labour. In: Recent Progress in Perinatal Medicine and Prevention of Congenital Anomaly. Tokyo Ministry of Health and Welfare Government of Japan, pp 77–96.

Carlson JM, Diehl JA, Sachtleben-Murray M, McRae M, Fenwick L, Friedman EA (1986). Maternal position during parturition in normal labor. Obstet Gynecol, 68: 443–447.

Caton D (1985). The secularization of pain. Anesthesiology, 62: 493–501.

Chapman CR (1984). New directions in the understanding and management of pain. Soc Sci Med, 19: 1261–1277.

Clark ME, McCorkle RR, Williams SB (1981). Music therapy-assisted labour and delivery. J Music Ther, 18: 88–100.

Council on Mental Health (1958). Medical use of hypnosis. JAMA, 168: 2.

Dick-Read G (1953). Childbirth Without Fear: The Original Approach to Natural Childbirth (4th edn). Wessel H, Ellis HE (eds). New York: Harper & Row.

Dolezal A, Hlavaty V (1970). Increase in uterine blood flow in the first stage of labor during abdominal decompression as measured with 131 I-HSA. Am J Obstet Gynecol, 106: 311–312.

Durham L, Collins M (1985). The effect of music as a conditioning aid in prepared childbirth education. J Obstet Gynecol Neonatal Nurs, 15: 268–270.

Editorial (1974). Abdominal decompression in pregnancy. Br Med J, 2: 238–239.

Ehrenreich B, English D (1973). Witches, Midwives and Nurses: a History of Women Healers. New York: The Feminist Press.

Englemann GJ (1882). Labor among Primitive Peoples. New York: AMS Press Inc.

Erkkola R, Pikkola P, Kanto J (1980). Transcutaneous nerve stimulation for pain relief during labour: a controlled study. Ann Chir Gynaecol, 69: 273–277.

Fenwick L, Simkin P (1987). Maternal positioning to prevent or alleviate dystocia in labor. Clin Obstet Gynecol 30: 83–89.

Fields HL, Levine JD (1984). Pain—mechanisms and management. (Medical Progress) West J Med, 141: 347–357.

Freeman RM, Macaulay AJ, Eve L, Chamberlain GVP (1986). Randomised trial of self hypnosis for analgesia in labour. Br Med J, 292: 657–658.

Gardner WJ, Licklider JCR, Weisz AZ (1960). Suppression of pain by sound. Science, 132: 32–33.

Gilman S, Winans S (eds) (1984). Essentials of Clinical Neuroanatomy and Neurophysiology (6th edn). Philadelphia: F A Davis, p 36.

Glass L (1964). Discussion following Burt and Korn's paper. Am J Obstet Gynecol, 88: 366.

Goldstein A (1980). Thrills in response to music and other stimuli. Physiol Psychol, 8: 126–129.

Grim LC, Morey SH (1985). Transcutaneous electrical nerve stimulation for relief of parturition pain: a clinical report. Phys Ther, 65: 337–339.

Hanser SB, Larson SC, O'Connell AS (1983). The effect of music on relaxation of expectant mothers during labour. J Music Ther, 20: 50–59.

Harrison RF, Woods T, Shore M, Mathews G, Unwin A (1986). Pain relief in labour using transcutaneous electrical nerve stimulation (TENS). A TENS/TENS placebo controlled study in two parity groups. Br J Obstet Gynaecol, 93: 739–746.

Hedstrom LW, Newton N (1986). Touch in labor: a comparison of cultures and eras. Birth, 13: 181–186.

Helms JM (1987). Acupuncture for the management of primary dysmenorrhea. Obstet Gynecol, 69: 51–56.

Heyns OS (1959). Abdominal decompression in the first stage of labour. J Obstet Gynaecol Br Empire, 66: 220–228.

Hilbers SM, Gennaro S (1986). Nonpharmaceutical pain relief. NAACOG Update Series, 5: 2–6.

Jensen D (1980). The Human Nervous System. New York: Appleton-Century-Crofts.

Jimenez SLM (1983). The Pregnant Woman's Comfort Guide. Englewood Cliffs, NJ: Prentice-Hall.

Jungman RG (1982). Education for Childbirth. A New Lamaze Handbook. San Antonio, USA: Education of Childbirth Inc.

Kitzinger S (1978). Pain in childbirth. J Med Ethics, 4: 119–121.

Krieger D (1975). Therapeutic touch: the imprimatur of nursing. Am J Nurs, 75: 784–787.

Krieger D, Peper E, Ancoli S (1979). Therapeutic touch: searching for evidence of physiologic change. Am J Nurs, 79: 660–662.

Ledergerber CP (1976). Electroacupuncture in obstetrics. Acupuncture Electro-Therapeutic Res Int J, 2(1–2): 105–118.

Lederman R, Lederman E, Work E, MacCann DS (1978). The relationship of maternal anxiety plasma catecholamines and plasma cortisol to progress in labor. Am J Obstet Gynecol, 132: 495.

Lieberman AB (1987). Easing Labor Pain. New York: Doubleday, pp 112–113.

Maslar PM (1986). The effect of music on the reduction of pain: a review of the literature. The Arts in Psychotherapy, 13: 215–219.

McCaffery M (1979). Nursing Management of the Patient with Pain. Philadelphia: Lippincott, p 119.

McDowell CR (1966). Obstetrical applications of audioanalgesia. Hosp Topics, 44: 102–104.

Melzack RD (1973). The Puzzle of Pain. New York: Basic Books.

Melzack R (1975). How acupuncture can block pain. In: Pain: Clinical and Experimental Perspectives. Weisenberg M (ed). St Louis: C V Mosby Co, pp 251–257.

Melzack R, Kinch R, Dobkin P, Lebrun M, Taenzer P (1984). Severity of labour pain: influence of physical as well as psychologic variables. Can Med Assoc J, 130: 579–584.

Miller Jones CMH (1980). Forum: transcutaneous nerve stimulation in labour. Anaesthesia, 35: 372–375.

Moir P (1939). The nature of the pain of labour. J Obstet Gynaecol Br Empire, 46: 409–424.

Moore WMO, McClure Browne JC, Hill ID (1965). Clinical trial of audioanalgesia in childbirth. J Obstet Gynaecol Br Commnwlth, 72: 626–629.

Morgan BM, Bulpitt CJ, Clifton P, Lewis PJ (1982). The consumer's attitude to obstetric care. Br J Obstet Gynaecol, 91: 624–628.

Nesheim B (1981). The use of transcutaneous nerve stimulation for pain relief during labour: a controlled clinical study. Acta Obstet Gynecol Scand, 60: 13–16

Norr KL, Block CR, Charles A, Meyering S, Meyers E (1977). Explaining pain and enjoyment in childbirth. J Health Soc Behav, 18: 260–275.

Odent M (1983). Birth under water. Lancet, ii: 1476–7.

Ohashi W, Hoover M (1983). Natural Childbirth the Eastern Way. New York: Ballantine Books.

Olson HA (1984). Hypnosis in the treatment of pain. Individual Psychol, 40: 412–423.

Omer H, Friedlander D, Palti Z (1986). Hypnotic relaxation in the treatment of premature labour. Psychosom Med, 48: 351–361.

Penny KS (1979). Postpartum perceptions of touch received during labour. Res Nurs Health, 2: 9–16.

Pomeranz B, Chiu D (1976). Naloxone blockade of acupuncture analgesia: endorphin implicated. Life Sci, 19: 1757–1762

Quinn LJ, McKeown RA (1962). Abdominal decompression during the first stage of labor. Am J Obstet Gynecol, 83: 458.

Robson JE (1979). Forum: transcutaneous nerve stimulation for pain relief in labour. Anaesthesia, 34: 357–360

Roberts JE, Mendez-Bauer C, Wodell DA (1983). The effects of maternal position on uterine contractility and efficiency. Birth, 10: 243–9.

Saltenis IJ (1962). Physical Touch and Nursing Support in Labor. Unpublished master's report. New Haven: Yale University.

Sammons LN (1984). The use of music by women during childbirth. J Nurse Midwifery, 29: 266–170.

Sandelowski M (1984). Pain Pleasure and American Childbirth. London: Greenwood Press.

Scott DB, Loudon JDO (1960). A method of abdominal decompression in labour. Lancet, i: 1181.

Shealy CN, Maurer D (1974). Transcutaneous nerve stimulation for control of pain. Surg Neurol, 2: 45–47.

Shulman H, Birnbaum SJ (1966). Evaluation of abdominal decompression during the first stage of labor. Am J Obstet Gynecol, 95: 421–425.

Simkin P (1986). Stress, pain, and catecholamines in labor: part 1. Birth, 13: 227–233.

Sjolund B, Terenius L, Eriksson M (1977). Increased cerebro-spinal fluid levels of endorphins after electro-acupuncture. Acta Physiol Scand, 100: 382–4.

Sjolund B, Eriksson M (1979). The influence of naloxone on analgesia produced by peripheral conditioning stimulation. Brain Res, 173: 295–301.

Smith (1987). The effect of warm tub bathing during labour. Presentation to the 3rd International Congress on Pre- and Perinatal Psychology. San Francisco, California July 9–12.

Sommer P (1979). Obstetrical patients' anxiety during transition of labor and the nursing intervention of touch. Abstract: doctoral dissertation. Texas Women's University.

Stewart P (1979). Transcutaneous nerve stimulation as a method of analgesia in labour. Anaesthesia, 34: 361–4.

Vardurro JF, Butts PA (1982). Reducing the anxiety and pain of childbirth through hypnosis. Am J Nurs, April: 620–623.

Wall PD (1978). The gate control theory of pain mechanisms: a re-examination and re-statement. Brain, 101: 1–18.

Werner WEF, Schauble PG, Knudson MS (1982). An argument for the revival of hypnosis in obstetrics. Am J Clin Hypnosis, 24: 149–171.

Wertz RW, Wertz DC, (1977). Lying-In: A History of Childbirth in America. New York: The Free Press.

Yang MMP, Kok SH (1979). Further study of the neurohumoral factor endorphin in the mechanism of acupuncture analgesia. Am J Clin Med, 7: 143–8.

Yang Z, Cai T, Wu J (1984). Psychological aspects of components of pain. J Psychol, 118: 135–146.

57 Pharmacological control of pain during labour

Kay Dickersin

1 Introduction

1.1 Pain and the history of anaesthesia in childbirth

The desire for pain relief for childbirth has spanned most, if not all, cultures for as long as human practices have been recorded. The use of opiates was mentioned in early Chinese writings, the drinking of wine was noted in the Persian literature, and wine, beer, and brandy were commonly self-administered in Europe during the Middle Ages. Various concoctions and potions have been used over time, some inhaled, some swallowed, and some applied to the labouring woman's skin. One such prescription, from colonial America, involved a lock of hair from a virgin half the age of the woman in labour, twelve ant eggs dried in an oven, ground to a powder and dissolved in a pint of red cow's milk or strong ale (Haggard 1929).

The pain associated with childbirth has, in Western society, been explained in a variety of ways. The most familiar explanation of its origins is the Biblical notion that physical suffering during birth is a punishment of womankind for Eve's temptation of Adam (Genesis 3:13–16). Other explanations have involved a personal responsibility for pain, as opposed to a universally shared responsibility for the original sin, although both approaches share the common view that pain is punish-

ment. Radical medical groups, such as the hydropaths in the nineteenth century, believed that obstetric pain was a direct result of leading an 'unnatural' life, as no natural process is painful if individuals lead healthy lives.

Not all people have seen pain as punishment. There have been many proponents of the view that pain is functional, a natural correlate of life itself, even necessary to the healing process. The observation that patients who feel little or no pain while undergoing unanaesthetized amputations or surgery do not recover well has suggested even a curative aspect to pain (Pernick 1985). The concept that pain plays a part in healing has extended not only to the physiologic processes, but also to emotional well-being. In obstetrics, this concept has been reflected in the belief that the suffering which a woman undergoes in labour is directly related to the love she feels for her offspring.

It is clear that if pain in childbirth is thought to be a punishment, either personal or for all of womankind, or if pain is thought to be an integral part of physiologic and emotional healing, then the advent of modern obstetric anaesthesia would be met not just with scepticism, but with tremendous opposition. It was, for these and other reasons (Pernick 1985).

In the mid-nineteenth century, when the use of anaesthesia for surgery was first described, modern medicine was at a turning point. In the United States, the effort to formalize a conservative branch of medicine, separate from the many existing medical sects, culminated in the formation of the American Medical Association (AMA) in 1847 (Kett 1968) and other influential local societies. The attempt to re-establish medicine as a profession was epitomized by American Medical Association efforts to control medical education, codes of ethics, as well as rules for consultation, fees, and etiquette. To the new 'orthodox' medical establishment, specialization within the field of medicine was synonymous with quackery.

In 1846, William Thompson Green Morton demonstrated ether anaesthesia at the Massachusetts General Hospital in Boston, Massachusetts, immediately creating an upheaval in surgery and medicine. As a dentist, Morton was subject to mistrust by members of the conservative medical groups. Furthermore, Morton's intent in demonstrating ether's use was commercial, and this was considered non-professional, partly because it allowed the public to have an opinion regarding its use. Finally, there was considerable public argument between Morton and his colleagues over who actually made the discovery. These facts contributed to extensive criticism by the medical profession of the use of anaesthesia.

Several months after Morton's demonstration, in 1847, James Young Simpson reported from Edinburgh on the use of ether on a woman in labour; later in the year he published his experiences using chloroform. He saw the use of anaesthesia as part of a humanitarian effort to end suffering. In response to religious critics, he argued that God intended humans to escape the pain of childbirth and surgery (Simpson 1847) and even suggested that for the birth of Eve, God may have been the first anaesthetist, 'And the Lord God caused a deep sleep to fall upon Adam, and he slept; and He took one of his ribs, and closed up the flesh instead thereof' (Genesis 2:21).

Simpson had an influence on John Snow, the English epidemiologist credited with identification and elimination of the source of cholera in London in 1854. It is generally reported that Snow administered chloroform to Queen Victoria for the birth of her eighth child, Prince Leopold, on April 7, 1853. This fact was established by a note in Snow's diary, summarized as follows: 'The inhalation lasted fifty three minutes. The chloroform was given on a handkerchief in fifteen minim doses, and the Queen expressed herself greatly relieved by the administration.' (Richardson 1858).

Interestingly, *The Lancet* published an article by Editor Thomas Wakley denouncing this 'rumour' and theorizing instead that what had occurred was the pretence of administering chloroform. The article admonished, 'In no case could it be justifiable to administer chloroform in perfectly ordinary labour' and

'Royal examples are followed with extraordinary readiness by a certain class of society in this country' (Wakley 1858). In fact, the trend followed as predicted, the phrase 'anaesthesia *à la reine*' being coined from Victoria's example. The difficulty of access to information regarding proper use, as well as the cost and lack of ease of administration, limited the routine use of anaesthesia for nonsurgical procedures. Clearly, though, the primary reason for its restricted use in obstetrics was the fact that at that time, most births took place at home. Nevertheless, the promise of possible relief from labour pain, concomitant with shifts in societal attitudes regarding the difficulty of childbirth, led to continued interest in pursuing pharmacologic methods of analgesia.

In the United States at the turn of the century, mortality resulting from childbirth was a leading cause of death for women aged 15–44. Women and men came to regard childbirth and death as inevitably connected. This was believed to be due, in part, to the fact that women of the middle and upper classes had become, over time, less capable for reproduction. According to this analysis, the problem arose as modern women directed more energy toward mental tasks and away from the physical self.

In 1902, 'twilight sleep' a morphine-scopolamine mixture, administered in a darkened, quiet setting, was introduced to obstetrics by Von Steinbuchel in Germany. In theory, the method allowed a woman to dissociate from her mental state (fear) and to proceed with childbirth in a 'natural' fashion. Although the method was initially rejected by United States physicians as too dangerous to both mother (delayed labour, postpartum haemorrhage) and child (overly narcotized babies) (DeLee 1905; DeLee *et al.* 1907), an article published in McClure's magazine in June, 1914 kindled a consumer movement which led to eventual widespread use. Women who had twilight sleep in Germany spearheaded a movement demanding its availability in the United States, charging the medical establishment with expropriation of the right to pain relief in labour (see Chapter 7). In a successful bid for power, this consumer movement changed obstetric practice and its relationship to the pharmacologic relief of pain forever. For one thing, twilight sleep necessitated moving childbirth from the home to the hospital, from the domain of midwives to the domain of physicians. Both women and physicians no longer saw pain as the inevitable corollary of childbirth, rather, they saw that the answer lay in use of specific drugs for relief.

Between the time when women first demanded the availability of twilight sleep and the beginning of the Natural Childbirth movement, in 1948 (Sandelowski 1984), drugs of all types were employed during labour and childbirth. These included narcotics, barbiturates and other sedatives, tranquillizers, and amnesiacs, given separately or in combination, and were administered in a variety of ways, including inhalant, oral, intravenous, intramuscular, and rectal. As pointed out by Sandelowski (1984), changes in DeLee's *The Principles and Practice of Obstetrics* reflect this situation. The 1915 edition stated that the author's experiences with pharmacologic means of pain relief in the first stage of labour had led him to forgo these means completely, except in unusual cases (DeLee 1915). In the 1920 edition, DeLee expressed the opinion that it was the duty of the physician to prevent labour pain and included information on the use of nitrous oxide and oxygen. In 1925, he stated that he usually gave morphine and scopolamine during labour, and in 1929, he described an increased array of drug regimens.

The Grantly Dick-Read method of 'natural' childbirth, in the 1930s, the first of many formal psychophysical approaches to preventing childbirth pain, was precipitated by a number of factors (Sandelowski 1984). Among them was an increasing interest by the medical establishment in a psychosomatic approach, a decrease in the mortality theretofore associated with childbirth, and a changing role for women in developed countries. The field of obstetrics has been considerably influenced by the status of women in a given society and by the level of political activity of women toward a change in that status. Dick-Read's writings became widely disseminated in the United States in the 1940s, a time when women had been 'wearing the pants' in the American family because of World War II. The postwar baby boom was thus influenced by the perception that women were capable and powerful—especially in their family roles. This mood no doubt influenced women's attitudes regarding their ability to reproduce and to labour without the help of pharmacologic pain relief. While many women continued to use various methods of analgesia or anaesthesia (e.g. rectal ether, narcotics, and inhalants), psychoprophylaxis never quite lost its hold, paving the way for Lamaze and other methods of 'natural' childbirth which became increasingly popular in the 1960s and 1970s (see Chapter 20).

The increased use of lumbar epidural analgesia in the 1970s and 1980s has reflected recent shifts in the modern women's movement. The concept that women have a choice with regard to lifestyle and occupation—marriage or not, homemaking or employment—has also influenced the field of obstetrics: the current dictum is that women who choose pharmacologic means of pain relief should not feel guilty. If history is any indication, the search for pain relief will continue for as long as women bear children.

As anaesthesia has become a relatively accepted component of the childbirth process, the field has advanced mainly by the development of new drugs and methods, but also by inquiries into the side-effects of particular procedures. Even in the early days of obstetric anaes-

thesia, workers such as Walter Channing and John Snow questioned the effect of anaesthesia on the infant, initiating work in an area still of prime concern in modern anaesthesiology.

The history of pain relief during childbirth is important today from a number of perspectives. First, an individual's perception as to the origins of obstetric pain determine the methods by which that person will attempt to conquer it. Clearly, the patient who believes pain to be a necessary corollary to health will approach anaesthesia differently from the person who believes pain to be a punishment. Similarly, the physician or midwife will be guided by his or her own views on the origins of pain. Second, the notion that patients do not have a place in decisions regarding obstetrical care is still rampant today, and this notion is perhaps the most grating of all to active consumer groups. The current attention focused on epidural analgesia in the lay literature reflects the patients' fear that there is more to the story than that which they know. Finally, there is no consensus amongst either consumers or caregivers as to the proper course of action regarding the status quo or new innovations. Introductions of new agents or techniques are met by both groups with a mixture of scepticism and open arms, reflecting anti-quackery feeling, fear that commercialism will dictate medical protocol, and the desire to be up to date.

Consumer groups have had a major effect in producing changes in both obstetrics in general, and obstetric anaesthesia in particular. From anaesthesia *à la reine*, to twilight sleep, to Lamaze birth, to epidural analgesia for caesarean section, the public has demanded and received various means of pain relief. They have also subtly transformed the way physicians practise. With the move of birth from home to hospital, a new specialty, obstetrics, became involved and midwives took a secondary role. Pain relief for labour was administered by obstetricians almost exclusively. With the increasing use of regional anaesthesia, again as much a response to consumers as to the medical community, a second specialty has become involved, anaesthesiology.

Responding responsibly to the changing demands of the consumer represents an overwhelming challenge to the practitioner. Reading and digestion of a voluminous literature is required to keep abreast of new developments. The published reports describe new anaesthetic agents, new methods of delivery of the agents, research in laboratory animals, surveys, epidemiologic studies comparing groups of patients receiving different types of care, and clinical trials comparing one formulation or method of administration to another. Yet, it is hard to feel with any certainty that what is thought to be true today will be conventional wisdom ten years from now. Recently, sentiments reflecting frustration with this complicated field were expressed by the president of a state society of anaesthesiologists in the United States:

'Obstetric anaesthesia, if it would just go away we would all be happy,' (Garrett 1984).

1.2 Focus of the chapter

1.2.1 Purpose

There have been more clinical trials done to study pharmacologic means of pain relief during labour and childbirth than any other subject in the perinatal field (National Perinatal Epidemiology Unit 1986). This chapter will review the data available from those trials, in addition to data from other sources, which concentrate on the pain of childbirth. This task will be approached so as to give most attention to modern methods of analgesia and anaesthesia, limiting the scope further to the major modern methods used in developed countries.

Advances in obstetric anaesthesiology, as gauged by the medical literature, are made in tiny overlapping increments. The nature of research dictates this fragmented accumulation of information, yet when the data are presented paper-by-paper, it is difficult to conceptualize the whole. In an effort to draw a complete picture and to synthesize appropriate conclusions, this chapter will group subsets of the published data by the research question being asked. For example, what is the difference in effect between lumbar epidural morphine and epidural bupivacaine?

Each subset that is described, however, is artificial and displays the available data in a form that sidesteps the real issues. Questions such as the effect of adding epinephrine to a local anaesthetic agent, or comparisons of individual but similar drugs are not the problems foremost in the practitioners' minds. While a comparison of a standard drug with, for example, a new drug, is a necessary element of medical progress, the questions of real importance are more general, and related to the fundamental question: 'are we doing more harm than good?'. The fact that pain during labour is usually not considered to be a medical problem adds to the difficulty of balancing the 'harm' and 'good'. In this context 'good' is primarily pain relief. The harm in the case of obstetric anaesthesia is a possible negative effect on the mother or infant. This could be, for the mother, drop in blood pressure, changes in respiration or uterine activity resulting in increased duration of labour, motor blockade, instrumental delivery, the required use of additional medications, change in heart rate, amnesia, nausea, vomiting, pruritus, drowsiness, shivering, or dizziness.

For the child, the ability to deal with a foreign substance such as anaesthetic or analgesic medication is of prime concern. Dealing with a drug potentially involves many physiological systems; those that have been looked at most closely are cardiovascular and respiratory function and blood gas balance. Potential neurobehavioural effects have always been of concern to investigators. However, they are difficult to measure, particularly because of confounding exposures and also because of the length of follow-up required.

Therefore, the question is not: is continuously administered epidural bupivacaine (at a particular concentration) 'superior' to epidural morphine? Rather, the question is: by what method can we achieve an acceptable level of pain relief in most labouring women, while least compromising the mother's and child's health? One cannot help but feel that the answer to this question lies buried in the already accumulated mass of evidence, but there are very few studies that confront it explicitly.

One of the implicit assumptions a reader may make in reviewing the data presented herein is that the findings contained in each publication are independent. It is unlikely that this is true. Much of the work in a given time period, for a given subject, has been done by a handful of researchers. Thus, the study design, analysis, and presentation of results for a majority of studies in a particular subset may have been guided by a single group of individuals. Therefore, these individuals, consciously or unconsciously, may have directed our thinking on a particular matter toward their point of view, and away from the 'truth' that investigators in the field are seeking.

1.2.2 Physiologic origins of obstetric pain

Before beginning a review of the literature, a brief comment on the origins of pain in labour (see also Chapter 56) is in order. It is necessary, as well, to provide definitions, for use in this chapter, of the terms 'anaesthesia' and 'analgesia' (Section 1.2.3).

The physiologic origins of labour pain are not completely understood, either physiologically or psychologically. A review by Bonica (1975) covers this topic in detail. Briefly, contributory factors to labour pain are, in first stage: dilatation and stretching of the cervix and lower uterine segments during uterine contraction, stretching of the peritoneum, compression of nerve ganglia in the cervix, compression of nerve ganglia in the lower uterus, and myometrial hypoxia. The pain which arises in the nociceptors of the uterus and cervix travels via afferent sensory nerves, accompanying sympathetic (efferent) fibres through the paracervical plexus, the pelvic, hypogastric, and aortic plexuses, and the lumbar and lower thoracic chain, to join the dorsal horn of the spinal cord at segments T10 through L1. These fibres synapse with ascending and descending fibres there, in particular with the interneurones of the substantia gelatinosa. Pain is referred to the skin dermatomes supplied by these spinal cord segments.

Later on, in late first stage and second stage, pain may be caused by distension and tearing of fasciae in the pelvis, vulva, and perineum, with impulses travelling via the lower lumbar and upper sacral nerves to the spinal cord and via the pudendal nerves to the second, third, and fourth sacral segments.

1.2.3 Definitions of anaesthesia and analgesia

The *Oxford Concise Medical Dictionary* (2nd edn, Oxford University Press, 1985) defines anaesthesia as a 'loss of feeling or sensation in a part or all of the body', and analgesia as the 'reduced sensibility to pain, without loss of consciousness and without the sense of touch necessarily being affected'. In this chapter, the term analgesia will refer to pain relief during labour and vaginal delivery and anaesthesia will refer to the administration of specific drugs for caesarean section.

2 Specific pharmacological methods of pain relief

2.1 Narcotics

As a class, the narcotics are chemically related to the opium alkaloids; some are derived directly or indirectly from the opium poppy and others are produced synthetically. Generally, they can provide reasonable pain relief for labour. Both maternal and neonatal depression are serious common problems associated with their use, the incidence of side effects increasing with higher doses. Because of the dose-related problems, complete analgesia during labour cannot be achieved; rather, narcotics are used to reduce pain.

There are other side-effects which are reportedly related to use of narcotics, about which investigators and practitioners have had some concern. Orthostatic hypotension (a result of peripheral vascular dilatation but less of a problem in obstetrics if women stay in bed) (Eckenhoff and Oech 1960), nausea and vomiting, dizziness, and a decrease in gastric motility (La Salvia and Steffan 1950; Nimmo *et al.* 1975) have all been embedded in the obstetric anaesthesia literature as potential problems related to administration of narcotics. There also exists some indication that labour progress, especially in early labour, can be slowed via a decrease in uterine activity and a slowing of cervical dilatation (Friedman 1971; James 1960) related to administration of narcotics. A shortening of labour has also been reported (DeVoe *et al.* 1969), and attributed to relief of anxiety.

There is ample evidence that narcotics cross the placenta (Moore *et al.* 1970; Moya and Thorndike 1962; Apgar *et al.* 1952). This may result in neonatal respiratory depression (Table 57.3), which more quickly follows intravenous than intramuscular administration (Bonica 1967).

Pethidine (meperidine, Demerol) is the most popular of the narcotics. Concern in terms of specific side-effects centres on neonatal depression, PaCO$_2$ increase,

duration of labour, fetal heart rate changes, neurobehavioural effects, and decreased Apgar score.

Pentazocine (Talwin) is chemically similar to pethidine but has both opiate agonist and weak antagonistic activity. In the mother it has been associated with less nausea, vomiting, and dizziness than pethidine (Moore and Ball 1974), and with regard to the fetus, it crosses to the placenta less easily than pethidine (Moore *et al.* 1970; Mowat and Garrey 1970). Hallucinations are often associated with use of the drug (Crawford 1978).

Alphaprodine (Nisentil) and butorphanol (Stadol), are newer narcotics currently of interest because of short time to onset and shorter duration of action than morphine or other drugs. The general problems associated with narcotics are relevant where these drugs are concerned as are additional problems specific to each compound.

Morphine, now rarely used in obstetrics, is perhaps the most effective drug for pain in labour, but has also been associated with unacceptable side-effects. Its long duration of action, when coupled with multiple doses and the sensitivity of the newborn's brain to morphine, may be related to the neonatal respiratory depression often seen with the drug.

Narcotic antagonists (Naloxone, nalorphine, or levallorphan) have been administered together with a narcotic to counteract the depressant effects of narcotics, either with each dose of narcotic or 10 to 15 minutes before delivery. Although the rationale is to provide analgesia with minimal respiratory depression, this does not make sense. Antagonists reverse the effects of pain relief (Girvan *et al.* 1976; Telford and Keats 1961) and do not necessarily counteract the depressant effect, as the antagonists may have depressant activity of their own (Rouge *et al.* 1969). Antagonists have also been tested with regard to their effect on gastric emptying. A trial of pethidine plus Naloxone versus pethidine plus placebo (Frame *et al.* 1984) found that a clinically significant increase in absorption of paracetamol (implying an increase in gastric emptying) occurred in patients given Naloxone. In summary, there is a role for administration of narcotic antagonists to narcotic-depressed neonates and, some believe, to mothers for whom delivery is unexpectedly precipitous.

In 1976, Moir stated: 'Despite the increasing use of epidural analgesia most British women have to depend on narcotic analgesics for pain relief in the first stage of labour', and in 1978 Crawford stated: 'In Britain, as elsewhere in the Western World, it is probable that pethidine continues to be the most commonly chosen systemically administered analgesic.'

Although these statements appear to many in the field as of historical interest only, both Albright *et al.* and Rosen confirmed this observation again in 1986: 'Meperidine [pethidine] is the most frequently used obstetric analgesic drug in Europe and North America,

Table 57.1a Selected trial design features: systemic narcotics versus saline

Authors, date country	Total n	Reported method of treatment assignment and masking	Funding source	Treatment groups	Top-ups?	Conclusions
Tournaire et al. (1980) France	58	Random, numbered ampoules; double-masked	?	(1) Pethidine (PETH) (1.25 mg/kg body wt) intramuscularly (IM) (2) Saline	?	Uterine tone increased w/PETH No difference in speed of dilatation of cervix, intensity, frequency, or number of contractions
Chang et al. (1976) Australia	(A) 48	Random, no method given; not masked	Felton Bequest	(1) PETH (1 mg/kg body wt) intravenously (IV) (2) Nalorphine (NAL) (0.1 mg/kg body wt) (IV) (3) Saline	?	Maternal, fetal pH lowest w/NAL Maternal pCO_2 highest w/NAL No differences in pH or pCO_2 between PETH and saline
	(B) 53	Random, no method given	Felton Bequest	(1) Morphine (MOR) (0.1 mg/kg body wt) (IV) (2) Heroin (0.1 mg/kg; IV) (3) Saline		Maternal, fetal pH lowest w/heroin Maternal pCO_2 highest w/heroin Fetal base excess level higher w/saline than MOR or heroin
Moore and Ball (1974) Ireland	460	Random, no method given; observer masked	Winthrop Labs	(1) PETH (50 mg) (2) PETH (100 mg) (3) Pentazocine (40 mg) (4) PETH (100 mg) + levallorphan (1.25 mg) (5) Saline	?	Patients not evenly distributed on prognostic factors Nausea, vomiting, dizziness, dysphoria, sweating, restlessness, increased w/narcotics Little pain relief w/saline, decreased relief w/PETH (50 mg)
DeKornfeld et al. (1964) US	335	Numbered ampoules; double-masked	NIH and American Cyanamid Co.	(1) PETH (75 mg) (2) Methotrimeprazine (15 mg) (3) Placebo	Yes; same drug or PETH	Labour longer in grps (1) and (2) Pain relief better in grps (1) and (2) up to 3 hrs, then all grps similar Drowsiness increased in grps (1) and (2) Apgar score decreased in grp (1)
Cullhed and Löfström (1961) Sweden	845	Date of admission used to decide injection or not; coded ampoules for type of drug; not masked	?	N_2O or trichloroethylene, if desired, for all women (1) 0.9% saline (2) PETH (50 mg) + scopolamine (SCOP) (0.2 mg/ml) (3) PETH (50 mg/ml) (4) SCOP (0.2 mg/ml)	 Yes Yes Yes Yes	Recall of severe pain least in PETH-SCOP grp Low Apgars in PETH-SCOP babies

Table 57.1(b) Observed effect of intervention on outcomes of interest: systemic narcotics versus saline

Authors, date (total *n*)	Number of pts. in each treatment group	Treatment groups	Good to excellent pain relief	Apgar score $\leqslant 6$ at 1 min
Tournaire *et al.* (1980) (*n* = 58)	29	(1) Pethidine (PETH)	NA*	NA
	29	(2) Saline	NA	NA
Chang *et al.* (1976) (A) (*n* = 48)	14	(1) PETH	NA	NA
(B) (*n* = 53)	17	(2) Nalorphine	NA	NA
	17	(3) Saline	NA	NA
	17	(1) Morphine	NA	NA
	15	(2) Heroin	NA	NA
	21	(3) Saline	NA	NA
Moore and Ball (1974) (*n* = 460)	45	(1) PETH (50 mg)	15/45	NA
	80	(2) PETH (100 mg)	54/80	NA
	240	(3) Pentazocine (40 mg)	156/240	NA
	65	(4) PETH (100 mg) + levallorphan (1.25 mg)	38/65	NA
	30	(5) Saline	2/30	NA
DeKornfeld *et al.* (1964) (*n* = 335)	112	(1) PETH (75 mg)	75/112	19/112
	111	(2) Methotrimeprazine (15 mg)	68/111	7/111
	112	(3) Placebo	36/112	10/112
Cullhed and Löfstrom (1961) (*n* = 845)	247	(1) No injection	178/247	9/245
	243	(2) Saline	149/243	12/241
	236	(3) PETH (50 mg) + scopolamine (SCOP) (0.2 mg/ml)	175/236	25/232
	67	(4) PETH (50 mg/ml)	35/67	NA
	53	(5) SCOP (0.2 mg/ml)	32/53	NA

*NA indicates 'Not available'.

even though no well controlled, double blind studies of different opiates in equianalgesic doses have established its superiority' (Albright *et al.* 1986a); '. . . in England and Wales more than 70 per cent of mothers receive meperidine during labour' (Rosen 1986). Rosen, however, commented that there seems to be some reluctance to use narcotic analgesia in the United States. It is indeed tempting to speculate that, at least in the United States, recent use of opiates such as pethidine for obstetric analgesia may have been affected as much by societal attitudes as by considerations of effectiveness.

The practitioner and researcher must turn to the question of evidence. Do opiates, administered systemically, relieve pain adequately and if so, at what cost in terms of short and long term effects on mother and child?

A large number of clinical trials, many in the 1960s, have been done which evaluate systemic narcotics; almost all include pethidine as a test group. There have been six trials of systemic narcotics versus a saline placebo control (Table 57.1), several with relatively large sample sizes. Although these trials indicate that pethidine is more effective than placebo in providing pain relief (Table 57.2), its effectiveness is far from complete. At what point does the delicate balance between adequate pain relief and potential side-effects tip far enough for a decision for or against a drug?

Only two of the trials collected data on Apgar score (DeKornfeld *et al.* 1964 Cullhed and Lofstrom, 1961). Both found lower scores in the group administered pethidine (Table 57.3). Tournaire *et al.* (1980) found increased uterine tone with pethidine, with no difference between groups in speed of dilatation of the cervix nor the intensity, frequency or number of contractions. Chang *et al.* (1976) looked at the effect of four narcotic agents on maternal blood pH and pCO_2 as well as pH and base excess in fetal scalp blood. They found that the narcotics caused a small decrease in maternal pH and concomitant increase in pCO_2, with decreases in fetal pH and base excess, when compared with the effect of saline. They felt this may be an indication of possible adverse metabolic side-effects on the fetus.

Table 57.2 Effect of systemic narcotics versus saline for analgesia in labour on inadequate pain relief

Study	EXPT		CTRL		Odds ratio	Graph of odds ratios and confidence intervals
	n	(%)	n	(%)	(95% CI)	0.01 0.1 0.5 1 2 10 100
DeKornfeld *et al.* (1964)	37/112	(33.04)	76/112	(67.86)	0.25 (0.15–0.42)	
Cullhed and Löfström (1961)	93/303	(30.69)	95/243	(39.09)	0.69 (0.48–0.98)	
Moore and Ball (1974)	167/430	(38.84)	28/30	(93.33)	0.11 (0.05–0.23)	
Typical odds ratio (95% confidence interval)					0.41 (0.31–0.54)	

Table 57.3 Effect of systemic narcotics versus saline for analgesia in labour on Apgar score <7 at 1 minute

Study	EXPT		CTRL		Odds ratio	Graph of odds ratios and confidence intervals
	n	(%)	n	(%)	(95% CI)	0.01 0.1 0.5 1 2 10 100
De Kornfeld *et al.* (1964)	19/112	(16.96)	10/112	(8.93)	2.03 (0.93–4.43)	
Cullhed and Löfstrom (1961)	25/232	(10.78)	22/486	(4.53)	2.77 (1.47–5.22)	
Typical odds ratio (95% confidence interval)					2.45 (1.50–4.00)	

Moore and Ball (1974) found increased nausea, vomiting, dizziness, dysphoria, sweating, and restlessness with the narcotics. Increased duration of labour and increased drowsiness were seen both in the pethidine and methotrimeprazine groups in the trial performed by DeKornfeld *et al.* (1964).

The DeKornfeld article makes a number of interesting methodologic observations. Comparison of the obstetricians' and mothers' evaluations of labour pain revealed that overall, for both placebo and active drug groups, physicians believed labour pain to be less severe than did the mother. This trial also tested the masking of the physicians to the identity of the anaesthetic. While they were capable of discerning between placebo and active drug, they were not as good at guessing which drug was being employed. Finally, they demonstrated that twenty-four hours postpartum, mothers are more likely to report effective pain relief (regardless of whether they had received any drug) than they were just after delivery.

In a randomized controlled trial of self-administered intravenous versus intramuscular pethidine, Robinson *et al.* (1980b) showed a trend towards increased pain relief in the self-administered intravenous group, for all stages of delivery, although mean total dose of pethidine was lower in the self-administered group. Forceps were used slightly more frequently in the self-administered group (9/41) than in the intramuscular group (9/48), but the small differences may easily reflect chance variation. Apgar scores were stated to be similar in the two groups, but no data were provided. Other side-effects of the analgesia were similar in both groups. These data indicate that self-administered intravenous pethidine is preferable to intramuscular pethidine, by virtue of the lower total dose.

2.2 Inhalation analgesia

Inhalation analgesia is used around the world to relieve pain during labour. In this chapter, the term 'inhalation anaesthesia' will be used to define a deeper effect than that of analgesia, an effect involving loss of consciousness; it is rarely, if ever, used today in a vaginal delivery, at least in the United States. (General anaesthesia for vaginal delivery was popular in the United States from the 1930s to at least the late 1960s and is still used in some places).

The agent used most often is nitrous oxide, although methoxyflurane, enflurane, isoflurane, and trichloroethylene have also been employed. These agents are either self-administered, or administered intermittently by an anaesthetist, using a mask. According to Cohen (1987), inhalation analgesia is still frequently used for vaginal delivery, perhaps because its administration requires less training than regional anaesthesia. Use of inhalation analgesia, however, has been decreasing over the years. A study published in 1970 by the American College of Obstetricians and Gynecologists indicated that inhalation analgesia was used in about one-third of all vaginal deliveries in the United States (American College of Obstetricians and Gynecologists 1970), and Crawford, in 1978, stated that 'undoubtedly, it is still the most popularly used technique in British obstetric practice . . .' (Crawford 1978). It has often been used in conjunction with other forms of analgesia (e.g. narcotics and tranquillizers), rather than alone. Inhalation analgesia is probably used today mainly at small non-teaching hospitals in the US and Canada. Recent data from the Canadian Institute of Child Health (personal communication, 1985) showed that Entonox was used in 17 per cent of the births at hospitals with 20–100 live births per year, 10 per cent at hospitals with 101–300 births, 0 per cent at those with 301–999 births, and 6 per cent at those with 1000 or more births.

Advantages to the use of inhalation analgesia are that the mother remains awake; that neither uterine activity nor 'bearing down' in second stage is affected; that the duration of effect is short and thus better control is possible; and that clinically obvious side-effects on the mother or fetus have not been noted. The main disadvantage is incomplete pain relief. This has to do both with the timing of the inhalation to match peak contraction pressure with peak analgesic effect and with the type of agent and apparatus used. Concern about long term effects of self-administered inhalation agents on medical personnel have also resulted in decreased use, at least in the United States. Issues surrounding a few specific inhalation agents (nitrous oxide, methoxyflurane, enflurane, isoflurane, trichloroethylene, and halothane) will be reviewed here briefly, and the reader is referred to other sources for more detailed reviews (Moir 1976; Cohen 1987).

Nitrous oxide has been in use for obstetric analgesia and anaesthesia for over 100 years. A mixture of 50 per cent nitrous oxide and 50 per cent air was the standard prescription. Administered by use of an apparatus designed by Minnitt (1934), this mixture was criticized for delivery of too little oxygen to the mother (a final concentration of about 10 per cent). In the 1960s the first machine (the Lucy Baldwin, named after the wife of a British prime minister who had led a campaign for improved pain relief for women in labour) capable of delivering an equal mixture (or other proportions if so desired) of nitrous oxide and oxygen was introduced. Later, Entonox, premixed nitrous oxide and oxygen, was made available; it is favoured in Great Britain and Canada but is not available in the United States. The ideal proportions of nitrous oxide and oxygen has been the subject of concern and debate over the years. Two

Medical Research Council trials (1970) showed no significant difference between 50 per cent and 70 per cent nitrous oxide mixtures in pain relief effected in normal labours, though mothers tended to lose consciousness more often in the 70 per cent group. The standard currently in use is 50 per cent.

Nitrous oxide has low lipid solubility, provides a rapid onset of analgesia, has no objectionable odour, and is inexpensive. Its effectiveness has been looked at formally in clinical trials (see Table 57.4) but Moir (1976) expressed what may be the prevailing medical opinion in Europe and the United States: 'There is now a willingness to admit that nitrous oxide analgesia is often inadequate and to accept that the explanation may lie with the agent and not always with the patient or the technique of administration. This more honest approach may be related to the wider availability of more effective analgesic methods such as epidural analgesia.'

Methoxyflurane is an extremely lipid soluble agent, producing a constant level of analgesia. One of the by-products of its metabolism—inorganic fluoride—has been reported to be responsible for the nephrotoxicity found to be associated with the use of this drug (Mazze *et al.* 1971). For this reason, it has not been used for the past ten or so years for obstetric anaesthesia (although it may still be used for analgesia, because smaller doses are used) and is considered to have no place in modern obstetrics.

Enflurane and isoflurane are more recently introduced inhalation agents and have not been studied as much as those previously mentioned, in terms of obstetric applications. They are not extensively metabolized and are of intermediate solubility. There is some debate as to whether enflurane provides good analgesia at subanaesthetic concentrations (Rolbin *et al.* 1978; Westmoreland *et al.* 1974; Devoghel 1974). Disadvantages may include reduced uterine contractility (Munson and Embro 1977).

Trichloroethylene is no longer available in the United States but has been quite popular in Great Britain and Canada. It is a potent analgesic and is very inexpensive. Its chemical interaction with soda lime, usually an integral part of the anaesthetic apparatus, and possible cardiac effects are disadvantages (Cohen 1987).

Halothane is not considered appropriate for use in labour because it has a poor analgesic effect and is a myometrial relaxant.

Administration of inhalation analgesia is typically by face mask or commercial inhaler. A study by Dolan and Rosen (1975) compared the acceptability of face mask versus mouthpiece for administration of analgesia in labouring patients. The mouthpiece was found to be more acceptable, because of factors relating to the freedom it confers: eyeglasses can be worn, the hands are free, there is no pressure on the face, etc.

Five clinical trials (Davies *et al.* 1975; Rosen at al. 1972; Bergsjø and Lindbaek 1971; Rosen *et al.* 1969; Jones *et al.* 1969) that compared methoxyflurane to nitrous oxide and oxygen are presented in Table 57.4. Sample sizes for four of the five studies ranged from 28 to 63, whereas one study included over 1200 women. Pain relief achieved with the two drugs appeared roughly the same: about 75 per cent of the time good to excellent pain relief was achieved (Table 57.5). Nitrous oxide use was associated with slightly more nausea and vomiting during labour and delivery than methoxyflurane (Table 57.6). It seems clear that the major drawback to inhalation analgesia is the fact that pain relief is incomplete. An additional factor is the risk of maternal mortality (Cohen 1987) due to accidental overdose resulting, for example, in aspiration of gastric contents.

Table 57.4(a) Selected trial design features: inhalation analgesia: N_2O-O_2 versus methoxyflurane (MF)

Authors, date country	Total n	Reported method of treatment assignment and masking	Funding source	Treatment groups	Conclusions
Davies *et al.* (1975) Wales	28	No method given, not masked	?	(1) 50% N_2O–50% O_2 (2) 0.35% MF	No difference between grps in inspired O_2 concentration
Rosen *et al.* (1972) Wales	50	Random, alternate weeks; not masked	?	(1) 50% N_2O–50% O_2 (2) 0.35% MF	No differences between grps for tests of renal function
Bergsjø and Lindbaek (1971) Norway	63	Random first use of inhalant, then other drugs, then by choice; not masked	Abbott Labs supplied MF	(1) 50% N_2O–50% O_2 (2) 0.25%–0.8% MF	Both agents gave good analgesia Patients preferred N_2O/O_2
Rosen *et al.* (1969) Wales	1257	Random plus free choice, method described; not masked	United Cardiff Hospitals; Abbott Labs supplied MF; Cyprane Ltd – vaporizers	(1) 50% N_2O–50% O_2 (2) 0.35% MF (3) 0.5% and 0.35% trichloroethylene	All agents gave good analgesia Nausea and vomiting for about 20% of each grp
Jones *et al.* (1969) Wales	48	Random, no method given; not masked	United Cardiff Hospitals; Abbott Labs supplied MF	(1) N_2O–O_2 (41%, mean) (2) MF (0.22%, mean), pethidine if desired	Satisfactory analgesia greater in grp (2) Nausea and vomiting less in grp (2)

Table 57.4(b) Observed effect of intervention on outcome: inhalation analgesia: N_2O-O_2 versus methoxyflurane (MF)

Authors, date (total n)	No. of pts in each treatment grp	Treatment groups	Good to excellent pain relief	Nausea in labour and delivery	Vomiting in labour and delivery
Davies *et al.* (1975) (28)	14	(1) 50% N_2O–50% O_2	NA*	NA	NA
	14	(2) 0.35% MF	NA	NA	NA
Rosen *et al.* (1972) (50)	25	(1) 50% N_2O–50% O_2	NA	NA	NA
	25	(2) 0.35% MF	NA	NA	NA
Bergsjø and Lindbaek (1971) (63, cross-over design)	63	(1) 50% N_2O–50% O_2	36/40 of those who preferred N_2O–O_2	4/63	3/63
	63	(2) 0.25–0.8% MF	21/22 of those who preferred MF	2/63	1/63
Rosen *et al.* (1969) (1257)	265	(1) 50% N_2O–50% O_2	190/265	50/265	20/265
	598	(2) 0.35% MF	421/598	138/598	9/598
	394	(3) 0.5% and 0.35% trichloroethylene	282/394	87/394	24/394
Jones *et al.* (1969) (48)	24	(1) N_2O–O_2 (40% mean)	19/ 22	8/24	4/24
	24	(2) MF (22% mean)	19/ 24	2/24	0/24

*NA indicates 'Not available'.

Finally, epidemiologic evidence of increased risk of spontaneous abortion to anaesthesia and nursing personnel has resulted in decreased interest in the method over the past decade (Ad hoc Committee on the Effect of Trace Anesthetics on the Health of Operating Room Personnel 1974).

2.3 Sedative-tranquillizers

Sedative-tranquillizers, generally useful in the first stage of labour, are either administered alone or in combination with a narcotic. Many clinicians feel that the use of a tranquillizer, especially in early labour, is helpful in reducing the woman's anxiety and in promoting sleep. One class of tranquillizers, the phenothiazines, is known for its antiemetic qualities, making it particularly attractive in certain cases. The drugs included in the sedative-tranquillizer category are the barbiturates, the phenothiazine derivatives, hydroxyzine, droperidol (abutyrophenone), and the benzodiazepines.

Although the barbiturates secobarbital, pentobarbital, and amobarbital are no longer popular for use in obstetrics, both because they seem to have no analgesic properties and because they may have a profound depressant effect on the newborn (Levinson and Shnider 1987), they are still used in the early latent phase of labour for their sedative effect.

The phenothiazine derivatives (promethazine, propiomazine, chlorpromazine, promazine, and prochlorperazine), as well as hydroxyzine, are, with the benzodiazepines diazepam and droperidol, the major tranquillizers currently used in obstetrics, at least in the United States (Albright *et al.* 1986a). They are often administered intramuscularly or intravenously in combination with narcotics. Known for their antiemetic as well as sedative properties, the phenothiazines have not been associated with neonatal depression.

Although the phenothiazines and phenothiazine derivatives have been compared to pethidine in a number of trials (Busacca *et al.* 1982; Treisser *et al.* 1981; Cosmi and Marx 1969; Malkasian *et al.* 1967; McQuitty 1967; Brelje and Garcia-Bunuel 1966; Spellacy *et al.* 1966; DeKornfeld *et al.* 1964; McDonald *et al.* 1964; Rowley *et al.* 1963; Powe *et al.* 1962; and Fromhagen and Carswell 1961), these will not be reviewed.

Droperidol, a major tranquillizer, can be used alone but is most often used in conjunction with the narcotic Fentanyl; the latter combination is marketed as Innovar. This combination is called neuroleptanalgesia, and is not used for childbirth because of the tendency to confer profound depressant effects on the newborn.

Diazepam rapidly appears in the fetal blood ten minutes after intravenous injection to the mother (Scher *et al.* 1972) and peaks at 60 minutes after

Table 57.5 Effect of methoxyflurane versus nitrous oxide/oxygen for analgesia in labour on inadequate pain relief

Study	EXPT		CTRL		Odds ratio	Graph of odds ratios and confidence intervals						
	n	(%)	n	(%)	(95% CI)	0.01	0.1	0.5	1	2	10	100
Rosen *et al.* (1969)	177/598	(29.60)	75/265	(28.30)	1.06 (0.77–1.46)							
Jones *et al.* (1969)	5/24	(20.83)	3/22	(13.64)	1.63 (0.36–7.39)							
Typical odds ratio (95% confidence interval)					1.08 (0.79–1.48)							

Table 57.6 Effect of methoxyflurane versus nitrous oxide/oxygen for analgesia in labour on nausea/vomiting

Study	EXPT		CTRL		Odds ratio	Graph of odds ratios and confidence intervals						
	n	(%)	n	(%)	(95% CI)	0.01	0.1	0.5	1	2	10	100
Bergsjø and Lindbaek (1971)	3/63	(4.76)	7/63	(11.11)	0.42 (0.12–1.53)							
Rosen *et al.* (1969)	114/598	(19.06)	61/265	(23.02)	0.78 (0.55–1.12)							
Jones *et al.* (1969)	2/24	(8.33)	8/24	(33.33)	0.23 (0.06–0.90)							
Typical odds ratio (95% confidence interval)					0.70 (0.50–0.98)							

intramuscular injection (Idanpaan-Heikkila *et al.* 1971); the fetal level of the drug is equal to (Scher *et al.* 1972) or greater than (DeSilva *et al.* 1964) the maternal blood level. Diazepam has a long half-life (21–37 hours) and concentrates in the fetal liver. It has been reported to be associated with respiratory depression in the neonate (Dalen *et al.* 1969; Catchlove and Kafer 1971), hypotonia and lethargy (Flowers *et al.* 1969; McCarthy *et al.* 1973), hypothermia (McAllister 1980), problems with temperature regulation, and loss of beat-to-beat variations during labour (Scher *et al.* 1972), and side-effects appear to be dose related.

Schiff *et al.* (1971) have raised the theoretical objection to use of diazepam in obstetrics that sodium benzoate, a buffer in which diazepam is dissolved, is a bilirubin–albumin uncoupler *in vitro*. To date, there is no evidence of increased kernicterus in neonates exposed to large doses of diazepam.

Trials that look at diazepam versus placebo (Table 57.7) are not, generally, very informative with regard to the above-mentioned potential problems. Holmskov and Schrøder (1975) did not show any shortening of labour, pain relief or amnesia when diazepam (maximum 30 mg) was compared with placebo for labour pain. In this study, neither asphyxia, hypotonia, nor Apgar score (Table 57.8) were any different in the two groups though instrumental delivery may have been reduced with diazepam. Aiken and Cope (1971) compared pethidine plus diazepam (20 mg) with pethidine plus placebo. Data were available only for neonatal drowsiness (Table 57.9), which was increased in the pethidine-diazepam group. Nisbet *et al.* (1967) employed a study design similar to that of Aiken and Cope and found that pain relief was better, but Apgar scores were lower, in the pethidine–diazepam group.

2.4 Regional analgesia

Over the past twenty years regional techniques of analgesia and anaesthesia have emerged as the major approach to pain relief in obstetrics, not only for vaginal and operative vaginal deliveries, but for caesarean section as well. There are many reasons for the popularity of regional anaesthesia.

The primary reason for use of analgesia and anaesthesia during labour and delivery is pain relief. Clearly, although general anaesthesia is effective in preventing a woman from feeling pain, its effect goes well beyond pain relief. This unnecessarily broad scope extends also to other methods of systemic analgesia such as tranquillizers, narcotics, and amnesiacs, where actual pain relief may not be effected. Clinical interest in minimizing the range of effect while maximizing the strength of the effect has directed the focus on regional analgesia. There, the attention has been increasingly on blocking only the regions of direct concern during labour and/or delivery. For example, spinal analgesia is not favoured

for labour and vaginal delivery, as it often does 'more' than necessary in the form of motor blockade, in addition to its other attendant dangers. Lumbar epidural block does not effect a motor blockade, unless improperly administered, and hence is the currently preferred method of providing regional analgesia. In addition to the implied benefits of blocking smaller areas, regional analgesia and anaesthesia do not affect the mother's consciousness.

Clinicians are perhaps less concerned than they should be about the dearth of good data on possible harmful effects. This may be in part because of the extremely positive aspects of epidural analgesia. In addition, common sense dictates that it is unlikely that a medication which provides complete pain relief yet presents absolutely no danger to mother or child will ever be identified.

2.4.1 Regional anaesthetics

Local anaesthetics fall into one of two main pharmacologic categories: those with an ester linkage and those with an amide linkage as integral to their molecular structure. Ester compounds (procaine, 2-chloroprocaine, tetracaine, and piperocaine) are generally rapidly hydrolysed in the bloodstream, while the amides (mepivacaine, bupivacaine, lidocaine, etidocaine, and propitocaine) are slowly broken down in the liver. Bupivacaine has emerged as the predominant agent in current use for lumbar epidurals owing to a general opinion that it confers relatively long duration of action and superior quality of analgesia. Recently, due to reports of cardiotoxicity from bupivacaine, lidocaine has re-emerged for use in caesarean section, but not for analgesia in labour.

2.4.2 Lumbar epidural analgesia

Use of lumbar epidural analgesia and anaesthesia (often called, simply, epidural block) seems to be increasing in developed countries, although national figures are difficult to come by. According to Hicks *et al.* (1976) it is currently the most commonly used regional technique in the United States. Gibbs *et al.* (1986), in a survey of a sample of 1200 United States hospitals, found that epidural anaesthesia was used in 16 per cent of the labours and 21 per cent of caesarean sections. In his survey, the only drugs used more often in labour were those classified broadly as narcotics/barbiturates/tranquillizers (49 per cent). Thirty-two per cent of the labours occurred without pain medication.

In 1978, Doughty reported on a personal survey of sixteen London teaching hospitals conducted in 1976 which revealed that the percentage of parturients receiving epidural anaesthesia at each hospital ranged from 5 per cent to 62 per cent; the median rate was 36 per cent.

Although the trend in Great Britain is toward increasing use of epidural block (May and DeVere

Table 57.7(a) Selected trial design features: diazepam versus placebo

Authors, date country	Total n	Reported method of treatment assignment and masking	Funding source	Treatment groups	Top-ups?	Conclusions
Holmskov and Schrøder (1975) Denmark	439	Random; double-masked	Roche	(1) Diazepam (10 mg) intramuscularly (IM) (2) Placebo (2 ml)	Yes	Duration of labour, Apgar scores, vacuum extractions same in both grps
Aiken and Cope (1971) UK	200	Numbered ampoules/boxes; double-masked	Roche Products, Ltd.	(1) Diazepam (20 mg) + pethidine (PETH) (100 mg) (2) Placebo + PETH (100 mg)		Duration of labour, operative intervention, postpartum haemorrhage, fetal depression, and pain relief similar for (1) and (2) Drowsiness increased in grp (1)
Nisbet et al (1967) US	204	Numbered packages of placebo or diazepam; double-masked	Hoffmann-LaRoche and Weinberger OB-GYN Fund	(1) Diazepam (10 mg) + PETH (2) Placebo + PETH	Yes	Greater pain relief in grp (1) Lower Apgars in grp (1)

Table 57.7(b) Observed effect of intervention on outcome: diazepam versus placebo

Authors, date (total n)	No. of pts in each treatment grp	Treatment groups	Apgar score <7 at 1 min	Instrumental delivery (forceps, vacuum)	Drowsiness
Holmskov and Schrøder (1975) (n = 439)	222 217	(1) Diazepam (10 mg) (IM) (2) Placebo (12 ml)	13/221* 13/218*	10/222 16/217	NA† NA
Aiken and Cope (1971) (n = 200)	? ?	(1) Diazepam (20 mg) + PETH (100 mg) (2) Placebo + PETH (100 mg)	NA NA	NA NA	38/91 22/89
Nisbet et al. (1967) (n = 204)	108 96	(1) Diazepam + PETH (2) Placebo + PETH	9/108 4/ 96	NA NA	NA NA

*Intentionally so written.
†NA indicates 'Not available'.

Table 57.8 Effect of diazepam in labour on Apgar score < 7 at 1 minute

Study	EXPT		CTRL		Odds ratio	Graph of odds ratios and confidence intervals
	n	(%)	n	(%)	(95% CI)	0.01 0.1 0.5 1 2 10 100
Nisbet *et al.* (1967)	9/108	(8.33)	4/96	(4.17)	2.00 (0.65–6.16)	
Holmskov and Schrøder (1975)	13/221	(5.88)	13/218	(5.96)	0.99 (0.45–2.18)	
Typical odds ratio (95% confidence interval)					1.25 (0.65–2.38)	

Table 57.9 Effect of diazepam in labour on neonatal drowsiness

Study	EXPT		CTRL		Odds ratio	Graph of odds ratios and confidence intervals
	n	(%)	n	(%)	(95% CI)	0.01 0.1 0.5 1 2 10 100
Aiken and Cope (1971)	38/91	(41.76)	22/89	(24.72)	2.14 (1.16–3.98)	
Typical odds ratio (95% confidence interval)					2.14 (1.16–3.98)	

1976; Bailey and Howard 1983), this is dependent on the availability of obstetric anaesthesia services. Recent surveys have shown that a 24-hour epidural anaesthesia service is still not universally available, even in units with more than 1000 deliveries per year (Reynolds 1986). Reports from Wales (Hibbard *et al.* 1979) have described a low use of obstetric epidural anaesthesia—about 3 per cent of all labouring women—also because of lack of available services, rather than lack of requests.

Unpublished 1985 data from the Canadian Institute of Child Health (personal communication) show that epidural anaesthesia (data are not available by stage of delivery) is available at 25 per cent of hospitals with 20–100 live births per year, 49 per cent of those with 101–300 births, 64 per cent of those with 301–999 births, and 86 per cent of those with 1000+ births. In general, hospitals performing a small number of births per year have a small proportion of women receiving epidurals, and hospitals performing a large number of births have a greater proportion of women receiving epidurals. Whether this is purely a matter of availability or a matter of different choices being made by the women and doctors is not known.

Lack of obstetric anaesthesia services can also be a problem in the United States: Gibbs *et al.* (1986) found that most anaesthesia for labour is provided by obstetricians, not anaesthetists, primarily because of lack of continuous coverage. (The reasons for this are complicated, and may be due to a low level of reimbursement for obstetric anaesthesia as compared with other areas of anaesthesia (Gibbs *et al.* 1986).

In Sweden, less common use of epidural anaesthesia may be due to the fact that pethidine and/or nitrous oxide/oxygen are the initial treatments administered. The National Swedish Board of Health and Welfare reported that about 12 per cent of mothers had epidural anaesthesia in 1978 (Bundsen *et al.* 1982). In summary, the desire for and use of epidural block seems to be increasing greatly, but this increase is limited by lack of availability of anaesthetic services.

Reynolds (1986) recently asked: 'Anaesthetists continue to advocate [epidural analgesia's] use: is it empire building or are there good reasons?'. The major reasons for the increase are practical, economic, and a matter of what's in style. First and foremost is the fact that lumbar epidural anaesthesia is usually effective and also allows the woman to remain awake and aware. It can also be used throughout parturition, even when caesarean section is required.

Second, there are economic reasons, though these are complicated by varying payment structures in different countries. The increased use of epidural anaesthesia in the United Kingdom was stimulated by the Central Midwives' Board of England and Wales decision in 1970 that midwives would be permitted to provide top-up injections of regional anaesthesia through a catheter sited by an anaesthetist (Doughty 1978). The additional prescription in 1972 that midwives should be trained in advanced methods may have also affected use of the technique in the United Kingdom. In the United States, anaesthetists or anaesthetist-supervised nurse anaesthetists administer most epidurals (Gibbs *et al.*

Table 57.10(a) Selected trial design features: lumbar epidural block versus systemic narcotics

Authors, date country	Total n	Reported method of treatment assignment and masking	Funding source	Treatment groups	Top-ups?	Conclusions
Ryhanen et al. (1985) Finland	10	Alternate assignment; not masked	Paulo Foundation	(1) segmental epidural 0.5% BV (4–6 ml) (2) PETH (IM) (50 mg) as necessary		Increased post-delivery leucocytes in mothers and infants w/ PETH Decreased T cells in mothers w/PETH No difference in duration of labour, Apgar scores
Robinson et al. (1980a); Revill et al. (1980) Wales	386	Random, no method given; not masked	Medical Research Council and the Welsh Office	(1) 0.5% BV (5–10 ml); Entonox (2) PETH (150 mg) + perphenazine 5 mg (IM); Entonox (3) PETH 0.25 mg/kg (0.19 ml/min) (IV) (self-administered); Entonox	Yes	More satisfactory analgesia in grp (1) Duration of labour similar in grps (1) and (2)
Jouppila et al (1980) Finland	28	Alternate assignment; not masked	?	(1) 0.5% BV-epi (4 ml) (2) PETH (50 mg) (IM), as necessary	Yes	Duration of labour longer w/ PETH No difference in Apgar Prolactin significantly decreased during labour in PETH group
Jouppila and Hollmen (1976); Jouppila (1976) Finland	28	Alternate assignment; not masked	?	(1) 0.5% BV (3–6 ml) (2) PETH (50 mg) (IM) as necessary	Yes	Duration of labour longer w/BV No difference in Apgar Maternal pH increased during labour w/PETH Umbilical creatinine phosphokinase higher w/BV
Thalme et al. (1974) Sweden	28	Random, no method given; not masked	Swedish Medical Research Council	(1) 0.25% BV-epi (6–8 ml) (2) PETH (100 mg) with chlorpromazine (12.5 mg); nitrous oxide	Yes	Less acidosis in grp (1) Bradycardia seen equally in grps (1) and (2)
Kurjak and Beazley (1974) UK	448	Random, no method given; not masked	?	(1) 0.5% BV-epi (8 ml) (2) PETH (150 mcg); promazine, promethazine, Entonox, MOR	Yes	Lower umbilical arterial pH in grp (1) Lower Apgar score in grp (2)
Buchan et al. (1973) Scotland	20	No method given; not masked	?	(1) 0.25% BV (2) PETH 150 mcg (IM)	Yes	Rise in maternal corticosteroid blocked in grp (1)
Noble et al. (1971) UK	245	Random, no method given; not masked	?	(1) 0.5% BV-epi (8 ml) (2) PETH 150 mg; Entonox, promazine, promethazine, MOR	Yes	Lower Apgar score in grp (2) Lower umbilical arterial pH in grp (2)

Table 57.10(b) Observed effect of intervention on outcomes of interest: lumbar epidural block versus systemic narcotics

Authors, date (total n)	No. of pts in each treatment grp	Treatment groups	Mean duration of analgesia (min) (SE)	Mean Apgar score (at 1 min)	Instrumental delivery (forceps, vacuum)	Duration 1st stage (hr)
Ryhanen (1984) (n = 10)	5	(1) 0.5% BV	NA*	8.6	NA	5.7
	5	(2) 50 mg PETH (IM) as necessary	NA	9.0	NA	5.3
Robinson et al. (1980a); Revill (1980) (n = 386 randomized; 93 analysed)	45	(1) 0.5% BV; Entonox	NA	NA	22/45	7.3
	48	(2) PETH (150 mg) + perphenazine (5 mg) (IM); Entonox	NA	NA	9/48	7.6
	47	(3) PETH 0.25 mg/kg (IV); Entonox	NA	NA	NA	NA
Jouppila et al. (1980) (n = 18)	8	(1) 0.5% BV	NA	8.9	NA	3.2
	10	(2) 50 mg PETH (IM) as necessary	NA	8.8	NA	5.5
Jouppila (1976); Jouppila and Hollmen (1976); (n = 28)	14	(1) 0.5% BV-epi	NA	9.0	1/14	6.7
	14	(2) 50 mg PETH (IM) as necessary	NA	8.8	1/14	4.0
Thalme et al. (1974) (n = 28)	14	(1) 0.25% BV-epi	NA	NA	6/12	11.3
	14	(2) PETH (100 mg) + chlorpromazine (12.5 mg) + N_2O-O_2 as needed	NA	NA	3/12	10.5
Kurjak and Beazley (1974) (n = 448)	224	(1) 0.5% BV-epi	NA	9.8 (at 5 min)	NA	NA
	224	(2) PETH (150 mg); promazine, Entonox, MOR	NA	9.6	NA	NA
Buchan (1973) (n = 20)	10	(1) 0.25% BV	NA	NA	5/10	NA
	10	(2) PETH (IM) (150 mg)	NA	NA	NA	NA
Noble et al. (1971) (n = 245)	125	(1) BV-epi	NA	9.8 (at 5 min)	30/100	NA
	120	(2) PETH; promazine, promethazine, Entonox, MOR	NA	9.4	6/102	NA

*NA indicates 'Not available'.

1986), while other analgesic procedures may not require their participation. Remuneration for these services by third party payers has probably contributed to increased rather than decreased popularity of epidurals, where service is available, although payment for obstetric anaesthesia lags far behind payment for anaesthesia in other areas.

Detailed descriptions of the technique used for lumbar epidural block may be found in Crawford 1978; Bromage 1978; Albright and Ferguson 1986; Covino and Scott 1985.

2.4.2.1 Epidural lumbar block versus systemic narcotics

The safety of lumbar epidural analgesia is not beyond question. Among the possible associated maternal complications are: hypotension resulting from sympathetic blockade, respiratory insufficiency, nausea and vomiting, shivering, prolonged labour, increased use of operative delivery, neurologic complications, bladder dysfunction, headache, backache, toxic drug reactions, maternal death, dural puncture, unblocked segments, and unilateral block. The fetus may also suffer complications as a result of maternal effects (e.g. hypotension) or direct drug toxicity.

Administration of epidural lumbar block has been compared with systemic narcotics in eight trials (Ryhanen 1984; Robinson 1980a, Revill 1980; Jouppila 1980; Joupilla 1980; Joupilla 1976a; Thalme 1974; Kurjak 1974; Buchan 1973; Noble 1971). Duration of first stage is not consistently affected by one method of analgesia or the other. Jouppila *et al.* (1980) found a shorter first stage with epidural bupivacaine but Jouppila and Hollmèn (1976) showed a shorter labour with systemic pethidine. Clearly, factors other than type of analgesia are playing a greater role in determining duration of labour.

The data provided show that epidural block is associated with an increased proportion of instrumental deliveries (Table 57.11). Robinson *et al.* (1980a),

Thalme *et al.* (1974), and Noble *et al.* (1971) report marked differences between groups receiving epidural bupivacaine and systemic pethidine. The increased risk of instrumental delivery associated with epidural block may well be reduced by careful timing of top-up doses and a liberal attitude to length of the second stage of labour.

A well-designed double-blind trial by Chestnut *et al.* (1987) compared the effect of continuing administration of bupivacaine 0.125 per cent by continuous infusion after 8 cm dilatation, with administration of a saline placebo. The continued bupivacaine had no effect on the adequacy of analgesia for the remainder of the first stage but did result in more adequate analgesia in the second stage (36/46 (78 per cent) versus 18/46 (39 per cent)). Caesarean section rates were identical in the two groups, but the use of continued bupivacaine resulted in prolongation of the second stage (124 ± 70 minutes versus 94 ± 54 minutes). Instrumental delivery was used for 21/40 (53 per cent) of the women with bupivacaine compared to 11/40 (28 per cent) of the women who received saline. Thus, the use of epidural anaesthesia after 8 cm dilatation can result in both prolongation of the second stage and increased use of instrumental vaginal delivery (Table 57.12).

Epidural analgesia can be administered either via intermittent 'top-up' doses by way of an indwelling catheter or continuous administration by one of a variety of infusion devices. Recently, a trial comparing the two methods has been completed (Smedstad and Morison 1988). Sixty primigravid women were randomized in unmasked fashion either to receive 8 ml 0.25 per cent bupivacaine per hour by continuous infusion or to receive 8 ml of 0.25 per cent bupivacaine per hour, as required and as determined by the nurse. Both groups received an initial dose of 12 ml of 0.25 per cent bupivacaine. Pain level was assessed using a vertical visual analogue scale before the epidural, one hour after its insertion, and one-half to one hour after delivery.

Table 57.11 Effect of lumbar epidural block versus systemic narcotics in labour on instrumental delivery

Study	EXPT		CTRL		Odds ratio	Graph of odds ratios and confidence intervals						
	n	(%)	n	(%)	(95% CI)	0.01	0.1	0.5	1	2	10	100
Noble *et al.* (1971)	30/100	(30.00)	6/102	(5.88)	5.15 (2.51–10.57)							
Robinson *et al.* (1980a)	22/45	(48.89)	9/48	(18.75)	3.83 (1.62–9.02)							
Jouppila (1976); Jouppila and Hollmén (1976)	1/14	(7.14)	1/14	(7.14)	1.00 (0.06–16.86)							
Thalme *et al.* (1974)	6/12	(50.00)	3/12	(25.00)	2.78 (0.55–14.02)							
Typical odds ratio (95% confidence interval)					4.12 (2.47–6.89)							

Table 57.12 Effect of epidural bupivacaine versus placebo after 8cm dilatation on inadequate analgesia during 1st stage

Study	EXPT		CTRL		Odds ratio	Graph of odds ratios and confidence intervals						
	n	(%)	*n*	(%)	(95% CI)	0.01	0.1	0.5	1	2	10	100
Chestnut *et al.* (1987)	2/46	(4.35)	1/46	(2.17)	1.98 (0.20–19.49)							
Typical odds ratio (95% confidence interval)					1.98 (0.20–19.49)							

Effect of epidural bupivacaine versus placebo after 8 cm dilatation on inadequate analgesia in 2nd stage

Chestnut *et al.* (1987)	8/46	(17.39)	26/46	(56.52)	0.19 (0.08–0.44)							
Typical odds ratio (95% confidence interval)					0.19 (0.08–0.44)							

Effect of epidural bupivacaine versus placebo after 8 cm dilatation on operative delivery

Chestnut *et al.* (1987)	27/46	(58.70)	17/46	(36.96)	2.37 (1.05–5.34)							
Typical odds ratio (95% confidence interval)					2.37 (1.05–5.34)							

Effect of epidural bupivacaine versus placebo after 8 cm dilatation on instrumental vaginal delivery

Chestnut *et al.* (1987)	21/46	(45.65)	11/46	(23.91)	2.58 (1.10–6.06)							
Typical odds ratio (95% confidence interval)					2.58 (1.10–6.06)							

Effect of epidural bupivacaine versus placebo after 8 cm dilatation on caesarean section

Chestnut et al. (1987)	6/46	(13.04)	6/46	(13.04)	1.00 (0.30–3.34)							
Typical odds ratio (95% confidence interval)					1.00 (0.30–3.34)							

Effect of epidural bupivacaine versus placebo after 8cm dilatation on Apgar score <7 at 1 minute

Chestnut *et al.* (1987)	6/46	(13.04)	10/46	(21.74)	0.55 (0.19–1.61)							
Typical odds ratio (95% confidence interval)					0.55 (0.19–1.61)							

Effect of epidural bupivacaine versus placebo after 8cm dilatation on Apgar score <7 at 5 minutes

Chestnut *et al.* (1987)	0/46	(0.00)	1/46	(2.17)	0.14 (0.00–6.82)							
Typical odds ratio (95% confidence interval)					0.14 (0.00–6.82)							

Not all patients were included in the analysis. Mothers administered the continuous block received a mean dose of bupivacaine that was almost twice as high as the mothers administered top-ups. Their labour was longer on the average (610 versus 499 minutes), and significantly more likely to require outlet forceps. Although there was a trend indicating greater pain relief with the continuous infusion, the difference was not statistically significant. If there had been a significant difference in pain relief, it would hardly have been surprising, given the greater total dose received by the infusion group.

In a trial comparing regular top-ups of epidural

analgesia at 90 minute intervals versus top-up on maternal demand (using concentrations of 0.5 per cent, 0.375 per cent, and 0.25 per cent), Purdy *et al.* (1987) found that episodes of severe pain were reported by 5/120 (4 per cent) of the women who received regular top-ups and 38/120 (32 per cent) of the women who had top-ups on demand. Moderate or severe pain was experienced by 17/120 (14 per cent) of the women in the regular top-up group compared to 103/120 (86 per cent) in the demand group. Eight of the 120 women (7 per cent) with regular top-ups felt that their analgesia was

less than good, as did 15 of the 120 women (13 per cent) with top-up on demand. Operative delivery rates and infant outcomes were similar in the two groups (Table 57.13).

Finally, two other trials (Vella *et al.* 1985; Justins *et al.* 1983) compared epidural administration of bupivacaine plus fentanyl versus epidural bupivacaine plus systemically administered fentanyl. In a meta-analysis of the results of these comparisons, Vella *et al.* (1985) report that a third trial of 'identical design' (Justins *et al.* 1982) has been carried out, but as far as this author

Table 57.13 Effect of epidural top-ups at maternal request versus scheduled top-ups on episodes of severe pain

Study	EXPT n	(%)	CTRL n	(%)	Odds ratio (95% CI)	Graph of odds ratios and confidence intervals
Purdy et al. (1987)	38/120	(31.67)	5/120	(4.17)	6.44 (3.33–12.44)	
Typical odds ratio (95% confidence interval)					6.44 (3.33–12.44)	

Effect of epidural top-ups at maternal request versus scheduled top-ups on episodes of moderate or severe pain

Purdy et al. (1987)	103/120	(85.83)	17/120	(14.17)	17.37 (10.48–28.78)	
Typical odds ratio (95% confidence interval)					17.37 (10.48–28.78)	

Effect of epidural top-ups at maternal request versus scheduled top-ups on poor quality of analgesia overall

Purdy et al. (1987)	15/120	(12.50)	8/120	(6.67)	1.96 (0.83–4.61)	
Typical odds ratio (95% confidence interval)					1.96 (0.83–4.61)	

Effect of epidural top-ups at maternal request versus scheduled top-ups on operative delivery

Purdy et al. (1987)	61/120	(50.83)	60/120	(50.00)	1.03 (0.62–1.71)	
Typical odds ratio (95% confidence interval)					1.03 (0.62–1.71)	

Effect of epidural top-ups at maternal request versus scheduled top-ups on instrumental vaginal delivery

Purdy et al. (1987)	42/120	(35.00)	47/120	(39.17)	0.84 (0.50–1.41)	
Typical odds ratio (95% confidence interval)					0.84 (0.50–1.41)	

Effect of epidural top-ups at maternal request versus scheduled top-ups on caesarean section

Purdy et al. (1987)	19/120	(15.83)	13/120	(10.83)	1.54 (0.73–3.23)	
Typical odds ratio (95% confidence interval)					1.54 (0.73–3.23)	

can determine, this study did not compare epidural with systemic administration of the drugs. Both Vella *et al.* (1985) and Justins *et al.* (1983) found that the combination of epidural bupivacaine plus fentanyl produced an increased duration of analgesia and may have increased the duration of the first stage of labour. Instrumental delivery was more frequent after epidural block. No clear difference was detected in respect of Apgar scores.

Of the 50 controlled trials published up to the end of 1987 that looked at lumbar epidural anaesthesia, 38 included the anaesthetic bupivacaine. What is presented below will focus on those trials that have studied bupivacaine: the effects of various doses, the effect of epinephrine, comparison with chloroprocaine, and comparison with narcotics used epidurally. Bupivacaine, lidocaine, and chloroprocaine are probably the drugs used most often today for epidural anaesthesia, at least in the United States, and there is interest in both drugs regarding dose and the effect of added epinephrine. In addition, there has been recent renewed interest in the use of narcotics, administered epidurally or in the subarachnoid space.

2.4.2.2 The effect of bupivacaine dosage   The results of six randomized trials comparing different bupivacaine concentrations have been published (Ewen *et al.* 1986; Li *et al.* 1985; Kenepp *et al.* 1983; Abouleish *et al.* 1982; Stainthorp *et al.* 1978; Challen *et al.* 1977; Purdy *et al.* 1987); these are summarized in Table 57.14. Only one (Abouleish *et al.* 1982) was double-blind. These trials were all small: the total sample sizes ranged from 18 to 98, with between 4 and 40 women per treatment group. In general, the main purpose of these trials was to look at the effect of bupivacaine concentration on pain relief. Total dose and side-effects (e.g. motor blockade, mode of delivery) were issues of subsidiary interest. A seventh trial (Covino *et al.* 1976) was described in an abstract, but no data were presented in that publication.

Data regarding the effect of various doses of bupivacaine on pain relief are presented in Table 57.13. The published data from the four remaining trials are not readily comparable. Data were collected at different times during labour and post-medication; individual differences in the progression of labour and the subjective measurement of pain are less serious analysis problems than the differences between studies of when, after administration of analgesia, pain was measured. Similarly, other aspects of these articles render quantitative comparisons between the reported data difficult if not impossible: use of different pain scales; undocumented meaning of pain scale values; and use of different methods of delivery of anaesthesia (continuous versus intermittent).

The data in Table 57.14 can be summarized as follows: there is evidence that higher, rather than lower,

concentrations of bupivacaine are effective in relieving labour pain. A decreased concentration of bupivacaine with an increased rate of infusion may be equally effective as the same total dosage per hour, infused at a higher concentration and slower rate. This summary assumes that the study populations are comparable, the data are unbiased and reliable, the experiments are repeatable, and the pain scales are valid. The data available give little or no guidance to the anaesthetist as to the optimal concentrations or rates of infusion of bupivacaine.

Recently, in a letter published in The Lancet, Turner *et al.* (1987) reported on a trial of 517 women, randomly allocated to 6–8 ml of 0.5 per cent, 10–14 ml of 0.25 per cent, or 6–8 ml of 0.25 per cent plain bupivacaine. The patients given low volume, low dose bupivacaine were less likely to require low or mid-forceps delivery. In response to this letter, Marcoux *et al.* (1987) reported a trial of 371 women randomized to receive 20 ml 0.375 per cent or 15 ml 0.5 per cent bupivacaine in a single shot. Midforceps delivery were applied in 22.5 per cent of deliveries in the 0.375 per cent group, and 42.9 per cent in the 0.5% group. Rotational forceps were used three times more often in the 0.5% bupivacaine group. Though little other data are available regarding the methods and results from these trials, they do provide evidence for increased use of forceps with higher doses of regional anaesthetic.

2.4.2.3 The effect of epinephrine   The effect of adding epinephrine (adrenaline) to an epidural anaesthetic, in particular bupivacaine, has been of great interest lately for two reasons: one concerns its use in a 'test' dose of anaesthetic, and the other its use as a method of prolonging the anaesthetic's action.

The former is primarily the result of several cases in the United States in which maternal death resulted from inadvertent intravenous delivery of large doses of bupivacaine (without added epinephrine) (Albright 1979). A number of investigators feel that addition of epinephrine to a bupivacaine test dose would prevent such an occurrence by allowing anaesthetists to detect the immediate increase in pulse rate if the epidural catheter were placed intravenously (Albright 1984; Marx 1984; Nicholas 1984). The test dose would in theory also detect a subarachnoid injection by a rapid onset of significant motor and sensory block.

Benefits of addition of epinephrine to the full dose of anaesthetic are not well established: the positive effects, protection against a myocardial effect (Moore and Scurlock 1983) and prolongation of action of the anaesthetic, may be outweighed by the possible adverse effects, particularly tachycardia, hypertension, and bradycardia (Leighton *et al.* 1987), and decreased uterine blood flow leading to fetal distress.

Although there is a plethora of literature debating

Table 57.14(a) Selected trial design features: lumbar epidural block using various dosages of bupivacaine (BV)

Authors, date country	Total *n*	Reported method of treatment assignment and masking	Funding source	Treatment groups	Top-ups?	Conclusions
Ewen *et al.* (1986) Scotland	53	Random, table of random numbers; not masked†	None*	(1) 0.08% BV (25 ml/hr) (2) 0.25% BV (8 ml/hr)	Yes	Intervention-free interval longer in grp (1) More top-ups in grp (2) Less motor block in grp (1)
Li *et al.* (1985) Wales	98	Random, no method given; not masked	Bioassays: Duncan Flockhart and Co.	(1) no infusion (2) 0.0625% BV (10 ml/hr) (3) 0.125% BV (5 ml/hr) (4) 0.125% BV (10 ml/hr) (5) 0.125% BV (15 ml/hr)	Yes	Greatest total dose BV for grp (5) Intervention-free interval longest in grps (4) and (5)
Kenepp *et al.* (1983) US	21	Random, no method given; not masked	?	(1) 0.125% BV (20 ml/hr) (2) 0.25% BV (20 mg/hr) (3) 0.5% BV (20 mg/hr) (4) 0.12% BV (10 mg/hr)	?	Highest number of dermatomes blocked in grp (1)
Abouleish *et al.* (1982) US	80	Random, no method given; double masked	Winthrop–Breon supplied drugs*	(1) 0.25% BV (8–11 ml) (2) 0.5% BV (8–11 ml)	Yes	Increased successful analgesia, longer duration, more spread in grp (2) No difference in side-effects
Stainthorp *et al.* (1978) UK Challen *et al.* (1977) UK	93	Random, no method given; not masked	?	(1) 0.125% BV (12 ml) (2) 0.25% BV (12 ml) (3) 0.375% BV (12 ml)	Yes	Least effective analgesia in grp (1) Mode of delivery, Apgars similar in all grps Increased total dosage with increased concentration BV Greater motor weakness in grp (3)
Purdy *et al.* (1987) Scotland	240	Random, no method given; not masked	?	(1) 0.5% BV (2) 0.375% BV (3) 0.25% BV	Yes	No significant differences

*Information obtained by contact with author.

these and other issues, there are apparently only five published trials comparing epidural anaesthetics with and without epinephrine (Abboud *et al.* 1984b, 1985; Broadfield *et al.* 1975; Moir *et al.* 1976; Reynolds *et al.* 1973; Reynolds and Taylor 1971); these are summarized in Table 57.15. Only one was double-blind (Reynolds and Taylor 1971), and no published report described the methods of randomization. Total sample size ranged from 13 to 70. For the most part, the studies were undertaken to explore the effect of epinephrine

added to bupivacaine for epidural anaesthesia: specifically, the umbilical venous:maternal venous ratio of bupivacaine concentration, toxic effects (primarily cardiovascular), and the duration of analgesic effect.

In terms of outcome, the mean duration of analgesia was increased for the bupivacaine–epinephrine groups in two of the three studies that made this measurement. However, the large difference seen in one of these (Abboud *et al.* 1984b, 1985) is so different from the others that it seems to decrease the reliability of such a

Table 57.14(b) Observed effect of intervention on outcome: lumbar epidural block using various dosages of bupivacaine (BV)

Authors, date (total n)	No. of pts in each treatment group	Treatment groups	Subjective pain score	Time of measurement	Method of anaesthetic delivery	Mean pain scores / % success
Ewen et al. (1986) (n = 53)	25	(1) 0.08% (25 ml/hr)	Worst pain during infusion: (0–3 score, 0 = none)	Postpartum interview	Injection and infusion (IJ/IF)	0.84 (mean pain score)
	28	(2) 0.25% (8 ml/hr)				1.36
Li, et al. (1985) (n = 98)	19	(1) Initial dose; no infusion;	Assessment of pain relief (10 cm linear analogue scale)	Postpartum interview	IJ/IF	30.2
	20	(2) 0.0625% (10 ml/hr)				34.5
	20	(3) 0.125% (5 ml/hr)				40.0
	19	(4) 0.125% (10 ml/hr)				45.3
	20	(5) 0.125% (15 ml/hr)				41.9
Kenepp et al. (1983) (n = 21)	?	(1) 0.5% (4 ml/hr)	NA*	20–30 min intervals during labour	IJ/IF	NA
		(2) 0.25% (8 ml/hr)				NA
		(3) 0.125% (16 ml/hr)				NA
		(4) 0.125% (8 ml/hr)				NA
Abouleish et al. (1982) (n = 80)	40	(1) 0.25% (8–11 ml)	Effect of epidural on pain (0–3 score, 0 = none)	Following each injection	Injection (IJ)	1.97
	40	(2) 0.5% (8–11 ml)				2.42
Stainthorp et al. (1978) (n = 93)	33	(1) 0.125% (12 ml)	Effective of first dose (% success)	20 min after first injection	IJ	61% (% success)
	29	(2) 0.25% (12 ml)				100%
	31	(3) 0.375% (12 ml)				94%
Purdy et al. (1987) (n = 240)	80	(1) 0.5%	Worst pain during infusion; adequate analgesia	Post partum interview	IJ	92%
	80	(2) 0.375%				89%
	80	(3) 0.25%				90%

*NA indicates 'not available'.

Table 57.15(a) Selected trial design features: lumbar epidural block using bupivacaine–plain (BV) versus bupivacaine–epinephrine (BV-epi)

Authors, date country	Total n	Reported method of treatment assignment and masking	Funding source	Treatment groups	Top-ups?	Conclusions
Abboud et al. (1984b, 1985) US	32	'Given in a random manner'; not masked	Bioassays: Astra Pharm. Co.	(1) 0.5% BV-epi (2) 0.5% BV	Yes	Hypotension less in grp (1) Duration of analgesia greater in grp (1) No increase in side-effects
Moir et al. (1976) UK	335	Random, no method given; not masked	?	(1) 0.5% BV (2) 0.5% BV-epi (3) 2% lidocaine (LC) (4) 2% LC-epi	Yes	Epinephrine did not affect pain Duration of analgesia greater in grp (2) Less hypotension in grp (2)
Broadfield et al. (1975) UK	13	Random, no method given; not masked	Beckwith–Smith	(1) 0.5% BV-epi (2) 0.5% BV (3) 0.25% BV-epi	Yes	Increased maternal heart rate in grp (2) Decreased central venous pressure in grp (2)
Reynolds et al. (1973) UK	70	Matched for age and parity; not masked	?	(1) 0.5% BV-epi (2) 0.5% BV	Yes	Greater mean maternal plasma BV concentration in grp (1)
Reynolds and Taylor (1971) UK	18	Method not given; double masked	BDH Pharm	(1) 0.5% BV-epi (2) 0.5% BV	Yes	Duration of analgesia not prolonged by epi

Table 57.15(b) Observed effect of intervention on outcome: lumbar epidural block using bupivacaine–plain (BV) versus bupivacaine–epinephrine (BV-epi)

Authors, date (total n)	No. of pts in each treatment group	BV treatment groups	Mean duration of analgesia (min)	Mean systolic blood pressure	UV:MV† BV ratio
Abboud et al. (1984b, 1985) (n = 32)	16 16	(1) 0.5% BV (2) 0.5% BV-epi	85 187	114 119	0.31 0.27
Moir et al. (1976) (n = 335)	91 80	(1) 0.5% BV (2) 0.5% BV-epi	122 145	NA* NA	NA NA
Broadfield et al. (1975) (n = 13)	?	(1) 0.5% BV (2) 0.5% BV-epi (3) 25% BV-epi	NA NA NA	132.3 136.5 131.4	NA NA NA
Reynolds et al. (1973) (n = 70)	35 35	(1) 0.5% BV (2) 0.5% BV-epi	139 164	NA NA	0.28 0.26
Reynolds and Taylor (1971) (n = 18)	9 9	(1) 0.5% BV (2) 0.5% BV-epi	146 136	NA NA	0.23 0.40

*NA indicates 'Not available'.
†UV: MV BV ratio is the ratio of umbilical venous to maternal venous bupivacaine concentration

generalization. Similarly, for systolic blood pressure, there was a small increase for the epinephrine group in the two trials that measured it, but the patient means were so different between the two studies that generalizing is difficult. The umbilical venous:maternal venous bupivacaine concentration ratio is fairly constant across studies.

All in all, randomized trials comparing epidural bupivacaine with and without epinephrine have not been of sufficient size to detect small to moderate differences in effect. With the exception of data from Abboud *et al.* (1984b, 1985) on duration of analgesic effect, there do not now appear to be large differences between the two types of solution.

2.4.2.4 Bupivacaine versus chloroprocaine   Four trials have been published which compare epidural bupivacaine with chloroprocaine (Table 57.15). All were reported to be double masked. The total sample sizes of these trials ranged from 24 to 150. Two studies (Abboud *et al.* 1984a; Cohen and Thurlow 1979) used combined injection and infusion methods to deliver the anaesthetic, while the other two used injection only. Two studies compared 2 per cent chloroprocaine with 0.5 per cent bupivacaine (Abboud *et al.* 1982a, 1984a). One compared 2 per cent chloroprocaine to 0.375 per cent bupivacaine (Allen and Johnson 1979), and one 3 per cent chloroprocaine to 0.5 per cent bupivacaine (Cohen and Thurlow 1979).

Overall, mean maternal systolic blood pressure did not seem to differ between the two groups, nor did Apgar score at one minute seem to be affected. In these studies, the duration of action of bupivacaine was greater than that of chloroprocaine. Two studies claimed to show increased late decelerations with bupivacaine. Caution must be exercised in interpreting differences between treatment groups for reasons already pointed out: small total sample, lack of information on those not included in the analyses, and the fact that multiple studies performed by a single research group cannot be considered as having independent findings.

2.4.2.5 Epidural bupivacaine versus epidural narcotics   A recent development in regional anaesthesia is epidural administration of narcotics. In 1979, Behar *et al.* described the successful use of epidural morphine in the treatment of acute and chronic pain. These authors did not observe sympathetic or motor blockade associated with this use, suggesting a possible use in obstetric continuous lumbar epidural anaesthesia. In Paris, Lassner *et al.* (1981) randomized thirty women in double-masked fashion to either 5 mg of morphine administered epidurally, or to a placebo (saline) epidural. Bupivacaine top-ups were administered to both groups as needed. The saline group received less total volume of bupivacaine than the morphine group, providing an additional indicator to confirm the study findings that morphine provided no better pain relief than placebo.

The results of five randomized controlled trials comparing administration of epidural narcotics to epidural bupivacaine for labour pain have been published (Table 57.17). Either morphine (Hughes *et al.* 1984; Writer *et al.* 1981) or fentanyl (Skerman *et al.* 1985; Youngstrom *et al.* 1984; Desprats *et al.* 1983; Justins *et al.* 1982) were the narcotics used in these trials, top-ups for both groups were the regional anaesthetics. The sample sizes ranged from 16 to 70. All studies were stated to be randomized, but only one report documented how this was achieved. Only two were double-masked.

There is some indication that the groups that received narcotics had a longer duration of analgesia than those receiving just bupivacaine. Whether this is an effect of the narcotics, *per se*, or the effect of an additional amount of anaesthetic is an open and pertinent question. Pruritus was increased with narcotic use in most studies (Hughes *et al.* 1984; Desprats *et al.* 1983; Justins *et al.* 1982; Muller *et al.* 1981), though the extent and severity of this symptom were not reported.

A sixth trial (Cohen *et al.* 1987) involving 82 parturients has been published, comparing 0.25 per cent bupivacaine (9 ml) to bupivacaine (9 ml)/fentanyl (50 µg), bupivacaine (9 ml)/fentanyl (100 µg), and bupivacaine (3 ml)/fentanyl (100 µg). No significant differences between groups were seen for time to onset of analgesia and pain relief. Duration of analgesia tended to be shorter for the low dose bupivacaine group when compared to the other bupivacaine/fentanyl groups, but not when compared to the bupivacaine-only group. Vomiting was seen solely in the bupivacaine-only group, though this group was the only one with no reports of pruritus. Urinary retention was highest in this group as well, though not significantly so.

2.4.3 Caudal epidural block

In recent years, the use of caudal epidural block has largely been supplanted by increased use of lumbar epidural block. There are several reasons: first, caudal administration requires a larger volume of anaesthetic to produce pain relief at an adequate level; second, caudal block results in more blocked spinal segments than the lumbar approach; third, the spread of the anaesthesia is easier to control with lumbar rather than with caudal administration; and fourth, it is possible for the anaesthetist to miss the caudal canal and insert the needle into the baby's scalp, a fatal event when anaesthetic is administered.

On the positive side for caudal block, the possibility of a dural tap is decreased using this approach, as the subarachnoid space ends at S2. Also, anaesthesia administered via the sacral hiatus is more able to reach

Table 57.16(a) Selected trial design features: lumbar epidural block using bupivacaine (BV) versus chloroprocaine (CP)

Authors, date country	Total n	Reported method of treatment assignment and masking	Funding source	Treatment groups	Top-ups?	Conclusions
Abboud et al. (1984a) US	61	Random, sealed envelopes; double-masked*	?	(1) 0.125% BV (14 ml/hr) (2) 0.75% CP (27 ml/hr) (3) 0.75% lidocaine (LC) (14 ml/hr)	Yes	Increased late and variable decelerations in grp (1) Baseline FHR, Apgar, uterine activity similar in all grps
Abboud et al. (1982a) US	150	Random, sealed envelopes; double-masked*	Pennwalt	(1) 0.5% BV (2) 2% CP (3) 1.5% LC	Yes	Increased late decelerations in grp (1) Baseline FHR, uterine activity similar in all grps
Allen and Johnson (1979) UK	24	Random, no method given; double-masked	Pennwalt	(1) 0.375% BV (10 ml) (2) 2% CP (10 ml)	Yes	Time to onset of analgesia shorter in grp (2) Duration of analgesia shorter in grp (2) Increased motor blockade in grp (2)
Cohen and Thurlow (1979) US	49	Random, no method given; double-masked	?	(1) 0.5% BV (8 ml) (2) 0.375% BV plus 1.5% CP (8 ml) (3) 3% CP (8 ml)	Yes	Duration of analgesia longest in grp (1) Time to onset of analgesia similar in all grps

*Information obtained by contact with author

Table 57.16(b) Observed effect of intervention on outcome: lumbar epidural block using bupivacaine (BV) versus chloroprocaine (CP)

Authors, date (total n)	No. of pts in each treatment grp	BV and CP treatment groups	Mean maternal systolic blood pressure	% Apgar ≤6 at 1 min	Mean duration of analgesia (min) (SE)	Fetal heart decelerations
Abboud et al. (1984a) (n = 61)	23	(1) 0.5% BV	115	19%	NA*	59%
	19	(2) 2% CP	117	12%	NA	56%
Abboud et al. (1982a) (n = 150)	50	(1) 0.5% BV	122	14%	115 (36)	24%
	50	(2) 2% CP	123	18%	46 (14)	6%
Allen and Johnson (1979) (n = 24)	12	(1) 0.375% BV	NA	NA	85 (2)	NA
	12	(2) 2% CP	NA	NA	48 (6)	NA
Cohen and Thurlow (1979) (n = 49)	19	(1) 0.5% BV	NA	5%	68 (6)	NA
	14	(2) 3% CP	NA	14%	50 (4)	NA

*NA indicates 'Not available'.

Table 57.17(a) Selected trial design features: lumbar epidural block using bupivacaine (BV) versus epidural narcotics

Authors, date country	Total n	Reported method of treatment assignment and masking	Funding source	Treatment groups	Top-ups?	Conclusions
Skerman et al. (1985) US	50	Random, no method given; not masked	?	(1) 0.25% BV, then 0.125% BV (10 ml/hr) (2) 0.25% BV + 5 mcg/ml fentanyl (FENT), then 0.125% BV + 2.5 mcg/ml FENT (10 m/hr) (epidurally)	Yes; 3% CP	Better analgesia in grp (2) No side-effects observed
Hughes et al. (1984) US	40	Random, no method given; selected observers masked	NIH; Anesthesia Research Foundation	(1) 0.5% BV (10 ml) (2) 2 mg morphine (MOR) (3) 5 mg MOR (4) 7.5 mg MOR	Yes; LC or BV	Analgesia unsatisfactory in grps (2) and (3) Additional relief for 2nd stage needed in grp (4) Apgar and neurologic scores similar in all groups Pruritis w/MOR
Youngstrom et al. (1984) US	65	Random, no method given; not masked	?	(1) 0.125% BV (10 ml) (2) 150 mgc FENT (10 ml) (3) 0.125% BV w/150 mgc FENT (10 ml)	Yes; BV or CP	Duration and effectiveness of analgesia greatest in grp (3); no difference between grps (1) and (2) Pruritis w/FENT
Desprats et al. (1983) France	60	Random, no method given; selected observers masked	?	(1) 0.25% BV (6 ml) (2) 0.25% BV plus 100 mg FENT (2 ml)	Yes; BV	Duration and effectiveness greatest in grp (2) Cardiovascular, respiratory and blood gas values similar in both grps
Justins et al. (1982) UK	70	Random, coded ampoules; double-masked	Janssen Pharmaceuticals	(1) 0.5% BV plus saline (2) 0.5% BV plus 80 mg FENT	Yes; BV	Number of 'supplements' greater in grp (1) Onset and duration of analgesia better in grp (2) Pruritis w/FENT
Writer et al. (1981) US	16	Random, no method given; double-masked	?	(1) 0.25% BV (2) 0.25% MOR	Yes; BV, MOR, or CP	Pain relief poor in grp (2) Skin T° increase in grp (1) Apgar and blood gas similar in both grps
Muller et al. (1981) Germany	45	No method given; double-masked	?	(1) 0.25% BV + NaCl (2) 0.25% BV + 0.05 mg/kg MOR	Yes; BV	Longer duration of analgesia in grp (2) Smaller total dosage in grp (2) Apgars similar in both grps

Table 57.17(b) Observed effect of intervention on outcome: lumbar epidural block using bupivacaine (BV) versus epidural narcotics

Authors, date (total *n*)	No. of pts in each treat- ment grp	Treatment groups	Mean duration of analgesia (min) (SE)	Good to excellent pain relief	Apgar $\leqslant 6$ at 1 minute
Skerman *et al.* (1985) (*n* = 50)	?	(1) 0.25% BV	NA*	NA	NA
		(2) 0.25% BV + FENT (5 mcg)	NA	NA	NA
Hughes *et al.* (1984) (*n* = 40)	10	(1) 0.5% BV	NA	100%	60%
	9	(2) 2 mg MOR	NA	20%	0%
	10	(3) 5 mg MOR	NA	0%	10%
	11	(4) 7.5 mg MOR	420 (192)	80%	9%
Youngstrom *et al.* (1984) (*n* = 65)	23	(1) 0.125% BV	69 (8.6)	NA	NA
	21	(2) 150 mcg FENT	93 (12.7)	NA	NA
	21	(3) 0.125% BV plus 150 mcg FENT	124 (12.8)	NA	NA
Desprats *et al.* (1983) (*n* = 60)	30	(1) 0.25% BV	65 (27)	40%	7% ($\leqslant 7$)
	30	(2) 0.25% BV plus 0.1 mg FENT	103 (32)	67%	13% ($\leqslant 7$)
Justins *et al.* (1982) (*n* = 70)	33	(1) 0.3% BV	80 (4)	82%	NA
	35	(2) 0.3% BV plus 80 µg FENT	142 (8)	94%	NA
					NA
Writer *et al.* (1981) (*n* = 16)	8	(1) 0.25% BV	NA	63%	NA
	8	(2) 0.025% MOR	NA	0%	NA
Muller *et al.* (1981) (*n* = 45)	25	(1) 0.25% BV + NaCl	90	NA	NA
	20	(2) 0.25% BV + 0.05 mg/kg MOR	170	NA	NA

*NA indicates 'Not available'.

the first sacral to the fifth lumbar segments, areas less easily reached when lumbar epidural anaesthesia is administered.

Failures (about 5–10 per cent, according to Crawford 1978, and Albright and Ferguson 1986) in caudal administration of epidural anaesthesia are mainly due to the difficulty of caudal punctures, owing to anatomic variation in the sacral hiatus and difficulties in identifying it. The reader is referred to other texts for detailed descriptions of the technique (Bromage 1978; Albright and Ferguson 1986; Ostheimer 1984).

Compared to lumbar epidural anaesthesia, the volume of drug required for caudal anaesthesia is large (5 ml for a test dose and 20–25 ml for the first therapeutic dose). A typical refill dose is 15–25 ml or 80 per cent of the initial total dose.

Trials of caudal analgesia will not be analysed here, as the results are primarily now of historical interest. The reader is referred to Gunther and Bellville 1972, Simcock 1970, Gunther and Bauman 1969, Bridenbaugh *et al.* 1969, Jacob and Rosen 1962, and Johnson 1957, if he or she wishes to review these trials, which mainly compare different anaesthetic agents.

2.4.4 Paracervical block

Paracervical block, popular in the 1950s and early 1960s, has fallen out of favour as a result of reports of fetal bradycardia, acidosis, and even death associated with its use (Nyirjesy *et al.* 1963; Rosefsky and Petersiel 1968; Rogers 1970). Nevertheless, Hicks *et al.* (1976) reported on a survey conducted in the United States in which 80 per cent of the respondents used paracervical block during the first stage of labour, at least occasionally.

The reported incidence of fetal bradycardia following paracervical block has varied from 2 per cent to 70 per cent (Shnider *et al.* 1970; Tafeen *et al.* 1968; Teramo and Widholm 1967). Estimations of this rate have used different definitions of bradycardia, have measured it using a variety of methods, and have been based on findings from studies employing different drugs at a variety of dosages. These different definitions are likely to be the primary reason for the wide disparity in the estimates.

It is generally accepted that fetal bradycardia associated with paracervical block occurs within 2 to 10 minutes after the block and usually disappears in 5 to 10 minutes, although the fetal heart rate can remain depressed for up to 30 minutes. This decrease in fetal heart rate happens very quickly, often during a uterine contraction. There is some feeling that the anaesthetics bupivacaine, mepivacaine, lidocaine, and chloroprocaine differ in the associated incidence of the phenomenon (Albright and Ferguson 1986; Shnider and Gildea 1973; Teramo and Widholm 1967), but this has not been tested in randomized controlled trials.

The aetiology of the reported bradycardia is unknown, but may be related either to an excessive concentration of the anaesthetic in the fetal bloodstream, resulting in bradycardia, or to hypoxia from decreased placental perfusion or constriction of the umbilical blood vessels. Paracervical block does result in high blood concentrations of local anaesthetics in both the fetus and mother. Reviews of the subject may be found in Albright and Ferguson (1986) and Thiery and Vroman (1972).

As indicated previously, it is mainly the issue of fetal bradycardia that has caused use of paracervical block to fall into disfavour. Yet currently the emphasis put on this risk seems to vary with locale. In 1983, Belfrage and Floberg stated: 'Paracervical block during labour is a relatively common form of analgesia in Sweden. According to the records of the National Board of Health it was given in about 9 per cent of all births in 1979.' Uleland stated: 'I know of no anesthetic technique that places the fetus at risk, be it transient or otherwise, at anywhere near the rate of that of paracervical block. It would be inappropriate to condone its continued use in obstetrics . . . Paracervical block analgesia has not been administered at Stanford University Medical Center to any patient in labour for pain relief since 1977' (Albright and Ferguson 1986).

One of the reasons paracervical block continues to be used in cases where a regional anaesthesia is desired is ease of administration and scarcity of obstetric anaesthetists.

The long nerve fibres that travel from the uterus and cervix to the spinal cord at the level of T11-T12 can be blocked at one of several levels to achieve anaesthesia in the first stage of labour. The block is produced either at the level of the uterovaginal plexus (the paracervical block), the paravertebral space (paravertebral block), the epidural space (epidural block), or the spinal canal (spinal block). The paracervical block is by far the simplest to perform. A detailed description of technique may be found in Gottschalk and Hamilton (1975).

There has been some renewed interest in paracervical block technique, in part because of the introduction of the regional anaesthetic agent chloroprocaine, a rapidly hydrolysed ester-linked agent, presumably less toxic than the amide-linked agents, bupivacaine and lidocaine. A major disadvantage to chloroprocaine, however, is its short duration of action. As the paracervical block is designed to relieve pain caused by dilatation of the cervix and is thus most useful during the active first stage of labour (dilatation of 4–6 cm), duration of action is an issue of importance in terms of total dosage the labouring woman receives.

Randomized trials of paracervical block are listed in Tables 57.18 (studies comparing paracervical block with saline or non-paracervical block controls) and 57.19 (studies comparing various anaesthetic agents). To summarize, trials have spanned roughly two decades, from the early 1960s to the early 1980s. While lidocaine was the drug most often used in the early studies, bupivacaine and chloroprocaine have been employed recently. With one exception, trials in the last ten years have tested the latter two anaesthetics exclusively and have taken place in Scandinavia or Finland, where paracervical blocks remain a popular method of analgesia for childbirth. In the United States the renewed interest may be because of the availability of chloroprocaine, or because of an underlying feeling that electronic fetal heart monitoring can help avert the bradycardia-associated deaths feared to be attributable to paracervical blocks, or perhaps because lack of sufficient obstetric anaesthesia services have necessitated its continued use.

As is true for the other regional anaesthetics, the questions remaining for the investigator are not whether paracervical block works in terms of pain relief—it does—but what the side-effects are and how commonly they occur. Fetal bradycardia has been identified as the main problem associated with paracervical block. Other effects that have been mentioned in the literature are lengthened or shortened labour, fetal acidosis, and low Apgar score. Because there are fewer trials of paracervical block than, say, of lumbar epidural anaesthesia and because these studies vary considerably in terms of treatments tested, it is difficult to group these studies in a way that is intuitively meaningful for an overview. For example, it may be the mode of delivery of the anaesthetic, not the drug itself, which is related to hypothesized subsequent side-effects. If this is the case, it is not drugs we should wish to compare, but method of effecting regional anaesthesia using a given drug. Or, it may be that depth of injection of the blocking agent or the total dosage is the factor of major comparative value. It is possible that the data summarized in an overview are of most value in presenting a 'natural history' of all patients given this type of anaesthesia, and that no effort should be made to analyse study results by treatment group. For these reasons the data contained in the reports of trials comparing a variety of regional anaesthetics for paracervical block will be summarized together in this review.

Where paracervical block with a regional anaesthetic is compared with a 'block' using saline (Table 57.18)

Table 57.18(a) Selected trial design features: paracervical block (PCB) versus non-PCB or saline-PCB controls

Authors, date country	Total n	Reported method of treatment assignment and masking	Funding source	Treatment groups	Top-ups?	Conclusions
Jensen F. et al. (1984) Denmark	117	Random, no method given; double masked	?	(1) 0.25% BV–PCB (12 ml) + saline (IM) (2) Saline–PCB/ (12 ml) + PETH (75 mg) (IM)	No	Pain relief better with BV-PCB, diminished by 90 min Lower umbilical pH, Apgar scores with pethidine Bradycardia in 3 infants, 2 w/ BV-PCB
Jenssen H. (1973, 1975) Norway	58	Random, no method given; not masked	?	(1) PCB: 0.25% BV-epi (16 ml) (2) Non-PCB: N_2O/O_2 or pethidine or N_2O/O_2 and pethidine or lumbar epidural block	?	Increased duration of labour, in non-PCB grp Decrease in frequency of contractions, uterine activity with PCB Amniotic pressure higher in PCB
Westholm et al. (1970a,b) Sweden	195	'Randomly selected', no method given; double-masked	AB Bofors, Nobel-Pharma	(1) 0.25% BV (20 ml) (2) 0.25% BV-epi (20 ml) (3) Saline (20 ml)	No	Analgesia effective for grps (1) and (2) Duration of analgesia same for grps (1) and (2) Increased uterine inertia in grp (2) Bradycardia in all 3 grps, increased in grp (2)
Teramo (1969) Finland	58	No method given; not masked	AB Bofors	(1) 0.25% BV (20 ml) (2) 0.25% BV-epi (20 ml) (3) 0.50% BV-epi (20 ml) (4) 0.9% NaCl (20 ml) and std analgesia if necessary	No	Increased fetal bradycardia with BV Increased acidosis with BV
Pitkin and Goddard (1963) US	268	5-phase study, coded ampoules; double-masked to end of each phase	?	(1) 1% lidocaine (LC) (2) 1% LC-epi $1:2 \times 10^5$ (3) 1% LC-epi $1:5 \times 10^5$ (4) 1% mepivacaine (MV) (5) 1% MV-epi (6) 1.5% MV (7) 0.05% tetracaine (8) Saline (9) Saline-epi	?	Complete analgesia in 82% of patients with PCB No measurable effect of concentration of anaesthetic Duration of analgesia greatest in grp (2), shortest in grp (1) Increased uterine inertia w/epinephrine Bradycardia in 5 infants in PCB grps
Seeds et al. (1962) US	100	Random, no method given; double-masked	?	(1) 1% LC (2) 1% MV (3) 0.1% tetracaine–1% LC mixture (4) Saline	Yes	Complete analgesia in 50% of pts w/PCB Duration of analgesia greatest in grp (2) Bradycardia in total of 7 infants, 6 w/PCB

Table 57.18(b) Observed effect of intervention on outcome: paracervical block (PCB) versus non-PCB or saline-PCB controls

Authors, date (total n)	No. of pts in each treatment grp	Treatment groups	Good to excellent pain relief	Mean duration of analgesia (min)	Incidence of bradycardia	Apgar < 7 at 5 min
Jensen F. et al. (1984) ($n = 117$)	55	(1) 0.25% BV (PCB) + Saline (IM)	70%	NA*	4%	5%
	62	(2) Saline (PCB) + PETH (75 mg) (IM)	26%	NA	2%	13%
Jenssen H (1973) ($n = 58$)	30	(1) 0.25% BV-epi	NA	NA	NA	NA
	28	(2) Non-PCB	NA	NA	NA	NA
Westholm et al. (1970) ($n = 195$)	64	(1) 0.25% BV	80%	125	3%	0%
	67	(2) 0.25% BV-epi	78%	125	6%	0%
	64	(3) Saline	23%	60	3%	0%
Teramo (1969) ($n = 58$)	14	(1) 0.25% BV	NA	NA		
	12	(2) 0.25% BV-epi	} 84%	NA	} 55%	} 8% (at 1 min)
	12	(3) 0.5% BV-epi	NA	NA		
	20	(4) Saline	0%	NA	15%	15%
Pitkin and Goddard (1963) ($n = 268$)	66	(1) 1% LC	97%	53	NA	NA
	40	(2) 1% LC-epi (1:2 × 10⁵)	78%	102	NA	NA
	14	(3) 1% LC-epi (1:5 × 10⁵)	93%	61	NA	NA
	62	(4) 1% MV	77%	78	} 2%	NA
	22	(5) 1% MV-epi	91%	82		NA
	22	(6) 1.5% MV	91%	78		NA
	17	(7) 0.05% Tetracaine	53%	61		NA
	15	(8) Saline	20%	NA	NA	NA
	10	(9) Saline-epi	30%	NA	NA	NA
Seeds et al. (1962) ($n = 100$)	25	(1) 1% LC	72%	57	4%	NA
	25	(2) 1% MV	80%	84	16%	NA
	25	(3) 1% Xylocaine + 0.11% Pontocaine	80%	76	4%	NA
	25	(4) Saline	12%	NA	4%	NA

*NA indicates 'Not available'.

Table 57.19(a) Selected trial design features: paracervical block comparing various agents

Authors, date country	Total n	Reported method of treatment assignment and masking	Funding source	Treatment groups	Top-ups?	Conclusions
Belfrage and Floberg (1983) Sweden	47	Random, no method given; not masked	Stiftelsen Allmänna Barnbordshusets Minnesfond	(1) 0.25% BV (12 ml) (2) 2% CP (12 ml)	Yes	Time of onset of analgesia, bradycardia similar in both grps Duration of analgesia shorter in grp (2)
Nesheim (1983) Norway	115	Random, coin toss; not masked	?	(1) 0.25% BV (20 ml) (2) 0.25% BV-epi (20 ml) (3) 2% CP (20 ml) (4) 2% CP-epi (20 ml)	?	Pain relief similar in all grps Duration of analgesia shortest in grp (3) Duration of labour increased in grp (2)
Weiss et al. (1983) US	60	Random, coded vials; double-masked	Pennwalt Pharm	(1) 1% LC (20 ml) (2) 2% CP (20 ml)	Yes	Adequacy and duration of analgesia similar in both grps Increased bradycardia in grp (1)
Hökegård (1969) Sweden	216	Random, no method given; double-masked	AB Bofors Nobel-Pharma	(1) 0.25% BV-epi (20 ml) (2) 1% MV-epi (20 ml)	Yes	Increased duration of analgesia in grp (1) Increased failure of analgesia in grp (1) Three fetal deaths (grp not specified)

Table 57.19(b). Observed effect of intervention on outcome: paracervical block comparing various agents

Authors, date (total n)	No. of pts in each treatment grp	Treatment groups	Good to excellent pain relief	Mean duration of analgesia (min) (SE)	Incidence of fetal bradycardia	Apgar ≤7 at 5 min
Belfrage and Floberg (1983) (n = 47)	24 23	(1) 0.25% BV (2) 2% CP	79% 87%	66 (28) 35 (10)	8% 4%	0% 4%
Neisheim (1983) (n = 115)	43 22 28 22	(1) 0.25% BV (2) 0.25% BV-epi (3) 2% CP (4) 2% CP-epi	94% 94.5% 96.5% 98.5%	105 120 40 75	2% 0% 7% 9%	0% 14% 4% 0%
Weiss et al. (1983) (n = 60)	31 29	(1) 1% LC (2) 2% CP	93% 97%	40 (15.2) 41 (10.0)	16% 3%	3% 0%
Hökegård (1969) (n = 216)	76 84	(1) 0.25% BV-epi (2) 1.0% MV-epi	82% 90%	120 (7) 99 (3)	0% 0%	NA* NA

*NA indicates 'Not available'.

(Jensen *et al.* 1984; Jenssen 1973, 1975; Westholm *et al.* 1970a, 1970b; Teramo 1969; Pitkin and Goddard 1963; Seeds *et al.* 1962) adequate pain relief attributable to the paracervical block was achieved at least 50 per cent of the time. When comparisons between various agents of pain relief were made (Belfrage and Floberg 1983; Nesheim 1983; Weiss *et al.* 1983; Hôkegård 1969), there was no clear advantage to any particular drug (Table 57.18). For duration of action, bupivacaine was superior to 2-chloroprocaine, mepivacaine superior to lidocaine.

One study that compared paracervical block with saline (Teramo 1969) showed an increased proportion of infants with bradycardia in the paracervical block group, while another (Westholm *et al.* 1970a) showed no difference. Seeds *et al.* (1962) showed an increase in bradycardia associated with mepivacaine as compared to saline and other anaesthetic agents. A possible trend of lower Apgar scores in the saline groups may reflect the effect of pethidine.

2.4.5 *Spinal anaesthesia*

The spinal, or subarachnoid, block was first administered inadvertently in 1885 when Leonard Corning of the United States accidentally injected cocaine in the subarachnoid space of a dog on which he was working. Bier in Germany, in 1899, first used the block for anaesthesia during surgery and a year later his countryman, Kreis, used the method for obstetric anaesthesia. Like other anaesthetic techniques in obstetrics, the spinal block has had ups and downs in terms of popularity. The introduction of better equipment and new local anaesthetics, as well as better understanding of the physiology has sparked renewed interest in the technique, at least for delivery, in the United States. Its use continues to be controversial in Europe and Great Britain.

Spinal anaesthesia is administered by injection directly into the subarachnoid space, usually at the level of the L3-L4 interspace, but not above L2-L3. Spinal anaesthesia is easier to perform than epidural anaesthesia because of the injection site and provides rapid and almost certain pain relief. Primarily because of the profound motor blockade induced, it is more useful in the second stage of labour or for caesarean section, while the patient is in the delivery room, rather than for control of pain in the first stage.

Advantages to the spinal block are that it is easy to administer, has a rapid onset, and has an extremely low failure rate. In addition, only a small amount of anaesthetic is injected, meaning that very little drug is transmitted to the fetus, and a toxic reaction in the mother is unlikely. The disadvantages of spinal anaesthesia are: a limited duration of action, profound motor blockade, and the associated possible side-effects of neurologic sequelae, hypotension, post-spinal head-ache, and respiratory insufficiency (seen at high levels of block).

Recently, a new approach to spinal anaesthesia in obstetrics has been taken: that is, the intrathecal injection of opiates. There has been one controlled clinical trial (Abboud *et al.* 1982b, 1984c) of 30 patients that compared two doses of morphine, 0.5 mg and 1.0 mg. Excellent analgesia for the first stage of labour was reported for both doses, but a high proportion of the mothers developed side-effects such as pruritus (80 per cent), nausea and/or vomiting (53 per cent), and urinary retention. The patients receiving the higher dose were more likely to experience these adverse effects. Use of beta-endorphin for intrathecal injection is another avenue being explored (Oyama *et al.* 1980).

As this chapter is primarily concerned with control of pain during first stage, spinal anaesthesia will not be discussed further. The reader is referred to Abouleish (1977), Albright *et al.* (1986a), and Shnider (1987) for additional general information.

3 Conclusions

3.1 Implications for current practice

Despite the fact that numerous clinical trials have been performed evaluating analgesia during labour, the available data for any one clinical problem may be meagre. The data presented in this chapter have emphasized the broad questions, generally those addressed by a majority of the trials in a particular area. The implications of the available results are briefly summarized here for the practitioner who is anxious to apply what has been learned using the controlled trial approach.

Systemic narcotics, most notably pethidine, are associated with maternal and perinatal depression. The effect is dose-related, thus the amount of analgesia achieved is limited by side effects of the drug. Trial data have confirmed that adequate pain relief can be realized with systemic narcotics, but have also shown lower Apgar scores in babies of mothers receiving pethidine or related drugs. Single trials have shown an increased duration of labour, increased uterine tone, and decreased maternal pH. Other data suggest that orthostatic hypotension, nausea, vomiting, dizziness, and a decrease in gastric motility are also associated with administration of narcotics in labour.

Systemic narcotics have been compared with lumbar epidural block in several clinical trials. This type of comparison offers an excellent opportunity to evaluate both the use of systemic narcotics and the epidural block as analgesic methods. The results have shown an increase in the duration of analgesia, an increase in second stage, and an increase in instrumental deliveries associated with epidural block. No difference has been seen between the two groups for Apgar score.

Inhalation analgesia, today used most often in conjunction with other forms of analgesia, does not offer reliable or complete pain relief. In addition, side-effects of nausea and vomiting, as well as the possibility of aspiration of gastric contents in cases of accidental overdose, decrease the usefulness of the method. Trial data comparing nitrous oxide with methoxyflurane have shown no difference in pain relief, although nitrous oxide has been associated with more nausea and vomiting.

Diazepam is known to have a long half-life and concentrate in the fetal liver. Associations between its use and neonatal respiratory depression, hypothermia, and loss of beat-to-beat variability have been reported. Clinical trials have been few, one showing lower Apgar scores and one showing increased neonatal drowsiness in the diazepam group.

Regional analgesia, particularly lumbar epidural analgesia, has recently surged in popularity. Numerous trials have been done to compare dosages of various anaesthetic agents, perhaps disproportionately so, in view of the relative importance of the safety and efficacy of the method versus the safety and efficacy of the dosage. Generally, trials have shown that higher volumes of bupivacaine at lower concentrations confer better pain relief than lower dosages, with added epinephrine conferring no obvious additional effect. Trials comparing bupivacaine and 2-chloroprocaine have shown no clear difference between the two, other than a longer duration of action for bupivacaine. When epidurally administered narcotics have been compared to bupivacaine, increased pruritus and a possible increased analgesic effect have been seen.

Caudal epidural blocks are rarely used now, requiring more anaesthetic, as well as resulting in more blocked segments and a less easily controlled spread than lumbar epidural analgesia.

Paracervical block is considered by many to be a risky technique, often resulting in fetal bradycardia, acidosis, and even death. Evidence from clinical trials has not shown clear trends for these and other potentially harmful effects, probably owing to small sample sizes. No particular drug used for paracervical block has been shown to be advantageous over any other agent.

Spinal anaesthesia is mainly used for the second stage of labour, although there has been recent interest in intrathecal opiates. Potential side effects of intrathecal opiate use that have emerged to date are maternal delayed respiratory depression, pruritus, nausea, vomiting, urinary retention, and drowsiness.

3.2 Implications for future research

The problem with the majority of available data on obstetric anaesthesia is that the questions being asked are too narrow to answer the question in the minds of both practitioner and consumer: by what method can we achieve an acceptable level of pain relief in most women while least compromising the mother's and child's health? The breadth of that question is not practical for the research investigator who must approach the problem in small steps, and hence the mountain of unique clinical trials, none answering any one question particularly well. In addition, many clinicians consider it possibly unethical, and certainly impractical, to conduct placebo-controlled trials in the obstetric setting. Trials comparing one method of analgesia to another method (e.g. lumbar epidural versus systemic narcotics) may appear similarly unethical to practitioners with a preference for one or the other.

Nevertheless, what is needed is a collaborative effort: first, to decide on the major outcomes of interest in studies of obstetric anaesthesia and second, to mount large trials with sufficiently long follow-up periods to address the outcome issues scientifically. The trials summarized in this chapter provide less information than they might have, primarily because of non-standardized design structure, but also for reasons of the quality of data collection, analysis, and reporting. The importance of standardized design is epitomized by the problems encountered in studying the side-effects of a given type of analgesia in that it may be the mode of delivery of the anaesthetic, not the drug itself, which is related to hypothesized subsequent side-effects. If this is the case, it is not the drugs we should wish to compare but the method of effecting regional anaesthesia, using a given drug.

What is truly needed, in terms of trial data for a given method and drug are:

(1) more data on minimum dosage for effective pain relief; and

(2) data on side-effects for the minimum dosage required for pain relief.

Achieving this will require a concerted effort on the part of the obstetric anaesthesia community to standardize trial protocols and to recruit large numbers of women.

While many will argue against this proposal on both practical and (what they feel to be) ethical grounds, the alternatives, the hit-or-miss and *laissez-faire* approaches, are neither practical nor ethical. The consumer movement has long had an influence on the conduct of childbirth practices. While there is nothing wrong with this, it would seem appropriate that the demand for a more scientific approach to the evaluation of methods of pain relief in childbirth be initiated by the practitioners themselves.

References

Abboud TK, Khoo SS, Miller F, Doan T, Henriksen EH (1982a). Maternal, fetal and neonatal responses after epidural anesthesia with bupivacaine, 2-chloroprocaine, or lidocaine. Anesth Analg (Cleve), 61: 638–644.

Abboud TK, Shnider SM, Dailey PA, Raya J, Khoo SS, Sarkis S, Desausa B, Baysinger CL, Miller F (1982b). Hyperbaric intrathecal morphine for the relief of labour pain. Anesthesiology (Suppl), 57: A384.

Abboud TK, Afrasiabi A, Sarkis F, Daftarian F, Nagappala S, Noueihed R, Kuhnert BR, Miller F (1984a). Continuous infusion epidural analgesia in parturients receiving bupivacaine, chloroprocaine, or lidocaine—maternal, fetal, and neonatal effects. Anesth Analg (Cleve), 63: 421–428.

Abboud TK, Sheik-ol-Eslam A, Yanagi T, Costandi J, Zakarian M, Hoffman D, Murakawa K, Kenriksen EH (1984b). Safety and efficacy of epinephrine added to bupivacaine for lumbar epidural analgesia in the parturient. Anesthesiology (Suppl), 61: 406.

Abboud TK, Shnider SM, Dailey PA, Raya JA, Sarkis F, Grobler NM, Sadri S, Khoo SS, DeSousa B, Baysinger CL, Miller F (1984c). Intrathecal administration of hyperbaric morphine for the relief of pain in labour. Br J Anaesth, 56: 1351–1359.

Abboud TK, Sheik-ol-Eslam A, Yanagi T, Murakawa K, Constandi J, Zakarian M, Hoffman D, Haroutunian S (1985). Safety and efficiency of epinephrine added to bupivacaine for lumbar epidural analgesia in obstetrics. Anesth Analg, 64: 585–591.

Abouleish E (1977). Pain Control in Obstetrics. Philadelphia: Lippincott.

Abouleish E, Pan P, Kang YG, De La Vega R, Harger J (1982). For epidural analgesia in labour, is 0.25% bupivacaine better than 0.5%? Anesthesiology (Suppl), 57: A399.

Ad hoc Committee on the Effect of Trace Anesthetics on the Health of Operating Room Personnel (1974). A national study. Anesthesiology, 41: 321–340.

Aiken RA, Cope E (1971). The value of promazine and diazepam as adjuncts to pethidine in labour. In: Psychosomatic Medicine in Obstetrics and Gynaecology. 3rd International Congress, London. Morris N, (ed). Basel: Karger pp 241–243.

Albright GA (1979). Cardiac arrest following regional anesthesia with etidocaine or bupivacaine (editorial). Anesthesiology, 51: 285–287.

Albright GA (1984). Epinephrine should be used with the therapeutic dose of bupivacaine in obstetrics. Anesthesiology, 61: 217–218.

Albright GA and Ferguson JE (1986). Paracervical, pudendal, and perineal field blocks. In: Anesthesia in Obstetrics. Albright GA, Ferguson JE, Joyce TH, Stevenson DK (eds). Boston, London: Butterworths.

Albright GA, Joyce TH, Stevenson DK (1986a). Systemic medication. In: Anesthesia in Obstetrics. Albright GA, Ferguson JE, Joyce TH, Stevenson DK (eds), Boston, London: Butterworths.

Albright GA, Ferguson JE, Joyce TH, Stevenson DK (1986b). Anesthesia in Obstetrics. Maternal, Fetal and Neonatal Aspects. Boston, London: Butterworths.

Allen PR, Johnson RW (1979). Extradural analgesia in labour. A comparison of 2-chloroprocaine hydrochloride and bupivacaine hydrochloride. Anaesthesia, 34: 839–843.

American College of Obstetricians and Gynecologists, Committee on Maternal Health (1970). National Study of Maternity Care. Survey of Obstetric Practice and Associated Services in Hospitals in the United States. Chicago.

Apgar V, Burns JJ, Brodie BB, Papper EM (1952). Transmission of meperidine across human placenta. Am J Obstet Gynecol, 64: 1368–1370.

Bailey PW, Howard FA (1983). Epidural analgesia and forceps delivery: laying a bogey. Anaesthesia, 38: 282–285.

Behar M, Magora F, Olshwang D, Davidson JT (1979). Epidural morphine in treatment of pain. Lancet, 1: 527.

Belfrage P, Floberg J (1983). Obstetrical paracervical block with chloroprocaine or bupivacaine. Acta Obstet Gynecol Scand, 62: 245–247.

Bergsjø P, Lindbaek E (1971). Comparison between nitrous oxide and methoxyflurane for obstetrical analgesia. Acta Obstet Gynecol Scand, 50: 285–290.

Bonica JJ (1967). Obstetric Analgesia and Anesthesia. Volume 2: Clinical Considerations. Philadelphia: Davis, p viii.

Bonica JJ (1972). Principles and Practice of Obstetric Analgesia and Anesthesia. Philadephia: FA Davis.

Bonica JJ (1975). The nature of pain and parturition. In: Obstetric Analgesia–Anesthesia. Recent Advances and Current Status. Bonica JJ (ed). Clin Obstet Gynecol, 2: 499–516.

Brelje MC, Garcia-Bunuel R (1966). Meperidine–hydroxyzine in obstetric analgesia. Obstet Gynecol, 27: 350–354.

Bridenbaugh PO, Bridenbaugh LD, Moore DC (1969). Methemoglobinemia and infant response to lidocaine and prilocaine in continuous caudal anesthesia: A double-blind study. Anesth Analg (Cleve), 48: 824–829.

Broadfield JB, Corall IM, Nicholson JR, Strunin L (1975). Cardiovascular changes in labour associated with extradural analgesia using bupivacaine. Br J Anaesth, 47: 1291–1295.

Bromage PR (1978). Epidural Analgesia. Philadelphia: W B Saunders.

Buchan PC, Milne MK, Browning MCK (1973). The effect of continuous epidural blockade on plasma 11-hydroxy-corticosteroid concentrations in labour. J Obstset Gynaecol Br Commonw, 80: 974–977.

Bundsen P, Peterson LE, Selstam U (1982). Pain relief during delivery. Acta Obstet Gynecol Scand, 61: 289–297.

Busacca M, Gementi P, Gambini E, Lenti C, Meschi F, Vionali M (1982). Neonatal effects of the administration of meperidine and promethazine to the mother in labour. Double blind study. J Perinat Med, 10: 48–53.

Canadian Institute of Child Health (1985). Unpublished data. Personal communication with Louise Hanvey.

Catchlove FH, Kafer ER (1971). The effects of diazepam on the ventilatory response to carbon dioxide and on steady-state gas exchange. Anesthesiology, 34: 9–13.

Challen PD, Stainthorp SF, Bradshaw EG, Tobias MA (1977). An assessment of low concentration bupivacaine for obstetric epidural analgesia. Anaesthesia, 32: 102.

Chang A, Wood C, Humphrey M, Gilbert M, Wagstaff C (1976). The effects of narcotics on fetal acid base status. Br J Obstet Gynaecol, 83: 56–61.

Chestnut DH, Vandewalker GE, Owen CL, Bates JN, Choi

WW (1987). The influence of continuous epidural bupivacaine analgesia on the second stage of labor and method of delivery in nulliparous women. Anesthesiology, 66: 774–780.

Cohen SE (1987). Inhalation analgesia and anesthesia for vaginal delivery. In: Anesthesia for Obstetrics. Shnider SM and Levinson G (eds). Baltimore: Williams & Wilkins.

Cohen SE, Thurlow A (1979). Comparison of a chloroprocaine–bupivacaine mixture with chloroprocaine and bupivacaine used individually for obstetric epidural analgesia. Anesthesiology, 51: 288–292.

Cohen SE, Tan S, Albright GA, Halpern J (1987). Epidural fentanyl/bupivacaine mixtures for obstetric analgesia. Anesthesiology, 67: 403–407.

Cosmi EV, Marx GF (1969). The effect of anesthesia on the acid–base status of the fetus. Anesthesiology, 30: 238–242.

Covino BG and Scott DB (1985). Handbook of Epidural Anaesthesia and Analgesia. Orlando: Grune & Stratton.

Covino B, Littlewood DG, Scott DB, Wilson J (1976). A comparative study of various local anaesthetics in epidural block in labour. (Obstet Anaesthetists Assoc Report). Anaesthesia, 31: 846–847.

Crawford JS (1978). Principles and Practice of Obstetric Anaesthesia. Oxford: Blackwell Scientific Publications.

Cullhed S, Löfström B (1961). Obstetric analgesia with pethidine and scopolamine. Lancet, 1: 75–77.

Dalen JE, Evans GL, Banas JS Jr, Brooks HL, Paraskos JA, Dexter L (1969). The hemodynamic and respiratory effects of diazepam (Valium). Anesthesiology, 30: 259–263.

Davies JM, Hogg M, Rosen M (1975). Maternal arterial oxygen tension during intermittent inhalation analgesia. Br J Anaesth, 47: 370–378.

DeKornfeld TJ, Pearson JW, Lasagna L (1964). Methotrimeprazine in the treatment of labour pain. N Engl J Med, 270: 391–394.

DeLee JB (ed) (1905). (Yearbook of) Obstetrics. Chicago: Yearbook Publishers.

DeLee JB (1915). The Principles and Practice of Obstetrics. Philadelphia: W B Saunders.

DeLee JB (1920). The Principles and Practice of Obstetrics. Philadelphia: W B Saunders.

DeLee JB (1925). The Principles and Practice of Obstetrics. Philadelphia: W B Saunders.

DeLee JB (1929). The Principles and Practice of Obstetrics. Philadelphia: W B Saunders.

DeLee JB, Roehler HD, Stowe HM (eds) (1907). (Yearbook of) Obstetrics. Chicago: Yearbook Publishers.

DeSilva JAF, D'Anconte L, and Kaplan J (1964). The determination of blood levels and the placental transfer of diazepam in humans. Curr Ther Res, 6: 115–121.

Desprats R, Mandry J, Grandjean H, Amar B, Pontonnier G, Lareng L (1983). The use of fentanyl and marcaine as compared with marcaine alone in epidural analgesia. J Gynecol Obstet Biol Reprod (Paris), 12: 901–905.

DeVoe ST, DeVoe K Jr, Rigsby WC, McDaniels BA (1969). Effect of meperidine on uterine contractility. Am J Obstet Gynecol, 105: 1004–1007.

Devoghel JC (1974). Enflurane (Ethrane) in obstetrics. Acta Anaesthesiol Belg, 2: 283–288.

Dolan PF, Rosen M (1975). Inhalational analgesia in labour: Face mask or mouthpiece. Lancet, 2: 1030–1031.

Doughty A (1978). Epidural analgesia in labour: the past, the present and the future. J R Soc Med, 71: 879–884.

Eckenhoff JE, Oech SK (1960). The effects of narcotics and antagonists upon respiration and circulation in man. Clin Pharmacol Ther, 1: 483–524.

Ewen A, McLeod DD, MacLeod DM, Campbell A, Tunstall ME (1986). Continuous infusion epidural analgesia in obstetrics. Anaesthesia, 41: 143–147.

Flowers CE, Rudolph AJ, Desmond MM (1969). Diazepam (Valium) as an adjunct in obstetric analgesia. Obstet Gynecol, 34: 6881.

Frame WT, Allison RH, Moir DD, Nimmo WS (1984). Effect of naloxone on gastric emptying during labour. Br J Anaesth, 56: 263–266.

Friedman EA (1971). The functional divisions of labour. Am J Obstet Gynecol, 109: 274–280.

Fromhagen C, Carswell AP (1961). Potentiation of analgesia during labour. A study of two tranquilizers. Obstet Gynecol, 18: 483–487.

Garrett LP (1984). Florida Society of Anesthesiologists' Newsletter, Feb.

Gibbs CP, Krischer J, Peckham BM, Sharp H, Kirschbaum TH (1986). Obstetric anesthesia: A national survey. Anesthesiology, 65: 298–306.

Girvan CB, Moore J, Dundee JW (1976). Pethidine compared with pethidine-naloxone administered during labour. Br J Anaesthesia, 48: 563–569.

Gottschalk W, Hamilton LA (1975). Regional anesthesia-II. Pudendal and paracervical blocks in obstetrics. In: Local Infiltration for Cesarean Section. Wynn R (ed). Obstetrics and Gynecology Annual. New York: Appleton-Century-Crofts.

Gunther RE, Bauman J (1969). Obstetrical caudal anesthesia: I. A randomized study comparing 1% mepivacaine with 1% lidocaine plus epinephrine. Anesthesiology, 31: 5–19.

Gunther RE, Bellville JW (1972). Obstetrical caudal anesthesia: II. A randomized study comparing 1% mepivacaine with 1% mepivacaine plus epinephrine. Anesthesiology, 37: 288–298.

Haggard HW (1929). Devils, Drugs, and Doctors. New York, London: Harper Bros.

Hibbard BM, Rees G, Rosen M (1979). Obstetric anaesthetic and analgesic services in Wales. Br Med J, 2: 698–700.

Hicks JS, Levinson G, Shnider SM (1976). Obstetric training centers in the USA—1975. Anesth Analg Curr Res, 55: 839–843.

Hökegård K (1969). Marcaine for paracervical anesthesia during labour. Am J Obstet Gynecol, 105: 278–279.

Holmskov A, Schrøder P (1975). Diazepam in obstetrics. A double-blind investigation to illustrate duration of labour, pain, Apgar score and complications. Ugeskr Laeger, 137: 734–737.

Hughes SC, Rosen MA, Shnider SM, Abboud TK, Stefani SJ, Norton M (1984). Maternal and neonatal effects of epidural morphine for labour and delivery. Anesth Analg (Cleve), 63: 319–324.

Idanpaan-Heikkila JE, Jouppila PI, Puolakka JO, Vorne MS (1971). Placental transfer and fetal metabolism of diazepam in early human pregnancy. Am J Obstet Gynecol, 109: 1011–1016.

Jacob J, Rosen M (1962). A clinical appraisal of four local

anesthetic agents used in caudal anesthesia in obstetrics by the double-blind method. A preliminary report. Anesth Analg (Cleve), 41: 546–551.

James LS (1960). The effect of pain relief for labour and delivery on the fetus and newborn. Anesthesiology, 21: 405–430.

Jensen F, Qvist I, Brocks V, Secher NJ, Westergaard LG (1984). Submucous paracervical blockade compared with intramuscular meperidine as analgesia during labour: a double-blind study. Obstet Gynecol, 64: 724–727.

Jenssen H (1973). The effect of paracervical block on cervical dilation and uterine activity. Acta Obstet Gynecol Scand, 52: 13–22.

Jenssen H (1975). The shape of the amniotic pressure curve before and after paracervical block during labour. Acta Obstet Gynecol Scand, 0: 1–29.

Johnson GT (1957). Prolonged labour: a clinical trial of continuous caudal analgesia. Br Med J, 2: 386–389.

Jones PL, Rosen M, Mushin WW, Jones EV (1969). Methoxyflurane and nitrous oxide as obstetric analgesics. I. A comparison by continuous administration. Br Med J, 3: 255–259.

Jouppila R (1976). The effect of segmental epidural analgesia on maternal growth hormone, insulin, glucose and free fatty acids during labour. Ann Chir Gynaecol, 65: 398–404.

Jouppila R, Hollmen A (1976). The effect of segmental epidural analgesia on maternal and foetal acid-base balance, lactate, serum potassium and creatine phosphokinase during labour. Acta Anaesthesiol Scand, 20: 259–268.

Jouppila R, Jouppila P, Moilanen K, Pakarinen A (1980). The effect of segmental epidural analgesia on maternal prolactin during labour. Br J Obstet Gynaecol, 87: 234–238.

Justins DM, Francis D, Houlton PG, Reynolds F (1982). A controlled trial of extradural fentanyl in labour. Br J Anaesth, 54: 409–414.

Justins DM, Knott C, Luthman J, Reynolds F (1983). Epidural versus intramuscular fentanyl. Anaesthesia, 38: 937–942.

Kenepp NB, Cheek TG, Gutsche BB (1983). Bupivacaine: continuous infusion epidural analgesia for labour. Anesthesiology (Suppl), 59: A407.

Kett JF (1968). The Formation of the American Medical Profession: The Role of Institutions 1780–1860. New Haven: Yale University Press.

Kurjak A, Beazley JM (1974). The effect of continuous lumbar epidural analgesia on the fetus, newborn child and the acid-base status of maternal blood. Acta Med Iugosl, 28: 15–26.

La Salvia LA, Steffan EA (1950). Delayed gastric emptying time in labour. Am J Obstet Gynecol, 59: 1075–1081.

Lassner J, Barrier G, Talafre ML, Durupty D (1981). Failure of extradural morphine to provide adequate pain relief in labour. Br J Anaesth, 53: 112P.

Leighton BL, Norris MC, Sosis M, Epstein R, Chayen B, Larijani GE (1987). Limitations of epinephrine as a marker of intravascular injection in laboring women. Anesthesiology, 66: 688–691.

Levinson G, Shnider SM (1987). Systemic medication for labour and delivery. In: Anesthesia for Obstetrics. Shnider SM and Levinson G (eds). Baltimore: Williams & Wilkins.

Li DF, Rees GAD, Rosen M (1985). Continuous extradural infusion of 0.0625% or 0.125% bupivacaine for pain relief in primigravid labour. Br J Anaesth, 57: 264–270.

Malkasian GD, Smith RA, Decker DG (1967). Comparison of hydroxyzine–meperidine and promethazine–meperidine for analgesia during labour. Obstet Gynecol, 30: 568–575.

Marcoux S, Mailloux J, Fontaine JY, LeClerc M (1987). Bupivacaine concentration and obstetric delivery. Lancet, 2: 330–331.

Marx GF (1984). Cardiotoxicity of local anesthetics—the plot thickens. Anesthesiology, 60: 3–5.

May DPL, DeVere RD (1976). Epidural analgesia in labour (letter). Br Med J, 2: 944.

Mazze RI, Toudell JR, Cousins MJ (1971). Methoxyflurane metabolism and renal dysfunction: Clinical correlation in man. Anesthesiology, 35: 247–252.

McAllister CB (1980). Placental transfer and neonatal effects of diazepam when administered to women just before delivery. Br J Anaesth, 52: 423–427.

McCarthy GT, O'Connell B, Robinson AE (1973). Blood levels of diazepam in infants of two mothers given large doses of diazepam during labour. J Obstet Gynecol Br Commwlth, 80: 349–352.

McDonald R, Shaw M, Craig C (1964). Effect of phenothiazines and analgesics given during labour on neonatal serum bilirubin. Br Med J, 5384: 677.

McQuitty FM (1967). Relief of pain in labour. A controlled double-blind trial comparing pethidine and various phenothiazine derivatives. J Obstet Gynaecol Br Commwlth, 74: 925–928.

Medical Research Council Committee on Nitrous Oxide and Oxygen Analgesia in Midwifery (1970). Clinical trials of different concentrations of oxygen and nitrous oxide for obstetric analgesia. Br Med J, 1: 709–713.

Minnitt RJ (1934). Self administered analgesia for the midwifery of general practice. Proc R Soc Med, 27: 1313–1318.

Moir DD (1976). Obstetric Anaesthesia and Analgesia. London: Baillière Tindall.

Moir DD, Slater PJ, Thorburn J, McLaren R, Moodie J (1976). Extradural analgesia in obstetrics: a controlled trial of carbonated lignocaine and bupivacaine hydrochloride with or without adrenaline. Br J Anaesth, 48: 129–135.

Moore DC, Scurlock JE (1983). Possible role of epinephrine in prevention or correction of myocardial depression associated with bupivacaine. Anesth Analg (Cleve), 62: 450–453.

Moore J, Ball HG (1974). A sequential study of intravenous analgesic treatment during labour. Br J Anaesth, 46: 365–372.

Moore J, Carson RM, Hunter RJ (1970). A comparison of the effects of pentazocine and pethidine administered during labour. J Obstet Gynaecol Br Commwlth, 77: 830–836.

Mowat J, Garrey MM (1970). Comparison of pentazocine and pethidine in labour. Br Med J, 2: 757–759.

Moya F, Thorndike V (1962). Passage of drugs across the placenta. Am J Obstet Gynecol, 84: 1778–1798.

Muller H, Brahler A, Stoyanov M, Borner U, Hempelmann G (1981). Epidural morphine as adjunct to epidural anaesthesia in obstetrics. Regional-Anaesthesie, 4: 42–45.

Munson ES, Embro WJ (1977). Enflurane, isoflurane and halothane and isolated human uterine muscle. Anesthesiology, 46: 11–14.

National Perinatal Epidemiology Unit (1986). A Classified Bibliography of Controlled Trials in Perinatal Medicine 1940–1984. Oxford: Oxford University Press.

Nesheim B-I (1983). Which local anesthetic is best suited for paracervical blocks? Acta Obstet Gynecol Scand, 62: 261–264.

Nesheim B-I, Lindbaek E, Storm-Mathisen I, Jenssen H (1979). Neurobehavioral response of infants after paracervical block during labour. Acta Obstet Gynecol Scand, 58: 41–44.

Nicholas ADG (1984). The optimal test dose for epidural anesthesia. Anesthesiology, 60: 79.

Nimmo WS, Wilson J, Prescott LF (1975). Narcotic analgesics and delayed gastric emptying during labour. Lancet, 1: 890–893.

Nisbet R, Boulas SH, Kantor HI (1967). Diazepam (Valium) during labour. Obstet Gynecol, 29: 726–729.

Noble AD, Craft IL, Bootes JAH, Edwards PA, Thomas DJ, Mills KLM (1971). Continuous lumbar epidural analgesia using bupivacaine: a study of the fetus and newborn child. J Obstet Gynaecol Br Commwlth, 78: 559–563.

Nyirjesy I, Hawks BLJ, Hopwood H, Falis H (1963). Hazards of use of paracervical block anesthesia in obstetrics. Am J Obstet Gynecol, 87: 231–235.

Ostheimer GW (ed) (1984). Manual of Obstetric Anesthesia. New York, London: Churchill Livingstone.

The Oxford Concise Medical Dictionary (1985). Second Edition, Oxford: Oxford University Press.

Oyama T, Matsuki A, Taneichi T, Ling N, Guillemin R (1980). Beta-endorphin in obstetric analgesia. Am J Obstet Gynecol, 137: 613–616.

Pernick MS (1985). A Calculus of Suffering. Pain, Professionalism, and Anesthesia in Nineteenth Century America. New York: Columbia University Press.

Pitkin RM, Goddard WB (1963). Paracervical and uterosacral block in obstetrics—a controlled, double-blind study. Obstet Gynecol, 21: 737–744.

Powe CE, Kiem IM, Fromhagen C, Cavanagh D (1962). Propiomazine hydrochloride in obstetrical analgesia. JAMA, 181: 290–294.

Purdy G, Currie J, Owen H (1987). Continuous extradural analgesia in labour: comparison between 'on demand' and regular top-up injections. Br J Anaesth, 59: 319–324.

Revill S (1980). Pain relief in labour; what the patient requires. Proceedings of the 1st European Congress of Obstetrical Anaesthesia and Analgesia. Birmingham, UK, 17–20 Sept. pp 1–16.

Reynolds F (1986). Obstetric anesthetic services. Br Med J, 293: 403–404.

Reynolds F, Taylor G (1971). Plasma concentrations of bupivacaine during continuous epidural analgesia in labour: the effect of adrenaline. Br J Anaesth, 43: 436–440.

Reynolds F, Hargrove RL, Wyman JB (1973). Maternal and foetal plasma concentrations of bupivacaine after epidural. Br J Anaesth, 45: 1049–1053.

Richardson BW (1858). In: On Chloroform and Other Anaesthetics. Snow J (ed). London: Churchill.

Robinson JO, Rosen M, Evans JM, Revill SI, David H, Rees GAD (1980a). Maternal opinion about analgesia for labour. A controlled trial between epidural block and intramuscular pethidine combined with inhalation. Anaesthesia, 35: 1173–1181.

Robinson JO, Rosen M, Evans JM, Revill SI, David H, Rees GAD (1980b). Self-administered intravenous and intramuscular pethidine -a controlled trial in labour. Anaesthesia, 35: 763–770.

Rogers RE (1970). Fetal bradycardia—associated with paracervical block anesthesia. Am J Obstet Gynecol, 106: 913–916.

Rolbin SH, Wright RG, Shnider SM, et al. (1978). Enflurane analgesia for vaginal delivery. In: Abstracts of Scientific Papers, Annual Meeting, Society for Obstetric Anesthesia and Perinatology, Memphis, p 53.

Rosefsky JB, Petersiel ME (1968). Perinatal deaths associated with mepivacaine paracervical block anesthesia in labour. N Engl J Med, 278: 530–533.

Rosen M (1986). Comment. In: Anesthesia in Obstetrics. Albright GA, Ferguson JE, Joyce TH, Stevenson DK (eds). Boston, London: Butterworths, p 176.

Rosen M, Mushin WW, Jones PL, Jones EV (1969). Methoxyflurane for obstetric analgesics. Br Med J, 4: 432–433.

Rosen M, Latto P, Asscher AW (1972). Kidney function after methoxyflurane analgesia during labour. Br Med J, 1: 81–83.

Rowley WF, Tannrikulu O, Grossman A, Hsia DY (1963). A controlled study on effect of promethazine hydrochloride and meperidine hydrochloride upon serum bilirubin levels in the newborn infant. J Pediatr, 62: 934–935.

Rouge JC, Banner MP, Smith TC (1969). Interactions of levallorphan and meperidine. Clin Pharmacol Ther, 10: 643.

Ryhanen P, Jouppila R, Lanning M, Jouppila P, Hollmen A, Kouvalainen K (1984). Effect of segmental epidural analgesia on changes in peripheral blood leucocyte counts, lymphocyte subpopulations, and in vitro transformation in healthy parturients and their newborns. Gynecol Obstet Invest, 17: 202–207.

Sandelowski M (1984). Pain Pleasure and American Childbirth. From Twilight Sleep to the Read Method, 1914–1960. Westport, Connecticut: Greenwood Press.

Scher J, Hailey DM, Beard RW (1972). The effects of diazepam on the fetus. J Obstet Gynaecol Br Commwlth, 79: 635–638.

Schiff D, Chan D, Stern L (1971). Fixed drug combinations and the displacement of bilirubin from albumin. Pediatrics, 48: 139–141.

Seeds AE Jr, Stein-Messinger P, Dorsey JH (1962). Paracervical blocks: results of a double-blind evaluation. Obstet Gynecol, 20: 462–467.

Shnider SM, Gildea J (1973). Paracervical block anesthesia in obstetrics. III. Choice of drug: Fetal bradycardia following administration of lidocaine, mepivacaine, and prilocaine. Am J Obstet Gynecol, 116: 320–325.

Shnider SM, Levinson G (1987). Anesthesia for Obstetrics. Baltimore, London: Williams & Wilkins.

Shnider SM, Asling JH, Joll JW, and Margolis AJ (1970). Paracervical block anesthesia in obstetrics. I. Fetal complications and neonatal morbidity. Am J Obstet Gynecol, 107: 619–625.

Simcock MJ (1970). Bupivacaine for regional analgesia in

labour. A double-blind comparison with lignocaine. Med J Austr, 1: 889–891.

Simpson JY (1847). Answer to Religious Objections Advanced Against the Employment of Anaesthetic Agents in Midwifery and Surgery.

Skerman JH, Thompson BA, Goldstein MT, Jacobs MA, Gupta A, Blass NH (1985). Combined continuous epidural fentanyl and bupivacaine in labour: a randomized study. Anesthesiology, 63: 449.

Smedstad KG, Morison DH (1988). A comparative study of continuous and intermittent epidural analgesia for labour and delivery (in press).

Spellacy WN, Shattuck CA, Loffer FD (1966). A double-blind study of the comparative effects of meperidine with secobarbital, hydroxyzine, or a placebo on labour and delivery. Obstet Gynecol, 27: 290–293.

Stainthorp SF, Bradshaw EG, Challen PD, Tobias MA (1978). 0.125% bupivacaine for obstetric analgesia. Anaesthesia, 33: 3–9.

Tafeen CH, Friedman HL, Harris H (1968). Combined continuous paracervical and continued pudendal nerve block anesthesia in labour. Am J Obstet Gynecol, 100: 55–62.

Telford J, Keats AS (1961). Narcotic–narcotic antagonist mixtures. Anesthesiology, 22: 465–484.

Teramo K (1969). Fetal acid-base balance and heart rate during labour with bupivacaine paracervical block anaesthesia. J Obstet Gynaecol Br Commwlth, 76: 881–892.

Teramo K and Widholm O (1967). Studies of the effects of anesthetics on foetus. I. The effect of paracervical block with mepivacaine upon fetal acid-base values. Acta Obstet Gynecol Scand, 46 (Suppl 2): 1–39.

Thalme B, Belfrage P, Raabe N (1974). Lumbar epidural analgesia in labour: I. Acid-base balance and clinical condition of mother, fetus and newborn child. Acta Obstet Gynecol Scand, 53: 27–35.

Thiery M and Vroman S (1972). Paracervical block analgesia during labor. Am J Obstet Gynecol, 113: 988–1033.

Tournaire M, Catinat-Ozil D, Breart G, Scherrer P, Baron JM, Leroy B (1980). The influence of pethidine on uterine activity and dilation of the cervix in spontaneous labour. J Gynecol Obstet Biol Reprod (Paris), 9: 261–266.

Treisser A, Breart G, Blum F, Jouhet P, Pigne A, Barrat J (1981). Dystocia at the onset of labour. An evaluation of the different treatments available. J Gynécol Obstet Biol Réprod (Paris), 10: 91–98.

Turner MJ, Silk J, Gordon H (1987). Bupivacaine concentration and mode of delivery. Lancet, 1: 1496–1497.

Vella LM, Willatts DG, Knott C, Lintin DJ, Justins DM, Reynolds F (1985). Epidural fentanyl in labour: An evaluation of the systemic contribution to analgesia. Anaesthesia, 40: 741–747.

Wakley T (1858). Administration of chloroform to the queen. Lancet, May 14: 453.

Weiss RR, Halevy S, Almonte RO, Gundersen K, Hinsvark ON, O'Brien JE (1983). Comparison of lidocaine and 2-chloroprocaine in paracervical block: clinical effects and drug concentrations in mother and child. Anesth Analg (Cleve), 62: 168–173.

Westholm H, Magno R, Berg AA (1970a). Experiences with paracervical block. A double blind study with bupivacaine (Marcaine). Acta Obstet Gynecol Scand (Suppl) 37: 276–281.

Westholm H, Magno R, Berg AA (1970b). Paracervical block in labour. Acta Obstet Gynecol Scand, 49: 335–341.

Westmoreland RT, Evans JA, and Chastain GM (1974). Obstetric use of enflurane (Ethrane). South Med J, 67: 527–530.

Writer WDR, James FM, Wheeler AS (1981). Double-blind morphine and bupivacaine for continuous epidural analgesia in labour. Anesthesiology, 54: 215–219.

Youngstrom P, Eastwood D, Patel H, Bhatia R, Cowan R, Sutheimer C (1984). Epidural fentanyl and bupivacaine in labour: double-blind study. Anesthesiology (Suppl), 61: 414.

58 Augmentation of labour

Marc J. N. C. Keirse

'Inefficient uterine action is far the most common complication of childbirth'
O'Driscoll and Meagher (1980).

1 Introduction

Protracted labour has been recognized for centuries and a wide variety of treatments has been proposed for its correction. One of the classical examples, depicted in a drawing by Dürer, involved opening doors and chests of drawers as an invitation to the cervix to do the same. Until the beginning of this century, a drink of holy water was recommended for this purpose in some parts of The Netherlands. In other parts of the country, the treatment was slightly more elaborate in that it required a suitable biblical text to be written in ink on a piece of paper, which was then washed, whereupon the 'fortified' water so produced was administered to the labouring woman (Naaktgeboren 1987).

Even in recent decades, treatments to accelerate labour have included a bewildering variety of approaches; these include various spasmolytic drugs (Samaya *et al.* 1966; Guerresi *et al.* 1981), homeopathic remedies (Coudert 1981), sparteine sulphate (Friedman and Sachtleben 1963; Edelstein 1964), oestrogens (Klopper and Dennis 1962), relaxin (Slate and Mengert 1960; Nesbitt and Cirigliano 1961), caulophyllum (Coudert 1981; Kewley 1986), dimenhydrate (Cooper 1963; Harkins *et al.* 1964; Klieger and Massart 1965), nipple stimulation (Van Lier 1987), intracervical injections of hyaluronidase (Green 1967), vibration of the cervix (Brant and Lachelin 1971), and acupuncture (Kewley 1986). Some investigators have also attempted to stop labour temporarily in the hope that it will progress more satisfactorily thereafter (Treisser *et al.* 1981). None of these approaches has been used as widely as amniotomy and intravenous oxytocin infusion, however.

In primigravidae, rates of oxytocin infusion during labour of spontaneous onset vary from about 5 per cent (Bidgood and Steer 1987a) to more than 40 per cent (Cardozo *et al.* 1982; Turner *et al.* 1986, 1988) among different institutions. In some centres, augmentation of labour is thus one of the most common interventions applied during spontaneous labour. In spite of its wide application, it is a subject that has been largely neglected by controlled research. Criteria for its use are often vague and poorly defined (see Chapter 53). Whatever criteria are used, however, the assumption is usually that 'inadequate' progress is bad, and that 'something should be done about it'.

2 General measures

Slow or inadequate progress obviously depends on what is considered to be normal and adequate progress (see Chapter 53) and on what is considered to be labour as opposed to so-called 'false labour', 'latent labour' or labour that is 'not established'.

O'Driscoll and Meagher (1980), who have been vigorous proponents of augmentation of labour in order to coerce the cervix to dilate at a rate of at least 1 cm per hour, mention that approximately 10 per cent of women who admit themselves 'in labour' are mistaken in their diagnosis. In their opinion 'it is a matter of paramount importance that these women be identified, before they are placed on a production line from which there is generally only one escape route' (O'Driscoll and Meagher 1980). Yet, the actual data published from the institution in which O'Driscoll and Meagher work show that 42 (40 per cent) of 103 primigravidae, who were supposedly mistaken in seeking admission in labour, actually returned to the delivery unit within 24 hours (O'Driscoll *et al.* 1973). One is forced to wonder whether these women were truly mistaken in their diagnosis or whether they merely had a narrow escape from a 'production line' geared to ensuring that delivery occurs within 12 hours of admission to the labour ward.

It would appear that there are a large number of situations in which augmentation of labour is not directed at correcting a perceived abnormality in a woman's labour, but at shortening the labour and commitment of her caregivers. It is highly unlikely that myometrial physiology, even in primigravidae, will differ so much as to account for augmentation rates ranging from 5 to 40 per cent in different countries or different areas of the same country. Many factors, however, can influence myometrial contractility and the progress in labour that results from it. Consequently, there are a number of measures that can obviate much of the need for augmentation of labour.

There is ample evidence from animal studies (Bontekoe *et al.* 1977) that environmental factors and the absence of perceived danger have marked influences on the process of labour (see Chapter 48). The available data suggest that environmental influences are important in human labour as well. The randomized trials of Doula support in labour (Sosa *et al.* 1980; Klaus *et al.* 1986), for instance, showed that the presence of a supportive companion was associated with a striking reduction in the length of labour and a lesser use of oxytocics for augmentation of labour (see Chapter 49).

Randomized trials of ambulation during the first stage of labour also demonstrated a lower use of oxytocics for augmentation of labour (Flynn *et al.* 1978; McManus and Calder 1978; Williams *et al.* 1980; Hemminki and Saarikoski 1983) without any evidence that this was accompanied by a lengthening of the duration of labour (see Chapter 55). Less well documented, but generally known to those who provide care in labour, is the observation that uterine contractility tends to subside temporarily upon transport from home to the hospital.

More often than not, allowing a woman and her companion(s) the necessary time to settle in and feel at home in the new environment will do considerably more good, at least in subjective terms, than a cascade of interventions aimed at procuring so-called 'adequate progress'.

Similarly, it would seem to be more appropriate to prevent ketosis by allowing free access to food and drink than to correct its alleged influence on labour progress with uterine stimulants and intravenous glucose infusions of unproven benefit and potential harm (see Chapter 52).

3 Increasing uterine contractility

The relationship between low levels of uterine contractility and slow progress in labour appears to be well established (Turnbull 1957; Steer *et al.* 1985a; Bidgood and Steer 1987b). There is also evidence that there is a subset of women in whom, despite an apparently normal onset of labour, (intra)uterine production of prostaglandins (the endogenous uterine stimulants) is substantially less than average, and that it is these women in particular who fail to progress later in labour (Keirse *et al.* 1977).

Means to increase uterine contractility may therefore be based either on the administration of uterine stimulants, such as oxytocin or prostaglandins, or on increasing the endogenous production of uterine stimulants. Stimulation of endogenous prostaglandin production within the uterus occurs in response to amniotomy (Mitchell *et al.* 1977; Sellers *et al.* 1984), possibly through disjunction between fetal membranes and uterine wall over a large surface area (Keirse *et al.* 1983). This is likely to be the mechanism responsible for the labour enhancing effect of amniotomy, although redirection of the forces acting on the uterine cervix may also need to be considered.

3.1 Amniotomy

Amniotomy has been used to augment labour for decades, but whether artificial rupture of the membranes confers more benefit than harm has been a topic of debate throughout the period of its use for this purpose. Friedman and Sachtleben (1963), reviewing the subject 25 years ago, observed that 'within the course of little more than a century, there are found equally vigorous condemnations of, and statements of praise for, amniotomy, the former because it is certain to produce among other problems, profound protraction of labour, the latter because just as infallibly it will enhance labour progress.' Commenting upon the prevailing belief of the time that amniotomy stimulates labour, they noted that 'earnest attempts to uncover the experimental evidences upon which this firm contention rests have yielded very little that can withstand critical objective scrutiny.'

To obtain such evidence they felt that an 'experiment should be embarked upon . . .' which 'basically entailed randomized selection of successive gravidas admitted in labour for assignment to categories in which the membranes were to be ruptured or left intact, respectively' (Friedman and Sachtleben 1963). Unfortunately they abandoned their attempt to implement the study they had recommended even before it started. Instead, they embarked on a study in which a permissive policy, which allowed the obstetrician complete freedom of choice as to whether or when membranes should be ruptured, was followed by a restrictive period, during which amniotomy was prohibited 'as completely as possible'. This was then followed by a third period during which permissive amniotomy was again instituted as a 'repeat of the first in the form of a double check' (Friedman and Sachtleben 1963).

For reasons that are predictable, data on the more than 1500 women entered in the study, however, provide no useful information on the effects of the policies. Most of the data were 'idealized' by excluding information relating to women who had received either uterine stimulation (more than 30 per cent in nulliparae), or heavy sedation (35 to 44 per cent in nulliparae), or caudal anaesthesia (20 per cent in nulliparae). Having professed that the wide swings of the pendulum of obstetric thinking for or against amniotomy 'bespeak a lack of considered, tempered judgement' the authors themselves reached a rather tempered, though not necessarily useful conclusion. 'It cannot be denied', they observed 'that in individual cases under special circumstances amniotomy may stimulate labour, and contrariwise it is apparently just as likely for inhibitory effects to follow in selected cases'.

Since this inauspicious beginning of the attempts to mount properly controlled evaluation of amniotomy, five studies using random or quasi-random allocation have investigated the influence of amniotomy during spontaneous labour on the length of labour (Wetrich 1970; Laros *et al.* 1972; Schwarcz *et al.* 1975; Guerresi *et al.* 1981; Stewart *et al.* 1982). These studies, summarized in Table 58.1, are of very variable methodological quality, however.

In the study of Laros *et al.* (1972), both nulliparae and multiparae allocated to the amniotomy group had statistically significantly longer latent phases of labour before randomization than those assigned to the control group. This indicates that the inherent labour patterns prior to randomization may have been slower in the amniotomy than in the control group. Since no data are given on the length of labour after randomization (at 5 to 8 cm; Table 58.1), the pre-existing differences in duration may well have masked differences that evolved after allocation to amniotomy or control.

The trial of Guerresi *et al.* (1981) reports on 50 nulliparous and 50 multiparous women who were matched for a number of parameters and 'randomly divided' into two equal subgroups in one of which amniotomy and an intravenous injection of 'placebo' were used at 4 cm dilation; women in the other group received the same placebo injection but were left to await spontaneous rupture of the membranes. Unfortunately, the authors applied a number of exclusion criteria after randomization. 'All cases in which other drugs had to be administered in the course of delivery or in which delivery became dystocic were excluded from the study' (Guerresi *et al.* 1981). It is thus unclear how the number of women retained in the analysis relates to the number entered in the trial. The largest trial (Table 58.1), was a collaborative study conducted in Latin America by Schwarcz and his colleagues (1975) in which 'alternate women' were said to have had early artificial rupture of the membranes at 4 to 5 cm dilatation, whereas in women in the control group the membranes were left intact (Caldeyro-Barcia *et al.* 1974; Schwarcz *et al.* 1975). Unfortunately, exclusions after allocation and the distribution of women among the groups with and without early amniotomy indicate that this study did not compare like with like, and does not allow unbiased comparisons between these groups. Despite 'alternate allocation' there was a difference of more than 10 per cent in the numbers of women in the two comparison groups (Caldeyro-Barcia *et al.* 1974; Schwarcz *et al.* 1975).

In at least two of the trials in Table 58.1 (Guerresi *et al.* 1981; Schwarcz *et al.* 1975), bias may thus have been large enough to warrant extreme caution in inferring

Table 58.1. Controlled studies of amniotomy during labour of spontaneous onset

Authors	Wetrich (1970)	Laros *et al.* (1972)	Schwarcz *et al.* (1975)	Guerresi *et al.* (1981)	Stewart *et al.* (1982)
Amniotomy vs. control					
No. of nulliparae	16 vs. 16	28 vs. 30	?	25 vs. 25	17 vs. 15
multiparae	—	42 vs. 25	?	25 vs. 25	17 vs. 15
all women	16 vs. 16	70 vs. 55	465 vs. 547	50 vs. 50	34 vs. 30
Timing of randomization	6 cm dilatation	5–8 cm dilatation	4–5 cm dilatation	4 cm dilatation	at admission cervix score $\geqslant 6$* dilatation $\leqslant 4$ cm
Type of allocation	'blind draw'	'randomly' not described	'alternate' total of 1124; exclusions after allocation for various reasons	'randomly' not described; dystocia and drug treatment excluded after randomization; number excluded not specified	'randomly' not described

*Score of Calder *et al.* (1974)

any causal relationship between amniotomy and the duration of labour. The data of the three other trials, however, indicate that labours progress more quickly if the membranes are ruptured than if they are left intact (Table 58.2). The large Latin American collaborative study also suggested a shortening of labour: the median duration of labour (from 4–5 cm to full dilatation) was 50 minutes shorter (95 per cent confidence interval: 30–70 minutes) in the group with early rupture (Schwarcz *et al.* 1975). Increases in uterine activity following amniotomy have been demonstrated by Van Praagh and Hendricks (1964) using intrauterine pressure measurements through transabdominal intrauterine catheters before and after amniotomy.

The effects of amniotomy during spontaneous labour on other labour and delivery outcomes, such as use of oxytocics to augment labour, malrotation of the fetal head to occipito-lateral or occipito-posterior positions, and operative delivery, were reported in only two of the controlled trials (Wetrich 1970; Stewart *et al.* 1982). As shown in Table 58.3, the small amount of data does not allow firm conclusions to be reached about the effects of amniotomy on any of these outcomes.

Confusion and contradiction about the effects of amniotomy has not been limited to its effect on the course and duration of labour. Caldeyro-Barcia and his co-workers in particular have suggested that amniotomy may have a variety of adverse effects (Caldeyro-Barcia *et al.* 1974). Based largely on data from the Latin American Collaborative Study mentioned above

(Schwarcz *et al.* 1975) they have argued that increased pressure differentials around the fetal skull, combined with a reduction in amniotic fluid volume after amniotomy, predispose to fetal skull deformity (Schwarcz *et al.* 1969), an increased incidence of early decelerations in fetal heart rate (Schwarcz *et al.* 1973), and acidosis of the infant at birth (Martell *et al.* 1976). They have suggested that more research should be carried out to establish what the long term consequences of amniotomy may be on the central nervous system of the infant (Schwarcz *et al.* 1973). Unfortunately, all of these data were obtained in investigations which do not allow unbiased comparisons between groups. The inequality in numbers despite 'alternate allocation' (Caldeyro-Barcia *et al.* 1974; Schwarcz *et al.* 1975) was mentioned earlier. In the study on fetal heart rate patterns (Schwarcz *et al.* 1973) 'the decision to perform or not (to perform) early amniotomy was made at random' (Schwarcz *et al.* 1973), but the two groups consisted of 17 women with early amniotomy between 4 and 5 cm dilatation on the one hand, and 20 women in whom early amniotomy was not performed and in whom 'the membranes remained intact at least until full cervical dilatation had been reached' (Schwarcz *et al.* 1973) on the other. As the decision not to perform early amniotomy does not guarantee that the membranes will remain intact until full dilatation (Schwarcz *et al.* 1975), this study too suggests strong selection bias. The study of acid–base balance at birth (Martell *et al.* 1976) contained 21 women with early amniotomy and 17

Table 58.2. Effect of amniotomy on the duration of spontaneous labour

		Duration of labour in min (mean ± SD)		
		Wetrich (1970)	Laros *et al.* (1972)	Stewart *et al.* (1982)
First stage defined as		from 6 cm to full dilatation	'active phase' of labour	admission to full dilatation
nulliparae	amniotomy	90.2	146 ± 97	
	control	151.7	186 ± 125	
	difference	− 61.5	− 40	
multiparae	amniotomy		124 ± 94	
	control		118 ± 65	
	difference		+ 6	
all women	amniotomy			294 ± 216
	control			420 ± 222
	difference			− 126
Second stage				
nulliparae	amniotomy	59.6	35 ± 17	
	control	69.1	61 ± 48	
	difference	− 9.5	− 26	
multiparae	amniotomy		16 ± 9	
	control		17 ± 8	
	difference		− 1	

Table 58.3 Effect of amniotomy to shorten spontaneous labour on use of oxytocin

Study	EXPT		CTRL		Odds ratio	Graph of odds ratios and confidence intervals
	n	(%)	*n*	(%)	(95% CI)	0.01　0.1　0.5　1　2　10　100
Wetrich (1970)	0/16	(0.00)	0/16	(0.00)	1.00 (1.00–1.00)	
Stewart *et al.* (1982)	8/34	(23.53)	14/30	(46.67)	0.36 (0.13–1.02)	
Typical odds ratio (95% confidence interval)					0.36 (0.13–1.02)	

Effect of amniotomy to shorten spontaneous labour on use of analgesia

Study	EXPT		CTRL		Odds ratio	Graph
Stewart *et al.* (1982)	31/34	(91.18)	25/30	(83.33)	2.03 (0.46–8.84)	
Typical odds ratio (95% confidence interval)					2.03 (0.46–8.84)	

Effect of amniotomy to shorten spontaneous labour on caesarean section

Study	EXPT		CTRL		Odds ratio	Graph
Wetrich (1970)	0/16	(0.00)	0/16	(0.00)	1.00 (1.00–1.00)	
Stewart *et al.* (1982)	0/34	(0.00)	0/30	(0.00)	1.00 (1.00–1.00)	
Typical odds ratio (95% confidence interval)					1.00 (1.00–1.00)	

Effect of amniotomy to shorten spontaneous labour on instrumental vaginal delivery

Study	EXPT		CTRL		Odds ratio	Graph
Wetrich (1970)	6/16	(37.50)	10/16	(62.50)	0.38 (0.10–1.48)	
Stewart *et al.* (1982)	9/34	(26.47)	13/30	(43.33)	0.48 (0.17–1.34)	
Typical odds ratio (95% confidence interval)					0.44 (0.19–1.00)	

Effect of amniotomy to shorten spontaneous labour on malrotation of the fetal head

Study	EXPT		CTRL		Odds ratio	Graph
Wetrich (1970)	5/15	(33.33)	8/16	(50.00)	0.52 (0.13–2.10)	
Typical odds ratio (95% confidence interval)					0.52 (0.13–2.10)	

without the intervention despite 'alternate allocation', since women in whom the membranes ruptured spontaneously during the first stage of labour were again excluded from the control group (Martell *et al.* 1976). Although these studies are frequently cited as providing evidence of harmful effects of amniotomy on the fetus and neonate, they do not permit unbiased assessments of the effects of amniotomy during labour on fetal or neonatal well-being.

Only one of the randomized trials reported thus far provides unbiased estimates of the effects of amniotomy during spontaneous labour on fetal and neonatal outcomes (Stewart *et al.* 1982). From the data shown in Table 58.4 there is no evidence of any significant effect on the outcomes studied, but the number of women included in the trial was so small that only dramatic differences would have been uncovered.

None of the studies discussed thus far specifically addressed the question of whether or not amniotomy is effective in augmenting slow or prolonged labour. As far as I am aware, this issue has never been addressed in a published report of a randomized controlled trial.

Table 58.4 Effect of amniotomy to shorten spontaneous labour on abnormal or suspect fetal heart rate

Study	EXPT		CTRL		Odds ratio	Graph of odds ratios and confidence intervals
	n	(%)	n	(%)	(95% CI)	0.01 0.1 0.5 1 2 10 100
Stewart *et al.* (1982)	6/34	(17.65)	7/30	(23.33)	0.71 (0.21–2.37)	
Typical odds ratio (95% confidence interval)					0.71 (0.21–2.37)	

Effect of amniotomy to shorten spontaneous labour on Apgar score <7 at 5 minutes

Stewart *et al.* (1982)	0/34	(0.00)	1/30	(3.33)	0.12 (0.00–6.02)	
Typical odds ratio (95% confidence interval)					0.12 (0.00–6.02)	

Effect of amniotomy to shorten spontaneous labour on jaundice

Stewart *et al.* (1982)	7/34	(20.59)	8/30	(26.67)	0.72 (0.23–2.26)	
Typical odds ratio (95% confidence interval)					0.72 (0.23–2.26)	

Effect of amniotomy to shorten spontaneous labour on admission to special care nursery

Stewart *et al.* (1982)	4/34	(11.76)	3/30	(10.00)	1.20 (0.25–5.69)	
Typical odds ratio (95% confidence interval)					1.20 (0.25–5.69)	

Given the evidence that is available from the controlled trials in spontaneous labour (Table 58.2) and from the data on induction of labour (see Chapter 62) it is highly unlikely, however, that amniotomy would not tend to enhance progress in prolonged labour.

3.2 Oxytocin

Intravenous infusion of synthetic oxytocin, usually after either spontaneous or artificial rupture of the membranes, is the most widely applied treatment to expedite labour when progress is deemed to be inadequate.

Four controlled trials have assessed the effects of early intervention with intravenous oxytocin infusion to expedite labour in case of poor progress. Comparison groups have involved either ambulation (Read *et al.* 1981; Hemminki *et al.* 1985) or no intervention (Bidgood and Steer 1987a,b; Cohen *et al.* 1987) until a further delay in progress occurred. The studies, details of which are summarized in Table 58.5, were rather heterogeneous, with average lengths of labour in the control groups ranging from a duration of 8 hours (Cohen *et al.* 1987), which can hardly be deemed to be

prolonged, to 27 hours (Bidgood and Steer 1987a,b) (Table 58.6). In three of the studies, the membranes had either ruptured spontaneously or been ruptured artificially before randomization; in the fourth study (Cohen *et al.* 1987), amniotomy was carried out at as a co-intervention in the oxytocin treated group, but not in the control group if the membranes were still intact when poor progress was diagnosed (Table 58.5).

Only three of the trials provide data on the length of labour and only two show a shorter mean duration in women allocated to early oxytocin augmentation compared with controls (Table 58.6). In both of the trials in which a shorter mean duration was observed, women in the control group received no intervention for at least 2 (Cohen *et al.* 1987) or 8 hours (Bidgood and Steer 1987). In the third trial (Hemminki *et al.* 1985), women in the control group were encouraged to get up and to move around, stand, or sit as they wished. The mean duration of labour was slightly, though not statistically significantly, shorter in the control group than in the augmented group (Table 58.6). These data are consistent with those of other controlled trials (Flynn *et al.* 1978; McManus and Calder 1978; Williams *et al.* 1980; Hemminki and Saarikoski 1983), which showed both a

Table 58.5. Controlled trials of early intervention with oxytocin infusion for poor progress in labour

Authors	Read *et al.* (1981)	Hemminki *et al.* (1985)	Bidgood and Steer (1987a)	Cohen *et al.* (1987)
No. of women oxytocin	6	27		75
low dose			21	
high dose			19	
control	8	30	20	75
Allocation	'random' not described	sealed envelope	sealed envelope	'alternately'
Entry criteria	no progress for ⩾ 1 hr + inadequate contractions	no progress in 2 hr on vag. examination; if membranes intact: amniotomy + wait 2 hr	cervix ⩾ 3 cm + active labour + rate of cervical dilatation ⩽ 0.5 cm/hr	uterine contractions + cervix ⩾ 3 cm or ruptured membranes + < 3 contractions of 40 sec per 10 min
Intervention	oxytocin titration	oxytocin titration	oxytocin titration (initial + increments) high dose: 7 mU/min low dose: 2 mU/min	amniotomy + oxytocin titration
Control treatment	intravenous fluids + ambulation	ambulation	oxytocin deferred for 8 hours	external monitoring
Oxytocin if necessary in control group	after the study period of 2 hr	or: − 4 hr no progress − delivery not imminent after 8 hr − wish of mother or caregiver	at discretion of clinicians after 8 hr	no dilatation for ⩾ 2 hr in 1st stage no descent for ⩾ 1 hr in 2nd stage
	(6 of 8)	(15 of 30)	(5 of 20)	(28 of 75)

58.6. Effect of early oxytocin augmentation on the duration of labour

Authors	Duration of labour in hours (mean ± SD)			
	Oxytocin group		Control group	Difference
Hemminki *et al.* (1985)	15.3 ± 5.3		14.4 ± 7.0	+ 0.9
Cohen *et al.* (1987)	7.8 ± 3.7		8.0 ± 3.3	− 0.2
Bidgood and Steer (1987a)	23.− ± 7.8 (high dose)	25.− ± 6.7 (low dose)	27.− ± 8.1	− 3.−

reduction in the use of oxytocin for augmentation of labour and a shortening of the first stage of labour when women were encouraged to be up and about during labour (see Chapter 55).

The available data on the rate of cervical dilatation show a similar pattern with a different trend between the studies in which ambulation was (Read *et al.* 1981) or was not (Bidgood and Steer 1987a; Cohen *et al.* 1987) prescribed in the control group (Table 58.7). The mean rate of cervical dilatation was slightly higher in women assigned to the ambulant group than in those assigned to oxytocin augmentation in the only ambulation study that provided data on this outcome (Read *et al.* 1981). Of the two studies without ambulation, one (Cohen *et al.* 1987) showed virtually no difference with oxytocin

treatment, but women in both groups had a rate of dilatation close to 2 cm per hour (Table 58.7), which would indicate that the diagnosis of poor progress in labour as an entry criterion was rather loosely applied in this study (see Chapter 53). Only the study of Bidgood and Steer (1987a) showed a statistically significant increase in the rate of cervical dilatation with oxytocin treatment (Table 58.7); this increase was more marked in the women receiving the high dose regimen than in those receiving the lower dose (see below).

In each of the four trials between 25 and 75 per cent of the women assigned to be controls ultimately received oxytocin for failure subsequently to meet the criteria of progress in labour set by the authors (Table 58.5). These studies therefore indicate that only

Table 58.7. Effect of early oxytocin augmentation on the rate of cervical dilatation during labour

Authors (time period)	Rate of dilatation (in cm/hr; mean ± SD)			
	Oxytocin group		Control group	Difference
Read et al. (1981) (within first 2 hr)	0.84		1.10	− 0.26
Cohen et al. (1987) (in active phase)	1.94 ± 1.22		2.05 ± 1.29	− 0.09
Bidgood and Steer (1987a)	0.93 ± 0.69 (high dose)	0.54 ± 0.41 (low dose)	0.41 ± 0.44	+ 0.13 + 0.52

Table 58.8 Effect of early oxytocin to shorten spontaneous labour on caesarean section

Study	EXPT		CTRL		Odds ratio	Graph of odds ratios and confidence intervals						
	n	(%)	n	(%)	(95% CI)	0.01	0.1	0.5	1	2	10	100
Bidgood and Steer (1987a)	12/40	(30.00)	9/20	(45.00)	0.52 (0.17–1.60)							
Hemminki et al. (1985)	0/27	(0.00)	3/30	(10.00)	0.14 (0.01–1.40)							
Cohen et al. (1987)	10/75	(13.33)	11/75	(14.67)	0.90 (0.36–2.25)							
Read et al. (1981)	2/6	(33.33)	1/8	(12.50)	3.16 (0.26–37.90)							
Typical odds ratio (95% confidence interval)					0.70 (0.36–1.35)							

between 25 and 75 per cent of the women, who are not primarily treated with oxytocin for inadequate progress, will be able to avoid receiving an oxytocin infusion before delivery.

Active management of labour with liberal use of amniotomy and oxytocin augmentation has been reputed to be instrumental in achieving low caesarean section rates (O'Driscoll et al. 1984; Turner et al. 1986). This may well be the case, but it is not demonstrated by the results of the four trials (Table 58.8). Obviously, the total number of women (n = 281) included in these four trials is too small to confidently indicate anything but a very dramatic effect on the caesarean section rate. However, they highlight the need for adequately controlled studies to assess the claims made on the basis of poorly controlled observational data (O'Driscoll et al. 1984; Turner et al. 1986).

Effects on instrumental vaginal delivery are shown in Table 58.9. The table merely indicates the need for further studies before any reliable conclusions can be drawn.

Only two of the trials provide categorical data on neonatal outcomes. Neither Apgar scores nor the incidence of admission to a special care nursery were detectably different between oxytocin augmentation and control groups (Table 58.10).

Only one of the studies (Hemminki et al. 1985) sought women's views on the augmentation procedures, and data are available only for a subsample of the women included in the trial so that some selection bias cannot entirely be excluded. Twelve of 23 women (52 per cent) asked about their opinion on the oxytocin treatment said that it was unpleasant and 14 (61 per cent) indicated that they would like to try without the drug when next giving birth. Nineteen (83 per cent) felt that it had increased the amount of pain that they had experienced, whereas only 4 of 21 women (19 per cent) in the ambulant group felt that way (Hemminki et al. 1985).

From the data available thus far, it does not appear that liberal use of oxytocin augmentation in labour is of benefit to the women and babies so treated. This does not imply, however, that there is no place for oxytocin augmentation in slow progress of labour; merely that other simple measures, such as allowing the woman freedom to move around (see Chapter 55), and to eat and drink as she pleases (see Chapter 52), may be at least as effective and certainly more pleasant for a sizeable proportion of women considered to be in need of augmentation of labour.

Situations will undoubtedly remain in which drug-induced augmentation will be necessary to correct

Table 58.9 Effect of early oxytocin to shorten spontaneous labour on instrumental vaginal delivery

Study	EXPT n	(%)	CTRL n	(%)	Odds ratio (95% CI)	Graph of odds ratios and confidence intervals
Bidgood and Steer (1987a)	17/40	(42.50)	8/20	(40.00)	1.11 (0.38–3.26)	
Hemminki et al. (1985)	3/27	(11.11)	1/30	(3.33)	3.23 (0.43–24.25)	
Cohen et al. (1987)	6/75	(8.00)	3/75	(4.00)	2.02 (0.53–7.75)	
Read et al. (1981)	2/6	(33.33)	3/8	(37.50)	0.84 (0.10–7.10)	
Typical odds ratio (95% confidence interval)					1.47 (0.71–3.06)	

Graph scale: 0.01 0.1 0.5 1 2 10 100

Table 58.10 Effect of early oxytocin to shorten spontaneous labour on Apgar score <7 at 1 minute

Study	EXPT n	(%)	CTRL n	(%)	Odds ratio (95% CI)	Graph of odds ratios and confidence intervals
Bidgood and Steer (1987a)	8/40	(20.00)	8/20	(40.00)	0.37 (0.11–1.22)	
Hemminki et al. (1985)	1/27	(3.70)	2/30	(6.67)	0.56 (0.06–5.61)	
Typical odds ratio (95% confidence interval)					0.40 (0.14–1.16)	

Graph scale: 0.01 0.1 0.5 1 2 10 100

Effect of early oxytocin to shorten spontaneous labour on Apgar score <7 at 5 minutes

Study	EXPT n	(%)	CTRL n	(%)	Odds ratio (95% CI)	
Bidgood and Steer (1987a)	1/40	(2.50)	1/20	(5.00)	0.47 (0.02–9.05)	
Hemminki et al. (1985)	0/27	(0.00)	0/30	(0.00)	1.00 (1.00–1.00)	
Typical odds ratio (95% confidence interval)					0.47 (0.02–9.05)	

Effect of early oxytocin to shorten spontaneous labour on admission to special care nursery

Study	EXPT n	(%)	CTRL n	(%)	Odds ratio (95% CI)	
Hemminki et al. (1985)	0/27	(0.00)	1/30	(3.33)	0.15 (0.00–7.58)	
Typical odds ratio (95% confidence interval)					0.15 (0.00–7.58)	

inadequate uterine activity in order to prevent maternal exhaustion and prolonged rupture of the membranes with its concomitant risks of fetal and maternal infection.

Logic would dictate that, in such circumstances, the smallest effective drug dose be given and this in the most effective manner. As individual sensitivity to oxytocin varies greatly from woman to woman (Turnbull and Anderson 1968; Bidgood and Steer 1987b) oxytocin titration by means of an intravenous infusion is the treatment of choice. It is less clear, however, what

the initial dose should be (recommendations vary from 1 mU (Seitchik and Castillo 1982) to 6 mU per minute (O'Driscoll et al. 1984)); how large the increments should be; and at what interval they should be implemented. Further questions relate to the type of equipment to be used. These range from gravity fed infusion systems, through infusion pumps, to fully automated infusion systems set to administer oxytocin doses in relation to a predetermined level of uterine activity (Steer et al. 1985b; Bidgood and Steer 1987a).

Bidgood and Steer (1987a,b) randomly allocated 19

women to high doses of oxytocin, starting at 7 mU/min and increasing the dose by 7 mU/min every 15 minutes until a contraction frequency of 7 per 15 minutes was reached, and 21 women to oxytocin administered by an automatic infusion system at an initial rate of 2 mU/min increased by 2 mU/min every 15 minutes until a stable phase of uterine activity or an activity in excess of 1500 kPa per 15 minutes was detected. As shown in Tables 58.6 and 58.7, the mean duration of labour was somewhat shorter and the mean rate of cervical dilatation higher in women receiving the higher oxytocin dose. However, 7 women in the high dose group (37 per cent) experienced hyperstimulation, defined as a contraction frequency of 7 or more in 15 minutes or an increase in basal tone above 1–33 kPa (10 mm Hg), compared with none in the low dose group. In 3 of these women hyperstimulation was severe enough to warrant withdrawal from the study protocol; in a fourth woman it was associated with late decelerations of the fetal heart rate, which prompted delivery by caesarean section.

Despite the fact that women were eligible for entry into the trial only if they had a progress in dilatation of less than 0.5 cm per hour during labour (defined as a cervical dilatation of 3 cm or more, regular contractions requiring analgesia and ruptured membranes; Table 58.5), 8 of the 21 women (38 per cent) assigned to the automated infusion system had levels of uterine activity in excess of 700 kPa per 15 minutes and therefore required no oxytocin (Bidgood and Steer 1987a). While this indicates that slow progress in cervical dilatation is not necessarily due to subnormal levels of uterine activity, the level of activity that is needed both to ensure adequate progress and to avoid hyperstimulation has not yet been established. Seitchik and Castillo (1983a) showed that half of the women (22 of 43) who received intravenous oxytocin for hypocontractility in spontaneous labour needed to achieve a level of uterine activity above the 95th centile of that observed in successful spontaneous first stage labour (Seitchik 1981) in order to accomplish cervical dilatation. In a series of experiments, these authors have argued that most women in dysfunctional labour will achieve progress in cervical dilatation with doses of oxytocin of 4 mU/min or less (Seitchik and Castillo 1982, 1983a; Seitchik et al. 1984). They consider an initial rate of 1 mU/min and increments no larger than 1 mU per 30 minutes as an ideal compromise between an unacceptably long interval to effect an adequate response on the one hand and excessive oxytocin doses on the other. Others, however, routinely administer at least 6 mU/min, increasing doses with 6 mU/min every 15 minutes up to 60 mU/min. Such dramatic variations in recommended practice and the strong feelings that are apparently held for some of these regimens (Turner and Gordon 1988; Stronge and Connolly 1988) would ap-

pear to offer excellent grounds for a trial of adequate size to determine the relative merits and hazards of these approaches.

4 Influencing cervical resistance

It is a truism that labour usually proceeds slower in a first than in a later birth. O'Driscoll and Meagher (1980) stated that 'these differences are so great that they warrant the statement that primigravidae and multigravidae behave as different biological species'. Although uterine activity does not appear to have been quantitated in the institution in which they work, they attributed these differences to the fact that inefficient uterine action is fare more common in nulliparae than in multiparae in whom the uterus is considered to be 'an efficient organ' (O'Driscoll and Meagher 1980). Consequently, they recommend liberal use of oxytocin augmentation as *the* logical approach to correct the inefficient nulliparous uterus (O'Driscoll and Meagher 1980; O'Driscoll et al. 1984).

More than 30 years ago, however, Turnbull (1957) suggested that the resistance of the cervix and pelvic tissues is much less in multiparae because these structures have been stretched in the previous childbirth. Since then, several authors have confirmed that, both in labour of spontaneous onset (Arulkumaran et al. 1984; Seitchik and Castillo 1983b; Fairlie et al. 1988) and in induced labour (Arulkumaran et al. 1985; Steer et al. 1985b), the total amount of uterine work needed to effect vaginal delivery is less in multiparae than in nulliparae. Moreover, as noted above, Seitchik and Castillo (1983a) have shown that half of the women treated for 'hypocontractility' had to achieve levels of uterine activity well above the 95th centile of those observed in 'normal' labour in order to achieve progress in cervical dilatation. A similar observation was made in the randomized trial of Bidgood and Steer (1987a) in that, as mentioned above, 8 of 21 women (38 per cent) assigned to automated oxytocin infusion system for slow progress in labour had levels of uterine activity that were judged to be adequate without oxytocin treatment.

High doses of oxytocin to augment uterine activity to levels well in excess of those encountered during normal spontaneous labour may be one way to overcome high resistance to dilatation. The other, and more logical, approach would be to reduce resistance. Several methods to influence resistance directly or indirectly in order to accelerate cervical dilatation have been tested in the past.

4.1 Relaxin

In 1926 Hisaw reported that an extract of the corpus luteum of sows contained a substance capable of relaxing the pelvic ligaments of the guinea pig. From this the compound apparently derived its name, relaxin, and the ovaries of pregnant sows are still the richest known natural source of it (MacLennan 1983). Following early investigations in experimental animals, relaxin was reported, in the 1950s, to forestall 'premature' labour in women (Abramson and Reid 1955; McCarthy *et al.* 1957), but also to facilitate term labour (Eisenberg 1957) and to reduce the length of labour when administered in combination with oxytocin (Birnberg and Abitbol 1957).

Between 1958 and 1961, four placebo-controlled trials were reported on the use of intravenous or intramuscular administration of porcine relaxin, generally at doses of 40 mg or between 3000 and 6000 'guinea pig units' for shortening labour (Decker *et al.* 1958; Dill and Chanatry 1958; Slate and Mengert 1960; Nesbitt and Cirigliano 1961). None of the trials specifically dealt with prolonged labour, but in all it was hoped that administration of relaxin in early established labour would favourably influence cervical dilatation and thence the duration of labour. The results of all four trials, which incorporated a total of 2365 women, indicated that relaxin did not shorten the duration of labour. As shown in Table 58.11, the trend would, if anything, support the reverse conclusion.

Only one of these studies provided information on the use of oxytocic drugs for (further) augmentation of labour (Decker *et al.* 1958); 2 of 109 women in the relaxin group required oxytocin compared with none of 107 women in the control group. The two studies (Decker *et al.* 1958; Slate and Mengert 1960) that provide data on the use of caesarean section and instrumental vaginal delivery in over 2200 women, showed no

advantages of relaxin treatment for either of these outcomes (Table 58.12).

Following these observations the use of relaxin largely disappeared from obstetrical practice. More recently, following achievement of a far higher purity of the compound (Sherwood and O'Byrne 1974), relaxin made a comeback for facilitating cervical ripening both on its own (MacLennan *et al.* 1980, 1986; Evans *et al.* 1983) and in combination with other drugs such as prostaglandins and oestrogens (MacLennan *et al.* 1981; see Chapter 61).

4.2 Hyaluronidase

Another approach to decreasing cervical resistance was followed by Green (1967). In the expectation that the enzyme hyaluronidase would cause lysis of mucopolysaccharides in the cervical stroma and thereby destabilize the collagen framework, he randomly assigned women to receive intracervical injections of hyaluronidase, saline or no injections. There was no apparent attempt at blinding; the numbers in the 3 groups are very unequal (respectively 82, 11, and 54); and it is not described how 'randomization' was achieved. The mean length of labour from 3 to 4 cm dilatation (the time when the injections were given) to delivery was significantly shorter in both nulliparous (3:15 ± 2:45 versus 5:31 ± 3:58; hr:min, mean ± SD) and parous (1:46 ± 1:24 versus 3:06 ± 2:30) women in the hyaluronidase group. No untoward effects were noted, although 3 of 39 hyaluronidase treated, and only 1 of 27 control nulliparae underwent caesarean section, all because of cephalopelvic disproportion. The author concluded that hyaluronidase injections shortened

Table 58.11. Effect of relaxin administration on the mean length of spontaneous labour (standard deviations not available)

Authors	Parity	Duration in hours (number of women)		
		Relaxin group	Control group	Difference
Dill and Chanatry (1958)	nulliparae	9.0 (n = 17)	9.0 (n = 7)	0
	multiparac	4.9 (n = 14)	4.2 (n = 9)	+ 0.7
Nesbitt and Cirigliano (1961)	nulliparae	8.2 (n = 8)	6.5 (n = 7)	+ 1.7
	multiparae	5.0 (n = 13)	4.8 (n = 11)	+ 0.2
Slate and Mengert (1960)	mixed	8.37 (n = 1000)	8.28 (n = 1000)	+ 0.09
Decker et al. (1958)	nulliparae	18.4 (n = 48)	18.9 (n = 40)	− 0.5
	multiparae	12.7 (n = 61)	11.5 (n = 67)	+ 1.2

Table 58.12 Effect of relaxin to shorten spontaneous labour on caesarean section

Study	EXPT		CTRL		Odds ratio	Graph of odds ratios and confidence intervals						
	n	(%)	n	(%)	(95% CI)	0.01	0.1	0.5	1	2	10	100
Decker *et al.* (1958)	1/109	(0.92)	3/107	(2.80)	0.36 (0.05–2.56)							
Slate and Mengert (1960)	9/1000	(0.90)	10/1000	(1.00)	0.90 (0.36–2.22)							
Typical odds ratio (95% confidence interval)					0.77 (0.34–1.74)							

Effect of relaxin to shorten spontaneous labour on instrumental vaginal delivery

Decker *et al.* (1958)	9/109	(8.26)	15/107	(14.02)	0.56 (0.24–1.30)							
Slate and Mengert (1960)	215/1000	(21.50)	204/1000	(20.40)	1.07 (0.86–1.33)							
Typical odds ratio (95% confidence interval)					1.03 (0.83–1.27)							

labour by an average of 2 hours (Green 1967), but no further evaluation of this approach has appeared in the literature.

4.3 Cervical vibration

In 1971, Brant and Lachelin reported the use of a cervical vibrator which had formerly been applied 'with success' in Japan. They stated that 'the technique was originally used by us only in nulliparous patients in whom there had been failure to progress in labour beyond half dilatation despite frequent strong contractions over a period of some hours, and in whom caesarean section seemed the only alternative. Latterly we have extended our indications and are using the technique in other situations when it seems desirable to expedite the first stage. Vibration of the cervix has led to a marked increase in cervical dilatation in every case.' Subsequently, they (Brant and Lachelin 1972) described a new apparatus for this purpose, stating that 'tolerance of the procedure varies, but unless epidural analgesia is being used it is advisable to give the patient a small dose of intravenous pethidine to help during the dilatation, and with the strong contractions which usually follow.'

No controlled trials of this technique in labour of spontaneous onset have been reported thus far. Beard *et al.* (1973), however, reported on its use in women in whom labour had been induced by amniotomy and intravenous oxytocin. Twenty-five of 50 women were randomly assigned to cervical vibration after the cervix had reached 4 cm dilatation (Beard *et al.* 1973). On average, the rate of cervical dilatation was almost twice as fast in the vibration group (3.1 cm/hour) than in the control group (1.7 cm/hr), but with a very wide varia-

tion (from 0.4 to 16.0 cm/hr in the vibrated group). Thirteen of the 25 women (52 per cent) had their cervix dilated to 7 cm by vibration, but the trial showed no statistically significant differences in the duration of labour, which averaged 11 hours 27 minutes in the vibrated group and 10 hours 23 minutes in the control group. Obviously, the trial was too small to show any real differences in the mode of delivery or in neonatal outcome (Table 58.13).

Observational studies have suggested that the technique is useful, particularly when cervical dilatation is delayed despite satisfactory uterine activity and absence of cephalopelvic disproportion (Dahlgren 1980) and that it is perinatally safe (Debruyne and Thiery 1982). On the whole, however, measures to reduce soft tissue resistance have hitherto been poorly explored.

5 Conclusions

5.1 Implications for current practice

Slow progress or lack of progress in the first stage of labour does not necessarily result from a level of uterine contractility that is inferior to that seen in uncomplicated labours. It may be due to a higher resistance in the soft parts of the birth canal or to cephalopelvic disproportion, although it will often be necessary to ensure that adequate uterine contractility exists, if necessary by oxytocic stimulation, in order to differentiate these different mechanisms.

The available evidence indicates that approximately half of the women judged to have slow labour or poor progress in cervical dilatation will progress equally well whether or not oxytocic drugs are administered. As it is

Table 58.13 Effect of cervical vibration to shorten spontaneous labour on caesarean section

Study	EXPT		CTRL		Odds ratio	Graph of odds ratios and confidence intervals
	n	(%)	n	(%)	(95% CI)	0.01 0.1 0.5 1 2 10 100
Beard *et al.* (1973)	1/25	(4.00)	1/25	(4.00)	1.00 (0.06–16.45)	
Typical odds ratio (95% confidence interval)					1.00 (0.06–16.45)	

Effect of cervical vibration to shorten spontaneous labour on instrumental vaginal delivery

Beard *et al.* (1973)	13/25	(52.00)	10/25	(40.00)	1.61 (0.53–4.83)	
Typical odds ratio (95% confidence interval)					1.61 (0.53–4.83)	

Effect of cervical vibration to shorten spontaneous labour on Apgar score <8 at 1 minute

Beard *et al.* (1973)	10/25	(40.00)	6/25	(24.00)	2.06 (0.63–6.67)	
Typical odds ratio (95% confidence interval)					2.06 (0.63–6.67)	

Effect of cervical vibration to shorten spontaneous labour on Apgar score <8 at 5 minutes

Beard *et al.* (1973)	2/25	(8.00)	1/25	(4.00)	2.00 (0.20–20.20)	
Typical odds ratio (95% confidence interval)					2.00 (0.20–20.20)	

Effect of cervical vibration to shorten spontaneous labour on resuscitation of neonate

Beard *et al.* (1973)	4/25	(16.00)	2/25	(8.00)	2.10 (0.39–11.37)	
Typical odds ratio (95% confidence interval)					2.10 (0.39–11.37)	

not easy to distinguish the women who will ultimately show adequate progress without oxytocin from those who will not, attention devoted to the prevention of the problem would seem to be at least as worthwhile as the attention which is usually devoted to its cure. Measures that have been demonstrated to be effective include allowing women to move about as they please and the provision of friendly support. Both of these may be seen as characteristics of a welcoming environment without unnecessary prohibitions and restrictions.

When augmentation becomes necessary, it would appear that the first approach should be to rupture the membranes. There are no controlled trials that have compared the use of oxytocin with or without amniotomy in these circumstances and these may be required to settle the question more satisfactorily than is possible on the basis of currently available data. Such data that are available, however, suggest that amniotomy will shorten the length of spontaneous labour and that it may forestall the need for oxytocin infusion in some of these women. Extrapolation of data obtained in trials of induction of labour (see Chapter 62) and cervical ripening (see Chapter 61) further suggests that the combination of amniotomy with oxytocin may provide a better stimulation of labour than oxytocin alone.

There is no evidence that high and fast escalating doses of oxytocin confer any advantage over a more moderate approach in which doses are increased at half-hourly intervals in response to uterine contractility. The risks of hyperstimulation and the relationship between strength of contractions and pain experience are worthy of consideration in this respect.

Other methods for augmenting dysfunctional or slow labour, including the use of prostaglandins, are certainly worth considering, but they have been inadequately explored up to the present time.

This review of the available literature found that most of the recommendations for augmenting labour in clinical practice, including the present recommendations, are built on thin ice. Changes in current practice based on such recommendations should, therefore, be implemented only within the context of well designed trials to establish whether or not the new policy actually leads to better care judged in less ambiguous terms than modest differences in average duration of labour.

5.2 Implications for future research

There is an almost appalling contrast between the frequency with which augmentation of labour is employed in obstetrical practice and the paucity of well controlled research data to judge the effectiveness of the interventions used for this purpose. Presumably, the need for and use of augmentation is often based on a desire to accommodate assumed maternal wishes for a relatively short labour and an agreeable 'birth experience'. Yet, there is an almost total lack of controlled research indicating whether or not women prefer a labour of shorter duration, even if this is achieved, by oxytocin titration to a (possibly longer) spontaneous labour.

Evidence from basic research, cited above, indicates that poor progress in the first stage of labour may be associated with lower uterine prostaglandin production, while other data indicate that prostaglandins influence both uterine contractility and cervical compliance (see Chapter 61). This would seem to provide a firm foundation for evaluating the use of these compounds for augmentation of labour, when needed, particularly since they may obviate the need for intravenous infusions (see Chapter 62) and may facilitate ambulation, which can also reduce the length of labour (see Chapter 55).

The paucity of evidence in favour of any of the current policies for augmentation of labour does not necessarily imply that such policies need to be abandoned. It does imply, however, that there is virtually no published evidence to justify a preference for any of the existing regimens over any newly proposed policy that appears to be based on (equally) sound principles. Provided that such a policy is implemented in the context of a well designed trial to investigate both the merits and the hazards of the new approach, it is likely to contribute more to effective care than continued use of some of the poorly evaluated augmentation schemes that are currently in use.

Outcomes such as perinatal mortality and severe maternal or neonatal morbidity associated with labour at term have become so rare that it will be very difficult to assess the relative merits of different augmention policies in these terms. Outcomes such as reductions in the mean length of labour or increases in the rate of cervical dilatation, on the other hand, although readily measured, provide little information on aspects that are of real importance for mothers and their babies. Some important issues, such as the effects on maternal satisfaction and use of the available resources, may well be answered in single institution trials. Others, however, such as the effects on the use of caesarean section and instrumental delivery, and on neonatal morbidity (as measured, for instance, in terms of admission to special care nurseries or extended hospital stay), are unlikely to be resolved within single centre trials; but they could easily be assessed through multicentre collaboration. There would seem to be a very strong case for such collaboration in order to resolve the many questions that have been touched upon, but remained unanswered, in this chapter.

References

Abramson D, Reid DE (1955). Use of relaxin in treatment of threatened premature labor. J Clin Endocrinol, 15: 206–209.

Arulkumaran S, Gibb DMF, Lun KC, Heng SH, Ratnam SS (1984). The effect of parity on uterine activity in labour. Br J Obstet Gynaecol, 91: 843–848.

Arulkumaran S, Gibb DMF, Ratnam SS, Lun KC, Heng SH (1985). Total uterine activity in induced labour—an index of cervical and pelvic tissue resistance. Br J Obstet Gynaecol, 92: 693–697.

Beard RJ, Boyd I, Holt E (1973). A study of cervical vibration in induced labour. J Obstet Gynaecol Br Commnwlth, 80: 966–969.

Bidgood KA, Steer PJ (1987a). A randomized control study of oxytocin augmentation of labour. 1. Obstetric outcome. Br J Obstet Gynaecol, 94: 512–517.

Bidgood KA, Steer PJ (1987b). A randomized control study of oxytocin augmentation of labour. 2. Uterine activity. Br J Obstet Gynaecol, 94: 518–522.

Birnberg CH, Abitbol MM (1957). Refined relaxin and length of labor: preliminary report. Obstet Gynecol, 10: 366–370.

Bontekoe EHM, Blacquière JF, Naaktgeboren C, Dieleman SJ, Willems PPM (1977). Influence of environmental disturbances on uterine motility during pregnancy and parturition in rabbit and sheep. Behavioural Processes, 2: 41–73

Brant HA, Lachelin GCL (1971). Vibration of the cervix to expedite first stage of labour. Lancet, ii: 686–688.

Brant HA, Lachelin GCL (1972). Cervix vibrator-dilator using the electromagnetic principle. Lancet, ii: 408–409.

Calder AA, Embrey MP, Hillier K (1974). Extra-amniotic prostaglandin E_2 for the induction of labour at term. J Obstet Gynaecol Br Commnwlth, 81: 39–46.

Caldeyro-Barcia R, Schwarcz R, Belizan JM, Martell M, Nieto F, Sabatino H, Tenzer SM (1974). Adverse perinatal effects of early amniotomy during labor. In: Modern Perinatal Medicine. Gluck L (ed). Chicago: Yearbook Publishers, pp 431–449.

Cardozo L, Gibb DMF, Studd JWW, Vasant RV, Cooper, DJ (1982). Predictive value of cervimetric labour patterns in primigravidae. Br J Obstet Gynaecol, 89: 33–38.

Cohen GR, O'Brien WF, Lewis L, Knuppel RA (1987). A

prospective randomized study of the aggressive management of early labor. Am J Obstet Gynecol, 157: 1174–1177.

Cooper K (1963). Failure of dimenhydrinate to shorten labor. Am J Obstet Gynecol, 86: 1041–1043.

Coudert M (1981). Étude expérimentale de l'action du caulophyllum dans le faux travail et la dystocie de démarrage. University of Limoges; MD thesis.

Dahlgren S (1980). Reduction of delivery time by cervical dilatation induced by vibrations. Acta Obstet Gynecol Scand, (Suppl) 93: 24.

Debruyne G, Thiery M (1982). Perinatal effects of cervical vibration. Z Geburtsh Perinatol, 186: 240–241.

Decker WH, Thwaite W, Bordat S, Kayser R, Harami T, Campbell J (1958). Some effects of relaxin in obstetrics. Obstet Gynecol, 12: 37–46.

Dill LV, Chanatry J (1958). Effect of relaxin on normal labour. JAMA, 167: 1910–1912.

Edelstein H (1964). Value of sparteine sulphate as an oxytocic: a preliminary report. S Afr J Obstet Gynaecol, 2: 9–14.

Eisenberg L (1957). Facilitation of full term labor with relaxin. J Am Osteopath, 57: 147–148.

Evans MI, Dougan MB, Moawad AH, Evans WJ, Bryant-Greenwood GD, Greenwood FC (1983). Ripening of the human cervix with porcine ovarian relaxin. Am J Obstet Gynecol, 147: 410–414.

Fairlie FM, Phillips GF, Andrews BJ, Calder AA (1988). An analysis of uterine activity in spontaneous labour using a microcomputer. Br J Obstet Gynaecol, 95: 57–64.

Flynn AM, Kelly J, Hollins G, Lynch PF (1978). Ambulation in labour. Br Med J, 2: 591–593.

Friedman EA, Sachtleben MR (1963). Amniotomy and the course of labor. Obstet Gynecol, 22: 755–770.

Green PS (1967). Intracervical injection of hyaluronidase. Effect on dilatation and length of labor. Am J Obstet Gynecol, 99: 337–340.

Guerresi E, Gori G, Beccari A, Farro M, Mazzanti C (1981). Influence of spasmolytic treatment and amniotomy on delivery times: a factorial clinical trial. Clin Ther, 3: 382–388.

Harkins JL, Van Praagh IG, Irwin NT (1964). A clinical evaluation of intravenous dimenhydrinate in labour. Can Med Assoc J, 91: 164–166.

Hemminki E, Saarikoski S (1983). Ambulation and delayed amniotomy in the first stage of labor. Eur J Obstet Gynecol Reprod Biol, 15: 129–139.

Hemminki E, Lenck M, Saarikoski S, Henriksson L (1985). Ambulation versus oxytocin in protracted labour: a pilot study. Eur J Obstet Gynecol Reprod Biol, 20: 199–208.

Hisaw FL (1926). Experimental relaxation of pubic ligaments of guinea pig. Proc Soc Exp Biol Med, 23: 661–663.

Keirse MJNC, Mitchell MD, Turnbull AC (1977): Changes in prostaglandin F and 13,14-dihydro-15-keto-prostaglandin F concentrations in amniotic fluid at the onset of and during labour. Br J Obstet Gynaecol, 84: 743–746.

Keirse MJNC, Thiery M, Parewijck W, Mitchell MD (1983): Chronic stimulation of uterine prostaglandin synthesis during cervical ripening before the onset of labor. Prostaglandins, 25: 671–682.

Kewley T (1986). Jimmy's birth. Association of Radical Midwives, newsletter no. 29: 15–16.

Klaus MH, Kennell JH, Robertson SS, Sosa R (1986). Effects of social support during parturition on maternal and infant morbidity. Br Med J, 293: 585–587.

Klieger JA, Massart JJ (1965). Clinical and laboratory survey into the oxytocic effects of dimenhydrinate in labor. Am J Obstet Gynecol, 92: 1–10.

Klopper AI, Dennis KJ (1962). Effect of oestrogens on myometrial contractions. Br Med J, 2: 1157–1159.

Laros RK, Work BA, Witting WC (1972). Amniotomy during the active phase of labor. Obstet Gynecol, 39: 702–704.

McManus TJ, Calder AA (1978). Upright posture and the efficiency of labour. Lancet, 1: 72–74.

MacLennan AH (1983). The role of relaxin in human reproduction. Clin Reprod Fertil, 2: 77–95.

MacLennan AH, Green RC, Bryant-Greenwood GD, Greenwood FC, Seamark RF (1980). Ripening of the human cervix and induction of labor with purified porcine relaxin. Lancet, i: 220–223.

MacLennan AH, Green RC, Bryant-Greenwood GD, Greenwood FC, Seamark RF (1981). Cervical ripening with combinations of vaginal prostaglandin $F_{2\alpha}$, estradiol and relaxin. Obstet Gynecol, 58: 601–604.

MacLennan AH, Green RC, Grant P, Nicolson R (1986). Ripening of the human cervix and induction of labor with intracervical purified porcine relaxin. Obstet Gynecol, 68: 598–601.

Martell M, Belizan JM, Nieto F, Schwarcz R (1976). Blood acid-base balance at birth in neonates from labors with early and late rupture of the membranes. J Pediatr, 89: 963–967.

McCarthy JJ, Erving HW, Laufe LE (1957). Preliminary report on the use of relaxin in the management of threatened premature labor. Am J Obstet Gynecol, 74: 134–138.

Mitchell MD, Keirse MJNC, Anderson ABM, Turnbull AC (1977): Evidence for a local control of prostaglandins within the pregnant human uterus. Br J Obstet Gynaecol, 84: 35–38.

Naaktgeboren C (1987). Wonder en realiteit in verleden en heden; een verkenning van de gedachten over zwangerschap en baring bij onze voorouders. In: Een kind onder het hart. Dupuis HM, Naaktgeboren C, Noordam DJ, Spanjer J, van der Waals FW (eds). Amsterdam: Meulenhof, pp 57–84.

Nesbitt REL, Cirigliano G (1961). Use of relaxin during parturition. NY State J Med, 61: 90–97.

O'Driscoll K, Meagher D (1980). Active Management of Labour. London: WB Saunders.

O'Driscoll K, Stronge J, Minogue M (1973). Active management of labour. Br Med J, 3: 135–137.

O'Driscoll K, Foley M, MacDonald D (1984). Active management of labor as an alternative to cesarean section for dystocia. Obstet Gynecol, 63: 485–490.

Read JA, Miller FC, Paul RH (1981). Randomized trial of ambulation versus oxytocin for labor enhancement: a preliminary report. Am J Obstet Gynecol, 139: 669–672.

Samaja BA, Frangipani GC, D'Aquino P (1966). Sperimentazione clinica di una nuova associazione analgesico-spasmolitico-ansiolitica (D-propossifene; Dimethil-n-ottil benzilato di etile ammonio bromuro; Clorodiazepossidе) in travaglio di parto. Minerva Ginecol, 18: 1136–1140.

Schwarcz R, Strada-Saenz G, Althabe O, Fernandez-Funes J, Caldeyro-Barcia R (1969). Pressure exerted by uterine contractions on the head of the human fetus during labour.

In: Perinatal Factors Affecting Human Development. Caldeyro-Barcia R (ed). Washington: Pan American Health Organization, pp 115–126.

Schwarcz R, Althabe O, Caldeyro-Barcia R, Belitsky R, Lanchares JL, Alvarez R, Berdaguer P, Capurro H, Belizan JM, Sabatino JH, Abusleme C (1973). Fetal heart rate patterns in labors with intact and with ruptured membranes. J Perinat Med, 1: 153–165.

Schwarcz R, Belízan JM, Nieto F, Tenzer SM (1975). La rotura precoz de las membranas ovulares y sus efectos sobre el parto y el neonato. Oficina Sanitaria Panamericana, 595: 1–80.

Seitchik J (1981). Quantitating uterine contractility in clinical context. Obstet Gynecol, 57: 453–457.

Seitchik J, Castillo M (1982). Oxytocin augmentation of dysfunctional labor. I. Clinical data. Am J Obstet Gynecol, 144: 899–905.

Seitchik J, Castillo M (1983a). Oxytocin augmentation of dysfunctional labor. II. Uterine activity data. Am J Obstet Gynecol, 145: 526–529.

Seitchik J, Castillo M (1983b). Oxytocin augmentation of dysfunctional labor. III. Multiparous patients. Am J Obstet Gynecol, 145: 777–780.

Seitchik J, Amico J, Robinson AG, Castillo M (1984). Oxytocin augmentation of dysfunctional labor. IV. Oxytocin pharmacokinetics. Am J Obstet Gynecol, 150: 225–228.

Sellers SM, Mitchell MD, Anderson ABM, Turnbull AC (1984): The influence of spontaneous and induced labour on the rise in prostaglandins at amniotomy. Br J Obstet Gynaecol, 91: 849–852.

Sherwood CD, O'Byrne EM (1974). Purification and characterisation of porcine relaxin. Arch Biochem Biophys, 160: 185–196.

Slate WG, Mengert WF (1960). Effect of the relaxing hormone on the laboring human uterus. Obstet Gynecol, 15: 409–414.

Sosa R, Kennell JH, Klaus M, Robertson S, Urrutia J (1980). The effect of a supportive companion on perinatal problems, length of labor and mother–infant interaction. New Engl J Med, 303: 597–600.

Steer PJ, Carter MC, Beard RW (1985a). The effect of oxytocin infusion on uterine activity levels in slow labour. Br J Obstet Gynaecol, 92: 1120–1126.

Steer PJ, Carter MC, Choong K, Hanson M, Gordon AJ, Pradhan P (1985b). A multicentre prospective randomized controlled trial of induction of labour with an automatic closed-loop feedback controlled oxytocin infusion system. Br J Obstet Gynaecol, 92: 1127–1133.

Stewart P, Kennedy JH, Calder AA (1982). Spontaneous labour: when should the membranes be ruptured? Br J Obstet Gynaecol, 89: 39–43.

Stronge J, Connolly R (1988). A randomized control study of oxytocin augmentation of labour: 1. Obstetric outcome. Br J Obstet Gynaecol, 95: 105–106.

Treisser A, Bréart G, Blum F, Jouhet P, Pigne A, Barrat J (1981). Dystocie de démarrage du travail. Evaluation des différentes thérapeutiques. J Gynécol Obstet Biol Réprod (Paris), 10: 91–98.

Turnbull AC (1957). Uterine contractions in normal and abnormal labour. J Obstet Gynaecol Br Empire, 64: 321–332.

Turnbull AC, Anderson ABM (1968). Uterine contractility and oxytocin sensitivity during human pregnancy in relation to the onset of labour. J Obstet Gynaecol Br Commnwlth, 75: 278–288.

Turner MJ, Gordon H (1988). A randomized control study of oxytocin augmentation of labour: 1. Obstetric outcome. Br J Obstet Gynaecol, 95: 104–105.

Turner MJ, Webb JB, Gordon H (1986). Active management of labour in primigravidae. J Obstet Gynaecol, 7: 79–83.

Turner MJ, Brassil M, Gordon H (1988). Active management of labor associated with a decrease in the cesarean section rate in nulliparas. Obstet Gynecol, 71: 150–154.

Van Lier DJ (1987). Nipple stimulation for augmentation of labor. Proceedings of 21st International Congress of International Confederation of Midwives, The Hague, The Netherlands, pp 9–12.

Van Praagh I, Hendricks CH (1964). The effect of amniotomy during labour in multiparas. Obstet Gynecol, 24: 258–265.

Wetrich DW (1970). Effect of amniotomy upon labor. Obstet Gynecol, 35: 800–806.

Williams RM, Thom MH, Studd JWW (1980). A study of the benefits and acceptability of ambulation in spontaneous labour. Br J Obstet Gynaecol, 87: 122–126.

Part VII

Initiating labour

59 The development of methods for inducing labour

Michel Thiery, Cornelia J. Baines, and Marc J. N. C. Keirse

1 Introduction

In describing the historical development of labour induction by artificial means it is difficult to adhere to a temporal sequence. Theory and practice were often distinctly different; several methods took decades to come of age clinically; and once-popular techniques, after first being abandoned, were often reintroduced, sometimes in combination with newly proposed methods. In the light of this complex picture, we begin this chapter with a chronologically organized overview of the development of induction of labour, and then go on to discuss the evolution of the specific methods we consider to be of particular historical or clinical importance.

2 A chronological overview

2.1 Developments prior to the twentieth century

Attempts to induce or augment labour have a long history. Induction of labour by manual dilatation of the cervix, mostly for pelvic deformity, was mentioned by Soranos of Ephesus in the second century AD. In the ninth and tenth centuries, Arab physicians devised instruments for the same purpose. In the sixteenth century, both Paré and his pupil Guillemeau induced labour by manual and instrumental dilatation in cases of severe uterine haemorrhage (Fasbender 1906), and Eucharius Rodion (Rhodion or Rösslin) gave an elaborate list of substances believed to facilitate labour

in the earliest printed obstetric textbook. These preparations, mostly plant decoctions, were ingested by the woman, but Rodion also mentions packing the genital tract with wool cloth soaked with the juices of *Ruta graveolens* and *Aristolochia* sp. (Rodion 1641). None of these writers, however, made a clear distinction between augmentation and genuine induction of labour, nor do they provide any evidence concerning the efficacy of these procedures or the extent to which they were actually carried out.

In the eighteenth century, packing the cervical canal was refined by using surgical tents (from the medieval Latin word *tenta*)—a cylinder of some material introduced into a canal or sinus to maintain its patency or dilate it (Stedman 1961). These were made of compressed sea-sponge or plant materials (laminaria and tupelo tents) and were introduced in the cervical canal where they swelled and slowly dilated the cervix.

The medical history of labour induction really starts in 1756, when George Macauley came upon the idea of preventing dystocia due to pelvic contraction by inducing labour before term in an attempt to circumvent the hazards of both caesarean section and fetal extraction with the crochet (Denman 1785).

Either low or high amniotomy were used in attempts to induce labour. The most influential promoter of low amniotomy (the so-called 'English operation') was Denman (1785), who was the 'doyen' of English obstetrics at that time. Through his influence, low amniotomy was adopted in Germany, Italy, and The Netherlands. In France, the method was at first opposed, possibly on religious grounds; but there too, it had been adopted or readopted by 1831. Indeed, low amniotomy had been used by the Parisian obstetrician François Mauriceau at the end of the seventeenth century to induce labour and control haemorrhage in placenta praevia (Cianfrani 1960).

High amniotomy, using a rubber catheter stiffened with silver wire, was introduced by Hamilton during the first half of the nineteenth century (Young 1963). Hamilton had begun his interest in induction of labour in 1810 when he had attempted to prevent the infection that not infrequently followed low amniotomy by trying to induce labour by simple digital separation of the membranes from the lower uterine segment without rupturing the membranes (Hamilton 1836). Soon after, he abandoned this technique in favour of high amniotomy. Both low and high amniotomy fell into disuse, however, only to be 'reinvented' in the present century.

Three other methods of induction were introduced during the first part of the nineteenth century, namely galvanism suggested by Herder in 1803 (Theobald 1973b), stimulation of the breasts (Merriman 1838), and installation of fluids into the vagina or the uterus. Efforts to induce labour using the third of these approaches were sometimes quite extreme. From 1844 to 1846, Kiwisch attempted repeated hot pressurized vaginal douches (reviewed by Brindeau 1926). Because the effect of this Teutonic approach to the induction of labour proved disappointing, some women fainting during treatment, Sarwey (1896) used large volumes (50 to 100 litres!) of lukewarm water every 3–4 hours in attempts to trigger the onset of labour, but to no avail.

According to Ovink (1896) it was Schweighaüser who first proposed extra-amniotic injection of fluids for induction of preterm labour in 1825. This method, however, came to bear the eponym of Cohen who published his method of instilling *aqua picea* between the uterine wall and the membranes in 1846 (reviewed by Ovink 1896). Other writers have substituted various fluids, for example Pelzer (1892), who suggested using 100 ml of sterile glycerin. Although uterine instillation of fluids to induce labour fell into disuse at the end of the nineteenth century, some obstetricians went on practising this method. As late as 1939, Aburel proposed intra-amniotic injection of distilled water for induction of labour, a method he termed 'artificial hydramnios', or 'uterine distension'.

Induction of labour, mostly preterm induction of labour, became progressively more popular during the later decades of the nineteenth century, and several new methods were introduced during this time. By far the most popular of these was insertion of a rubber bougie between the membranes and the uterine wall, a procedure introduced by Krause in 1855.

About the same time as Krause introduced his bougie method, the idea of using inflatable rubber bags was floated. At first these contraptions were inserted in the vagina (*colpeurynter*), but because of lack of effectiveness they were soon replaced by intrauterine bags, or *metreurynters* (reviewed by Biermer 1899). In 1851, Carl Braun used a rubber toy balloon intravaginally both to induce preterm labour and to check 3rd-trimester vaginal haemorrhage (Biermer 1899). In 1862, Tarnier had a balloon catheter for insertion into the lower segment (the '*dilatateur intra-utérin*' or '*excitateur utérin*') constructed by Charrière in Paris (Charrière 1862). In the same year Barnes introduced his fiddle-shaped device which could be adjusted to fit both the cervical canal and the lower uterine segment. In 1883, Schauta was the first to insert Braun's original intravaginal balloon into the uterus. In 1878, Tarnier's pupil Champetier de Ribes (1888) introduced the ultimate metreurynter: a conical intracorporeal bag in several sizes made of rubber fortified by silk which was both impermeable and inextensible. Metreurynters seem to have been quite efficient and their effectiveness in triggering uterine activity could be increased by putting weight on the device.

2.2 Developments during the twentieth century

In 1913, an entirely new approach to labour induction was proposed by Benjamin Watson (Watson 1922). Basically, this method (which the author called 'medical induction' to distinguish it from surgical intervention), involved administering castor oil and quinine, to which pituitary extract was later added. Although the Watson regimen did not fulfil its early promise, it continued to be used, mainly in Europe, until the 1950s. The principle of medical induction had come to stay, however. The modern era of labour induction was initiated in 1928 by the clinical introduction of purified posterior pituitary extract for medical induction (Kamm *et al.* 1928); it became established in 1955, when synthetically prepared oxytocin was made available commercially (Boissonas *et al.* 1955).

Although the exact role of oxytocin in human parturition is still discussed, its introduction had a profound influence on the practice of induction of labour. At first, highly diluted solutions ('the oxytocin drip') were used (Theobald *et al.* 1948); by 1968, intravenous infusion of escalating doses ('titrated' against uterine contractions) was introduced by Turnbull and Anderson (1968) to reduce the rate of failed induction after amniotomy. Other developments in obstetrics made this evolution possible. These include the quantitation of the spontaneous contractility of the gravid uterus (Alvarez and Caldeyro-Barcia 1950); the elucidation of the uterine response to oxytocin (Caldeyro-Barcia and Heller 1961); the introduction of semi-quantitative systems for the prediction of inducibility (Bishop 1964); graphic analysis of the progress of labour (Friedman 1954,

1978); the availability of commercial equipment for electronic recording of (intra)uterine pressure variations and fetal heart rate patterns; biochemical assessment of the fetus during labour (Saling 1966); and the refinement of methods for the relief of labour pain.

Since 1968, however, oxytocin has had a rival for labour induction—the prostaglandins. Since Karim first reported success with intravenous infusion of prostaglandin $F_{2\alpha}$ (Karim *et al.* 1968), both this compound and prostaglandin E_2 have been used widely for this purpose. Several reasons explain the explosion of interest in prostaglandins. By the 1960s, a sound pharmacological basis had been established for administering oxytocin and this was readily extended to provide a rationale for the use of prostaglandins. Due to the unique effect of prostaglandins on the uterine cervix, however, they offered a solution to the problem presented by women who, on account of their unfavourable cervix, had remained poor candidates for 'conventional' induction using oxytocin. Furthermore, because prostaglandins are effective when administered either locally or systemically, the choice of alternative routes of administration increased their attractiveness. Uterine administration has the attendant advantage of requiring much lower doses of prostaglandin and therefore helped to address the problem of untoward side-effects provoked by intravenous prostaglandin administration. Finally, the recent commercial availability of stable preparations of PGE_2, mainly vaginal tablets and gels, boosted the clinical use of prostaglandins both for priming the cervix and for inducing labour (see Chapters 61–63).

Throughout the period during which the use of oxytocin and the prostaglandins has been refined, older methods were being reassessed and new ones were being tried. These included high amniotomy (Smythe 1931), nipple stimulation (Lorand and Asbot 1952), electrical induction (Theobald and Lundborg 1962), cervical vibration (Tokuyama and Fujimoto 1968), and acupuncture (Tsuei and Lai 1974).

In the early 1970s, Theobald (1974) summarized the state of the art as follows: 'Approximately all women within two weeks of term will have an 80 per cent chance of going into labour within 24 hours of amniotomy, and of these more than 90 per cent will be delivered within that time. A further 14 per cent will go into labour after having a physiological oxytocin drip for nine hours'. He concluded that 'the real problem is to detect and treat the remaining 6 per cent in whom there is difficulty in establishing labour'. A few years later, the problem presented by the uncompromising cervix was also solved.

Unfortunately, the development of successful methods for achieving induction of labour resulted in a dramatic increase in induced labour in some countries (Chalmers and Richards 1977). In the same year that

Theobald (1974) had published his review, for example, there was a public outcry in the United Kingdom against the use of induction of labour for trivial indications (Chalmers 1976), particularly as the harmful effects of this liberal use of induction came to be recognized (Chalmers *et al.* 1978). As the twentieth century draws to a close, the most important question is no longer *how* to induce labour, but *when* is inducing labour likely to do more good than harm.

3 Mechanical methods

Introduction of devices into the cervical canal, the extra-ovular space, or the amniotic cavity was referred to as 'mechanical induction' by our predecessors. Mechanical methods have never been completely abandoned and, even today, publications devoted to a new instrument appear from time to time in the literature. Furthermore, several mechanical methods have contemporary relevance to attempts to ripen the cervix (see Chapter 61).

In fact, we now know that the effectiveness of so-called 'mechanical' methods for induction is due to enhanced local synthesis of uterotonic prostaglandins. *In vitro* (Klöck and Jung 1973; Hillier and Coad 1982) and *in vivo* studies (Manabe *et al.* 1985) have demonstrated that stretching of myometrial and cervical tissues results in the release of prostaglandins. Immediately following the insertion of a Foley catheter into the extra-ovular space, maternal plasma levels of 13,14-dihydro-15-keto-$PGF_{2\alpha}$, a main prostaglandin metabolite in the circulation, soar and remain high for several hours thereafter (Keirse *et al.* 1983). The designation of the induction methods discussed in this section as 'mechanical' has, however, been retained for historical reasons.

3.1 Bougies and tents

Although the bougies introduced by Albert Krause in 1855 were still being used to induce labour in French obstetric departments in the 1960s (Pigeaud and Favier 1964), they appear to have been abandoned in the early 1970s (Brémond *et al.* 1978). As mentioned above, however, gradual stretching of the cervical canal is a related approach to induction and one which is still relevant in contemporary attempts to prepare the cervix for induction (see Chapter 61). Prepared sea-sponges and tupelo tents (sponge wood, *Nyssa* sp.) were gradually replaced by *stipes laminaria*, but the technique fell into disuse in the 1920s, apparently because of problems with infection. In the 1970s, as modern methods of sterilization reduced this danger, they were reintroduced (Newton 1972; Cross and Pitkin 1978; Lackritz *et al.* 1979). In recent years sponges made of synthetic hydrophilic materials (*Lamicel*®) were made commercially available (Nicolaides *et al.* 1983) and

Lippert (personal communication) in Germany is currently investigating the use of *Lamicel®* sponges containing prostaglandin for priming the cervix and induction of labour.

3.2 Catheters, metreurynters, and balloons

At the end of the nineteenth century, gastric sounds and Nélaton's urethral catheters were equally popular devices for the induction of labour (Fasbender 1906). Views about the Champetier de Ribes metreurynter have varied. It was considered to be unsatisfactory by some obstetricians because it ruptured easily at the seams. Because of this tendency, James Voorhees, at the Sloane Hospital for Women in New York, had the device improved in 1900 and the Voorhees bag occupied a prominent place in the armamentarium of the American obstetrician for decades thereafter (Speert 1980). The use of the Champetier de Ribes metreurynter was still taught to medical students in the late 1950s at the University of Gent in Belgium, however, and Veyre and colleagues (1974) reported the results of 84 cases treated during the early 1970s in Dijon, France, complaining that the bag had become increasingly difficult to obtain.

Balloon catheters have also been used throughout most of this century. In the late 1920s, Karel de Snoo in Utrecht in The Netherlands, following a lead from Mensinga, produced a homemade device consisting of a condom tied tightly on to a urinary catheter (Kloosterman 1947). Having inserted the condom between the membranes and the uterine wall, it could be filled with water, using the catheter. In 1947, Kloosterman considered this device the most effective and safest method for labour induction.

Balloon catheters were also inserted into the amniotic cavity, and the use of one such device was encouraged as late as the 1950s (Huber 1955). In the 1960s, dissatisfaction with the results of the then generally used repeat oxytocin infusion for ripening the cervix, resulted in a reintroduction of intrauterine balloons (Theobald and Lundborg 1962; Embrey and Mollison 1967). An indwelling Foley catheter with a 50 ml balloon capacity was introduced just above the cervical isthmus.

Just as traction was used in conjunction with metreurynters in attempts to improve their effectiveness in the nineteenth century, so also has it been used with balloons and other mechanical devices. In 1966, Dwyer had a sort of miniature metal umbrella constructed which was inserted into the lower uterine segment, unfolded and brought under traction to elicit contractions or correct poor uterine activity. Similarly, in 1979, Lippert and Peters described a *Ballonbelastung der Zervix* for labour induction after fetal death: after positioning an extra-amniotic Foley catheter and filling its balloon with 50 ml of water, the device is secured to the foot of the bed via a pulley and loaded with a 300–500 g weight.

4 Surgical methods

Advocacy of low (or forewater) amniotomy to induce preterm labour dates from the mid-eighteenth century (Denman 1785). The procedure was discarded early in the nineteenth century and for a hundred years or so, was little used. In 1928, Jackson revived interest in low amniotomy, which he combined with subcutaneous injections of posterior pituitary extract, mostly for elective induction of labour (Titus 1945). In 1932, Slemons expressed his preference for a combination of castor oil and quinine, followed by artificial rupture of the membranes and then intranasal administration of pituitary extract (Titus 1945). This method was still being advocated by Titus in the 1945 edition of his classic textbook *The Management of Obstetric Difficulties*.

The renaissance of low amniotomy was at first slow. Like their predecessors almost two centuries previously, many obstetricians were hesitant to puncture the membranes because, according to classical teaching, the bag of waters served as the main hydrostatic wedge and its integrity was considered imperative for the progress of cervical dilatation. They were also concerned about the risk of cord prolapse (notwithstanding the demonstration by Van Der Hoeven in 1908 that this was directly related to the degree of cervical dilatation at the time of spontaneous rupture of the membranes).

In the early 1930s however, the previous obsession with 'dry labour' was dispelled by suggestive evidence that amniotomy accelerated the first stage of labour (Eastman 1938; see Chapter 58). Once low amniotomy became used more widely, the efficacy of surgical induction of labour in most cases became self-evident. More importantly, the cases in which amniotomy failed to induce and establish labour taught obstetricians to recognize the contraindications for its use. They began to realize that to perform surgical induction on a woman with 'unfavourable' prospects for induction was to ask for trouble (Eastman 1938). Although the importance of cervical 'readiness' for the course of labour following amniotomy had been demonstrated during the 1930s, it took some time for this factor to be generally appreciated. It was not until the 1960s that risk factors for predicting the likely success of surgically-induced labour were formally combined in a quantitative manner (Bishop 1964; see Chapter 61).

No details are available concerning the technique originally used for piercing the forewaters, probably because Denman (1785) thought that the minutiae of the 'English Operation' were common knowledge. After the revival of low amniotomy in this century, a variety of surgical instruments (for example, Kocher or dressing forceps, a long clamp, one blade of a disarticulated volsellum, or even a pair of long scissors) were used to hook, grasp, and then disrupt the ovular sac. Besides these, an array of 'membrane perforators' was introduced, such as Currie's 'induction catheter'

(Thackray 1935) and Titus' 'special perforator' (Titus 1951). New amniotomy devices continue to be proposed occasionally, the latest being the Amnicot® (Samco Industries Inc., Stoughton, MA, USA), a latex fingercot provided with a small hook.

An alternative technique for surgical induction is the so-called high (or hindwater) amniotomy. This was originally proposed by Hamilton in 1836 and reintroduced by Drew Smythe of Bristol in the 1930s (Smythe 1931). To puncture the membranes beyond the fetal head, Smythe devised a double curved silver catheter with a blunt-ended stylet (Smythe 1949; Titus 1951). Although this once-popular instrument fell into disuse in the 1960s, it is still sometimes used in special circumstances, such as with hydramnios, or when there is a floating fetal head and induction is required.

According to Theobald (1974), artificial rupture of the membranes is 'the most efficacious single procedure for inducing labour' and has remained the backbone of the 'conventional' induction method (Turnbull and Anderson 1968). Amniotomy causes a rise of prostaglandin levels in amniotic fluid (Mitchell *et al.* 1976) and of prostaglandin metabolite levels in maternal plasma, which is continuous and increases further with the progress of labour (Keirse 1979). The recent finding that if labour does not ensue, the rise of prostaglandin metabolite levels tends to be transient, suggests a biochemical explanation for the failures and main contraindication (unripe cervix) of surgical induction (Sellers *et al.* 1981, Husslein *et al.* 1983).

5 Medical methods

Administration of chemical substances is both an age-old and a modern method for induction and augmentation of labour (Ploss and Bartels 1899). Up to the start of this century, Chinese women used to ingest a strong concoction of ginseng (*Panax ginseng*) to correct desultory labour (Kleiweg de Zwaan 1917). For the same indication the Aztecs used a brew of their native *zoapatle* (*Cihuapatli*) plant (Speert 1973), and research has shown that some isolates of *Montanoa tomentosa* do indeed have uterotonic effects (Waller *et al.* 1987). In Rwanda, one of us has witnessed the lethal effects (through uterine rupture) of *ichuli*, a watery extract of unidentified plants, administered by witchdoctors to women in obstructed labour (Thiery 1968). Western obstetric texts are replete with the names of uterine stimulants (ecbolics) and the nicknames given to some of these substances leave no doubt about their association with the birthing process. Thus, for ages borax has been known as *sal uterinum* (Klein 1910), and ergot of rye was dubbed *'pulvis ad partum'* by nineteenth-century physicians (Stearns 1808).

The modern era of medicinal induction of labour was initiated early in this century with the introduction of a combination of physical and chemical approaches to the induction of labour proposed by Benjamin Watson in 1913 (Watson 1922). The original proposal involved the use of castor oil, quinine, subcutaneous injections of pituitary extract, a hot bath, and a hot soap enema. Over the years, variations of Watson's 'labour regimen' were described, mainly by Stein and Dover in 1917 who recommended injection of smaller doses of pituitary extract over longer periods to avoid uterine hyperstimulation (Stein 1934).

In the 1940s, an alkaloid (sparteine) extracted from broom (*Cytisus scoparius*) was adopted enthusiastically in France as an oxytocic (Speert 1980). Sparteine sulphate was used briefly in the United States for induction of labour, but then discarded because of its erratic and often delayed effects, sometimes causing uterine hyperstimulation (Cibils and Hendricks 1969).

Pituitary extract was to become the forerunner of oxytocin, which was synthesized in the 1950s, and progressively widely used during the 1960s and 1970s.

The latest addition to this list of medical methods for inducing labour are the uterotonic prostaglandins which were introduced into clinical practice during the 1960s and 1970s.

5.1 Ergot

Known in the Far East for millennia as an abortifacient, powdered ergot (*Claviceps purpurea, Secale cornutum*) was used briefly by French obstetricians in the mid-eighteenth century for treating women with prolonged labour. Because it was misused by midwives and physicians, however, it became known as *'pulvis ad necem pronis'* and *'pulvis ad mortuum'* (Mérat de Lens 1831). Experience in France did not prevent the New York physician John Stearns, in 1808, from learning of the 'virtues' of a decoction of *secale* powder from the local midwife, and he introduced ergot into orthodox medicine again. In 1813 his colleague Prescott published a dissertation entitled 'The Natural History and Medicinal Effects of the Secale Cornutum, or Ergot' (Speert 1980) and due to the wide circulation of this text, medical interest in ergot was stimulated in Europe for the second time. Clinical experience again revealed the dangers inherent in the use of this potent uterine stimulant before and during labour, but this time it took more than half a century before obstetric use of ergot (apart from its use to control postpartum haemorrhage) was branded as constituting malpractice by the profession. The rise and fall in medical opinion which occurred in this period of time is illustrated by Michell's prediction in 1828 that 'As soon it (ergot) is generally known in female practice, it will supersede the necessity for male practitioners' (Michell 1828), and Engelmann's statement, half a century later, that 'The injury done by this powerful drug is so great that I would condemn its use altogether' (Engelmann 1883).

As chemical technology developed during the twentieth century, a number of complex alkaloid components of ergot were identified. All of them were uterine stimulants, but obviously different from the specific and rapidly acting uterotonic agent present in liquid extracts of ergot. Ergometrin was finally discovered simultaneously by Davis in America (Davis *et al.* 1935) and by Dudley and Moir (1935) in England. The fascinating story of the isolation of this oxytocic alkaloid has been recorded by one of the key figures in its discovery (Moir 1974).

Renewed interest in the use of ergot derivatives for induction of labour manifested itself for the third time in the 1940s and oral preparations continued to be advocated until the 1950s. Tocographic studies during the 1960s, however, showed that these substances mainly promote the frequency of contractions and are prone to induce uterine hypertonicity (Smyth 1961; Cibils and Hendricks 1969).

5.2 The Watson–Stein labour regimen

During the first half of this century the standard method for medical induction of labour was the Watson–Stein labour regimen. This consisted of a hot soap enema and a hot bath, oral administration of castor oil and quinine, and subcutaneous injections of pituitary extract (Eastman 1938; Kloosterman 1947; Titus 1945). By 1956, Chassar Moir was stating that the ritual was an utter 'waste of time, energy and suffering' and ascribed the relative success of the method to the pituitary extract which had been its last addition (Moir 1956); yet the method was still being mentioned in Reid's *Obstetrics* in 1962.

The rationale behind the elements which comprise the Watson–Stein labour regimen is rather commonplace. That heat increases uterine contractility had been suspected for ages. Even in Paré's time doctors forbade pregnant women at term to take a hot bath 'lest the child become too hot within the womb, and craving the more temperate air without, come forth before its time' (Guttmacher 1936). Hot enemas have been used by physicians to enhance labour contractions for several centuries; indeed, in 1722, de La Motte reported using them to distinguish false from true labour. No formal assessment of these physical adjuvants for labour induction was made until the late 1950s, however, when Mathie and Dawson (1959), using Smyth's guard ring tocograph (Smyth 1954), showed that administration of a hot soap enema to women at term produced a slight but significant increase in uterine contractility, while a hot bath produced no changes.

The administration of purging doses of castor oil for stimulating uterine contractions has been used for generations, earning it the name '*wonderolie*' ('miracle oil') in Dutch. Only in the late 1950s, however, was the effect of this substance on uterine contractility demonstrated by external tocography (Mathie and Dawson 1959). Because castor oil is only active after it has been hydrolized into ricinoleic acid in the gut, the uterine activity that it stimulated was believed to be an indirect result of the purgative effects of castor oil. It has since been demonstrated that this acid contracts strips of human myometrium (Abraham and Hawkins 1967) and therefore has direct uterotonic properties.

The use of quinine sulphate as an abortifacient was first proposed by Petitjean of Lyons, France, in the mid-nineteenth century (Plantard 1875). Sixteen years later, Monteverdi advocated using this drug for the induction of labour and to promote expulsion of the placenta (Plantard 1875). From the end of the nineteenth century onwards, oral and rectal administration of quinine salts became a widely used approach for the medical induction of labour. Quinine freely crosses the placenta and affects almost every tissue in the body, earning it the name of 'general protoplasmic poison'. A concern gradually emerged among obstetricians that it might be toxic to the fetus and instances of fetal death were attributed to the drug (Titus 1945). These concerns, together with doubts about the effectiveness of quinine for labour induction (Theobald 1959; Baumgarten 1967) led to it gradually being dropped from the Watson–Stein labour regimen.

5.3 Pituitary extract and oxytocin

The discovery of the uterotonic effect of oxytocin dates back to the start of this century when the *in vitro* effect of posterior pituitary extract was reported by Dale (1906), and its effect on the pregnant animal uterus was reported by Frankl-Hochwart and Fröhlich (1909). Clinical use of crude extracts from animal pituitary glands was introduced, first for management of postpartum haemorrhage (Bell 1909), but later for the induction of labour as well (Hofbauer 1911). Because these extracts contained antidiuretic hormone in addition to oxytocin, they were not altogether safe. They were later purified to remove the vasopressor–antidiuretic compound as far as possible (Kamm *et al.* 1928). Thus, from the early 1930s onwards, virtually pure preparations of oxytocin were available for obstetric use.

Following elucidation of the structure of oxytocin independently in 1953 by Vincent du Vigneaud in New York (du Vigneaud *et al.* 1953b) and Tuppy and Michl (1953) in Vienna, this hormone has been prepared synthetically (du Vigneaud *et al.* 1953a), largely using the procedure developed by Boissonas (Boissonas *et al.* 1955), a chemist working in the laboratories of the Sandoz Company. Synthetic oxytocin, which soon replaced pituitary extract in clinical practice (Bainbridge *et al.* 1956), still has a weak antidiuretic effect and high intravenous dosages of this hormone produce water retention (Abdul-Karim and Assali 1961). The most recent development has been the synthesis of oxytocin analogues, which, because they are not destroyed by oxytocinase, have a more prolonged uterotonic effect.

For decades pituitary extract was administered subcutaneously, intramuscularly or by the intranasal route. It was not until the 1940s that the more easily controlled intravenous drip infusion was introduced (Page 1943; Theobald *et al.* 1948). Theobald, as one of the pioneers of this method, used what he considered to be a 'physiologic' amount of pituitary extract (equivalent to 2.5 mU/min of synthetic oxytocin) for labour induction. He used antidiuretic hormone as a yardstick, suggesting that 'just as ADH is a fine regulator of renal water metabolism, so oxytocin is a fine regulator of uterine activity during labour, operating primarily in the interest of the foetus' (Theobald 1973a; Theobald *et al.* 1956).

Theobald fiercely defended the philosophical basis of his method (Theobald 1974), even after alternative approaches had been adopted in the light of greater understanding about the effects of oxytocin on the pregnant human uterus. This understanding came through the pioneering work of Alvarez and Caldeyro-Barcia (1950) who, by recording intrauterine pressure changes, provided the first quantitative assessment of the spontaneous contractility of the uterus. Likewise, Caldeyro-Barcia and his colleagues were first to describe the dose-related response of the uterus at term to oxytocin infused intravenously (reviewed by Caldeyro-Barcia and Heller 1961). This knowledge was of key significance in attempts to mimic spontaneous labour activity, and forms the basis for the current use of oxytocin in obstetrics. The main conclusions derived from Caldeyro-Barcia's finding of a dose–response relation between dose of oxytocin and uterine contractility were first, that the individual sensitivity of the uterus for oxytocin varies widely at term, and second, that this sensitivity changes during the course of labour. In clinical terms, this meant that the 'physiological' dose of hormone is neither uniform nor constant and must be assessed individually when attempting labour induction. Others had intuitively sensed this basic principle and proposed a two-step incremental dose infusion of pituitary extract as more effective for inducing labour (Hellman 1949). But it was Turnbull and Anderson, in 1968, who gave the method its final touch by combining intravenous oxytocin 'titration' with artificial rupture of the membranes, an adjunct to medical induction with oxytocin which had originally been proposed by Jackson in 1928 (Titus 1945) and popularized in the 1950s (Theobald *et al.* 1948).

5.4 Prostaglandins

Prostaglandins are known to play an important role in the physiology of human labour and it is likely that the last step in the complicated series of events preceding the onset of labour is an increase in the endogenous release of these substances (Keirse 1979). The use of uterotonic prostaglandins was assessed for the induction of labour in the late 1960s. The development of the prostaglandin method is a long story, though. The oxytocic properties of these substances had been known long before the prostaglandins were identified as such. In the eighteenth century, Dutch whalers had observed that pregnant Eskimo women ingested the fat from the claws of the polar bear (which has a high content of prostaglandin precursors) in an attempt to initiate labour (Mertens 1710). From time immemorial, sexual intercourse (semen is the richest natural source of uterotonic prostaglandins) had been practised to induce and facilitate labour, and in many population groups coitus is taboo during pregnancy, possibly because of the risk of stimulating preterm labour (Ploss and Bartels 1899). In 1930, the uterotonic effects of fresh human semen were confirmed *in vitro* (Kurzrock and Lieb 1930). Shortly afterwards, substances capable of provoking contraction of smooth muscle fibres were found in seminal fluid (Goldblatt 1933; von Euler 1934). Von Euler (1935) showed these substances to be fat-soluble acids and named them (incorrectly) prostaglandins. It took more than 20 years before the isolation of the first prostaglandin (PGF_{1a}) was achieved (Bergström and Sjövall 1957). From that moment, however, development accelerated. In 1964, the identification and biosynthesis of several uterotonic prostaglandins was achieved (Bergström *et al.* 1964; Van Dorp *et al.* 1964), and in the same year Bygdeman (1964) reassessed the effects of prostaglandins on the human myometrium. Because of Bygdeman's tentative conclusions that these compounds were unfit for practical use, however, his *in vitro* studies were not followed immediately by the clinical introduction of uterotonic prostaglandins. The obstetric breakthrough resulted from the work of Pickles, who, in 1959, had postulated that the uterine colic which characterizes spastic dysmenorrhea was caused by the presence in the menstrual fluid of a potent uterotonic substance which the author termed 'menstrual stimulant'. Six years later Pickles identified this to be a mixture of prostaglandins E and F (Pickles *et al.* 1965). Karim, noting a similarity between uterine colic and labour pains, identified PGE_2 and PGF_{2a} in liquor amnii and showed that the concentration of these substances increased during early labour (Karim and Devlin 1967). The stage was thus set for the first clinical experiment; in 1968, Karim announced the successful induction of labour at term by constant-dose intravenous infusion of PGF_{2a} (Karim *et al.* 1968). The next year, Embrey (1969) suggested that equipotent doses of PGE_2 were equally useful for elective induction of labour.

Two problems had to be solved before large-scale clinical testing of prostaglandins could be achieved, however. First, the amounts of prostaglandins obtained from sheep seminal vesicles by biosynthesis were much too small to cover clinical demands (Pike 1971). This problem was solved in 1972, when Light and Samuelsson stumbled upon a more profitable natural source, the sea-coral *Plexaura homomalla*, for the semi-synthesis of these substances before total chemical synthesis became available. The second problem was the lack of shelf stability of PGE_2, but this too was soon solved.

It thus took virtually 40 years before prostaglandins were incorporated into obstetric practice, first for the induction of labour and later for ripening the cervix prior to 'conventional' induction with oxytocin (see Chapter 61).

6 Miscellaneous methods

6.1 Electrical pulses and acupuncture

For almost two centuries excitation of the uterine muscle by electricity has been explored. According to Theobald (1973b), Herder first suggested the use of a galvanic current for the induction of labour in 1803, and this method was employed sporadically in Germany, Great Britain, and France during the nineteenth century. Interest in electrical induction of labour seems to have been revived since the 1960s, mainly in England (Theobald and Lundborg 1962; Theobald 1973b), Japan (Sawazaki and Fujimoto 1966; Fujimoto and Tokuyama 1973) and Russia (Osnos and Stupko 1973; Chiladze and Budzhiashvili 1973).

In 1966 Sawazaki and Fujimoto reported their method of inducing labour by passing an electric current though the cervix for short periods, but the results were equivocal. By moving the electrode towards the cervical canal Theobald and Lundborg (1962) appeared to improve the success rate, but the fact that the presence of any foreign body in the cervix often succeeds in starting labour makes it difficult to assess the part played by the electric current. In the early 1970s, Theobald modified the Transistor Pulse Generator used in the original experiment and devised the Belt Transistor Pulse Generator, an external contraption which, worn by the woman as an out-patient, was expected to trigger labour activity (Theobald 1973b). Although preliminary results showed that the 'electric bikini' was easy to use and apparently safe for mother and child, the clinical possibilities offered by this device do not seem to have been explored further.

For more than 3000 years acupuncture has been used in the Far East to alleviate labour pains (Fu Weikang 1985). More recently, it has also been used both to inhibit labour (Tsuei *et al.* 1977) and in an attempt to induce labour (Fouques Duparc *et al.* 1979; Tsuei and Lai 1974), sometimes in combination with electrical stimulation. There is no evidence of any continuing interest in acupuncture as a method of inducing labour.

6.2 Cervical vibration

The application of mechanical low-frequency vibrations to the cervix to induce labour or expedite dilatation was first proposed by Tokuyama and Fujimoto in 1968 in Japan. Although Tokuyama and Fujimoto (1968) and Chimura *et al.* (1969) reported that they were able to achieve induction of labour in this way, European investigators have only applied this technique to shorten the first stage of labour (Dahlgren 1972; Dahlgren 1976; Brandt and Lachelin 1971; Brandt and Lachelin 1974; Beard *et al.* 1973; see also Chapter 58). Apparently, these instruments (Cervilator®, and Svedia Cervix Dilator®) did not awaken interest outside Japan, England, and Scandinavia, and clinical trials of vibration induction seem not to have been pursued since the 1970s.

6.3 Stimulating endogenous oxytocin and prostaglandin release

Although the relationship between nipple stimulation and uterine contractility, which was well known to Hippocrates and Soranus, has been used to prevent postpartum haemorrhage by putting the neonate at the breast immediately following delivery (Ploss and Bartels 1899), antepartum breast stimulation to cause the uterus to contract seems to be a relatively recent innovation. About 150 years ago, Merriman (1838) recommended 'consensual' stimulation of the nipples and areolae to 'introduce' labour. In 1849, Friedrich discussed the use of vesicants for breast stimulation, and Scanzoni (1849) advocated the use of cupping glasses on the breasts for augmenting labour. It was not until 1952, however, that Lorand and Asbot actually recorded the effect of massaging the nipples on uterine contractility. They noted a doubling of the intensity and duration of uterine contractions in all the women they studied.

Mechanical nipple stimulation induces uterine contractility through release of oxytocin from the maternal pituitary gland (Salzmann 1971), and there have been several reports of clinicians attempting to make use of this effect (Leinzinger and Rainer 1954; Salzmann 1971; Elliott and Flaherty 1984; Fragner and Miyazaki 1987). Although the uterine contractility induced by nipple stimulation is currently believed to remain within physiological ranges (Lazaro 1973), there have been several reports suggesting that it had caused uterine hypertonus, sometimes resulting in profound fetal bradycardia (Viegas *et al.* 1986; see also Chapter 61).

Finally, according to folklore, indulging in coital activity in late pregnancy is said to facilitate labour (Ploss and Bartels 1899). The suggestion that female orgasm is accompanied by the release of oxytocin and uterine contractility (Goodlin *et al.* 1971; Goodlin *et al.* 1972; Pystynen and Nummi 1974), the knowledge that seminal fluid is a concentrated source of prostaglandins and that intravaginal prostaglandin administration successfully ripens the cervix and/or induces labour (Chapters 61 and 62), all render it plausible that orgasmic coitus and intravaginal ejaculation may indeed induce labour in some women. So far, we are not aware of any formal attempt to assess whether this might offer a practicable approach to achieving induction of labour.

7 Conclusions

Throughout the ages there has been no shortage of 'trial and error' in attempts to gain control over the timing of childbirth. The great diversity of means and methods deployed are testimony to the inventiveness of practitioners in their attempts to control this important event. It must also reflect their frustration with the 'erratic' nature of pregnancy, which refuses to yield the secret of when it is about to end.

At first sight there appears to be little coherence among these methods, and many of them were apparently applied with little insight as to whether and how they might work. Yet, nearly all of them were intended to influence one or both of the two mechanisms that are currently still regarded as the main determinants of successful induction namely, uterine contractility and cervical resistance.

Throughout the history of attempts to induce labour,

invention and development of methods appear to have received far greater priority than the development of means and methods to assess and quantitate their effects. Thus methods have not only been invented, introduced and abandoned; some of them have been 'reinvented' or, at least, reintroduced. Possibly they may also be re-abandoned before solid evidence on their effects has become available.

In contrast with the 'trial and error' approach that characterized innovation in this field during most of its history, properly controlled evaluation has now become increasingly common. This development has resulted in more efficient refinement of the methods used for induction, as well as more valid assessment of their effects. Had these research designs been applied more systematically in earlier years, many women and babies would have been protected more efficiently from ineffective and often dangerous methods. If proper methods of evaluation continue to become used more frequently, it is likely that further refinements will be achieved efficiently.

Over the years that methods of induction have evolved, the indications for induction have changed dramatically. In the present era, induction of labour has been used on a far wider scale than ever before. This development underscores the need, not for vast improvements in methods of induction, but for careful assessment of the circumstances in which induction of labour is more likely to do good than harm.

References

Abdul-Karim R, Assali N (1961). Renal function in human pregnancy. J Lab Clin Med, 57: 522–532.

Abrahams OL, Hawkins DF (1967). Lipid-soluble uterine muscle stimulants in human amniotic fluid. J Obstet Gynaecol Br Commnwlth, 74: 235–246.

Aburel E (1939). Le déclenchement du travail par injection intra-amniotique. Rev Médicochir Iasi (Roumanie), 20: 310–320.

Alvarez H, Caldeyro-Barcia R (1950). Contractility of the human uterus recorded by new methods. Surg Gynecol Obstet, 91: 1–13.

Bainbridge MN, Nixon WCW, Schild HO, Smyth CN (1956). Synthetic oxytocin. Br Med J, 1: 1133–1135.

Baumgarten K (1967). Die Beeinflussung der Uterusmotilität. Vienna: Brüder Hollinek.

Beard R, Boyd I, Holt E (1973). A study of cervical vibration in induced labour. J Obstet Gynaecol Br Commnwlth, 80: 966–969.

Bell WB (1909). The pituitary body. Br Med J, 2: 1609–1613.

Bergström S, Sjövall J (1957). The isolation of prostaglandin. Acta Chem Scand, 11: 1086.

Bergström S, Danielsson H, Samuelsson B (1964). The enzymatic formation of PGE2 from arachidonic acid. Biochim Biophys Acta, 90: 207–210.

Biermer H (1899). Der Kolpeurynter. Seine Geschichte und Anwendung in der Geburtshilfe. Wiesbaden: Bergmann.

Bishop E (1964). Pelvic scoring for elective induction. Obstet Gynecol, 24: 266–268.

Boissonas RA, Guttman S, Jacquenod PA, Waller JP (1955). Une nouvelle synthèse de l'oxytocine. Helv Chim Acta, 38: 1491–1501.

Brant HA, Lachelin GCL (1971). Vibration of the cervix to expedite first stage of labour. Lancet, 2: 686–688.

Brandt HA, Lachelin GCL (1974). Vibration of the cervix in labour. J Obstet Gynaecol Br Commnwlth, 81: 278–281.

Brémond A, Dominici J, Magnin P (1978). L'induction artificielle du travail. Etude comparée de trois méthodes à propos de 334 observations. Rev Franç Gynécol, 73: 673–676.

Brindeau A (1926). La pratique de l'Art des Accouchements, Vol. IV. Paris: Vigot, pp 36–40.

Bygdeman M (1964). The effect of different prostaglandins on human myometrium in vitro. Acta Physiol Scand (Suppl), 242: 1–78.

Caldeyro-Barcia R, Heller H (1961). Oxytocin. New York: Pergamon Press.

Chalmers I (1974). British debate on obstetric practice. Pediatrics, 58: 308–312.

Chalmers I, Richards MPM (1977). Intervention and causal inference in obstetric practice. In: Benefits and Hazards of the New Obstetrics. Chard T, Richards MPM (eds). Clinics in Developmental Medicine No.64. London: Spastics International Medical Publications, Heinemann Medical Books, pp 34–61.

Chalmers I, Dauncey ME, Verrier-Jones ER, Dodge JA, Gray OP (1978). Respiratory distress syndrome in infants of Cardiff residents during 1965–1975. Br Med J, 2: 1119–1121.

Champetier de Ribes (1988). De l'accouchement provoqué. Dilatation du canal génital à l'aide de ballons introduits dans la cavité utérin pendant la grossesse. Annal Gynécol Obstét (Paris), 30: 401–438.

Charrière MJ (1862). Note au sujet du dilatateur intra-utérin de M. Tarnier. Gazette des Hôpitaux, 135: 220.

Chiladze ZA, Budzhiasvili ON (1973). Electrical induction and stimulation of uterine contractions. Seventh World Congress of Obstetrics and Gynecology, Moscow, August 1973. Amsterdam: Excerpta Medica No. 279, p 58.

Chimura T, Nagametsu K, Watabe T, Watanabe T (1969). Results obtained with the 'cervilator' and discussion of its clinical aspects. Jap J Obstet Gynaecol, 36: 901–905.

Cianfrani T (1960). A Short History of Obstetrics and Gynecology. Springfield, Ill: Thomas.

Cibils LA, Hendricks CH (1969). Effect of ergot derivatives and sparteine sulfate upon the human uterus. J Reprod Med, 2: 147–167.

Cross WG, Pitkin RM (1978). Laminaria as an adjunct in induction of labor. Obstet Gynecol, 51: 606–608.

Dahlgren S (1972). Reduction of foetal trauma during labour with the aid of low frequency vibrations. In: Proceedings of the International Symposium on the Treatment of Foetal Risks. Baumgarten K, Wesselius de Casparis A (eds). Vienna: University Press, pp 118–120.

Dahlgren S (1976). Shortening of labour especially the period of dilatation with low frequency vibrations against the cervix. A clinical study. Acta Obstet Gynecol Scand (Suppl), 55: 1–103.

Dale HH (1906). On some physiological actions of ergot. J Physiol, 34: 163–205.

Davis ME, Adair EL, Rogers G, Kharasch MS, Legault RR (1935). A new active principle in ergot and its effects in uterine motility. Am J Obstet Gynecol, 29: 155–167.

de La Motte G (1722). Traité complet des Acouchements Naturels, non Naturels, et contre Nature, etc., Paris.: -Ch Dowry.

Denman T (1785). Principles of Midwifery on Puerperal Medicine. London: E Cox.

Dudley HW, Moir JC (1935). The substance responsible for the traditional clinical effect of ergot. Br Med J, 1: 520–523.

Du Vigneaud V, Ressler C, Swan JM, Roberts CW, Katsoyannis PG, Gordon S (1953a). The synthesis of an octapeptide amide with the hormonal activity of oxytocin. J Am Chem Soc, 75: 4879–4880.

Du Vigneaud V, Ressler C, Trippett S (1953b). The sequence of amino-acids in oxytocin with a proposal for the structure of oxytocin. J Biol Chem, 205: 949–957.

Dwyer G (1966). The acceleration of the first stage of labour: A new instrument. J Obstet Gynaecol Br Commnwlth, 73: 672–678.

Eastman NJ (1938). The induction of labor. Am J Obstet Gynecol, 35: 721–730.

Elliott JP, Flaherty JT (1984). The use of breast stimulation to prevent postdate pregnancy. Am J Obstet Gynecol, 149: 628–632.

Embrey MP (1969). The effect of prostaglandins on the human pregnant uterus. J Obstet Gynaecol Br Commnwlth, 76: 783–789.

Embrey MP, Mollison, BG (1967). The unfavorable cervix and induction of labour using a cervical balloon. J Obstet Gynaecol Br Commnwlth, 74: 44–48.

Engelmann GJ (1883). Ergot: The use and abuse of this dangerous drug. Trans Am Gynecol Soc, 8: 235–244.

Fasbender H (1906). Geschichte der Geburtshilfe. Stuttgart: Fischer.

Fouques Duparc V, Herlicoviez M, Lévy G (1979). Le déclenchement du travail par électrostimulation acuponcturale. J Gynécol Obstét Biol Réprod, 8: 755–760.

Fragner NB, Miyazaki FS (1987). Intrauterine monitoring of contractions during breast stimulation. Obstet Gynecol, 69: 767–769.

Frankl-Hochwart L, Fröhlich A (1909). Zur Kenntnis der Wirkung des Hypophysins auf das sympatische und autonome Nervensystem. Wien Klin Wochenschr, 22: 982–983.

Friedman E (1954). The graphic analysis of labor. Am J Obstet Gynecol, 68: 1568–1575.

Friedman E (1978). Evolution of graphic analysis of labor. Am J Obstet Gynecol, 132, 824–827.

Freidrich R (1839). De nova quodam partus praematurus celebrandi methoddo. Rostock: Inaugural dissertation.

Fu Weikang (1985). Traditional Chinese Medicine and Pharmacology. Beijing: Foreign Languages Press.

Fujimoto J, Tokuyama T (1973). New technique for the electrical induction of labor (increasing the labor score). Seventh World Congress of Obstetrics and Gynecology, Moscow, August 1973. Amsterdam: Excerpta Medica No. 279, p 36.

Goldblatt MW (1933). A depressor substance in seminal fluid. J Soc Chem Ind, 52: 1056–1059.

Goodlin RC, Keller DW, Raffin M (1971). Orgasm during late pregnancy: Possible deleterious effects. Obstet Gynecol, 38: 916–920.

Goodlin RC, Schmidt W, Creevy DC (1972). Uterine tension and heart rate during maternal orgasm. Obstet Gynecol, 39: 125–127.

Guttmacher AF (1936). Ambroise Paré does a delivery. Bull Inst Hist Med, 4: 703–717.

Hamilton J (1836). Practical Observations on Various Subjects Relating to Midwifery. Part II. London, p. 179.

Hellman LM (1949). Factors influencing posterior pituitary treatment of functional uterine dystocia with particular consideration of its intravenous administration. Am J Obstet Gynecol, 57: 364–369.

Hillier K, Coad N (1982). Synthesis of prostaglandins by the human uterine cervix *in vitro* during passive mechanical stretch. J Pharm Pharmacol, 34: 262–263.

Hofbauer J (1911). Hypophysenextrakt als Wehenmittel. Zbl Gynäkol, 35: 137–141.

Hofbauer JI, Hoerner JK (1927). The nasal application of pituitary extract for induction of labor. Am J Obstet Gynecol, 14: 137–148.

Huber R (1955). Geburtseinleitung mit dem Verweilkatheter. Zbl Gynäkol, 77: 540–546.

Husslein P, Kopler E, Rasmussen AB, Sumulong L, Fuchs A, Fuchs F (1983). Oxytocin and the initiation of human parturition. IV. Plasma concentrations of oxytocin and 13,14-dihydro-15-keto-PGF$_{2\alpha}$ during induction of labor by artificial rupture of the membranes. Am J Obstet Gynecol, 147: 503–507.

Kamm O, Aldrich TB, Grite IW, Rowe LW, Bugbee EP (1928). The active principles of the posterior lobe of the pituitary gland. J Am Chem Soc, 50: 573–601.

Karim SMM, Devlin, J (1967). PG content of amniotic fluid during pregnancy and labour. J Obstet Gynaecol Br Commnwlth, 74: 230–234.

Karim SMM, Trussell RR, Patel RC, Hillier K (1968). Response of pregnant human uterus to PGF$_{2\alpha}$-induction of labour. Br Med J, 4: 621–623.

Keirse MJNC (1979). Endogenous prostaglandins in human parturition. In: Human Parturition. Keirse MJNC, Anderson ABM, Bennebroek Gravenhorst J (eds). The Hague: Leiden University Press, pp 101–142.

Keirse MJNC, Thiery M, Parewijck W, Mitchell MD (1983). Chronic stimulation of uterine prostaglandin synthesis during cervical ripening before the onset of labor. Prostaglandins, 25: 671–682.

Klein G (1910). Eucharius Rösslin's Rosengarten, gedruckt im Jahre 1513. Munich: Carl Kuhn.

Kleiweg de Zwaan JP (1917). Völkerkundliches und Geschichtliches über die Heilkunde der Chinesen und Japanern. Haarlem: Van Erven Loosjes.

Klöck FK, Jung H (1973). In vitro release of prostaglandins from human myometrium under the influence of stretching. Am J Obstet Gynecol, 115: 1066–1069.

Kloosterman GJ (1947). Over het kunstmatig opwekken der baring in de tweede helft der zwangerschap door middel van een condoomcatheter. Ned Tijdschr Verlosk Gynaecol, 47: 19–62.

Krause A (1855). Die künstliche Frühgeburt. Breslau: Trewendt Granier.

Kurzrok R, Lieb CC (1930). Biochemical studies of human semen. Proc Soc Exp Biol Med, 28: 268–272.

Lackritz R, Gibson M, Frigoletto FD (1979). Preinduction use of laminaria for the unripe cervix. Am J Obstet Gynecol, 134, 349–350.

Lazaro JL (1973). Induction of labor with the help of suction to the mammary glands. Seventh World Congress of Obstetrics and Gynecology, Moscow, August 1973. Amsterdam: Excerpta Medica No. 279, p 49.

Leinzinger E, Rainier A (1954). Die bilaterale Selbstfriktion der Brustwarzenbereiches zur Anregung der Wehentätigkeit. Klin Med, 3: 127–131.

Light RJ, Samuelsson B (1972). Identification of prostaglandins in the Gorgonian, Plexaura homomalla. Eur J Biochem, 28: 232–240.

Lippert T, Peters F (1979). Geburtseinleitung bei intrauterinem Fruchttod durch Ballonbelastung der Zervix und Oxytocin-titration. Geburtshilfe Frauenheilkd, 39: 699–703.

Lorand S, Asbot J (1952). Über die durch Reizung der Brustwarze angeregten reflektorischen Uteruskontraktionen. Zbl Gynäkol, 74: 345–352.

Manabe Y, Yoshimura S, Mori T, Aso T (1985). Plasma levels of 13,14-dihydro-15-keto-PGF$_{2\alpha}$, estrogens and progesterone during stretch-induced labor at term. Prostaglandins, 30: 141–152.

Mathie JG, Dawson BH (1959). Effect of castor oil, soap enema, and hot bath on the pregnant human uterus near term. A tocographic study. Br Med J, 1: 1162–1165.

Mérat de Lens (1831). Ergot de seigle. In: Dictionnaire, Vol. 3. Paris: pp 134–137.

Merriman S (1838). A Synopsis of the Various Kinds of Difficult Parturition. London: Churchill Livingstone.

Mertens F (1710). Vojagie naar Groenland of Spitsbergen. Amsterdam: de Groot, p 254.

Michell W (1828). On Difficult Cases of Parturition and the Use of Ergot of Rye. London: Underwood.

Mitchell MD, Keirse MJNC, Anderson ABM, Turnbull AC (1977). Evidence for a local control of prostaglandins within the pregnant human uterus. Br J Obstet Gynaecol, 84: 35–38.

Moir JC (1956). Munro Kerr's Operative Obstetrics (2nd edn). London: Baillière, Tindall & Cox, p 626.

Moir J (1974). Ergot: From 'St. Anthony's Fire' to the isolation of its active principle, ergometrine (ergonovine). Am J Obstet Gynecol, 120: 291–296.

Newton BW (1972). Laminaria tent: Relic of the past or modern medical device? Am J Obstet Gynecol, 113: 442–448.

Nicolaides KH, Welch CC, MacPherson MBA, Johnson IR, Filshie GM (1983). Lamicel: A new technique for cervical dilatation for first trimester abortion. Br J Obstet Gynaecol, 90: 475–479.

Osnos GM, Stupko AI (1973). Electric excitation and electric stimulation of labour. Seventh World Congress of Obstetrics and Gynecology, Moscow, August 1973. Amsterdam: Excerpta Medica No. 279, p 57.

Ovink WS (1896). Over Intrauterine Injecties ter Opwekking van Vroeggeboorte. Amsterdam: MD thesis.

Page EW (1943). Response of human pregnant uterus to Pitocin tannate in oil. Proc Soc Exp Biol Med, 52: 195–197.

Pelzer F (1892). Über Einleitung der künstlichen Frühgeburt. Zbl Gynäkol, 16: 35–36.

Pickles VR (1959). A plain-muscle stimulant in the menstruum. Nature, 180: 1198–1199.

Pickles VR, Hall WJ, Best FA, Smith GN (1965). Prostaglandins in endometrium and menstrual fluid from normal and dysmenorrheic subjects. J Obstet Gynaecol Br Commnwlth, 72: 185–192.

Pigeaud H, Favier JP (1964). Cinq cents observations d'accouchements provoqués à l'aide d'une bougie de Krause. Gynécol Obstét (Paris), 63: 621–636.

Pike JE (1971). Prostaglandins. Scient Am, 225: 84–92.

Plantard JM (1875). De l'Emploi du Sulfate de Quinine pendant la Grossesse. Paris: MD thesis.

Ploss H, Bartels M (1899). Das Weib in der Natur- und Völkerkunde. Leipzig: Grieben.

Pystynen P, Nummi S (1974). Beziehung des Koitus zu Beginn der Uteruswehen und der Geburt gegen Ende der Schwangerschaft. Zbl Gynäkol, 96: 430–432.

Reid DE (1962). Obstetrics. Philadelphia: W B Saunders.

Rodion E (1641). Des Divers Travaux et Enfantemens des Femmes. Rouen: Guillaume Iore.

Saling E (1966). Das Kind im Bereich der Geburtshilfe. Stuttgart: Georg Thieme.

Salzmann K (1971). An untapped source of oxytocin. J R Coll Gen Pract, 21: 282–286.

Sarwey O (1896). Die künstliche Frühgeburt bei Beckenenge. Berlin: August Hirschwald.

Sawazaki C, Fujimoto J (1966). The induction of labour pains by electrical stimulation apparatus. Sanfujui Jissai, 15: 6–9.

Scanzoni FW (1849). Lehrbuch der Geburtshilfe, Vol. 1. Vienna: Seidel.

Schauta F (1883). Über intrauterine Colpeuryse. Centralblatt für die gesammte Therapie, 1: 1–9.

Sellers SM, Mitchell MD, Anderson ABM, Turnbull AC (1981). The relation between the release of prostaglandins at amniotomy and the subsequent onset of labour. Br J Obstet Gynaecol, 88: 1211–1216.

Smyth CN (1954). Apparatus used in the study of the forces of labour and their effect on the welfare of the foetus. First FIGO Congress Genève. Basel: Exposition Scientifique Item 79, Sandoz.

Smyth CN (1961). A comparison of the effects of oxytocin and ergometrine on the human uterus. In: Oxytocin. Caldeyro-Barcia R, Heller H (eds). New York: Pergamon Press, pp 281–294.

Smythe HJD (1931). Indications for the induction of premature labour. Br Med J, 1: 1018–1020.

Smythe HJD (1949). Surgical induction of labour. J Obstet Gynaecol Br Empire, 56: 431–438.

Speert H (1973). Iconographia Gyniatrica. Philadelphia: F A Davis.

Speert H (1980). Obstetrics and Gynecology in America. A History. Chicago: College of Obstetricians and Gynecologists, pp 181–182.

Stearns J (1808). Account of the pulvis parturiens, a remedy for quickening child-birth. Med Repository, 11: 308–309.

Stedman's Medical Dictionary (1961). Baltimore: Williams & Wilkins.

Stein A (1934). The use of small dosages of pituitary extract in obstetrics. Surg Gynecol Obstet, 59: 872–875.

Thackray CF (1935). A Catalogue of Surgical Instruments. London: p 117.

Theobald GW (1959). The choice between death from postmaturity or prolapsed cord and life from induction of labour. Lancet, 1: 59–65.

Theobald G (1973a). Endocrine Control of Uterine Innervation. London: Butterworths.

Theobald GW (1973b). The Electrical Induction of Labour. London: Butterworths.

Theobald GW (1974). The induction of labour. In: Obstetric Therapeutics. Clinical Pharmacology and Therapeutics in Obstetric Practice. Hawkins DF (ed). London: Baillière Tindall, pp 341–379.

Theobald GW, Lundborg RA (1962). The electrical induction of labour with the Transistor Pulse Generator and Pulse Current Measuring Device. J Obstet Gynaecol Br Commnwlth, 69: 434–442.

Theobald GW, Graham A, Campbell J, Gange PD, Driscoll WJ (1948). The use of post-pituitary extract in physiological amounts in obstetrics. A preliminary report. Br Med J, 2: 123–127.

Theobald GW, Kelsey HA, Muirhead JMB (1956). The pitocin drip. J Obstet Gynaecol Br Commnwlth, 63: 641–662.

Thiery M (1968). The clinical use of oxytocic substances. Ned Tijdschr Geneeskd, 20: 1021–1024.

Titus P (1945). The Management of Obstetric Difficulties. St Louis: Mosby, pp 621–622.

Tokuyama T, Fujimoto J (1968). A new method for dilatation of the cervical canal by vibration. Japan J Obstet Gynaecol, 35: 31–34.

Tsuei JJ, Lai YF (1974). Induction of labor by acupuncture and electrical stimulation. Obstet Gynecol, 43: 337–342.

Tsuei JJ, Lai YF, Sharma SD (1977). The influence of acupuncture stimulation during pregnancy. Obstet Gynecol, 50: 479–488.

Tuppy H, Michl H (1953). Ueber die chemische Struktur des Oxytocins. Monatsh Chem, 84: 1011–1020.

Turnbull A, Anderson A (1968). Induction of labour. III. Results with amniotomy and oxytocin 'titration'. J Obstet Gynaecol Br Commnwlth, 75: 32–41.

Van Der Hoeven PCT (1908). De Betekenis van het Breken der Vliezen bij de Baring. Leiden: Van Doesburgh.

Van Dorp DA, Beerthuis RK, Nugteren DH, Vonkeman H (1964). The biosynthesis of prostaglandins. Biochim Biophys Acta, 90: 204–207.

Veyre JF, Laumosne J, Mavel A, Feldman JP, Pélikan P, Michiels Y (1974). Le ballon de Boissard. Antiquité ou moyen moderne de déclenchement? Rev Franç Gynécol, 69: 535–539.

Viegas OAC, Adaikan PG, Singh K, Arulkumaran S, Kottegoda SR, Ratnam GS (1986). Intrauterine response to nipple stimulation in late pregnancy. Gynecol Obstet Invest, 22: 128–133.

Voorhees JD (1900). Dilatation of the cervix by means of a modified Champetier de Ribes balloon. Med Rec, 58: 361–366.

von Euler US (1934). Zur Kenntnis der pharmakologischen Wirkungen von Nativsekreten und Extrakten männlicher accessorischer Geschlechtsdrüsen. Arch Pharmacol Exper Pathol, 175: 78–91.

von Euler US (1935). Ueber die spezifische blutdrucksenkende Substanz des menschlichen Prostata- und Samenblasensekretes. Klin Wochenschr, 14: 1182–1183.

Waller DP, Martin A, Oshima Y, Fong HHS (1987). Studies on zoapatle. Contraception, 35: 147–153.

Watson BP (1922). Further experience with pituitary extract in the induction of labor. Am J Obstet Gynecol, 4: 603–608.

Young JH (1963). James Hamilton, obstetrician and controversialist. Med Hist, 7: 62–73.

60 Evaluating elective delivery

Iain Chalmers and Marc J. N. C. Keirse

1 Introduction

'A large element of potential danger is averted by inducing labour when the end of profitable intrauterine life has been accomplished and a continuance thereof can only be an indifference, if not an invocation to all those dangers, morbidities and mortalities which are so familiar to us ... By this judiciously timed procedure, the contractions of labour may be inaugurated when the child is ripe ... The mother is spared from four to six hours of suffering, as well as serious operative trauma, and she rises from her confinement quickly and with unimpaired vitality ... The knowledge that the gestation will terminate on a definite date is both a mental and a financial relief to the patient and a marked convenience to the doctor.'

Reed (1920)

'The spontaneous onset of labour is a robust and effective mechanism which is preceded by the maturation of several fetal systems, and should be given every opportunity to operate on its own. We should only induce labour when we are sure that we can do better.'

Turnbull (1976)

Decisions to bring pregnancy to an end prior to the spontaneous onset of labour constitute one of the most fundamental ways of intervening in the 'natural history' of pregnancy and childbirth. The indications for such 'elective deliveries' (which may be achieved either by inducing labour or by elective caesarean section) range from those that are life-saving, to those that are trivial.

In this chapter, the term 'elective delivery' is used to imply that onset of the process of childbirth (whether by uterine contractions or by rupture of the membranes) has not occurred naturally, but has been brought about by some deliberate action on the part of the caregiver. Others (e.g. Amy et al. 1976; Vierhout et al. 1985) have suggested that the term 'elective induction' should be restricted to circumstances in which induction of labour is used in women, at term, with a clinically normal pregnancy and no maternal or fetal pathology. In proposing a 'set of working definitions

and criteria applicable to induction of labour', Amy and his colleagues (1976) recommended that the term 'therapeutic induction of labour' be used to refer to induction in all other circumstances. In their view then, 'therapeutic induction' implies the existence of an anomaly that may affect fetal or maternal well-being (Amy et al. 1976). By implication, however, this terminology suggests that 'therapeutic induction' will 'treat' the maternal or fetal pathology. Although this may sometimes be the case (for example, in pregnancy-induced hypertension; see Chapter 33), in many circumstances it clearly is not. Induction of labour based on a firm maternal wish to end pregnancy for psychological or social reasons, for example, is more likely to be truly 'therapeutic' than induction based on many of the medical indications that are currently accepted (without good supporting evidence) as reasonable practice.

The term 'elective delivery' as used in this chapter then, simply refers to a deliberate attempt to terminate pregnancy either by inducing labour, or by performing an elective caesarean section. The use of elective delivery by those providing care during pregnancy and childbirth, like so many other aspects of their practice, has been shown to vary widely both from place to place, and over time. During the mid-1970s, for example, the proportion of births following induced labour ranged from just over 10 per cent in Norway to nearly 40 per cent in England and Wales (Chalmers and Richards 1977); within England, the regional rates ranged from just over 20 per cent to nearly 50 per cent of births (Chalmers 1979).

Trends in the overall rate of elective delivery have also been dramatic. As far as England is concerned, the rate of induced labour rose steeply during the late 1960s and early 1970s, and then levelled off for two or three years, before declining at the beginning of the current decade (Macfarlane and Mugford 1984). The rise in the use of elective delivery reflected poorly substantiated opinions that certainty about the date of delivery had medical, psychological, and social advantages (Tacchi 1971; Jeffcoate 1976; McNay et al. 1977; Hillemans et *al.* 1977; Gitsch *et al.* 1978; Richter *et al.* 1979; Wulf 1979; Lampe 1980; Hendry 1981). In at least one population, the gestational age (and weight) distribution of births was shifted downwards as elective delivery became more widespread (Newcombe and Chalmers 1977), and the complications associated with relative immaturity became more prevalent (Chalmers *et al.* 1978). Then, as the use of elective delivery declined as concerns about its adverse effects became more widespread, the gestational age distribution reverted to its previous pattern (Newcombe 1983).

In Britain, it was eventually public criticism of this massive and poorly controlled obstetric experiment in newspapers and the broadcasting media which provoked explicit debate within the professions about the validity of the poorly substantiated claims that had fuelled the 'epidemic' of elective delivery (Chalmers 1976). The polar extremes of this professional debate can be illustrated by contrasting quotations similar to those with which this chapter began. On the one hand, a senior professor of obstetrics maintained that 'induction rates of 20 to 50 per cent are reported from most major maternity units, these being shown to give the best maternal and fetal results' (Jeffcoate 1976), and, in the same vein, the 1975 edition of the standard British midwifery textbook suggested that 'there are distinct maternal and fetal advantages in not permitting pregnancy to continue beyond 40 weeks ... Induction has been proved a safe procedure for mother and fetus' (Myles 1975). On the other hand, a *Lancet* editorial (1974) from the same era noted that 'the timing of spontaneous delivery is controlled by complex mechanisms which are still incompletely understood despite intensive research', and went on to ask whether it was correct to advocate 'wholesale interference with this delicately balanced physiological process'. It ended by characterizing induction on the grounds of social convenience as a 'pernicious practice which has no place in modern obstetric care' (*Lancet* 1974).

In part, these variations in opinion and practice reflect differences of opinion about the place of elective delivery in the presence of markers of increased fetal risk, or frank evidence of fetal compromise. They also reflect differences in people's assessments of the risks associated with elective delivery. Lastly, however, the variations reflect the extent to which elective delivery is used as a way of timing births for the convenience of those providing or those receiving care (Oakley and Richards 1990). In a survey of British obstetricians, for example, about half stated that the increased use of induction of labour had improved their job satisfaction and made the running of maternity departments easier (Cartwright 1979). The use of elective delivery to influence the timing of births was reflected in a disruption of the previously random pattern of births by day of the week; as elective delivery became more common,

a relative deficit of births at weekends and on public holidays became apparent (Macfarlane and Mugford 1984).

It would not be unreasonable to describe the picture that emerges as chaotic. The data and quotations cited above suggest that there is considerable collective uncertainty about the circumstances in which elective delivery is more likely to do good than harm. It is important that the effects of elective delivery should be assessed more carefully than they have been in the past. Neither induction of labour nor elective caesarean section are free of hazard, and those who advocate a more liberal use of elective delivery should thus be required to provide the evidence to justify an extended use of this policy in the variety of circumstances where disagreement exists about its merits.

2 Assessing the place of elective delivery

Although the desirability of elective delivery in any particular circumstances cannot be assessed without considering the efficacy and safety of the methods through which it may be achieved, research in this field has concentrated almost exclusively on evaluating methods of induction. As is clear from the marked variations in the use of elective delivery, relatively little is known about the circumstances in which it is a preferable alternative to waiting for the spontaneous onset of labour.

In some circumstances the advantages of elective delivery are clear from documented case series without formal controls: a woman who is psychologically distressed by her continued carriage of a dead fetus, for example, can be helped by using either a natural prostaglandin or a prostaglandin analogue to induce labour and effect the delivery of her dead baby (see Chapter 65). Similarly, elective delivery may become necessary to avoid the serious maternal morbidity which can result from fulminating pre-eclampsia (see Chapter 33). The debates about the place of elective delivery, however, relate to its use in circumstances in which it is less clear that it confers advantages compared with a more conservative approach. It is in these circumstances— where differential effects of active and conservative policies are likely to be relatively modest—that control of biases and random errors in the evaluative studies become most crucial.

One of the earliest examples of a randomized controlled trial to assess the value of elective delivery related to its use in Rhesus haemolytic disease (Mollison and Walker 1952; Armitage and Mollison 1953). This demonstrated that the not uncommon practice of elective preterm induction of labour in this situation was associated with a *higher* perinatal death rate than that associated with a policy of waiting for the spontaneous onset of labour (see also Chapter 35). Had the policy of elective delivery of diabetic mothers before term also been evaluated in similar randomized trials, the now widespread practice of allowing these women to have as normal a pregnancy as possible might have come into effect much earlier, and the outcome of diabetic pregnancy, in particular the incidence of respiratory distress syndrome among infants of diabetic mothers, might have begun to improve earlier than it did (see Chapter 36).

A clear demonstration of frank fetal pathology, such as Rhesus haemolytic disease, provides a more secure starting point for randomized trials of elective delivery than the less concrete diagnoses of 'fetal compromise' that result from clinical, biochemical, and biophysical investigations of the fetus (see Chapters 26–30). So far, the only circumstances in which controlled trials of elective delivery have suggested any protective effect against perinatal death in these circumstances are those in which fetal compromise has been suggested either by abnormally reduced fetal movements (see Chapter 28); by abnormal ultrasonographic placentography (see Chapter 27); or by abnormal fetal haemodynamics diagnosed using Doppler ultrasound (see Chapter 27). All of this evidence is tentative and an adequate basis for clinical practice must await the results of further controlled studies.

The only area of practice in which there have been substantial numbers of controlled trials comparing elective delivery with a more conservative policy relate to pregnancies that have continued past term. Although there is an increased risk of fetal and neonatal morbidity and mortality associated with these pregnancies, it is still not clear whether this can be reduced by elective delivery (see Chapters 46 and 47). Although a total of nearly 4000 women have participated in trials of elective delivery for post-term pregnancy, no beneficial effects of elective delivery on the risk of fetal heart rate abnormalities, depressed Apgar scores or perinatal mortality have been detected. The only effects of the more active policies which have been detected have been a reduction in the incidence of meconium-stained liquor (not surprisingly), and an increase in the rate of instrumental vaginal delivery (see Chapter 47). The very large sample sizes required to evaluate whether induction of labour confers more benefit than harm in most of the situations where there is professional uncertainty has been reinforced by analyses using observational data derived from very large databases (Chalmers *et al.* 1976a,b; Yudkin 1976).

In summary, there remain many circumstances in which elective delivery may either result in an increase or a decrease in maternal or perinatal morbidity. These uncertainties are reflected in widely differing uses of elective delivery and they cannot be resolved without

substantially more evidence derived from properly controlled and sufficiently large trials.

3 Comparing different methods of achieving elective delivery

There is little purpose in assessing the relative merits of different ways of achieving elective delivery if there is no need for it in the first place. This has not prevented a vast amount of research in which different methods for achieving elective delivery have been compared (see Chapters 61–65, below). None of these studies has compared the two main methods of effecting elective delivery—induction of labour and elective caesarean section. All of the controlled trials thus involve comparisons of alternative ways of inducing labour, with or without preparation of the cervix for induction.

The main limitation of this enormous body of literature is that means have often been confused with ends. Little information is provided on substantive outcomes, the studies concentrating almost exclusively on intermediate outcome measures, like mean duration of labour, or induction to delivery intervals. These surrogate outcome measures are difficult to interpret for a variety of reasons. They often relate only to those women in whom induction was considered to be successful (however 'success' was defined). Thus women in whom a second induction attempt was made and women undergoing caesarean section have sometimes been excluded from the data presented.

Potentially important adverse effects, like 'uterine hypertonus' or 'hyperstimulation', have often been poorly defined. Even when authors have described what they mean by these terms, there has been little resemblance between the criteria used by different authors. Not surprisingly, incidences of 'uterine hypertonus', 'hyperstimulation', or 'excessive uterine contractility' (which all refer to a situation that has prompted concern that uterine relaxation may be inadequate to allow adequate exchange of oxygen and nutrients from mother to fetus) have varied widely among studies that appear very similar in other respects. The same applies to outcomes such as fetal heart rate 'abnormalities', which have included both severe and very modest deviations from fetal heart rate patterns considered to be 'normal'. Although the significance for the well-being of the baby of these modest deviations from normal is unclear (see Chapter 54), they are not insignificant for the mother if they prompt a variety of other interventions, including caesarean section.

The important outcomes of any procedure to induce labour or to prepare the cervix for induction are not increases in cervical compliance or mean lengths of labour, but reductions in maternal and fetal morbidity. This is not to say that the ease with which induction can be implemented, or the creation of greater comfort in elective delivery for the caregiver is unimportant. On the contrary, such considerations may weigh heavily, not only for their own sake, but also because they are likely to have a great influence on the way in which care will be provided for and experienced by the mother. Similarly, short induction to delivery intervals are more likely to allow for continuity of care during labour and childbirth than long intervals, and this continuity is known to increase maternal satisfaction with care (see Chapters 8 and 49). None of the above implies, however, that 'outcome measures' such as changes in cervical resistance and induction–delivery intervals, important as they may be, have any value in themselves. Any value they have derives from the extent to which they contribute to an improved outcome and experience of labour and delivery for all concerned.

As far as maternal outcomes are concerned, important information has simply not been collected or not been reported by the majority of clinical investigators in this field. Indeed, one of the reasons for the public outcry at the epidemic of induced labours in Britain in the early 1970s was that professionals appeared to be unaware that women who had previously experienced spontaneous labours found that induced labours in subsequent pregnancies were more painful (Oakley and Richards 1990). Survey data collected at that time showed that, in contrast to their wishes in respect of other elements of care, a majority of women who had experienced induction did not wish labour to be induced in a subsequent pregnancy (Cartwright 1979). Although these negative responses to induced labour may partly reflect inadequate provision of information about induction (*British Medical Journal* 1976), they seem likely to reflect more fundamental concerns of women that they were not in control of what was happening to them during childbirth (Oakley and Richards 1990).

The results of a study conducted in The Netherlands demonstrate the importance of taking into account women's preferences about elective delivery (Out 1983). Of 66 women who had opted for and experienced elective delivery, 45 said that they would choose the same for a subsequent birth. However, of 32 women who had opted for elective delivery but started labour spontaneously (either before arrangements had been made for elective delivery or before the planned date), only 7 said that they would choose induction of labour again in a subsequent pregnancy; the vast majority (25 of 32) said that they would prefer to await the spontaneous onset of labour in a subsequent pregnancy (Out 1983).

The chapters reviewing alternative methods of inducing labour which follow this chapter will concentrate on trying to assess their relative merits in terms of substantive maternal outcomes. Such assessments are often difficult to make from the available published evidence. For example, the amount of pain and discomfort suffered during labour is a main concern of women (see Chapter 8) and a concern that ranked high among the reasons for dissatisfaction with liberal induction policies in the United Kingdom in the mid-1970s (Kitzinger 1975; Stewart 1979). Among alternative policies for inducing labour, it would appear essential to choose those methods that are least likely to be painful and uncomfortable. Yet, few controlled comparisons have addressed this issue specifically, and those that did concentrated almost exclusively on the provision of pain relief. For example, of 35 reports on controlled comparisons between prostaglandins and oxytocin for induction of labour, only 5 (14 per cent) provide data on the number of women who received analgesia during labour (Chapter 63). Moreover, the provision of pain relief is not necessarily an adequate reflection of the amount of pain experienced by the woman. Unless the caregivers are blinded to the nature of the treatment given for induction of labour, the provision of analgesia may depend on their knowledge of treatment allocation and their expectations of (real or assumed) drug effects, or drug interactions with the oxytocic agents.

In the chapters that follow, the relative effects of alternative methods for inducing labour will be assessed as far as possible in terms of the chances of delivery (preferably vaginal delivery) within a reasonable time interval. There is likely to be general agreement that induced labour, and the strain which it imposes on the mother and those who support her during labour, should last no longer than 24 hours and should preferably lead to vaginal delivery within 12 hours. Again, only a minority of the studies evaluating alternative policies for induction of labour have provided data on these substantive outcomes (see Chapters 61–63).

Surprisingly, some of the published reports on controlled comparisons of alternative procedures for inducing labour even fail to mention how many women actually experienced the outcome that the policy was intended to achieve: vaginal delivery. Others appear to disregard completely the fate of women who failed to respond 'adequately' to the procedures inflicted upon them. Occasionally, the presentation of results only for women who were 'successfully induced' (whatever that may mean) even creates the impression that the least 'successful' treatment actually provides the best outcome in terms of substantive outcomes such as caesarean section and instrumental vaginal delivery. To use one from many possible examples, Westergaard and his colleagues (1983) reported a caesarean section rate of 7 per cent among 133 women induced with oral PGE_2 without amniotomy, compared with a rate of 3 per cent among 131 women induced with buccal desaminooxytocin. However, 18 per cent of the PGE_2-treated women and 36 per cent of the oxytocin-treated women were reported as 'failures' to whom only scant reference is made in the published report. Further (unpublished) information kindly provided by the authors reveals that 25 per cent of the 72 'failures' were subsequently delivered by caesarean section. The total caesarean section rates among PGE_2-induced and oxytocin-induced women were thus 11 per cent and 13 per cent respectively, figures that convey a very different message from that presented in the published report.

Because labour is rarely induced for maternal indications, only substantive indicators of fetal and neonatal outcome will be examined in the chapters which follow. Apart from depressed Apgar scores, on which more information is available than on any other infant outcomes, these include the need for resuscitation at birth; neonatal convulsions; admission to a special care nursery; the development of hyperbilirubinaemia (or use of phototherapy or exchange transfusion); and perinatal death. Although information has also been sought about maternal morbidity postpartum, particularly pyrexia and postpartum haemorrhage leading to blood transfusion, data on such outcomes, which affect the mother's well-being and her interaction with the baby in the first days or weeks after childbirth, are only encountered in a minority of the reports of controlled research on alternative methods of induction.

As this body of evidence is reviewed, it will become clear just how inadequate it remains for answering substantive questions about the relative merits of alternative ways of effecting elective delivery. Vast amounts of time, money, and equipment have been used with few clear dividends in terms of clinically useful results. Table 60.1, derived from Chapter 61, provides an example to illustrate this situation. It lists all of the published reports of controlled evaluations of vaginally administered PGE_2 for cervical ripening. As can be seen in the table, each of the arms of the trials contained only between 12 and 41 women; the largest number of women treated with PGE_2 in any of these studies was

Table 60.1 Characteristics of controlled comparisons of vaginally administered PGE_2 for cervical ripening

Authors and dates	No. of women treated	PGE_2 dose (mg)	Vehicle type	Cervical score		Control*	Parity†	Data available on		
				Type used	Cut-off			Caesarean section	Resucitation newborn	Admission to special care unit
MacKenzie and Embrey (1977)	12	2	Carboxymethyl cellulose	Calder	<4	Pla.	N	yes	no	no
MacKenzie and Embrey (1979)	16	5	Tylose gel	Calder	<4	Pla.	N	yes	no	no
Lewis (1983)	22	3	Witepsol pessary	Other	<5 of 15	NT	N + M	yes	no	no
Prins et al. (1983)	15	5	Tylose gel	Calder	<5	Pla.	N + M	yes	no	no
Walker and Gordon (1983)	15	4	Tylose gel	Other	<4 of?	Pla.	N	cross over	no	no
Buchanan et al. (1984)	38	3	Suppository	Bishop	<5	Pla.	N + M	yes	no	no
Jagani et al. (1984)	15	2–3	Suppositories	Bishop	<5	NT	N + M	yes	no	no
Lorenz et al. (1984)	21	2	Hydroxyethyl cellulose	Calder	not stated	Pla.	N + M	yes	yes	no
Thiery et al. (1984)	41	2	Vaginal tablet‡	Bishop	<6	Pla.‡	N + M	yes	no	no
Graves et al. (1985)	20 20 20	1 2 3	Triacetin gel	Bishop	<5	Pla.	N + M	yes	no	no
Ulmsten et al. (1985)	19	2	Suppository	Other	<6 of 10	Pla.	N	yes	yes	no
Williams et al. (1985)	20 20	3 5	Cellulose	Bishop	<6	Pla.	N + M	yes	no	no

* Pla: placebo; NT: no treatment
† N: nulliparae; M: multiparae
‡ These women also received an endocervical placebo gel

60, and these 60 were divided among three groups with different doses of the drug. The state of the cervix at entry into these twelve trials was assessed with different scores; the doses used ranged from 1 mg to 5 mg, and the vehicles in which PGE_2 was administered varied widely. In addition, the periods allowed for achieving ripening ranged from 12 hours to 24 hours, and there were differences in the methods used to pursue induction after the end of this period. Only two of the trials provided information on substantive indicators of perinatal morbidity.

4 Conclusions

The frequency with which birth follows elective delivery shows wide variations from place to place, as well as increases and decreases over time. These variations reflect the many uncertainties that exist about the circumstances in which elective delivery is more likely to do good than harm. There is a need for research to address these uncertainties, because it is clear that unjustified use of elective delivery in the past has had harmful effects, and because it is also clear that there are

some circumstances in which elective delivery may be beneficial. If elective delivery is to be assessed in terms of outcomes that matter to parents, a fundamental reorientation is required. First, investigators must begin to assess the maternal outcomes that matter to women themselves; second, they must collaborate in order to obtain more precise estimates of the effects of elective delivery on substantive indicators of maternal, fetal, and neonatal morbidity.

Although the effects of elective delivery are inevitably bound up with the effects of the methods used to achieve it, comparisons within the plethora of different methods available should be seen as a secondary goal of research in this field. Pursuit of this goal too, however, will require multicentre collaboration if the research is to provide useful estimates of the relative merits of alternative methods. There is encouraging evidence that such collaboration is becoming more common and good reason to hope, therefore, that future research in this field will be more productive and yield more useful information than the currently available evidence. This is essential if there is to be a more rational basis for clinical practice.

References

Amy JJ, Thiery M, Crawford JS, Kerenyi TD, Bygdeman M, Karim SMM (1976). A suggested set of working definitions and criteria applicable to induction of labour. Int J Gynaecol Obstet, 14: 379–383.

Armitage P, Mollison PL (1953). Further analysis of controlled trials of treatment of haemolytic disease of the newborn. J Obstet Gynaecol Br Empire, 60: 605–620.

British Medical Journal (1976). Induction of labour. Br Med J, 1: 729–730.

Buchanan D, Macer J, Yonekura ML (1984). Cervical ripening with prostaglandin E_2 vaginal suppositories. Obstet Gynecol, 63: 659–663.

Cartwright A (1979). The Dignity of Labour? London: Tavistock.

Chalmers I (1976) British debate on obstetric practice. Pediatrics, 58: 308–312.

Chalmers I (1979) The epidemiology of perinatal practice. J Matern Child Health, November, p 435–436.

Chalmers I, Richards MPM (1977). Intervention and causal inference in obstetric practice. In: Benefits and Hazards of the New Obstetrics. Chard T, Richards MPM (eds). Clinics in Developmental Medicine No. 64. London: Spastics International Medical Publications, Heinemann Medical Books, pp 34–61.

Chalmers I, Zlosnik JE, Johns KA, Campbell H (1976a). Obstetric practice and outcome of pregnancy in Cardiff residents, 1965–1973. Br Med J, 1: 735–738.

Chalmers I, Lawson JG, Turnbull AC (1976b). Evaluation of different approaches to obstetric care. Parts I and II. Br J Obstet Gynaecol, 83: 921–933.

Chalmers I, Dauncey ME, Verrier Jones ER, Dodge JA, Gray OP (1978). Respiratory distress syndrome in infants of

Cardiff residents during 1965–1975. Br Med J, 2: 1119–1121.

Gitsch E, Reinold E, Tulzer H (1978). Programmierte Geburt. Wien Med Wochenschr, 21: 669–672.

Graves GR, Baskett TF, Gray JH, Luther ER (1985). The effect of vaginal administration of various doses of prostaglandin E_2 gel on cervical ripening and induction of labour. Am J Obstet Gynecol, 151: 178–181.

Hendry RA (1981). The weekend—a dangerous time to be born? Br J Obstet Gynaecol, 80:1200–1203.

Hillemans HG, Mross F, Sneller H, Steiner H (1977). Die programmierte Geburt. Geburtshilfe Frauenheilk, 37: 373–386.

Jagani N, Schulman H, Fleischer A, Mitchell J, Blattner P (1984). Role of prostaglandin-induced cervical changes in labor induction. Obstet Gynecol, 63: 225–229.

Jeffcoate TNA (1976). Medicine versus surgery. J R Coll Surg Edinburgh, 21: 263–277.

Kitzinger S (1975). Some Mothers' Experiences of Induced Labour. London: National Childbirth Trust.

Lampe LG (1980). Selective planned induction of labour. Acta Chir Acad Sci Hung, 21: 43–53.

Lancet (1974) A time to be born (editorial). Lancet, 2: 1183.

Lewis GJ (1983). Cervical ripening before induction of labour with prostaglandin E_2 pessaries or a Foley's catheter. J Obstet Gynaecol, 3: 173–176.

Lorenz RP, Botti JJ, Chez RA, Bennett N (1984). Variations of biologic activity of low-dose prostaglandin E_2 on cervical ripening. Obstet Gynecol, 64: 123–127.

Macfarlane AJ, Mugford M (1984). Birth Counts. London: Her Majesty's Stationery Office.

MacKenzie IZ, Embrey MP (1977). Cervical ripening with intravaginal prostaglandin E_2 gel. Br Med J, 2: 1381–1384.

MacKenzie IZ, Embrey MP (1979). A comparison of PGE_2

and PGF$_{2a}$ vaginal gel for ripening the cervix before induction of labour. Br J Obstet Gynaecol, 86: 167–170.

McNay MB, McIlwaine GM, Howie PW, Macnaughton MC (1977). Perinatal deaths: analysis by clinical cause to assess value of induction of labour. Br Med J, 1: 347–350.

Mollison PL, Walker W (1952). Controlled trials of the treatment of haemolytic disease of the newborn. Lancet, 1: 429–433.

Myles MF (1975). Textbook for Midwives. Edinburgh: Churchill Livingstone.

Newcombe RG (1983). Reversal of changes in distribution of gestational age and birth weight among firstborn infants of Cardiff residents. Br Med J, 287: 1095–1097.

Newcombe RG, Chalmers (1977). Changes in distribution of gestational age and birthweight among first born infants of Cardiff residents. Br Med J, 2: 925–926.

Oakley A, Richards MPM (1990). Womens' experiences of caesarean delivery. In: The Politics of Maternity Care. Garcia J, Kilpatrick R, Richards M (eds). Oxford: Oxford University Press, pp 183–201.

Out JJ (1983). De Electieve Inleiding van de Baring. Een Prospectief Obstetrisch en Psychologisch Onderzoek. Rotterdam: MD thesis.

Prins RP, Bolton RN, Mark C, Neilson DR, Watson P (1983). Cervical ripening with intravaginal prostaglandin E$_2$ gel. Obstet Gynecol, 61: 459–462.

Reed CB (1920). The induction of labour at term. Am J Obstet Gynecol, 1: 24–33.

Richter D, Steiner H, Hillemans HG (1979). The advantage of elective induction of labour by a psychosomatic approach. In: Emotion and Reproduction. 5th International Congress of Psychosomatic Obstetrics and Gynecology. Carenza L, Zichella L (eds). London: Academic Press, pp 887–892.

Stewart P (1979). Patient's attitudes to induction of labour. Br Med J, 2: 749–752.

Tacchi D (1971). Towards easier childbirth. Lancet, 2: 1134–1136.

Thiery M, De Coster JM, Parewijck W, Noah ML, Derom R, Van Kets H, Defoort P, Aertsens W, Debruyne G, De Geest K, Vandekerckhove F (1984). Endocervical prostaglandin E$_2$ gel for preinduction cervical softening. Prostaglandins, 27: 429–439.

Turnbull AC (1976). Cited in Nowlan D (1976). Obstetricians welcome reversal of trend in cases of induced labour. Irish Times, 30 June, p 3.

Ulmsten U, Ekman G, Belfrage P, Bygdeman M, Nyberg C (1985). Intracervical vs intravaginal PGE$_2$ for induction of labor at term in patients with an unfavorable cervix. Arch Gynecol, 236: 243–248.

Vierhout ME, Out JJ, Wallenburg HCS (1985). Elective induction of labor: a prospective clinical study, I: Obstetric and neonatal effects. J Perinat Med, 13: 155–162.

Walker E, Gordon AJ (1983). Length of exposure to prostaglandin E$_2$ and cervical ripening in primigravidae. J Obstet Gynaecol, 4: 88–89.

Westergaard JG, Lange AP, Pedersen GT, Secher NJ (1983). Oral oxytocics for induction of labor. Acta Obstet Gynecol Scand, 62: 103–110.

Williams JK, Wilkerson WG, O'Brien WF, Knuppel RA (1985). Use of prostaglandin E$_2$ topical cervical gel in high-risk patients: a critical analysis. Obstet Gynecol, 66: 769–773.

Wulf KH (1979). Die programmierte Geburt. Arch Gynäkol, 228: 57–66.

Yudkin P (1976). Problems in assessing the effects of induction of labour on perinatal mortality. Br J Obstet Gynaecol, 83: 603–607.

61 Preparing the cervix for induction of labour

Marc J. N. C. Keirse and A. Carla C. van Oppen

1 Introduction

In order to be successful, induction of labour must result in what is defined as 'labour', namely adequate uterine contractions and progressive dilatation of the uterine cervix. Although these two processes—adequate uterine contractions and cervical dilatation—are usually concurrent, they are in fact distinct. Yet, the total amount of uterine contractility required to achieve cervical dilatation is very dependent on the state of the cervix (Burnhill *et al.* 1962; Arulkumaran *et al.* 1985). A firm and rigid (unripe) cervix may require a total quantity of uterine work that is three to four times greater than that needed when the cervix is softer and more yielding (ripe) (Burnhill *et al.* 1962).

The consequences of this for the induction of labour have been known for a long time (Cockx 1955). Many of the early reports on induction emphasized that the state of the cervix was the most important predictor of success (Burnhill *et al.* 1962; Embrey and Anselmo 1962; Turnbull and Anderson 1967, 1968), a finding that has been confirmed in more recent observations (Calder 1979; Lamberti and Nowak 1983).

Realization of the importance of the state of the cervix for induction has led, first, to the development of various methods to assess cervical 'ripeness' and their use to predict the outcome of induction (Bishop 1964; Burnett 1966; Fields 1966; Friedman *et al.* 1967) and,

second, to the search for methods that decrease cervical resistance prior to induction.

This chapter assesses the effectiveness and limitations of the various procedures that have been used in attempts to influence the cervix with the purpose of facilitating subsequent induction of labour.

2 Aims of cervical ripening

Ripening of the cervix aims to increase cervical compliance. An 'unripe' cervix fails to dilate as well as it ought to do in response to induction of labour, and this results in high failure rates of induction. These failures are characterized by protracted and exhausting labours, a high incidence of caesarean section, and, depending on the method of induction used, high rates of a variety of complications (Calder 1979). Foremost among these are pyrexia and intrauterine infection when amniotomy is a component of the procedure, and uterine hypertonus and drug-induced side-effects (due to the high doses needed) when oxytocics are used.

In as much as an unripe cervix indicates low cervical compliance, it is logical to assume that increasing cervical compliance will make it yield more easily in response to uterine contractions. As such, increasing cervical compliance should be beneficial. Provided that the procedure to achieve it does no harm and is not prohibitively expensive, it may be felt to require little evidence of effectiveness before being considered a worthy element of care. Before one accepts this view, however, two important qualifiers need to be taken into account.

First, boosting cervical compliance is only a means to an end. There is little purpose in artificially augmenting cervical compliance when there is no need for the cervix to dilate. The important outcomes, therefore, are not so much the increases in cervical compliance, but improvements in the outcome of labour and delivery. The latter, and thus also the effects of cervical ripening to facilitate these processes, need to be assessed in terms of maternal and infant morbidity and the degree of discomfort experienced by the mother. As mentioned elsewhere (see Chapter 60), this does not mean that the ease with which induction can be implemented is unimportant. It merely implies that changes in cervical compliance derive any value that they have from the extent to which they improve outcome and experience of labour and delivery for all concerned. Unfortunately, the extent to which these fundamental objectives have been achieved is not always obvious from the many studies that have been conducted on cervical ripening. Many of these studies confuse the means with the end, concentrating almost exclusively on surrogate measures such as absolute or relative increases in cervical ripeness. This might be less of a problem if there was good evidence that an increase in cervical ripeness brought about by pharmacological or mechanical means has exactly the same prognostic significance as an increase occurring physiologically. No such evidence exists, however.

A second issue concerns whether the promotion of cervical ripening must be achieved without provoking a degree of uterine contractility higher than what would be present if no measures to ripen the cervix were undertaken. There are two contrary views on this question and both can be defended on theoretical grounds. On the one hand, cervical ripening aims to promote successful labour and delivery. An increase in uterine contractility up to the extent of clinically recognized labour might thus be seen as beneficial. In these circumstances, the desired labour would have started without any further formal interventions to induce it. The primary intervention of cervical ripening can then be seen as having resulted in 'no need for formal induction of labour' and in what may, rightly or wrongly, be referred to as 'spontaneous' labour.

On the other hand, since cervical ripening is undertaken because the cervix has been judged to be insufficiently compliant to respond adequately to uterine contractility, it would seem logical to avoid an increase in contractility until greater cervical compliance has been achieved (Hillier and Wallis 1978). Thus, Ellwood and his colleagues (1979) proposed that 'a clear distinction must be made between cervical ripening by pre-treatment before induction and treatments which cause changes in cervical state by inducing labour'. With this view, the onset of uterine contractions during the ripening process (and particularly when they are uncomfortable or painful for the mother) becomes a negative, not a positive, outcome.

Important as these theoretical considerations may be, the fundamental question with regard to care is not whether cervical ripening influences uterine contractility or not, but whether or not it improves the substantive outcomes that are of interest to mother and baby.

3 Assessment of the cervix

The capacity of the cervix to remain closed throughout most of pregnancy depends largely on its rigidity, a property that derives from the collagen fibres which make up the bulk of the cervical stroma. The firm cervical connective tissue consists mainly of collagen and its matrix of large proteoglycan molecules. The cervix was formerly thought to be relatively inert, with changes resulting merely from increasing uterine pressure, but it is now well recognized to be a dynamic structure that undergoes many changes, particularly in late pregnancy (Ellwood and Anderson 1981; Ulmsten 1986). Along with biochemical changes in the proteoglycan matrix and collagen degradation, there is an increase in vascularity, an accumulation of interstitial fluid, and migration of white cells and macrophages into the cervical tissue. These changes lead, in turn, to changes in the biophysical characteristics of the cervix and result in a greater compliance and less resistance to dilatation. The increase in compliance is most readily recognized in the palpable differences between the firm, rigid cervix at the beginning of pregnancy, and the soft, oedematous structure felt at term.

Unfortunately, digital assessment of the cervix is highly subjective, and even experienced examiners may differ in their appraisal of cervical features. Several cervical scoring systems have been developed in an attempt to overcome this problem, and to establish more comparable guidelines for cervical assessment. The best known of these is the score proposed by Bishop (1964), which rates five different qualities (cervical effacement, cervical dilatation, cervical consistency, position of the cervix relative to the axis of the pelvis, and descent of the fetal presenting part) on a total score from 0 to 13 (Table 61.1). Not all elements in Bishop's score relate directly to the condition of the cervix. Three of a possible 13 marks refer to descent of the presenting part, a feature that is present in most 'cervical scores' (Fig. 61.1). It is interesting to note that Bishop originally referred to 'pelvic' and not to 'cervical' scoring. He suggested that this 'pelvic score' could be applied to elective induction of labour in multiparae with a fetus, presenting cephalically, within 3 weeks of

Table 61.1 Bishop's 'pelvic score' for assessment of cervical ripeness (after Bishop 1964)

Criteria	Number of marks awarded			
	0	1	2	3
Cervical dilatation (cm)	0	1–2	3–4	5–6
Cervical effacement (%)	0–30	40–50	60–70	≥80
Cervical consistency	firm	medium	soft	
Cervical position	posterior	central	anterior	
Station (in relation to the spines)	3 cm above	2 cm above	1–0 cm above	1–2 cm below

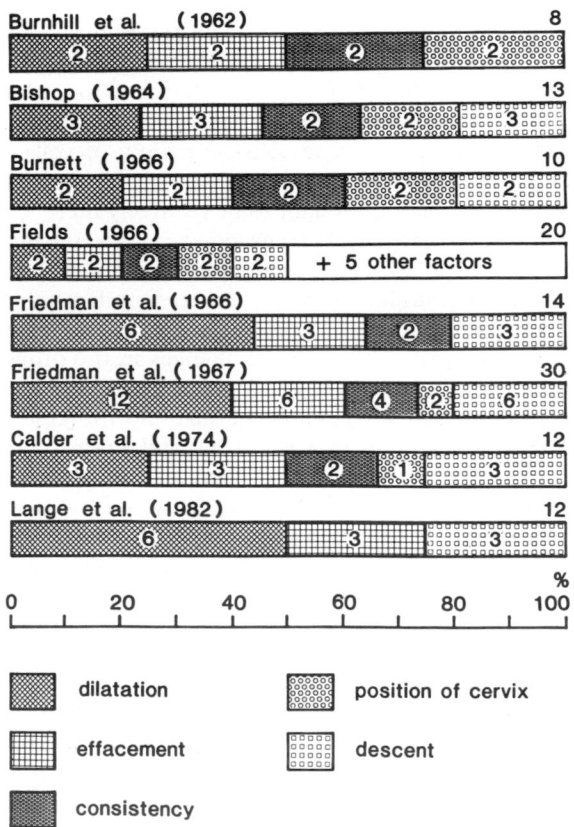

Fig. 61.1 Comparison of various scores and their components used for assessment of the cervix prior to induction of labour. The number of marks assigned to individual components of the score is indicated in the bars, while the maximal number that can be achieved in the total score is indicated above the bars.

term; but he estimated that '. . . owing to the unpredictability of the duration of labour in the nullipara, even in the presence of apparently favorable circumstances, induction of labour brings little advantage for either obstetrician or patient' (Bishop 1964).

Although Bishop (1964) did not refer to an earlier report in which he had related cervical dilatation, effacement, and descent of the fetal presenting part to the duration of induced labour in multiparae (Bishop 1955), it is logical to assume that the earlier study influenced the construction of his score. In that earlier study, he had concluded 'that before elective induction of labour is considered, the cervix should be not less than 3 cm dilated and not less than 60 per cent effaced with the presenting part at station −1 or lower' (Bishop 1955). This recommendation was based on his acceptance of the idea that 4 hours was the ideal duration of labour. While, in general, inducibility (i.e. the ability to achieve active, progressive labour) and duration of labour will be interrelated, these cannot be seen as synonymous, and each may to some extent be determined by different factors.

In the published report, Bishop (1964) placed the emphasis mainly on the view that use of the score would permit elective delivery, whether by elective induction or elective caesarean section, 'in close proximity to the time when spontaneous onset of labour would naturally occur', 'thus almost eliminating the elective delivery of a premature infant' (Bishop 1964). In essence, his aim was therefore to 'estimate the expected date of delivery more accurately than by the traditional methods' (Bishop 1964). He also reported, however, that with a score of 9 or more 'we have had no failures in induction, and the average duration of labour has been less than 4 hr. While . . . induction can be performed successfully under less favorable circumstances . . . interference under such circumstances is associated with increased hazard, longer than ideal duration of labour, and a decreased chance for success' (Bishop 1964). Unfortunately, these important qualifications stated clearly by Bishop are widely ignored. The Bishop score is employed as frequently in nulliparae as in multiparae, and at gestational ages that are no longer confined to those above 36 weeks.

Several other scoring systems have been derived empirically and introduced into clinical practice. With few exceptions, they are all based on the same characteristics of consistency, length, position, and dilatation of the cervix and descent of the presenting part; they merely accord different weights to the individual characteristics (Fig. 61.1). Many elements of the scores are interrelated. Thus a cervix that is partially dilated will usually be softer and more effaced than one which is closed. These various components may well have different predictive values (Friedman *et al.* 1966; Lange *et al.* 1982), and this appears to be one of the main reasons why new scoring systems have been introduced. More often than not, new scores, as well as the large number of so-called 'modified Bishop scores' that are encountered in the literature, have originated from an intuitive clinical feeling that relatively more or less weight should be attributed to particular component factors in the total score.

Few comparisons of the performance of different scores are available (Hughey *et al.* 1976; Lange *et al.* 1982). None of these has involved prospective evaluation of the utility of one score against another for predicting the outcome of induction. Thus far, the main, and possibly only, effect of the wide variety of scoring systems used has been that it is extremely difficult to assess whether different studies of cervical ripening have included women with roughly similar cervical characteristics. This difficulty is further aggravated by the large number of studies in which cervical assessment was stated to be based on a 'modified Bishop score' without any indication as to what the modification entailed. As can be seen in Fig. 61.1, even a standard subdivision within the scores based on whether, for example, 20 or 40 per cent of the maximal score result was obtained, results in largely incomparable groups of women being selected with different scoring systems.

4 Prostaglandins for cervical ripening

A few years after the introduction of prostaglandins for inducing labour in the late 1960s, doses which by themselves were insufficient to induce labour successfully were found to effect a marked softening of the uterine cervix (Calder and Embrey 1973; Embrey 1975). This phenomenon is not only observed at term; marked cervical softening and changes in the shape of the lower uterine pole are phenomena that are well-known to those experienced with prostaglandin-induced terminations of pregnancy in the 2nd trimester. In experimental animals it has been shown that this softening results from a direct effect of prostaglandins on the cervix, which need not be mediated by uterine contractility (Liggins 1978), and there is now a substantial body of evidence on the influence of both endogenous and exogenous prostaglandins on biochemical and biophysical characteristics of the cervix (Ellwood and Anderson 1981; Conrad and Ueland 1983; Ulmsten 1986).

4.1 Controlled comparisons with placebo or 'no treatment'

From the mid-1970s onwards there has been a large number of investigations on the effects of prostaglandins for ripening the cervix prior to induction of labour. Most of the controlled studies have dealt with prostaglandin E_2 (PGE_2); some have used prostaglandin $F_{2\alpha}$ ($PGF_{2\alpha}$) because it is the only prostaglandin available in some countries (e.g. Australia); and one (Roberts *et al.* 1986) apparently used prostaglandin E_1 (PGE_1). These studies have used a wide range of doses, vehicles, and routes of administration. In some studies the prostaglandin was administered only once; in others the administration was repeated either once or several times. The entry criteria have varied widely: some studies have involved only nulliparous women; both nulliparous and parous women have participated in others. Several cervical scoring systems have been applied, and within these scores different cut-off points have been used to select candidates for cervical ripening. The time interval allowed for achieving a ripening effect before the next step (induction of labour) was undertaken has also differed among studies. Finally, there have been differences in the way in which induction of labour was implemented; in some studies it was attempted in all women; in others only in those judged to have achieved an adequate degree of cervical ripening.

Although this large number of variations among controlled studies might imply that it is inadvisable to consider them together, there is little point in examining secondary questions about doses, routes, or vehicles for prostaglandin administration, without first assessing whether prostaglandins are effective in achieving the objectives of cervical ripening. We have therefore examined all controlled comparisons in which any dose of any prostaglandin was administered by any route, and was compared with either placebo or 'no treatment' to ripen the cervix prior to induction of labour. Only those studies have been included in which all other interventions, including the procedure for inducing labour, were similar in the prostaglandin-treated and the control groups. The numbers of trials represented in Tables 61.2 to 61.17 vary because some data items were not always available from every trial, and because data that were not available from some reports on multicentre trials were, on occasions, available from separate publications from the participating centres. Some of the data that were lacking in the report of Noah and his colleagues (1987), for example, could thus be obtained from six other related reports (Keirse *et al.* 1985; Bung *et al.* 1986; Kieback *et al.* 1986; Kristoffersen *et al.* 1986; Pulle *et al.* 1986; Zahradnik *et al.* 1987).

With only two exceptions (Friedman and Sachtleben 1975; Prins *et al.* 1983), all 27 trial reports that provided data on the frequency of labour occurring before the

Table 61.2 Effect of any prostaglandin (any route) vs. placebo (no treatment) for cervical ripening on labour onset during ripening

Study	EXPT n	(%)	CTRL n	(%)	Odds ratio (95% CI)	Graph of odds ratios and confidence intervals
Friedman and Sachtleben (1975)	3/15	(20.00)	3/15	(20.00)	1.00 (0.17–5.81)	
Pearce (1977)	5/25	(20.00)	1/23	(4.35)	4.06 (0.75–22.10)	
Williams *et al.* (1985)	18/40	(45.00)	0/20	(0.00)	8.22 (2.57–26.28)	
Nimrod *et al.* (1984)	13/30	(43.33)	1/15	(6.67)	5.33 (1.42–20.02)	
MacKenzie and Embrey (1979)	13/32	(40.63)	0/16	(0.00)	7.50 (1.97–28.52)	
MacLennan and Green (1979)	20/40	(50.00)	3/40	(7.50)	7.76 (2.96–20.31)	
Hutchon *et al.* (1980)	16/32	(50.00)	3/35	(8.57)	7.45 (2.59–21.42)	
Quinn *et al.* (1981)	4/15	(26.67)	0/15	(0.00)	9.31 (1.17–73.76)	
Prins *et al.* (1983)	3/15	(20.00)	3/15	(20.00)	1.00 (0.17–5.81)	
Walker and Gordon (1983)	3/15	(20.00)	0/15	(0.00)	8.57 (0.82–89.45)	
MacKenzie and Embrey (1977)	4/12	(33.33)	0/12	(0.00)	9.97 (1.22–81.60)	
Laube *et al.* (1986)	8/30	(26.67)	0/15	(0.00)	5.95 (1.20–29.57)	
Bernstein *et al.* (1987)	83/206	(40.29)	16/202	(7.92)	5.80 (3.69–9.11)	
Wingerup *et al.* (1978)	8/10	(80.00)	0/10	(0.00)	23.73 (4.15–99.99)	
Fenton *et al.* (1985)	8/15	(53.33)	1/15	(6.67)	8.57 (1.85–39.79)	
Thiery *et al.* (1984)	14/81	(17.28)	1/40	(2.50)	3.86 (1.23–12.12)	
Heinzl *et al.* (1980)	20/60	(33.33)	4/60	(6.67)	5.22 (2.14–12.73)	
Buchanan *et al.* (1984)	26/38	(68.42)	4/39	(10.26)	11.18 (4.50–27.78)	
Lorenz *et al.* (1984)	2/21	(9.52)	1/23	(4.35)	2.22 (0.22–22.56)	
Graves *et al.* (1985)	16/60	(26.67)	0/20	(0.00)	5.19 (1.47–18.23)	
Murphy *et al.* (1980)	19/165	(11.52)	7/100	(7.00)	1.66 (0.72–3.83)	
Lucas *et al.* (1986)	9/27	(33.33)	1/23	(4.35)	5.90 (1.49–23.38)	
Noah *et al.* (1987)	240/416	(57.69)	20/403	(4.96)	11.37 (8.47–15.25)	
Valentine (1977)	4/30	(13.33)	0/15	(0.00)	5.00 (0.58–43.09)	
Trofatter *et al.* (1985)	11/30	(36.67)	1/29	(3.45)	7.50 (2.13–26.38)	
Lewis (1983)	14/22	(63.64)	0/22	(0.00)	17.58 (5.01–61.62)	
Jagani *et al.* (1984)	4/15	(26.67)	2/16	(12.50)	2.41 (0.42–13.91)	
Typical odds ratio (95% confidence interval)					7.32 (6.12–8.77)	

Graph axis: 0.01   0.1   0.5   1   2   10   100

start of induction (during the period allocated for cervical ripening) showed that this occurred more often in women receiving prostaglandins for cervical ripening than in those receiving placebo or no treatment (Table 61.2). In most of the individual trials (19 of 27; 70 per cent), the difference between the two groups was statistically significant and there was not a single trial in which more women went into labour with placebo or no treatment than with prostaglandin administration (Table 61.2). The typical odds ratio was 7.32 with a 95 per cent confidence interval of 6.12 to 8.77 (Table 61.2).

All trials that provided data on the number of women delivered during the period of cervical ripening and before induction of labour was to be undertaken, reported more deliveries in prostaglandin-treated women than in controls. This difference reached statistical significance in 14 of the 17 trials (82 per cent)

reporting this outcome, yielding a typical odds ratio of 6.15 (95 per cent confidence interval 4.59–8.25; Table 61.3).

Twelve trials provided data on the number of women who had either 'no increase', or 'too small an increase', in cervical score with cervical ripening. All but one (Friedman and Sachtleben 1975) of these trials showed a statistically significant difference between the prostaglandin and control groups, no increase or poor increase in cervical score being less frequent in prostaglandin-treated women (Table 61.4), resulting in a typical odds ratio of 0.14 (95 per cent confidence interval 0.10–0.18).

Fifteen reports provided data on what the authors had (variously) described as 'induction failure' or 'unsuccessful induction', indicating that the whole process of cervical ripening and subsequent induction of

Table 61.3 Effect of any prostaglandin (any route) vs. placebo (no treatment) for cervical ripening on delivered during ripening

Study	EXPT n	(%)	CTRL n	(%)	Odds ratio (95% CI)
Ulmsten et al. (1985)	15/38	(39.47)	2/20	(10.00)	4.05 (1.24–13.16)
Golbus and Creasy (1977)	6/25	(24.00)	1/25	(4.00)	5.09 (1.05–24.77)
MacLennan and Green (1979)	13/40	(32.50)	3/40	(7.50)	4.68 (1.57–13.90)
MacKenzie and Embrey (1977)	3/12	(25.00)	0/12	(0.00)	8.94 (0.84–95.49)
Laube et al. (1986)	8/30	(26.67)	0/15	(0.00)	5.95 (1.20–29.57)
Wingerup et al. (1978)	8/10	(80.00)	0/10	(0.00)	23.73 (4.15–99.99)
Weiss et al. (1975)	9/32	(28.13)	1/24	(4.17)	4.97 (1.26–19.56)
Heinzl et al. (1980)	20/60	(33.33)	4/60	(6.67)	5.22 (2.14–12.73)
Cabrol et al. (1988)	47/108	(43.52)	14/105	(13.33)	4.35 (2.40–7.87)
Keirse et al. (1985)	10/25	(40.00)	0/25	(0.00)	11.59 (2.94–45.70)
Kieback et al. (1986)	16/50	(32.00)	3/50	(6.00)	5.33 (1.97–14.39)
Kristoffersen et al. (1986)	10/25	(40.00)	0/25	(0.00)	11.59 (2.94–45.70)
Yonekura et al. (1985)	3/25	(12.00)	0/23	(0.00)	7.43 (0.73–75.21)
Valentine (1977)	1/30	(3.33)	0/15	(0.00)	4.48 (0.07–99.99)
Trofatter et al. (1985)	6/30	(20.00)	0/29	(0.00)	8.60 (1.61–45.90)
Pulle et al. (1986)	10/25	(40.00)	0/25	(0.00)	11.59 (2.94–45.70)
Bung et al. (1986)	18/41	(43.90)	1/39	(2.56)	9.53 (3.42–26.52)
Typical odds ratio (95% confidence interval)					6.15 (4.59–8.25)

Table 61.4 Effect of any prostaglandin (any route) vs. placebo (no treatment) for cervical ripening on poor increase in cervix score

Study	EXPT		CTRL		Odds ratio	Graph of odds ratios and confidence intervals
	n	(%)	n	(%)	(95% CI)	0.01 0.1 0.5 1 2 10 100
Friedman and Sachtleben (1975)	4/15	(26.67)	4/15	(26.67)	1.00 (0.20–4.91)	
Nimrod *et al.* (1984)	2/30	(6.67)	6/15	(40.00)	0.11 (0.02–0.53)	
MacKenzie and Embrey (1979)	11/32	(34.38)	12/16	(75.00)	0.20 (0.06–0.67)	
MacLennan and Green (1979)	3/40	(7.50)	20/40	(50.00)	0.13 (0.05–0.34)	
Wingerup *et al.* (1978)	0/10	(0.00)	10/10	(100.0)	0.02 (0.00–0.12)	
Thiery *et al.* (1984)	44/81	(54.32)	32/40	(80.00)	0.34 (0.15–0.73)	
Heinzl *et al.* (1980)	13/60	(21.67)	41/60	(68.33)	0.15 (0.08–0.32)	
Cabrol *et al.* (1988)	43/104	(41.35)	75/104	(72.12)	0.29 (0.17–0.50)	
Keirse *et al.* (1985)	3/25	(12.00)	23/25	(92.00)	0.04 (0.01–0.13)	
Shepherd *et al.* (1976)	1/15	(6.67)	15/15	(100.0)	0.03 (0.01–0.11)	
Valentine (1977)	0/30	(0.00)	15/15	(100.0)	0.01 (0.00–0.05)	
Lewis (1983)	2/22	(9.09)	22/22	(100.0)	0.03 (0.01–0.09)	
Typical odds ratio (95% confidence interval)					0.14 (0.10–0.18)	

labour had been rather unsatisfactory in terms of achieving the aims that had been set. With only one exception (Graves *et al.* 1985), 'induction failure' tended to occur less frequently in the prostaglandin-treated than in the control groups. Overall the difference was highly statistically significant, with a typical odds ratio of 0.33 and a 95 per cent confidence interval ranging from 0.26 to 0.41 (Table 61.5).

Ten of the trial reports provided data on the incidence of 'uterine hypertonus' or 'uterine hyperstimulation' either during cervical ripening, or during the subsequent induction of labour. The typical odds ratio of 1.70 with a 95 per cent confidence interval of 1.06 to 2.72 showed that this occurred statistically significantly more often in prostaglandin-treated women than with placebo or no treatment prior to induction (Table 61.6). Whether for this or for other reasons, the incidence of fetal heart rate abnormalities in the 14 trial reports that provided this information also tended to be higher with the prostaglandin treatment, although the difference compared to placebo or no treatment was not statistically significant (typical odds ratio 1.29; 95 per cent confidence interval 0.97–1.70; Table 61.7).

Very few reports provide data on the incidence of analgesia or epidural analgesia in the active treatment and control groups (Table 61.8). In those that do, the incidence of epidural analgesia is statistically significantly lower among prostaglandin-treated women than among women in the control group (typical odds ratio 0.60; 95 per cent confidence interval 0.41–0.86; Table 61.8).

The data shown in Tables 61.9 and 61.10, although referring to relatively few trials (most of which were small), indicate that the likelihood of not being delivered within 12 or 24 hours after the start of induction (Table 61.9), and of not having a vaginal delivery within 12 or 24 hours after the start of induction (Table 61.10), was considerably reduced in prostaglandin-treated women. The typical odds ratios for all of these outcomes ranged between 0.13 and 0.27, with 95 per cent confidence intervals that never reached an upper limit higher than 0.57 for any of these outcomes (Tables 61.9 and 61.10).

Data on the incidence of caesarean section relate to more than 3500 women included in the various trials. None of these trials showed a statistically significant influence of prostaglandin treatment on the incidence of this important outcome (Table 61.11). Overall, how-

Table 61.5 Effect of any prostaglandin (any route) vs. placebo (no treatment) for cervical ripening on 'induction failure'

Study	EXPT		CTRL		Odds ratio	Graph of odds ratios and confidence intervals
	n	(%)	n	(%)	(95% CI)	0.01 0.1 0.5 1 2 10 100
Friedman and Sachtleben (1975)	3/15	(20.00)	4/15	(26.67)	0.70 (0.13–3.68)	
Golbus and Creasy (1977)	9/25	(36.00)	9/25	(36.00)	1.00 (0.32–3.14)	
Pearce (1977)	1/25	(4.00)	1/23	(4.35)	0.92 (0.06–15.16)	
Williams et al. (1985)	4/40	(10.00)	2/20	(10.00)	1.00 (0.17–5.90)	
Prins et al. (1983)	2/15	(13.33)	8/15	(53.33)	0.18 (0.04–0.78)	
Laube et al. (1986)	1/30	(3.33)	2/15	(13.33)	0.21 (0.02–2.42)	
Bernstein et al. (1988)	9/108	(8.33)	20/110	(18.18)	0.43 (0.20–0.93)	
Wingerup et al. (1978)	0/10	(0.00)	7/10	(70.00)	0.05 (0.01–0.32)	
Buchanan et al. (1984)	2/38	(5.26)	12/39	(30.77)	0.18 (0.06–0.58)	
Cabrol et al. (1988)	7/108	(6.48)	13/105	(12.38)	0.50 (0.20–1.26)	
Graves et al. (1985)	19/60	(31.67)	6/20	(30.00)	1.08 (0.36–3.19)	
Roberts et al. (1986)	1/27	(3.70)	10/24	(41.67)	0.11 (0.03–0.42)	
Noah et al. (1987)	66/413	(15.98)	170/403	(42.18)	0.28 (0.21–0.38)	
Yonekura et al. (1985)	1/25	(4.00)	3/25	(12.00)	0.34 (0.05–2.61)	
Valentine (1977)	1/30	(3.33)	4/15	(26.67)	0.10 (0.01–0.70)	
Typical odds ratio (95% confidence interval)					0.33 (0.26–0.41)	

ever, the trials show a modest, but statistically significant decrease in the caesarean section rate with prostaglandin treatment as compared with placebo or no treatment, the typical odds ratio being 0.83 (95 per cent confidence interval 0.69–0.99; Table 61.11). A similar, but more marked effect was seen on the incidence of instrumental vaginal delivery (Table 61.12). Although these data relate to a considerably smaller number of women than the data on caesarean section, the typical odds ratio was 0.71 with a 95 per cent confidence interval of 0.56 to 0.91 (Table 61.12). Both of these statistically significant trends led to a sizeable and statistically highly significant reduction in the incidence of operative delivery overall (Table 61.13). The typical odds ratio for operative delivery was 0.67 with a 95 per cent confidence interval ranging from 0.54 to 0.82. From Tables 61.11 to 61.13 it will be noted that for some trials the total number of women for whom caesarean section rates were calculated differs from the number on which instrumental vaginal deliveries and operative deliveries are based. This is due to the fact that some investigators (for example, Lorenz et al. 1984) reported only whether women with failed induction of labour were ultimately delivered by caesarean section or vaginally, and not whether they had had a spontaneous or an instrumental vaginal delivery.

Only 7 trial reports (incorporating just over 500 women) provided data on the incidence of postpartum haemorrhage and/or the use of blood transfusion. None of the individual trials showed any statistically significant effect of the active policy. Overall, the data do not suggest that these outcomes are influenced by the use of prostaglandins for cervical ripening, but the confidence

Table 61.6 Effect of any prostaglandin (any route) vs. placebo (no treatment) for cervical ripening on hypertonus–hyperstimulation

Study	EXPT		CTRL		Odds ratio	Graph of odds ratios and confidence intervals
	n	(%)	n	(%)	(95% CI)	0.01 0.1 0.5 1 2 10 100
Friedman and Sachtleben (1975)	0/15	(0.00)	2/15	(13.33)	0.13 (0.01–2.12)	
Golbus and Creasy (1977)	2/25	(8.00)	1/25	(4.00)	2.00 (0.20–20.20)	
Laube *et al.* (1986)	1/30	(3.33)	0/15	(0.00)	4.48 (0.07–99.99)	
Bernstein *et al.* (1988)	3/206	(1.46)	7/202	(3.47)	0.43 (0.12–1.51)	
Weiss *et al.* (1975)	5/32	(15.63)	1/24	(4.17)	3.24 (0.59–17.68)	
Thiery *et al.* (1984)	1/81	(1.23)	1/40	(2.50)	0.46 (0.02–8.90)	
Noah *et al.* (1987)	32/416	(7.69)	12/404	(2.97)	2.53 (1.38–4.65)	
Yonekura *et al.* (1985)	2/25	(8.00)	1/23	(4.35)	1.84 (0.18–18.64)	
Trofatter *et al.* (1985)	1/30	(3.33)	1/29	(3.45)	0.97 (0.06–15.83)	
Lewis (1983)	0/22	(0.00)	0/22	(0.00)	1.00 (1.00–1.00)	
Typical odds ratio (95% confidence interval)					1.70 (1.06–2.72)	

interval is wide (typical odds ratio 0.89; 95 per cent confidence interval 0.47–1.71; Table 61.14).

Categorical data on Apgar scores at 1 and 5 minutes after birth, although available from relatively few trial reports, relate to about a thousand infants born after prostaglandin-induced cervical ripening. The typical odds ratios for both of these outcomes show no statistically significant influence of the prostaglandin treatment (Table 61.15). Although the trend is for a slight reduction in the incidence of low Apgar scores at 5 minutes after birth, this effect is compatible with chance (typical odds ratio 0.84; 95 per cent confidence interval 0.33–1.25). Extremely few trial reports provide data on the more substantive infant outcome measures, such as resuscitation of the newborn, admission to a special care nursery, and perinatal death (Tables 61.16 and 61.17). None of these outcome measures suggested any influence, good or bad, of cervical ripening, but the estimates are very imprecise. The 95 per cent confidence interval of the typical odds ratio for perinatal death, for example, ranged from 0.12 to 3.92 (Table 61.17). Only one of the many reports provided data on the incidence of neonatal hyperbilirubinaemia; the trial comprised only 48 infants and the outcome occurred with a similar frequency among infants born from mothers with and without prostaglandin administration (Table 61.16).

In summary, and with the reservations that should be

borne in mind, the data thus indicate that administration of prostaglandins for cervical ripening does indeed ripen the cervix. The treatment is also more likely than either placebo or no treatment to start labour; to obviate the need for formal induction with oxytocin; and to effect delivery within the period set for ripening the cervix.

The few data that are available do not suggest any consistent effect of prostaglandin pretreatment of the cervix before induction of labour on the use of analgesia.

On the negative side, administration of prostaglandins for cervical ripening increases the likelihood of (variously defined) 'uterine hypertonus' or 'hyperstimulation'. It may also increase the likelihood of fetal heart rate abnormalities, although this is not reflected in the pattern of operative deliveries.

Overall, cervical ripening with prostaglandins markedly reduces the likelihood of not being delivered within 12 hours from the start of induction, which is a major advantage with regard to providing continuity of care during labour and delivery (see Chapters 8 and 49). Also, fewer women will experience induction–delivery intervals in excess of 24 hours after prostaglandin treatment than without such treatment. Moreover, the likelihood of experiencing a vaginal delivery within 24 and within 48 hours after being induced is considerably higher in women pretreated with prostaglandins than in

Table 61.7 Effect of any prostaglandin (any route) vs. placebo (no treatment) for cervical ripening on fetal heart rate 'abnormalities'

Study	EXPT		CTRL		Odds ratio	Graph of odds ratios and confidence intervals
	n	(%)	*n*	(%)	(95% CI)	0.01 0.1 0.5 1 2 10 100
Friedman and Sachtleben (1975)	2/15	(13.33)	1/15	(6.67)	2.05 (0.20–21.36)	
Williams *et al.* (1985)	0/40	(0.00)	0/20	(0.00)	1.00 (1.00–1.00)	
Hutchon *et al.* (1980)	13/32	(40.63)	10/35	(28.57)	1.69 (0.62–4.61)	
Quinn *et al.* (1981)	1/15	(6.67)	0/15	(0.00)	7.39 (0.15–99.99)	
Bernstein *et al.* (1988)	11/206	(5.34)	3/202	(1.49)	3.19 (1.10–9.26)	
Weiss *et al.* (1975)	0/32	(0.00)	0/24	(0.00)	1.00 (1.00–1.00)	
Thiery *et al.* (1984)	7/81	(8.64)	5/40	(12.50)	0.65 (0.18–2.30)	
Heinzl *et al.* (1980)	6/60	(10.00)	4/60	(6.67)	1.54 (0.42–5.60)	
Buchanan *et al.* (1984)	4/38	(10.53)	2/35	(5.71)	1.88 (0.36–9.87)	
Cabrol *et al.* (1988)	37/110	(33.64)	35/107	(32.71)	1.04 (0.59–1.83)	
Graves *et al.* (1985)	3/60	(5.00)	0/20	(0.00)	3.93 (0.28–55.42)	
Roberts *et al.* (1986)	1/27	(3.70)	1/24	(4.17)	0.89 (0.05–14.65)	
Noah *et al.* (1987)	55/416	(13.22)	47/404	(11.63)	1.16 (0.76–1.75)	
Valentine (1977)	1/30	(3.33)	0/15	(0.00)	4.48 (0.07–99.99)	
Typical odds ratio (95% confidence interval)					1.29 (0.97–1.70)	

Table 61.8 Effect of any prostaglandin (any route) vs. placebo (no treatment) for cervical ripening on use of analgesia

Study	EXPT		CTRL		Odds ratio	Graph of odds ratios and confidence intervals
	n	(%)	*n*	(%)	(95% CI)	0.01 0.1 0.5 1 2 10 100
MacLennan and Green (1979)	25/40	(62.50)	21/40	(52.50)	1.50 (0.62–3.62)	
Lorenz *et al.* (1984)	7/21	(33.33)	11/23	(47.83)	0.56 (0.17–1.83)	
Hirse *et al.* (1985)	23/25	(92.00)	19/25	(76.00)	3.21 (0.72–14.35)	
Typical odds ratio (95% confidence interval)					1.29 (0.68–2.45)	

Table 61.8—*continued* Effect of any prostaglandin (any route) vs. placebo (no treatment) for cervical ripening on use of epidural analgesia

Study	EXPT		CTRL		Odds ratio	Graph of odds ratios and confidence intervals						
	n	(%)	n	(%)	(95% CI)	0.01	0.1	0.5	1	2	10	100
MacKenzie and Embrey (1979)	18/32	(56.25)	13/16	(81.25)	0.34 (0.10–1.19)							
MacLennan and Green (1979)	12/40	(30.00)	15/40	(37.50)	0.72 (0.29–1.80)							
Cabrol et al. (1988)	25/110	(22.73)	34/107	(31.78)	0.63 (0.35–1.15)							
Murphy et al. (1980)	21/165	(12.73)	19/100	(19.00)	0.61 (0.31–1.23)							
Keirse et al. (1985)	8/25	(32.00)	12/25	(48.00)	0.52 (0.17–1.60)							
Typical odds ratio (95% confidence interval)					0.60 (0.41–0.86)							

Table 61.9 Effect of any prostaglandin (any route) vs. placebo (no treatment) for cervical ripening on not delivered 12 hours after induction

Study	EXPT		CTRL		Odds ratio	Graph of odds ratios and confidence intervals						
	n	(%)	n	(%)	(95% CI)	0.01	0.1	0.5	1	2	10	100
MacLennan and Green (1979)	3/40	(7.50)	0/40	(0.00)	7.78 (0.79–77.04)							
Wingerup et al. (1978)	0/10	(0.00)	9/10	(90.00)	0.03 (0.01–0.18)							
Heinzl et al. (1980)	40/60	(66.67)	56/60	(93.33)	0.19 (0.08–0.47)							
Lorenz et al. (1984)	12/21	(57.14)	13/23	(56.52)	1.03 (0.31–3.34)							
Keirse et al. (1985)	2/25	(8.00)	20/25	(80.00)	0.06 (0.02–0.17)							
Valentine (1977)	12/30	(40.00)	13/15	(86.67)	0.16 (0.05–0.54)							
Bung et al. (1986)	9/41	(21.95)	16/39	(41.03)	0.42 (0.16–1.07)							
Typical odds ratio (95% confidence interval)					0.24 (0.15–0.37)							

Effect of any prostaglandin (any route) vs. placebo (no treatment) for cervical ripening on not delivered 24 hours after induction

Study	EXPT		CTRL		Odds ratio							
Pearce (1977)	1/25	(4.00)	1/23	(4.34)	0.92 (0.06–15.16)							
Wingerup et al. (1978)	0/10	(0.00)	7/10	(70.00)	0.05 (0.01–0.32)							
Weiss et al. (1975)	3/32	(9.38)	6/24	(25.00)	0.32 (0.08–1.34)							
Heinzl et al. (1980)	18/60	(30.00)	47/60	(78.33)	0.15 (0.07–0.30)							
Keirse et al. (1985)	2/25	(8.00)	17/25	(68.00)	0.08 (0.03–0.26)							
Valentine (1977)	3/30	(10.00)	8/15	(53.33)	0.10 (0.02–0.42)							
Typical odds ratio (95% confidence interval)					0.13 (0.08–0.22)							

Table 61.10 Effect of any prostaglandin (any route) vs. placebo (no treatment) for cervical ripening on no vaginal delivery within 12 hours after induction

Study	EXPT		CTRL		Odds ratio	Graph of odds ratios and confidence intervals
	n	(%)	n	(%)	(95% CI)	0.01 0.1 0.5 1 2 10 100
Wingerup et al. (1978)	0/10	(0.00)	9/10	(90.00)	0.03 (0.01–0.18)	
Lorenz et al. (1984)	15/21	(71.43)	14/23	(60.87)	1.58 (0.46–5.44)	
Keirse et al. (1985)	4/25	(16.00)	20/25	(80.00)	0.08 (0.03–0.24)	
Valentine (1977)	16/30	(53.33)	15/15	(100.0)	0.12 (0.03–0.45)	
Lewis (1983)	3/22	(13.64)	14/22	(63.64)	0.13 (0.04–0.42)	
Typical odds ratio (95% confidence interval)					0.16 (0.09–0.29)	

Effect of any prostaglandin (any route) vs. placebo (no treatment) for cervical ripening on no vaginal delivery within 12 hours after induction

Study	EXPT		CTRL		Odds ratio	Graph
Walker and Gordon (1983)	4/15	(26.67)	2/15	(13.33)	2.24 (0.39–13.00)	
Wingerup et al. (1978)	0/10	(0.00)	7/10	(70.00)	0.05 (0.01–0.32)	
Valentine (1977)	9/30	(30.00)	12/15	(80.00)	0.14 (0.04–0.48)	
Lewis (1983)	3/22	(13.64)	6/22	(27.27)	0.44 (0.10–1.88)	
Typical odds ratio 95% confidence interval)					0.27 (0.13–0.57)	

women who received no such treatment. The caesarean section rate among prostaglandin-treated women was statistically significantly reduced in comparison with women in the control groups, although this reduction in odds may be from as little as 1 per cent to as much as 30 per cent. The need for instrumental vaginal delivery was reduced even more, so that the overall odds of operative delivery were reduced by between 15 and 45 per cent.

4.2 Type of prostaglandin

More than 80 per cent of the trials (and about 95 per cent of the women involved in them) discussed in the preceding section have dealt with prostaglandin E_2. Only one study (Roberts et al. 1986) dealt with PGE_1, and there is no evidence that this compound acts differently from PGE_2 on either the pregnant cervix or myometrium (Keirse 1975). Five trials included in the preceding section dealt with prostaglandin $F_{2\alpha}$; it is, therefore, useful to examine whether the conclusions reached in respect of any prostaglandin also apply to this particular compound.

In the early days of the clinical application of prostaglandins in obstetrics, most studies were conducted with $PGF_{2\alpha}$, which was the first prostaglandin compound tested for induction of labour (Karim et al. 1968). Later, especially after the initial problems of shelf instability of PGE_2 had been overcome, $PGF_{2\alpha}$ was largely replaced by PGE_2, which has a uterotonic potency nearly 10 times greater than $PGF_{2\alpha}$ and is therefore less likely to cause side-effects through influences on other organ systems (see Chapter 62). Cervical ripening as an objective was pursued later than induction of labour and most studies were therefore conducted with PGE_2. In some countries, however, only $PGF_{2\alpha}$ and not PGE_2 is available for clinical use in obstetrics. It is therefore pertinent to examine whether similar effects can be obtained with $PGF_{2\alpha}$.

Five controlled trials have compared $PGF_{2\alpha}$ with placebo or no treatment for ripening of the unfavourable cervix prior to induction of labour (MacKenzie and Embrey 1979; MacLennan and Green 1979; Heinzl et al. 1980; Murphy et al. 1980; Quinn et al. 1981). The characteristics of these studies, which have used dif-

Table 61.11 Effect of any prostaglandin (any route) vs. placebo (no treatment) for cervical ripening on caesarean section

Study	EXPT n	(%)	CTRL n	(%)	Odds ratio (95% CI)	Graph of odds ratios and confidence intervals
MacKenzie and Embrey (1979)	4/32	(12.50)	3/16	(18.75)	0.61 (0.11–3.29)	
MacLennan and Green (1979)	2/40	(5.00)	3/40	(7.50)	0.66 (0.11–3.97)	
Hutchon et al. (1980)	11/32	(34.38)	13/35	(37.14)	0.89 (0.33–2.40)	
Quinn et al. (1981)	1/15	(6.67)	2/10	(20.00)	0.30 (0.03–3.32)	
Prins et al. (1983)	4/15	(26.67)	7/15	(46.67)	0.43 (0.10–1.87)	
MacKenzie and Embrey (1977)	0/12	(0.00)	0/12	(0.00)	1.00 (1.00–1.00)	
Laube et al. (1986)	8/30	(26.67)	1/15	(6.67)	3.39 (0.73–15.71)	
Bernstein et al. (1988)	55/206	(26.70)	67/202	(33.17)	0.74 (0.48–1.12)	
Ulmsten et al. (1985)	10/38	(26.32)	6/20	(30.00)	0.83 (0.25–2.77)	
Golbus and Creasy (1977)	1/25	(4.00)	2/25	(8.00)	0.50 (0.05–5.03)	
Pearce (1977)	1/25	(4.00)	1/23	(4.35)	0.92 (0.06–15.16)	
Williams et al. (1985)	13/40	(32.50)	7/20	(35.00)	0.90 (0.29–2.77)	
Nimrod et al. (1984)	4/30	(13.33)	0/15	(0.00)	5.00 (0.58–43.09)	
Wingerup et al. (1978)	0/10	(0.00)	3/10	(30.00)	0.11 (0.01–1.17)	
Heinzl et al. (1980)	3/60	(5.00)	6/60	(10.00)	0.49 (0.13–1.89)	
Fenton et al. (1985)	2/15	(13.33)	5/15	(33.33)	0.34 (0.06–1.79)	
Weiss et al. (1975)	1/32	(3.13)	1/24	(4.17)	0.74 (0.04–12.55)	
Thiery et al. (1984)	1/81	(1.23)	0/39	(0.00)	4.40 (0.07–99.99)	
Buchanan et al. (1984)	15/38	(39.47)	17/39	(43.59)	0.85 (0.34–2.08)	
Cabrol et al. (1988)	30/110	(27.27)	23/107	(21.50)	1.37 (0.74–2.53)	
Lorenz et al. (1984)	10/21	(47.62)	7/23	(30.43)	2.03 (0.61–6.75)	
Murphy et al. (1980)	10/165	(6.06)	9/100	(9.00)	0.64 (0.25–1.68)	
Graves et al. (1985)	16/60	(26.67)	3/20	(15.00)	1.89 (0.58–6.16)	
Roberts et al. (1986)	3/27	(11.11)	8/24	(33.33)	0.28 (0.07–1.04)	
Noah et al. (1987)	67/413	(16.22)	84/403	(20.84)	0.74 (0.52–1.05)	
Yonekura et al. (1985)	10/25	(40.00)	6/25	(24.00)	2.06 (0.63–6.67)	
Trofatter et al. (1985)	8/30	(26.67)	9/29	(31.03)	0.81 (0.27–2.48)	
Lewis (1983)	3/22	(13.64)	6/22	(27.27)	0.44 (0.10–1.88)	
Jagani et al. (1984)	5/15	(33.33)	2/16	(12.50)	3.17 (0.60–16.62)	
Shepherd et al. (1976)	1/15	(6.67)	1/15	(6.67)	1.00 (0.06–16.79)	
Valentine (1977)	7/30	(23.33)	7/15	(46.67)	0.34 (0.09–1.30)	
Typical odds ratio (95% confidence interval)					0.83 (0.69–0.99)	

Graph scale markers: 0.01, 0.1, 0.5, 1, 2, 10, 100

Table 61.12 Effect of any prostaglandin (any route) vs. placebo (no treatment) for cervical ripening on instrumental vaginal delivery

Study	EXPT		CTRL		Odds ratio	Graph of odds ratios and confidence intervals
	n	(%)	*n*	(%)	(95% CI)	0.01 0.1 0.5 1 2 10 100
Ulmsten *et al.* (1985)	7/38	(18.42)	6/20	(30.00)	0.52 (0.14–1.88)	
MacLennan and Green (1979)	12/40	(30.00)	16/40	(40.00)	0.65 (0.26–1.61)	
Quinn *et al.* (1981)	6/15	(40.00)	7/10	(70.00)	0.32 (0.07–1.51)	
Bernstein *et al.* (1988)	49/206	(23.79)	51/202	(25.25)	0.92 (0.59–1.45)	
Wingerup *et al.* (1978)	0/10	(0.00)	1/10	(10.00)	0.14 (0.00–6.82)	
Heinzl *et al.* (1980)	5/60	(8.33)	5/60	(8.33)	1.00 (0.28–3.63)	
Buchanan *et al.* (1984)	1/38	(2.63)	2/38	(5.26)	0.50 (0.05–5.00)	
Lorenz *et al.* (1984)	2/18	(11.11)	6/19	(31.58)	0.31 (0.07–1.45)	
Murphy *et al.* (1980)	32/165	(19.39)	33/100	(33.00)	0.48 (0.27–0.86)	
Keirse *et al.* (1985)	5/25	(20.00)	6/25	(24.00)	0.80 (0.21–2.99)	
Kieback *et al.* (1986)	5/50	(10.00)	10/50	(20.00)	0.46 (0.15–1.37)	
Yonekura *et al.* (1985)	1/25	(4.00)	4/24	(16.67)	0.26 (0.04–1.61)	
Shepherd *et al.* (1976)	8/15	(53.33)	7/15	(46.67)	1.29 (0.32–5.29)	
Valentine (1977)	11/30	(36.67)	4/15	(26.67)	1.55 (0.42–5.70)	
Trofatter *et al.* (1985)	6/30	(20.00)	8/29	(27.59)	0.66 (0.20–2.18)	
Kristoffersen *et al.* (1986)	7/25	(28.00)	5/25	(20.00)	1.54 (0.43–5.56)	
Pulle *et al.* (1986)	1/25	(4.00)	2/25	(8.00)	0.50 (0.05–5.03)	
Sung *et al.* (1986)	8/41	(19.51)	7/39	(17.95)	1.11 (0.36–3.38)	
Typical odds ratio (95% confidence interval)					0.71 (0.56–0.91)	

ferent doses and different routes of administration, are shown in Table 61.18. The data shown in Table 61.19) indicate that $PGF_{2\alpha}$ administered by various routes does indeed affect cervical ripening, in that the typical odds ratio for a poor increase in cervical score was 0.18 (95 per cent confidence interval 0.10–0.30), a finding which is similar to that observed for all prostaglandins (Table 61.4). The active treatment also resulted in a higher incidence of both labour and delivery occurring before formal induction of labour was undertaken (Table 61.19). Likewise, the incidence of not being delivered within 12 and within 24 hours after induction

of labour was statistically significantly lower in $PGF_{2\alpha}$-treated women than in controls (Table 61.19). As observed with any prostaglandin (Table 61.6), use of $PGF_{2\alpha}$ for cervical ripening before induction also resulted in a statistically significantly higher incidence of 'uterine hypertonus' or 'hyperstimulation' (Table 61.19).

All five studies using $PGF_{2\alpha}$ reported fewer caesarean sections among women treated with $PGF_{2\alpha}$ than among controls (Table 61.20). This is consistent with the data on any prostaglandin used for cervical ripening (Table 61.11), although the data did not reach statistical sig-

Table 61.13 Effect of any prostaglandin (any route) vs. placebo (no treatment) for cervical ripening on operative delivery

Study	EXPT n	(%)	CTRL n	(%)	Odds ratio (95% CI)	Graph of odds ratios and confidence intervals
Ulmsten et al. (1985)	17/38	(44.74)	12/20	(60.00)	0.55 (0.19–1.61)	
MacLennan and Green (1979)	14/40	(35.00)	19/40	(47.50)	0.60 (0.25–1.46)	
Quinn et al. (1981)	7/15	(46.67)	9/10	(90.00)	0.16 (0.03–0.84)	
Bernstein et al. (1988)	104/206	(50.49)	118/202	(58.42)	0.73 (0.49–1.07)	
Wingerup et al. (1978)	0/10	(0.00)	4/10	(40.00)	0.09 (0.01–0.79)	
Heinzl et al. (1980)	8/60	(13.33)	11/60	(18.33)	0.69 (0.26–1.83)	
Buchanan et al. (1984)	16/38	(42.11)	19/38	(50.00)	0.73 (0.30–1.79)	
Lorenz et al. (1984)	12/18	(66.67)	13/19	(68.42)	0.93 (0.24–3.60)	
Murphy et al. (1980)	42/165	(25.45)	42/100	(42.00)	0.47 (0.27–0.80)	
Keirse et al. (1985)	7/25	(28.00)	8/25	(32.00)	0.83 (0.25–2.75)	
Kieback et al. (1986)	10/50	(20.00)	16/50	(32.00)	0.54 (0.22–1.31)	
Yonekura et al. (1985)	11/25	(44.00)	10/24	(41.67)	1.10 (0.36–3.37)	
Shepherd et al. (1976)	9/15	(60.00)	8/15	(53.33)	1.30 (0.31–5.38)	
Valentine (1977)	18/30	(60.00)	11/15	(73.33)	0.57 (0.16–2.04)	
Trofatter et al. (1985)	14/30	(46.67)	17/29	(58.62)	0.62 (0.23–1.72)	
Kristoffersen et al. (1986)	11/25	(44.00)	8/25	(32.00)	1.65 (0.53–5.10)	
Pulle et al. (1986)	4/25	(16.00)	5/25	(20.00)	0.77 (0.18–3.20)	
Bung et al. (1986)	8/41	(19.51)	7/39	(17.95)	1.11 (0.36–3.38)	
Typical odds ratio (95% confidence interval)					0.67 (0.54–0.82)	

Table 61.14 Effect of any prostaglandin (any route) vs. placebo (no treatment) for cervical ripening on postpartum haemorrhage

Study	EXPT n	(%)	CTRL n	(%)	Odds ratio (95% CI)	Graph of odds ratios and confidence intervals
Thiery et al. (1984)	1/81	(1.23)	0/40	(0.00)	4.45 (0.07–99.99)	
Cabrol et al. (1988)	4/110	(3.64)	1/107	(0.93)	3.30 (0.56–19.38)	
Buchanan et al. (1984)	5/38	(13.16)	3/35	(8.57)	1.59 (0.37–6.84)	
Keirse et al. (1985)	8/25	(32.00)	10/25	(40.00)	0.71 (0.23–2.23)	
Yonekura et al. (1985)	3/25	(12.00)	5/23	(21.74)	0.50 (0.11–2.26)	
Kristoffersen et al. (1986)	1/25	(4.00)	3/25	(12.00)	0.34 (0.05–2.61)	
Pulle et al. (1986)	0/25	(0.00)	1/25	(4.00)	0.14 (0.00–6.82)	
Typical odds ratio (95% confidence interval)					0.89 (0.47–1.71)	

Graph axis: 0.01 0.1 0.5 1 2 10 100

Table 61.15 Effect of any prostaglandin (any route) vs. placebo (no treatment) for cervical ripening on low Apgar score at 1 minute

Study	EXPT n	(%)	CTRL n	(%)	Odds ratio (95% CI)	Graph of odds ratios and confidence intervals
Golbus and Creasy (1977)	4/25	(16.00)	2/25	(8.00)	2.10 (0.39–11.37)	
Pearce (1977)	7/25	(28.00)	8/23	(34.78)	0.73 (0.22–2.46)	
MacKenzie and Embrey (1979)	2/32	(6.25)	2/16	(12.50)	0.45 (0.05–3.85)	
Bernstein et al. (1988)	10/206	(4.85)	11/202	(5.45)	0.89 (0.37–2.13)	
Thiery et al. (1984)	14/81	(17.28)	12/40	(30.00)	0.47 (0.19–1.19)	
Cabrol et al. (1988)	19/110	(17.27)	21/107	(19.63)	0.86 (0.43–1.70)	
Lorenz et al. (1984)	5/21	(23.81)	7/22	(31.82)	0.68 (0.18–2.53)	
Murphy et al. (1980)	5/165	(3.03)	3/100	(3.00)	1.01 (0.24–4.30)	
Noah et al. (1987)	53/401	(13.22)	38/397	(9.57)	1.43 (0.93–2.22)	
Yonekura et al. (1985)	4/25	(16.00)	6/23	(26.09)	0.55 (0.14–2.18)	
Lewis (1983)	0/22	(0.00)	1/22	(4.55)	0.14 (0.00–6.82)	
Typical odds ratio (95% confidence interval)					0.98 (0.74–1.30)	

Graph axis: 0.01 0.1 0.5 1 2 10 100

Table 61.15—*continued* Effect of any prostaglandin (any route) vs. placebo (no treatment) for cervical ripening on low Apgar score at 5 minutes

Study	EXPT		CTRL		Odds ratio	Graph of odds ratios and confidence intervals
	n	(%)	n	(%)	(95% CI)	0.01 0.1 0.5 1 2 10 100
Ulmsten *et al.* (1985)	0/38	(0.00)	0/20	(0.00)	1.00 (1.00–1.00)	
Golbus and Creasy (1977)	2/25	(8.00)	0/25	(0.00)	7.70 (0.47–99.99)	
Pearce (1977)	2/25	(8.00)	4/23	(17.39)	0.43 (0.08–2.35)	
Prins *et al.* (1983)	0/14	(0.00)	0/15	(0.00)	1.00 (1.00–1.00)	
Bernstein *et al.* (1988)	1/206	(0.49)	0/202	(0.00)	7.25 (0.14–99.99)	
Wingerup *et al.* (1978)	0/10	(0.00)	0/10	(0.00)	1.00 (1.00–1.00)	
Weiss *et al.* (1975)	0/32	(0.00)	0/24	(0.00)	1.00 (1.00–1.00)	
Thiery *et al.* (1984)	4/81	(4.94)	4/40	(10.00)	0.44 (0.10–2.02)	
Heinzl *et al.* (1980)	0/60	(0.00)	0/60	(0.00)	1.00 (1.00–1.00)	
Buchanan *et al.* (1984)	0/38	(0.00)	1/35	(2.86)	0.12 (0.00–6.28)	
Lorenz *et al.* (1984)	1/21	(4.76)	1/22	(4.55)	1.05 (0.06–17.36)	
Graves *et al.* (1985)	2/60	(3.33)	1/20	(5.00)	0.63 (0.04–8.94)	
Noah *et al.* (1987)	5/401	(1.25)	7/397	(1.76)	0.71 (0.23–2.21)	
Yonekura *et al.* (1985)	0/25	(0.00)	2/23	(8.70)	0.12 (0.01–1.96)	
Shepherd *et al.* (1976)	0/15	(0.00)	0/15	(0.00)	1.00 (1.00–1.00)	
Lewis (1983)	0/22	(0.00)	0/22	(0.00)	1.00 (1.00–1.00)	
Typical odds ratio (95% confidence interval)					0.64 (0.33–1.25)	

Table 61.16 Effect of any prostaglandin (any route) vs. placebo (no treatment) for cervical ripening on resuscitation of newborn

Study	EXPT		CTRL		Odds ratio	Graph of odds ratios and confidence intervals
	n	(%)	n	(%)	(95% CI)	0.01 0.1 0.5 1 2 10 10
Ulmsten *et al.* (1985)	0/38	(0.00)	0/20	(0.00)	1.00 (1.00–1.00)	
Friedman and Sachtleben (1975)	0/15	(0.00)	0/15	(0.00)	1.00 (1.00–1.00)	
Lorenz *et al.* (1984)	7/21	(33.33)	9/22	(40.91)	0.73 (0.21–2.47)	
Keirse *et al.* (1985)	1/25	(4.00)	2/25	(8.00)	0.50 (0.05–5.03)	
Typical odds ratio (95% confidence interval)					0.67 (0.23–1.98)	

Table 61.16—*continued* Effect of any prostaglandin (any route) vs. placebo (no treatment) for cervical ripening on admission to special care nursery

Study	EXPT		CTRL		Odds ratio	Graph of odds ratios and confidence intervals
	n	(%)	n	(%)	(95% CI)	0.01 0.1 0.5 1 2 10 100
Friedman and Sachtleben (1975)	0/15	(0.00)	0/15	(0.00)	1.00 (1.00–1.00)	
Nimrod et al. (1984)	1/30	(3.33)	2/15	(13.33)	0.21 (0.02–2.42)	
Typical odds ratio (95% confidence interval)					0.21 (0.02–2.42)	

Effect of any prostaglandin (any route) vs. placebo (no treatment) for cervical ripening on jaundice–hyperbilirubinaemia

	EXPT		CTRL		Odds ratio	
Yonekura et al. (1985)	2/25	(8.00)	2/23	(8.70)	0.91 (0.12–6.95)	
Typical odds ratio (95% confidence interval)					0.91 (0.12–6.95)	

Table 16.17 Effect of any prostaglandin (any route) vs. placebo (no treatment) for cervical ripening on perinatal death (excluding lethal malformations)

Study	EXPT		CTRL		Odds ratio	Graph of odds ratios and confidence intervals
	n	(%)	n	(%)	(95% CI)	0.01 0.1 0.5 1 2 10 100
...msten et al. (1985)	0/38	(0.00)	0/20	(0.00)	1.00 (1.00–1.00)	
...iedman and Sachtleben (1975)	0/15	(0.00)	0/15	(0.00)	1.00 (1.00–1.00)	
...arce (1977)	0/25	(0.00)	0/23	(0.00)	1.00 (1.00–1.00)	
...mrod et al. (1984)	0/30	(0.00)	0/14	(0.00)	1.00 (1.00–1.00)	
...inn et al. (1981)	1/15	(6.67)	0/15	(0.00)	7.39 (0.15–99.99)	
...ns et al. (1983)	0/14	(0.00)	0/15	(0.00)	1.00 (1.00–1.00)	
...cKenzie and Embrey (1977)	0/12	(0.00)	0/12	(0.00)	1.00 (1.00–1.00)	
...abe et al. (1986)	0/30	(0.00)	0/15	(0.00)	1.00 (1.00–1.00)	
...tchon et al. (1980)	0/31	(0.00)	1/35	(2.86)	0.15 (0.00–7.70)	
...nstein et al. (1988)	1/206	(0.49)	0/202	(0.00)	7.25 (0.14–99.99)	
...ery et al. (1984)	0/81	(0.00)	0/40	(0.00)	1.00 (1.00–1.00)	
...nzl et al. (1980)	0/60	(0.00)	0/60	(0.00)	1.00 (1.00–1.00)	
...rol et al. (1988)	0/110	(0.00)	1/107	(0.93)	0.13 (0.00–6.63)	
...th et al. (1987)	0/406	(0.00)	1/404	(0.25)	0.13 (0.00–6.79)	
...pherd et al. (1976)	0/15	(0.00)	0/15	(0.00)	1.00 (1.00–1.00)	
...ical odds ratio (...% confidence interval)					0.68 (0.12–3.92)	

Table 61.18 Characteristics of the controlled evaluations of prostaglandin $F_{2\alpha}$ for cervical ripening

Authors and dates	Allocation	Treatments compared dose of $PGF_{2\alpha}$ and type of gel used	No. treated PG	No. treated Placebo	Cervix score + cut-off	Interval to induction + method of induction
MacKenzie and Embrey (1979)	double-blind	25 mg vs. placebo gel methylhydroxyethyl cellulose vaginally	16 : nulliparae	16	Calder <4	15½ hours amniotomy + oxytocin
MacLennan and Green (1979)	sealed envelopes	50 mg vs. placebo gel methyl cellulose vaginally	40 : mixed parity	40	Calder not stated	15 hours by persons unaware of treatment received
Heinzl et al. (1980)	double-blind	5 mg vs. placebo gel endocervically in home-made gel	31 : nulliparae 31 : multiparae	32 30	Calder <4	12 hours oxytocin if 'feasible' others were sent home
Murphy et al. (1980)	double-blind	1.5 mg vs. placebo gel 3.0 mg 10 mg methylhydroxyethyl cellulose vaginally	55 : 55 : 55 : mixed parity	100	Calder <4	12 hours amniotomy + oxytocin
Quinn et al. (1981)	double-blind	10 mg vs. placebo gel extra-amniotically in methylhydroxyethyl cellulose gel	15 : nulliparae	10	Calder <4	12 hours amniotomy + oxytocin

Table 61.19 Effect of $PGF_{2\alpha}$ (any route) for cervical ripening on poor increase in cervix score

Study	EXPT n	EXPT (%)	CTRL n	CTRL (%)	Odds ratio (95% CI)	Graph of odds ratios and confidence intervals
MacKenzie and Embrey (1979)	11/16	(68.75)	12/16	(75.00)	0.74 (0.16–3.38)	
MacLennan and Green (1979)	3/40	(7.50)	20/40	(50.00)	0.13 (0.05–0.34)	
Heinzl et al. (1980)	13/60	(21.67)	41/60	(68.33)	0.15 (0.08–0.32)	
Typical odds ratio (95% confidence interval)					0.18 (0.10–0.30)	

Effect of $PGF_{2\alpha}$ (any route) for cervical ripening on labour onset during ripening

MacKenzie and Embrey (1979)	2/16	(12.50)	0/16	(0.00)	7.90 (0.47–99.99)	
MacLennan and Green (1979)	20/40	(50.00)	3/40	(7.50)	7.76 (2.96–20.31)	
Quinn et al. (1981)	4/15	(26.67)	0/10	(0.00)	6.72 (0.79–57.01)	
Heinzl et al. (1980)	20/60	(33.33)	4/60	(6.67)	5.22 (2.14–12.73)	
Murphy et al. (1980)	19/165	(11.52)	7/100	(7.00)	1.66 (0.72–3.83)	
Typical odds ratio (95% confidence interval)					3.99 (2.44–6.52)	

Graph scale: 0.01 0.1 0.5 1 2 10 100

Table 61.19—*continued* Effect of PGF$_{2\alpha}$ (any route) for cervical ripening on delivered during ripening

Study	EXPT		CTRL		Odds ratio	Graph of odds ratios and confidence intervals
	n	(%)	*n*	(%)	(95% CI)	0.01 0.1 0.5 1 2 10 100
MacLennan and Green (1979)	13/40	(32.50)	3/40	(7.50)	4.68 (1.57–13.90)	
Heinzl *et al.* (1980)	20/60	(33.33)	4/60	(6.67)	5.22 (2.14–12.73)	
Typical odds ratio (95% confidence interval)					5.00 (2.51–9.96)	

Effect of PGF$_{2\alpha}$ (any route) for cervical ripening on hypertonus and/or hyperstimulation

MacKenzie and Embrey (1979)	1/16	(6.25)	0/16	(0.00)	7.39 (0.15–99.99)	
Quinn *et al.* (1981)	1/15	(6.67)	0/10	(0.00)	5.29 (0.10–99.99)	
Heinzl *et al.* (1980)	6/60	(10.00)	0/60	(0.00)	8.07 (1.57–41.38)	
Typical odds ratio (95% confidence interval)					7.57 (1.84–31.06)	

Effect of PGF$_{2\alpha}$ (any route) for cervical ripening on use of epidural analgesia

MacKenzie and Embrey (1979)	11/16	(68.75)	13/16	(81.25)	0.52 (0.11–2.53)	
MacLennan and Green (1979)	12/40	(30.00)	15/40	(37.50)	0.72 (0.29–1.80)	
Murphy *et al.* (1980)	21/165	(12.73)	19/100	(19.00)	0.61 (0.31–1.23)	
Typical odds ratio (95% confidence interval)					0.63 (0.38–1.07)	

Effect of PGF$_{2\alpha}$ (any route) for cervical ripening on not delivered within 12 hours

MacKenzie and Embrey (1979)	7/16	(43.75)	10/16	(62.50)	0.48 (0.12–1.89)	
MacLennan and Green (1979)	3/40	(7.50)	0/40	(0.00)	7.78 (0.79–77.04)	
Heinzl *et al.* (1980)	40/60	(66.67)	56/60	(93.33)	0.19 (0.08–0.47)	
Typical odds ratio (95% confidence interval)					0.35 (0.17–0.71)	

Effect of PGF$_{2\alpha}$ (any route) for cervical ripening on not delivered within 24 hours

Heinzl *et al.* (1980)	18/60	(30.00)	47/60	(78.33)	0.15 (0.07–0.30)	
Typical odds ratio (95% confidence interval)					0.15 (0.07–0.30)	

Table 61.20 Effect of PGF$_{2a}$ (any route) for cervical ripening on caesarean section

Study	EXPT		CTRL		Odds ratio	Graph of odds ratios and confidence intervals
	n	(%)	n	(%)	(95% CI)	0.01 0.1 0.5 1 2 10 100
MacKenzie and Embrey (1979)	2/16	(12.50)	3/16	(18.75)	0.63 (0.10–4.13)	
MacLennan and Green (1979)	2/40	(5.00)	3/40	(7.50)	0.66 (0.11–3.97)	
Quinn et al. (1981)	1/15	(6.67)	2/10	(20.00)	0.30 (0.03–3.32)	
Heinzl et al. (1980)	3/60	(5.00)	6/60	(10.00)	0.49 (0.13–1.89)	
Murphy et al. (1980)	10/165	(6.06)	9/100	(9.00)	0.64 (0.25–1.68)	
Typical odds ratio (95% confidence interval)					0.57 (0.30–1.09)	

Effect of PGF$_{2a}$ (any route) for cervical ripening on instrumental vaginal delivery

MacLennan and Green (1979)	12/40	(30.00)	16/40	(40.00)	0.65 (0.26–1.61)	
Quinn et al. (1981)	6/15	(40.00)	7/10	(70.00)	0.32 (0.07–1.51)	
Heinzl et al. (1980)	5/60	(8.33)	5/60	(8.33)	1.00 (0.28–3.63)	
Murphy et al. (1980)	32/165	(19.39)	33/100	(33.00)	0.48 (0.27–0.86)	
Typical odds ratio (95% confidence interval)					0.54 (0.35–0.84)	

Table 61.21 Effect of PGF$_{2a}$ (any route) for cervical ripening on low Apgar score at 1 minute

Study	EXPT		CTRL		Odds ratio	Graph of odds ratios and confidence intervals
	n	(%)	n	(%)	(95% CI)	0.01 0.1 0.5 1 2 10 100
MacKenzie and Embrey (1979)	1/16	(6.25)	2/16	(12.50)	0.49 (0.05–5.09)	
Murphy et al. (1980)	5/165	(3.03)	3/100	(3.00)	1.01 (0.24–4.30)	
Typical odds ratio (95% confidence interval)					0.83 (0.24–2.83)	

Effect of PGF$_{2a}$ (any route) for cervical ripening on low Apgar score at 5 minutes

Heinzl et al. (1980)	0/60	(0.00)	0/60	(0.00)	1.00 (1.00–1.00)	
Typical odds ratio (95% confidence interval)					1.00 (1.00–1.00)	

Effect of PGF$_{2a}$ (any route) for cervical ripening on fetal death post entry

Quinn et al. (1981)	1/15	(6.67)	0/10	(0.00)	5.29 (0.10–99.99)	
Heinzl et al. (1980)	0/60	(0.00)	0/60	(0.00)	1.00 (1.00–1.00)	
Typical odds ratio (95% confidence interval)					5.29 (0.10–99.99)	

Table 61.22 Effect of vaginal PGE vs. PGF for cervical ripening on labour onset during ripening

Study	EXPT n	(%)	CTRL n	(%)	Odds ratio (95% CI)	Graph of odds ratios and confidence intervals (0.01 0.1 0.5 1 2 10 100)
MacKenzie and Embrey (1979)	11/16	(68.75)	2/16	(12.50)	9.57 (2.39–38.39)	
Typical odds ratio (95% confidence interval)					9.57 (2.39–38.39)	

Effect of vaginal PGE vs. PGF for cervical ripening on failed induction

Study	EXPT n	(%)	CTRL n	(%)	Odds ratio (95% CI)	
Neilson et al. (1983)	4/38	(10.53)	8/37	(21.62)	0.44 (0.13–1.51)	
Typical odds ratio (95% confidence interval)					0.44 (0.13–1.51)	

Effect of vaginal PGE vs. PGF for cervical ripening on caesarean section

Study	EXPT n	(%)	CTRL n	(%)	Odds ratio (95% CI)	
MacKenzie and Embrey (1979)	2/16	(12.50)	2/16	(12.50)	1.00 (0.13–7.86)	
Neilson et al. (1983)	9/38	(23.68)	9/37	(24.32)	0.97 (0.34–2.77)	
Typical odds ratio (95% confidence interval)					0.97 (0.38–2.48)	

Effect of vaginal PGE vs. PGF for cervical ripening on instrumental vaginal delivery

Study	EXPT n	(%)	CTRL n	(%)	Odds ratio (95% CI)	
Neilson et al. (1983)	17/38	(44.74)	25/37	(67.57)	0.40 (0.16–0.99)	
Typical odds ratio (95% confidence interval)					0.40 (0.16–0.99)	

Effect of vaginal PGE vs. PGF for cervical ripening on operative delivery

Study	EXPT n	(%)	CTRL n	(%)	Odds ratio (95% CI)	
Neilson et al. (1983)	28/38	(73.68)	34/37	(91.89)	0.29 (0.09–0.94)	
Typical odds ratio (95% confidence interval)					0.29 (0.09–0.94)	

Effect of vaginal PGE vs. PGF for cervical ripening on low Apgar score at 1 minute

Study	EXPT n	(%)	CTRL n	(%)	Odds ratio (95% CI)	
MacKenzie and Embrey (1979)	1/16	(6.25)	1/16	(6.25)	1.00 (0.06–16.74)	
Typical odds ratio (95% confidence interval)					1.00 (0.06–16.74)	

Effect of vaginal PGE vs. PGF for cervical ripening on low Apgar score at 5 minutes

Study	EXPT n	(%)	CTRL n	(%)	Odds ratio (95% CI)	
Neilson et al. (1983)	2/38	(5.26)	0/37	(0.00)	7.39 (0.45–99.99)	
Typical odds ratio (95% confidence interval)					7.39 (0.45–99.99)	

nificance for $PGF_{2\alpha}$ (Table 61.20). The effect on instrumental vaginal delivery was also consistent with that observed for all prostaglandin studies, showing a statistically significantly lower incidence with $PGF_{2\alpha}$ treatment than in the control groups (typical odds ratio 0.54; 95 per cent confidence interval 0.35–0.84; Table 61.20). Unfortunately, very few infant outcomes were available from these trial reports, and as shown in Table 61.21, those that were available never related to more than two of the five trials.

Only two direct, comparisons of PGE_2 and $PGF_{2\alpha}$ for ripening the unfavourable cervix have been reported in the literature (MacKenzie and Embrey 1979; Neilson *et al.* 1983). Both were double-blind and compared vaginal administration of 5 mg PGE_2 in a methylhydroxyethyl cellulose (Tylose®) gel with either 25 mg (MacKenzie and Embrey 1979) or 40 mg (Neilson *et al.* 1983) $PGF_{2\alpha}$ suspended in the same Tylose gel. Labour was induced 14 to 15 hours later with intravenous oxytocin (Neilson *et al.* 1983) or by amniotomy combined with intravenous oxytocin (MacKenzie and Embrey 1979). One of the studies (MacKenzie and Embrey 1979) involved only nulliparae with a cervical score (Calder *et al.* 1974; see Fig. 61.1) of less than 4; the other (Neilson *et al.* 1983) included women of various parities who had scored an average of 4 using the same cervical score.

In the study which used the lower dose of $PGF_{2\alpha}$

(MacKenzie and Embrey 1979), statistically significantly more women went into labour with PGE_2 than with $PGF_{2\alpha}$ (Table 61.22). The other study (Neilson *et al.* 1983) provided no data on this outcome, but suggested a reduction (not statistically significant) in the incidence of failed induction, and a statistically significantly reduced incidence of instrumental vaginal delivery and operative delivery with PGE_2 compared with $PGF_{2\alpha}$ (Table 61.22). All of these data are based on a small number of investigations, however, and none of the other outcomes showed any difference between the two prostaglandins used (Table 61.22).

In summary, there is thus no convincing evidence, either from direct comparisons or indirect from the placebo-controlled studies, that these two prostaglandins, PGE_2 and $PGF_{2\alpha}$, have clinically important differential effects on cervical ripening when used in equipotent doses.

4.3 Route of administration

4.3.1 Oral prostaglandins

Between 1975 and 1977, five randomized trials were reported in which oral PGE_2 was compared with either placebo or no treatment for cervical ripening (Friedman and Sachtleben 1975; Weiss *et al.* 1975; Golbus and Creasy 1977; Pearce 1977; Valentine 1977). All of the

Table 61.23 Characteristics of the controlled evaluations of oral PGE_2 for cervical ripening

| Authors and dates | Random method | Treatments compared | | Bishop score at entry | No. of nulliparae: multiparae | | Interval to and method of induction |
		PGE₂	Control		PGE₂	Control	
Friedman and Satchleben (1975)	double-blind	1 mg every 3 hours (3 doses)	placebo tablets	<6	7:8	7: 8	8–12 hours; intravenous oxytocin
Weiss *et al.* (1975)	double-blind	1 mg every 3 hours (3 doses)	placebo tablets	means 4.5–5.0	0:15	0:24	14 hours; intravenous oxytocin without amniotomy
		1 mg first, then depending on contractions (3 doses)	placebo tablets		0:17		
Golbus and Creasy (1977)	double-blind	1 mg every 3 hours (3 doses)	placebo tablets	means 4.5–5.6	6:19	7:18	15–20 hours; intravenous oxytocin
Pearce (1977)	double-blind	0.5 mg per hour for 10 hours	placebo tablets	<6	12:13	14: 9	10 hours; amniotomy + intravenous oxytocin
Valentine (1977)	random not described	0.5 mg per hour for 10 hours	no treatment	<5	12: 3	12: 3	24 hours; intravenous oxytocin + amniotomy if possible
		1 mg per hour for 10 hours			13: 2		

trials were small. Each of them reported results on between 30 and 60 women, and a total of only 229 women were entered in these 5 trials. Moreover, entry criteria, doses of PGE_2, the time allowed for the ripening effect, and the methods of induction all varied among these trials (Table 61.23).

Only three of the trial reports (Friedman and Sachtleben 1975; Pearce 1977; Valentine 1977) mention whether women went into labour during the ripening period before the induction of labour; the results (Table 61.24) are consistent with those derived from the overview of all trials (Table 61.2). The other two trials (Weiss *et al.* 1975; Golbus and Creasy 1977) indicated that women assigned to prostaglandin treatment were more likely to be delivered within the ripening period than women assigned to the control groups (typical odds ratio 5.02; 95 per cent confidence interval 1.78–14.15; Table 61.24). The incidence of 'failed induction', although variously defined, was not statistically significantly different between the PGE_2 and the control groups for the four trials that provided data on this outcome (Friedman and Sachtleben 1975; Golbus and Creasy 1977; Pearce 1977; Valentine 1977). Although this difference did not reach statistical significance (95 per cent confidence interval 0.27–1.38), the three trials which reported on the number of women not delivered within 24 hours after the start of formal induction of labour, indicate that this occurred less frequently in PGE_2-treated women than in the control groups (typical odds ratio 0.22; 95 per cent confidence interval 0.08–0.56; Table 61.24). All other outcome measures on which categorical data were available failed to detect effects of oral PGE_2 pretreatment, but the precision of these estimates is low (Table 61.24).

Overall, the data do not indicate that oral PGE_2 is a suitable approach to ripening of the cervix. The drug apparently needs to be administered repeatedly over a period of several hours in order to have effects that, on the whole, are not very impressive.

4.3.2 Vaginal prostaglandins

Thirteen (12 published and 1 unpublished) controlled trials have compared vaginal administration of PGE_2 with either placebo (11 trials) or no treatment groups (2 trials; Table 61.25). One of the placebo-controlled trials (Walker and Gordon 1983), however, was a crossover study in which women received either 4 mg PGE_2 in Tylose® gel (methylhydroxyethyl cellulose) 24 hours before and Tylose® gel alone 12 hours before the planned induction, or the placebo gel 24 hours before and the PGE_2 gel 12 hours before the induction. True comparison of PGE_2 with placebo is therefore only possible for outcomes that occurred within the first 12 hours of the trial. In two of the placebo-controlled trials (Thiery *et al.* 1984; Ulmsten *et al.* 1985), all women allocated to either vaginal PGE_2 or placebo also received placebo gel endocervically, because these trials compared both vaginal and endocervical PGE_2 with placebo in three trial arms. In yet another of the placebo-controlled trials (Jagani *et al.* 1984), both the PGE_2 and the placebo group had an extra-amniotic catheter inserted at the start of the ripening period, which may have stimulated endogenous prostaglandin production in both groups (Keirse *et al.* 1983).

Each of the arms of the trials contained between 12 and 41 women (Table 61.25); the largest number of women treated with prostaglandins in any of these studies was 60, and these 60 were divided among three groups with different doses of the drug (Graves *et al.* 1985). The doses used ranged from 0.5 mg to 5 mg in the 11 trials in which a single dose was administered, and from 2 to 3 mg in the one study (Jagani *et al.* 1984) that used two doses, separated by an interval of 4 hours. The vehicle in which PGE_2 was administered also varied widely among studies. Four used a vaginal tablet or suppository (Thiery *et al.* 1984; Jagani *et al.* 1984; Buchanan *et al.* 1984; Ulmsten *et al.* 1985), and one a Witepsol-based pessary (Lewis 1983). In 7 of the trials, PGE_2 was administered in a gel. The gel was methylhydroxyethyl cellulose (Tylose®) in 3 studies (MacKenzie and Embrey 1979; Prins *et al.* 1983; Walker and Gordon 1983); triacetin in 2 studies (Graves *et al.* 1985; Hayashi R, unpublished); and carboxymethyl cellulose (MacKenzie and Embrey 1977), cellulose (Williams *et al.* 1985), and hydroxyethyl cellulose (Lorenz *et al.* 1984) in 1 of each of the remaining 3 trials (Table 61.25).

The state of the cervix at entry into these 13 trials was assessed with four different scores, although 6 studies used the Bishop score (1964), and 4 the modification of Calder *et al.* (1974). The entry criteria for those who used the Bishop score (Bishop 1964) were a score of less than 5 or 6; for those using the modification of Calder and his colleagues (1974), they were either less than 4 or 5, or not described. Six studies allowed for a ripening period of 12 hours (Williams *et al.* 1985; Lorenz *et al.* 1984; Thiery *et al.* 1984; Jagani *et al.* 1984; Buchanan *et al.* 1984; Hayashi R, unpublished); 4 for a period of between 12 and 16 hours (Graves *et al.* 1985; MacKenzie and Embrey 1979; Lewis 1983; Prins *et al.* 1983); one for a period of 16 to 18 hours (MacKenzie and Embrey 1977); and one (in which the aim clearly was to induce labour as well as achieve cervical softening) allowed an interval of 24 hours before a formal induction attempt with either endocervical PGE_2 or oxytocin was undertaken (Ulmsten *et al.* 1985). In all studies, induction of labour after the ripening period was by oxytocin infusion, except that in two of them this depended on the state of the cervix at the end of the ripening period (Ulmsten *et al.* 1985; Thiery *et al.* 1984). In some of the trials, amniotomy was systematically performed at the start of the oxytocin infusion (MacKenzie and Embrey 1979; Walker and Gordon

Table 61.24 Effect of oral PGE$_2$ for cervical ripening on labour onset during ripening

Study	EXPT n	(%)	CTRL n	(%)	Odds ratio (95% CI)	Graph of odds ratios and confidence intervals
Friedman and Sachtleben (1975)	3/15	(20.00)	3/15	(20.00)	1.00 (0.17–5.81)	
Pearce (1977)	5/25	(20.00)	1/23	(4.35)	4.06 (0.75–22.10)	
Valentine (1977)	4/30	(13.33)	0/15	(0.00)	5.00 (0.58–43.09)	
Typical odds ratio (95% confidence interval)					2.56 (0.89–7.41)	

Effect of oral PGE$_2$ for cervical ripening on delivered during ripening

Study	EXPT n	(%)	CTRL n	(%)	Odds ratio (95% CI)	
Golbus and Creasy (1977)	6/25	(24.00)	1/25	(4.00)	5.09 (1.05–24.77)	
Weiss *et al.* (1975)	9/32	(28.13)	1/24	(4.17)	4.97 (1.26–19.56)	
Typical odds ratio (95% confidence interval)					5.02 (1.78–14.15)	

Effect of oral PGE$_2$ for cervical ripening on hypertonus–hyperstimulation

Study	EXPT n	(%)	CTRL n	(%)	Odds ratio (95% CI)	
Friedman and Sachtleben (1975)	0/15	(0.00)	2/15	(13.33)	0.13 (0.01–2.12)	
Golbus and Creasy (1977)	3/25	(12.00)	1/25	(4.00)	2.90 (0.38–21.94)	
Weiss *et al.* (1975)	5/32	(15.63)	1/24	(4.17)	3.24 (0.59–17.68)	
Typical odds ratio (95% confidence interval)					1.77 (0.54–5.76)	

Effect of oral PGE$_2$ for cervical ripening on fetal heart rate abnormalities

Study	EXPT n	(%)	CTRL n	(%)	Odds ratio (95% CI)	
Friedman and Sachtleben (1975)	2/15	(13.33)	1/15	(6.67)	2.05 (0.20–21.36)	
Golbus and Creasy (1977)	1/25	(4.00)	3/25	(12.00)	0.34 (0.05–2.61)	
Weiss *et al.* (1975)	0/32	(0.00)	0/24	(0.00)	1.00 (1.00–1.00)	
Typical odds ratio (95% confidence interval)					0.74 (0.16–3.41)	

Effect of oral PGE$_2$ for cervical ripening on failed induction

Study	EXPT n	(%)	CTRL n	(%)	Odds ratio (95% CI)	
Friedman and Sachtleben (1975)	3/15	(20.00)	4/15	(26.67)	0.70 (0.13–3.68)	
Golbus and Creasy (1977)	9/25	(36.00)	9/25	(36.00)	1.00 (0.32–3.14)	
Pearce (1977)	1/25	(4.00)	1/23	(4.35)	0.92 (0.06–15.16)	
Valentine (1977)	1/30	(3.33)	4/15	(26.67)	0.10 (0.01–0.70)	
Typical odds ratio (95% confidence interval)					0.61 (0.27–1.38)	

Table 61.24—*continued* Effect of oral PGE_2 for cervical ripening on not delivered within 24 hours

Study	EXPT n	(%)	CTRL n	(%)	Odds ratio (95% CI)	Graph of odds ratios and confidence intervals
Pearce (1977)	1/25	(4.00)	1/23	(4.35)	0.92 (0.06–15.16)	
Weiss et al. (1975)	3/32	(9.38)	6/24	(25.00)	0.32 (0.08–1.34)	
Valentine (1977)	3/30	(10.00)	8/15	(53.33)	0.10 (0.02–0.42)	
Typical odds ratio (95% confidence interval)					0.22 (0.08–0.56)	

Effect of oral PGE_2 for cervical ripening on caesarean section

Study	EXPT n	(%)	CTRL n	(%)	Odds ratio (95% CI)	
Golbus and Creasy (1977)	1/25	(4.00)	2/25	(8.00)	0.50 (0.05–5.03)	
Pearce (1977)	1/25	(4.00)	1/23	(4.35)	0.92 (0.06–15.16)	
Weiss et al. (1975)	1/32	(3.13)	1/24	(4.17)	0.74 (0.04–12.55)	
Valentine (1977)	7/30	(23.33)	7/15	(46.67)	0.34 (0.09–1.30)	
Typical odds ratio (95% confidence interval)					0.46 (0.17–1.24)	

Effect of oral PGE_2 for cervical ripening on low Apgar score at 1 minute

Study	EXPT n	(%)	CTRL n	(%)	Odds ratio (95% CI)	
Golbus and Creasy (1977)	4/25	(16.00)	2/25	(8.00)	2.10 (0.39–11.37)	
Pearce (1977)	7/25	(28.00)	8/23	(34.78)	0.73 (0.22–2.46)	
Typical odds ratio (95% confidence interval)					1.05 (0.39–2.80)	

Effect of oral PGE_2 for cervical ripening on low Apgar score at 5 minutes

Study	EXPT n	(%)	CTRL n	(%)	Odds ratio (95% CI)	
Golbus and Creasy (1977)	2/25	(8.00)	0/25	(0.00)	7.70 (0.47–99.99)	
Pearce (1977)	2/25	(8.00)	4/23	(17.39)	0.43 (0.08–2.35)	
Weiss et al. (1975)	0/32	(0.00)	0/24	(0.00)	1.00 (1.00–1.00)	
Typical odds ratio (95% confidence interval)					0.93 (0.22–3.98)	

1983; MacKenzie and Embrey 1977); in others amniotomy was systematically not performed at induction (Williams *et al.* 1985; Graves *et al.* 1985; Prins *et al.* 1983; Buchanan *et al.* 1984); in others it was only carried out 'if possible' (Lewis 1983).

A fourteenth trial dealt with PGE_1 administered in a viscous gel and placed vaginally 'against the cervix' (Roberts *et al.* 1986), and three further trials, one of which also investigated PGE_2 (MacKenzie and Embrey 1979), dealt with $PGF_{2\alpha}$ administered in a viscous gel.

Some of the characteristics of all these trials are listed in Table 61.25.

Fourteen of the total of 16 trials reported on the onset of labour during the period of cervical ripening (Table 61.26). In all but one (Prins *et al.* 1983), this occurred more often in women receiving prostaglandin than in control women; the typical odds ratio of 4.93 (95 per cent confidence interval 3.45–7.05) showed this to be statistically highly significant (Table 61.26). Consequently, more women in the prostaglandin-treated

Table 61.25 Characteristics of the controlled evaluations of vaginally administered prostaglandins for cervical ripening

Authors and dates	No. of women treated	PG dose (mg)	Vehicle type	Cervical score		Control treatment	Nulliparae and/or multiparae
				Type used*	Cut-off		
Prostaglandin E₂							
MacKenzie and Embrey (1977)	12	2	carboxymethyl cellulose	Calder	<4	placebo	nulli
MacKenzie and Embrey (1979)	16	5	Tylose gel	Calder	<4	placebo	nulli
Lewis (1983)	22	3	Witepsol pessary	Other score	<5 of 15	no treatment	nulli + multi
Prins *et al.* (1983)	15	5	Tylose gel	Calder	<5	placebo	nulli + multi
Walker and Gordon (1983)	15	4	Tylose gel	Other score	<4 of ?	placebo	nulli
Buchanan *et al.* (1984)	38	3	suppository	Bishop	<5	placebo	nulli + multi
Jagani *et al.* (1984)†	15	2–3	suppositories	Bishop	<5	no treatment	nulli + multi
Lorenz *et al.* (1984)	21	2	hydroxyethyl cellulose	Calder	not stated	placebo	nulli + multi
Thiery *et al.* (1984)†	41	2	vaginal tablet	Bishop	<6	placebo	nulli + multi
Graves *et al.* (1985)	20 20 20	1 2 3	triacetin gel	Bishop	<5	placebo	nulli + multi
Ulmsten *et al.* (1985)†	19	2	suppository	Other score	<6 of 10	placebo	nulli
Williams *et al.* (1985)	20 20	3 5	cellulose	Bishop	<6	placebo	nulli + multi
Hayashi (unpub.)	15 15 15	½ 1 1½	triacetin gel	Bishop	<6	placebo	nulli + multi
Prostaglandin E₁							
Roberts *et al.* (1986)	27	3	Tylose gel	Bishop	<5	no treatment	nulli + multi
Prostaglandin PGF₂ₐ							
MacKenzie and Embrey (1979)	16	25	Tylose gel	Calder	<4	placebo	nulli
MacLennan and Green (1979)	40	50	methyl cellulose	Calder	not stated	placebo	nulli + multi
Murphy *et al.* (1980)	55	1½ 3 10	Tylose gel	Calder	not stated	placebo	nulli + multi

* See Fig. 61.1 for scores.
† Women in both treatment and control groups in the trial of Jagani *et al.* (1984) had an extra-amniotic catheter inserted; in the trials of Thiery *et al.* (1984) and Ulmsten *et al.* (1985) they all received an endocervical placebo gel.

group were ultimately delivered without requiring formal induction of labour (typical odds ratio 5.52; 95 per cent confidence interval 3.35–9.10; Table 61.26). Also, the rate of 'failed induction', as defined by the investigators, was statistically significantly lower in prostaglandin-treated women than in controls (typical odds ratio 0.21; 95 per cent confidence interval 0.10–0.41; Table 61.26). On the negative side, however, there was a statistically significantly higher incidence of 'uterine hypertonus' or 'hyperstimulation' in the women treated with vaginal prostaglandin than in women receiving placebo or no treatment (typical odds ratio 5.67; 95 per cent confidence interval 1.86–17.33; Table 61.26).

The incidence of caesarean section, which was available for all trials, showed a tendency to be lower with vaginal prostaglandin treatment. This effect may be due to chance, however; although the typical odds ratio was 0.88, its 95 per cent confidence interval ranged from 0.62 to 1.25 (Table 61.27). As observed with other routes of prostaglandin administration, the incidence of

Table 61.26 Effect of vaginal prostaglandins vs. placebo (or no treatment) for cervical ripening on labour onset during ripening

Study	EXPT n	(%)	CTRL n	(%)	Odds ratio (95% CI)	Graph of odds ratios and confidence intervals
MacKenzie and Embrey (1979)	3/32	(9.38)	0/16	(0.00)	4.79 (0.41–55.70)	
Prins *et al.* (1983)	3/15	(20.00)	3/15	(20.00)	1.00 (0.17–5.81)	
Walker and Gordon (1983)	3/15	(20.00)	0/15	(0.00)	8.57 (0.82–89.45)	
MacKenzie and Embrey (1977)	4/12	(33.33)	0/12	(0.00)	9.97 (1.22–81.60)	
Williams *et al.* (1985)	15/40	(37.50)	0/20	(0.00)	7.15 (2.09–24.43)	
Hayashi (unpub)	8/45	(17.78)	1/15	(6.67)	2.36 (0.46–11.94)	
MacLennan and Green (1979)	20/40	(50.00)	3/40	(7.50)	7.76 (2.96–20.31)	
Thiery *et al.* (1984)	5/41	(12.20)	1/40	(2.50)	4.04 (0.77–21.10)	
Buchanan *et al.* (1984)	26/38	(68.42)	4/39	(10.26)	11.18 (4.50–27.78)	
Lorenz *et al.* (1984)	2/21	(9.52)	1/23	(4.35)	2.22 (0.22–22.56)	
Graves *et al.* (1985)	16/60	(26.67)	0/20	(0.00)	5.19 (1.47–18.23)	
Murphy *et al.* (1980)	19/165	(11.52)	7/100	(7.00)	1.66 (0.72–3.83)	
Lewis (1983)	14/22	(63.64)	0/22	(0.00)	17.58 (5.01–61.62)	
Jagani *et al.* (1984)	4/15	(26.67)	2/16	(12.50)	2.41 (0.42–13.91)	
Typical odds ratio (95% confidence interval)					4.93 (3.45–7.05)	

Scale: 0.01 0.1 0.5 1 2 10 100

Effect of vaginal prostaglandins vs. placebo (or no treatment) for cervical ripening on no need for formal induction of labour

Study	EXPT n	(%)	CTRL n	(%)	Odds ratio (95% CI)	Graph
MacKenzie and Embrey (1979)	12/32	(37.50)	0/16	(0.00)	7.09 (1.80–27.93)	
MacKenzie and Embrey (1977)	4/12	(33.33)	0/12	(0.00)	9.97 (1.22–81.60)	
Hayashi (unpub)	10/45	(22.22)	1/15	(6.67)	2.78 (0.62–12.42)	
MacLennan and Green (1979)	30/40	(75.00)	14/40	(35.00)	4.93 (2.06–11.84)	
Buchanan *et al.* (1984)	15/38	(39.47)	2/39	(5.13)	7.17 (2.46–20.92)	
Graves *et al.* (1985)	16/60	(26.67)	0/20	(0.00)	5.19 (1.47–18.23)	
Typical odds ratio (95% confidence interval)					5.52 (3.35–9.10)	

Table 61.26—*continued* Effect of vaginal prostaglandins vs. placebo (or no treatment) for cervical ripening on failed induction

Study	EXPT n	(%)	CTRL n	(%)	Odds ratio (95% CI)	Graph of odds ratios and confidence intervals
Prins *et al.* (1983)	2/15	(13.33)	8/15	(53.33)	0.18 (0.04–0.78)	
Williams *et al.* (1985)	4/40	(10.00)	2/20	(10.00)	1.00 (0.17–5.90)	
Buchanan *et al.* (1984)	2/38	(5.26)	12/39	(30.77)	0.18 (0.06–0.58)	
Roberts *et al.* (1986)	1/27	(3.70)	10/24	(41.67)	0.11 (0.03–0.42)	
Typical odds ratio (95% confidence interval)					0.21 (0.10–0.41)	

Effect of vaginal prostaglandins vs. placebo (or no treatment) for cervical ripening on hypertonus and/or hyperstimulation

Study	EXPT n	(%)	CTRL n	(%)	Odds ratio (95% CI)	Graph
MacKenzie and Embrey (1979)	2/32	(6.25)	0/16	(0.00)	4.63 (0.24–90.41)	
Hayashi (unpub)	1/45	(2.22)	0/15	(0.00)	3.79 (0.04–99.99)	
Thiery *et al.* (1984)	0/41	(0.00)	1/40	(2.50)	0.13 (0.00–6.65)	
Buchanan *et al.* (1984)	3/38	(7.89)	0/35	(0.00)	7.21 (0.73–71.75)	
Graves *et al.* (1985)	7/20	(35.00)	0/20	(0.00)	10.63 (2.12–53.21)	
Lewis (1983)	0/22	(0.00)	0/22	(0.00)	1.00 (1.00–1.00)	
Typical odds ratio (95% confidence interval)					5.67 (1.86–17.33)	

Graph axis (odds ratios): 0.01 0.1 0.5 1 2 10 100

instrumental vaginal delivery was statistically significantly reduced, yielding a typical odds ratio of 0.51 (95 per cent confidence interval 0.33–0.79; Table 61.27). This was also reflected in the rate of operative delivery, which showed a typical odds ratio of 0.59 (95 per cent confidence interval 0.41–0.85; Table 61.27).

None of the infant outcomes (Table 61.28) suggested any effect, good or bad, of the treatment. This is hardly surprising since all prostaglandin treatments considered together (see Tables 61.15 to 61.17 above) failed to show any effect on parameters of infant outcome.

The analysis of these trials of vaginal prostaglandins for cervical ripening also reveals that the risks associated with induction of labour, particularly in women with pregnancy complications, do not start at the time of induction, but with the start of cervical ripening. Indeed, during the time interval allowed for cervical ripening, caesarean section was performed more frequently in prostaglandin-treated women than in controls (typical odds ratio 3.61; 95 per cent confidence interval 1.26–10.35; Table 61.29). Thus, overall, 7 per cent of prostaglandin-treated women (divided over 8 trials; Table 61.29) underwent caesarean section during the cervical ripening period, as opposed to only 1.3 per cent of the women who received either placebo or no treatment. This higher incidence of caesarean section during cervical ripening was apparently compensated for by a lower caesarean section rate during induced labour, since the overall caesarean section rate tended to be lower rather than higher with the prostaglandin treatment. Nevertheless, these data indicate that the use of vaginal prostaglandins for ripening the cervix is not a harmless procedure. On the basis of this evidence it is certainly inappropriate to administer prostaglandins for cervical ripening for trivial reasons and without careful monitoring of maternal and fetal well-being.

4.3.3 Endocervical prostaglandins

Endocervical administration in a viscous gel (injected in the cervical canal) is the method of prostaglandin administration for cervical ripening that has been explored most thoroughly in controlled comparisons. Both the number of controlled comparisons reported and the number of women included in these comparisons is larger than for any other cervical ripening

Table 61.27 Effect of vaginal prostaglandins vs. placebo (or no treatment) for cervical ripening on caesarean section

Study	EXPT n	(%)	CTRL n	(%)	Odds ratio (95% CI)	Graph of odds ratios and confidence intervals
MacKenzie and Embrey (1979)	4/32	(12.50)	3/16	(18.75)	0.61 (0.11–3.29)	
Prins et al. (1983)	4/15	(26.67)	7/15	(46.67)	0.43 (0.10–1.87)	
Ulmsten et al. (1985)	7/19	(36.84)	6/20	(30.00)	1.35 (0.36–5.03)	
Williams et al. (1985)	13/40	(32.50)	7/20	(35.00)	0.90 (0.29–2.77)	
Hayashi (unpub)	12/45	(26.67)	4/15	(26.67)	1.00 (0.27–3.71)	
MacLennan and Green (1979)	2/40	(5.00)	3/40	(7.50)	0.66 (0.11–3.97)	
MacKenzie and Embrey (1977)	0/12	(0.00)	0/12	(0.00)	1.00 (1.00–1.00)	
Thiery et al. (1984)	0/41	(0.00)	0/40	(0.00)	1.00 (1.00–1.00)	
Buchanan et al. (1984)	15/38	(39.47)	17/39	(43.59)	0.85 (0.34–2.08)	
Lorenz et al. (1984)	10/21	(47.62)	7/23	(30.43)	2.03 (0.61–6.75)	
Graves et al. (1985)	16/60	(26.67)	3/20	(15.00)	1.89 (0.58–6.16)	
Murphy et al. (1980)	10/165	(6.06)	9/100	(9.00)	0.64 (0.25–1.68)	
Roberts et al. (1986)	3/27	(11.11)	8/24	(33.33)	0.28 (0.07–1.04)	
Lewis (1983)	3/22	(13.64)	6/22	(27.27)	0.44 (0.10–1.88)	
Jagani et al. (1984)	5/15	(33.33)	2/16	(12.50)	3.17 (0.60–16.62)	
Typical odds ratio (95% confidence interval)					0.88 (0.62–1.25)	

Effect of vaginal prostaglandins vs. placebo (or no treatment) for cervical ripening on instrumental vaginal delivery

Study	EXPT n	(%)	CTRL n	(%)	Odds ratio (95% CI)	Graph of odds ratios and confidence intervals
Ulmsten et al. (1985)	4/19	(21.05)	6/20	(30.00)	0.63 (0.15–2.62)	
MacLennan and Green (1979)	12/40	(30.00)	16/40	(40.00)	0.65 (0.26–1.61)	
Buchanan et al. (1984)	1/38	(2.63)	2/38	(5.26)	0.50 (0.05–5.00)	
Lorenz et al. (1984)	2/18	(11.11)	6/19	(31.58)	0.31 (0.07–1.45)	
Murphy et al. (1980)	32/165	(19.39)	33/100	(33.00)	0.48 (0.27–0.86)	
Typical odds ratio (95% confidence interval)					0.51 (0.33–0.79)	

Scale (graph): 0.01 0.1 0.5 1 2 10 100

Table 61.27—*continued* Effect of vaginal prostaglandins vs. placebo (or no treatment) for cervical ripening on operative delivery

Study	EXPT		CTRL		Odds ratio	Graph of odds ratios and confidence intervals
	n	(%)	n	(%)	(95% CI)	0.01 0.1 0.5 1 2 10 100
Ulmsten *et al.* (1985)	11/19	(57.89)	12/20	(60.00)	0.92 (0.26–3.24)	
MacLennan and Green (1979)	14/40	(35.00)	19/40	(47.50)	0.60 (0.25–1.46)	
Buchanan *et al.* (1984)	16/38	(42.11)	19/38	(50.00)	0.73 (0.30–1.79)	
Lorenz *et al.* (1984)	12/18	(66.67)	13/19	(68.42)	0.93 (0.24–3.60)	
Murphy *et al.* (1980)	42/165	(25.45)	42/100	(42.00)	0.47 (0.27–0.80)	
Typical odds ratio (95% confidence interval)					0.59 (0.41–0.85)	

Table 61.28 Effect of vaginal prostaglandins vs. placebo (or no treatment) for cervical ripening on low Apgar score at 1 minute

Study	EXPT		CTRL		Odds ratio	Graph of odds ratios and confidence intervals
	n	(%)	n	(%)	(95% CI)	0.01 0.1 0.5 1 2 10 100
MacKenzie and Embrey (1979)	2/32	(6.25)	2/16	(12.50)	0.45 (0.05–3.85)	
Prins *et al.* (1983)	0/14	(0.00)	0/15	(0.00)	1.00 (1.00–1.00)	
Hayashi (unpub)	5/45	(11.11)	1/15	(6.67)	1.63 (0.24–11.21)	
Thiery *et al.* (1984)	9/41	(21.95)	12/40	(30.00)	0.66 (0.25–1.78)	
Lorenz *et al.* (1984)	5/21	(23.81)	7/22	(31.82)	0.68 (0.18–2.53)	
Murphy *et al.* (1980)	5/165	(3.03)	3/100	(3.00)	1.01 (0.24–4.30)	
Lewis (1983)	0/22	(0.00)	1/22	(4.55)	0.14 (0.00–6.82)	
Typical odds ratio (95% confidence interval)					0.73 (0.40–1.36)	

Effect of vaginal prostaglandins vs. placebo (or no treatment) for cervical ripening on low Apgar score at 5 minutes

Study	EXPT		CTRL		Odds ratio	Graph of odds ratios and confidence intervals
Prins *et al.* (1983)	0/14	(0.00)	0/15	(0.00)	1.00 (1.00–1.00)	
Ulmsten *et al.* (1985)	0/19	(0.00)	0/20	(0.00)	1.00 (1.00–1.00)	
Hayashi (unpub)	0/45	(0.00)	0/15	(0.00)	1.00 (1.00–1.00)	
Thiery *et al.* (1984)	2/41	(4.88)	4/40	(10.00)	0.48 (0.09–2.50)	
Buchanan *et al.* (1984)	0/38	(0.00)	1/35	(2.86)	0.12 (0.00–6.28)	
Lorenz *et al.* (1984)	1/21	(4.76)	1/22	(4.55)	1.05 (0.06–17.36)	
Graves *et al.* (1985)	2/60	(3.33)	1/20	(5.00)	0.63 (0.04–8.94)	
Lewis (1983)	0/22	(0.00)	0/22	(0.00)	1.00 (1.00–1.00)	
Typical odds ratio (95% confidence interval)					0.52 (0.16–1.70)	

Table 61.28—*continued* Effect of vaginal prostaglandins vs. placebo (or no treatment) for cervical ripening on resuscitation of newborn

Study	EXPT		CTRL		Odds ratio	Graph of odds ratios and confidence intervals						
	n	(%)	n	(%)	(95% CI)	0.01	0.1	0.5	1	2	10	100
Ulmsten et al. (1985)	0/19	(0.00)	0/20	(0.00)	1.00 (1.00–1.00)							
Lorenz *et al.* (1984)	7/21	(33.33)	9/22	(40.91)	0.73 (0.21–2.47)							
Typical odds ratio (95% confidence interval)					0.73 (0.21–2.47)							

Table 61.29 Effect of vaginal prostaglandins vs. placebo (or no treatment) for cervical ripening on caesarean section during ripening

Study	EXPT		CTRL		Odds ratio	Graph of odds ratios and confidence intervals						
	n	(%)	n	(%)	(95% CI)	0.01	0.1	0.5	1	2	10	100
MacKenzie and Embrey (1979)	2/32	(6.25)	0/16	(0.00)	4.63 (0.24–90.41)							
Walker and Gordon (1983)	0/15	(0.00)	0/15	(0.00)	1.00 (1.00–1.00)							
MacKenzie and Embrey (1977)	0/12	(0.00)	0/12	(0.00)	1.00 (1.00–1.00)							
Hayashi (unpub)	2/45	(4.44)	0/15	(0.00)	3.88 (0.15–97.95)							
Buchanan *et al.* (1984)	4/38	(10.53)	2/39	(5.13)	2.10 (0.40–10.99)							
Graves *et al.* (1985)	3/60	(5.00)	0/20	(0.00)	3.93 (0.28–55.42)							
Lewis (1983)	3/22	(13.64)	0/22	(0.00)	8.15 (0.80–82.71)							
Jagani *et al.* (1984)	0/15	(0.00)	0/16	(0.00)	1.00 (1.00–1.00)							
Typical odds ratio (95% confidence interval)					3.61 (1.26–10.35)							

method. All except one of these investigations have dealt with PGE_2; the one exception used 5 mg $PGF_{2\alpha}$ in a home-made gel, on basis of methylhydroxyethyl cellulose, glycerine, and chlorhexidine (Heinzl *et al.* 1980).

Most of the investigations have been conducted with 0.5 mg PGE_2 (Table 61.30), a dose that is much smaller than those used with either the oral (Table 61.23) or vaginal (Table 61.25) routes of administration. Most of the data relate to a preparation of 0.5 mg PGE_2 in a 2.5 ml triacetin gel; and these data include results from three multicentre studies conducted in Europe (Noah *et al.* 1987; Cabrol *et al.* 1988) and Canada (Bernstein *et al.* 1988), which all used the same dose regimen and together involved more than 1400 women (Table 61.30). Not surprisingly, therefore, the results of the endocervical trials closely resemble those presented earlier for any prostaglandin administered by any route (Tables 61.2 to 61.17). Only one trial (Heinzl *et al.*

1980), presented in Tables 61.18 to 61.21, dealt with endocervical administration of $PGF_{2\alpha}$, which was used in a dose (5 mg) 10 times higher than the usual endocervical dose of PGE_2 (0.5 mg).

The data specifically for endocervical administration of PGE_2 show that the treatment is more likely than either placebo or no treatment to result in uterine activity; in the onset of labour; in a reduction of the need for formal induction of labour at the end of the ripening period, which in most trials lasted for 12 hours; and in delivery during the ripening period (Table 61.31). However, as observed with the vaginal administration of prostaglandins, more women underwent caesarean section during the ripening period in the prostaglandin-treated groups (4.2 per cent) than in the control groups (1.4 per cent) of the trials which provided that information (Table 61.31).

The incidence of 'ripening and induction failure'

Table 61.30 Characteristics of the controlled evaluations of endocervical PGE_2 for cervical ripening

Authors and dates	Random method	No. of women PG : control	Treatments compared PG dose and control + type of gel used	Cervix score + cut-off	Hours to and method of induction
Wingerup et al. (1978)	double-blind	10 : 10	1 mg placebo hydroxypropylmethyl cellulose	other <6/10	24 hours oxytocin no amniotomy
Hutchon et al. (1980)	double-blind	14 : 35 18	0.45 mg placebo 0.65 mg methylhydroxyethyl cellulose	Calder <5	'one night' amniotomy
Nimrod et al. (1984)	double-blind	15 15 : 15	0.25 mg placebo 0.50 mg gel type not stated	other <4/?	12 hours at discretion of obstetrician
Thiery et al. (1984)	double-blind	40 : 40	0.5 mg placebo triacetin	Bishop <6	12 hours amniotomy + oxytocin if cervix ripe
Keirse et al. (1985)	sealed envelopes	25 : 25	part of multicentre study of Noah et al. (1987)		
Trofatter et al. (1985)	random not described	30 : 29	0.5 mg catheter triacetin no gel inserted	Bishop <5	12 hours oxytocin
Ulmsten et al. (1985)	double-blind	19 : 20	0.5 mg placebo triacetin	other <6/10	24 hours oxytocin if cervix ripe
Yonekura et al. (1985)	sealed envelopes	25 : 25	0.5 mg placebo triacetin	Bishop <5	12 hours oxytocin
Bernstein et al. (1986)	double-blind	52 : 52	part of multicentre study of Bernstein et al. (1988)		
Bung et al. (1986)	list of numbers	41 : 39	part of multicentre study of Noah et al. (1987)		
Christilaw and King (1986)	double-blind	32 : 34	part of multicentre study of Bernstein et al. (1988)		
Kieback et al. (1986)	list of numbers	50 : 50	same data as Zahradnik et al. (1987) part of multicentre study of Noah et al. (1987)		
Kristoffersen et al. (1986)	list of numbers	25 : 25	part of multicentre study of Noah et al. (1987)		
Laube et al. (1986)	double-blind	15 : 15 15	0.25 mg placebo 0.50 mg	Bishop <5	12 hours oxytocin if cervix ripe
Lucas et al. (1986)	random not described	27 : 23	0.5 mg no triacetin treatment	Bishop not stated	12 hours oxytocin
Pulle et al. (1986)	list of numbers	25 : 25	part of multicentre study of Noah et al. (1987)		
Bernstein et al. (1987)	double-blind	52 : 55	part of multicentre study of Bernstein et al. (1988)		
Noah et al. (1987)	list of numbers	416 : 403	0.5 mg no triacetin treatment	Bishop <6	12 hours oxytocin no amniotomy
Zahradnik et al. (1987)	list of numbers	50 : 50	same data as Kieback et al. (1986) part of multicentre study of Noah et al. (1987)		
Bernstein et al. (1988)	double-blind	206 : 202	0.5 mg placebo triacetin	Bishop <6	12 hours oxytocin
Cabrol et al. (1988)	double-blind	110 : 107	0.5 mg placebo triacetin	Bishop <6	12 hours oxytocin

Table 61.31 Effect of endocervical PGE$_2$ for cervical ripening on uterine activity during ripening

Study	EXPT		CTRL		Odds ratio	Graph of odds ratios and confidence intervals
	n	(%)	n	(%)	(95% CI)	0.01 0.1 0.5 1 2 10 100
Laube *et al.* (1986)	23/30	(76.67)	2/15	(13.33)	12.28 (3.58–42.16)	
Bernstein *et al.* (1988)	84/108	(77.78)	47/110	(42.73)	4.28 (2.49–7.36)	
Wingerup *et al.* (1978)	10/10	(100.0)	2/10	(20.00)	23.73 (4.15–99.99)	
Cabrol *et al.* (1988)	83/110	(75.45)	51/107	(47.66)	3.23 (1.87–5.57)	
Keirse *et al.* (1985)	23/25	(92.00)	1/25	(4.00)	31.66 (10.56–94.97)	
Yonekura *et al.* (1985)	16/25	(64.00)	2/23	(8.70)	10.08 (3.17–32.07)	
Kristoffersen *et al.* (1986)	21/25	(84.00)	1/25	(4.00)	24.09 (7.97–72.78)	
Ulle *et al.* (1986)	24/25	(96.00)	0/25	(0.00)	43.35 (14.45–99.99)	
Typical odds ratio (95% confidence interval)					7.35 (5.44–9.95)	

Effect of endocervical PGE$_2$ for cervical ripening on labour onset during ripening

Study	EXPT		CTRL		Odds ratio	Graph of odds ratios and confidence intervals
Nimrod *et al.* (1984)	13/30	(43.33)	1/15	(6.67)	5.33 (1.42–20.02)	
Hutchon *et al.* (1980)	16/32	(50.00)	3/35	(8.57)	7.45 (2.59–21.42)	
Laube *et al.* (1986)	8/30	(26.67)	0/15	(0.00)	5.95 (1.20–29.57)	
Bernstein *et al.* (1988)	83/206	(40.29)	16/202	(7.92)	5.80 (3.69–9.11)	
Wingerup *et al.* (1978)	8/10	(80.00)	0/10	(0.00)	23.73 (4.15–99.99)	
Thiery *et al.* (1984)	9/40	(22.50)	1/40	(2.50)	6.08 (1.63–22.71)	
Lucas *et al.* (1986)	9/27	(33.33)	1/23	(4.35)	5.90 (1.49–23.38)	
Noah *et al.* (1987)	240/416	(57.69)	20/403	(4.96)	11.37 (8.47–15.25)	
Trofatter *et al.* (1985)	11/30	(36.67)	1/29	(3.45)	7.50 (2.13–26.38)	
Typical odds ratio (95% confidence interval)					8.86 (7.10–11.05)	

Table 61.31—*continued* Effect of endocervical PGE$_2$ for cervical ripening on delivered during ripening

Study	EXPT		CTRL		Odds ratio	Graph of odds ratios and confidence intervals						
	n	(%)	n	(%)	(95% CI)	0.01	0.1	0.5	1	2	10	100
Ulmsten et al. (1985)	11/19	(57.89)	2/20	(10.00)	8.17 (2.19–30.41)							
Laube et al. (1986)	8/30	(26.67)	0/15	(0.00)	5.95 (1.20–29.57)							
Wingerup et al. (1978)	8/10	(80.00)	0/10	(0.00)	23.73 (4.15–99.99)							
Cabrol et al. (1988)	47/108	(43.52)	14/105	(13.33)	4.35 (2.40–7.87)							
Keirse et al. (1985)	10/25	(40.00)	0/25	(0.00)	11.59 (2.94–45.70)							
Kieback et al. (1986)	16/50	(32.00)	3/50	(6.00)	5.33 (1.97–14.39)							
Yonekura et al. (1985)	3/25	(12.00)	0/23	(0.00)	7.43 (0.73–75.21)							
Kristoffersen et al. (1986)	10/25	(40.00)	0/25	(0.00)	11.59 (2.94–45.70)							
Trofatter et al. (1985)	6/30	(20.00)	0/29	(0.00)	8.60 (1.61–45.90)							
Pulle et al. (1986)	10/25	(40.00)	0/25	(0.00)	11.59 (2.94–45.70)							
Bung et al. (1986)	18/41	(43.90)	1/39	(2.56)	9.53 (3.42–26.52)							
Typical odds ratio (95% confidence interval)					6.98 (4.93–9.89)							

Effect of endocervical PGE$_2$ for cervical ripening on no need for formal induction of labour

Study	EXPT		CTRL		Odds ratio	
Nimrod et al. (1984)	13/30	(43.33)	1/15	(6.67)	5.33 (1.42–20.02)	
Bernstein et al. (1987)	30/52	(57.69)	10/55	(18.18)	5.32 (2.44–11.61)	
Wingerup et al. (1978)	8/10	(80.00)	0/10	(0.00)	23.73 (4.15–99.99)	
Cabrol et al. (1988)	47/108	(43.52)	14/105	(13.33)	4.35 (2.40–7.87)	
Keirse et al. (1985)	17/25	(68.00)	1/25	(4.00)	15.21 (4.85–47.73)	
Kieback et al. (1986)	28/50	(56.00)	4/50	(8.00)	8.88 (3.85–20.49)	
Yonekura et al. (1985)	16/25	(64.00)	2/23	(8.70)	10.08 (3.17–32.07)	
Kristoffersen et al. (1986)	10/25	(40.00)	0/25	(0.00)	11.59 (2.94–45.70)	
Pulle et al. (1986)	11/25	(44.00)	0/25	(0.00)	12.34 (3.28–46.42)	
Bung et al. (1986)	18/41	(43.90)	1/39	(2.56)	9.53 (3.42–26.52)	
Typical odds ratio (95% confidence interval)					7.37 (5.40–10.05)	

Table 61.31—*continued* Effect of endocervical PGE₂ for cervical ripening on caesarean section during ripening

Study	EXPT		CTRL		Odds ratio	Graph of odds ratios and confidence intervals
	n	(%)	*n*	(%)	(95% CI)	0.01 0.1 0.5 1 2 10 100
Bernstein *et al.* (1988)	2/206	(0.97)	2/202	(0.99)	0.98 (0.14–7.01)	
Wingerup *et al.* (1978)	0/10	(0.00)	0/10	(0.00)	1.00 (1.00–1.00)	
Cabrol *et al.* (1988)	12/110	(10.91)	3/107	(2.80)	3.50 (1.23–9.98)	
Keirse *et al.* (1985)	2/25	(8.00)	0/25	(0.00)	7.70 (0.47–99.99)	
Yonekura *et al.* (1985)	0/25	(0.00)	0/23	(0.00)	1.00 (1.00–1.00)	
Trofatter *et al.* (1985)	1/30	(3.33)	0/29	(0.00)	7.15 (0.14–99.99)	
Bung *et al.* (1986)	2/41	(4.88)	1/39	(2.56)	1.88 (0.19–18.66)	
Typical odds ratio (95% confidence interval)					2.89 (1.29–6.44)	

Table 61.32 Effect of endocervical PGE₂ for cervical ripening on hypertonus

Study	EXPT		CTRL		Odds ratio	Graph of odds ratios and confidence intervals
	n	(%)	*n*	(%)	(95% CI)	0.01 0.1 0.5 1 2 10 100
Laube *et al.* (1986)	1/30	(3.33)	0/15	(0.00)	4.48 (0.07–99.99)	
Bernstein *et al.* (1988)	3/206	(1.46)	7/202	(3.47)	0.43 (0.12–1.51)	
Thiery *et al.* (1984)	1/40	(2.50)	1/40	(2.50)	1.00 (0.06–16.27)	
Noah *et al.* (1987)	32/416	(7.69)	12/404	(2.97)	2.53 (1.38–4.65)	
Yonekura *et al.* (1985)	2/25	(8.00)	1/23	(4.35)	1.84 (0.18–18.64)	
Trofatter *et al.* (1985)	1/30	(3.33)	1/29	(3.45)	0.97 (0.06–15.83)	
Typical odds ratio (95% confidence interval)					1.76 (1.06–2.93)	

Effect of endocervical PGE₂ for cervical ripening on fetal heart rate abnormalities

Bernstein *et al.* (1988)	11/206	(5.34)	3/202	(1.49)	3.19 (1.10–9.26)	
Thiery *et al.* (1984)	3/40	(7.50)	5/40	(12.50)	0.58 (0.14–2.47)	
Cabrol *et al.* (1988)	37/110	(33.64)	35/107	(32.71)	1.04 (0.59–1.83)	
Noah *et al.* (1987)	55/416	(13.22)	47/404	(11.63)	1.16 (0.76–1.75)	
Typical odds ratio (95% confidence interval)					1.18 (0.87–1.62)	

Table 61.32—*continued* Effect of endocervical PGE$_2$ for cervical ripening on failed induction

Study	EXPT n	(%)	CTRL n	(%)	Odds ratio (95% CI)	Graph of odds ratios and confidence intervals
Laube *et al.* (1986)	1/30	(3.33)	2/15	(13.33)	0.21 (0.02–2.42)	
Bernstein *et al.* (1988)	9/108	(8.33)	20/110	(18.18)	0.43 (0.20–0.93)	
Wingerup *et al.* (1978)	0/10	(0.00)	7/10	(70.00)	0.05 (0.01–0.32)	
Cabrol *et al.* (1988)	7/108	(6.48)	13/105	(12.38)	0.50 (0.20–1.26)	
Noah *et al.* (1987)	66/413	(15.98)	170/403	(42.18)	0.28 (0.21–0.38)	
Yonekura *et al.* (1985)	1/25	(4.00)	3/25	(12.00)	0.34 (0.05–2.61)	
Typical odds ratio (95% confidence interval)					0.30 (0.23–0.39)	

Effect of endocervical PGE$_2$ for cervical ripening on not delivered 12 hours after induction

Study	EXPT n	(%)	CTRL n	(%)	Odds ratio (95% CI)	Graph
Wingerup *et al.* (1978)	0/10	(0.00)	9/10	(90.00)	0.03 (0.01–0.18)	
Keirse *et al.* (1985)	2/25	(8.00)	20/25	(80.00)	0.06 (0.02–0.17)	
Bung *et al.* (1986)	9/41	(21.95)	16/39	(41.03)	0.42 (0.16–1.07)	
Typical odds ratio (95% confidence interval)					0.14 (0.07–0.27)	

Effect of endocervical PGE$_2$ for cervical ripening on not delivered 24 hours after induction

Study	EXPT n	(%)	CTRL n	(%)	Odds ratio (95% CI)	Graph
Wingerup *et al.* (1978)	0/10	(0.00)	7/10	(70.00)	0.05 (0.01–0.32)	
Keirse *et al.* (1985)	2/25	(8.00)	17/25	(68.00)	0.08 (0.03–0.26)	
Typical odds ratio (95% confidence interval)					0.07 (0.03–0.19)	

(variously defined even among the three multicentre trials) was statistically significantly reduced with endocervical prostaglandin treatment (Table 61.32). Consequently, the number of women who were not delivered within 12 hours and within 24 hours after the end of the ripening period and the beginning of induction was statistically significantly reduced in the few trials that provided data on this outcome (Table 61.32).

The trends with regard to the incidence of caesarean section, instrumental vaginal delivery, and overall rate of operative delivery were consistent with those observed with any prostaglandin, administered by any route. Only the lower incidence of operative delivery, however, reached statistical significance in the overview of this subgroup of trials (typical odds ratio 0.72; 95 per cent confidence interval 0.55–0.95; Table 61.33). The incidences of caesarean section and of instrumental vaginal delivery yielded 95 per cent confidence intervals of respectively 0.69–1.08 and 0.58–1.10; Table 61.33).

As with the global results for all prostaglandins administered by any route, there was a higher incidence of 'uterine hypertonus' and 'uterine hyperstimulation' (typical odds ratio 1.76; 95 per cent confidence interval 1.06–2.93; (Table 61.32) and a tendency for fetal heart rate abnormalities to be more frequent with than without endocervical prostaglandin administration, which was not statistically significant (typical odds ratio 1.18; 95 per cent confidence interval 0.87–1.62; (Table 61.32). Neither of these apparently resulted in an increased use of obstetric interventions, such as caesarean section or instrumental vaginal delivery; nor was there any evidence that this resulted in a higher inci-

Table 61.33 Effect of endocervical PGE$_2$ for cervical ripening on caesarean section

Study	EXPT n	(%)	CTRL n	(%)	Odds ratio (95% CI)	Graph of odds ratios and confidence intervals
Ulmsten et al. (1985)	3/19	(15.79)	6/20	(30.00)	0.46 (0.11–2.00)	
Nimrod et al. (1984)	4/30	(13.33)	0/15	(0.00)	5.00 (0.58–43.09)	
Hutchon et al. (1980)	11/32	(34.38)	13/35	(37.14)	0.89 (0.33–2.40)	
Laube et al. (1986)	8/30	(26.67)	1/15	(6.67)	3.39 (0.73–15.71)	
Bernstein et al. (1988)	55/206	(26.70)	67/202	(33.17)	0.74 (0.48–1.12)	
Wingerup et al. (1978)	0/10	(0.00)	3/10	(30.00)	0.11 (0.01–1.17)	
Thiery et al. (1984)	1/40	(2.50)	0/39	(0.00)	7.21 (0.14–99.99)	
Cabrol et al. (1988)	30/110	(27.27)	23/107	(21.50)	1.37 (0.74–2.53)	
Noah et al. (1987)	67/413	(16.22)	84/403	(20.84)	0.74 (0.52–1.05)	
Yonekura et al. (1985)	10/25	(40.00)	6/25	(24.00)	2.06 (0.63–6.67)	
Trofatter et al. (1985)	8/30	(26.67)	9/29	(31.03)	0.81 (0.27–2.48)	
Typical odds ratio (95% confidence interval)					0.87 (0.69–1.08)	

Effect of endocervical PGE$_2$ for cervical ripening on instrumental vaginal delivery

Study	EXPT n	(%)	CTRL n	(%)	Odds ratio (95% CI)	Graph
Ulmsten et al. (1985)	3/19	(15.79)	6/20	(30.00)	0.46 (0.11–2.00)	
Bernstein et al. (1988)	49/206	(23.79)	51/202	(25.25)	0.92 (0.59–1.45)	
Wingerup et al. (1978)	0/10	(0.00)	1/10	(10.00)	0.14 (0.00–6.82)	
Keirse et al. (1985)	5/25	(20.00)	6/25	(24.00)	0.80 (0.21–2.99)	
Sieback et al. (1986)	5/50	(10.00)	10/50	(20.00)	0.46 (0.15–1.37)	
Yonekura et al. (1985)	1/25	(4.00)	4/23	(17.39)	0.25 (0.04–1.54)	
Kristoffersen et al. (1986)	7/25	(28.00)	5/25	(20.00)	1.54 (0.43–5.56)	
Trofatter et al. (1985)	6/30	(20.00)	8/29	(27.59)	0.66 (0.20–2.18)	
Olle et al. (1986)	1/25	(4.00)	2/25	(8.00)	0.50 (0.05–5.03)	
ang et al. (1986)	8/41	(19.51)	7/39	(17.95)	1.11 (0.36–3.38)	
Typical odds ratio (95% confidence interval)					0.80 (0.58–1.10)	

Table 61.33—*continued* Effect of endocervical PGE$_2$ for cervical ripening on operative delivery

Study	EXPT n	(%)	CTRL n	(%)	Odds ratio (95% CI)	Graph of odds ratios and confidence intervals
Ulmsten *et al.* (1985)	6/19	(31.58)	12/20	(60.00)	0.33 (0.09–1.14)	
Bernstein *et al.* (1988)	104/206	(50.49)	118/202	(58.42)	0.73 (0.49–1.07)	
Wingerup *et al.* (1978)	0/10	(0.00)	4/10	(40.00)	0.09 (0.01–0.79)	
Keirse *et al.* (1985)	7/25	(28.00)	8/25	(32.00)	0.83 (0.25–2.75)	
Kieback *et al.* (1986)	10/50	(20.00)	16/50	(32.00)	0.54 (0.22–1.31)	
Yonekura *et al.* (1985)	11/25	(44.00)	9/23	(39.13)	1.22 (0.39–3.79)	
Kristoffersen *et al.* (1986)	11/25	(44.00)	8/25	(32.00)	1.65 (0.53–5.10)	
Trofatter *et al.* (1985)	14/30	(46.67)	17/29	(58.62)	0.62 (0.23–1.72)	
Pulle *et al.* (1986)	4/25	(16.00)	5/25	(20.00)	0.77 (0.18–3.20)	
Bung *et al.* (1986)	13/41	(31.71)	13/39	(33.33)	0.93 (0.37–2.36)	
Typical odds ratio (95% confidence interval)					0.72 (0.55–0.95)	

Graph scale: 0.01 0.1 0.5 1 2 10 100

dence of low 1-minute and 5-minute Apgar scores (Table 61.34).

4.3.4 Extra-amniotic prostaglandins

Only 3 placebo-controlled trials have been reported on extra-amniotic administration of a prostaglandin for cervical ripening; 2 dealt with PGE$_2$ (Shepherd *et al.* 1976; Fenton *et al.* 1985), and 1 with PGF$_{2\alpha}$ (Quinn *et al.* 1981). The characteristics of these trials, each of which included only 15 women in the actively treated group, are summarized in Table 61.35.

Only three categorical outcome measures were available for all 3 trials: the number of women who went into labour during ripening, the incidence of caesarean section, and the number of babies born alive (Table 61.36).

There was one fetal death among the 45 prostaglandin-treated women (Table 61.36). This death (reported separately by Quinn and Murphy 1981) occurred (before amniotomy) after insertion of an extra-amniotic dose of 10 mg PGF$_{2\alpha}$, which can be considered as excessive for extra-amniotic administration.

Overall, there are too few data to permit adequate judgement of either the merits or the hazards of extra-amniotic prostaglandin administration for ripening the unfavourable cervix.

4.4 Direct comparisons between different routes of administration

Seven English-language reports on controlled comparisons between various routes of prostaglandin administration have been published (Ulmsten *et al.* 1985; Thiery *et al.* 1984; Wilson 1978; Davey and MacNab 1979; Toplis and Sims 1979; Stewart *et al.* 1983; Parewijck and Thiery 1986). They have involved comparisons between oral and vaginal administration (Wilson 1978; Davey and MacNab 1979); between oral and extra-amniotic administration (Wilson 1978); between vaginal and endocervical administration (Ulmsten *et al.* 1985; Thiery *et al.* 1984); between vaginal and extra-amniotic administration (Wilson 1978; Toplis and Sims 1979; Stewart *et al.* 1983); and between endocervical and extra-amniotic administration (Parewijck and Thiery 1986). Only two of these comparisons, both of them comparing the endocervical and vaginal routes of administration have been conducted in a double-blind manner (Ulmsten *et al.* 1985; Thiery *et al.* 1984). The other investigators all used either alternate allocation or did not describe their method of random or quasi-random allocation. There is thus potential for bias in all except two of these trials (Ulmsten *et al.* 1985; Thiery *et al.* 1984). Moreover, the total numbers of women included in these comparisons are small. In addition, they have occasionally been divided over several

Table 61.34 Effect of endocervical PGE$_2$ for cervical ripening on low Apgar score at 1 minute

Study	EXPT		CTRL		Odds ratio	Graph of odds ratios and confidence intervals
	n	(%)	n	(%)	(95% CI)	0.01 0.1 0.5 1 2 10 100
Bernstein et al. (1988)	10/206	(4.85)	11/202	(5.45)	0.89 (0.37–2.13)	
Thiery et al. (1984)	5/40	(12.50)	12/40	(30.00)	0.36 (0.12–1.03)	
Cabrol et al. (1988)	19/110	(17.27)	21/107	(19.63)	0.86 (0.43–1.70)	
noah et al. (1987)	53/401	(13.22)	38/397	(9.57)	1.43 (0.93–2.22)	
Yonekura et al. (1985)	4/25	(16.00)	6/23	(26.09)	0.55 (0.14–2.18)	
Typical odds ratio (95% confidence interval)					1.02 (0.74–1.39)	

Effect of endocervical PGE$_2$ for cervical ripening on low Apgar score at 5 minutes

Ulmsten et al. (1985)	0/19	(0.00)	0/20	(0.00)	1.00 (1.00–1.00)	
Bernstein et al. (1988)	1/206	(0.49)	0/202	(0.00)	7.25 (0.14–99.99)	
Wingerup et al. (1978)	0/10	(0.00)	0/10	(0.00)	1.00 (1.00–1.00)	
Thiery et al. (1984)	2/40	(5.00)	4/40	(10.00)	0.49 (0.09–2.56)	
Cabrol et al. (1988)	3/110	(2.73)	1/107	(0.93)	2.68 (0.37–19.30)	
Noah et al. (1987)	5/401	(1.25)	7/397	(1.76)	0.71 (0.23–2.21)	
Yonekura et al. (1985)	0/25	(0.00)	2/23	(8.70)	0.12 (0.01–1.96)	
Typical odds ratio (95% confidence interval)					0.77 (0.35–1.70)	

Effect of endocervical ripening on perinatal death excluding lethal malformation

Ulmsten et al. (1985)	0/19	(0.00)	0/20	(0.00)	1.00 (1.00–1.00)	
Nimrod et al. (1984)	0/30	(0.00)	0/15	(0.00)	1.00 (1.00–1.00)	
Hutchon et al. (1980)	0/31	(0.00)	1/35	(2.86)	0.15 (0.00–7.70)	
Laube et al. (1986)	0/30	(0.00)	0/15	(0.00)	1.00 (1.00–1.00)	
Bernstein et al. (1988)	1/206	(0.49)	0/202	(0.00)	7.25 (0.14–99.99)	
Cabrol et al. (1988)	0/110	(0.00)	1/107	(0.93)	0.13 (0.00–6.63)	
Noah et al. (1987)	0/416	(0.00)	1/404	(0.25)	0.13 (0.00–6.62)	
Typical odds ratio (95% confidence interval)					0.37 (0.05–2.64)	

Table 61.35 Characteristics of controlled evaluations of extra-amniotic prostaglandins for cervical ripening

Authors and dates	Allocation	Treatments compared and type of gel used	No. treated PG : Placebo	Cervix score + cut-off	Interval to induction + method of induction
Shepherd *et al.* (1976)	alternate	0.25 mg vs. placebo PGE$_2$ gel methylhydroxyethyl cellulose	nulliparae 9 : 11 multiparae 6 : 4	Bishop <5	14½ hours method not reported
Quinn *et al.* (1981)	double-blind	10 mg vs. placebo PGF$_{2\alpha}$ gel methylhydroxyethyl cellulose	nulliparae 15 : 10	Calder <4	12 hours amniotomy + oxytocin
Fenton *et al.* (1985)	double-blind	0.4 mg vs. placebo PGE$_2$ gel hydroxymethyl cellulose	nulliparae 15 : 15	Bishop <5	12 hours amniotomy + oxytocin

Table 61.36 Effect of extra-amniotic prostaglandis for cervical ripening on labour onset during ripening

Study	EXPT n	(%)	CTRL n	(%)	Odds ratio (95% CI)	Graph of odds ratios and confidence intervals
Quinn *et al.* (1981)	4/15	(26.67)	0/10	(0.00)	6.72 (0.79–57.01)	
Fenton *et al.* (1985)	8/15	(53.33)	1/15	(6.67)	8.57 (1.85–39.79)	
Shepherd *et al.* (1976)	8/15	(53.33)	1/15	(6.67)	8.57 (1.85–39.79)	
Typical odds ratio (95% confidence interval)					8.15 (3.10–21.46)	

Effect of extra-amniotic prostaglandins for cervical ripening on caesarean section

Quinn *et al.* (1981)	1/15	(6.67)	2/10	(20.00)	0.30 (0.03–3.32)	
Fenton *et al.* (1985)	2/15	(13.33)	5/15	(33.33)	0.34 (0.06–1.79)	
Shepherd *et al.* (1976)	1/15	(6.67)	1/15	(6.67)	1.00 (0.06–16.79)	
Typical odds ratio (95% confidence interval)					0.40 (0.12–1.38)	

Effect of extra-amniotic prostaglandins for cervical ripening on instrumental delivery

Quinn *et al.* (1981)	6/15	(40.00)	7/10	(70.00)	0.32 (0.07–1.51)	
Shepherd *et al.* (1976)	8/15	(53.33)	7/15	(46.67)	1.29 (0.32–5.29)	
Typical odds ratio (95% confidence interval)					0.69 (0.24–1.97)	

Table 61.36—*continued* Effect of extra-amniotic prostaglandins for cervical ripening on operative delivery

Study	EXPT		CTRL		Odds ratio	Graph of odds ratios and confidence intervals
	n	(%)	*n*	(%)	(95% CI)	0.01 0.1 0.5 1 2 10 100
Quinn *et al.* (1981)	7/15	(46.67)	9/10	(90.00)	0.16 (0.03–0.84)	
Shepherd *et al.* (1976)	9/15	(60.00)	8/15	(53.33)	1.30 (0.31–5.38)	
Typical odds ratio (95% confidence interval)					0.53 (0.18–1.56)	

Effect of extra-amniotic prostaglandins for cervical ripening on fetal death after randomization

Quinn *et al.* (1981)	1/15	(6.67)	0/10	(0.00)	5.29 (0.10–99.99)	
Fenton *et al.* (1985)	0/15	(0.00)	0/15	(0.00)	1.00 (1.00–1.00)	
Shepherd *et al.* (1976)	0/15	(0.00)	0/15	(0.00)	1.00 (1.00–1.00)	
Typical odds ratio (95% confidence interval)					5.29 (0.10–99.99)	

Effect of extra-amniotic prostaglandins for cervical ripening on low Apgar score at 5 minutes

Shepherd *et al.* (1976)	0/15	(0.00)	0/15	(0.00)	1.00 (1.00–1.00)	
Typical odds ratio (95% confidence interval)					1.00 (1.00–1.00)	

groups. For example, Davey and MacNab (1979) reported controlled comparisons in which a total of 33 women were 'randomized' to 5 different dose regimens of PGE$_2$, 3 of which were administered vaginally and 2 orally. The data derived from these comparisons are therefore unlikely to be helpful.

The results of the two reasonably well conducted double-blind trials of endocervical vs. vaginal PGE$_2$ for cervical ripening (Ulmsten *et al.* 1985; Thiery *et al.* 1984), details of which have been shown in Tables 61.25 and 61.30, are presented in Table 61.37). They suggest some superiority of the endocervical over the vaginal approach in terms of the number of women going into labour during ripening (if this is considered to be a desirable outcome); the number delivered during ripening; and the rate of caesarean section. The precision of these estimates is such that firm conclusions regarding the differential effects of these routes of administration will have to await the results of further larger trials. One such multicentre trial is currently being conducted in The Netherlands.

The three trials which compared extra-amniotic with vaginal administration (Wilson 1978; Toplis and Sims 1979; Stewart *et al.* 1983) showed that labour was more likely to occur during ripening when the intrauterine rather than the vaginal route of administration was selected (typical odds ratio 2.71; 95 per cent confidence interval 1.34–5.51; Table 61.38). None of the other outcome measures on which data were available indicated any differential effect between these two routes of administration (Table 61.38), but the precision of these estimates is low.

The results of the single trial which has reported on a comparison between extra-amniotic and endocervical administration (Parewijck and Thiery 1986) show that 75 per cent of women receiving the PGE$_2$ extra-amniotically went into labour as opposed to 32 per cent of those who received the drug endocervically (Table 61.39). This would suggest that the extra-amniotic route, if at all used, should be reserved for women in whom immediate induction of labour is warranted.

Table 61.37 Effect of endocervical vs. vaginal PGE$_2$ for cervical ripening on labour onset during ripening

Study	EXPT n	(%)	CTRL n	(%)	Odds ratio (95% CI)	Graph of odds ratios and confidence intervals
Thiery *et al.* (1984)	9/40	(22.50)	5/41	(12.20)	2.04 (0.65–6.40)	
Typical odds ratio (95% confidence interval)					2.04 (0.65–6.40)	

Effect of endocervical vs. vaginal PGE$_2$ for cervical ripening on delivered during ripening

Ulmsten *et al.* (1985)	11/19	(57.89)	4/19	(21.05)	4.49 (1.24–16.20)	
Typical odds ratio (95% confidence interval)					4.49 (1.24–16.20)	

Effect of endocervical vs. vaginal PGE$_2$ for cervical ripening on excessive uterine activity

Thiery *et al.* (1984)	1/40	(2.50)	0/41	(0.00)	7.58 (0.15–99.99)	
Typical odds ratio (95% confidence interval)					7.58 (0.15–99.99)	

Effect of endocervical vs. vaginal PGE$_2$ for cervical ripening on fetal heart rate abnormalities

Thiery *et al.* (1984)	3/40	(7.50)	4/41	(9.76)	0.75 (0.16–3.52)	
Typical odds ratio (95% confidence interval)					0.75 (0.16–3.52)	

Effect of endocervical vs. vaginal PGE$_2$ for cervical ripening on gastrointestinal side-effects

Ulmsten *et al.* (1985)	0/19	(0.00)	0/19	(0.00)	1.00 (1.00–1.00)	
Thiery *et al.* (1984)	6/40	(15.00)	7/41	(17.07)	0.86 (0.26–2.79)	
Typical odds ratio (95% confidence interval)					0.86 (0.26–2.79)	

Effect of endocervical vs. vaginal PGE$_2$ for cervical ripening on caesarean section

Ulmsten *et al.* (1985)	3/19	(15.79)	7/19	(36.84)	0.35 (0.08–1.44)	
Thiery *et al.* (1984)	1/40	(2.50)	0/41	(0.00)	7.58 (0.15-99.99)	
Typical odds ratio (95% confidence interval)					0.50 (0.15–99.99)	

Effect of endocervical vs. vaginal PGE$_2$ for cervical ripening on low Apgar score at 5 minutes

Ulmsten *et al.* (1985)	0/19	(0.00)	0/19	(0.00)	1.00 (1.00–1.00)	
Thiery *et al.* (1984)	2/40	(5.00)	2/41	(4.88)	1.03 (0.14–7.57)	
Typical odds ratio (95% confidence interval)					1.03 (0.14–7.57)	

Table 61.38 Effect of extra-amniotic vs. vaginal PGE$_2$ for cervical ripening on labour onset during ripening

Study	EXPT		CTRL		Odds ratio	Graph of odds ratios and confidence intervals
	n	(%)	n	(%)	(95% CI)	0.01 0.1 0.5 1 2 10 100
Wilson (1978)	5/15	(33.33)	3/15	(20.00)	1.93 (0.39–9.49)	
Toplis and Sims (1979)	6/20	(30.00)	9/40	(22.50)	1.48 (0.43–5.07)	
Stewart *et al.* (1983)	17/32	(53.13)	5/30	(16.67)	4.79 (1.71–13.46)	
Typical odds ratio (95% confidence interval)					2.71 (1.34–5.51)	

Effect of extra-amniotic vs. vaginal PGE$_2$ for cervical ripening on no need for formal induction of labour

Toplis and Sims (1979)	12/20	(60.00)	17/40	(42.50)	1.99 (0.69–5.78)	
Stewart *et al.* (1983)	10/32	(31.25)	13/30	(43.33)	0.60 (0.22–1.67)	
Typical odds ratio (95% confidence interval)					1.07 (0.51–2.23)	

Effect of extra-amniotic vs. vaginal PGE$_2$ for cervical ripening on failed induction

Toplis and Sims (1979)	1/20	(5.00)	5/40	(12.50)	0.44 (0.07–2.60)	
Typical odds ratio (95% confidence interval)					0.44 (0.07–2.60)	

Effect of extra-amniotic vs. vaginal PGE$_2$ for cervical ripening on hypertonus and/or hyperstimulation

Wilson (1978)	0/15	(0.00)	0/15	(0.00)	1.00 (1.00–1.00)	
Toplis and Sims (1979)	0/20	(0.00)	0/40	(0.00)	1.00 (1.00–1.00)	
Typical odds ratio (95% confidence interval)					1.00 (1.00–1.00)	

Effect of extra-amniotic vs. vaginal PGE$_2$ for cervical ripening on pyrexia in labour

Wilson (1978)	0/15	(0.00)	0/15	(0.00)	1.00 (1.00–1.00)	
Toplis and Sims (1979)	5/20	(25.00)	3/40	(7.50)	4.43 (0.93–21.22)	
Typical odds ratio (95% confidence interval)					4.43 (0.93–21.22)	

Effect of extra-amniotic vs. vaginal PGE$_2$ for cervical ripening on caesarean section

Wilson (1978)	1/15	(6.67)	3/15	(20.00)	0.33 (0.04–2.60)	
Toplis and Sims (1979)	1/20	(5.00)	7/40	(17.50)	0.35 (0.07–1.65)	
Stewart *et al.* (1983)	5/32	(15.63)	5/30	(16.67)	0.93 (0.24–3.55)	
Typical odds ratio (95% confidence interval)					0.54 (0.22–1.35)	

Table 61.38—*continued* Effect of extra-amniotic vs. vaginal PGE$_2$ for cervical ripening on instrumental vaginal delivery

Study	EXPT		CTRL		Odds ratio	Graph of odds ratios and confidence intervals						
	n	(%)	n	(%)	(95% CI)	0.01	0.1	0.5	1	2	10	100
Wilson (1978)	4/15	(26.67)	3/15	(20.00)	1.43 (0.27–7.57)							
Toplis and Sims (1979)	10/20	(50.00)	22/40	(55.00)	0.82 (0.28–2.39)							
Stewart *et al.* (1983)	11/32	(34.38)	12/30	(40.00)	0.79 (0.28–2.19)							
Typical odds ratio (95% confidence interval)					0.88 (0.45–1.74)							

Effect of extra-amniotic vs. vaginal PGE$_2$ for cervical ripening on operative delivery

Study	EXPT		CTRL		Odds ratio							
Wilson (1978)	5/15	(33.33)	6/15	(40.00)	0.76 (0.18–3.26)							
Toplis and Sims (1979)	11/20	(55.00)	29/40	(72.50)	0.46 (0.15–1.43)							
Stewart *et al.* (1983)	16/32	(50.00)	17/30	(56.67)	0.77 (0.29–2.07)							
Typical odds ratio (95% confidence interval)					0.64 (0.33–1.25)							

Effect of extra-amniotic vs. vaginal PGE$_2$ for cervical ripening on neonatal infection

Study	EXPT		CTRL		Odds ratio							
Toplis and Sims (1979)	0/20	(0.00)	0/40	(0.00)	1.00 (1.00–1.00)							
Typical odds ratio (95% confidence interval)					1.00 (1.00–1.00)							

Effect of extra-amniotic vs. vaginal PGE$_2$ for cervical ripening on low Apgar score at 5 minutes

Study	EXPT		CTRL		Odds ratio							
Stewart *et al.* (1983)	1/32	(3.13)	0/30	(0.00)	6.94 (0.14–99.99)							
Typical odds ratio (95% confidence interval)					6.94 (0.14–99.99)							

Table 61.39 Effect of extra-amniotic vs. endocervical PGE$_2$ for cervical ripening on labour onset during ripening

Study	EXPT		CTRL		Odds ratio	Graph of odds ratios and confidence intervals						
	n	(%)	n	(%)	(95% CI)	0.01	0.1	0.5	1	2	10	10
Parewijck and Thiery (1986)	75/101	(74.26)	30/93	(32.26)	5.38 (3.06–9.46)							
Typical odds ratio (95% confidence interval)					5.38 (3.06–9.46)							

Effect of extra-amniotic vs. endocervical PGE$_2$ for cervical ripening on intrauterine infection

Study	EXPT		CTRL		Odds ratio							
Parewijck and Thiery (1986)	0/101	(0.00)	0/93	(0.00)	1.00 (1.00–1.00)							
Typical odds ratio (95% confidence interval)					1.00 (1.00–1.00)							

Table 61.39—*continued* Effect of extra-amniotic vs. endocervical PGE_2 for cervical ripening on caesarean section

Study	EXPT		CTRL		Odds ratio	Graph of odds ratios and confidence intervals
	n	(%)	*n*	(%)	(95% CI)	0.01 0.1 0.5 1 2 10 100
Parewijck and Thiery (1986)	1/101	(0.99)	2/93	(2.15)	0.47 (0.05–4.57)	
Typical odds ratio (95% confidence interval)					0.47 (0.05–4.57)	

5 Other methods for cervical ripening

5.1 Oestrogens

Ten trials have been reported in which an oestrogen was administered for cervical ripening (Gordon and Calder 1977; Thiery *et al.* 1979; Luther *et al.* 1980; Quinn *et al.* 1981; Tromans *et al.* 1981; Stewart *et al.* 1981; Pedersen *et al.* 1981; Sasaki *et al.* 1982; MacLennan *et al.* 1981; Magnani and Cabrol 1986). Three of these compared extra-amniotic or vaginal administra-tion of oestradiol with either prostaglandins (Tromans *et al.* 1981; Stewart *et al.* 1981), or with various combi-nations consisting of oestradiol, prostaglandin $F_{2\alpha}$, and relaxin (MacLennan *et al.* 1981). Seven trials compared the administration of an oestrogen with placebo (Gor-don and Calder 1977; Thiery *et al.* 1979; Luther *et al.* 1980; Pedersen *et al.* 1981; Quinn *et al.* 1981; Sasaki *et al.* 1982; Magnani and Cabrol 1986). The characteris-tics of these seven trials, most of which have tested extra-amniotic oestrogen administration, are shown in Table 61.40. Four of the trials included a

Table 61.40 Characteristics of the placebo-controlled evaluations of oestrogens for cervical ripening

Authors and dates	Random method	Treatments compared		No. of women		Method of induction
		Oestrogens	Placebo	Oestro-gens	Placebo	
Gordon and Calder (1977)	random not described	150 mg oestradiol in Tylose gel extra-amniotically	Tylose gel extra-amniotically	25 nulliparae	25	amniotomy + oxytocin after 16 hours
Thiery *et al.* (1978, 1979)	random not described	180 mg oestradiol in Tylose gel extra-amniotically	Tylose gel extra-amniotically	35	35	amniotomy + oxytocin after 12 hours, only if cervix favourable
		250 mg oestriol in Tylose gel extra-amniotically		35 all parities		
Luther *et al.* (1980)	double-blind	10 mg oestradiol in sesame oil intramuscularly	identical appearing placebo intramuscularly	51 all parities	49	oral PGE_2 after 48 hours
Pedersen *et al.* (1981)	double-blind	115 mg oestradiol extra-amniotically	0.9% saline solution extra-amniotically	25 nulliparae	25	oxytocin tablets every 30 min for 5 hours started immediately
Quinn *et al.* (1981)	double-blind	15 mg oestriol in Tylose gel extra-amniotically	Tylose gel extra-amniotic	15 nulliparae	10	amniotomy + oxytocin after 12 hours
Sasaki *et al.* (1982)	double-blind	100 mg dehydro-epiandrosterone sulphate intravenously twice a week from 38 weeks until delivery	10 ml glucose 5% intravenous twice a week from 38 weeks until delivery	44 all parities	40	not applicable (no induction of labour)
Magnani and Cabrol (1986)	double-blind	150 mg oestradiol in Tylose gel intracervically	Tylose gel intracervically	10 nulliparae	10	no information available
	double-blind	150 mg oestradiol in Tylose gel vaginally	Tylose gel vaginally	14 all parities	15	0.5 mg PGE_2 extra-amniotic after 24 hours

Table 61.41 Effect of oestrogens for cervical ripening on labour onset during ripening

Study	EXPT		CTRL		Odds ratio	Graph of odds ratios and confidence intervals
	n	(%)	*n*	(%)	(95% CI)	0.01 0.1 0.5 1 2 10 100
Quinn *et al.* (1981)	1/15	(6.67)	0/10	(0.00)	5.29 (0.10–99.99)	
Magnani and Cabrol (1986)	0/13	(0.00)	0/13	(0.00)	1.00 (1.00–1.00)	
Gordon and Calder (1977)	1/25	(4.00)	1/25	(4.00)	1.00 (0.06–16.45)	
Typical odds ratio (95% confidence interval)					1.73 (0.17–17.16)	

Effect of oestrogens for cervical ripening on delivered during ripening

Study	EXPT		CTRL		Odds ratio	
Luther *et al.* (1980)	7/51	(13.73)	7/49	(14.29)	0.95 (0.31–2.94)	
Pedersen *et al.* (1981)	15/25	(60.00)	17/25	(68.00)	0.71 (0.23–2.23)	
Magnani and Cabrol (1986)	0/13	(0.00)	0/13	(0.00)	1.00 (1.00–1.00)	
Typical odds ratio (95% confidence interval)					0.83 (0.37–1.84)	

Effect of oestrogens for cervical ripening on hypertonus and/or hyperstimulation

Study	EXPT		CTRL		Odds ratio	
Quinn *et al.* (1981)	0/15	(0.00)	0/10	(0.00)	1.00 (1.00–1.00)	
Thiery *et al.* (1979)	0/70	(0.00)	0/35	(0.00)	1.00 (1.00–1.00)	
Gordon and Calder (1977)	0/25	(0.00)	0/25	(0.00)	1.00 (1.00–1.00)	
Typical odds ratio (95% confidence interval)					1.00 (1.00–1.00)	

Effect of oestrogens for cervical ripening on not delivered within 12 hours

Study	EXPT		CTRL		Odds ratio	
Luther *et al.* (1980)	38/51	(74.51)	36/49	(73.47)	1.05 (0.43–2.57)	
Typical odds ratio (95% confidence interval)					1.05 (0.43–2.57)	

Effect of oestrogens for cervical ripening on caesarean section

Study	EXPT		CTRL		Odds ratio	
Luther *et al.* (1980)	6/51	(11.76)	10/49	(20.41)	0.53 (0.18–1.53)	
Quinn *et al.* (1981)	1/15	(6.67)	2/10	(20.00)	0.30 (0.03–3.32)	
Sasaki *et al.* (1982)	0/44	(0.00)	0/40	(0.00)	1.00 (1.00–1.00)	
Magnani and Cabrol (1986)	2/13	(15.38)	3/13	(23.08)	0.62 (0.09–4.21)	
Thiery *et al.* (1979)	1/70	(1.43)	2/35	(5.71)	0.22 (0.02–2.45)	
Gordon and Calder (1977)	3/25	(12.00)	7/25	(28.00)	0.38 (0.10–1.48)	
Typical odds ratio (95% confidence interval)					0.44 (0.22–0.88)	

Table 61.41—*continued* Effect of oestrogens for cervical ripening on instrumental vaginal delivery

Study	EXPT		CTRL		Odds ratio	Graph of odds ratios and confidence intervals
	n	(%)	n	(%)	(95% CI)	0.01 0.1 0.5 1 2 10 100
...inn *et al.* (1981)	6/15	(40.00)	7/10	(70.00)	0.32 (0.07–1.51)	
...gnani and Cabrol (1986)	5/13	(38.46)	3/13	(23.08)	2.00 (0.39–10.26)	
...pical odds ratio (...% confidence interval)					0.77 (0.25–2.37)	

Effect of oestrogens for cervical ripening on pyrexia in labour

...rdon and Calder (1977)	0/25	(0.00)	5/25	(20.00)	0.11 (0.02–0.71)	
...pical odds ratio (...% confidence interval)					0.11 (0.02–0.71)	

Effect of oestrogens for cervical ripening on low Apgar score at 1 minute

...gnani and Cabrol (1986)	0/13	(0.00)	0/13	(0.00)	1.00 (1.00–1.00)	
...rdon and Calder (1977)	0/25	(0.00)	3/25	(12.00)	0.12 (0.01–1.25)	
...pical odds ratio (...% confidence interval)					0.12 (0.01–1.25)	

Effect of oestrogens for cervical ripening on perinatal death

...ery *et al.* (1979)	0/70	(0.00)	0/35	(0.00)	1.00 (1.00–1.00)	
...rdon and Calder (1977)	0/25	(0.00)	0/25	(0.00)	1.00 (1.00–1.00)	
...pical odds ratio (...% confidence interval)					1.00 (1.00–1.00)	

Effect of oestrogens for cervical ripening on neonatal jaundice

...ersen *et al.* (1981)	13/25	(52.00)	4/25	(16.00)	4.82 (1.51–15.34)	
...pical odds ratio (...% confidence interval)					4.82 (1.51–15.34)	

treatment group receiving oestradiol extra-amniotically and two included a group receiving oestriol extra-amniotically (Table 61.40). Since there is no evidence that these two oestrogens act differently, the results of these trials have been considered together. In comparing these studies it should be realized, however, that the oestrogenic potency of oestriol is about 10 times lower than that of oestradiol. In two of the trials the oestrogenic substance was administered systemically; one used 10 mg oestradiol intramuscularly (Luther *et al.* 1980); and the other (Sasaki *et al.* 1982) used intravenous dehydroepiandrosterone sulphate, which is trans-

formed into oestrogens in the fetoplacental unit (Flint 1979).

Much of the interest in oestrogens for cervical ripening has been derived from the idea that these agents might ripen the cervix without concomitant effects on uterine contractility (Gordon and Calder 1977; Hillier and Wallis 1978; Ellwood *et al.* 1979; Stewart *et al.* 1981). Nevertheless, of the 7 placebo-controlled trials, only 3 provided data on the frequency with which labour started during the treatment period reserved for achieving cervical ripening (Table 61.41), and, overall, there were only 53 oestrogen-treated women in these 3 trials. One of these three trials, and two others in addition, also provided data on the number of women who delivered during the ripening period. Data for this outcome were available on 89 oestrogen-treated women, of whom 13 were already represented in the data on onset of labour during cervical ripening. The pooled overviews (Table 61.41) offer no suggestion that labour is more likely to start or delivery more likely to occur during oestrogen treatment than it is with placebo treatment. No case of 'uterine hypertonus' or 'hyperstimulation' was reported (among 110 oestrogen-treated women) in the three trials that referred to this complication (Table 61.41).

Calder and his colleagues, who introduced oestrogen treatment for ripening the cervix (Gordon and Calder 1977), have suggested that 'the value of oestradiol may be reduced by the relative insensitivity of the uterus to subsequent forewater amniotomy and oxytocin for the induction of labour' (Stewart and Calder 1981). Unfortunately, only one trial (Luther *et al.* 1980) provided information on the number of women who were delivered within 12 hours after induction of labour following oestrogen pretreatment; there was no difference with the control group (Table 61.41).

Notwithstanding the apparent lack of contraction-enhancing activity of the oestrogen treatment, it was associated with a statistically significant reduction in the incidence of caesarean section (Table 61.41). All of the trials which provided data on the incidence of caesarean section showed either no caesarean sections or fewer caesarean sections in the oestrogen-treated than in the placebo group and the typical odds ratio was 0.44 (with a 95 per cent confidence interval of 0.22 to 0.88; Table 61.41). Only one trial (Gordon and Calder 1977) provided data on the incidence of pyrexia during labour and both groups of women had received an extra-amniotic gel (Table 61.41). However, pyrexia was statistically significantly less common in women receiving oestradiol than in women receiving placebo (Table 61.41), suggesting that the addition of oestradiol to the gel vehicle lowered the likelihood of infection. Other side-effects were apparently not observed, or at least not reported in any of the trials.

Categorical data on infant outcomes are lacking in most of the reports. Only two of the reports (Gordon and Calder 1977; Thiery *et al.* 1979) mention perinatal deaths; there were none. This may well apply also to the other trials, but there is no certainty from the reports that this is indeed the case. The two trials (Gordon and Calder 1977; Magnani and Cabrol 1986) that provided categorical data on low 1-minute Apgar scores suggest a decrease with oestrogen treatment, but this reduction is compatible with chance (95 per cent confidence interval 0.01–1.25; Table 61.41). Pedersen *et al.* (1981) noted a statistically significantly higher incidence of phototherapy in the oestradiol-treated group (Table 61.41) than in the placebo group. None of the other trials provided data on this outcome, and it is therefore uncertain whether this constitutes a real effect.

5.2 Oxytocin

Five trials have investigated the value of oxytocin for cervical ripening (Pentecost 1973; Valentine 1977; Jagani *et al.* 1982, 1984; Roberts *et al.* 1986). Together they included only 90 oxytocin-treated women and 89 control women, and in all but one of the trials (Pentecost 1973) these women were of mixed parity (Table 61.42). In 4 of the trials, intravenous oxytocin was

Table 61.42 Characteristics of the controlled evaluations of oxytocin for cervical ripening

Authors and dates	Random method	Oxytocin treatment	Control treatment	No. of women	Interval to induction	Method of induction
Pentecost (1973)	double-blind	buccal oxytocin citrate 100–400 Units every 30 min for 7½ hours	placebo tablets	25:25 nulliparae	24 hours	not described (amniotomy and/or oxytocin infusion)
Valentine (1977)	random not described	30 U oxytocin intravenously for 10 hours	no treatment	15:15 mixed parity	24 hours	amniotomy if possible + intravenous oxytocin
Jagani *et al.* (1982)	case record number	oxytocin IV until adequate contractility	no treatment	10:10 mixed parity	12 hours	amniotomy + intravenous oxytocin
		– both groups had an extra-amniotic catheter inserted –				
Jagani *et al.* (1984)	case record number	oxytocin IV dose not specified	no treatment	16:16 mixed parity	12 hours	amniotomy + intravenous oxytocin
		– both groups had an extra-amniotic catheter inserted –				
Roberts *et al.* (1986)	sealed envelopes	1 mU oxytocin per min for 12 hours	no treatment	25:24 mixed parity	12 hours	intravenous oxytocin

compared with no treatment; in the fifth the comparison was between buccal oxytocin and placebo tablets (Table 61.42). Three of these trials also contained (small) comparison groups receiving Foley catheters, laminaria, amniotomy, or prostaglandins for cervical ripening (Roberts *et al.* 1986; Jagani 1982, 1984).

The combined data of all 5 trials incorporated too few women to allow firm conclusions to be drawn. Pentecost (1973), who intended to enter 200 women in his trial, stopped his study after 50 had been entered (two of whom were subsequently excluded because of 'technical problems') because 'results were such that there seemed no point in pursuing the study any further'. Each of the other trials included only between 10 and 16 oxytocin-treated women. Remarkably, the overall results of the trials indicate that women with an unripe cervix (defined as a Bishop score below 5 in all trials except that of Pentecost (1973) who used a score of his own) were no more likely to go into labour during cervical ripening with oxytocin than occurred normally without such treatment (Table 61.43). The two studies which assessed whether or not amniotomy was possible after the ripening regimen showed no statistically significant differences between the treated and the control groups (Table 61.43).

The incidence of caesarean section in oxytocin-treated women was similar to that found in the control group, with a typical odds ratio of 0.87 (95 per cent confidence interval 0.43–1.74; Table 61.43). The data shown in Table 61.43 are consistent with other data derived from trials comparing prostaglandins with oxytocin for cervical ripening, and from the 'no treatment' arms of controlled trials in which prostaglandin or no treatment for cervical ripening was followed by oxytocin infusion without concomitant amniotomy. The results of some of these trials have indicated that labour is more likely to ensue during a 12-hour period of cervical ripening with prostaglandins than it is during a similar period of 'no treatment' followed by a 12-hour course of oxytocin infusion (Keirse *et al.* 1987). All the information currently available indicates that oxytocin administration to ripen the cervix (rather than to induce labour), whether administered intravenously or through the mucosae, serves no useful purpose. Oxytocin infusions for prolonged periods of time (as is usually the case when the aim is to ripen the cervix) are unpleasant, limit the woman's mobility, and may lead to water intoxication when administered in large doses (Burt *et al.* 1969). This practice should be abandoned.

5.3 Mechanical methods

In recent years, mechanical devices such as catheters and tents, which were formerly used for induction of labour (see Chapter 59) and termination of pregnancy, have also been applied in attempts to achieve cervical ripening. In the 1960s, dissatisfaction with the repeat oxytocin infusions that were used when the cervix was unfavourable led to the introduction of balloon catheters inserted in the extra-amniotic space (Embrey and Mollison 1967; see also Chapter 59). Laminaria tents, which had apparently disappeared into obscurity (see Chapter 59), were reintroduced first as an adjunct to methods for terminating pregnancy (Newton 1972; Eaton *et al.* 1972; Lischke and Goodlin 1973; Duenhoelter *et al.* 1976), and subsequently to ripen the cervix in term pregnancies (Cross and Pitkin 1978; Lackritz *et al.* 1979).

In addition to laminaria tents, new synthetic hydrophylic materials were developed with the same aims in mind. Only one of these, Lamicel®, a polyvinyl alcohol polymer sponge that behaves like a synthetic laminaria tent, has thus far been tested in controlled comparisons for ripening the cervix prior to induction. Lamicel® is impregnated with 450 mg of magnesium sulphate and compressed to form a rigid cylindrical tent 5 mm in diameter and 77 mm long. When inserted into the cervical canal, it absorbs water and swells to four times its original size while changing from a rigid cylinder to a soft sponge. The controlled comparison has been with other ripening agents, however, rather than with no treatment (MacPherson 1984; Johnson *et al.* 1985).

The mechanism by which the various mechanical methods influence cervical compliance may differ according to whether the insertion is extra-amniotic (as it is for Foley catheters and other types of balloons), or mainly endocervical (as for Lamicel® and laminaria). The latter may exert any effect they have by a gradual process of mechanical distension of the cervix. The former, which do not distend the cervical canal, are likely to achieve their effects in a more general manner, either by uterine stimulation, or by enhancing the production of substances which induce cervical softening (Keirse *et al.* 1983). It may therefore not be entirely appropriate to include the results of controlled comparisons of these devices in a single overview. The separate analyses (not shown) provided no indications, however, that the conclusions reached in respect of any one of these methods were not applicable to all of them.

Six controlled trials, each involving between 12 and 74 women, have examined the clinical effects of mechanical methods on cervical ripening before induction of labour. Four have dealt with laminaria (Cross and Pitkin 1978; Roberts *et al.* 1986; Lackritz *et al.* 1979; Gower *et al.* 1982); one with the insertion of a Foley catheter (Lewis 1983); and the sixth with both of these procedures (Jagani *et al.* 1982). None of the trials is above suspicion with regard to the possibility of selection bias, either at or after allocation.

One further trial (Manabe *et al.* 1982) has been excluded from the overview because it was uncertain whether contemporary controls had been used. This trial reported on 200 'randomly selected cases', 100

Table 61.43 Effect of oxytocin vs. no treatment for unripe cervix on labour onset during ripening

Study	EXPT n	(%)	CTRL n	(%)	Odds ratio (95% CI)	Graph of odds ratios and confidence intervals
Pentecost (1973)	2/24	(8.33)	3/24	(12.50)	0.65 (0.10–4.04)	
Valentine (1977)	2/15	(13.33)	0/15	(0.00)	7.94 (0.47–99.99)	
Jagani et al. (1982)	0/10	(0.00)	2/10	(20.00)	0.12 (0.01–2.09)	
Jagani et al. (1984)	2/16	(12.50)	2/16	(12.50)	1.00 (0.13–7.86)	
Typical odds ratio (95% confidence interval)					0.85 (0.27–2.62)	

Effect of oxytocin vs. no treatment for unripe cervix on amniotomy impossible/not performed

Study	EXPT n	(%)	CTRL n	(%)	Odds ratio (95% CI)	
Pentecost (1973)	5/24	(20.83)	9/24	(37.50)	0.45 (0.13–1.56)	
Valentine (1977)	8/15	(53.33)	8/15	(53.33)	1.00 (0.24–4.10)	
Typical odds ratio (95% confidence interval)					0.64 (0.25–1.62)	

Effect of oxytocin vs. no treatment for unripe cervix on caesarean section

Study	EXPT n	(%)	CTRL n	(%)	Odds ratio (95% CI)	
Pentecost (1973)	2/24	(8.33)	5/24	(20.83)	0.37 (0.08–1.83)	
Roberts et al. (1986)	6/25	(24.00)	8/24	(33.33)	0.64 (0.19–2.18)	
Valentine (1977)	4/15	(26.67)	7/15	(46.67)	0.43 (0.10–1.87)	
Jagani et al. (1982)	3/10	(30.00)	0/10	(0.00)	9.35 (0.85–99.99)	
Jagani et al. (1984)	5/16	(31.25)	2/16	(12.50)	2.89 (0.56–15.07)	
Typical odds ratio (95% confidence interval)					0.87 (0.43–1.74)	

Effect of oxytocin vs. no treatment for unripe cervix on instrumental vaginal delivery

Study	EXPT n	(%)	CTRL n	(%)	Odds ratio (95% CI)	
Pentecost (1973)	4/24	(16.67)	2/24	(8.33)	2.11 (0.39–11.46)	
Valentine (1977)	7/15	(46.67)	4/15	(26.67)	2.30 (0.53–9.90)	
Typical odds ratio (95% confidence interval)					2.22 (0.73–6.69)	

Effect of oxytocin vs. no treatment for unripe cervix on operative delivery

Study	EXPT n	(%)	CTRL n	(%)	Odds ratio (95% CI)	
Pentecost (1973)	6/24	(25.00)	7/24	(29.17)	0.81 (0.23–2.87)	
Valentine (1977)	11/15	(73.33)	11/15	(73.33)	1.00 (0.20–4.91)	
Typical odds ratio (95% confidence interval)					0.88 (0.33–2.36)	

Table 61.44 Effect of mechanical methods for cervical ripening on poor increase in cervical score

Study	EXPT		CTRL		Odds ratio	Graph of odds ratios and confidence intervals
	n	(%)	*n*	(%)	(95% CI)	0.01 0.1 0.5 1 2 10 100
Lewis (1983)	7/22	(31.82)	22/22	(100.0)	0.05 (0.02–0.18)	
Typical odds ratio (95% confidence interval)					0.05 (0.02–0.18)	

Effect of mechanical methods for cervical ripening on labour onset during ripening

Study	EXPT		CTRL		Odds ratio	
Lackritz *et al.* (1979)	1/7	(14.29)	0/5	(0.00)	5.55 (0.10–99.99)	
Lewis (1983)	2/22	(9.09)	0/22	(0.00)	7.75 (0.47–99.99)	
Magani *et al.* (1982)	1/20	(5.00)	2/10	(20.00)	0.20 (0.02–2.40)	
Cross and Pitkin (1978)	6/35	(17.14)	1/39	(2.56)	5.36 (1.14–25.23)	
Typical odds ratio (95% confidence interval)					2.86 (0.91–8.95)	

Effect of mechanical methods for cervical ripening on delivered during ripening

Study	EXPT		CTRL		Odds ratio	
Lewis (1983)	2/22	(9.09)	0/22	(0.00)	7.75 (0.47–99.99)	
Cross and Pitkin (1978)	6/35	(17.14)	1/39	(2.56)	5.36 (1.14–25.23)	
Typical odds ratio (95% confidence interval)					5.84 (1.51–22.67)	

Effect of mechanical methods for cervical ripening on no vaginal delivery within 12 hours

Study	EXPT		CTRL		Odds ratio	
Lackritz *et al.* (1979)	7/7	(100.0)	5/5	(100.0)	1.00 (1.00–1.00)	
Lewis (1983)	7/22	(31.82)	14/22	(63.64)	0.29 (0.09–0.93)	
Typical odds ratio (95% confidence interval)					0.29 (0.09–0.93)	

Effect of mechanical methods for cervical ripening on no vaginal delivery within 48 hours

Study	EXPT		CTRL		Odds ratio	
Lackritz *et al.* (1979)	2/7	(28.57)	3/5	(60.00)	0.31 (0.03–2.84)	
Lewis (1983)	7/22	(31.82)	6/22	(27.27)	1.24 (0.34–4.45)	
Typical odds ratio (95% confidence interval)					0.87 (0.29–2.66)	

Table 61.44—*continued* Effect of mechanical methods for cervical ripening on caesarean section

Study	EXPT		CTRL		Odds ratio	Graph of odds ratios and confidence intervals
	n	(%)	n	(%)	(95% CI)	0.01 0.1 0.5 1 2 10 100
Gower *et al.* (1982)	11/26	(42.31)	6/22	(27.27)	1.90 (0.59–6.16)	
Roberts *et al.* (1986)	5/28	(17.86)	8/24	(33.33)	0.45 (0.13–1.55)	
Lackritz *et al.* (1979)	2/7	(28.57)	3/5	(60.00)	0.31 (0.03–2.84)	
Lewis (1983)	7/22	(31.82)	6/22	(27.27)	1.24 (0.34–4.45)	
Jagani *et al.* (1982)	4/20	(20.00)	0/10	(0.00)	5.33 (0.59–47.88)	
Typical odds ratio (95% confidence interval)					1.08 (0.57–2.06)	

Effect of mechanical methods for cervical ripening on pyrexia in labour/puerperium

Study	EXPT		CTRL		Odds ratio	
Gower *et al.* (1982)	3/23	(13.04)	3/20	(15.00)	0.85 (0.15–4.71)	
Roberts *et al.* (1986)	7/28	(25.00)	10/24	(41.67)	0.48 (0.15–1.50)	
Cross and Pitkin (1978)	3/29	(10.34)	3/38	(7.89)	1.34 (0.25–7.21)	
Typical odds ratio (95% confidence interval)					0.70 (0.31–1.61)	

Effect of mechanical methods for cervical ripening on low Apgar score at 1 minute

Study	EXPT		CTRL		Odds ratio	
Lewis (1983)	2/22	(9.09)	1/22	(4.55)	2.01 (0.20–20.43)	
Cross and Pitkin (1978)	3/29	(10.34)	2/38	(5.26)	2.06 (0.33–12.81)	
Typical odds ratio (95% confidence interval)					2.04 (0.49–8.58)	

Effect of mechanical methods for cervical ripening on low Apgar score at 5 minutes

Study	EXPT		CTRL		Odds ratio	
Lewis (1983)	0/22	(0.00)	0/22	(0.00)	1.00 (1.00–1.00)	
Cross and Pitkin (1978)	0/29	(0.00)	0/38	(0.00)	1.00 (1.00–1.00)	
Typical odds ratio (95% confidence interval)					1.00 (1.00–1.00)	

nulliparous and 100 parous women, who had a 7–8 mm by 30 mm elastic rubber bougie inserted in the extra-amniotic space under antibiotic cover (1 to 1.5 g oral cephalosporin per day) before having labour induced, 18 hours later, by removal of the bougie and artificial rupture of the membranes. The authors reported that 6 women were excluded because of inadvertent rupture of the membranes upon insertion of the bougie, but these women did apparently not belong to the 200 'randomly selected cases' on whom results are reported (Manabe *et al.* 1982). 'For control purposes', these 200 women were compared with a same number of 'randomly selected' parous and nulliparous women. The results indicate that 56 per cent of nulliparous and 68 per cent of parous women went into labour within 18 hours of bougie insertion as compared with 2 per cent of the 'randomly selected' control nulliparae and 4 per cent of the multiparae. Four per cent of the bougie-treated nulliparae and 8 per cent of the parae delivered within 18 hours, but other outcomes on labour, delivery, or the infant are not reported.

Data on the other trials are shown in Table 61.44. Only one of the reports (Lewis 1983) provided categorical data on increases in cervical score and the data indicate an effect of the procedure (extra-amniotic insertion of a Foley catheter) on cervical ripening Table 61.44. This procedure in particular has been shown to cause a chronic stimulation of uterine prostaglandin production (Keirse *et al.* 1983). All four of the trials provided data on the onset of labour during the ripening period; three of them indicated that this occurred more often in the cervical ripening group than in the control group, but the overall data show no statistically significant effect (Table 61.44). Nevertheless, the two trials which indicated whether women actually delivered during the ripening procedure showed that this occurred statistically significantly more often in the ripening than in the control group (typical odds ratio 5.84; 95 per cent confidence interval 1.51–22.67; Table 61.44). Categorical data on vaginal delivery within 12 and within 48 hours were available for only 27 women in receipt of the active treatment in two trials; these data are certainly too limited to allow meaningful conclusions (Table 61.44).

The cumulative data from all 5 trials do not suggest that applying mechanical methods for ripening the cervix results in a lower rate of caesarean section (Table 61.44). The typical odds ratio was close to 1 (1.08), but had a wide 95 per cent confidence interval (0.57–2.06). The trials which provided information on pyrexia occurring either during labour or in the puerperium did not suggest that its incidence was increased with the use of mechanical methods to ripen the cervix (Table 61.44). Only two groups of investigators (Cross and Pitkin 1978; Lewis 1983) provided information on the incidence of low Apgar scores at 1 and 5 minutes;

neither showed marked differences between the two groups and none of the infants had low 5-minute scores (Table 61.44). The same investigators (Cross and Pitkin 1978; Lewis 1983) are the only ones to have reported on perinatal deaths; but none actually occurred in their study.

Overall the data, limited as they are, do not suggest that the insertion of various mechanical devices into the cervix, or the extra-amniotic space, is a useful approach to ripening the cervix prior to induction of labour.

5.4 Relaxin

Porcine relaxin, a polypeptide hormone extracted from corpora lutea of sows and capable of relaxing the pelvic ligaments of the guinea-pig (Hisaw 1926), was first thought to be involved in remodelling the collagenous structure of the cervix in the 1950s (Porter 1981). In 1956, Eichner and his associates claimed that 45 000 guinea-pig units of relaxin induced 'extreme softening' of the cervix in 'almost all' of 32 women. Around the same time, relaxin was reported as forestalling 'premature' labour in women (Abramson and Reid 1955; McCarthy *et al.* 1957) and, on the other hand, facilitating term labour (Eisenberg 1957) and reducing the length of oxytocin-stimulated labour (Birnberg and Abitbol 1957). Placebo-controlled trials conducted shortly thereafter (Decker *et al.* 1958; Dill and Chanatry 1958; Slate and Mengert 1960; Nesbitt and Cirigliano 1961) failed to reveal a shortening of labour following the administration of relaxin (see Chapter 58), and the use of relaxin disappeared from obstetric practice.

Following the introduction of new extraction processes, which resulted in a far higher purity of the compound (Sherwood and O'Byrne 1974), relaxin made a comeback for cervical ripening. Three controlled trials (MacLennan *et al.* 1980; Evans *et al.* 1983; MacLennan *et al.* 1986) have compared relaxin with placebo for cervical ripening. Relaxin was administered vaginally (2 mg relaxin in Tylose® gel) in one trial (MacLennan *et al.* 1980) and endocervically in doses of 1, 2, and 4 mg in the other two trials (Evans *et al.* 1983; MacLennan *et al.* 1986). A further trial (MacLennan *et al.* 1981) reported comparisons between various combinations of 2 mg relaxin, 10 mg oestradiol, and 25 mg prostaglandin $F_{2\alpha}$ in a vaginal gel, given to ripen the cervix to groups of 10 women of mixed parity. All of these trials are small; they were conducted in women of mixed parity; and the outcomes that are of interest have not always been reported in a similar manner. Moreover, the women included in the studies of MacLennan and his colleagues (1980, 1981, 1986) already had rather high cervical scores at the time of entry into the trials. These factors limit not only the conclusions that can be drawn, but also their generalizability.

The only differences that reached statistical significance in any of the individual placebo-controlled trials were a greater increase in Bishop score and a higher incidence of labour starting during relaxin treatment than that observed in the control groups. All 3 trials appear to indicate a lower incidence of caesarean section with than without relaxin treatment, but these observations are compatible with the play of chance (Table 61.45). Although theoretically the merits of the treatment might be to enhance cervical softening without a concomitant effect on uterine contractility, the sparse data that are available do not suggest that this actually occurs in practice. The data show that about 25 per cent of women will go into labour during ripening with relaxin treatment (Table 61.45). The few categorical data on infant outcome measures that are available from these 3 trials offer no suggestive evidence for any effect, good or bad (Table 61.45).

The available evidence does not suggest that relaxin is a worthwhile treatment for ripening the cervix prior to induction of labour. It should not be adopted into clinical practice unless larger, properly controlled trials show that it does more good than harm.

Table 61.45 Effect of relaxin for cervical ripening on labour onset during ripening

Study	EXPT		CTRL		Odds ratio	Graph of odds ratios and confidence intervals
	n	(%)	n	(%)	(95% CI)	0.01 0.1 0.5 1 2 10 100
MacLennan et al. (1980)	10/30	(33.33)	0/30	(0.00)	10.59 (2.76–40.71)	
MacLennan et al. (1986)	11/48	(22.92)	1/23	(4.35)	3.68 (0.99–13.74)	
Typical odds ratio (95% confidence interval)					6.17 (2.41–15.82)	

Effect of relaxin for cervical ripening on caesarean section

Study	EXPT		CTRL		Odds ratio	Graph
MacLennan et al. (1980)	1/30	(3.33)	3/30	(10.00)	0.35 (0.05–2.61)	
MacLennan et al. (1986)	6/48	(12.50)	4/23	(17.39)	0.67 (0.16–2.77)	
Evans et al. (1983)	5/49	(10.20)	9/46	(19.57)	0.48 (0.15–1.48)	
Typical odds ratio (95% confidence interval)					0.51 (0.23–1.14)	

Effect of relaxin for cervical ripening on resuscitation of the newborn

Study	EXPT		CTRL		Odds ratio	Graph
MacLennan et al. (1980)	2/30	(6.67)	4/30	(13.33)	0.48 (0.09–2.57)	
Typical odds ratio (95% confidence interval)					0.48 (0.09–2.57)	

Effect of relaxin for cervical ripening on low Apgar score at 1 minute

Study	EXPT		CTRL		Odds ratio	Graph
MacLennan et al. (1986)	10/48	(20.83)	7/23	(30.43)	0.59 (0.19–1.89)	
Typical odds ratio (95% confidence interval)					0.59 (0.19–1.89)	

Effect of relaxin for cervical ripening on low Apgar score at 5 minutes

Study	EXPT		CTRL		Odds ratio	Graph
MacLennan et al. (1986)	0/48	(0.00)	0/23	(0.00)	1.00 (1.00–1.00)	
Typical odds ratio (95% confidence interval)					1.00 (1.00–1.00)	

Table 61.46 Effect of breast stimulation for cervical ripening on labour onset during ripening

Study	EXPT		CTRL		Odds ratio	Graph of odds ratios and confidence intervals						
	n	(%)	n	(%)	(95% CI)	0.01	0.1	0.5	1	2	10	100
Salmon *et al.* (1986)	18/50	(36.00)	0/50	(0.00)	11.19 (4.05–30.87)							
Elliott and Flaherty (1983)	19/42	(45.24)	2/36	(5.56)	7.32 (2.70–19.85)							
Typical odds ratio (95% confidence interval)					9.02 (4.43–18.37)							

5.5 Breast stimulation

In an attempt to explore 'natural' methods for ripening the cervix, two groups of investigators (Salmon *et al.* 1986; Elliott and Flaherty 1983) have investigated the effects of breast stimulation in a controlled manner. In each of these trials, the intervention consisted of self-applied gentle massage of the breasts for 3 hours a day (spread over 2 to 3 sessions) on 3 consecutive days. The control group was instructed to avoid breast stimulation. All of the women were asked to abstain from sexual intercourse during the study period. One of the trials required the stimulation to be carried out with a warm, moist cloth (Elliott and Flaherty 1983); the other required gentle massage of 'alternate breasts, especially around the nipples, using alternate hands', while moist towels, powder, or cream could be used according to individual preferences (Salmon *et al.* 1986). Only women with a normal uncomplicated pregnancy at term were entered into these studies. None of the studies investigated the effect on subsequent induction of labour or on the mode of delivery. Both trials report that women allocated to breast stimulation were more likely to go into labour during the intervention period than those allocated to the control group (Table 61.46). Both studies reported statistically significant increases in the mean Bishop score in the 3 days of breast stimulation, but neither of the two reports mentions whether this resulted in easier labour or delivery.

Some concern has been expressed that breast stimulation, or more correctly stimulation of the nipple and the areola, may cause hypertonic uterine contractions, sometimes resulting in fetal bradycardia (Hill *et al.* 1984; Lenke and Nemes 1984; Viegas *et al.* 1984; Viegas *et al.* 1986). No instances of uterine hypertonus were observed in the study of Salmon *et al.* (1986) and they attribute the absence of this complication to their insistence that only one nipple be stimulated at any one time.

From these two studies it would appear that labour is more likely to ensue during a 3-day course of breast stimulation at term than it is when no such stimulation is applied. Although the authors report that the proced-ure will also ripen the cervix, there is no evidence that either of these effects favourably influenced the course of labour, whether spontaneous or induced, or that it influenced the mode of delivery.

6 Prostaglandins vs. other methods

A number of controlled comparisons have been conducted in which prostaglandins have been compared with alternative methods, such as oxytocin or oestrogen administration, or the endocervical or extra-amniotic insertion of mechanical devices. Most of these comparisons have involved small numbers of women.

6.1 Prostaglandins vs. oestrogens

Four controlled trials have compared prostaglandins with oestrogens for cervical ripening; the characteristics of these trials are shown in Table 61.47. Two of the trials used the vaginal route and two the extra-amniotic route of administration; the oestrogen used was oestradiol in three trials and oestriol in one; the prostaglandin used was PGE_2 in two trials and $PGF_{2\alpha}$ in the other two, one of which combined 2 mg relaxin with both the $PGF_{2\alpha}$ and oestradiol treatments.

The data from these four trials are summarized in (Table 61.48) and they are consistent with the evidence derived from indirect comparisons (prostaglandins vs. no treatment and oestrogens vs. no treatment) discussed above. All four trials indicated that women were more likely to experience labour during cervical ripening with a prostaglandin than with oestradiol, yielding a typical odds ratio of 7.29 (95 per cent confidence interval 3.17–16.76); Table 61.48. Otherwise there were no differences between both treatment groups, but data on the different outcomes were only available for some of the trials and all estimates lack precision (Table 61.48).

Earlier reference has been made to the one perinatal death shown in Table 61.48; it occurred in the trial of Quinn *et al.* (1981) between insertion of the extra-amniotic prostaglandin gel and amniotomy. As men-

Table 61.47 Characteristics of the controlled comparisons between prostaglandins and oestrogens for cervical ripening

Authors and dates	Random method	Treatments compared		No. of women in each arm	Method of induction
		Prostaglandin	Oestrogens		
MacLennan et al. (1981)	double-blind	25 mg $PGF_{2\alpha}$ + 2 mg relaxin in Tylose gel vaginally	150 mg oestradiol + 2 mg relaxin in Tylose gel vaginally	10:10 all parities	amniotomy + oxytocin after 15 hours
Quinn et al. (1981)	double-blind	10 mg $PGF_{2\alpha}$ in Tylose gel extra-amniotically	15 mg oestriol in Tylose gel extra-amniotically	15:15 nulliparae	amniotomy + oxytocin after 12 hours
Stewart et al. (1981)	alternate	0.45 mg PGE_2 in Tylose gel extra-amniotically	150 mg oestradiol in Tylose gel extra-amniotically	30:30 nulliparae	amniotomy + oxytocin after 12–16 hours
Tromans et al. (1981)	date of birth	4 mg PGE_2 in Tylose gel vaginally	150 mg oestradiol in Tylose gel vaginally	30:30 all parities	amniotomy + oxytocin if Bishop score > 3
		both treatments were repeated after 12 hours if the Bishop score was < 4			

Table 61.48 Effect of prostaglandins vs. oestrogens for cervical ripening on uterine activity during ripening

Study	EXPT		CTRL		Odds ratio	Graph of odds ratios and confidence intervals						
	n	(%)	n	(%)	(95% CI)	0.01	0.1	0.5	1	2	10	100
Tromans et al. (1981)	25/30	(83.33)	5/30	(16.67)	13.77 (5.05–37.56)							
Typical odds ratio (95% confidence interval)					13.77 (5.05–37.56)							

Effect of prostaglandins vs. oestrogens for cervical ripening on labour onset during ripening

Study	EXPT		CTRL		Odds ratio	
Quinn et al. (1981)	4/15	(26.67)	1/15	(6.67)	4.02 (0.61–26.58)	
MacLennan et al. (1981)	4/10	(40.00)	1/10	(10.00)	4.57 (0.64–32.89)	
Tromans et al. (1981)	2/30	(6.67)	0/30	(0.00)	7.65 (0.47–99.99)	
Stewart et al. (1981)	15/30	(50.00)	1/30	(3.33)	10.45 (3.36–32.51)	
Typical odds ratio (95% confidence interval)					7.29 (3.17–16.76)	

Effect of prostaglandins vs. oestrogens for cervical ripening on poor increase in cervical score

Study	EXPT		CTRL		Odds ratio	
MacLennan et al. (1981)	1/10	(10.00)	3/10	(30.00)	0.30 (0.04–2.58)	
Tromans et al. (1981)	7/30	(23.33)	7/30	(23.33)	1.00 (0.31–3.28)	
Typical odds ratio (95% confidence interval)					0.76 (0.27–2.13)	

Table 61.48—*continued* Effect of prostaglandins vs. oestrogens for cervical ripening on fetal heart rate abnormalities

Study	EXPT		CTRL		Odds ratio	Graph of odds ratios and confidence intervals						
	n	(%)	n	(%)	(95% CI)	0.01	0.1	0.5	1	2	10	100
Quinn *et al.* (1981)	1/15	(6.67)	2/15	(13.33)	0.49 (0.05–5.10)							
Tromans *et al.* (1981)	2/30	(6.67)	0/30	(0.00)	7.65 (0.47–99.99)							
Typical odds ratio (95% confidence interval)					1.52 (0.25–9.18)							

Effect of prostaglandins vs. oestrogens for cervical ripening on use of epidural analgesia

Study	EXPT		CTRL		Odds ratio	Graph
Tromans *et al.* (1981)	21/30	(70.00)	24/30	(80.00)	0.59 (0.19–1.89)	
Typical odds ratio (95% confidence interval)					0.59 (0.19–1.89)	

Effect of prostaglandins vs. oestrogens for cervical ripening on caesarean section

Study	EXPT		CTRL		Odds ratio	Graph
Quinn *et al.* (1981)	1/15	(6.67)	1/15	(6.67)	1.00 (0.06–16.79)	
Tromans *et al.* (1981)	7/30	(23.33)	8/30	(26.67)	0.84 (0.26–2.68)	
Stewart *et al.* (1981)	3/30	(10.00)	9/30	(30.00)	0.29 (0.08–1.03)	
Typical odds ratio (95% confidence interval)					0.55 (0.24–1.23)	

Effect of prostaglandins vs. oestrogens for cervical ripening on instrumental vaginal delivery

Study	EXPT		CTRL		Odds ratio	Graph
Quinn *et al.* (1981)	6/15	(40.00)	6/15	(40.00)	1.00 (0.24–4.21)	
Typical odds ratio (95% confidence interval)					1.00 (0.24–4.21)	

Effect of prostaglandins vs. oestrogens for cervical ripening on operative delivery

Study	EXPT		CTRL		Odds ratio	Graph
Quinn *et al.* (1981)	7/15	(46.67)	7/15	(46.67)	1.00 (0.24–4.10)	
Typical odds ratio (95% confidence interval)					1.00 (0.24–4.10)	

Effect of prostaglandins vs. oestrogens for cervical ripening on low Apgar score at 1 minute

Study	EXPT		CTRL		Odds ratio	Graph
Stewart *et al.* (1981)	0/30	(0.00)	3/30	(10.00)	0.13 (0.01–1.26)	
Typical odds ratio (95% confidence interval)					0.13 (0.01–1.26)	

Effect of prostaglandins vs. oestrogens for cervical ripening on perinatal death

Study	EXPT		CTRL		Odds ratio	Graph of odds ratios and confidence intervals						
	n	(%)	*n*	(%)	(95% CI)	0.01	0.1	0.5	1	2	10	100
Quinn *et al.* (1981)	1/15	(6.67)	0/15	(0.00)	7.39 (0.15–99.99)							
MacLennan *et al.* (1981)	0/10	(0.00)	0/10	(0.00)	1.00 (1.00–1.00)							
Tromans *et al.* (1981)	0/30	(0.00)	0/30	(0.00)	1.00 (1.00–1.00)							
Typical odds ratio (95% confidence interval)					7.39 (0.15–99.99)							

Table 61.49 Characteristics of controlled comparisons between prostaglandins and oxytocin for cervical ripening

Authors and dates	Allocation	Treatments compared		No. of women		Interval to + method of induction
				Prosta-glandin	Oxy-tocin	
Valentine (1977)	random not described	0.5 (*n* = 15) *or* 1.0 (*n* = 15) mg oral PGE$_2$ per hour for 10 hours	incremental dose of intravenous oxytocin (total: 30 U) for 10 hours	15 : 15 : mixed parity	15	24 hours oxytocin + amniotomy if possible
Jagani *et al.* (1984)	case record	1 mg PGE$_2$ in vaginal suppository followed by 1 or 2 mg after 4 hours depending on contractions	intravenous oxytocin for 12 hours	15 : mixed parity	16	
Sorensen *et al.* (1985)	double-blind	0.57 mg PGE$_2$ in oxipropylmethyl cellulose endocervically + buccal placeto tablets	50 U demoxytocin buccal tablets every ½ hour for 5 hours + endocervical placebo gel	53 : mixed parity	50	24 hours repeat of same regime if not in labour
Wilson *et al.* (1985)	random not described	0.4 mg PGE$_2$ in methylhydroxyethyl cellulose extra-amniotically *or* 1 mg oral PGE$_2$ per hour for 10 hours *or* 2 mg PGE$_2$ in vaginal tablet	intravenous oxytocin in escalating doses for 8 hours	15 : mixed parity 15 : mixed parity 15 : mixed parity	15	amniotomy + oxytocin infusion
Roberts *et al.* (1986)	sealed envelopes	3 mg PGE$_2$ in methylhydroxyethyl cellulose gel vaginally against cervix	intravenous oxytocin 1 mU/min for 12 hours	27 : mixed parity	24	12 hours oxytocin by 'standard protocol'

tioned earlier, these investigators used an excessively high extra-amniotic dose of $PGF_{2\alpha}$. For example, in comparison with the study of Stewart and his colleagues (1981), who also used the extra-amniotic approach (Table 61.48), their prostaglandin dose was more than twice as high when expressed in terms of uterotonic potency, and their oestrogen dose was 100 times lower in terms of oestrogenic potency. These and other differences among the four small trials do not allow to draw conclusions with any degree of confidence.

6.2 Prostaglandins vs. oxytocin

Five trials have compared prostaglandins (always PGE_2) with oxytocin for cervical ripening. As shown in Table 61.49, all of these trials have been small and have included various routes of prostaglandin administration. Moreover, the largest trial (Sorensen *et al.* 1985) is probably more appropriately classified as an induction of labour trial, since women in whom cervical ripening failed to produce labour underwent another attempt with the same regimen before being induced. In addition, only two categorical outcome measures were available in all five trial reports; these relate to the onset of labour during ripening, and to caesarean section.

Despite the paucity of data, the results are consistent with what could be predicted from indirect comparisons of placebo or 'no treatment' controlled trials discussed above. There was thus a statistically signifi-cantly greater likelihood of labour starting during cervical ripening with the prostaglandin preparation than with oxytocin (typical odds ratio 2.29; 95 per cent confidence interval 1.24–4.23; Table 61.50). Also, statistically significantly more women were delivered during ripening with PGE_2 than with oxytocin (typical odds ratio 2.35; 95 per cent confidence interval 1.19–4.67; Table 61.50). Thus, the number of women who were not delivered within 24 hours and within 48 hours after induction of labour was statistically significantly smaller in prostaglandin-treated than in oxytocin-treated women (Table 61.50). The number of caesarean sections, although tending to be smaller with prostaglandin than with oxytocin treatment (typical odds ratio 0.62), was not statistically significantly different, yielding a 95 per cent confidence interval of 0.30 to 1.27 (Table 61.50).

Overall, the data lend further support to our earlier conclusion that oxytocin is not an effective treatment for ripening the cervix prior to induction of labour.

6.3 Prostaglandins vs. mechanical methods

Randomized comparisons between prostaglandins and mechanical devices such as laminaria (Jeeva and Dommisse 1982; Roberts *et al.* 1986), Foley catheter (Lewis 1983) and Lamicel (Johnson *et al.* 1985) have been conducted by four groups of investigators. In each of these trials, the comparison was with a vaginally administered prostaglandin, either PGE_2 or (in one

Table 61.50 Effect of prostaglandin E_2 vs. oxytocin for cervical ripening on labour onset during ripening

Study	EXPT		CTRL		Odds ratio	Graph of odds ratios and confidence intervals
	n	(%)	*n*	(%)	(95% CI)	0.01　0.1　0.5　1　2　10　100
Sorensen *et al.* (1985)	29/53	(54.72)	17/50	(34.00)	2.29 (1.06–4.97)	
Jagani *et al.* (1984)	4/15	(26.67)	2/16	(12.50)	2.41 (0.42–13.91)	
Valentine (1977)	4/30	(13.33)	2/15	(13.33)	1.00 (0.16–6.07)	
Wilson (1978)	8/45	(17.78)	0/15	(0.00)	4.54 (0.83–24.96)	
Typical odds ratio (95% confidence interval)					2.29 (1.24–4.23)	

Effect of prostaglandin E_2 vs. oxytocin for cervical ripening on delivered during ripening

Study	EXPT		CTRL		Odds ratio	Graph of odds ratios and confidence intervals
Sorensen *et al.* (1985)	29/53	(54.72)	17/50	(34.00)	2.29 (1.06–4.97)	
Wilson (1978)	8/45	(17.78)	0/15	(0.00)	4.54 (0.83–24.96)	
Valentine (1977)	1/30	(3.33)	1/15	(6.67)	0.46 (0.02–9.08)	
Typical odds ratio (95% confidence interval)					2.35 (1.19–4.67)	

Table 61.50—*continued* Effect of prostaglandin E₂ vs. oxytocin for cervical ripening on more than one induction attempt

Study	EXPT		CTRL		Odds ratio	Graph of odds ratios and confidence intervals						
	n	(%)	n	(%)	(95% CI)	0.01	0.1	0.5	1	2	10	100
Sorensen *et al.* (1985)	24/53	(45.28)	33/50	(66.00)	0.44 (0.20–0.94)							
Typical odds ratio (95% confidence interval)					0.44 (0.20–0.94)							

Effect of prostaglandin E₂ vs. oxytocin for cervical ripening on not delivered within 24 hours

Study	EXPT		CTRL		Odds ratio							
Sorensen *et al.* (1985)	24/53	(45.28)	33/50	(66.00)	0.44 (0.20–0.94)							
Valentine (1977)	3/30	(10.00)	7/15	(46.67)	0.13 (0.03–0.55)							
Typical odds ratio (95% confidence interval)					0.33 (0.17–0.66)							

Effect of prostaglandin E₂ vs. oxytocin for cervical ripening on not delivered within 48 hours

Study	EXPT		CTRL		Odds ratio							
Sorensen *et al.* (1985)	9/50	(18.00)	16/42	(38.10)	0.37 (0.15–0.92)							
Valentine (1977)	0/30	(0.00)	2/15	(13.33)	0.05 (0.00–0.91)							
Typical odds ratio (95% confidence interval)					0.31 (0.13–0.74)							

Effect of prostaglandin E₂ vs. oxytocin for cervical ripening on caesarean section

Study	EXPT		CTRL		Odds ratio							
Roberts *et al.* (1986)	3/27	(11.11)	6/25	(24.00)	0.41 (0.10–1.72)							
Valentine (1977)	7/30	(23.33)	4/15	(26.67)	0.84 (0.20–3.49)							
Wilson (1978)	8/45	(17.78)	5/15	(33.33)	0.41 (0.10–1.66)							
Jagani *et al.* (1984)	5/15	(33.33)	5/16	(31.25)	1.10 (0.25–4.83)							
Typical odds ratio (95% confidence interval)					0.62 (0.30–1.27)							

trial) PGE₁. Overall, the data involve 123 prostaglandin-treated women and 132 women who had any one of these mechanical devices. The only outcome data that are available for all of these women relate to the incidence of caesarean section. For all other outcomes of interest, data were never available from more than three of the five trials (Table 61.51).

From the trials from which data are available, it appears that no or poor increase in cervical ripeness is less likely with vaginal prostaglandin administration than with endocervical or intrauterine insertion of these mechanical devices (Table 61.51). The data further indicate that prostaglandin administration is more likely to result in the onset of labour and to require no formal induction of labour at the end of the ripening period, than is the insertion of these mechanical devices

(Table 61.51). Of the three trials that provided information on the incidence of 'fetal distress' (as defined by the authors), two detected no difference in incidence and one found the incidence to be statistically significantly higher in prostaglandin-treated women than in women receiving Lamicel® (Table 61.51). It is therefore difficult to judge whether this represents a real difference between the two type of methods, particularly since the dose of PGE₂ (4 mg in cellulose gel) used in that study may be considered high for the objective of cervical ripening.

There is no evidence for any differential effects in other maternal outcomes on which data were reported (such as the incidences of caesarean section, instrumental vaginal delivery and pyrexia during labour and the puerperium), but all of these estimates are rather

Table 61.51 Effect of prostaglandins vs. mechanical methods for cervical ripening on poor increase in cervical score

Study	EXPT n	(%)	CTRL n	(%)	Odds ratio (95% CI)	Graph of odds ratios and confidence intervals
Lewis (1983)	2/22	(9.09)	7/22	(31.82)	0.26 (0.06–1.09)	
Thomas *et al.* (1986)	5/25	(20.00)	14/31	(45.16)	0.33 (0.11–1.00)	
Typical odds ratio (95% confidence interval)					0.30 (0.13–0.73)	

Effect of prostaglandins vs. mechanical methods for cervical ripening on labour onset during ripening

Study	EXPT n	(%)	CTRL n	(%)	Odds ratio (95% CI)	
Johnson *et al.* (1985)	22/40	(55.00)	0/40	(0.00)	15.24 (5.75–40.43)	
Lewis (1983)	14/22	(63.64)	2/22	(9.09)	10.01 (2.97–33.72)	
Jeeva and Dommisse (1982)	4/10	(40.00)	2/10	(20.00)	2.47 (0.38–15.94)	
Typical odds ratio (95% confidence interval)					10.21 (5.05–20.64)	

Effect of prostaglandins vs. mechanical method for cervical ripening on no need for formal induction of labour

Study	EXPT n	(%)	CTRL n	(%)	Odds ratio (95% CI)	
Lewis (1983)	14/22	(63.64)	2/22	(9.09)	10.01 (2.97–33.72)	
Jeeva and Dommisse (1982)	6/10	(60.00)	8/10	(80.00)	0.40 (0.06–2.61)	
Typical odds ratio (95% confidence interval)					3.85 (1.39–10.65)	

Effect of prostaglandins vs. mechanical methods for cervical ripening on hypertonus

Study	EXPT n	(%)	CTRL n	(%)	Odds ratio (95% CI)	
Johnson *et al.* (1985)	1/40	(2.50)	0/40	(0.00)	7.39 (0.15–99.99)	
Jeeva and Dommisse (1982)	0/10	(0.00)	0/10	(0.00)	1.00 (1.00–1.00)	
Thomas *et al.* (1986)	10/24	(41.67)	11/32	(34.38)	1.36 (0.46–4.01)	
Typical odds ratio (95% confidence interval)					1.53 (0.54–4.35)	

Effect of prostaglandins vs. mechanical methods for cervical ripening on fetal distress

Study	EXPT n	(%)	CTRL n	(%)	Odds ratio (95% CI)	
Roberts *et al.* (1986)	1/27	(3.70)	1/28	(3.57)	1.04 (0.06–17.04)	
Johnson *et al.* (1985)	20/40	(50.00)	8/40	(20.00)	3.68 (1.48–9.16)	
Jeeva and Dommisse (1982)	0/10	(0.00)	0/10	(0.00)	1.00 (1.00–1.00)	
Typical odds ratio (95% confidence interval)					3.26 (1.37–7.76)	

Table 61.51—*continued* Effect of prostaglandins vs. mechanical methods for cervical ripening on pyrexia in labour/puerperium

Study	EXPT n	(%)	CTRL n	(%)	Odds ratio (95% CI)	Graph of odds ratios and confidence intervals
Roberts *et al.* (1986)	5/27	(18.52)	7/28	(25.00)	0.69 (0.19–2.45)	
Johnson *et al.* (1985)	0/40	(0.00)	1/40	(2.50)	0.14 (0.00–6.82)	
Jeeva and Dommisse (1982)	0/10	(0.00)	0/10	(0.00)	1.00 (1.00–1.00)	
Typical odds ratio (95% confidence interval)					0.59 (0.18–1.97)	

Graph scale: 0.01 0.1 0.5 1 2 10 100

Effect of prostaglandins vs. mechanical methods for cervical ripening on no vaginal delivery within 24 hours

Study	EXPT n	(%)	CTRL n	(%)	Odds ratio (95% CI)	
Lewis (1983)	3/22	(13.64)	7/22	(31.82)	0.36 (0.09–1.47)	
Typical odds ratio (95% confidence interval)					0.36 (0.09–1.47)	

Effect of prostaglandins vs. mechanical methods for cervical ripening on no vaginal delivery within 48 hours

Study	EXPT n	(%)	CTRL n	(%)	Odds ratio (95% CI)	
Lewis (1983)	3/22	(13.64)	7/22	(31.82)	0.36 (0.09–1.47)	
Typical odds ratio (95% confidence interval)					0.36 (0.09–1.47)	

Effect of prostaglandins vs. mechanical methods for cervical ripening on caesarean section

Study	EXPT n	(%)	CTRL n	(%)	Odds ratio (95% CI)	
Roberts *et al.* (1986)	3/27	(11.11)	5/28	(17.86)	0.59 (0.13–2.59)	
Johnson *et al.* (1985)	10/40	(25.00)	6/40	(15.00)	1.85 (0.62–5.51)	
Lewis (1983)	3/22	(13.64)	7/22	(31.82)	0.36 (0.09–1.47)	
Jeeva and Dommisse (1982)	3/10	(30.00)	4/10	(40.00)	0.66 (0.11–3.95)	
Thomas *et al.* (1986)	7/24	(29.17)	7/32	(21.88)	1.47 (0.44–4.92)	
Typical odds ratio (95% confidence interval)					0.96 (0.53–1.75)	

Effect of prostaglandins vs. mechanical methods for cervical ripening on instrumental vaginal delivery

Study	EXPT n	(%)	CTRL n	(%)	Odds ratio (95% CI)	
Johnson *et al.* (1985)	21/40	(52.50)	15/40	(37.50)	1.82 (0.76–4.37)	
Thomas *et al.* (1986)	3/24	(12.50)	4/32	(12.50)	1.00 (0.20–4.88)	
Typical odds ratio (95% confidence interval)					1.58 (0.74–3.40)	

Effect of prostaglandins vs. mechanical methods for cervical ripening on low Apgar score at 1 minute

Study	EXPT n	(%)	CTRL n	(%)	Odds ratio (95% CI)	
Lewis (1983)	0/22	(0.00)	2/22	(9.09)	0.13 (0.01–2.13)	
Typical odds ratio (95% confidence interval)					0.13 (0.01–2.13)	

Table 61.51—*continued* Effect of prostaglandins vs. mechanical methods for cervical ripening on low Apgar score at 5 minutes

Study	EXPT		CTRL		Odds ratio	Graph of odds ratios and confidence intervals
	n	(%)	n	(%)	(95% CI)	0.01 0.1 0.5 1 2 10 100
Johnson *et al.* (1985)	1/40	(2.50)	1/40	(2.50)	1.00 (0.06–16.27)	
Lewis (1983)	0/22	(0.00)	0/22	(0.00)	1.00 (1.00–1.00)	
Typical odds ratio (95% confidence interval)					1.00 (0.06–16.27)	

imprecise (Table 61.51). The same applies to infant outcomes, for which very few data were available (Table 61.51).

7 Hazards of cervical ripening

From the evidence reviewed for this chapter it is clear that ripening of the cervix, with any of the methods that have been used for this purpose, is not a trivial intervention. The risks of the ripening intervention itself include a (small) danger of intrauterine infection with mechanical procedures and extra-amniotic drug administration; an increased likelihood of 'uterine hypertonus' and of fetal heart rate 'abnormalities'; and a non-negligible degree of discomfort and inconvenience for the mother. Some of these hazards, uterine 'hypertonus' and fetal heart rate 'abnormalities' in particular, are ill-defined and of unclear significance for the baby. Yet, they are known to have prompted caesarean sections during cervical ripening and are therefore not insignificant to the mother.

There is no evidence of serious maternal morbidity or mortality in the totality of the information derived from the controlled trials, apart from a report of placental abruption in a woman who had received prostaglandins (Laube *et al.* 1986), and a maternal death of a woman who was assigned to a 'no prostaglandin' group (Noah *et al.* 1987). However, events such as these are rare in any circumstances and it is difficult to be certain that cervical ripening has no influence on these important outcomes. Certainly there have been case reports which have been influential in practice. For example, the death of a woman with proteinuric hypertension from amniotic fluid embolism after vaginal administration of 3 mg of PGE_2 for induction with an unfavourable cervix (National Maternity Hospital Dublin 1986) raised concern about the safety of these compounds in respect of these very rare, but catastrophic outcomes.

Perhaps the most important hazard of all, however, is that the risks of cervical ripening are not limited to those of the intervention itself, but include those associated with other aspects of induction of labour. In our view, the greatest hazard is that awareness among clinicians that it is possible to 'ripen' the cervix will result in unnecessary induction of labour in women for whom an artificial ending of pregnancy would not otherwise have been contemplated. This can only increase the numbers of women exposed to any serious hazards of these procedures without a concomitant expectation of benefit.

8 Conclusions

8.1 Implications for current practice

The state of the cervix at the time that induction of labour is attempted is the most important determinant of the subsequent duration of labour. An unripe cervix increases the likelihood that induced labour will be prolonged and that it will end in operative delivery. Because rates of maternal and perinatal morbidity increase importantly with longer durations of induced labour, a variety of methods have been used in attempts to influence the success of induction by modifying ('ripening') the state of the cervix (Table 61.52).

None of the methods that are successful in ripening the unripe cervix is a trivial intervention. None of them acts exclusively on the cervix, and all of them tend to increase myometrial contractility. Making a distinction between cervical and myometrial effects is a nice concept in theory, but the evidence currently available does not show it to be a realistic proposition in clinical practice. It is therefore illogical to view cervical ripening as anything other than the first step in induction of labour. This implies that it should not be used unless there are valid grounds for ending pregnancy artificially.

The occasional need to induce labour in the presence of an unripe cervix requires methods that have not only been shown to increase cervical compliance, but which increase the likelihood of spontaneous vaginal delivery of a healthy baby within a reasonable period of time. Of the various interventions used, only the prostaglandins, which have also been the most extensively studied, have so far approached this goal. Use of prostaglandins in these circumstances decreases the likelihood of 'failed induction', decreases the incidence of labour lasting

Table 61.52 Interventions to ripen the uterine cervix prior to the induction of labour that have been compared in controlled trials with random or quasi-random allocation of subjects

Type of intervention	Route of administration
Prostaglandin E$_2$	oral
	vaginal
	endocervical
	extra-amniotic
Prostaglandin E$_1$	vaginal
Prostaglandin F$_{2\alpha}$	vaginal
	endocervical
	extra-amniotic
Oestradiol	intramuscular
	vaginal
	endocervical
	extra-amniotic
Oestriol	extra-amniotic
Dehydroepiandrosterone sulphate	intravenous
Oxytocin	buccal
	intravenous
Relaxin	vaginal
	endocervical
Placebo tablets and gels	oral
	buccal
	vaginal
	endocervical
	extra-amniotic
Foley catheter	extra-amniotic
Bougie	endocervical
Laminaria	endocervical
Lamicel	endocervical
Nipple stimulation	breasts

more than 12 and more than 24 hours, and increases the chances of a spontaneous vaginal delivery. Despite a plethora of studies on the use of prostaglandins for preinduction cervical ripening, however, there are still insufficient data to allow any confident statements about the effects of this form of care on the infant.

There are currently insufficient data to permit firm conclusions about the relative merits of E and F prostaglandins for this indication. However, the much lower drug dose needed for PGE$_2$ would suggest this compound may be superior to PGF$_{2\alpha}$. Oral administration of prostaglandins, in order to have any effect, requires repeat administration over a long period of time and may be associated with unpleasant maternal side-effects; it no longer has any place in cervical ripening. Apart from this, there is currently no basis for believing that any one of the other routes of adminstration (vaginal, extra-amniotic, or endocervical) that have been used, is clinically superior to any other route. It is, of course, essential that doses be adapted to take into account the particular route of administration. On balance and in the light of current evidence, the most appropriate route would be the one that entails least discomfort for the mother. When choice of the extra-amniotic route involves use of an indwelling Foley catheter, for example, the discomfort and inconvenience experienced by the mother might be sufficient reason to choose either endocervical or vaginal administration.

Of the other approaches to cervical ripening, only oestrogens, and oestradiol in particular, have been studied with any consistency. Although they are known to affect cervical compliance, the available evidence does not allow confident conclusions about their effects on substantive outcomes. In particular, it is unclear whether oestrogen pretreatment actually increases the likelihood that women will be delivered within a reasonable time interval after induction of labour.

There is even less information to allow an assessment of the possible place of relaxin, the mechanical methods, and breast stimulation. Neither of these can currently be recommended in the care for women with an unripe cervix for whom there is a need to bring pregnancy to an end. The same applies to the use of oxytocin for ripening the cervix before a formal induction attempt is undertaken; the procedure is troublesome and unpleasant for the mother, and no benefits have been demonstrated. The direct randomized comparisons between prostaglandins and these other methods are consistent with these observations and suggest that prostaglandins currently represent the approach of choice for ripening the unfavourable cervix.

8.2 Implications for future research

Considering the vast amount of resources that have been used to study methods of cervical ripening, many important questions remain unanswered. In particular, there is only scanty information on the effects of any of these methods on the substantive outcomes that really matter. Too many of the studies even failed to mention whether the babies born after these procedures were at least alive at birth.

There is no need for any further small studies using different devices or different drugs, in different doses and by different routes. Future studies must be sufficiently large to enable evaluation to be conducted not in terms of small differences in induction–delivery intervals or mean Apgar scores, but in terms of substantive outcomes. Placebo-controlled trials are unlikely to have any further place, unless they are of sufficiently large size to enable evaluation of important infant outcomes. If comparisons with 'no active treatment' are undertaken, they should be designed to address questions of the form 'Is induction in the presence of an unripe cervix (with a particular agent or approach) preferable to no induction?'

In view of the data presented in this chapter, there may still be a place for a large trial to compare the relative merits of oestrogens and prostaglandins for cervical ripening directly. As far as prostaglandins are concerned, the main priorities are to assess the relative merits of different routes of administration. In particular, it would be helpful to know whether endocervical administration is superior to vaginal administration.

References

Abramson D, Reid DE (1955). Use of relaxin in treatment of threatened premature labor. J Clin Endocrinol, 15: 206–209.

Arulkumaran S, Gibb DMF, Ratnam SS, Lun KC, Heng SH (1985). Total uterine activity in induced labour—an index of cervical and pelvic resistance. Br J Obstet Gynaecol, 92: 693–697.

Bernstein EP, Leyland N, Gurland P, Gare D (1986). Effect of administration of PGE$_2$ gel and placebo gel into the cervical canal on cervical softening and induction of labour. Proceedings of Annual Meeting of Society of Obstetricians and Gynaecologists of Canada, p 108.

Bernstein EP, Leyland N, Gurland P, Gare D (1987). Cervical ripening and labor induction with prostaglandin E$_2$ gel: a placebo-controlled study. Am J Obstet Gynecol, 156: 336–340.

Bernstein EP, Gauthier RJ, King JF, Hunter DJS, Jasmin Y, Manning FA, Gare DJ, Fawcett PD, D'Alton M (1988). Prostaglandin E$_2$ gel for cervical ripening and labour induction: a Canadian multi-centre placebo controlled trial. (In preparation.)

Birnberg CH, Abitbol MM (1957). Refined relaxin and length of labor: preliminary report. Obstet Gynecol, 10: 366–370.

Bishop EH (1955). Elective induction of labor. Obstet Gynecol, 5: 519-527.

Bishop EH (1964). Pelvic scoring for elective induction. Obstet Gynecol, 24: 266–268.

Buchanan D, Macer J, Yonekura ML (1984). Cervical ripening with prostaglandin E$_2$ vaginal suppositories. Obstet Gynecol, 63: 659–663.

Bung P, Baer S, Djahanschahi D, Huch R, Huch A, Huber JF, Extermann P, Beguin F, Delaloye JF, Germond M, Bossart H, De Grandi P, Pfister A, Ehrsam A, Haller U (1986). Multizentrische Erfahrungen bei intrazervikaler Applikation eines neuen PGE$_2$-Gels bei Geburtseinleitung. Geburtshilfe Frauenheilkd, 46: 93–97.

Burnett JE (1966). Preinduction scoring: An objective approach to induction of labor. Obstet Gynecol, 28: 479–483.

Burnhill MS, Danezis J, Cohen J (1962). Uterine contractility during labor studied by intra-amniotic fluid pressure recordings. Am J Obstet Gynecol, 83: 561–571.

Burt RL, Oliver KL, Whitener DL (1969). Water intoxication complicating elective induction of labour at term. Obstet Gynecol, 34: 212–214.

Cabrol D, Bernard N, Chouraqui A, Domenichi Y, Lemaire P, Lopes P, Morelli E, Remes JM, Treisser A, Uzan S (1988). Maturation du col utérin à terme par application unique d'un gel de prostaglandine E$_2$ intracervical. J Gynécol Obstet Biol Réprod (Paris), 17: 527–534.

Calder AA (1979). The management of the unripe cervix. In: Human Parturition. Keirse MJNC, Anderson ABM, Bennebroek Gravenhorst J (eds). The Hague: Leiden University Press, pp 201–217.

Calder AA, Embrey MP (1973). Prostaglandins and the unfavourable cervix. Lancet, 2: 1322–1323.

Calder AA, Embrey MP, Hillier K (1974). Extra-amniotic prostaglandin E$_2$ for the induction of labour at term. J Obstet Gynaecol Br Commnwlth, 81: 39–46.

Christilaw J, King JF (1986). A randomised, placebo controlled trial to determine the effect of intracervical prostaglandin gel on the unripe cervix, prior to induction of labour. Proceedings of Annual Meeting of Society of Obstetricians and Gynaecologists of Canada, 107.

Cockx DP (1955). Significance of initial condition of cervix uteri to subsequent course of labour. Br Med J, 1: 327–328.

Conrad J, Ueland K (1983). Physical characteristics of the cervix. Clin Obstet Gynecol, 26: 27–36.

Cross WG, Pitkin RM (1978). Laminaria as an adjunct in induction of labor. Obstet Gynecol, 51: 606–608.

Davey DA, MacNab M (1979). Oral and intravaginal prostaglandin E$_2$ for cervical ripening and induction of labour. S Afr Med J, 55: 837–842.

Decker WH, Thwaite W, Bordat S, Kayser R, Harami T, Campbell J (1958). Some effects of relaxin in obstetrics. Obstet Gynecol, 12: 37–46.

Dill LV, Chanatry J (1958). Effect of relaxin on normal labour. J Am Med Assoc, 167: 1910–1912.

Duenhoelter JH, Gant NF, Jimenez JM (1976). Concurrent use of prostaglandin F$_2$ and laminaria tents for induction of midtrimester abortion. Obstet Gynecol, 47: 469–472.

Eaton CJ, Cohen F, Bollinger CC (1972). Laminaria tent as a cervical dilator prior to aspiration-type therapeutic abortion. Obstet Gynecol, 39: 533–537.

Eichner E, Waltner C, Goodman M, Post S (1956). Relaxin, the third ovarian hormone: its experimental use in women. Am J Obstet Gynecol, 71: 1035–1048.

Eisenberg L (1957). Facilitation of full term labor with relaxin. J Am Osteopath, 57: 147–148.

Ekman G, Forman A, Marsal K, Ulmsten U (1983). Intravaginal versus intracervical application of prostaglandin E$_2$ in viscous gel for cervical priming and induction of labor at term in patients with an unfavorable cervical state. Am J Obstet Gynecol, 147: 657–661.

Elliott JP, Flaherty JF (1983). The use of breast stimulation to ripen the cervix in term pregnancies. Am J Obstet Gynecol, 145: 553–556.

Ellwood DA, Anderson ABM (1981). The Cervix in Pregnancy and Labour. Edinburgh: Churchill Livingstone.

Ellwood DA, Mitchell MD, Anderson ABM, Turnbull AC (1979). Oestrogens, prostaglandins, and cervical ripening. Lancet, 1: 376–377.

Embrey MP (1975). The Prostaglandins in Human Reproduction. Edinburgh: Churchill Livingstone.

Embrey MP, Anselmo JF (1962). J Obstet Gynaecol Br Commnwlth, 69: 918–923.

Embrey MP, Mollison BG (1967). The unfavourable cervix and induction of labour using a cervical balloon. J Obstet Gynaecol Br Commnwlth, 74: 44–48.

Evans MI, Dougan MB, Moawad AH, Evans WJ, Bryant-Greenwood GD, Greenwood FC (1983). Ripening of the human cervix with porcine ovarian relaxin. Am J Obstet Gynecol, 147: 410–414.

Fenton DW, Speedie J, Duncan SLB (1985). Does cervical ripening with PGE_2 affect subsequent uterine activity in labour? Acta Obstet Gynecol Scand, 64: 27–30.

Fields H (1966). Induction of labor. Readiness for induction. Am J Obstet Gynecol, 95: 426–429.

Flint APF (1979). Role of progesterone and oestrogens in the control of the onset of labour in man: a continuing controversy. In: Human Parturition. Keirse MJNC, Anderson ABM, Bennebroek Gravenhorst J (eds). The Hague: Leiden University Press, pp 85–100.

Friedman EA, Sachtleben MR (1975). Preinduction priming with oral prostaglandin E_2. Am J Obstet Gynecol, 121: 521–523.

Friedman EA, Niswander KR, Bayonet-Rivera NP, Sachtleben MR (1966). Relation of prelabor evaluation to inducibility and the course of labor. Obstet Gynecol, 28: 495–501.

Friedman EA, Niswander KR, Bayonet-Rivera NP, Sachtleben MR (1967). Prelabor status evaluation. II. Weighted score. Obstet Gynecol, 29: 539–44.

Golbus MS, Creasy RK (1977). Uterine priming with oral prostaglandin E_2 prior to elective induction with oxytocin. Prostaglandins, 14: 577–581.

Gordon AJ, Calder AA (1977). Oestradiol applied locally to ripen the unfavourable cervix. Lancet, 2: 1319–1321.

Gower RH, Toraya J, Miller JM (1982). Laminaria for preinduction cervical ripening. Obstet Gynecol, 60: 617–619.

Graves GR, Baskett TF, Gray JH, Luther ER (1985). The effect of vaginal administration of various doses of prostaglandin E_2 gel on cervical ripening and induction of labour. Am J Obstet Gynecol, 151: 178–181.

Hayashi R (unpublished). PGE_2 gel (Prepidil gel) for preinduction cervical softening.

Heinzl S, Ramzin MS, Schneider M, Luescher KP (1980). Priming der Zervix mit Prostaglandin-Gel bei unreifer Geburtssituation am Termin. Z Geburtsh Perinatol, 184: 395–400.

Hill WC, Moenning RK, Katz M, Kitzmiller JL (1984). Characteristics of uterine activity during the breast stimulation test. Obstet Gynecol, 64: 489–492.

Hillier K, Wallis R (1978). Oestrogens and the unfavourable cervix. Lancet, 2: 1377–1378.

Hisaw FL (1926). Experimental relaxation of pubic ligaments of guinea pig. Proc Soc Exp Biol Med, 23: 661–663.

Hughey MJ, McElin TW, Bird CC (1976). An evaluation of preinduction scoring systems. Obstet Gynecol, 48: 635–641.

Hutchon DJR, Geirsson R, Patel NB (1980). A double-blind controlled trial of PGE_2 gel in cervical ripening. Int J Gynaecol Obstet, 17: 604–607.

Jagani N, Schulman H, Fleischer A, Mitchell J, Randolph G (1982). Role of the cervix in the induction of labor. Obstet Gynecol, 59: 21–26.

Jagani N, Schulman H, Fleischer A, Mitchell J, Blattner P (1984). Role of prostaglandin-induced cervical changes in labor induction. Obstet Gynecol, 63: 225–229.

Jeeva MA, Dommisse J (1982). Laminaria tents or vaginal prostaglandins for cervical ripening. S Afr Med J, 61: 402–403.

Johnson IR, Macpherson MBA, Welch CC, Filshie GM (1985). A comparison of Lamicel and prostaglandin E_2 vaginal gel for cervical ripening before induction of labor. Am J Obstet Gynecol, 151: 604–607.

Karim SMM, Trussell RR, Patel RC, Hillier K (1968). Response of pregnant human uterus to prostaglandin $F_{2\alpha}$-induction of labour. Br Med J, 4: 621–623.

Keirse MJNC (1975). Studies on Prostaglandins in Relation to Human Parturition. University of Oxford: D Phil thesis.

Keirse MJNC, Thiery M, Parewijck W, Mitchell MD (1983). Chronic stimulation of uterine prostaglandin synthesis during cervical ripening before the onset of labor. Prostaglandins, 25: 671–682.

Keirse MJNC, Kanhai HHH, Verwey RA, Bennebroek Gravenhorst J (1985). European multi-centre trial of intracervical PGE_2 in triacetin gel: report on the Leiden data. In: The role of prostaglandins in labour. Wood C (ed). London: RSM Services Limited, pp 93–100.

Keirse MJNC, Schulpen MAGT, Corbeij RSACM, Oosterbaan HP (1987). The Dutch experience in cervical ripening with prostaglandin gel. In Priming and Induction of Labour by Prostaglandins. Keirse MJNC, de Koning Gans HJ (eds). Leiden: Boerhaave Committee for Postacademic Medical Education, pp 53–77.

Kieback DG, Zahradnik HP, Quaas L, Kroner-Fehmel EE, Lippert TH (1986). Clinical evaluation of endocervical prostaglandin E_2-triacetin-gel for preinduction cervical softening in pregnant women at term. Prostaglandins, 32: 81–85.

Kristoffersen M, Sande HA, Sande OS (1986). Ripening of the cervix with prostaglandin E_2-gel. A randomized study with a new ready-to-use compound of triacetin-prostaglandin-E_2-gel. Int J Gynaecol Obstet, 24: 297–300.

Lackritz R, Gibson M, Frigoletto FD (1979). Preinduction use of laminaria for the unripe cervix. Am J Obstet Gynecol, 134: 349–350.

Lamberti G, Nowak J (1983). Zur Geburtsreife der Zervix. III. Abhängigkeit von Geburtsverlauf und -dauer von den Zervixkriterien. Z Geburtsh Perinatol, 187: 88–94.

Lange AP, Secher NJ, Westergaard JG, Skovgard I (1982). Prelabor evaluation of inducibility. Obstet Gynecol, 60: 137–147.

Laube DW, Zlatnik FJ, Pitkin RM (1986). Preinduction cervical ripening with prostaglandin E_2 intracervical gel. Obstet Gynecol, 68: 54–57.

Leiberman JR, Piura B, Chaim W, Cohen A (1977). The cervical balloon method for induction of labor. Acta Obstet Gynecol Scand, 56: 499–503.

Lenke RR, Nemes JR (1984). Use of nipple stimulation to obtain contraction stress test. Obstet Gynecol, 63: 345–348.

Lewis GJ (1983). Cervical ripening before induction of labour with prostaglandin E_2 pessaries or a Foley's catheter. J Obstet Gynaecol, 3: 173–176.

Liggins GC (1978). Ripening of the cervix. Seminars Perinatol, 2: 261–272.

Lischke JH, Goodlin RC (1973). Use of laminaria tents with hypertonic saline amnioinfusion. Am J Obstet Gynecol, 116: 586–587.

Lorenz RP, Botti JJ, Chez RA, Bennett N (1984). Variations

of biologic activity of low-dose prostaglandin E₂ on cervical ripening. Obstet Gynecol, 64: 123–127.

Lucas MJ, Leveno KJ, Williams M Lynne, Brewster S (1986). Efficacy of prostaglandin-E₂ gel in cervical ripening: preliminary results. Proceedings of 6th Annual Meeting of the Society of Perinatal Obstetricians, San Antonio, Texas, USA, 240: 256.

Luther ER, Roux J, Popat R, Gardner A, Gray J, Soubiran E, Korcaz Y (1980). The effect of estrogen priming on induction of labor with prostaglandins. Am J Obstet Gynecol, 137: 351–357.

MacKenzie IZ, Embrey MP (1977). Cervical ripening with intravaginal prostaglandin E₂ gel. Br Med J, 2: 1381–1384.

MacKenzie IZ, Embrey MP (1979). A comparison of PGE₂ and PGF₂ₐ vaginal gel for ripening the cervix before induction of labour. Br J Obstet Gynaecol, 86: 167–170.

MacLennan AH, Green RC (1979). Cervical ripening and induction of labour with intravaginal prostaglandin F₂ₐ. Lancet, 1: 117–119.

MacLennan AH, Green RC (1980). A double blind dose trial of intravaginal prostaglandin F₂ₐ for cervical ripening and induction of labour. Aust NZ J Obstet Gynaecol, 20: 80–83.

MacLennan AH, Green RC, Bryant-Greenwood GD, Greenwood FC, Seamark RF (1980). Ripening of the human cervix and induction of labor with purified porcine relaxin. Lancet, 1: 220–223.

MacLennan AH, Green RC, Bryant-Greenwood GD, Greenwood FC, Seamark RF (1981). Cervical ripening with combinations of vaginal prostaglandin F₂ₐ, estradiol and relaxin. Obstet Gynecol, 58: 601–604.

MacLennan AH, Green RC, Grant P, Nicolson R (1986). Ripening of the human cervix and induction of labor with intracervical purified porcine relaxin. Obstet Gynecol, 68: 598–601.

MacPherson M (1984). Comparison of Lamicel with prostaglandin E₂ gel as a cervical ripening agent before the induction of labour. J Obstet Gynaecol, 4: 205–206.

Magnani M, Cabrol D (1986). Déclenchement artificiel du travail par la prostaglandine E₂ après maturation du col par l'estradiol. In: Control and Management of Parturition. Paris: INSERM, 151: 109–118.

Manabe Y, Manabe A, Sagawa N (1982). Stretch-induced cervical softening and initiation of labor at term. A possible correlation with prostaglandins. Acta Obstet Gynecol Scand, 61: 279–280.

McCarthy JJ, Erving HW, Laufe LE (1957). Preliminary report on the use of relaxin in the management of threatened premature labor. Am J Obstet Gynecol, 74: 134–138.

Murphy AJ, Jalland M, Pepperell RJ, Quinn MA (1980). Use of vaginal prostaglandin gel before induction of labour. Austral NZ J Obstet Gynaecol, 20: 84–86.

National Maternity Hospital Dublin (1986). Clinical Report for the Year 1985, p 43.

Neilson DR, Prins RP, Bolton RN, Mark C, Watson P (1983). A comparison of prostaglandin E₂ gel and prostaglandin F₂ₐ gel for preinduction cervical ripening. Am J Obstet Gynecol, 146: 526–532.

Nesbitt REL, Cirigliano G (1961). Use of relaxin during parturition. NY State J Med, 61: 90–97.

Newton, BW (1972). Laminaria tent : Relic of the past or modern medical device ? Am J Obstet Gynecol, 113, 442–448.

Nimrod C, Currie J, Yee J, Dodd G, Persaud D (1984). Cervical ripening and labor induction with intracervical triacetin base prostaglandin E₂ gel: a placebo-controlled study. Obstet Gynecol, 64: 476–479.

Noah ML, Thiery M, Parewijck W, De Coster JM (1985). Assessment of a two dose scheme of PGE₂ gel for preinduction cervical softening. Prostaglandins, 30: 305–311.

Noah ML, De Coster JM, Fraser TJ, Orr JD (1987). Preinduction cervical softening with endocervical PGE₂ gel. Acta Obstet Gynecol Scand, 66: 3–7.

Parewijck W, Thiery M (1986). Cervical ripening: randomized comparative study of extra-amniotic vs intracervical PGE₂ gel. In: Proceedings of 10th European Congress of Perinatal Medicine, Leipzig, Germany, 165.

Pearce DJ (1977). Pre-induction priming of the uterine cervix with oral prostaglandin E₂ and a placebo. Prostaglandins, 14: 571–576.

Pedersen S, Moller-Petersen J, Aegidius J (1981). Comparison of oestradiol and prostaglandin E₂ vaginal gel for ripening the unfavourable cervix. Br Med J, 282: 1395.

Pentecost AF (1973). The effect of buccal 'Pitocin' on the unripe cervix. Curr Med Res Opin, 1: 482–484.

Porter DG (1981). Relaxin and cervical softening: a review. In: The Cervix in Pregnancy and Labour. Ellwood DA, Anderson ABM (eds). Edinburgh: Churchill Livingstone, pp 85–99.

Prins RP, Bolton RN, Mark C, Neilson DR, Watson P (1983). Cervical ripening with intravaginal prostaglandin E₂ gel. Obstet Gynecol, 61: 459–462.

Pulle C, Granese D, Panama S, Celona A (1986). Cervical ripening and induction of labour by single intracervical PGE₂-gel application. Acta Therapeutica, 12: 5–12.

Quinn MA, Murphy AJ (1981). Fetal death following extra-amniotic prostaglandin gel: report of two cases. Br J Obstet Gynaecol, 88: 650–651.

Quinn MA, Murphy AJ, Kuhn RJP, Robinson HP, Brown JB (1981). A double blind trial of extra-amniotic oestriol and prostaglandin F₂ₐ gels in cervical ripening. Br J Obstet Gynaecol, 88: 644–649.

Roberts WE, North DH, Speed JE, Martin JN, Palmer SM, Morrison JC (1986). Comparative study of prostaglandin, laminaria, and minidose oxytocin for ripening of the unfavorable cervix prior to induction of labor. J Perinatol, 6: 16–19.

Salmon YM, Kee WH, Tan SL, Jen SW (1986). Cervical ripening by breast stimulation. Obstet Gynecol, 67: 21–24.

Sasaki K, Nakano R, Kadoya Y, Iwao M, Shima K, Sowa M (1982). Cervical ripening with dehydroepiandrosterone sulphate. Br J Obstet Gynaecol, 89: 195–198.

Shepherd J, Sims CD, Craft I (1976). Extra-amniotic prostaglandin E₂ and the unfavourable cervix. Lancet, 2: 709–710.

Sherwood CD, O'Byrne EM (1974). Purification and characterisation of porcine relaxin. Arch Biochem Biophys, 160: 185–196.

Slate WG, Mengert WF (1960). Effect of the relaxing hormone on the laboring human uterus. Obstet Gynecol, 15: 409–414.

Sorensen SS, Brocks V, Lenstrup C (1985). Induction of labor and cervical ripening by intracervical prostaglandin E₂. Obstet Gynecol, 65: 110–114.

Stewart P, Calder AA (1981). Correspondence. Br J Obstet Gynaecol, 88: 1071–1072.

Stewart P, Kennedy JH, Barlow DH, Calder AA (1981). A comparison of oestradiol and prostaglandin E₂ for ripening the cervix. Br J Obstet Gynaecol, 88: 236–239.

Stewart P, Kennedy JH, Hillan E, Calder AA (1983). The unripe cervix: management with vaginal or extra-amniotic prostaglandin E₂. J Obstet Gynaecol, 4: 90–93.

Thiery M, De Gezelle H, Van Kets H, Voorhoof L, Verheugen C, Smis B, Gerris J, Martens G (1978). Extra-amniotic oestrogens for the unfavourable cervix. Lancet, 2: 835–836.

Thiery M, De Gezelle H, Van Kets H, Voorhoof L, Verheugen C, Smis B, Gerris J, Derom R, Martens G (1979). The effect of locally administered estrogens on the human cervix. Z Geburtsh Perinatol, 183: 448–451.

Thiery M, De Coster JM, Parewijck W, Noah ML, Derom R, Van Kets H, Defoort P, Aertsens W, Debruyne G, De Geest K, Vandekerckhove F (1984). Endocervical prostaglandin E₂ gel for preinduction cervical softening. Prostaglandins, 27: 429–439.

Thomas IL, Chenoweth JN, Tronc GN, Johnson IR (1986). Preparation for induction of labour of the unfavourable cervix with Foley catheter compared with vaginal prostaglandin. Austral NZ J Obstet Gynaecol, 26: 30–35.

Toplis PJ, Sims CD (1979). Prospective study of different methods and routes of administration of prostaglandin E₂ to improve the unripe cervix. Prostaglandins, 18: 127–136.

Trofatter K, Bowers D, Gall SA, Killam AP (1985). Preinduction cervical ripening with prostaglandin E₂ (prepidil) gel. Am J Obstet Gynecol, 153: 268–271.

Tromans PM, Beazley JM, Shenouda PI (1981). Comparative study of oestradiol and prostaglandin E₂ vaginal gel for ripening the unfavourable cervix before induction of labour. Br Med J, 282: 679–681.

Turnbull AC, Anderson ABM (1967). Induction of labour. Part I: Results Amniotomy. J Obstet Gynaecol Br Commnwlth, 74: 849.

Turnbull A, Anderson A (1968). Induction of labour. Part III: Results with amniotomy and oxytocin 'titration'. J Obstet Gynaecol Br Commnwlth, 75: 32–41.

Ulmsten U (1986). The cervix. In: Prostaglandins and their Inhibitors in Clinical Obstetrics and Gynaecology. Bygdeman M, Berger GS, Leith LG (eds). Lancaster: MTP Press, pp 29–57.

Ulmsten U, Ekman G, Belfrage P, Bygdeman M, Nyberg C (1985). Intracervical vs intravaginal PGE₂ for induction of labor at term in patients with an unfavorable cervix. Arch Gynecol, 236: 243–248.

Valentine BH (1977). Intravenous oxytocin and oral prostaglandin E₂ for ripening of the unfavourable cervix. Br J Obstet Gynaecol, 84: 846–854.

Varma TR, Norman J (1984). Comparison of three dosages of prostaglandin E₂ pessaries for ripening the unfavourable cervix prior to induction of labor. Acta Obstet Gynecol Scand, 63: 17–21.

Viegas OAC, Adaikan PG, Singh K, Arulkumaran S, Kottegoda SR, Ratnam GS (1986). Intrauterine response to nipple stimulation in late pregnancy. Gynecol Obstet Invest, 22: 128–133.

Viegas OAC, Arulkumaran S, Ratnam GS (1984). Nipple stimulation in late pregnancy causing uterine hyperstimulation and profound bradycardia. Br J Obstet Gynaecol, 91: 364–366.

Walker E, Gordon AJ (1983). Length of exposure to prostaglandin E₂ and cervical ripening in primigravidae. J Obstet Gynaecol, 4: 88–89.

Weiss RR, Tejani N, Israeli I, Evans MI, Bhakthavathsalan A, Mann LI (1975). Priming of the uterine cervix with oral prostaglandin E₂ in the term multigravida. Obstet Gynecol, 46: 181–184.

Williams JK, Wilkerson WG, O'Brien WF, Knuppel RA (1985). Use of prostaglandin E₂ topical cervical gel in high-risk patients: a critical analysis. Obstet Gynecol, 66: 769–773.

Wilson PD (1978). A comparison of four methods of ripening the unfavourable cervix. Br J Obstet Gynaecol, 85: 941–944.

Wingerup L, Andersson KE, Ulmsten U (1978). Ripening of the uterine cervix and induction of labour at term with prostaglandin E₂ in viscous gel. Acta Obstet Gynecol Scand, 57: 403–406.

Yonekura ML, Songster G, Smith-Wallace T (1985). Preinduction cervical priming with PGE₂ intracervical gel. Am J Perinatol, 2: 305–310.

Zahradnik HP, Quaas L, Kroner-Fehmel EE, Kieback DG, Lippert TH (1987). Medikamentöse Zervixreifung vor Oxytocin-Geburtseinleitung. Geburtshilfe Frauenheilkd, 47: 190–192.

62 Methods for inducing labour

Marc J. N. C. Keirse and Iain Chalmers

1 Introduction

A wide variety of approaches have been used in attempts to induce labour (see Chapter 59). Some methods, for instance sparteine sulphate and intrauterine bags and balloons, although still occasionally reported in the current literature (Leiberman *et al.* 1977; Manabe *et al.* 1982), have generally been abandoned. Although there is some information from controlled evaluations of these older and less frequently used methods (Aickin 1966; Van Voorhis *et al.* 1966; Leiberman *et al.* 1977; Manabe *et al.* 1982), they are not considered here because their relevance to current clinical practice is minimal.

For practical purposes, modern obstetric practice uses only three broad approaches to the induction of labour; namely, stripping (sweeping) of the membranes, amniotomy, and oxytocic drugs (either oxytocin itself or one of the prostaglandins). This chapter considers the available evidence about these three modalities for inducing labour. The next chapter will review direct comparisons between prostaglandins and oxytocin for inducing labour.

2 Sweeping (stripping) the membranes

Sweeping (stripping) the membranes from the lower uterine segment, which was apparently introduced by Hamilton in 1810 (see Chapter 59), has been widely used to induce labour (Swann 1958). Although it is now rarely considered as a formal method of inducing labour, the procedure is still frequently applied at term in the hope that it will at least circumvent the need to induce labour formally with either amniotomy, oxytocic drugs, or both.

Sweeping the membranes has been shown to increase prostaglandin production to such an extent that it results in a statistically significant elevation of the levels of prostaglandin metabolites in the maternal circulation (Mitchell *et al.* 1977). Moreover, the magnitude of the increase in intrauterine prostaglandin production seems to relate to the surface area of the detachment between the membranes and the uterine wall (Keirse *et al.* 1983). In view of the pivotal role of prostaglandins in the initiation and maintenance of labour (Keirse *et al.* 1987a), there thus are good theoretical reasons for predicting that stripping the membranes from the lower uterine segment may induce labour.

Despite its long history and its wide use, we are aware of only one formal attempt to assess the effects of digital stripping of the membranes at term (Swann 1958). The resident staff were instructed 'to strip in every third patient if there were no contraindications'. The other two patients were assigned to either a 'finger control' group (in whom an examining finger was introduced in the cervix without stripping the membranes) or a 'plain control' group (in whom no intervention was used). Despite this form of allocation, 147 women underwent stripping, while only 29 were assigned to the 'finger control' group and 45 to the 'plain control' group.

Of the 147 women who had the membranes stripped daily for three days, 69 per cent went into labour within

24 hours following the third stripping, compared with only 19 of 74 women (26 per cent) who served as controls. The author felt that the apparent success of the method in inducing labour was counteracted by the unpredictable interval between stripping and the onset of labour, and by 'a definite increase in maternal morbidity' (Swann 1958). The available data indicate that 'one day fever' occurred in 11.5 per cent of the stripped group and in 8.4 per cent of the controls, and that (undefined) morbidity affected 8.1 per cent of the stripped and 10.8 per cent of the control groups.

Although these data tend to confirm the widespread belief that stripping the membranes can induce labour, the gross imbalance in the sizes of the comparison groups in this study does not suggest that it was a properly controlled trial. It is remarkable that such a commonly performed procedure has been the subject of such little interest among researchers. Randomized trials could easily be mounted to assess its effects more satisfactorily than is possible using the scanty available data.

3 Amniotomy

3.1 Low amniotomy and high amniotomy

There are basically two ways of rupturing the membranes artificially: low amniotomy ('forewater' rupture), and high amniotomy ('hindwater' rupture). Low amniotomy, that is, rupture of the 'forewaters' lying below the presenting fetal part, is by far the more commonly used of the two approaches. It has been performed using a variety of different devices (see Chapter 59), but any instrument capable of piercing the membranes without damaging the birth canal or the baby should be suitable. Disposable plastic instruments such as the 'amniohook' (which resembles a small crochet hook on the end of a rigid plastic shaft) are widely used. In addition to the 'blind' use of instruments, low amniotomy is sometimes performed under direct vision through an amnioscope. Several advantages have been claimed for this approach, such as timely recognition and avoidance of fetal vessels in the membranes, a reduced risk of damage to the cervix and the ease of the intervention (Saling 1966; Barham 1973). None of these claims has been assessed adequately, however.

High amniotomy ('hindwater rupture'), initially introduced in the nineteenth century (see Chapter 59), was popularized by Drew Smythe (1931), who devised a curved, metal instrument especially for this purpose. The Drew Smythe catheter, which was widely used at one stage (Quinlivan 1968), was introduced through the cervix and then slid posteriorly between the membranes and the uterine wall, well above the presenting part. An interior stilette was then advanced to puncture the membranes.

A number of advantages have been claimed for high amniotomy, including reduced risks of infection and cord prolapse by preservation of the 'forewaters'; controlled release of amniotic fluid; and the possibility of rupturing the membranes when the cervix is too firmly closed to allow forewater rupture. None of these claims have been assessed in randomized comparisons, and it may well be that 'advantages' such as the ability to rupture the membranes through a long and closed cervix are more likely to be disadvantageous than useful. Furthermore, the procedure can undoubtedly cause damage to the fetus, the placenta, and the genital tract of the mother (Russell *et al.* 1956; Parker 1957; Husslein and Baumgarten 1962). High amniotomy, if it is to be used at all, should be reserved for those situations in which there is polyhydramnios in addition to a firm indication for induction of labour.

3.2 Amniotomy used alone

Although there continues to be debate about whether amniotomy performed *during* labour increases or decreases uterine contractility (see Chapter 58), there has never been much doubt that this procedure, when performed *before* the onset of labour, can induce labour. Ever since it was introduced (in the mid-eighteenth century) for inducing labour before term in order to avert the risk of cephalopelvic disproportion at term (see Chapter 59), amniotomy has had its ups and downs in popularity. This is not surprising since it represents one of the most irrevocable interventions in pregnancy. Once the membranes have been ruptured, there is no way back; irrespective of whether labour ensues or not, the damage cannot be repaired. Amniotomy thus constitutes obstetric interference of the most profound nature. More than any other intervention currently used to induce labour, it embodies a firm commitment to delivery.

The main disadvantage of amniotomy for the induction of labour is the occasional, unpredictably long interval to the onset of labour-like uterine activity, and thus to delivery (Setna *et al.* 1967; Turnbull and Anderson 1967; Bradford and Gordon 1968). In one fairly typical study, for example, only 55 per cent (44 of 80) of primigravidae and 59 per cent (71 of 120) of multigravidae were in established labour within 12 hours of amniotomy, and 15 per cent of the primigravidae and 22 per cent of the multigravidae were not in established labour even 24 hours after amniotomy (Patterson 1971).

3.3 Amniotomy with oxytocic drugs vs. amniotomy alone

Because of the low success rate of amniotomy used alone, oxytocic drugs have been started either at the time that the membranes are ruptured, or after an interval of a few hours if labour has not started. This policy has been evaluated in three controlled trials (Patterson 1971; Saleh 1975; Sivasuriya *et al.* 1978), the characteristics of which are shown in Table 62.1. One of the trials reported only on neonatal serum bilirubin levels (Sivasuriya *et al.* 1978). The two other trials showed that women who received oxytocics from the time of amniotomy were statistically significantly more likely to be delivered within 12 hours and within 24 hours than those who had amniotomy alone (Table 62.2), and less likely to be delivered by caesarean section or forceps (Table 62.2). Furthermore, fewer women in the early than in the late oxytocin group had operative deliveries performed in the presence of maternal pyrexia and foul-smelling liquor (Patterson 1971). This might be expected to increase the maternal morbidity associated with these interventions. The only trial to report rates of puerperal pyrexia shows a trend in this direction (Saleh 1975), although the differences do not achieve statistical significance (Table 62.2).

In the trial of Saleh (1975), all women were offered (and accepted) epidural analgesia once labour was established (Table 62.2). Patterson (1971) reported that both primigravidae and multigravidae in the group with the early oxytocin administration required statistically significantly less sedation and less 'units' of analgesia than those having late oxytocin administration. This need not necessarily mean that induction of labour was less painful in these women; it may simply have been a reflection of the shorter interval between amniotomy and delivery. In both of the trials for which data are available, the incidence of postpartum haemorrhage was lower when amniotomy was followed by early oxytocin administration (Table 62.2).

As for the condition of the infant, the incidence of depressed Apgar scores was lower following the policy of using oxytocin from the time of amniotomy, although this difference was only statistically significantly different in one of the two trials reporting this outcome (Table 62.2). The available data (from two trials) provide no clear evidence of a differential effect on neonatal hyperbilirubinaemia (Table 62.2).

3.4 Amniotomy with oxytocic drugs vs. oxytocic drugs alone

There has been only one controlled trial that has compared a policy of using amniotomy routinely at the time that oxytocic drugs to induce labour are started with a policy in which the membranes were left intact. 'By drawing a slip of paper at random from a box', women were allocated either to receive an oxytocic drug and simultaneous amniotomy, or to receive the drug alone (Ratnam *et al.* 1974). The oxytocic drug regimen consisted of either intravenous infusion of oxytocin (doubling the dose every 30 minutes until adequate uterine contractions were recorded), or oral PGE_2 tablets (0.5 to 2 mg per hour until labour was established). The only observed effect of concurrent amniotomy was that, compared with women who had received the oxytocic drug alone, a higher proportion of women were in established labour within 6 hours of the start of the induction procedure. No significant differences were detected in the proportions of women delivered within 24 and 48 hours, however, nor in the incidences of caesarean section (Table 62.3).

This trial, despite involving just over 200 women, may have been too small to detect clinically important differences between the two policies compared. Observational data derived from studies conducted in the

Table 62.1 Characteristics of the controlled comparisons of amniotomy with early vs. late oxytocin infusion for induction of labour

Authors and dates	Allocation	Treatments compared		Additional information
		(Number allocated : analysed)		
		Early oxytocin	Late oxytocin	
Patterson (1971)	random not described	amniotomy + IV oxytocin started simultaneously (200 : 200) +4	amniotomy + IV oxytocin after 24 hrs if not in labour (200 : 200) +7	11 women (4 with early; 7 with late oxytocin) who had a caesarean section were replaced in the trial by 'the next patient' to ensure equal numbers of vaginal deliveries.
Saleh (1975)	random not described	amniotomy + IV oxytocin started simultaneously (50 : 50)	amniotomy + IV oxytocin after 24 hrs if not in labour (50 : 50)	only primigravidae were included
Sivasuriya *et al.* (1978)	'in rotation'	amniotomy + IV oxytocin started simultaneously	amniotomy alone (no data on whether/when IV oxytocin was added)	number of women allocated to each group not stated (all conditions related with an increased incidence of jaundice excluded after treatment allocation)

Table 62.2 Effect of amniotomy plus early vs. late oxytocin infusion for induction of labour on not delivered within 12 hours

Study	EXPT		CTRL		Odds ratio	Graph of odds ratios and confidence intervals
	n	(%)	*n*	(%)	(95% CI)	0.01 0.1 0.5 1 2 10 100
Saleh (1975)	8/50	(16.00)	34/50	(68.00)	0.12 (0.05–0.27)	
Patterson (1971)	29/200	(14.50)	148/200	(74.00)	0.09 (0.06–0.13)	
Typical odds ratio (95% confidence interval)					0.10 (0.07–0.14)	

Effect of amniotomy plus early vs. late oxytocin infusion for induction of labour on not delivered within 24 hours

Saleh (1975)	0/50	(0.00)	16/50	(32.00)	0.09 (0.03–0.27)	
Patterson (1971)	0/200	(0.00)	73/200	(36.50)	0.09 (0.05–0.14)	
Typical odds ratio (95% confidence interval)					0.09 (0.06–0.14)	

Effect of amniotomy plus early vs. late oxytocin infusion for induction of labour on caesarean section

Saleh (1975)	1/50	(2.00)	4/50	(8.00)	0.29 (0.05–1.71)	
Typical odds ratio (95% confidence interval)					0.29 (0.05–1.71)	

Effect of amniotomy plus early vs. late oxytocin infusion for induction of labour on instrumental vaginal delivery

Saleh (1975)	25/50	(50.00)	25/50	(50.00)	1.00 (0.46–2.18)	
Patterson (1971)	31/205	(15.12)	59/205	(28.78)	0.45 (0.28–0.72)	
Typical odds ratio (95% confidence interval)					0.56 (0.37–0.83)	

Effect of amniotomy plus early vs. late oxytocin infusion for induction of labour on operative delivery

Saleh (1975)	35/209	(16.75)	66/212	(31.13)	0.46 (0.29–0.71)	
Patterson (1971)	26/50	(52.00)	29/50	(58.00)	0.79 (0.36–1.72)	
Typical odds ratio (95% confidence interval)					0.52 (0.35–0.77)	

Effect of amniotomy plus early vs. late oxytocin infusion for induction of labour on use of analgesia

Saleh (1975)	50/50	(100.0)	50/50	(100.0)	1.00 (1.00–1.00)	
Patterson (1971)	152/200	(76.00)	165/200	(82.50)	0.67 (0.42–1.09)	
Typical odds ratio (95% confidence interval)					0.67 (0.42–1.09)	

Table 62.2–*continued* Effect of amniotomy plus early vs. late oxytocin infusion for induction of labour on use of epidural analgesia

Study	EXPT		CTRL		Odds ratio	Graph of odds ratios and confidence intervals						
	n	(%)	*n*	(%)	(95% CI)	0.01	0.1	0.5	1	2	10	100
Saleh (1975)	50/50	(100.0)	50/50	(100.0)	1.00 (1.00–1.00)							
Typical odds ratio (95% confidence interval)					1.00 (1.00–1.00)							

Effect of amniotomy plus early vs. late oxytocin infusion for induction of labour on pyrexia in the puerperium

Study	EXPT		CTRL		Odds ratio	
Saleh (1975)	1/50	(2.00)	4/50	(8.00)	0.29 (0.05–1.71)	
Typical odds ratio (95% confidence interval)					0.29 (0.05–1.71)	

Effect of amniotomy plus early vs. late oxytocin infusion for induction of labour on postpartum haemorrhage

Study	EXPT		CTRL		Odds ratio	
Saleh (1975)	2/50	(4.00)	5/50	(10.00)	0.40 (0.09–1.85)	
Patterson (1971)	6/200	(3.00)	13/200	(6.50)	0.46 (0.18–1.16)	
Typical odds ratio (95% confidence interval)					0.45 (0.20–0.98)	

Effect of amniotomy plus early vs. late oxytocin infusion for induction of labour on low Apgar score at 1 minute

Study	EXPT		CTRL		Odds ratio	
Patterson (1971)	16/203	(7.88)	33/202	(16.34)	0.45 (0.25–0.82)	
Typical odds ratio (95% confidence interval)					0.45 (0.25–0.82)	

Effect of amniotomy plus early vs. late oxytocin infusion for induction of labour on low Apgar score at 5 minutes

Study	EXPT		CTRL		Odds ratio	
Saleh (1975)	2/50	(4.00)	5/50	(10.00)	0.40 (0.09–1.85)	
Typical odds ratio (95% confidence interval)					0.40 (0.09–1.85)	

Effect of amniotomy plus early vs. late oxytocin infusion for induction of labour on jaundice and/or hyperbilirubinaemia

Study	EXPT		CTRL		Odds ratio	
Saleh (1975)	3/50	(6.00)	3/50	(6.00)	1.00 (0.19–5.17)	
Sivasuriya *et al.* (1978)	2/31	(6.45)	1/26	(3.85)	1.67 (0.17–16.90)	
Typical odds ratio (95% confidence interval)					1.19 (0.31–4.53)	

Table 62.3 Effect of oxytocic agents with amniotomy vs. oxytocics alone for induction of labour on not in established labour within 6 hours

Study	EXPT		CTRL		Odds ratio	Graph of odds ratios and confidence intervals						
	n	(%)	n	(%)	(95% CI)	0.01	0.1	0.5	1	2	10	100
Ratnam et al. (1974)	0/103	(0.00)	34/104	(32.69)	0.09 (0.04–0.19)		▬					
Typical odds ratio (95% confidence interval)					0.09 (0.04–0.19)		▬					

Effect of oxytocics with or without amniotomy for induction of labour on not delivered within 24 hours

Ratnam et al. (1974)	12/103	(11.65)	9/104	(8.65)	1.39 (0.56–3.41)				▬▬			
Typical odds ratio (95% confidence interval)					1.39 (0.56–3.41)				▬▬			

Effect of oxytocic agents with or without amniotomy for induction of labour on not delivered within 48 hours

Ratnam et al. (1974)	0/103	(0.00)	0/104	(0.00)	1.00 (1.00–1.00)							
Typical odds ratio (95% confidence interval)					1.00 (1.00–1.00)							

Effect of oxytocic agents with amniotomy vs. oxytocics alone for induction of labour on caesarean section

Ratnam et al. (1974)	9/103	(8.74)	8/104	(7.69)	1.15 (0.43–3.09)				▬▬			
Typical odds ratio (95% confidence interval)					1.15 (0.43–3.09)				▬▬			

Table 62.4 Number of women not delivered within 24 hours among women receiving intravenous oxytocin without concomitant amniotomy in all controlled comparisons between prostaglandins and oxytocin for induction of labour that provide data on this outcome

Authors	No. of women	Not delivered within 24 hours	
		No.	Per cent
Beazley and Gillespie (1971)*	146	27	18.4
Blackburn et al. (1973)	12	0	0
Naismith et al. (1973)*	20	0	0
Ratnam et al. (1974)	50	2	4.0
Scher et al. (1972)	23	0	0
Secher et al. (1981)	119	47	39.5
Ulmsten et al. (1979)**	50	22	44.0
Vakhariya and Sherman (1972)*	50	0	0

* Amniotomy performed only when in established labour and (**) if the cervix was also 4 cm or more dilated.

1960s suggest that about a third of women in whom induction of labour is attempted with oxytocin administration alone, without concurrent amniotomy, will remain undelivered 2 to 3 days after the start of the induction attempt (Lilienthal and Ward 1971; Hellfer-ich and Favier 1972). Table 62.4 presents data derived from controlled comparisons between prostaglandins and oxytocin, showing that variable, but often large proportions of women with intact membranes remained undelivered 24 hours after the induction attempt began. Data from trials (of cervical ripening) conducted in women with unripe cervices further substantiate these observations. A higher proportion of women remained undelivered after 12 hours of oxytocin infusion without ruptured membranes than after a single administration of prostaglandins to ripen the cervix (Keirse et al. 1987b; see Chapter 61). Not surprisingly, in the light of these observations, amniotomy has come to be used routinely at the time that oxytocic drugs to induce labour are started.

3.5 Timing of amniotomy in relation to oxytocic drug administration

One 'randomized' trial attempted to assess whether induction of labour should start with oxytocin infusion followed by amniotomy if necessary, or by amniotomy followed by oxytocin if necessary (Bakos and Bäckström 1987). Using dates of birth, the investigators assigned 223 women to receive either amniotomy, or an oxytocin infusion. If, four hours later, regular uterine contractions lasting 40 to 60 seconds with an interval of 3 minutes or less had become established, progress was considered to be acceptable and no further action was taken. If labour had not become established by this time, women who had been assigned to the amniotomy group received intravenous oxytocin, and those assigned to the oxytocin group had an amniotomy performed. Forty per cent of the women who had been assigned to oxytocin required amniotomy after 4 hours; 67 per cent of those induced by amniotomy required oxytocin supplementation. These observations would have been interesting were it not for the fact that both the allocation of women to the amniotomy or oxytocin groups, and the judgements that a further intervention was needed, were almost certainly biased (Keirse 1988).

3.6 Hazards of amniotomy

Apart from the special hazards associated with the use of instruments for high amniotomy, a number of undesirable consequences have been attributed to artificial rupture of the membranes (see also Chapter 58). These include intrauterine infection (occasionally leading to septicaemia); early decelerations in the fetal heart rate; umbilical cord prolapse; and bleeding, either from fetal vessels in the membranes, from the cervix, or from the placental site.

It must be assumed that any instrument (or finger) passing up the vagina in order to rupture the amniotic sac will carry some of the vaginal bacterial flora with it. It has long been known, however, that the risk of clinically significant intrauterine infection ensuing from these procedures is largely dependent on the interval until delivery (Shubeck *et al.* 1966; Muldoon 1968; Patterson 1971).

There is no unanimity as to whether amniotomy for induction of labour is responsible for decelerations of the fetal heart rate, other than when these are associated with umbilical cord complications (Jung *et al.* 1974; Hofer 1974; Steer *et al.* 1976). The view that amniotomy does predispose to fetal heart rate decelerations is largely based on the results of a study of its use in labour of spontaneous onset (Schwarcz *et al.* 1973, 1974, 1975; Caldeyro-Barcia *et al.* 1974). As discussed in Chapter 58, however, there was considerable potential for bias in this study and the results are therefore impossible to interpret with any confidence.

As far as the risk of umbilical cord prolapse is concerned, observational studies that have included at least 1000 women have indicated a risk of cord prolapse ranging from 0.1 to 0.4 per thousand (Kettel *et al.* 1958; Fields 1960; Niswander and Patterson 1963; d'Esopo *et al.* 1964; Setna *et al.* 1967; Pinkerton and Carson 1968; MacDonald 1970). As observed with spontaneous rupture of the membranes before the onset of labour

(see Chapter 43), this does not always occur at the time of amniotomy, but may supervene when labour eventually starts.

There is obviously also a risk that amniotomy may provoke bleeding from either vasa praevia or placenta praevia, conditions that will cause bleeding even if amniotomy is not performed. This complication occurred in 1 woman in a series of 1000 inductions reported by MacDonald (1970), and in one woman in a series of 3130 inductions reported by Setna *et al.* (1967).

4 Oxytocin

4.1 Routes and methods of administration

Intravenous infusion of oxytocin is currently the most widely used method for inducing labour. It was not until the 1940s, however, that the administration of oxytocin by intravenous drip was introduced (Page 1943; Theobald *et al.* 1948). Before that time, pituitary extract, and later oxytocin, had been administered either subcutaneously, intramuscularly, or by the intranasal route (see Chapter 59).

Much of the current understanding on the dose-related response of the uterus to oxytocin came from the pioneering work of Alvarez and Caldeyro-Barcia (reviewed by Caldeyro-Barcia and Heller 1961). They were the first investigators to record intrauterine pressure changes and thus provide quantitative assessments of uterine contractility. Using the knowledge derived from these physiological studies, Turnbull and Anderson, in a series of classic studies in Aberdeen, 'titrated' oxytocin in response to uterine contractions and thus introduced the principle on which the clinical use of oxytocin is now usually based (Turnbull and Anderson 1967, 1968a,b; Anderson *et al.* 1968).

Unfortunately, none of the early studies used properly controlled comparisons to provide more substantive evidence on the effects of oxytocin, and alternative doses, routes and methods of administration. In fact, prior to the introduction of prostaglandins, a total of only six controlled evaluations involving oxytocin administration had been reported. These compared natural with synthetic oxytocin (Danezis *et al.* 1962); buccal with nasal administration of oxytocin (Bergsjø and Jenssen 1969a, 1969b; Sjöstedt 1969); and intramuscular injections of oxytocin with sparteine sulphate (Van Voorhis *et al.* 1966). None of these comparisons revealed any striking differences between the drugs and routes of administration compared. No formal comparisons between intravenous infusions of oxytocin and other routes of administration have been reported.

Intravenous oxytocin has been administered in a variety of different ways. These range from simple, gravity-fed infusion systems adjusted manually; through mechanically or electronically controlled infusion systems and pumps; to fully automated closed loop feedback systems in which the dose of oxytocin is regulated by the intensity of uterine contractions. Gravity-fed systems have the disadvantage that the amount of oxytocin infused may be difficult to regulate accurately and may vary with the position of the woman. A further disadvantage of both gravity-fed and mechanically or electronically controlled infusion systems is that the amount of diluent fluid administered intravenously may be large, and may thus increase the risk of water intoxication (Abdul-Karim and Assali 1961; Burt *et al.* 1969; Schwartz and Jones 1978). Infusion pumps, by contrast, deliver oxytocin at a well-regulated rate, in a small volume of diluent fluid. Automatic oxytocin infusion equipment was introduced by Francis *et al.* (1970), and has been developed further during the years since then (Butterworth 1974; Parsons 1980; Carter and Steer 1980). In theory it should optimize efficacy and safety during oxytocin administration.

The only formal comparisons of different methods for administering oxytocin to induce labour are two trials comparing automatic oxytocin infusion systems with 'standard' infusions, using either manually (Steer *et al.* 1985) or electronically (Thomas and Blackwell 1974) controlled infusion systems or infusion pumps (Steer *et al.* 1985). A total of only 131 women were studied in these two trials, and it is not surprising that no differences were detected in any of the substantive outcomes available from these reports (Table 62.5). Steer and his colleagues (1985) reported that both the mean infusion rate and the total dose of oxytocin were reduced with the automatic feedback controlled system. It is logical to assume, as they suggested (Steer *et al.* 1985), that this would decrease the incidence of side-effects, but no evidence to that effect has been presented thus far in either controlled (Steer *et al.* 1985) or uncontrolled observations (Gibb *et al.* 1985). Observations based on experience with the early versions of the

Table 62.5 Effect of automated vs. standard oxytocin infusion for induction of labour on use of more than one induction attempt

Study	EXPT		CTRL		Odds ratio	Graph of odds ratios and confidence intervals						
	n	(%)	n	(%)	(95% CI)	0.01	0.1	0.5	1	2	10	100
Steer *et al.* (1985)	0/46	(0.00)	0/49	(0.00)	1.00 (1.00–1.00)							
Thomas and Blackwell (1974)	0/17	(0.00)	0/19	(0.00)	1.00 (1.00–1.00)							
Typical odds ratio (95% confidence interval)					1.00 (1.00–1.00)							

Effect of automated vs. standard oxytoxin infusion for induction of labour on use of analgesia

Steer *et al.* (1985)	34/40	(85.00)	40/44	(90.91)	0.57 (0.15–2.13)							
Thomas and Blackwell (1974)	16/17	(94.12)	18/19	(94.74)	0.89 (0.05–14.91)							
Typical odds ratio (95% confidence interval)					0.62 (0.19–2.04)							

Effect of automated vs. standard oxytocin infusion for induction of labour on use of epidural analgesia

Steer *et al.* (1985)	24/40	(60.00)	31/44	(70.45)	0.63 (0.26–1.55)							
Thomas and Blackwell (1974)	3/17	(17.65)	5/19	(26.32)	0.61 (0.13–2.90)							
Typical odds ratio (95% confidence interval)					0.63 (0.29–1.36)							

Effect of automated vs. standard oxytocin infusion for induction of labour on hyperstimulation

Thomas and Blackwell (1974)	7/17	(41.18)	8/19	(42.11)	0.96 (0.26–3.57)							
Typical odds ratio (95% confidence interval)					0.96 (0.26–3.57)							

Table 62.5—*continued* Effect of automated vs. standard oxytocin infusion for induction of labour on not delivered within 12 hours

Study	EXPT		CTRL		Odds ratio	Graph of odds ratios and confidence intervals						
	n	(%)	n	(%)	(95% CI)	0.01	0.1	0.5	1	2	10	100
Steer *et al.* (1985)	11/46	(23.91)	10/49	(20.41)	1.22 (0.47–3.21)							
Thomas and Blackwell (1974)	7/17	(41.18)	3/19	(15.79)	3.42 (0.81–14.45)							
Typical odds ratio (95% confidence interval)					1.68 (0.75–3.75)							

Effect of automated vs. standard oxytocin infusion for induction of labour on caesarean section

Study	EXPT		CTRL		Odds ratio	Graph
Steer *et al.* (1985)	6/46	(13.04)	4/49	(8.16)	1.67 (0.45–6.15)	
Thomas and Blackwell (1974)	4/17	(23.53)	3/19	(15.79)	1.62 (0.32–8.25)	
Typical odds ratio (95% confidence interval)					1.65 (0.60–4.57)	

Effect of automated vs. standard oxytocin infusion for induction of labour on instrumental vaginal delivery

Study	EXPT		CTRL		Odds ratio	Graph
Steer *et al.* (1985)	9/46	(19.57)	18/49	(36.73)	0.43 (0.18–1.05)	
Thomas and Blackwell (1974)	6/17	(35.29)	6/19	(31.58)	1.18 (0.30–4.62)	
Typical odds ratio (95% confidence interval)					0.58 (0.28–1.23)	

automated infusion systems have indicated a sufficiently high frequency of problems (Goodlin *et al.* 1974; Thomas and Blackwell 1974; Correy *et al.* 1975; Neves dos Santos *et al.* 1976) to warrant a more thorough evaluation of their merits and risks relative to conventional methods of administration before trying to assess their place, if any, in clinical practice.

One randomized controlled trial has been reported in which women were allocated to receive either continuous or 'pulsed' oxytocin infusion (whereby oxytocin was infused during only one in every 10 minutes) (Pavlou *et al.* 1978). It is unclear from the report how many women were 'randomly' assigned to the two treatment arms. Only 26 women were studied and (not surprisingly) no differences in substantive outcomes were detected. The authors suggested several advantages of pulsed administration, ranging from a reduced risk of oxytocin overdose to financial savings in the use of oxytocin and infusion fluids (Pavlou *et al.* 1978), but these remain to be substantiated by good evidence.

4.2 Hazards of oxytocin administration

The possible hazards of oxytocin itself must be distinguished from the hazards associated with any attempt to end pregnancy artificially before the sponta-neous onset of labour, and those that are associated with any artificial stimulation of uterine contractions, whether before or during labour. The extensive literature documenting and trying to explain the association between use of oxytocin and neonatal hyperbilirubinae-mia illustrates the problems in reaching confident conclusions in this kind of situation.

A relation between oxytocin administration in labour and the subsequent development of neonatal jaundice in 'mature' neonates was first observed in 1971 (Mast *et al.* 1971; Quakernack and Mast 1971). It was a letter to the *Lancet* in 1972 (Ghosh and Hudson 1972), however, that suddenly stimulated interest in this association, particularly in Britain where induction rates at the time were probably the highest in the world. This letter stimulated considerable research activity (O'Driscoll 1972; Davidson *et al.* 1973; Davies *et al.* 1973; Calder *et al.* 1974b; Gould *et al.* 1974; Gray and Mitchell 1974; Campbell *et al.* 1975; Chalmers *et al.* 1975; Sims and Neligan 1975; Thiery *et al.* 1975; Chalmers *et al.* 1976; Friedman and Sachtleben 1976; Chalmers 1977; Chew and Swann 1977; Chew 1977; Jeffares 1977; Friedman *et al.* 1978; D'Souza *et al.* 1979). Except for the smaller studies, most of this research confirmed the association between the use of oxytocin and neonatal hyperbilirubinaemia. Explanations for the association, however, included direct, toxic effects of the drug; pre-existent pathology, which had been the reason for using oxytocin in the first place; instrumental delivery; relative immaturity of bilirubin conjugation in the neonate; analgesia in labour; and increased haemolysis as a result of direct effects on the red cell membrane.

The balance of evidence suggests that induction of labour with oxytocin increases the incidence of neonatal hyperbilirubinaemia. This increase is probably more a reflection of relative immaturity of the neonate as a result of earlier termination of pregnancy than a reflection of the use of oxytocin *per se*. Nevertheless, the limited data available from controlled trials comparing prostaglandins with oxytocin for inducing labour (see Chapter 63), suggest that hyperbilirubinaemia is less likely to occur when labour is induced with prostaglandins than when it is induced with oxytocin (typical odds ratio 0.54), although the difference does not quite reach conventional levels of statistical significance (95 per cent confidence interval 0.28–1.04).

The antidiuretic effect of oxytocin, which is always observed to some (recognizable) extent when infusion rates exceed 45 mU per minute, is more plausibly attributable to the drug than to elective delivery, or the indications for elective delivery (Abdul-Karim and Assali 1961; Burt *et al.* 1969; Schwartz and Jones 1978). The antidiuretic action results in water retention and hyponatraemia, and may lead to coma, convulsions and (ultimately) maternal death (Hatch 1969). These risks are mainly associated with oxytocin infusions at relatively early stages of pregnancy, when uterine sensitivity to oxytocin is far less than it is at term (Hendricks and Brenner 1964), and when relatively large doses are therefore required to stimulate uterine contractions. In women with an already reduced urinary output the danger of water intoxication is an important consideration regardless of the stage of gestation.

Logically, any factor that causes uterine contractions, whether it be a drug such as oxytocin and the prostaglandins, or other factors such as nipple stimulation, may also cause excessive uterine contractility. Whenever the contraction force in the myometrium exceeds the levels of venous pressure, the venous circulation through the myometrium will become compromised, and flow from and to the placenta will be affected. Excessive uterine contractility (whether it is labelled 'uterine hypertonus' or 'uterine hyperstimulation') may thus lead to inadequate fetal oxygenation. Uterine rupture is a further, though much rarer consequence of excessive stimulation of uterine activity. These hazards will be minimized firstly, by restricting the use of elective delivery to circumstances in which it can be justified, and secondly, by appropriate regulation of uterine contractility, regardless of the method through which it is stimulated artificially.

5 Prostaglandins

Prostaglandins were first introduced for the induction of labour in the late 1960s, but their oxytocic properties were known long before the substances themselves were identified (see Chapter 59). The first reports dealt with prostaglandin F_{2a} (Karim *et al.* 1968). In 1967, Karim and Devlin still believed E prostaglandins had relaxing rather than stimulating effects on the uterus, and, one year later, Bygdeman and his colleagues suggested (1968), albeit for different reasons, that E prostaglandins would never be suitable for the induction of labour. Yet, as early as 1969, clinical research conducted by Embrey (1969) suggested that equipotent doses of PGE_2 were as useful as PGF_{2a} for induction of labour. Much of the early clinical research was conducted with PGF_{2a}, both because it was thought to be more specifically uterotonic (an incorrect view that is still occasionally heard), and because several years were needed to overcome the problems of the 'shelf instability' of PGE_2.

Since 1971, a large number of controlled evaluations of prostaglandins for inducing labour have been conducted, using not only the two main prostaglandins, but several different vehicles and routes of administration (Table 62.6). At first, these involved controlled comparisons between intravenous prostaglandins and intravenous oxytocin (see Chapter 63). Later, with the advent of other routes of prostaglandin administration, the controlled comparisons have been with placebo treatments; with intravenous and buccal oxytocin; and between different routes and doses of prostaglandins.

Table 62.6 Routes and methods of administering prostaglandins E and F in controlled trials with random or quasi-random allocation of subjects

Type of drug	Form of administration
Prostaglandin E_2	intravenous (infusion oral (tablets, solutions) buccal (tablets) rectal (tablets) vaginal (tablets, pessaries, gels) endocervical extra-amniotic (solutions, gels)
Prostaglandin F_{2a}	intravenous (infusion) oral (tablets) vaginal endocervical extra-amniotic

5.1 Comparisons with placebo

Seven studies, all conducted between 1978 and 1984, have compared prostaglandins (administered in various doses, formulations and routes) with placebo treatments that were identical except for the added prostaglandin (Wingerup *et al.* 1978; Gordon-Wright and

Elder 1979; Liggins 1979; MacLennan and Green 1980; MacKenzie *et al.* 1981; Ulmsten *et al.* 1982; Campbell 1984). The characteristics of these seven studies, six of which dealt with PGE_2 and one with PGF_{2a}, are shown in Table 62.7. As could be anticipated, the 'failure' rate of induction and the proportion of women needing a second induction attempt were statistically significantly lower following prostaglandin administration in all of the trials that provided data on these outcomes (Table 62.8). Not surprisingly in the light of these findings, the proportions of women who had not delivered vaginally within 12 hours and within 24 hours were also statistically significantly lower in the prostaglandin treated groups in those trials that provided data on these outcomes (Table 62.8).

Five of the trials provided data on the number of caesarean sections. In one, there were no caesarean sections (Ulmsten *et al.* 1982); in the other four, there were fewer caesarean sections in the prostaglandin than in the placebo groups, yielding a typical odds ratio of 0.45 with a 95 per cent confidence interval of 0.23 to 0.87 (Table 62.8). The incidence of instrumental vaginal delivery (available from 3 trials) showed no striking differences between the prostaglandin and placebo groups (Table 62.8).

As far as side-effects of the prostaglandin induction are concerned, six of the seven trials mentioned specifically that 'uterine hypertonus' and/or 'uterine hyperstimulation' were not observed (Table 62.8). Five trials specifically sought data on the incidence of gastrointestinal side-effects, such as vomiting and diarrhoea, but only one woman out of a total of 197 women receiving prostaglandins in these trials was reported as having experienced gastrointestinal side-effects; she had diarrhoea after receiving 50 mg PGF_{2a} vaginally (Table 62.8). Only two trials make specific mention of pyrexia during labour or the puerperium, but this side-effect was not observed in either trial (MacLennan and Green 1980; Ulmsten *et al.* 1982).

Very few infant outcomes were reported in any of these trials, and, among those in which they were reported, none showed any differences between the prostaglandin and placebo groups (Table 62.8). One instance of fetal death occurred in the trial reported by Liggins (1979). A woman who had not started labour after receiving 0.2 mg vaginal PGE_2 suppositories was

Table 62.7 Characteristics of the placebo-controlled trials of prostaglandins for induction of labour

Authors and dates	Prostaglandin preparation	Number of women		Further details on study design
		PG	Placebo	
Campbell (1984)	3 mg PGE_2 in polyethylene glycol pessary vaginally	96	105	Membranes were ruptured when labour became established; second pessary when not in labour after 8 hours; if labour did not occur within 24 hours –> other method of induction
Wingerup *et al.* (1978)	1 mg PGE_2 in hydroxypropyl-methyl cellulose gel endocervically	10	10	If not in established labour –> oxytocin infusion the next day (after 24 hours)
Gordon-Wright *et al.* (1979)	1 mg PGE_2 in a vaginal tablet	50	27	Administered in the evening; if not delivered the next morning –> amniotomy; aims of the study included both cervical ripening and induction of labour.
Liggins (1979)	0.2 mg or 0.4 mg mg PGE_2 in a Witepsol pessary vaginally every 2 hours	26 (0.2 mg) 26 (0.4 mg)	32	Treatment from 09:00 hours until onset of labour or 21:00 hr; treatment resumed next morning at 7:00 and continued until 15 tablets had been inserted; amniotomy only performed when labour established and cervix at least 4 cm dilated; if no labour within 48 hours after first suppository –> amniotomy and intravenous oxytocin.
MacLennan and Green (1980)	25 mg or 50 mg PGF_{2a} in methyl-hydroxyethyl cellulose gel vaginally	30 (50 mg) 30 (50 mg)	30	Treatment given at 17:00 hr; reassessment the next day at 8:00 hr following which treatment was at discretion of the attending obstetrician.
MacKenzie *et al.* (1981)	2.5 mg PGE_2 in a Witepsol pessary vaginally	21	21	Amniotomy was performed 3 hours later, followed another 5 hours later by intravenous oxytocin if necessary.
Ulmsten *et al.* (1982)	0.5 mg PGE_2 in starch polymer gel endocervically	25	25	Amniotomy not performed before cervix was 4 cm dilated; women not in labour were reassessed after 24 hours; form of care in women undelivered after 24 hours not reported.

subsequently induced by amniotomy, which revealed clear liquor. The fetus developed severe bradycardia 2 hours later and died soon afterwards. The death was attributed to acute intrauterine asphyxia (Liggins 1979). Perinatal deaths were mentioned in only two other trials (Gordon-Wright and Elder 1979; MacKenzie *et al.* 1981), but only to confirm that none had occurred.

5.2 Prostaglandin E vs. prostaglandin F

Both E and F prostaglandins stimulate uterine contractility. Among these two series of prostaglandins, only PGE_2 and PGF_{2a} (which are also naturally formed from arachidonic acid during spontaneous labour; Keirse 1979) have been used to any extent for the induction of labour. As mentioned previously, most of the early studies (using the intravenous route of administration) dealt with PGF_{2a}. Currently PGE_2 is used almost

Table 62.8 Effect of any prostaglandin vs. placebo for induction of labour on 'induction failure'

Study	EXPT		CTRL		Odds ratio	Graph of odds ratios and confidence intervals						
	n	(%)	n	(%)	(95% CI)	0.01	0.1	0.5	1	2	10	100
Liggins (1979)	13/52	(25.00)	29/32	(90.63)	0.07 (0.03–0.18)							
MacLennan and Green (1980)	41/60	(68.33)	30/30	(100.0)	0.15 (0.05–0.44)							
Wingerup *et al.* (1978)	0/10	(0.00)	8/10	(80.00)	0.04 (0.01–0.24)							
Campbell (1984)	43/95	(45.26)	90/104	(86.54)	0.16 (0.09–0.28)							
Typical odds ratio (95% confidence interval)					0.12 (0.08–0.19)							

Effect of any prostaglandin vs. placebo for induction of labour on use of more than one induction attempt

MacLennan and Green (1980)	27/60	(45.00)	23/30	(76.67)	0.28 (0.12–0.68)							
MacKenzie *et al.* (1981)	5/21	(23.81)	12/21	(57.14)	0.26 (0.08–0.88)							
Wingerup *et al.* (1978)	2/10	(20.00)	10/10	(100.0)	0.04 (0.01–0.24)							
Typical odds ratio (95% confidence interval)					0.21 (0.11–0.40)							

Effect of any prostaglandin vs. placebo for induction of labour on no vaginal delivery within 12 hours

MacLennan and Green (1980)	9/60	(15.00)	30/30	(100.0)	0.03 (0.01–0.08)							
Ulmsten *et al.* (1982)	17/25	(68.00)	25/25	(100.0)	0.10 (0.02–0.43)							
Wingerup *et al.* (1978)	2/10	(20.00)	10/10	(100.0)	0.04 (0.01–0.24)							
Typical odds ratio (95% confidence interval)					0.04 (0.02–0.09)							

Effect of any prostaglandin vs. placebo for induction of labour on no vaginal delivery within 24 hours

Ulmsten *et al.* (1982)	14/25	(56.00)	23/25	(92.00)	0.16 (0.05–0.56)							
Wingerup *et al.* (1978)	2/10	(20.00)	10/10	(100.0)	0.04 (0.01–0.24)							
Typical odds ratio (95% confidence interval)					0.10 (0.04–0.28)							

Table 62.8—*continued* Effect of any prostaglandin vs. placebo for induction of labour on caesarean section

Study	EXPT		CTRL		Odds ratio	Graph of odds ratios and confidence intervals						
	n	(%)	*n*	(%)	(95% CI)	0.01	0.1	0.5	1	2	10	100
Liggins (1979)	7/52	(13.46)	9/32	(28.13)	0.39 (0.13–1.19)							
MacLennan and Green (1980)	3/60	(5.00)	3/30	(10.00)	0.45 (0.08–2.59)							
Ulmsten *et al.* (1982)	0/25	(0.00)	0/25	(0.00)	1.00 (1.00–1.00)							
Wingerup *et al.* (1978)	0/10	(0.00)	3/10	(30.00)	0.11 (0.01–1.17)							
Campbell (1984)	6/95	(6.32)	10/104	(9.62)	0.64 (0.23–1.78)							
Typical odds ratio (95% confidence interval)					0.45 (0.23–0.87)							

Effect of any prostaglandin vs. placebo for induction of labour on instrumental vaginal delivery

Study	EXPT		CTRL		Odds ratio							
Liggins (1979)	11/52	(21.15)	5/32	(15.63)	1.43 (0.47–4.35)							
MacLennan and Green (1980)	19/60	(31.67)	15/30	(50.00)	0.46 (0.19–1.14)							
Campbell (1984)	14/95	(14.74)	13/104	(12.50)	1.21 (0.54–2.72)							
Typical odds ratio (95% confidence interval)					0.90 (0.53–1.53)							

Effect of any prostaglandin vs. placebo for induction of labour on operative delivery

Study	EXPT		CTRL		Odds ratio							
Liggins (1979)	18/52	(34.62)	14/32	(43.75)	0.68 (0.28–1.68)							
MacLennan and Green (1980)	22/60	(36.67)	18/30	(60.00)	0.39 (0.16–0.94)							
Campbell (1984)	20/95	(21.05)	23/104	(22.12)	0.94 (0.48–1.84)							
Typical odds ratio (95% confidence interval)					0.68 (0.43–1.08)							

Effect of any prostaglandin vs. placebo for induction of labour on hypertonus/hyperstimulation

Study	EXPT		CTRL		Odds ratio							
Gordon-Wright and Elder (1979)	0/50	(0.00)	0/27	(0.00)	1.00 (1.00–1.00)							
Liggins (1979)	0/52	(0.00)	0/32	(0.00)	1.00 (1.00–1.00)							
Ulmsten *et al.* (1982)	0/25	(0.00)	0/25	(0.00)	1.00 (1.00–1.00)							
MacLennan and Green (1980)	0/60	(0.00)	0/30	(0.00)	1.00 (1.00–1.00)							
Wingerup *et al.* (1978)	0/10	(0.00)	0/10	(0.00)	1.00 (1.00–1.00)							
Campbell (1984)	0/95	(0.00)	0/104	(0.00)	1.00 (1.00–1.00)							
Typical odds ratio (95% confidence interval)					1.00 (1.00–1.00)							

Effect of any prostaglandin vs. placebo for induction of labour on gastrointestinal side-effects

Study	EXPT n	(%)	CTRL n	(%)	Odds ratio (95% CI)	Graph
Gordon-Wright and Elder (1979)	0/50	(0.00)	0/27	(0.00)	1.00 (1.00–1.00)	
MacLennan and Green (1980)	1/60	(1.67)	0/30	(0.00)	4.48 (0.07–99.99)	
Ulmsten et al. (1982)	0/25	(0.00)	0/25	(0.00)	1.00 (1.00–1.00)	
Liggins (1979)	0/52	(0.00)	0/32	(0.00)	1.00 (1.00–1.00)	
Wingerup et al. (1978)	0/10	(0.00)	0/10	(0.00)	1.00 (1.00–1.00)	
Typical odds ratio (95% confidence interval)					4.48 (0.07–99.99)	

Effect of any prostaglandin vs. placebo for induction of labour on low Apgar score at 1 minute

Study	EXPT n	(%)	CTRL n	(%)	Odds ratio (95% CI)	Graph
Liggins (1979)	6/52	(11.54)	6/32	(18.75)	0.56 (0.16–1.95)	
Typical odds ratio (95% confidence interval)					0.56 (0.16–1.95)	

Effect of any prostaglandin vs. placebo for induction of labour on low Apgar score at 5 minutes

Study	EXPT n	(%)	CTRL n	(%)	Odds ratio (95% CI)	Graph
Gordon-Wright and Elder (1979)	3/50	(6.00)	0/27	(0.00)	4.86 (0.44–53.78)	
Wingerup et al. (1978)	0/10	(0.00)	0/10	(0.00)	1.00 (1.00–1.00)	
Typical odds ratio (95% confidence interval)					4.86 (0.44–53.78)	

Table 62.9 Effect of oral PGE_2 vs. oral $PGF_{2\alpha}$ for induction of labour on gastrointestinal side-effects

Study	EXPT n	(%)	CTRL n	(%)	Odds ratio (95% CI)	Graph of odds ratios and confidence intervals 0.01 0.1 0.5 1 2 10
Yeung et al. (1977)	17/84	(20.24)	30/89	(33.71)	0.51 (0.26–0.99)	
Typical odds ratio (95% confidence interval)					0.51 (0.26–0.99)	

Effect of oral PGE_2 vs. oral $PGF_{2\alpha}$ for induction of labour on drug discontinued due to side-effects

Study	EXPT n	(%)	CTRL n	(%)	Odds ratio (95% CI)	Graph
Yeung et al. (1977)	5/84	(5.95)	11/89	(12.36)	0.47 (0.17–1.31)	
Typical odds ratio (95% confidence interval)					0.47 (0.17–1.31)	

Table 62.9—*continued* Effect of oral PGE_2 vs. oral $PGF2_\alpha$ for induction of labour on labour not established within 12 hours

Yeung *et al.* (1977)	7/84	(8.33)	21/89	(23.60)	0.33 (0.15–0.73)	
Typical odds ratio (95% confidence interval)					0.33 (0.15–0.73)	

Effect of oral PGE_2 vs. oral $PGF_{2\alpha}$ for induction of labour on caesarean section

Yeung *et al.* (1977)	7/84	(8.33)	11/89	(12.36)	0.65 (0.25–1.72)	
Typical odds ratio (95% confidence interval)					0.65 (0.25–1.72)	

Effect of oral PGE_2 vs. oral $PGF_{2\alpha}$ for induction of labour on instrumental vaginal delivery

Yeung *et al.* (1977)	19/84	(22.62)	23/89	(25.84)	0.84 (0.42–1.68)	
Typical odds ratio (95% confidence interval)					0.84 (0.42–1.68)	

Effect of oral PGE_2 vs. oral $PGF_{2\alpha}$ for induction of labour on operative delivery

Yeung *et al.* (1977)	26/84	(30.95)	34/89	(38.20)	0.73 (0.39–1.36)	
Typical odds ratio (95% confidence interval)					0.73 (0.39–1.36)	

exclusively, except in countries where it has not been made available. Comparisons between the effects of these two prostaglandins are confounded by changes in the routes of administration that have occurred during the history of their use for inducing labour. Furthermore, differences in their oxytocic potencies render these comparisons difficult to interpret unless they are conducted with equipotent doses.

There have been only two direct comparisons between PGE_2 and $PGF_{2\alpha}$ for formal induction of labour. The first of these compared intravenous administration of the two prostaglandins, but the trial involved a total of only 20 women and was too small to detect any differential effects, except for a higher incidence of pyrexia during labour induced with PGE_2 (Naismith *et al.* 1973). The other trial involved 173 women and compared oral administration of either PGE_2 or $PGF_{2\alpha}$ (Yeung and Pang 1977). After the membranes had been ruptured artificially, the women received hourly doses of 1–2 mg PGE_2 or 5–10 mg $PGF_{2\alpha}$ until uterine contractility was firmly established. The results indicate that PGE_2 is superior to $PGF_{2\alpha}$ in all of the aspects for which categorical data are available (Table 62.9). In addition, the authors reported the mean induction to delivery intervals to be statistically significantly shorter with oral PGE_2 than with the 10 times higher dose of $PGF_{2\alpha}$, both in nulliparous and in multiparous women.

The results of this trial are consistent with observational data (Thiery and Amy 1975; Embrey 1975; Amy and Thiery 1979). Most of these data relate to the (now superseded) intravenous route of administration, but the inferences drawn from them will also apply to some extent to other routes of administration. Thus it appears, first, that in order to achieve a similar effect on uterine contractility, $PGF_{2\alpha}$ needs to be administered in a dose which is about eight to ten times as large as that needed when PGE_2 is used. Second, this difference in potency, which applies to the stimulating properties of these compounds on the myometrium, does not apply to the same extent to the effects of these agents on other organ systems, most notably the gastrointestinal tract. Consequently, for a comparable uterotonic effect, the incidence of other, undesired effects tends to be larger with $PGF_{2\alpha}$ than with PGE_2. This was stated graphically by one investigator when he wrote (about oral $PGF_{2\alpha}$) that 'ten cases were acutely miserable on account of diarrhoea amounting to virtual incontinence, and by the end of our 50 cases we could not persuade one other patient to take these capsules' (Barr 1973).

There appear to be only two exceptions to the general rule that PGE_2 is preferable to $PGF_{2\alpha}$ as far as side-effects are concerned, namely, that hyperthermia and venous erythema are more often observed with PGE_2 than with $PGF_{2\alpha}$ administration (Thiery and Amy 1975; Embrey 1975). Venous erythema in particular, which is associated exclusively with intravenous administration and relates to dilatation of the vasa vasorum of the venous system, is seen virtually only with PGE_2 infusions; although on occasions quite dramatic from a visual point of view, it is entirely painless and disappears after the end of the infusion period.

5.3 Routes and methods of administration

5.3.1 Intravenous, oral, and vaginal administration

Early studies of prostaglandins for the induction of labour used the intravenous route of administration. From these studies, which were comprehensively reviewed by Thiery and Amy (1975) and summarized by Embrey (1975) in the mid-1970s, few, if any, advantages of using prostaglandins for induction of labour emerged. Compared with oxytocin they appeared to offer no advantage and were considerably more expensive. They tended to produce bothersome side-effects, mainly vomiting and diarrhoea (which were particularly prominent with $PGF_{2\alpha}$), but also hyperthermia (especially with the use of PGE_2). Finally, they appeared to require an even more careful determination of the infused dose than oxytocin, because of the small margin between doses that would stimulate uterine contractions adequately and those that would cause 'hyperstimulation'. Indeed, between 1971 and 1973, eight controlled comparisons of intravenous prostaglandins with intravenous oxytocin for the induction of labour (Beazley and Gillespie 1971; Rangarajan *et al.* 1971; Le Maire *et al.* 1972; Scher *et al.* 1972; Vakhariya and Sherman 1972; Vroman *et al.* 1972; Blackburn *et al.* 1973; Naismith *et al.* 1973) were reported; and none (on its own) provided any evidence supporting adoption of prostaglandins (see Chapter 63).

In 1971, Karim and Sharma reported on the oral administration of PGE_2 for induction. From then on, oral administration of PGE_2 (in doses increasing from 0.5 to 2 mg) became widely used as an alternative to intravenous infusions of prostaglandins for inducing labour, particularly when combined with amniotomy (Ratnam *et al.* 1974) and in women with a favourable cervix (see Chapter 63). Thiery and his colleagues (1977), in a randomized controlled comparison involving 50 women, showed that it was not necessary for the prostaglandin tablets to be swallowed: there were no differences detected in any of the outcome measures between the 25 women who received PGE_2 orally in doses of 0.5 to 3 mg, and the 25 women who were instructed to let the tablets melt away under the tongue.

Because of its gastrointestinal side-effects, $PGF_{2\alpha}$ is entirely unsuited for oral administration. Even with oral PGE_2, however, gastrointestinal side-effects occur, although they are usually mild and mostly confined to one or two episodes of vomiting. In a few reports, these side-effects have been reported to affect between 20 and 50 per cent of women, depending on the doses used (Thiery *et al.* 1977; Friedman and Sachtleben 1974; Friedman *et al.* 1975). In nearly all of the controlled comparisons, however, the incidence of gastrointestinal side-effects with oral PGE_2 has been reported to be at or below 10 per cent (Lykkesfeldt and Osler 1981; Westergaard *et al.* 1983; Bremme and Bygdeman 1980; Read and Martin 1974; Ratnam *et al.* 1974; Haeri *et al.* 1976; Beard *et al.* 1975).

Probably the most widely adopted mode of administration of PGE_2 (and of $PGF_{2\alpha}$ in countries where PGE_2 is not available; MacLennan and Green 1980) has become the vaginal route. Five of the seven placebo-controlled trials discussed earlier employed this route of administration (Gordon-Wright and Elder 1979; Liggins 1979; MacLennan and Green 1980; MacKenzie *et al.* 1981; Campbell 1984). The formulations used in clinical practice have encompassed, among others, vaginal administration of oral tablets; vaginal tablets; pessaries based on wax, starch, glyceride, and lactose; and a variety of commercial and home made viscous gels. Apart from the studies mentioned earlier and a few controlled comparisons between different doses of vaginal PGE_2 (Hunter and Hammad 1982; Hunter *et al.* 1984; Liggins 1979), there have been no controlled evaluations of these different formulations.

5.3.2 Endocervical and extra-amniotic administration

Because intravenous, oral, and vaginal administration of prostaglandins all lead to high levels of these drugs in the blood, or the gastrointestinal tract, or both, localized, intrauterine routes of administration have been used in attempts to reduce the side-effects associated with the other routes. Extra-amniotic infusion of a solution of PGE_2 was shown to be effective for inducing labour in 1974 (Calder *et al.* 1974a), but as the procedure is rather cumbersome and inconvenient for the mother, it was later replaced by extra-amniotic injection of PGE_2 suspended in viscous gel (Calder *et al.* 1977).

There have been only two controlled comparisons of the extra-amniotic route with other routes of prostaglandin administration. One of these (Iskander 1978) compared extra-amniotic infusion of PGE_2 (0.325 microgram per minute, increased with 0.15 microgram per minute every 20 minutes until satisfactory uterine contractions were obtained) with an intravenous infusion of PGE_2 (from 0.25 up to 1 microgram per minute).

Table 62.10 Effect of extra-amniotic PGE$_2$ vs. other route for induction of labour on failed induction

Study	EXPT		CTRL		Odds ratio	Graph of odds ratios and confidence intervals						
	n	(%)	n	(%)	(95% CI)	0.01	0.1	0.5	1	2	10	100
Clarke *et al.* (1980)	80/133	(60.15)	61/128	(47.66)	1.65 (1.02–2.68)							
Iskander (1978)	1/20	(5.00)	0/20	(0.00)	7.39 (0.15–99.99)							
Typical odds ratio (95% confidence interval)					1.69 (1.04–2.73)							

Effect of extra-amniotic PGE$_2$ vs. other route for induction of labour on hypertonus

Study	EXPT		CTRL		Odds ratio							
Clarke *et al.* (1980)	0/133	(0.00)	0/128	(0.00)	1.00 (1.00–1.00)							
Iskander (1978)	1/20	(5.00)	0/20	(0.00)	7.39 (0.15–99.99)							
Typical odds ratio (95% confidence interval)					7.39 (0.15–99.99)							

Effect of extra-amniotic PGE$_2$ vs. other route for induction of labour on vomiting

Study	EXPT		CTRL		Odds ratio							
Clarke *et al.* (1980)	0/133	(0.00)	0/128	(0.00)	1.00 (1.00–1.00)							
Iskander (1978)	0/20	(0.00)	1/20	(5.00)	0.14 (0.00–6.82)							
Typical odds ratio (95% confidence interval)					0.14 (0.00–6.82)							

Effect of extra-amniotic PGE$_2$ vs. other route for induction of labour on caesarean section

Study	EXPT		CTRL		Odds ratio							
Iskander (1978)	1/20	(5.00)	0/20	(0.00)	7.39 (0.15–99.99)							
Typical odds ratio (95% confidence interval)					7.39 (0.15–99.99)							

Effect of extra-amniotic PGE$_2$ vs. other route for induction of labour on instrumental vaginal delivery

Study	EXPT		CTRL		Odds ratio							
Iskander (1978)	2/20	(10.00)	2/20	(10.00)	1.00 (0.13–7.69)							
Typical odds ratio (95% confidence interval)					1.00 (0.13–7.69)							

Effect of extra-amniotic PGE$_2$ vs. other route for induction of labour on low Apgar score at 5 minutes

Study	EXPT		CTRL		Odds ratio							
Iskander (1978)	0/20	(0.00)	0/20	(0.00)	1.00 (1.00–1.00)							
Typical odds ratio (95% confidence interval)					1.00 (1.00–1.00)							

The other (Clarke *et al.* 1980) compared PGE$_2$ (0.3 mg) placed extra-amniotically with PGE$_2$ (2 mg) given vaginally, both being administered in a methylhydroxyethyl cellulose (Tylose®) gel. Neither of the two trials showed any advantage of the more invasive extra-amniotic route, but the precision of the estimates derived from these trials is very low (Table 62.10). One further controlled trial (Thiery *et al.* 1981) assigned 91 women to receive extra-amniotic PGE$_2$ in Tylose® gel, removing the catheter in 43 of them and leaving it in the extra-amniotic space in the remaining 48; no difference in any substantive outcomes were detected between the two policies.

Another route of local administration, endocervical injection of PGE$_2$ in a viscous gel, was introduced in 1978 (Wingerup *et al.* 1978), but it has been used mainly for ripening the cervix for induction (see Chapter 61). Two of the placebo-controlled trials presented in Tables 62.7 and 62.8 have used this approach (Wingerup *et al.* 1978; Ulmsten *et al.* 1982). As discussed in Chapter 61, several controlled comparisons with placebo or 'no treatment' in women with unfavourable cervical features have further demonstrated that this intervention will frequently initiate labour. However, the relative merits and hazards in comparison to other routes of administration have not yet been adequately assessed.

5.4 Hazards of prostaglandin administration

The specific hazards attributable to prostaglandins *per se* relate mainly to their effects on the gastrointestinal tract. The small number of placebo-controlled trials of prostaglandins for induction of labour provides little evidence of these effects. Important additional evidence, however, is available from the larger number of trials in which prostaglandins have been compared with oxytocin for the induction of labour (Table 62.11; see also Chapter 63). These effects are minimal when the drugs are administered endocervically or extra-amniotically, and maximal when routes of administration (intravenous, oral, and vaginal) are used that lead to high levels of these drugs in either the blood or the gastrointestinal tract. As mentioned previously, controlled comparisons which have involved the use of oral PGE$_2$ indicate that these problems may affect up to about 10 per cent of women.

Pyrexia also results from a direct effect of prostaglandins on thermoregulating centres in the brain. This is particularly a problem of prostaglandin E$_2$ administration and may give rise to concern that intrauterine infection has supervened. This concern may be further fuelled by a rise in the leucocyte count, which can also be stimulated by prostaglandin administration (Keirse

and Bennebroek Gravenhorst 1977; Wallenburg *et al.* 1980). If the membranes are intact and labour has been of relatively short duration, however, pyrexia is almost always due to an effect of prostaglandin E$_2$ rather than to incipient uterine infection.

Important though it is to consider the specific hazards of prostaglandins, it should not be forgotten that they pale into insignificance when considered against the far more worrying indirect hazards associated with their use. These are first, that the availability of these drugs will prompt obstetricians to embark on elective delivery for trivial reasons, and second, that even when they are being administered for good reasons, inadequate attention will be paid to careful monitoring of uterine contractility.

6 Conclusions

6.1 Implications for current practice

The most important decisions to be made in relation to induction of labour do not relate to the methods used to achieve it, but to the justification for pre-empting the spontaneous onset of labour. Furthermore, whatever method is chosen to implement a justified decision to induce labour, there is a clear need for careful monitoring of uterine contractility and maternal and fetal well-being.

The available evidence indicates that amniotomy alone is often inadequate to induce labour. In addition, the administration of oxytocic drugs, especially oxytocin, without amniotomy is also associated with a unacceptable failure rate of induction attempts. These observations indicate, first, that if amniotomy is used to induce labour and fails to result in adequate uterine contractility, oxytocic drugs should be administered promptly. Second, although the only controlled trial provides little evidence to support the policy, the weight of evidence indicates that oxytocin infusion is likely to be more effective in achieving delivery within a reasonable time if it is combined with amniotomy, than when it is used alone.

If prostaglandins are used to induce labour, the selection of prostaglandin E$_2$ rather than prostaglandin F$_{2\alpha}$ is likely to lead to fewer gastrointestinal side-effects. Indeed, the use of oral prostaglandin F$_{2\alpha}$ should be abandoned completely. Assuming that the cervix is 'ripe' and that a decision has been made to use prostaglandins to induce labour, the two main alternatives are oral or vaginal administration of prostaglandin E$_2$. There is currently no satisfactory evidence on which to base a rational choice between these two routes of administration.

6.2 Implications for future research

Sweeping (stripping) the membranes is a commonly used intervention which has received virtually no systematic attention from clinical researchers. Its effects on the onset of labour and on maternal and perinatal morbidity should be evaluated in randomized controlled trials.

A variety of automatic infusion systems for administering oxytocin have become available, but their advantages, if any, compared with more conventional methods for administering the drug have not been demonstrated. They should be subjected to proper

evaluation in order to assess whether there are any benefits to offset against the substantial cost of installing these machines.

The available research comparing different doses and routes of administration of prostaglandins for induction of labour is characterized by a plethora of small and very diverse studies, most of which provide no helpful guidance for clinical practice. Clinical researchers should agree on the most important questions in this field and collaborate in the design and execution of studies that will answer them.

References

Abdul-Karim R, Assali N (1961). Renal function in human pregnancy. J Lab Clin Med, 57: 522–532.

Aickin DR (1966). Sparteine sulphate and synthetic oxytocin: A comparative study. Austral NZ J Obstet Gynaecol, 6: 85–94.

Amy JJ, Thiery M (1979). Induction of labour with prostaglandins. In Practical Applications of Prostaglandins and their Synthesis. Karim SMM (ed). Lancaster: MTP Press, pp 437–446.

Anderson ABM, Turnbull AC, Baird D (1968). The influence of induction of labour on caesarean section rate, duration of labour and perinatal mortality in Aberdeen primigravidae between 1938 and 1966. J Obstet Gynaecol Br Commnwlth, 75: 800–811.

Andreasson B, Bock JE, Larsen J (1985). Induction of labour. A double-blind randomized controlled study of prostaglandin E₂ vaginal suppositories compared with intranasal oxytocin and with sequential treatment. Acta Obstet Gynecol Scand, 64: 157–161.

Bakos O, Bäckström T (1987). Induction of labor: a prospective, randomized study into amniotomy and oxytocin as induction methods in a total unselected population. Acta Obstet Gynecol Scand, 66: 537–541.

Barham K (1973). Amnioscopy anmiotomy: A look at surgical induction of labor. Am J Obstet Gynecol, 117: 35-38.

Barr W (1973). Induction of labor by prostaglandin E₂. In: The Prostaglandins. Clinical Application in Human Reproduction. Southern EM (ed). Mount Kisco: Futura, pp 219–222.

Beard RJ, Harrison R, Kiriakidis J, Underhill R, Craft I (1975). A clinical and biochemical assessment of the use of oral prostaglandin E₂ compared with intravenous oxytocin for labor induction in multiparous patients. Eur J Obstet Gynecol Reprod Biol, 5: 203–207.

Beazley JM, Gillespie A (1971). Double-blind trial of prostaglandin E₂ and oxytocin in induction of labour. Lancet, 1: 152–155.

Bergsjø P, Jenssen H (1969a). Comparison between intranasal and transbuccal oxytocin for the induction of labour. Acta Obstet Gynecol Scand, 470: 134–136.

Bergsjø P, Jenssen H (1969b). Nasal and buccal oxytocin for the induction of labour: a clinical trial. J Obstet Gynaecol Br Commnwlth, 76: 131–136.

Blackburn MG, Mancusi-Unbaro HR, Orzalesi MM, Hobbins JC, Anderson GG (1973). Effects on the neonate of the induction of labor with prostaglandin F₂alpha and oxytocin. Am J Obstet Gynecol, 116: 847–853.

Bradford WP, Gordon G (1968). Induction of labour by amniotomy and simultaneous Syntocinon infusion. J Obstet Gynaecol Br Commnwlth, 75: 698–701.

Bremme K, Bygdeman M (1980). Induction of labor by oxytocin or prostaglandin E₂. Acta Obstet Gynecol Scand, 11–21.

Burt RL, Oliver KL, Whitener DL (1969). Water intoxication complicating elective induction of labour at term. Obstet Gynecol, 34: 212–214.

Butterworth MJ (1974). Automated incremental oxytocin infusion in the induction of labor. Obstet Gynecol, 44: 238–245.

Bygdeman M, Kwon SU, Mukherjee T, Wiqvist N (1968). Effect of intravenous infusion of prostaglandin E₁ and E₂ on motility of the pregnant human uterus. Am J Obstet Gynecol, 102: 317–326.

Calder AA, Embrey MP, Hillier K (1974a). Extra-amniotic prostaglandin E₂ for the induction of labour at term. J Obstet Gynaecol Br Commnwlth, 81: 39–46.

Calder AA, Moar VA, Ounsted MK, Turnbull AC (1974b). Increased bilirubin levels in neonates after induction of labour by intravenous prostaglandin E₂ or oxytocin. Lancet, 2: 1339–1342.

Calder AA, Embrey MP, Tait T (1977). Ripening of the cervix with extra-amniotic PGE₂ in viscous gel before induction of labour. Br J Obstet Gynaecol, 84: 264–268.

Caldeyro-Barcia R, Heller H (1961). Oxytocin. New York: Pergamon Press.

Caldeyro-Barcia R, Schwarcz R, Belizan JM, Martell M, Nieto F, Sabatino H, Tenzer SM (1974). Adverse perinatal effects of early amniotomy during labor. In: Modern Perinatal Medicine. Gluck L (ed). Chicago: Yearbook Publishers, pp 431–449.

Campbell JM (1984). Induction of labour using prostaglandin E₂ pessaries. Clin Exp Obst Gyn, 11: 1–5.

Campbell N, Harvey D, Norman AP (1975). Increased frequency of neonatal jaundice in a maternity hospital. Br Med J, 2: 548–552.

Carter MC, Steer PJ (1980). An automatic infusion system for the measurement and control of uterine activity. Med Instrum, 14: 169–173.

Chalmers I (1977). Epidemiological surveillance in perinatal practice. In: Epidemiological Evaluation of Drugs. Colombo F, Tognoni G (eds). Amsterdam: Elsevier/North Holland Biomedical Press. pp 249–255.

Chalmers I, Campbell H, Turnbull AC (1975). Use of oxytocin and incidence of neonatal jaundice. Br Med J, 1: 116–118.

Chalmers I, Campbell H, Turnbull AC (1976). Oxytocin and neonatal jaundice. Br Med J, 1: 647–648.

Chew WC (1977). Neonatal hyperbilirubinaemia: a comparison between prostaglandin E_2 and oxytocin inductions. Br Med J, 2: 679–680.

Chew WC, Swann IL (1977). Influence of simultaneous low amniotomy and oxytocin infusion and other maternal factors on neonatal jaundice: a prospective study. Br Med J, 1: 72–73.

Clarke GA, Letchworth AT, Noble AD (1980). Comparative trial of extra-amniotic and vaginal prostaglandin E_2 in tylose gel for induction of labor. J Perinat Med, 8: 236–240.

Correy JF, Tait TG, Fullerton R (1975). A critical assessment of the induction and maintenance of labour using the Cardiff infusion system. Austral NZ J Obstet Gynaecol, 15: 136–144.

D'Souza SW, Black P, Macfarlane T, Richards B (1979). The effect of oxytocin in induced labour on neonatal jaundice. Br J Obstet Gynaecol, 86: 133–138.

Danezis J, Cohen J, Burnhill MS (1962). A comparison of synthetic and natural oxytocin as determined by intra-amniotic fluid pressure recordings. Am J Obstet Gynecol, 83: 770–773.

Davidson DC, Ford JA, McIntosh W (1973). Neonatal jaundice and maternal oxytocin infusion. Br Med J, 4: 106–107.

Davies DP, Gomersall R, Robertson R, Gray OP, Turnbull AC (1973). Neonatal jaundice and maternal oxytocin infusion. Br Med J, 3: 476–477.

Ekman G, Granstrom L, Ulmsten U (1986). Induction of labor with intravenous oxytocin or vaginal PGE_2 suppositories. Acta Obstet Gynecol Scand, 65: 857–859.

D'Esopo DA, Moore DB, Lenzi E (1964). Elective induction of labor. Am J Obstet Gynecol 89: 561–567.

Embrey MP (1969). The effect of prostaglandins on the human pregnant uterus. J Obstet Gynaecol Br Commnwlth, 76: 783–798.

Embrey MP (1975). The Prostaglandins in Human Reproduction. Edinburgh: Churchill Livingstone.

Fields H (1960). Complications of Elective Induction. Obstet Gynecol 15: 476–480.

Francis JG, Turnbull AC, Thomas FF (1970). Automatic oxytocin infusion equipment for induction of labour. J Obstet Gynaecol Br Commnwlth, 77: 594–602.

Friedman EA, Sachtleben MR (1974). Oral prostaglandin E_2 for induction of labor at term. Obstet Gynecol, 43: 178–185.

Friedman EA, Sachtleben MR (1976). Neonatal jaundice in association with oxytocin stimulation of labour and operative delivery. Br Med J, 1: 198–199.

Friedman EA, Sachtleben MR, Green W (1975). Oral prostaglandin E_2 for induction of labor at term. II. Comparison of two low-dosage regimens. Am J Obstet Gynecol, 123: 671–674.

Friedman L, Lewis PJ, Clifton P, Bulpitt CJ (1978). Factors influencing the incidence of neonatal jaundice. Br Med J, 1: 1235–1237.

Ghosh A, Hudson FP (1972). Oxytocin and neonatal hyperbilirubinaemia (letter). Lancet, 2: 823.

Gibb DMF, Arulkumaran S, Ratnam SS (1985). A comparative study of methods of oxytocin administration for induction of labour. Br J Obstet Gynaecol, 92: 688–692.

Goodlin RC, Lowe EW, Douglas R (1974). Instruments and methods: clinical trial with alarm system labor monitors. Obstet Gynecol, 44: 281–285.

Gordon-Wright AP, Elder MG (1979). Prostaglandin E_2 tablets used intravaginally for the induction of labour. Br J Obstet Gynaecol, 86: 32–36.

Gould SR, Mountrose U, Brown DJ, Whitehouse WL, Barnardo DE (1974). Influence of previous oral contraception and maternal oxytocin infusion on neonatal jaundice. Br Med J, 3: 228–230.

Gray HG, Mitchell R (1974). Neonatal hyperbilirubinaemia and oxytocin. Lancet, 2: 1144.

Haeri AD, Scher J, Davey DA, Leader M (1976). Comparison of oral prostaglandin E_2 and intravenous oxytocin for induction of labor. S Afr Med J, 50: 516–518.

Hatch MC (1969). Maternal deaths associated with induction of labor. NY State J Med, 69: 599–602.

Hellferich M, Favier J (1972). Inleiding van de baring met behulp van een oxytocine-druppelinfusie. Ned Tijdschr Geneeskd, 116: 221–226.

Hendricks CH, Brenner WE (1964). Patterns of increasing uterine activity in late pregnancy and the development of uterine responsiveness to oxytocin. Am J Obstet Gynecol, 90: 485–492.

Hofer U (1974). Ist die Künstliche Blasensprengung gefärlich?. Z Geburtsh Perinatol, 178: 273–278.

Hunter IWE, Hammad MK (1982). Induction of labour using prostaglandin pessaries of varying strength. Ulster Med J, 51: 141–145.

Hunter IWE, Cato E, Ritchie JWK (1984). Induction of labor using high-dose or low-dose prostaglandin vaginal pessaries. Obstet Gynecol, 63: 418–420.

Husslein H, Baumgarten K (1962). Die tiefe Blasensprengung zur Geburtseinleitung. Geburtshilfe Frauenheilkd, 22: 1202–1205.

Iskander MN (1978). A comparison of the efficacy and safety of extra-amniotic prostaglandin E_2 and intravenous prostaglandin E_2 for the induction of labour in patients with unripe cervices. J Int Med Res, 6: 144–146.

Jeffares MJ (1977). A multifactorial survey of neonatal jaundice. Br J Obstet Gynaecol, 84: 452–455.

Jung H, Lamberti G, Austermann R, Closs HP (1974). Die Programmierte Geburt. Z Geburtsh Perinatol, 178: 265–272.

Karim SMM, Devlin, J (1967). Prostaglandin content of

amniotic fluid during pregnancy and labour. J Obstet Gynaecol Br Commnwlth, 74: 230–234.

Karim SMM, Sharma SD (1971). Oral administration of prostaglandins for the induction of labour. Br Med J, 1: 260–262.

Karim SMM, Trussell, RR, Patel, RC, Hillier, K (1968). Response of pregnant human uterus to prostaglandin F_{2a}-induction of labour. Br Med J, 4: 621–623.

Keettel WC, Randall JH, Donnelly MM (1958). The hazards of elective induction of labor. Am J Obstet Gynecol 75: 496–510.

Keirse MJNC (1979). Endogenous prostaglandins in human parturition. In: Human Parturition. Keirse MJNC, Anderson ABM, Bennebroek Gravenhorst J (eds). The Hague: Leiden University Press, pp 101–142.

Keirse MJNC (1988). Amniotomy or oxytocin for induction of labor: re-analysis of a randomized controlled trial. Acta Obstet Gynecol Scand, 67: 731–735.

Keirse MJNC, Bennebroek Gravenhorst J (1979). Het inleiden van de baring bij intra-uteriene vruchtdood. Ned Tijdschr Geneeskd, 123: 1195–1199.

Keirse MJNC, Thiery M, Parewijck W, Mitchell MD (1983). Chronic stimulation of uterine prostaglandin synthesis during cervical ripening before the onset of labor. Prostaglandins, 25: 671–682.

Keirse MJNC, Noort W, Erwich JJHM (1987a) The role of prostaglandins and prostaglandin synthesis in the pregnant uterus. In: Priming and Induction of Labour by Prostaglandins. Keirse MJNC, de Koning Gans HJ (eds). Leiden: Boerhaave Committee for Postacademic Medical Education, pp 1–25.

Keirse MJNC, Schulpen MAGT, Corbeij RSACM, Oosterbaan HP (1987b). The Dutch experience in cervical ripening with prostaglandin gel. In: Priming and Induction of Labour by Prostaglandins. Keirse MJNC, de Koning Gans HJ (eds). Leiden: Boerhaave Committee for Postacademic Medical Education, pp 53–77.

Le Maire WJ, Spellacy WN, Shevach AB, Gall SA (1972). Changes in plasma estriol and progesterone during labor induced with prostaglandin F_{2a} or oxytocin. Prostaglandins, 2: 93–101.

Leiberman JR, Piura B, Chaim W, Cohen A (1977). The cervical balloon method for induction of labor. Acta Obstet Gynecol Scand, 56: 499–503.

Liggins GC (1979). Controlled trial of induction of labor by vaginal suppositories containing prostaglandin E_2. Prostaglandins, 18: 167–172.

Lilienthal CM, Ward JP (1971). Medical induction of labour. J Obstet Gynaecol Br Commnwlth, 78: 317–321.

Lykkesfeldt G, Osler M (1979). A comparison of three methods for inducing labor: oral prostaglandin E_2, buccal desaminooxytocin, intravenous oxytocin. Acta Obstet Gynecol Scand, 58: 321–325.

Lykkesfeldt G, Osler M (1981). Induction of labor with oral prostaglandin E_2 and buccal demoxytocin without amniotomy. Acta Obstet Gynecol Scand, 60: 429–430.

MacDonald D (1970). Surgical induction of labor. Am J Obstet Gynecol, 107: 908–911.

MacKenzie IZ, Bradley S, Embrey MP (1981). A simpler approach to labor induction using lipid-based prostaglandin E_2 vaginal suppository. Am J Obstet Gynecol, 141: 158–162.

MacLennan AH, Green RC (1980). A double blind dose trial of intravaginal prostaglandin F_{2a} for cervical ripening and induction of labour. Austral NZ J Obstet Gynaecol, 20: 80–83.

Macer J, Buchanan D, Yonekura ML (1984). Induction of labor with prostaglandin E_2 vaginal suppositories. Obstet Gynecol, 63: 664–668.

Manabe Y, Manabe A, Sagawa N (1982). Stretch-induced cervical softening and initiation of labor at term. A possible correlation with prostaglandins. Acta Obstet Gynecol Scand, 61: 279–280.

Mast H, Quakernack K, Lenfers M, Hagen C (1971). Der Einflusz des Geburtsverlaufes auf den Ikterus neonatorum. Geburtshilfe Frauenheilkd, 31: 443–453.

Mitchell MD, Flint APF, Bibby J, Brunt J, Anderson ABM, Turnbull AC (1977). Rapid increases in plasma prostaglandin concentrations after vaginal examination and amniotomy. Br Med J, 2: 1183–1185.

Muldoon MJ (1968). A prospective study of intrauterine infection following surgical induction of labour. J Obstet Gynaecol Br Commnwlth, 75: 1144–1150.

Naismith WCMK, Barr W, MacVicar J (1973). Comparison of intravenous prostaglandins F_2alpha and E_2 with intravenous oxytocin in the induction of labour. J Obstet Gynaecol Br Commnwlth, 80: 531–535.

Neves dos Santos LM, Odendaal HJ, Crawford JW, Henry MJ (1976). Investigation of some problems associated with the Cardiff infusion pump. Br J Obstet Gynaecol, 83: 225–228.

Niswander KR, Patterson RJ (1963). Hazards of elective induction of labor. Obstet Gynecol, 22: 228–233.

O'Driscoll D (1972). Oxytocic agents and neonatal hyperbilirubinaemia. Lancet, 2: 1150.

Page EW (1943). Response of human pregnant uterus to Pitocin tannate in oil. Proc Soc Exp Biol Med, 52: 195–197.

Parker RB (1957). The results of surgical induction of labour. J Obstet Gynaecol Br Commnwlth, 64: 94–112.

Parsons RJ (1980). Oxytocin infusion control in labour with the MP40 automatic pump. In Fetal and Neonatal Physiological Measurements. Rolfe P (ed). Bath: Pitman Medical, pp 158–176.

Patterson WM (1971). Amniotomy, with or without simultaneous oxytocin infusion. J Obstet Gynaecol Br Commnwlth, 78: 310–316.

Pavlou C, Barker GH, Roberts A, Chamberlain GVP (1978). Pulsed oxytocin infusion in the induction of labour. Br J Obstet Gynaecol, 85: 96–100.

Pinkerton JHM, Carson M (1968). Caesarean section after surgical induction of labour. J Obstet Gynaecol Br Commnwlth, 75: 1287–1290.

Quakernack K, Mast H (1971). Der Einflusz der Wehenmittel auf den Ikterus neonatorum. Arch Gynäkol, 31: 144–146.

Quinlivan WLG (1968). Instrument and method. Obstet Gynecol, 31: 734–735.

Rangarajan NS, La Croix GE, Moghissi KS (1971). Induction of labor with prostaglandin. Obstet Gynecol, 38: 546–550.

Ratnam SS, Khew KS, Chen C, Lim TC (1974). Oral prostaglandin E₂ in induction of labour. Austral NZ J Obstet Gynaecol, 14: 26–30.

Read MD, Martin RH (1974). A comparison between intravenous oxytocin and oral prostaglandin E₂ for the induction of labour in parous patients. Curr Med Res Opin, 2: 236–239.

Russell JK, Smith DF, Yule R (1956). Foetal exsanguination associated with surgical induction of labour. Br Med J, 2: 1414–1415.

Saleh YZ (1975). Surgical induction of labour with and without oxytocin infusion. A prospective study. Austral NZ J Obstet Gynaecol, 15: 80–83.

Saling E (1966). Das Kind im Bereich der Geburtshilfe. Stuttgart: Georg Thieme.

Scher J, Davey DA, Baillie P, Friend J, Friend DM (1972). A comparison of prostaglandin F₂ₐ and oxytocin in the induction of labour. S Afr Med J, 46: 2009–2012.

Schwarcz R, Althabe O, Caldeyro-Barcia R, Belitsky R, Lanchares JL, Alvarez R, Berdaguer P, Capurro H, Belizan JM, Sabatino JH, Abusleme C (1973). Fetal heart rate patterns in labors with intact and with ruptured membranes. J Perinat Med, 1: 153–165.

Schwarcz R, Belizan JM, Cifuentes JR, Cuadro JC, Marques MB, Caldeyro-Barcia R (1974). Fetal and maternal monitoring in spontaneous labors and in elective inductions. Am J Obstet Gynecol, 120: 356–362.

Schwarcz R, Belizan JM, Nieto F, Tenzer SM (1975). La rotura precoz de las membranas ovulares y sus efectos sobre el parto y el neonato. Oficina Sanitaria Panamericana, 595: 1–80.

Schwartz RH, Jones RWA (1978). Transplacental hyponatraemia due to oxytocin. Br Med J, 1: 152–153.

Secher NJ, Lange AP, Hassing Nielsen F, Thomson Pedersen G, Westergaard JG (1981). Induction of labor with and without primary amniotomy. A randomized study of prostaglandin E₂ tablets and intravenous oxytocin. Acta Obstet Gynecol Scand, 60: 237–241.

Setna F, Chatterjee TK, Black MD (1967). An assessment of the safety of surgical induction of labour. J Obstet Gynaecol Br Commnwlth, 74: 262–265.

Shubeck F, Benson RC, Clark WW, Berendes H, Weiss W, Deutschberger J (1966). Fetal hazard after rupture of the membranes. Obstet Gynecol, 28: 22–31.

Sims DG, Neligan GA (1975). Factors affecting the increasing incidence of severe non-haemolytic neonatal jaundice. Br J Obstet Gynaecol, 82: 863–867.

Sivasuriya M, Tan KL, Salmon YM, Karim SMM (1978). Neonatal serum bilirubin levels in spontaneous and induced labour. Br J Obstet Gynaecol, 85: 619–623.

Sjöstedt S (1969). Induction of labour. A comparison of intranasal and transbuccal administration of oxytocin. Acta Obstet Gynecol Scand, 48: 1–17.

Smythe HJD (1931). Indications for the induction of premature labour. Br Med J, 1: 1018–1020.

Steer PJ, Little DJ, Lewis NL, Kelly MCME, Beard RW (1976). The effect of membrane rupture on fetal heart rate in induced labour. Br J Obstet Gynaecol, 83: 454–459.

Steer PJ, Carter MC, Choong K, Hanson M, Gordon AJ, Pradhan P (1985). A multicentre prospective randomized controlled trial of induction of labour with an automatic closed-loop feedback controlled oxytocin infusion system. Br J Obstet Gynaecol, 92: 1127–1133.

Swann RO (1958). Induction of labour by stripping membranes. Obstet Gynecol, 11: 74–78.

Theobald GW, Graham A, Campbell J, Gange PD, Driscoll WJ (1948). The use of post-pituitary extract in physiological amounts in obstetrics. A preliminary report. Br Med J, 2: 123–128.

Thiery M, Amy JJ (1975). Induction of labour with prostaglandins. In: Prostaglandins and Reproduction. Karim SMM (ed). Lancaster: MTP Press, pp 149–228.

Thiery M, de Hemptinne D, Schuddinck L, Martens G (1975). Neonatal jaundice after induction of labour. Lancet, 1: 161.

Thiery M, Benijts G, Martens G, Yo Le Sian A, Amy JJ, Derom R (1977). A comparison of buccal (oromucosal) and oral prostaglandin E₂ for the elective induction of labor. Prostaglandins, 14: 371–379.

Thiery M, Parewijck W, Martens G, Derom R, Van Kets H (1981). Extra-amniotic prostaglandin E₂ gel versus amniotomy for elective induction of labour. Z Geburtsh Perinatol, 185: 323–326.

Thomas G, Blackwell RJ (1974). A controlled trial of the Cardiff automatic infusion system in the management of induced labour. Br J Clin Pract, 28: 203–206.

Turnbull AC, Anderson ABM (1967). Induction of labour. Part I. Amniotomy. J Obstet Gynaecol Br Commnwlth, 74: 849–854.

Turnbull AC, Anderson ABM (1968a). Induction of labour. Part II. Intravenous oxytocin infusion. J Obstet Gynaecol Br Commnwlth, 75: 24–31.

Turnbull AC, Anderson ABM (1968b). Induction of labour. III. Results with amniotomy and oxytocin 'titration'. J Obstet Gynaecol Br Commnwlth, 75: 32–41.

Ulmsten U, Wingerup L, Andersson KE (1979). Comparison of prostaglandin E₂ and intravenous oxytocin for induction of labor. Obstet Gynecol, 54: 581–584.

Ulmsten U, Wingerup L, Belfrage P, Ekman G, Wiqvist N (1982). Intracervical application of prostaglandin gel for induction of term labor. Obstet Gynecol, 59: 336–339.

Vakhariya VR, Sherman AI (1972). Prostaglandin F₂ₐ for induction of labor. Am J Obstet Gynecol, 113: 212–222.

Van Voorhis LW, Dunn LJ, Heggen O (1966). Effect of sparteine sulfate on amniotomy induction. A double blind evaluation. Am J Obstet Gynecol, 94: 230–233.

Vroman S, Thiery M, Yo Le Sian A, Depiere M, Vanderheyden C, Derom R, Van Kets H, Brouckaert J (1972). A double blind comparative study of prostaglandin F₂ₐ and oxytocin for the elective induction of labor. Eur J Obstet Gynecol Reprod Biol, 4: 115–123.

Wallenburg HCS, Keirse MJNC, Freie HMP, Blacquière JF (1980). Intramuscular administration of 15(S)-15-methyl prostaglandin F₂ₐ for induction of labour in patients with fetal death. Br J Obstet Gynaecol, 87: 203–209.

Westergaard JG, Lange AP, Pedersen GT, Secher NJ (1983). Oral oxytocics for induction of labor. Acta Obstet Gynecol Scand, 62: 103–110.

Wildemeersch DA, Schellen AMCM (1976). Double-blind trial of prostaglandin $F_{2\alpha}$ and oxytocin in the induction of labour. Curr Med Res Opin, 4: 263–266.

Wingerup L, Andersson KE, Ulmsten U (1978). Ripening of the uterine cervix and induction of labour at term with prostaglandin E_2 in viscous gel. Acta Obstet Gynecol Scand, 57: 403–406.

Yeung KK, Pang JCK (1977). Oral prostaglandins E_2 and $F_{2\alpha}$ in the induction of labour. Austral NZ J Obstet Gynaecol, 17: 32–35.

63 Comparison of prostaglandins and oxytocin for inducing labour

Marc J. N. C. Keirse and A. Carla C. van Oppen

1 Introduction

Oxytocin administration, combined with amniotomy, remains the most widely used approach to the induction of labour. During recent years, however, prostaglandins have become more widely used for induction, particularly when the cervix is 'unripe'. Ways of achieving cervical ripening have already been considered in Chapter 61. In Chapter 62, the available methods for achieving induction of labour more formally were reviewed. In this chapter we review evidence derived from controlled trials in which direct comparisons have been made between prostaglandins and oxytocin for the induction of labour.

Perhaps the most important single question that can be posed about the relative merits of prostaglandins and oxytocin for the induction of labour is the question that can be formulated most simply, namely, 'Are prostaglandins, on balance, superior to oxytocin for the induction of labour?' We begin this chapter by addressing this important question, in an attempt to obtain a broadly generalizable answer. In subsequent analyses, we shall attempt to ask more specific questions, and thus refine and qualify the general conclusion resulting from our initial analysis.

A large number of controlled comparisons of prostaglandins with oxytocin for induction of labour have been reported. As shown in Table 63.1, both prostaglandin E_2 and prostaglandin $F_{2\alpha}$ have been used in these studies; they have been administered by intravenous, oral, vaginal, and endocervical routes; the com-

parisons have been not only with intravenous oxytocin, but also with intranasal drops and with buccally administered desamino-oxytocin; the total drug doses and their rates of administration have varied; in some of the trials artificial rupture of the membranes was performed routinely at the onset of the induction, in others it was not performed at all, or only after uterine contractions had become firmly established; and the exclusion criteria, indications for induction, parity of the participating women, and degree of cervical ripeness at entry all varied among trials. Indeed, these trials are, on the face of it, probably more heterogeneous than any other body of research reviewed in this book.

It could be argued that there is no useful purpose in conducting an analysis based on all these diverse data considered together. There are, however, several important counter-arguments to this point of view (see also Chapter 2). First, if the simple but important question posed above is to be addressed, an analysis based on all the controlled comparisons of prostaglandins and oxytocin for the induction of labour is the most appropriate analysis for producing a widely generalizable answer. The wide variety of populations studied is unlikely to be any more diverse than the individual women requiring induction of labour in clinical practice. Similarly, differences in the prostaglandin preparations used within this body of research are unlikely to be more marked than the existing choice among different formulations of prostaglandins, which is limited in most countries by the availability of alternative preparations. Seen in this light, the lack of

Table 63.1 Nature of the treatments used in controlled comparisons between prostaglandins and oxytocin for induction of labour conducted by investigators in various countries

Comparisons with amniotomy in both treatment arms

Intravenous prostaglandin E$_2$ vs. intravenous oxytocin
Calder and Embrey (1975)	England

Oral prostaglandin E$_2$ vs. intravenous oxytocin
Ratnam *et al.* (1974)	Singapore
Read and Martin (1974)	England
Beard *et al.* (1975)	England
Miller *et al.* (1975)	England
Haeri *et al.* (1976)	South Africa
Kennedy *et al.* (1978)	Scotland
Sivasuriya *et al.* (1978)	Singapore
Bremme and Bygdeman (1980a)	Sweden
Bremme and Bygdeman (1980b)*	Sweden
Bremme and Eneroth (1980)*	Sweden
Secher *et al.* (1981)	Denmark
Bremme *et al.* (1984)	Sweden

Oral prostaglandin E$_2$ vs. buccal oxytocin
Mathews *et al.* (1976)	England
Westergaard *et al.* (1983)	Denmark

Vaginal prostaglandin PGF$_{2\alpha}$ vs. intravenous oxytocin
MacLennan and Green (1980)	Australia

Comparisons without amniotomy in either treatment arm

Intravenous prostaglandin E$_2$ vs. intravenous oxytocin
Beazley and Gillespie (1971)	England
Naismith *et al.* (1973)	Scotland
Gowenlock *et al.* (1975)	England

Intravenous prostaglandin F$_{2\alpha}$ vs. intravenous oxytocin
Rangarajan *et al.* (1971)	United States
Anderson *et al.* (1972)	United States
Le Maire *et al.* (1972)	United States
Scher *et al.* (1972)	South Africa
Vakhariya and Sherman (1972)	United States
Vroman *et al.* (1972)	Belgium
Blackburn *et al.* (1973)†	United States
Naismith *et al.* (1973)	Scotland
Spellacy *et al.* (1973)	United States
Gowenlock *et al.* (1975)	England
Wildemeersch and Schellen (1976)	Netherlands
Baxi *et al.* (1980)	United States

Oral prostaglandin E$_2$ vs. intravenous oxytocin
Ratnam *et al.* (1974)	Singapore
Secher *et al.* (1981)	Denmark
Somell and Larsson (1983)	Sweden

Oral prostaglandin E$_2$ vs. buccal oxytocin
Lykkesfeldt and Osler (1979)	Denmark
Ulstein *et al.* (1979)	Norway
Lykkesfeldt and Osler (1981)	Denmark
Westergaard *et al.* (1983)	Denmark

Endocervical prostaglandin E$_2$ vs. intravenous oxytocin
Ulmsten *et al.* (1979)	Sweden

Vaginal prostaglandin E$_2$ vs. nasal oxytocin
Andreasson *et al.* (1985)	Denmark

Vaginal prostaglandin E$_2$ vs. intravenous oxytocin
Macer *et al.* (1984)	United States
Ekman *et al.* (1986)	Sweden

* Subpopulation of Bremme and Bygdeman (1980a).
† Subpopulation of Anderson *et al.* (1972).

uniformity among these studies is actually a strength, and increases the likelihood that any patterns that emerge in the analyses will have at least some bearing on the reality of daily clinical practice.

The second reason for conducting and presenting an analysis based on all controlled comparisons of prostaglandins with oxytocin for induction of labour is that it is unrealistic to expect large differential effects of these two classes of oxytocic agents. Sample sizes that are much larger than those offered by the individual trials available for analysis (or by more specific subgroupings of trials) are required if there is to be any hope of detecting important differential effects on the (relatively rare) adverse outcomes that really matter (see Chapter 60).

Lastly, even if the estimates of differential effects generated by the analyses presented below are not acceptable to some as a basis for guiding clinical practice, they can and should inform future research, both in terms of the hypotheses to be addressed, and in terms of the size of samples that will be required to test them.

2 Any type or route of prostaglandin vs. any route of oxytocin

2.1 Effects on time and mode of delivery

Although there is no doubt that both oxytocin and prostaglandins (whether it be prostaglandin E$_2$ or prostaglandin F$_{2\alpha}$) stimulate uterine contractility, the main purpose of administering them is not so much to cause uterine contractions or labour, but to effect delivery. For the sake of maternal comfort as well as for the provision of social support and continuity of care (see Chapter 49), delivery should occur within a reasonable period of time. Although this is well recognized by most of the investigators who have conducted controlled comparisons of prostaglandins and oxytocin (Table 63.1), the majority of them have reported average intervals between the start of induction and either full cervical dilatation, or delivery. These outcomes are difficult to interpret for a variety of reasons. They often relate only to those women in whom induction was considered to have been successful (however 'success' was defined); in some studies women undergoing caesarean section or in whom a first induction attempt failed have been included, but they have been excluded from others; for women who underwent more than one induction attempt, the interval calculations have sometimes included only the last induction attempt, but sometimes both, with or without the time interval between them being added.

Only a minority of investigators reported categorical data on the proportion of women who were not delivered within certain time intervals, and, unfortunately,

Table 63.2 Effect of any prostaglandin (by any route) vs. oxytocin (any route) for induction of labour on not delivered within 12 hours

Study	EXPT n	(%)	CTRL n	(%)	Odds ratio (95% CI)	Graph of odds ratios and confidence intervals
Baxi *et al.* (1980)	2/25	(8.00)	2/25	(8.00)	1.00 (0.13–7.56)	
Mathews *et al.* (1976)	18/50	(36.00)	9/50	(18.00)	2.47 (1.03–5.95)	
MacLennan and Green (1980)	3/30	(10.00)	6/30	(20.00)	0.46 (0.11–1.89)	
Ulmsten *et al.* (1979)	34/50	(68.00)	42/50	(84.00)	0.42 (0.17–1.05)	
Blackburn *et al.* (1973)	0/11	(0.00)	0/12	(0.00)	1.00 (1.00–1.00)	
Naismith *et al.* (1973)	14/20	(70.00)	8/20	(40.00)	3.26 (0.95–11.16)	
Haeri *et al.* (1976)	3/50	(6.00)	5/50	(10.00)	0.58 (0.14–2.46)	
Scher *et al.* (1972)	6/20	(30.00)	10/23	(43.48)	0.57 (0.17–1.94)	
Typical odds ratio (95% confidence interval)					0.98 (0.63–1.52)	

Effect of any prostaglandin (by any route) vs. oxytocin (any route) for induction of labour on not delivered within 24 hours

Study	EXPT n	(%)	CTRL n	(%)	Odds ratio (95% CI)	
Vakhariya and Sherman (1972)	0/50	(0.00)	0/50	(0.00)	1.00 (1.00–1.00)	
Beazley and Gillespie (1971)	21/146	(14.38)	27/146	(18.49)	0.74 (0.40–1.38)	
Mathews *et al.* (1976)	9/50	(18.00)	3/50	(6.00)	3.08 (0.93–10.23)	
MacLennan and Green (1980)	0/30	(0.00)	0/30	(0.00)	1.00 (1.00–1.00)	
Ulmsten *et al.* (1979)	14/50	(28.00)	22/50	(44.00)	0.50 (0.22–1.13)	
Blackburn *et al.* (1973)	0/11	(0.00)	0/12	(0.00)	1.00 (1.00–1.00)	
Naismith *et al.* (1973)	1/20	(5.00)	0/20	(0.00)	7.39 (0.15–99.99)	
Ratnam *et al.* (1974)	14/107	(13.08)	7/100	(7.00)	1.94 (0.79–4.78)	
Kennedy *et al.* (1978)	0/30	(0.00)	0/30	(0.00)	1.00 (1.00–1.00)	
Haeri *et al.* (1976)	0/50	(0.00)	0/50	(0.00)	1.00 (1.00–1.00)	
Lykkesfeldt and Osler (1981)	32/40	(80.00)	38/45	(84.44)	0.74 (0.24–2.24)	
Scher *et al.* (1972)	0/20	(0.00)	0/23	(0.00)	1.00 (1.00–1.00)	
Secher *et al.* (1981)	51/179	(28.49)	47/165	(28.48)	1.00 (0.63–1.60)	
Lykkesfeldt and Osler (1979)	55/77	(71.43)	66/87	(75.86)	0.80 (0.40–1.60)	
Westergaard *et al.* (1983)	48/133	(36.09)	69/131	(52.67)	0.51 (0.32–0.83)	
Ekman *et al.* (1986)	2/19	(10.53)	11/19	(57.89)	0.13 (0.03–0.48)	
Typical odds ratio (95% confidence interval)					0.77 (0.61–0.97)	

Table 63.2—*continued* Effect of any prostaglandin (by any route) vs. oxytocin (any route) for induction of labour on not delivered within 48 hours

Study	EXPT		CTRL		Odds ratio	Graph of odds ratios and confidence intervals
	n	(%)	n	(%)	(95% CI)	0.01 0.1 0.5 1 2 10 100
Andreasson *et al.* (1985)	18/100	(18.00)	30/100	(30.00)	0.52 (0.27–0.99)	
Vakhariya and Sherman (1972)	0/50	(0.00)	0/50	(0.00)	1.00 (1.00–1.00)	
MacLennan and Green (1980)	0/30	(0.00)	0/30	(0.00)	1.00 (1.00–1.00)	
Ulmsten *et al.* (1979)	8/50	(16.00)	22/50	(44.00)	0.27 (0.11–0.63)	
Bremme and Bygdeman (1980a)	0/104	(0.00)	0/96	(0.00)	1.00 (1.00–1.00)	
Blackburn *et al.* (1973)	0/20	(0.00)	0/20	(0.00)	1.00 (1.00–1.00)	
Naismith *et al.* (1973)	0/20	(0.00)	0/20	(0.00)	1.00 (1.00–1.00)	
Ratnam *et al.* (1974)	0/107	(0.00)	0/100	(0.00)	1.00 (1.00–1.00)	
Kennedy *et al.* (1978)	0/30	(0.00)	0/30	(0.00)	1.00 (1.00–1.00)	
Lykkesfeldt and Osler (1981)	22/40	(55.00)	28/45	(62.22)	0.74 (0.32–1.76)	
Scher *et al.* (1972)	0/20	(0.00)	0/23	(0.00)	1.00 (1.00–1.00)	
Secher *et al.* (1981)	21/179	(11.73)	19/165	(11.52)	1.02 (0.53–1.97)	
Haeri *et al.* (1976)	0/50	(0.00)	0/50	(0.00)	1.00 (1.00–1.00)	
Westergaard *et al.* (1983)	24/181	(13.26)	48/206	(23.30)	0.52 (0.31–0.86)	
Lykkesfeldt and Osler (1979)	42/77	(54.55)	51/87	(58.62)	0.85 (0.46–1.57)	
Typical odds ratio (95% confidence interval)					0.62 (0.47–0.81)	

few were able to provide such information from their unpublished files (if these were still available). Others, whose reports included several study populations (for example, trial arms with and without concomitant amniotomy) were able to provide this information for some, but not for all of the trial arms. For these reasons, in the tables presented in this chapter, different denominators may be encountered for data originating from the same studies.

Data on the proportions of women who remained undelivered within 12 hours of the start of induction were available from 8 studies; these proportions were similar for women induced with prostaglandins to those induced with oxytocin (typical odds ratio 0.98; 95 per cent confidence interval 0.63–1.52; Table 63.2). Data on delivery within 24 hours were available from 16 studies; 6 of these found that fewer women remained undelivered 24 hours after the induction attempt when they had been induced with prostaglandins than when they had been induced with oxytocin. The effect across

the 16 trials was statistically significant (typical odds ratio 0.77; 95 per cent confidence interval 0.61–0.97; Table 63.2). The proportion of women who remained undelivered after 48 hours (for which data are available from 15 trials) showed an even larger difference in favour of prostaglandins (typical odds ratio 0.62; 95 per cent confidence interval 0.47–0.81; Table 63.2). However, only 6 of the 15 trials with data on this outcome involved women in whom the first induction attempt, and any intervention that followed it, had not resulted in delivery within 48 hours. All of these 6 trials were conducted in Scandinavian countries, and all but one, which was conducted in Sweden (Ulmsten *et al.* 1979; 1979), originated from Denmark (Lykkesfeldt and Osler 1979, 1981; Secher *et al.* 1981; Westergaard *et al.* 1983; Andreasson *et al.* 1985).

From the data shown in Table 63.2 it cannot necessarily be concluded that, overall, the immediate goal of labour induction (to effect delivery) is achieved more

Table 63.3 Effect of any prostaglandin (by any route) vs. oxytocin (any route) for induction of labour on no vaginal delivery within 12 hours

Study	EXPT		CTRL		Odds ratio	Graph of odds ratios and confidence intervals
	n	(%)	n	(%)	(95% CI)	0.01 0.1 0.5 1 2 10 100
Baxi et al. (1980)	2/25	(8.00)	2/25	(8.00)	1.00 (0.13–7.56)	
Spellacy et al. (1973)	36/115	(31.30)	36/107	(33.64)	0.90 (0.51–1.58)	
Vakhariya and Sherman (1972)	4/50	(8.00)	4/50	(8.00)	1.00 (0.24–4.21)	
MacLennan and Green (1980)	3/30	(10.00)	6/30	(20.00)	0.46 (0.11–1.89)	
Ulmsten et al. (1979)	34/50	(68.00)	42/50	(84.00)	0.42 (0.17–1.05)	
Blackburn et al. (1973)	0/11	(0.00)	0/12	(0.00)	1.00 (1.00–1.00)	
Naismith et al. (1973)	14/20	(70.00)	8/20	(40.00)	3.26 (0.95–11.16)	
Haeri et al. (1976)	3/50	(6.00)	5/50	(10.00)	0.58 (0.14–2.46)	
Scher et al. (1972)	6/20	(30.00)	10/23	(43.48)	0.57 (0.17–1.94)	
Typical odds ratio (95% confidence interval)					0.80 (0.56–1.16)	

Effect of any prostaglandin (by any route) vs. oxytocin (any route) for induction of labour on no vaginal delivery within 24 hours

Study	EXPT		CTRL		Odds ratio	Graph of odds ratios and confidence intervals
Andreasson et al. (1985)	29/100	(29.00)	58/100		0.31 (0.18–0.54)	
Vakhariya and Sherman (1972)	1/50	(2.00)	1/50	(2.00)	1.00 (0.06–16.22)	
MacLennan and Green (1980)	0/30	(0.00)	1/30	(0.00)	1.14 (0.00–6.82)	
Ulmsten et al. (1979)	15/50	(30.00)	22/50	(44.00)	0.55 (0.25–1.24)	
Blackburn et al. (1973)	0/11	(0.00)	0/12	(0.00)	1.00 (1.00–1.00)	
Naismith et al. (1973)	1/20	(5.00)	0/20	(5.00)	1.00 (0.06–16.58)	
Kennedy et al. (1978)	2/30	(6.67)	1/30	(3.33)	1.99 (0.20–19.94)	
Haeri et al. (1976)	2/50	(4.00)	8/50	(16.00)	0.27 (0.07–0.98)	
Scher et al. (1972)	0/20	(0.00)	0/23	(0.00)	1.00 (1.00–1.00)	
Secher et al. (1981)	1/57	(1.75)	2/46	(4.35)	0.40 (0.04–4.02)	
Westergaard et al. (1983)	55/133	(41.35)	72/131	(54.96)	0.58 (0.36 0.94)	
Ekman et al. (1986)	2/19	(10.53)	12/19	(63.16)	0.11 (0.03–0.41)	
Typical odds ratio (95% confidence interval)					0.43 (0.32–0.58)	

Table 63.3—*continued* Effect of any prostaglandin (by any route) vs. oxytocin (any route) for induction of labour on no vaginal delivery within 48 hours

Study	EXPT		CTRL		Odds ratio	Graph of odds ratios and confidence intervals						
	n	(%)	*n*	(%)	(95% CI)	0.01	0.1	0.5	1	2	10	100
Andreasson *et al.* (1985)	20/100	(20.00)	32/100	(32.00)	0.54 (0.29–1.01)							
Vakhariya and Sherman (1972)	1/50	(2.00)	1/50	(2.00)	1.00 (0.06–16.22)							
MacLennan and Green (1980)	0/30	(0.00)	1/30	(3.33)	0.14 (0.00–6.82)							
Ulmsten *et al.* (1979)	9/50	(18.00)	22/50	(44.00)	0.30 (0.13–0.70)							
Bremme and Bygdeman (1980a)	6/104	(5.77)	10/96	(10.42)	0.53 (0.19–1.48)							
Blackburn *et al.* (1973)	0/11	(0.00)	0/12	(0.00)	1.00 (1.00–1.00)							
Naismith *et al.* (1973)	0/20	(0.00)	1/20	(5.00)	0.14 (0.00–6.82)							
Ratnam *et al.* (1974)	12/107	(11.21)	5/100	(5.00)	2.27 (0.84–6.12)							
Kennedy *et al.* (1978)	2/30	(6.67)	1/30	(3.33)	1.99 (0.20–19.94)							
Haeri *et al.* (1976)	2/50	(4.00)	8/50	(16.00)	0.27 (0.07–0.98)							
Lykkesfeldt and Osler (1981)	25/40	(62.50)	32/45	(71.11)	0.68 (0.28–1.67)							
Scher *et al.* (1972)	0/20	(0.00)	0/23	(0.00)	1.00 (1.00–1.00)							
Secher *et al.* (1981)	1/57	(1.75)	2/46	(4.35)	0.40 (0.04–4.02)							
Westergaard *et al.* (1983)	33/133	(24.81)	52/131	(39.69)	0.51 (0.30–0.85)							
Typical odds ratio (95% confidence interval)					0.56 (0.42–0.74)							

readily when prostaglandins rather than oxytocin are used to stimulate uterine contractions. If prostaglandins were, for example, more likely to lead to complications that required caesarean section they could readily be shown to result in a larger proportion of women being delivered within a short interval of the start of the induction. Data from the trials which provided information on the number of women who did not have a *vaginal* delivery within these 12, 24, and 48 hours' intervals indicate that this is not the case, however. If anything, the differential effects of prostaglandins and oxytocin for induction of labour, although they are available for somewhat fewer trials, appear to be more striking (Table 63.3). Thus a statistically significantly higher proportion of women induced with prostaglandins delivered vaginally within 24 hours (typical odds ratio 0.43; 95 per cent confidence interval 0.32–0.58), and within 48 hours (typical odds ratio 0.56; 95 per cent confidence interval 0.42–0.74; Table 63.3).

Data on the incidence of caesarean section were available from 29 trials. Regrettably, in the published reports, these data were sometimes available only for women who delivered within a certain time period after the start of the induction. This applied in particular to trials (mostly originating from the Scandinavian countries) in which large proportions of women who had had an induction of labour apparently remained undelivered for a considerable length of time. On occasions, the published data could therefore not be interpreted reliably without further information from the principal investigators. If it was available, that information was carefully assessed and the combined published and unpublished data were used in the construction of tables on the mode of delivery. Sometimes the information was available for the incidence of caesarean section, but not for the number of instrumental vaginal deliveries. This explains the different denominators that may be encountered in the tables dealing with these outcomes. In other instances, even the extra information (kindly provided by the investigators) was unfortunately not sufficiently comprehensive for inclusion in the overviews. To take one example from a number of

Table 63.4 Effect of any prostaglandin (by any route) vs. oxytocin (any route) for induction of labour on caesarean section

Study	EXPT		CTRL		Odds ratio	Graph of odds ratios and confidence intervals
	n	(%)	n	(%)	(95% CI)	
Vroman et al. (1972)	0/25	(0.00)	0/25	(0.00)	1.00 (1.00–1.00)	
Vakhariya and Sherman (1972)	1/50	(2.00)	1/50	(2.00)	1.00 (0.06–16.22)	
Calder and Embrey (1975)	5/50	(10.00)	7/50	(14.00)	0.69 (0.21–2.28)	
Baxi et al. (1980)	1/25	(4.00)	1/25	(4.00)	1.00 (0.06–16.45)	
Spellacy et al. (1973)	9/115	(7.83)	0/107	(0.00)	7.41 (1.96–28.07)	
Andreasson et al. (1985)	9/100	(9.00)	13/100	(13.00)	0.67 (0.28–1.61)	
Lange et al. (1984)	16/99	(16.16)	19/103	(18.45)	0.85 (0.41–1.77)	
Mathews et al. (1976)	1/50	(2.00)	0/50	(0.00)	7.39 (0.15–99.99)	
MacLennan and Green (1980)	0/30	(0.00)	1/30	(3.33)	0.14 (0.00–6.82)	
Bremme et al. (1984)	4/44	(9.09)	3/39	(7.69)	1.20 (0.26–5.59)	
Bremme and Bygdeman (1980a)	6/104	(5.77)	10/96	(10.42)	0.53 (0.19–1.48)	
Anderson et al. (1972)	0/46	(0.00)	1/27	(3.70)	0.07 (0.00–3.88)	
Ratnam et al. (1974)	12/107	(11.21)	5/100	(5.00)	2.27 (0.84–6.12)	
Kennedy et al. (1978)	2/30	(6.67)	1/30	(3.33)	1.99 (0.20–19.94)	
Haeri et al. (1976)	2/50	(4.00)	8/50	(16.00)	0.27 (0.07–0.98)	
Beard et al. (1975)	0/22	(0.00)	0/20	(0.00)	1.00 (1.00–1.00)	
Scher et al. (1972)	0/20	(0.00)	0/23	(0.00)	1.00 (1.00–1.00)	
Somell and Larsson (1983)	1/52	(1.92)	2/30	(6.67)	0.26 (0.02–2.86)	
Lykkesfeldt and Osler (1981)	3/18	(16.67)	4/17	(23.53)	0.66 (0.13–3.38)	
Secher et al. (1981)	11/161	(6.83)	6/146	(4.11)	1.68 (0.63–4.47)	
Read and Martin (1974)	1/99	(1.01)	0/88	(0.00)	6.61 (0.13–99.99)	
Naismith et al. (1973)	0/20	(0.00)	1/20	(5.00)	0.14 (0.00–6.82)	
Ulstein et al. (1979)	5/134	(3.73)	10/129	(7.75)	0.47 (0.17–1.34)	
Gowenlock et al. (1975)	0/50	(0.00)	1/25	(4.00)	0.05 (0.00–3.18)	
Lykkesfeldt and Osler (1979)	12/77	(15.58)	9/87	(10.34)	1.59 (0.64–3.98)	
Miller et al. (1975)	6/100	(6.00)	2/51	(3.92)	1.51 (0.34–6.77)	
Westergaard et al. (1983)	14/133	(10.53)	17/131	(12.98)	0.79 (0.37–1.67)	
Ekman et al. (1986)	0/19	(0.00)	1/19	(5.26)	0.14 (0.00–6.82)	
Macer et al. (1984)	2/45	(4.44)	2/40	(5.00)	0.88 (0.12–6.53)	
Typical odds ratio (95% confidence interval)					0.93 (0.72–1.21)	

Graph scale: 0.01 0.1 0.5 1 2 10 100

Table 63.4—*continued* Effect of any prostaglandin (by any route) vs. oxytocin (any route) for induction of labour on instrumental vaginal delivery

Study	EXPT		CTRL		Odds ratio	Graph of odds ratios and confidence intervals
	n	(%)	n	(%)	(95% CI)	0.01 0.1 0.5 1 2 10 100
Calder and Embrey (1975)	34/50	(68.00)	33/50	(66.00)	1.09 (0.48–2.51)	
Andreasson *et al.* (1985)	9/100	(9.00)	10/100	(10.00)	0.89 (0.35–2.29)	
Mathews *et al.* (1976)	2/50	(4.00)	1/50	(2.00)	1.97 (0.20–19.43)	
MacLennan and Green (1980)	8/30	(26.67)	12/30	(40.00)	0.55 (0.19–1.61)	
Bremme and Bygdeman (1980a)	29/104	(27.88)	23/96	(23.96)	1.23 (0.65–2.30)	
Blackburn *et al.* (1973)	4/11	(36.36)	8/12	(66.67)	0.31 (0.06–1.55)	
Read and Martin (1974)	3/99	(3.03)	8/88	(9.09)	0.34 (0.10–1.14)	
Somell and Larsson (1983)	8/52	(15.38)	7/30	(23.33)	0.59 (0.19–1.88)	
Naismith *et al.* (1973)	14/20	(70.00)	10/20	(50.00)	2.25 (0.65–7.86)	
Ulstein *et al.* (1979)	9/134	(6.72)	14/129	(10.85)	0.60 (0.25–1.40)	
Kennedy *et al.* (1978)	6/30	(20.00)	10/30	(33.33)	0.51 (0.16–1.59)	
Haeri *et al.* (1976)	0/50	(0.00)	3/50	(6.00)	0.13 (0.01–1.28)	
Beard *et al.* (1975)	5/22	(22.73)	6/20	(30.00)	0.69 (0.18–2.70)	
Lykkesfeldt and Osler (1981)	4/18	(22.22)	2/17	(11.76)	2.04 (0.36–11.57)	
Secher *et al.* (1981)	18/161	(11.18)	23/146	(15.75)	0.67 (0.35–1.30)	
Lykkesfeldt and Osler (1979)	8/77	(10.39)	15/87	(17.24)	0.57 (0.24–1.37)	
Macer *et al.* (1984)	3/45	(6.67)	3/40	(7.50)	0.88 (0.17–4.61)	
Typical odds ratio (95% confidence interval)					0.77 (0.60–0.99)	

Table 63.4—*continued* Effect of any prostaglandin (by any route) vs. oxytocin (any route) for induction of labour on operative delivery

Study	EXPT n	(%)	CTRL n	(%)	Odds ratio (95% CI)	Graph of odds ratios and confidence intervals
Calder and Embrey (1975)	39/50	(78.00)	40/50	(80.00)	0.89 (0.34–2.31)	
Andreasson et al. (1985)	18/100	(18.00)	23/100	(23.00)	0.74 (0.37–1.46)	
Mathews et al. (1976)	3/50	(6.00)	1/50	(2.00)	2.80 (0.38–20.52)	
MacLennan and Green (1980)	8/30	(26.67)	13/30	(43.33)	0.49 (0.17–1.39)	
Bremme and Bygdeman (1980a)	35/104	(33.65)	33/96	(34.38)	0.97 (0.54–1.74)	
Blackburn et al. (1973)	4/11	(36.36)	8/12	(66.67)	0.31 (0.06–1.55)	
Read and Martin (1974)	4/99	(4.04)	8/88	(9.09)	0.43 (0.13–1.39)	
Somell and Larsson (1983)	9/52	(17.31)	9/30	(30.00)	0.48 (0.16–1.42)	
Naismith et al. (1973)	14/20	(70.00)	11/20	(55.00)	1.87 (0.53–6.61)	
Ulstein et al. (1979)	14/134	(10.45)	24/129	(18.60)	0.52 (0.26–1.03)	
Kennedy et al. (1978)	8/30	(26.67)	11/30	(36.67)	0.63 (0.22–1.87)	
Haeri et al. (1976)	2/50	(4.00)	11/50	(22.00)	0.21 (0.06–0.66)	
Beard et al. (1975)	5/22	(22.73)	6/20	(30.00)	0.69 (0.18–2.70)	
Lykkesfeldt and Osler (1981)	7/18	(38.89)	6/17	(35.29)	1.16 (0.30–4.49)	
Secher et al. (1981)	29/161	(18.01)	29/146	(19.86)	0.89 (0.50–1.57)	
Lykkesfeldt and Osler (1979)	20/77	(25.97)	24/87	(27.59)	0.92 (0.46–1.84)	
Macer et al. (1984)	5/45	(11.11)	5/40	(12.50)	0.88 (0.24–3.26)	
Typical odds ratio (95% confidence interval)					0.74 (0.59–0.92)	

possible instances to illustrate the problem, Ulmsten and his colleagues (Ulmsten et al. 1979) reported a controlled comparison in which 50 women were induced with PGE_2 and 50 induced with oxytocin; one of the 70 women delivered within 48 hours underwent a caesarean section, but nothing was known, not even about the route of delivery, for 8 women induced with PGE_2 and 22 women induced with oxytocin who failed to deliver within 48 hours.

Data from all 29 trials on which information on the number of caesarean sections was thus available are considered together in Table 63.4. The data provided no evidence for a differential effect of prostaglandins and oxytocin, yielding a typical odds ratio of 0.93 with a 95 per cent confidence interval ranging from 0.72 to 1.21.

The incidence of instrumental vaginal delivery (on which information was available from 17 trials) showed that a smaller proportion of women induced with prostaglandins required delivery by forceps or vacuum extraction, than of women induced with oxytocin (typical odds ratio 0.77; 95 per cent confidence interval 0.60–0.99; Table 63.4). The overall incidence of operative delivery was thus statistically significantly reduced in women induced with prostaglandins compared with oxytocin (typical odds ratio 0.74; 95 per cent confidence interval 0.59–0.92; Table 63.4).

2.2 Effects on the mother

As discussed in Chapter 62, there are some major differences between the effects of these two classes of drugs on organ systems other than the uterus. The controlled comparisons thus showed that a larger proportion of women experienced gastrointestinal side-effects when prostaglandins rather than oxytocin were used for the induction of labour. Eighteen trials provided information on the incidence of vomiting. In none of the trials were there more women who vomited with oxytocin than with prostaglandin administration. The typical odds ratio was 2.51 with a 95 per cent confidence interval ranging from 1.55 to 4.05 (Table 63.5). A similar trend was observed for the incidence of diarrhoea (for which data were available from 13 trials). In none of the trials were there fewer women experienc-ing diarrhoea among those induced with prostaglandins than among those induced with oxytocin (Table 63.5). The overall incidence of gastrointestinal side-effects (available for 12 trials) thus yielded a typical odds ratio of 4.36 with a 95 per cent confidence interval from 2.62 to 7.23; Table 63.5).

The incidence of pyrexia during labour was reported for 8 trials. In 5 of these, each involving between 40 and 200 women, pyrexia was not observed; in one trial, pyrexia was observed in only one woman in each group (Macer *et al.* 1984); in the remaining two trials pyrexia was observed more frequently with prostaglandin than with oxytocin administration (Naismith *et al.* 1973;

Table 63.5 Effect of any prostaglandin (by any route) vs. oxytocin (any route) for induction of labour on vomiting

Study	EXPT		CTRL		Odds ratio	Graph of odds ratios and confidence intervals
	n	(%)	n	(%)	(95% CI)	
Vroman *et al.* (1972)	2/25	(8.00)	2/25	(8.00)	1.00 (0.13–7.56)	
Vakhariya and Sherman (1972)	1/50	(2.00)	0/50	(0.00)	7.39 (0.15–99.99)	
Calder and Embrey (1975)	5/50	(10.00)	3/50	(6.00)	1.71 (0.41–7.21)	
Andreasson *et al.* (1985)	0/100	(0.00)	0/100	(0.00)	1.00 (1.00–1.00)	
Hauth *et al.* (1977)	1/50	(2.00)	0/50	(0.00)	7.39 (0.15–99.99)	
Bremme and Bygdeman (1980a)	11/104	(10.58)	7/96	(7.29)	1.49 (0.57–3.92)	
Mathews *et al.* (1976)	4/50	(8.00)	3/50	(6.00)	1.36 (0.29–6.25)	
Ulmsten *et al.* (1979)	0/50	(0.00)	0/50	(0.00)	1.00 (1.00–1.00)	
MacLennan and Green (1980)	0/30	(0.00)	0/30	(0.00)	1.00 (1.00–1.00)	
Read and Martin (1974)	2/99	(2.02)	0/88	(0.00)	6.68 (0.41–99.99)	
Ratnam *et al.* (1974)	2/107	(1.87)	0/100	(0.00)	6.99 (0.43–99.99)	
Haeri *et al.* (1976)	5/50	(10.00)	1/50	(2.00)	4.07 (0.79–21.04)	
Beard *et al.* (1975)	1/22	(4.55)	0/20	(0.00)	6.75 (0.13–99.99)	
Ulstein *et al.* (1979)	4/134	(2.99)	1/129	(0.78)	3.26 (0.56–19.06)	
Lykkesfeldt and Osler (1981)	6/40	(15.00)	0/45	(0.00)	9.58 (1.83–50.03)	
Wildemeersch and Schellen (1976)	0/14	(0.00)	0/14	(0.00)	1.00 (1.00–1.00)	
Westergaard *et al.* (1983)	6/181	(3.31)	3/206	(1.46)	2.26 (0.60–8.49)	
Ekman *et al.* (1986)	1/19	(5.26)	0/19	(0.00)	7.39 (0.15–99.99)	
Typical odds ratio (95% confidence interval)					2.51 (1.55–4.05)	

Graph scale: 0.01　0.1　0.5　1　2　10　100

Table 63.5—*continued* Effect of any prostaglandin (by any route) vs. oxytocin (any route) for induction of labour on diarrhoea

Study	EXPT		CTRL		Odds ratio	Graph of odds ratios and confidence intervals
	n	(%)	n	(%)	(95% CI)	0.01 0.1 0.5 1 2 10 100
Vroman et al. (1972)	0/25	(0.00)	0/25	(0.00)	1.00 (1.00–1.00)	
Andreasson et al. (1985)	0/100	(0.00)	0/100	(0.00)	1.00 (1.00–1.00)	
Mathews et al. (1976)	2/50	(4.00)	0/50	(0.00)	7.54 (0.47–99.99)	
Ulmsten et al. (1979)	0/50	(0.00)	0/50	(0.00)	1.00 (1.00–1.00)	
MacLennan and Green (1980)	0/30	(0.00)	0/30	(0.00)	1.00 (1.00–1.00)	
Bremme and Bygdeman (1980a)	2/104	(1.92)	0/96	(0.00)	6.91 (0.43–99.99)	
Ulstein et al. (1979)	3/134	(2.24)	1/129	(0.78)	2.65 (0.37–19.01)	
Ratnam et al. (1974)	8/107	(7.48)	0/100	(0.00)	7.41 (1.81–30.37)	
Beard et al. (1975)	0/22	(0.00)	0/20	(0.00)	1.00 (1.00–1.00)	
Wildemeersch and Schellen (1976)	0/14	(0.00)	0/14	(0.00)	1.00 (1.00–1.00)	
Westergaard et al. (1983)	14/181	(7.73)	4/206	(1.94)	3.68 (1.43–9.49)	
Miller et al. (1975)	0/100	(0.00)	0/51	(0.00)	1.00 (1.00–1.00)	
Ekman et al. (1986)	0/19	(0.00)	0/19	(0.00)	1.00 (1.00–1.00)	
Typical odds ratio (95% confidence interval)					4.52 (2.28–8.97)	

Effect of any prostaglandin (by any route) vs. oxytocin (any route) for induction of labour on gastrointestinal side-effects

Study	EXPT		CTRL		Odds ratio	Graph of odds ratios and confidence intervals
Vroman et al. (1972)	2/25	(8.00)	2/25	(8.00)	1.00 (0.13–7.56)	
Andreasson et al. (1985)	0/100	(0.00)	0/100	(0.00)	1.00 (1.00–1.00)	
Ulmsten et al. (1979)	0/50	(0.00)	0/50	(0.00)	1.00 (1.00–1.00)	
MacLennan and Green (1980)	0/30	(0.00)	0/30	(0.00)	1.00 (1.00–1.00)	
Beard et al. (1975)	1/22	(4.55)	0/20	(0.00)	6.75 (0.13–99.99)	
Secher et al. (1981)	14/182	(7.69)	3/165	(1.82)	3.52 (1.33–9.32)	
Wildemeersch and Schellen (1976)	0/14	(0.00)	0/14	(0.00)	1.00 (1.00–1.00)	
Westergaard et al. (1983)	20/181	(11.05)	3/206	(1.46)	5.54 (2.38–12.87)	
Lykkesfeldt and Osler (1979)	6/77	(7.79)	0/87	(0.00)	9.00 (1.77–45.87)	
Lykkesfeldt and Osler (1979)	6/77	(7.79)	0/87	(0.00)	9.00 (1.77–45.87)	
Macer et al. (1984)	3/45	(6.67)	2/40	(5.00)	1.35 (0.22–8.14)	
Ekman et al. (1986)	1/19	(5.26)	0/19	(0.00)	7.39 (0.15–99.99)	
Typical odds ratio (95% confidence interval)					4.36 (2.62–7.23)	

Calder and Embrey 1975). Both these trials had used prostaglandin E_2 intravenously, and in one of them the difference compared to oxytocin reached statistical significance (Calder and Embrey 1975). Overall, the data indicate that pyrexia is more likely to occur with prostaglandins than with oxytocin (typical odds ratio 3.71; 95 per cent confidence interval 1.75–7.87; Table 63.6), although all of the differential effect derived from the controlled comparisons appears to be attributable to intravenous PGE_2 (Table 63.6).

Only 4 trials provided information on whether women received analgesia during labour (Beard *et al.* 1975; Calder and Embrey 1975; Bremme and Bygdeman 1980a; MacLennan and Green 1980), and in one of these all the women studied had had epidural analgesia (Calder and Embrey 1975). The use of analgesia was statistically significantly less common among women induced with prostaglandins than among those induced with oxytocin (typical odds ratio 0.28; 95 per cent

confidence interval 0.14–0.56; Table 63.6). These differential effects in respect of this particular outcome need to be interpreted with caution, however, because the investigators were not blinded to the oxytocic drug administered.

Twenty of the trials mentioned that 'uterine hypertonus' and/or 'uterine hyperstimulation' had been sought as an outcome. Although there was a wide variation in the ways in which investigators used these terms, the high proportion of investigators who mentioned them suggests that most considered them to be important. Of the 20 trials that provided data on 'uterine hypertonus' and/or 'uterine hyperstimulation', 13 (involving a total of 1700 women) reported that this complication was not observed. Of the 7 trials in which it was observed, 5 reported its incidence to be higher among women who had been induced with prostaglandins than among those who had been induced using oxytocin (Rangarajan *et al.* 1971; Vakhariya and Sherman 1972; Vroman

Table 63.6 Effect of any prostaglandin (by any route) vs. oxytocin (any route) for induction of labour on pyrexia during labour

Study	EXPT		CTRL		Odds ratio	Graph of odds ratios and confidence intervals
	n	(%)	*n*	(%)	(95% CI)	
Calder and Embrey (1975)	22/50	(44.00)	7/50	(14.00)	4.23 (1.79–9.99)	
Andreasson *et al.* (1985)	0/100	(0.00)	0/100	(0.00)	1.00 (1.00–1.00)	
Ulmsten *et al.* (1979)	0/50	(0.00)	0/50	(0.00)	1.00 (1.00–1.00)	
Mathews *et al.* (1976)	0/50	(0.00)	0/50	(0.00)	1.00 (1.00–1.00)	
MacLennan and Green (1980)	0/30	(0.00)	0/30	(0.00)	1.00 (1.00–1.00)	
Naismith *et al.* (1973)	4/20	(20.00)	1/20	(5.00)	3.81 (0.60–24.23)	
Macer *et al.* (1984)	1/45	(2.22)	1/40	(2.50)	0.89 (0.05–14.50)	
...kman *et al.* (1986)	0/19	(0.00)	0/19	(0.00)	1.00 (1.00–1.00)	
Typical odds ratio (95% confidence interval)					3.71 (1.75–7.87)	

Effect of any prostaglandin (by any route) vs. oxytocin (any route) for induction of labour on use of analgesia

Study	EXPT		CTRL		Odds ratio	Graph
Calder and Embrey (1975)	50/50	(100.0)	50/50	(100.0)	1.00 (1.00–1.00)	
MacLennan and Green (1980)	14/30	(46.67)	26/30	(86.67)	0.17 (0.06–0.49)	
Bremme and Eneroth (1980)	23/37	(62.16)	29/37	(78.38)	0.46 (0.17–1.25)	
Beard *et al.* (1975)	20/22	(90.91)	20/20	(100.0)	0.14 (0.01–2.35)	
Typical odds ratio (95% confidence interval)					0.28 (0.14–0.56)	

Table 63.6—*continued* Effect of any prostaglandin (by any route) vs. oxytocin (any route) for induction of labour on hypertonus–hyperstimulation

Study	EXPT		CTRL		Odds ratio	Graph of odds ratios and confidence intervals
	n	(%)	n	(%)	(95% CI)	0.01 0.1 0.5 1 2 10 100
Calder and Embrey (1975)	27/50	(54.00)	9/50	(18.00)	4.70 (2.08–10.59)	
Baxi *et al.* (1980)	0/25	(0.00)	0/25	(0.00)	1.00 (1.00–1.00)	
Andreasson *et al.* (1985)	0/100	(0.00)	0/100	(0.00)	1.00 (1.00–1.00)	
Vroman *et al.* (1972)	2/25	(8.00)	0/25	(0.00)	7.70 (0.47–99.99)	
Vakhariya and Sherman (1972)	8/50	(16.00)	1/50	(2.00)	5.43 (1.39–21.23)	
Mathews *et al.* (1976)	0/50	(0.00)	0/50	(0.00)	1.00 (1.00–1.00)	
MacLennan and Green (1980)	0/30	(0.00)	0/30	(0.00)	1.00 (1.00–1.00)	
Ulmsten *et al.* (1979)	0/50	(0.00)	0/50	(0.00)	1.00 (1.00–1.00)	
Bremme and Bygdeman (1980a)	3/63	(4.76)	0/61	(0.00)	7.39 (0.75–72.45)	
Rangarajan *et al.* (1971)	8/20	(40.00)	1/20	(5.00)	7.08 (1.63–30.65)	
Ulstein *et al.* (1979)	0/140	(0.00)	0/140	(0.00)	1.00 (1.00–1.00)	
Ratnam *et al.* (1974)	0/107	(0.00)	0/100	(0.00)	1.00 (1.00–1.00)	
Kennedy *et al.* (1978)	0/30	(0.00)	0/30	(0.00)	1.00 (1.00–1.00)	
Haeri *et al.* (1976)	7/50	(14.00)	8/50	(16.00)	0.86 (0.29–2.55)	
Lykkesfeldt and Osler (1981)	0/40	(0.00)	0/45	(0.00)	1.00 (1.00–1.00)	
Scher *et al.* (1972)	0/20	(0.00)	0/23	(0.00)	1.00 (1.00–1.00)	
Wildemeersch and Schellen (1976)	0/14	(0.00)	0/14	(0.00)	1.00 (1.00–1.00)	
Westergaard *et al.* (1983)	0/181	(0.00)	0/206	(0.00)	1.00 (1.00–1.00)	
Lykkesfeldt and Osler (1979)	0/77	(0.00)	0/87	(0.00)	1.00 (1.00–1.00)	
Macer *et al.* (1984)	1/45	(2.22)	2/40	(5.00)	0.45 (0.05–4.43)	
Typical odds ratio (95% confidence interval)					3.22 (1.94–5.36)	

et al. 1972; Calder and Embrey 1975; Bremme and Bygdeman 1980a,b), and these 5 trials were of somewhat better methodological quality than the two in which the opposite trend was observed (Haeri *et al.* 1976; Macer *et al.* 1984). Overall, the incidence of this complication was statistically significantly higher with prostaglandin than with oxytocin administration (typical odds ratio 3.22; 95 per cent confidence interval 1.94–5.36; Table 63.6). 'Hypertonus–uterine hyperstimulation' may have lead to a variety of interventions, rang-

ing from innocuous changes in position, through fetal scalp blood sampling, to administration of betamimetic agents and caesarean section. Irrespective of whether or not 'hypertonus–uterine hyperstimulation' actually jeopardized either the mother or the fetus, therefore, it is clear that it may often have affected maternal comfort during labour.

Very few data were available on measures of maternal morbidity after delivery of the baby. These include the incidence of retained placenta (available from 8 trials),

Table 63.7 Effect of any prostaglandin (by any route) vs. oxytocin (any route) for induction of labour on retained placenta

Study	EXPT		CTRL		Odds ratio	Graph of odds ratios and confidence intervals
	n	(%)	*n*	(%)	(95% CI)	0.01 0.1 0.5 1 2 10 100
Vroman *et al.* (1972)	1/25	(4.00)	0/25	(0.00)	7.39 (0.15–99.99)	
Vakhariya and Sherman (1972)	1/50	(2.00)	0/50	(0.00)	7.39 (0.15–99.99)	
Mathews *et al.* (1976)	1/50	(2.00)	2/50	(4.00)	0.51 (0.05–4.98)	
MacLennan and Green (1980)	1/30	(3.33)	0/30	(0.00)	7.39 (0.15–99.99)	
Ulmsten *et al.* (1979)	0/50	(0.00)	0/50	(0.00)	1.00 (1.00–1.00)	
Bremme and Bygdeman (1980a)	4/106	(3.77)	4/96	(4.17)	0.90 (0.22–3.70)	
Read and Martin (1974)	2/99	(2.02)	2/88	(2.27)	0.89 (0.12–6.42)	
Lykkesfeldt and Osler (1979)	2/77	(2.60)	4/87	(4.60)	0.57 (0.11–2.90)	
Typical odds ratio (95% confidence interval)					0.98 (0.43–2.20)	

Effect of any prostaglandin (by any route) vs. oxytocin (any route) for induction of labour on postpartum haemorrhage

Study	EXPT		CTRL		Odds ratio	Graph
Vakhariya and Sherman (1972)	2/50	(4.00)	1/50	(2.00)	1.97 (0.20–19.43)	
Mathews *et al.* (1976)	1/49	(2.04)	2/50	(4.00)	0.52 (0.05–5.09)	
MacLennan and Green (1980)	0/30	(0.00)	1/29	(3.45)	0.13 (0.00–6.59)	
Ulmsten *et al.* (1979)	1/50	(2.00)	3/50	(6.00)	0.36 (0.05–2.61)	
Bremme and Bygdeman (1980a)	26/104	(25.00)	18/96	(18.75)	1.44 (0.74–2.80)	
Read and Martin (1974)	0/99	(0.00)	0/88	(0.00)	1.00 (1.00–1.00)	
Ratnam *et al.* (1974)	7/107	(6.54)	2/100	(2.00)	2.97 (0.78–11.25)	
Lecher *et al.* (1981)	5/182	(2.75)	11/165	(6.67)	0.41 (0.15–1.12)	
Vildemeersch and Schellen (1976)	0/14	(0.00)	0/14	(0.00)	1.00 (1.00–1.00)	
Macer *et al.* (1984)	8/45	(17.78)	9/40	(22.50)	0.75 (0.26–2.15)	
Typical odds ratio (95% confidence interval)					0.98 (0.64–1.51)	

Effect of any prostaglandin (by any route) vs. oxytocin (any route) for induction of labour on pyrexia postpartum

Study	EXPT		CTRL		Odds ratio	Graph
Andreasson *et al.* (1985)	0/100	(0.00)	0/100	(0.00)	1.00 (1.00–1.00)	
Vroman *et al.* (1972)	1/25	(4.00)	0/25	(0.00)	7.39 (0.15–99.99)	
MacLennan and Green (1980)	0/30	(0.00)	0/30	(0.00)	1.00 (1.00–1.00)	
Ulmsten *et al.* (1979)	0/50	(0.00)	0/50	(0.00)	1.00 (1.00–1.00)	
Typical odds ratio (95% confidence interval)					7.39 (0.15–99.99)	

the incidence of postpartum haemorrhage (available from 10 trials), and the incidence of pyrexia during the puerperium (available from only 4 trials). None of these outcomes showed any differential effects of prostaglandins and oxytocin (Table 63.7).

2.3 Effects on the infant

In view of the increased incidence of 'uterine hyperstimulation' associated with induction using prostaglandins it is important to note that the incidence of fetal heart rate 'abnormalities' was similar among the fetuses of women receiving prostaglandins and those in the oxytocin group (typical odds ratio 0.97; 95 per cent confidence interval 0.54–1.72; Table 63.8), but only 6 trials provided data on this outcome.

Unfortunately, very few trials provided data on substantive infant outcomes, such as resuscitation of the newborn, admission to a special care nursery, or early neonatal convulsions. Even data on perinatal death were only available from half of the trials. From the 5 trials that provided data on the need for resuscitation of the newborn, and the 3 trials with data on admission to a special care nursery, no differential effects of prostaglandins and oxytocin emerged. However, the precision of these estimates is extremely low, yielding 95 per cent confidence intervals that ranged respectively from 0.51 to 10.61 and from 0.00 to 6.82 (Table 63.9).

Somewhat more data were available on the incidence of low 1-minute and 5-minute Apgar scores. Of the 10 trials with categorical data on low 1-minute Apgar scores (which usually, but not always referred to a score of less than 7), 3 had no infants with low Apgar scores, but the 7 other trials all found slightly more infants with low 1-minute Apgar scores after prostaglandin than after oxytocin inductions. Nevertheless, when considered together the differential effect may still be

due to chance, yielding a typical odds ratio of 1.41 with a 95 per cent confidence interval ranging from 0.96 to 2.07; Table 63.10). Thirteen trials, only 4 of which are included in the overview of 1-minute Apgar scores (Table 63.10), provided data on 5-minute Apgar scores, but no differential effects of prostaglandins compared with oxytocin were detected on this outcome (typical odds ratio 1.09; 95 per cent confidence interval 1.09–2.06; Table 63.10).

In only 15 out of the total of 35 trials was there any reference to perinatal deaths among the infants born to the women involved in these studies (Table 63.11). It would be unwise to assume that there were no deaths in those trials that provided no information on this important outcome. The investigators may, rightly or wrongly, have considered any deaths that occurred as 'incidental', and not causally related to either induction of labour or the method used to implement it.

Among the total of 1912 infants for whom this outcome is recorded, there were six deaths from causes other than lethal anomalies. Five of these deaths occurred among infants whose mothers had been induced with prostaglandins, compared with only one death among infants of mothers who had been induced with oxytocin (Table 63.11).

Five of the trials specifically mentioned whether the infants had hyperbilirubinaemia or jaundice, but these data relate to no more than 180 infants born to mothers who had been induced with prostaglandins and to 181 born to mothers who had been induced with oxytocin. The incidence of neonatal hyperbilirubinaemia was lower among infants born after induction of labour with prostaglandins than among those born after induction with oxytocin (typical odds ratio 0.54), but the difference is compatible with chance (95 per cent confidence interval 0.28–1.04; Table 63.9).

Table 63.8 Effect of any prostaglandin (by any route) vs. oxytocin (any route) for induction of labour on fetal heart rate 'abnormalities'

Study	EXPT		CTRL		Odds ratio	Graph of odds ratios and confidence intervals
	n	(%)	n	(%)	(95% CI)	0.01 0.1 0.5 1 2 10 10
Vroman *et al.* (1972)	8/25	(32.00)	6/25	(24.00)	1.48 (0.43–5.01)	
Mathews *et al.* (1976)	3/50	(6.00)	1/50	(2.00)	2.80 (0.38–20.52)	
Scher *et al.* (1972)	0/20	(0.00)	0/23	(0.00)	1.00 (1.00–1.00)	
Secher *et al.* (1981)	11/182	(6.04)	15/165	(9.09)	0.65 (0.29–1.43)	
Wildemeersch and Schellen (1976)	0/14	(0.00)	0/14	(0.00)	1.00 (1.00–1.00)	
Lykkesfeldt and Osler (1979)	4/77	(5.19)	4/87	(4.60)	1.14 (0.27–4.70)	
Typical odds ratio (95% confidence interval)					0.97 (0.54–1.72)	

3 Intravenous prostaglandins vs. intravenous oxytocin

The earliest form of prostaglandin administration for the induction of labour was intravenous infusion (Karim *et al.* 1968; Embrey 1969; see also Chapter 62). Between 1971 and 1980, 13 controlled trials were reported in which intravenous prostaglandins had been compared with intravenous oxytocin for the induction of labour (Table 63.1). We have considered these trials separately because the comparisons involved a single route of administration for the two types of oxytocic agent, and because they offered an opportunity for double-blind investigations. Only 7 of these trials actually used a double-blind approach, however (Calder and Embrey 1975; Beazley and Gillespie 1971; Le Maire *et al.* 1972; Vakhariya and Sherman 1972; Vroman *et al.* 1972; Spellacy *et al.* 1973; Baxi *et al.* 1980). One further trial, on which two reports are available (Anderson *et al.* 1972; Blackburn *et al.* 1973), was claimed to have been conducted in a double-blind manner, but the strength of the prostaglandin infusion was changed on three occasions during the course of the

Table 63.9 Effect of any prostaglandin (by any route) vs. oxytocin (any route) for induction of labour on resuscitation of newborn

Study	EXPT		CTRL		Odds ratio	Graph of odds ratios and confidence intervals
	n	(%)	n	(%)	(95% CI)	0.01 0.1 0.5 1 2 10 100
Vakhariya and Sherman (1972)	1/50	(2.00)	0/50	(0.00)	7.39 (0.15–99.99)	
MacLennan and Green (1980)	1/30	(3.33)	1/30	(3.33)	1.00 (0.06–16.37)	
Ulmsten *et al.* (1979)	0/50	(0.00)	0/50	(0.00)	1.00 (1.00–1.00)	
Beard *et al.* (1975)	3/22	(13.64)	1/20	(5.00)	2.66 (0.35–20.42)	
Wildemeersch and Schellen (1976)	0/14	(0.00)	0/14	(0.00)	1.00 (1.00–1.00)	
Typical odds ratio (95% confidence interval)					2.32 (0.51–10.61)	

Effect of any prostaglandin (by any route) vs. oxytocin (any route) for induction of labour on admission to special care nursery

Study	EXPT		CTRL		Odds ratio	Graph
Vakhariya and Sherman (1972)	0/50	(0.00)	0/50	(0.00)	1.00 (1.00–1.00)	
MacLennan and Green (1980)	0/30	(0.00)	1/30	(3.33)	0.14 (0.00–6.82)	
Ulmsten *et al.* (1979)	0/50	(0.00)	0/50	(0.00)	1.00 (1.00–1.00)	
Typical odds ratio (95% confidence interval)					0.14 (0.00–6.82)	

Effect of any prostaglandin (by any route) vs. oxytocin (any route) for induction of labour on jaundice–hyperbilirubinaemia

Study	EXPT		CTRL		Odds ratio	Graph
MacLennan and Green (1980)	2/30	(6.67)	7/30	(23.33)	0.28 (0.07–1.13)	
Ulmsten *et al.* (1979)	0/50	(0.00)	0/50	(0.00)	1.00 (1.00–1.00)	
Keri *et al.* (1976)	9/50	(18.00)	13/50	(26.00)	0.63 (0.25–1.62)	
Beard *et al.* (1975)	2/22	(9.09)	5/20	(25.00)	0.33 (0.07–1.63)	
Jayasuriya *et al.* (1978)	3/28	(10.71)	2/31	(6.45)	1.72 (0.28–10.59)	
Typical odds ratio (95% confidence interval)					0.54 (0.28–1.04)	

Table 63.10 Effect of any prostaglandin (by any route) vs. oxytocin (any route) for induction of labour on low Apgar score at 1 minute

Study	EXPT		CTRL		Odds ratio	Graph of odds ratios and confidence intervals
	n	(%)	n	(%)	(95% CI)	0.01 0.1 0.5 1 2 10 100
Baxi et al. (1980)	0/25	(0.00)	0/25	(0.00)	1.00 (1.00–1.00)	
Spellacy et al. (1973)	14/71	(19.72)	13/79	(16.46)	1.25 (0.54–2.86)	
Vakhariya and Sherman (1972)	6/50	(12.00)	5/50	(10.00)	1.22 (0.35–4.26)	
Beazley and Gillespie (1971)	38/101	(37.62)	32/105	(30.48)	1.37 (0.77–2.44)	
Mathews et al. (1976)	0/41	(0.00)	0/47	(0.00)	1.00 (1.00–1.00)	
Blackburn et al. (1973)	0/11	(0.00)	0/12	(0.00)	1.00 (1.00–1.00)	
Somell and Larsson (1983)	5/51	(9.80)	1/27	(3.70)	2.34 (0.41–13.30)	
Naismith et al. (1973)	9/20	(45.00)	8/20	(40.00)	1.22 (0.35–4.21)	
Beard et al. (1975)	4/22	(18.18)	2/20	(10.00)	1.92 (0.35–10.61)	
Lykkesfeldt and Osler (1981)	3/18	(16.67)	1/17	(5.88)	2.81 (0.36–21.94)	
Typical odds ratio (95% confidence interval)					1.41 (0.96–2.07)	

Effect of any prostaglandin (by any route) vs. oxytocin (any route) for induction of labour on low Apgar score at 5 minutes

Study	EXPT		CTRL		Odds ratio	
Spellacy et al. (1973)	4/71	(5.63)	4/79	(5.06)	1.12 (0.27–4.64)	
Andreasson et al. (1985)	0/100	(0.00)	0/100	(0.00)	1.00 (1.00–1.00)	
Vroman et al. (1972)	1/25	(4.00)	0/25	(0.00)	7.39 (0.15–99.99)	
Beazley and Gillespie (1971)	9/101	(8.91)	8/105	(7.62)	1.19 (0.44–3.19)	
MacLennan and Green (1980)	0/30	(0.00)	0/30	(0.00)	1.00 (1.00–1.00)	
Ulmsten et al. (1979)	0/50	(0.00)	0/50	(0.00)	1.00 (1.00–1.00)	
Bremme and Bygdeman (1980a)	0/104	(0.00)	1/96	(1.04)	0.12 (0.00–6.30)	
Blackburn et al. (1973)	0/11	(0.00)	0/12	(0.00)	1.00 (1.00–1.00)	
Read and Martin (1974)	0/99	(0.00)	0/88	(0.00)	1.00 (1.00–1.00)	
Naismith et al. (1973)	3/20	(15.00)	2/20	(10.00)	1.56 (0.25–9.94)	
Haeri et al. (1976)	4/50	(8.00)	4/50	(8.00)	1.00 (0.24–4.21)	
Beard et al. (1975)	0/22	(0.00)	1/20	(5.00)	0.12 (0.00–6.20)	
Macer et al. (1984)	0/45	(0.00)	0/40	(0.00)	1.00 (1.00–1.00)	
Typical odds ratio (95% confidence interval)					1.09 (0.58–2.06)	

Table 63.11 Effect of any prostaglandin (by any route) vs. oxytocin (any route) for induction of labour on perinatal death

Study	EXPT		CTRL		Odds ratio	Graph of odds ratios and confidence intervals						
	n	(%)	n	(%)	(95% CI)	0.01	0.1	0.5	1	2	10	100
Spellacy *et al.* (1973)	1/115	(0.87)	0/107	(0.00)	6.89 (0.14–99.99)							
Andreasson *et al.* (1985)	0/100	(0.00)	0/100	(0.00)	1.00 (1.00–1.00)							
Baxi *et al.* (1980)	1/25	(4.00)	0/25	(0.00)	7.39 (0.15–99.99)							
Vroman *et al.* (1972)	0/25	(0.00)	0/25	(0.00)	1.00 (1.00–1.00)							
MacLennan and Green (1980)	0/30	(0.00)	0/30	(0.00)	1.00 (1.00–1.00)							
Ulmsten *et al.* (1979)	0/50	(0.00)	0/50	(0.00)	1.00 (1.00–1.00)							
Bremme and Bygdeman (1980a)	0/104	(0.00)	0/96	(0.00)	1.00 (1.00–1.00)							
Blackburn *et al.* (1973)	0/11	(0.00)	0/12	(0.00)	1.00 (1.00–1.00)							
Naismith *et al.* (1973)	0/20	(0.00)	0/20	(0.00)	1.00 (1.00–1.00)							
Ratnam *et al.* (1974)	1/107	(0.93)	1/100	(1.00)	0.93 (0.06–15.06)							
Haeri *et al.* (1976)	0/50	(0.00)	0/50	(0.00)	1.00 (1.00–1.00)							
Lykkesfeldt and Osler (1981)	0/40	(0.00)	0/45	(0.00)	1.00 (1.00–1.00)							
Scher *et al.* (1972)	0/20	(0.00)	0/23	(0.00)	1.00 (1.00–1.00)							
Westergaard *et al.* (1983)	2/181	(1.10)	0/206	(0.00)	8.53 (0.53–99.99)							
Lykkesfeld and Osler (1979)	0/77	(0.00)	0/87	(0.00)	1.00 (1.00–1.00)							
Typical odds ratio (95% Confidence interval)					3.85 (0.77–19.14)							

trial, so that it is uncertain whether that claim is justified.

In only one of the trials (which used PGE₂) was the administration of the oxytocic drug routinely combined with artificial rupture of the membranes (Calder and Embrey 1975). Of the remaining trials, 9 dealt with PGF$_{2\alpha}$ (Rangarajan *et al.* 1971; Anderson *et al.* 1972; Le Maire *et al.* 1972; Scher *et al.* 1972; Vakhariya and Sherman 1972; Vroman *et al.* 1972; Spellacy *et al.* 1973; Wildemeersch and Schellen 1976; Baxi *et al.* 1980); one with PGE₂ (Beazley and Gillespie 1971); and two with both PGE₂ and PGF$_{2\alpha}$ (Naismith *et al.* 1973; Gowenlock *et al.* 1975).

Data on the incidence of delivery within 12 hours (available for 4 trials) and of vaginal delivery within 12 hours (available for 5 trials) did not reveal any differential effects of prostaglandins and oxytocin (Table 63.12). Neither was a differential effect detected in the incidence of delivery within 24 hours (data not shown).

Incidences of caesarean section (available for 9 trials), instrumental vaginal delivery (available for 3 trials), and operative delivery (available for 3 trials) showed no evidence of any differential effect of prostaglandins and oxytocin (Table 63.12).

The only differential effects detected when these trials are considered together relate to the proportion of women who experienced side-effects of the uterine stimulants during their induction of labour (Table 63.13). Eight of the trial reports mentioned whether 'uterine hypertonus' and/or 'uterine hyperstimulation' were observed: in half of these it was not; in the other four it always occurred more frequently with prostaglandins than with oxytocin, yielding a typical odds ratio of 5.33 with a 95 per cent confidence interval of 2.88 to 9.85 (Table 63.13).

Overall, the proportion of women, who vomited during the administration of the oxytocic agents, was not statistically significantly different between those

Table 63.12 Effect of intravenous prostaglandins vs. oxytocin for induction of labour on not delivered within 12 hours

Study	EXPT n	(%)	CTRL n	(%)	Odds ratio (95% CI)	Graph of odds ratios and confidence intervals
Beazley et al. (1971)	50/146	(34.25)	65/146	(44.52)	0.65 (0.41–1.04)	
Blackburn et al. (1973)	0/11	(0.00)	0/12	(0.00)	1.00 (1.00–1.00)	
Naismith et al. (1973)	14/20	(70.00)	8/20	(40.00)	3.26 (0.95–11.16)	
Scher et al. (1972)	6/20	(30.00)	10/23	(43.48)	0.57 (0.17–1.94)	
Typical odds ratio (95% confidence interval)					0.77 (0.51–1.16)	

Effect of intravenous prostaglandins vs. oxytocin for induction of labour on no vaginal delivery within 12 hours

Study	EXPT n	(%)	CTRL n	(%)	Odds ratio (95% CI)	
Baxi et al. (1980)	2/25	(8.00)	2/25	(8.00)	1.00 (0.13–7.56)	
Spellacy et al. (1973)	36/115	(31.30)	36/107	(33.64)	0.90 (0.51–1.58)	
Vakhariya and Sherman (1972)	4/50	(8.00)	4/50	(8.00)	1.00 (0.24–4.21)	
Blackburn et al. (1973)	0/11	(0.00)	0/12	(0.00)	1.00 (1.00–1.00)	
Naismith et al. (1973)	8/20	(40.00)	8/20	(40.00)	1.00 (0.29–3.49)	
Scher et al. (1972)	6/20	(30.00)	10/23	(43.48)	0.57 (0.17–1.94)	
Typical odds ratio (95% confidence interval)					0.87 (0.56–1.35)	

Effect of intravenous prostaglandins vs. oxytocin for induction of labour on caesarean section

Study	EXPT n	(%)	CTRL n	(%)	Odds ratio (95% CI)	
Baxi et al. (1980)	1/25	(4.00)	1/25	(4.00)	1.00 (0.06–16.45)	
Spellacy et al. (1973)	9/115	(7.83)	0/107	(0.00)	7.41 (1.96–28.07)	
Vroman et al. (1972)	0/25	(0.00)	0/25	(0.00)	1.00 (1.00–1.00)	
Vakhariya and Sherman (1972)	1/50	(2.00)	1/50	(2.00)	1.00 (0.06–16.22)	
Calder and Embrey (1975)	5/50	(10.00)	7/50	(14.00)	0.69 (0.21–2.28)	
Blackburn et al. (1973)	0/11	(0.00)	0/12	(0.00)	1.00 (1.00–1.00)	
Naismith et al. (1973)	0/20	(0.00)	1/20	(5.00)	0.14 (0.00–6.82)	
Scher et al. (1972)	0/20	(0.00)	0/23	(0.00)	1.00 (1.00–1.00)	
Gowenlock et al. (1975)	0/50	(0.00)	1/25	(4.00)	0.05 (0.00–3.18)	
Typical odds ratio (95% confidence interval)					1.41 (0.65–3.09)	

Table 63.12—*continued* Effect of intravenous prostaglandins vs. oxytocin for induction of labour on instrumental vaginal delivery

Study	EXPT n	(%)	CTRL n	(%)	Odds ratio (95% CI)	Graph of odds ratios and confidence intervals
Calder and Embrey (1975)	34/50	(68.00)	33/50	(66.00)	1.09 (0.48–2.51)	
Blackburn *et al.* (1973)	4/11	(36.36)	8/12	(66.67)	0.31 (0.06–1.55)	
Naismith *et al.* (1973)	14/20	(70.00)	10/20	(50.00)	2.25 (0.65–7.86)	
Typical odds ratio (95% confidence interval)					1.08 (0.57–2.04)	

Effect of intravenous prostaglandins vs. oxytocin for induction of labour on operative delivery

Study	EXPT n	(%)	CTRL n	(%)	Odds ratio (95% CI)	Graph
Calder and Embrey (1975)	39/50	(78.00)	40/50	(80.00)	0.89 (0.34–2.31)	
Blackburn *et al.* (1973)	4/11	(36.36)	8/12	(66.67)	0.31 (0.06–1.55)	
Naismith *et al.* (1973)	14/20	(70.00)	11/20	(55.00)	1.87 (0.53–6.61)	
Typical odds ratio (95% confidence interval)					0.91 (0.46–1.82)	

Table 63.13 Effect of intravenous prostaglandins vs. oxytocin for induction of labour on hyperstimulation–hypertonus

Study	EXPT n	(%)	CTRL n	(%)	Odds ratio (95% CI)	Graph of odds ratios and confidence intervals
Roman *et al.* (1972)	2/25	(8.00)	0/25	(0.00)	7.70 (0.47–99.99)	
Zakhariya and Sherman (1972)	8/50	(16.00)	1/50	(2.00)	5.43 (1.39–21.23)	
Baxi *et al.* (1980)	0/25	(0.00)	0/25	(0.00)	1.00 (1.00–1.00)	
Calder and Embrey (1975)	27/50	(54.00)	9/50	(18.00)	4.70 (2.08–10.59)	
Beazley *et al.* (1971)	0/146	(0.00)	0/146	(0.00)	1.00 (1.00–1.00)	
Fisher *et al.* (1972)	0/20	(0.00)	0/23	(0.00)	1.00 (1.00–1.00)	
Rangarajan *et al.* (1971)	8/20	(40.00)	1/20	(5.00)	7.08 (1.63–30.65)	
Vildemeersch and Schellen (1976)	0/14	(0.00)	0/14	(0.00)	1.00 (1.00–1.00)	
Typical odds ratio (95% confidence interval)					5.33 (2.88–9.85)	

Table 63.13—*continued* Effect of intravenous prostaglandins vs. oxytocin for induction of labour on vomiting

Study	EXPT		CTRL		Odds ratio	Graph of odds ratios and confidence intervals
	n	(%)	*n*	(%)	(95% CI)	0.01 0.1 0.5 1 2 10 100
Vroman *et al.* (1972)	2/25	(8.00)	2/25	(8.00)	1.00 (0.13–7.56)	
Vakhariya and Sherman (1972)	1/50	(2.00)	0/50	(0.00)	7.39 (0.15–99.99)	
Calder and Embrey (1975)	5/50	(10.00)	3/50	(6.00)	1.71 (0.41–7.21)	
Wildemeersch and Schellen (1976)	0/14	(0.00)	0/14	(0.00)	1.00 (1.00–1.00)	
Typical odds ratio (95% confidence interval)					1.64 (0.53–5.03)	

Effect of intravenous prostaglandins vs. oxytocin for induction of labour on pyrexia during labour

Calder and Embrey (1975)	22/50	(44.00)	7/50	(14.00)	4.23 (1.79–9.99)	
Naismith *et al.* (1973)	4/20	(20.00)	1/20	(5.00)	3.81 (0.60–24.23)	
Typical odds ratio (95% confidence interval)					4.15 (1.90–9.06)	

Effect of intravenous prostaglandins vs. oxytocin for induction of labour on venous erythema

Baxi *et al.* (1980)	1/25	(4.00)	0/25	(0.00)	7.39 (0.15–99.99)	
Vroman *et al.* (1972)	0/25	(0.00)	0/25	(0.00)	1.00 (1.00–1.00)	
Calder and Embrey (1975)	30/50	(60.00)	1/50	(2.00)	14.65 (6.30–34.05)	
Naismith *et al.* (1973)	1/20	(5.00)	0/20	(0.00)	7.39 (0.15–99.99)	
Wildemeersch and Schellen (1976)	0/14	(0.00)	0/14	(0.00)	1.00 (1.00–1.00)	
Typical odds ratio (95% confidence interval)					13.82 (6.17–30.98)	

receiving prostaglandins and those receiving oxytocin, but this information was available for only 4 trials and the precision of the estimate is very low (95 per cent confidence interval 0.53–5.03; Table 63.13).

A statistically significantly larger proportion of women developed pyrexia during labour with prostaglandin administration than with oxytocin (Table 63.13). The only two trials with data on this outcome reported 26 cases (37 per cent) of pyrexia among a total of 70 prostaglandin-treated women; 25 of these women belonged to a group of 60 who had received PGE_2 and one belonged to the 10 women who had received $PGF_{2\alpha}$.

Venous erythema, a fairly specific effect of PGE_2 (see Chapter 62), occurred statistically significantly more

often among prostaglandin than among oxytocin-treated women; all but one of the 32 instances observed in the 4 trials with data on this outcome were associated with the use of PGE_2 (Table 63.13).

Three of the perinatal deaths mentioned earlier (see Table 63.11) occurred among infants whose mothers had received intravenous prostaglandins for inducing labour (Table 63.14). There were no deaths among infants whose mothers had received oxytocin in the 8 trials that provided information on perinatal mortality. No differential effects were detected for any of the other infant outcomes reported, which included resuscitation of the newborn, admission to a special care nursery, and 1-minute and 5-minute Apgar scores (Table 63.14).

Table 63.14 Effect of intravenous prostaglandins vs. oxytocin for induction of labour on resuscitation of the newborn

Study	EXPT		CTRL		Odds ratio	Graph of odds ratios and confidence intervals
	n	(%)	*n*	(%)	(95% CI)	0.01 0.1 0.5 1 2 10 100
Vakhariya and Sherman (1972)	1/50	(2.00)	0/50	(0.00)	7.39 (0.15–99.99)	
Calder and Embrey (1975)	3/50	(6.00)	6/50	(12.00)	0.48 (0.12–1.89)	
Wildemeersch and Schellen (1976)	0/14	(0.00)	0/14	(0.00)	1.00 (1.00–1.00)	
Typical odds ratio (95% confidence interval)					0.65 (0.18–2.35)	

Effect of intravenous prostaglandins vs. oxytocin for induction of labour on low Apgar score at 1 minute

Baxi *et al.* (1980)	0/25	(0.00)	0/25	(0.00)	1.00 (1.00–1.00)	
Spellacy *et al.* (1973)	14/71	(19.72)	13/79	(16.46)	1.25 (0.54–2.86)	
Vroman *et al.* (1972)	5/25	(20.00)	1/25	(4.00)	4.41 (0.82–23.89)	
Beazley *et al.* (1971)	38/101	(37.62)	32/105	(30.48)	1.37 (0.77–2.44)	
Blackburn *et al.* (1973)	0/11	(0.00)	0/12	(0.00)	1.00 (1.00–1.00)	
Naismith *et al.* (1973)	9/20	(45.00)	8/20	(40.00)	1.22 (0.35–4.21)	
Typical odds ratio (95% confidence interval)					1.42 (0.93–2.18)	

Effect of intravenous prostaglandins vs. oxytocin for induction of labour on low Apgar score at 5 minutes

Spellacy *et al.* (1973)	4/71	(5.63)	4/79	(5.06)	1.12 (0.27–4.64)	
Vroman *et al.* (1972)	1/25	(4.00)	0/25	(0.00)	7.39 (0.15–99.99)	
Beazley *et al.* (1971)	9/101	(8.91)	8/105	(7.62)	1.19 (0.44–3.19)	
Blackburn *et al.* (1973)	0/11	(0.00)	0/12	(0.00)	1.00 (1.00–1.00)	
Naismith *et al.* (1973)	3/20	(15.00)	2/20	(10.00)	1.56 (0.25–9.94)	
Typical odds ratio (95% confidence interval)					1.30 (0.63–2.70)	

Effect of intravenous prostaglandins vs. oxytocin for induction of labour on admission to intensive neonatal care

Vakhariya and Sherman (1972)	0/50	(0.00)	1/50	(2.00)	0.14 (0.00–6.82)	
Typical odds ratio (95% confidence interval)					0.14 (0.00–6.82)	

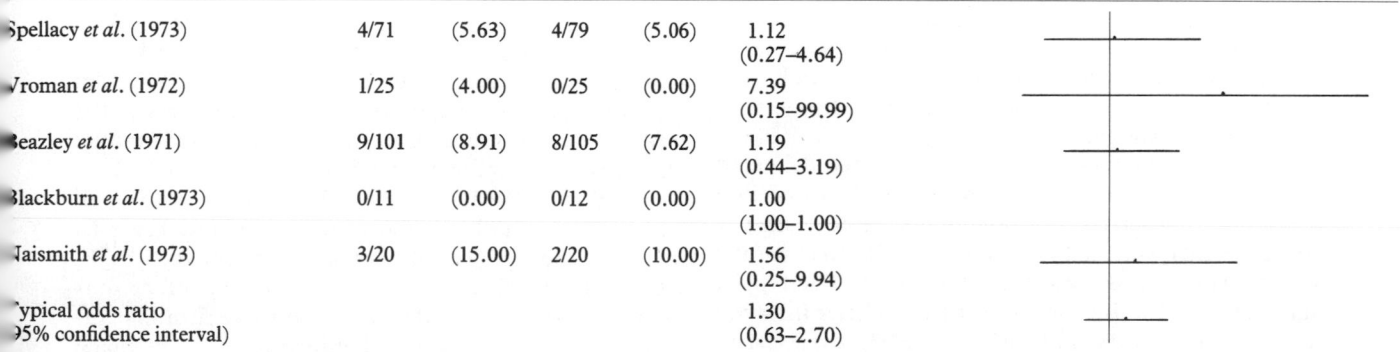

Table 63.14—*continued* Effect of intravenous prostaglandins vs. oxytocin for induction of labour on perinatal death (excluding malformations)

Study	EXPT		CTRL		Odds ratio	Graph of odds ratios and confidence intervals						
	n	(%)	n	(%)	(95% CI)	0.01	0.1	0.5	1	2	10	100
Spellacy et al. (1973)	1/115	(0.87)	0/107	(0.00)	6.89 (0.14–99.99)							
Baxi et al. (1980)	1/25	(4.00)	0/25	(0.00)	7.39 (0.15–99.99)							
Calder et al. (1975)	0/50	(0.00)	0/50	(0.00)	1.00 (1.00–1.00)							
Vakhariya and Sherman (1972)	0/50	(0.00)	0/50	(0.00)	1.00 (1.00–1.00)							
Beazley et al. (1971)	2/146	(1.37)	0/146	(0.00)	7.44 (0.46–99.99)							
Blackburn et al. (1973)	0/11	(0.00)	0/12	(0.00)	1.00 (1.00–1.00)							
Naismith et al. (1973)	0/20	(0.00)	0/20	(0.00)	1.00 (1.00–1.00)							
Scher et al. (1972)	0/20	(0.00)	0/23	(0.00)	1.00 (1.00–1.00)							
Typical odds ratio (95% confidence interval)					7.29 (1.02–51.83)							

4 Oral prostaglandins vs. oxytocin

4.1 Oral prostaglandins vs. buccal oxytocin

Five controlled comparisons have been conducted in which both the prostaglandin (always PGE_2) and oxytocin were administered by mouth (Table 63.1). Three of these were conducted in women with intact membranes (Lykkesfeldt and Osler 1979; Ulstein et al. 1979; Lykkesfeldt and Osler 1981); in one the membranes were artificially ruptured at the beginning of the induction (Mathews et al. 1976); and one contained a group of women who had amniotomy at the start of the induction and a group of women in whom the membranes were left intact (Westergaard et al. 1983).

The proportions of women who had not delivered within 24 hours (in 4 trials) and within 48 hours (in 3 trials) after the start of the induction were both smaller among women who had received oral PGE_2 than among women who had received buccal oxytocin. The typical odds ratios (with their 95 per cent confidence interval) were 0.70 (0.49–1.00) and 0.65 (0.45–0.93) respectively. Also, the proportions of women who failed to deliver vaginally within 24 hours and within 48 hours were both statistically significantly less with oral PGE_2 than with buccal oxytocin, although these data were available from fewer trials (Table 63.15). The incidences of caesarean section, instrumental vaginal delivery, and operative delivery, however, were similar among prostaglandin and among oxytocin-induced women (Table 63.15).

All 5 trials sought 'uterine hypertonus' and/or 'uterine hyperstimulation', but these complications were not

observed in any of them. Gastrointestinal side-effects were statistically significantly more common among women who received PGE_2 than among those who had received oxytocin. The typical odds ratio for vomiting (available for 4 trials) was 2.91, with a 95 per cent confidence interval from 1.35 to 6.29; that for diarrhoea (available for 3 trials) was 3.70, with a 95 per cent confidence interval from 1.64 to 8.37.

Only three of the trials provided categorical data on 1-minute Apgar scores (Mathews et al. 1976; Lykkesfeldt and Osler 1979; Lykkesfeldt and Osler 1981), and in only one of them (Lykkesfeldt and Osler 1979) did the data relate to all infants born to all mothers in the two treatment arms. Categorical data on 5-minute Apgar scores were available from only one trial (Westergaard et al. 1983), and these data did not relate to all infants of the mothers who were entered into this trial either. Although no differential effects between PGE_2 and oxytocin were detected, the data on infant outcomes are scanty and do not permit any firm conclusions. Three trials provided information on perinatal death (Lykkesfeldt and Osler 1979; Lykkesfeldt and Osler 1981; Westergaard et al. 1983). There was only one death (from intracranial haemorrhage and respiratory distress syndrome due to 'prematurity'), and this occurred in an infant whose mother had received oral PGE_2.

4.2 Oral prostaglandins vs. intravenous oxytocin

Intravenous oxytocin, with or without amniotomy, is currently the most commonly employed method of

Table 63.15 Effect of oral PGE$_2$ vs. buccal oxytocin for induction of labour on no vaginal delivery within 24 hours

Study	EXPT		CTRL		Odds ratio	Graph of odds ratios and confidence intervals
	n	(%)	n	(%)	(95% CI)	0.01 0.1 0.5 1 2 10 100
Westergaard *et al.* (1983)	55/133	(41.35)	72/131	(54.96)	0.58 (0.36–0.94)	
Typical odds ratio (95% confidence interval)					0.58 (0.36–0.94)	

Effect of oral PGE$_2$ vs. buccal oxytocin for induction of labour on no vaginal delivery within 48 hours

Lykkesfeldt and Osler (1981)	25/40	(62.50)	32/45	(71.11)	0.68 (0.28–1.67)	
Westergaard *et al.* (1983)	35/181	(19.34)	57/206	(27.67)	0.63 (0.40–1.01)	
Typical odds ratio (95% confidence interval)					0.64 (0.42–0.97)	

Effect of oral PGE$_2$ vs. buccal oxytocin for induction of labour on instrumental vaginal delivery

Mathews *et al.* (1976)	2/50	(4.00)	1/50	(2.00)	1.97 (0.20–19.43)	
Ulstein *et al.* (1979)	9/134	(6.72)	14/129	(10.85)	0.60 (0.25–1.40)	
Westergaard *et al.* (1983)	18/153	(11.76)	22/143	(15.38)	0.73 (0.38–1.43)	
Lykkesfeldt and Osler (1979)	12/77	(15.58)	9/87	(10.34)	1.59 (0.64–3.98)	
Typical odds ratio (95% confidence interval)					0.87 (0.55–1.35)	

Effect of oral PGE$_2$ vs. buccal oxytocin for induction of labour on operative delivery

Mathews *et al.* (1976)	3/50	(6.00)	1/50	(2.00)	2.80 (0.38–20.52)	
Ulstein *et al.* (1979)	14/134	(10.45)	24/129	(18.60)	0.52 (0.26–1.03)	
Lykkesfeldt and Osler (1979)	20/77	(25.97)	24/87	(27.59)	0.92 (0.46–1.84)	
Typical odds ratio (95% confidence interval)					0.75 (0.47–1.20)	

Effect of oral PGE$_2$ vs. buccal oxytocin for induction of labour on vomiting

Mathews *et al.* (1976)	4/50	(8.00)	3/50	(6.00)	1.36 (0.29–6.25)	
Ulstein *et al.* (1979)	4/134	(2.99)	1/129	(0.78)	3.26 (0.56–19.06)	
Lykkesfeldt and Osler (1981)	6/40	(15.00)	0/45	(0.00)	9.58 (1.83–50.03)	
Westergaard *et al.* (1983)	6/181	(3.31)	3/206	(1.46)	2.26 (0.60–8.49)	
Typical odds ratio (95% confidence interval)					2.91 (1.35–6.29)	

Table 63.16 Effect of oral PGE$_2$ vs. intravenous oxytocin for induction of labour on no vaginal delivery within 24 hours

Study	EXPT n	(%)	CTRL n	(%)	Odds ratio (95% CI)	Graph of odds ratios and confidence intervals
Haeri et al. (1976)	2/50	(4.00)	8/50	(16.00)	0.27 (0.07–0.98)	
Kennedy et al. (1978)	1/30	(3.33)	2/30	(6.67)	0.50 (0.05–5.02)	
Ratnam et al. (1974)	14/107	(13.08)	7/100	(7.00)	1.94 (0.79–4.78)	
Secher et al. (1981)	1/57	(1.75)	2/46	(4.35)	0.40 (0.04–4.02)	
Typical odds ratio (95% confidence interval)					0.89 (0.45–1.74)	

Effect of oral PGE$_2$ vs. intravenous oxytocin for induction of labour on no vaginal delivery within 48 hours

Study	EXPT n	(%)	CTRL n	(%)	Odds ratio (95% CI)	Graph of odds ratios and confidence intervals
Haeri et al. (1976)	2/50	(4.00)	8/50	(16.00)	0.27 (0.07–0.98)	
Kennedy et al. (1978)	1/30	(3.33)	2/30	(6.67)	0.50 (0.05–5.02)	
Ratnam et al. (1974)	12/107	(11.21)	5/100	(5.00)	2.27 (0.84–6.12)	
Secher et al. (1981)	1/57	(1.75)	2/46	(4.35)	0.40 (0.04–4.02)	
Typical odds ratio (95% confidence interval)					0.88 (0.43–1.80)	

Effect of oral PGE$_2$ vs. intravenous oxytocin for induction of labour on caesarean section

Study	EXPT n	(%)	CTRL n	(%)	Odds ratio (95% CI)	Graph of odds ratios and confidence intervals
Bremme et al. (1984)	4/44	(9.09)	5/39	(12.82)	0.68 (0.17–2.71)	
Bremme and Bygdeman (1980a)	6/104	(5.77)	10/96	(10.42)	0.53 (0.19–1.48)	
Read and Martin (1974)	1/99	(1.01)	0/88	(0.00)	6.61 (0.13–99.99)	
Secher et al. (1981)	1/57	(1.75)	2/46	(4.35)	0.40 (0.04–4.02)	
Beard et al. (1975)	0/22	(0.00)	0/20	(0.00)	1.00 (1.00–1.00)	
Haeri et al. (1976)	2/50	(4.00)	8/50	(16.00)	0.27 (0.07–0.98)	
Ratnam et al. (1974)	12/107	(11.21)	5/100	(5.00)	2.27 (0.84–6.12)	
Somell and Larsson (1983)	1/52	(1.92)	2/30	(6.67)	0.26 (0.02–2.86)	
Kennedy et al. (1978)	2/30	(6.67)	1/30	(3.33)	1.99 (0.20–19.94)	
Miller et al. (1975)	6/100	(6.00)	2/51	(3.92)	1.51 (0.34–6.77)	
Typical odds ratio (95% confidence interval)					0.84 (0.52–1.37)	

Table 63.16—*continued* Effect of oral PGE$_2$ vs. intravenous oxytocin for induction of labour on instrumental vaginal delivery

Study	EXPT		CTRL		Odds ratio	Graph of odds ratios and confidence intervals
	n	(%)	*n*	(%)	(95% CI)	
Bremme and Bygdeman (1980a)	29/104	(27.88)	23/96	(23.96)	1.23 (0.65–2.30)	
Read and Martin (1974)	3/99	(3.03)	8/88	(9.09)	0.34 (0.10–1.14)	
Haeri *et al.* (1976)	0/50	(0.00)	3/50	(6.00)	0.13 (0.01–1.28)	
Beard *et al.* (1975)	5/22	(22.73)	6/20	(30.00)	0.69 (0.18–2.70)	
Secher *et al.* (1981)	8/57	(14.04)	3/46	(6.52)	2.18 (0.62–7.63)	
Somell and Larsson (1983)	8/52	(15.38)	7/30	(23.33)	0.59 (0.19–1.88)	
Kennedy *et al.* (1978)	6/30	(20.00)	10/30	(33.33)	0.51 (0.16–1.59)	
Typical odds ratio (95% confidence interval)					0.82 (0.54–1.23)	

Effect of oral PGE$_2$ vs. intravenous oxytocin for induction of labour on operative delivery

Study	EXPT		CTRL		Odds ratio	Graph of odds ratios and confidence intervals
Bremme and Bygdeman (1980a)	35/104	(33.65)	33/96	(34.38)	0.97 (0.54–1.74)	
Read and Martin (1974)	4/99	(4.04)	8/88	(9.09)	0.43 (0.13–1.39)	
Haeri *et al.* (1976)	2/50	(4.00)	11/50	(22.00)	0.21 (0.06–0.66)	
Beard *et al.* (1975)	5/22	(22.73)	6/20	(30.00)	0.69 (0.18–2.70)	
Secher *et al.* (1981)	9/57	(15.79)	5/46	(10.87)	1.51 (0.49–4.68)	
Kennedy *et al.* (1978)	8/30	(26.67)	11/30	(36.67)	0.63 (0.22–1.87)	
Somell and Larsson (1983)	9/52	(17.31)	9/30	(30.00)	0.48 (0.16–1.42)	
Typical odds ratio (95% confidence interval)					0.69 (0.48–0.99)	

inducing labour. Apart from the controlled comparisons with intravenous prostaglandins, which have been discussed earlier, only one route of prostaglandin administration has been extensively investigated against this 'standard' form of treatment, namely, oral administration of prostaglandin E$_2$. Eleven controlled comparisons between these two treatments have been reported in which the state of the membranes was identical in both treatment arms. In 8 of these the membranes were left intact (Read and Martin 1974; Beard *et al.* 1975; Miller *et al.* 1975; Haeri *et al.* 1976; Kennedy *et al.* 1978; Sivasuriya *et al.* 1978; Bremme and Bygdeman 1980a; Bremme *et al.* 1984); in one the membranes were ruptured artificially (Somell and Larsson 1983); and two involved two groups of women, one with and one without amniotomy (Ratnam *et al.* 1974; Secher *et al.* 1981).

Only 4 of the 11 trials provided data on the proportion of women who were not delivered within 24 hours after starting induction (Ratnam *et al.* 1974; Haeri *et al.* 1976; Kennedy *et al.* 1978; Secher *et al.* 1981). A total of 470 women were included in these 4 trials. Twenty-one (5 per cent) of them were undelivered 24 hours after the start of induction, but all of these were in one of the four trials (Ratnam *et al.* 1974), and no differential effects between oral PGE$_2$ and intravenous oxytocin were detected. As far as the proportion of women who did not deliver vaginally within 24 or 48 hours is concerned, data were available from all four trials, but again, no differential effects of the two drugs were detected (Table 63.16). All trials provided information on the incidence of caesarean section. In one, however, this information was only available for the women who had amniotomy at the start of the induction, while the

Table 63.17 Effect of oral PGE$_2$ vs. intravenous oxytocin for induction of labour on use of analgesia

Study	EXPT n	(%)	CTRL n	(%)	Odds ratio (95% CI)	Graph of odds ratios and confidence intervals
Bremme et al. (1984)	35/44	(79.55)	37/39	(94.87)	0.27 (0.08–0.95)	
Bremme and Eneroth (1980)	23/37	(62.16)	29/37	(78.38)	0.46 (0.17–1.25)	
Beard et al. (1975)	20/22	(90.91)	20/20	(100.0)	0.14 (0.01–2.35)	
Typical odds ratio (95% confidence interval)					0.35 (0.17–0.74)	

Effect of oral PGE$_2$ vs. intravenous oxytocin for induction of labour on vomiting

Study	EXPT n	(%)	CTRL n	(%)	Odds ratio (95% CI)	
Bremme and Bygdeman (1980a)	11/104	(10.58)	7/96	(7.29)	1.49 (0.57–3.92)	
Read and Martin (1974)	2/99	(2.02)	0/88	(0.00)	6.68 (0.41–99.99)	
Ratnam et al. (1974)	2/107	(1.87)	0/100	(0.00)	6.99 (0.43–99.99)	
Haeri et al. (1976)	5/50	(10.00)	1/50	(2.00)	4.07 (0.79–21.04)	
Beard et al. (1975)	1/22	(4.55)	0/20	(0.00)	6.75 (0.13–99.99)	
Typical odds ratio (95% confidence interval)					2.43 (1.15–5.17)	

Effect of oral PGE$_2$ vs. intravenous oxytocin for induction of labour on diarrhoea

Study	EXPT n	(%)	CTRL n	(%)	Odds ratio (95% CI)	
Bremme and Bygdeman (1980a)	2/104	(1.92)	0/96	(0.00)	6.91 (0.43–99.99)	
Ratnam et al. (1974)	8/107	(7.48)	0/100	(0.00)	7.41 (1.81–30.37)	
Haeri et al. (1976)	8/50	(16.00)	0/50	(0.00)	8.60 (2.04–36.23)	
Beard et al. (1975)	0/22	(0.00)	0/20	(0.00)	1.00 (1.00–1.00)	
Miller et al. (1975)	0/100	(0.00)	0/51	(0.00)	1.00 (1.00–1.00)	
Typical odds ratio (95% confidence interval)					7.84 (3.04–20.21)	

Effect of oral PGE$_2$ vs. intravenous oxytocin for induction of labour on postpartum haemorrhage

Study	EXPT n	(%)	CTRL n	(%)	Odds ratio (95% CI)	
Bremme and Bygdeman (1980a)	18/104	(17.31)	13/96	(13.54)	1.33 (0.62–2.86)	
Secher et al. (1981)	5/182	(2.75)	11/165	(6.67)	0.41 (0.15–1.12)	
Read and Martin (1974)	0/97	(0.00)	0/86	(0.00)	1.00 (1.00–1.00)	
Ratnam et al. (1974)	7/107	(6.54)	2/100	(2.00)	2.97 (0.78–11.25)	
Typical odds ratio (95% confidence interval)					1.07 (0.61–1.86)	

Table 63.17—*continued* Effect of oral PGE$_2$ vs. intravenous oxytocin for induction of labour on placental retention

Study	EXPT		CTRL		Odds ratio	Graph of odds ratios and confidence intervals
	n	(%)	n	(%)	(95% CI)	0.01 0.1 0.5 1 2 10 100
Bremme and Bygdeman (1980a)	4/104	(3.85)	4/96	(4.17)	0.92 (0.22–3.78)	
Read and Martin (1974)	2/99	(2.02)	2/88	(2.27)	0.89 (0.12–6.42)	
Typical odds ratio (95% confidence interval)					0.91 (0.29–2.87)	

Table 63.18 Effect of oral PGE$_2$ vs. intravenous oxytocin for induction of labour on resuscitation of the newborn

Study	EXPT		CTRL		Odds ratio	Graph of odds ratios and confidence intervals
	n	(%)	n	(%)	(95% CI)	0.01 0.1 0.5 1 2 10 100
Beard et al. (1975)	3/22	(13.64)	1/20	(5.00)	2.66 (0.35–20.42)	
Typical odds ratio (95% confidence interval)					2.66 (0.35–20.42)	

Effect of oral PGE$_2$ vs. intravenous oxytocin for induction of labour on low Apgar score at 1 minute

Study	EXPT		CTRL		Odds ratio	
Beard et al. (1975)	4/22	(18.18)	2/20	(10.00)	1.92 (0.35–10.61)	
Somell and Larsson (1983)	0/51	(0.00)	0/27	(0.00)	1.00 (1.00–1.00)	
Kennedy et al. (1978)	5/30	(16.67)	3/30	(10.00)	1.76 (0.40–7.72)	
Typical odds ratio (95% confidence interval)					1.83 (0.60–5.59)	

Effect of oral PGE$_2$ vs. intravenous oxytocin for induction of labour on low Apgar score at 5 minutes

Study	EXPT		CTRL		Odds ratio	
Bremme (1984)	0/44	(0.00)	0/39	(0.00)	1.00 (1.00–1.00)	
Bremme and Bygdeman (1980a)	0/104	(0.00)	1/96	(1.04)	0.12 (0.00–6.30)	
Haeri et al. (1976)	4/50	(8.00)	4/50	(8.00)	1.00 (0.24–4.21)	
Beard et al. (1975)	0/22	(0.00)	1/20	(5.00)	0.12 (0.00–6.20)	
Somell and Larsson (1983)	0/51	(0.00)	0/27	(0.00)	1.00 (1.00–1.00)	
Read and Martin (1974)	0/99	(0.00)	0/88	(0.00)	1.00 (1.00–1.00)	
Typical odds ratio (95% confidence interval)					0.64 (0.18–2.30)	

Table 63.18—*continued* Effect of oral PGE$_2$ vs. intravenous oxytocin for induction of labour on perinatal death (excluding malformations)

Study	EXPT		CTRL		Odds ratio	Graph of odds ratios and confidence intervals
	n	(%)	n	(%)	(95% CI)	0.01 0.1 0.5 1 2 10 100
Bremme and Bygdeman (1980a)	0/104	(0.00)	0/96	(0.00)	1.00 (1.00–1.00)	
Ratnam et al. (1974)	1/107	(0.93)	1/100	(1.00)	0.93 (0.06–15.06)	
Haeri et al. (1976)	0/50	(0.00)	0/50	(0.00)	1.00 (1.00–1.00)	
Miller et al. (1975)	1/100	(1.00)	0/51	(0.00)	4.53 (0.07–99.99)	
Typical odds ratio (95% confidence interval)					1.52 (0.15–15.34)	

mode of delivery is unknown for the women whose membranes were left intact and who did not deliver within two days (Secher *et al.* 1981). The data from these 10 trials were unable to detect any difference in caesarean section rate between women induced with oral PGE$_2$ and those induced with intravenous oxytocin (Table 63.16). Nor was a difference detected in the rate of instrumental vaginal delivery (available for 7 trials; Table 63.16). Although both showed a slight tendency to be lower with oral PGE$_2$ than with intravenous oxytocin, the total operative delivery rate (available for 7 trials) was not statistically significantly different between the two treatment arms (Table 63.16).

Only 3 trials provided data on the proportion of women receiving analgesia during labour (Beard *et al.* 1975; Bremme and Eneroth 1980; Bremme *et al.* 1984), and one of these reported this outcome only for a subpopulation of the women entered into the larger trial (Bremme and Bygdeman 1980a). Fewer PGE$_2$-treated than oxytocin-treated women received analgesia, yielding a typical odds ratio of 0.35 (95 per cent confidence interval 0.17–0.74; Table 63.17). Data on the incidence of vomiting and of diarrhoea were available from five trials. Both of these outcomes occurred in a statistically significantly larger proportion of women who had been induced with PGE$_2$ (Table 63.17). The typical odds ratios (with their 95 per cent confidence intervals) for vomiting and for diarrhoea were 2.43 (1.15–5.17) and 7.84 (3.04–20.21) respectively. Only 2 trials make specific mention of 'uterine hypertonus' and/or 'uterine hyperstimulation' (Ratnam *et al.* 1974; Kennedy *et al.* 1978); but these complications were not observed. Data on the incidence of postpartum haemorrhage and placental retention, available from 4 and 2 trials respectively, did not suggest any differential effects of the two drugs (Table 63.17).

No differences in any of the infant outcomes that are available from these trials were detected (Table 63.18).

5 Vaginal prostaglandins vs. oxytocin

Among the controlled trials comparing prostaglandins with oxytocin for the induction of labour (listed in Table 63.1), there is one further series that can be considered together, namely, those comparing vaginal administration of prostaglandins with oxytocin administration. Even when trials in which amniotomy was performed in one treatment arm but not in the other (e.g. Egarter *et al.* 1987) are excluded, and although they have been among the most recently conducted, these trials show a far wider diversity than any of the categories discussed earlier (Table 63.1).

Of the 4 trials available, three have used PGE$_2$ and one PGF$_{2\alpha}$; 3 were conducted without amniotomy, and the fourth with simultaneous amniotomy; in three studies, the comparison was with intravenous oxytocin, in the other it was with intranasally administered oxytocin; and so forth (MacLennan and Green 1980; Macer *et al.* 1984; Andreasson *et al.* 1985; Ekman *et al.* 1986). All 4 trials together involved only 194 women induced with prostaglandins and 189 induced with oxytocin.

Categorical data on the interval between the start of induction and delivery were not available for all trials; 3 provided data on the number of women who had no vaginal delivery within 12 hours of being induced (MacLennan and Green 1980; Andreasson *et al.* 1985; Ekman *et al.* 1986), and two of these (MacLennan and Green 1980; Andreasson *et al.* 1985) also provide data on the number of women who had not delivered vaginally within 48 hours (Table 63.19). Only delivery within 12 hours of being induced occurred statistically significantly more frequently among women induced with prostaglandins than among those induced with oxytocin. In all 4 trials there were fewer caesarean sections in the prostaglandin than in the oxytocin groups; but, overall, the difference is compatible with chance variation (Table 63.19). The 3 trials that provided these data did not suggest that there were any

Table 63.19 Effect of vaginal prostaglandins vs. oxytocin for induction of labour on no vaginal delivery within 12 hours

Study	EXPT n	(%)	CTRL n	(%)	Odds ratio (95% CI)	Graph of odds ratios and confidence intervals
						0.01 0.1 0.5 1 2 10 100
Andreasson *et al.* (1985)	29/100	(29.00)	58/100	(58.00)	0.31 (0.18–0.54)	
MacLennan and Green (1980)	3/30	(10.00)	6/30	(20.00)	0.46 (0.11–1.89)	
Ekman *et al.* (1986)	2/19	(10.53)	12/19	(63.16)	0.11 (0.03–0.41)	
Typical odds ratio (95% confidence interval)					0.28 (0.17–0.46)	

Effect of vaginal prostaglandins vs. oxytocin for induction of labour on no vaginal delivery within 48 hours

Study	EXPT n	(%)	CTRL n	(%)	Odds ratio (95% CI)	
Andreasson *et al.* (1985)	20/100	(20.00)	32/100	(32.00)	0.54 (0.29–1.01)	
MacLennan and Green (1980)	0/30	(0.00)	1/30	(3.33)	0.14 (0.00–6.82)	
Typical odds ratio (95% confidence interval)					0.52 (0.28–0.97)	

Effect of vaginal prostaglandins vs. oxytocin for induction of labour on caesarean section

Study	EXPT n	(%)	CTRL n	(%)	Odds ratio (95% CI)	
Andreasson *et al.* (1985)	9/100	(9.00)	13/100	(13.00)	0.67 (0.28–1.61)	
MacLennan and Green (1980)	0/30	(0.00)	1/30	(3.33)	0.14 (0.00–6.82)	
Macer *et al.* (1984)	2/45	(4.44)	2/40	(5.00)	0.88 (0.12–6.53)	
Ekman *et al.* (1986)	0/19	(0.00)	1/19	(5.26)	0.14 (0.00–6.82)	
Typical odds ratio (95% confidence interval)					0.61 (0.28–1.33)	

Effect of vaginal prostaglandins vs. oxytocin for induction of labour on instrumental vaginal delivery

Study	EXPT n	(%)	CTRL n	(%)	Odds ratio (95% CI)	
Andreasson *et al.* (1985)	9/100	(9.00)	10/100	(10.00)	0.89 (0.35–2.29)	
MacLennan and Green (1980)	8/30	(26.67)	12/30	(40.00)	0.55 (0.19–1.61)	
Macer *et al.* (1984)	3/45	(6.67)	3/40	(7.50)	0.88 (0.17–4.61)	
Typical odds ratio (95% confidence interval)					0.75 (0.39–1.43)	

differences in the rate of instrumental vaginal deliveries in the prostaglandin and oxytocin groups (MacLennan and Green 1980; Macer *et al.* 1984; Andreasson *et al.* 1985; (Table 63.19)).

Vomiting, on which 3 trials provided data (MacLennan and Green 1980; Andreasson *et al.* 1985; Ekman *et al.* 1986), occurred in only one of 149 prostaglandin-induced women and in none of the oxytocin-induced women. Diarrhoea, on which data were available from the same 3 trials, was not observed. All 4 trials provided data on pyrexia during labour; this occurred in only one woman who had received PGE_2 (Macer *et al.* 1984) and in none who had received oxytocin. Whether 'uterine hypertonus' and/or 'uterine hyperstimulation' occurred or not was reported for all trials; it occurred in 1 woman who had received prostaglandins and in 2 women who had received oxytocin, all 3 cases being observed in the same trial (Macer *et al.* 1984).

No differential effects in substantive infant outcomes were detected.

6 Conclusions

6.1 Implications for current practice

The first point to note about the trials comparing prostaglandins with oxytocin for induction of labour is the apparent lack of any coherent research strategy to evaluate the relative merits of these broad approaches for inducing labour (see Table 63.1). The second point to note is that it is clear that many of the women entered into these trials did not have pressing indications for induction of labour, as evidenced by the high proportions of women who remained undelivered several days after the induction had started. A third point is that selective under-reporting of important outcomes is almost certain to have occurred. It is highly implausible, for example, that there were no more than 6 perinatal deaths among well over 3000 infants born to mothers entered into these trials, from 1971 onwards.

In the light of these reservations what are the implications of these data for current practice? It would appear that prostaglandins are likely to reduce the incidence of operative delivery associated with induction of labour, a conclusion that is consistent with evidence derived from the trials reviewed in Chapter 61 (which dealt more specifically with the unripe cervix). Prostaglandins may also increase the likelihood that vaginal delivery will occur within a reasonable length of time after the start of the induction. The extent to which this may be a reflection of the greater mobility possible with some forms of prostaglandin administration than with intravenously administered oxytocin is unknown.

These positive effects of prostaglandins must be considered in the light of their definite and possible negative effects. Depending on the routes, type, and dose of prostaglandin used, between 5 and 20 per cent of women will experience troublesome gastrointestinal side-effects, or pyrexia. With the types and formulations of the drugs that are currently available, there is

also an important difference in the cost of prostaglandin and oxytocin inductions. As far as the baby is concerned there is quite simply too little evidence to allow any judgement about whether prostaglandins are more or less safe than oxytocin.

With regard to routes of administration, the evidence reviewed for this chapter is consistent with data reviewed in the preceding chapter (Chapter 62). It is difficult to envisage any advantage of administering prostaglandins rather than oxytocin by the intravenous route. If, for some women, the apparent benefits of prostaglandins are felt to outweigh their disadvantages, they should probably be administered orally or vaginally.

6.2 Implications for future research

There is clearly too little good evidence to allow confident conclusions about the relative merits of prostaglandins and oxytocin for inducing labour. This is not due to a lack of research activity, but to the lack of any perceptible strategy in the research efforts that have been reported so far. Induction of labour is one of the most important and irrevocable interventions in obstetric practice. It is therefore very important to discover which of these two categories of oxytocic drugs should predominate when induction of labour is necessary. If better answers to this important question are to be obtained, the first priority would seem to be the development of a more coherent research strategy. This will undoubtedly require multicentre collaboration in trials of sufficient size to detect important differential effects on substantive outcomes. If the research is to generate results which are relevant to clinical practice, the women participating in these trials should have genuine indications for induction of labour. Furthermore, their views of the alternative approaches to induction, which have thus far been largely neglected, should be assessed systematically. It would seem sensible to give priority to a comparison of oxytocin administered in the most efficient way (intravenously, with concomitant amniotomy) with prostaglandins given by routes that allow maternal mobility during labour, which is known to have positive effects (see Chapter 55).

References

Anderson GG, Hobbins JC, Speroff L (1972). Intravenous prostaglandins E_2 and $F_{2\alpha}$ for the induction of term labor. Am J Obstet Gynecol, 112: 382–386.

Andreasson B, Bock JE, Larsen J (1985). Induction of labour. A double-blind randomized controlled study of prostaglandin E_2 vaginal suppositories compared with intranasal oxytocin and with sequential treatment. Acta Obstet Gynecol Scand, 64: 157–161.

Baxi LV, Petrie RH, Caritis SN (1980). Induction of labor with low-dose prostaglandin $F_{2\alpha}$ and oxytocin. Am J Obstet Gynecol, 136: 28–31.

Beard RJ, Harrison R, Kiriakidis J, Underhill R, Craft I (1975). A clinical and biochemical assessment of the use of oral prostaglandin E_2 compared with intravenous oxytocin for labor induction in multiparous patients. Eur J Obstet Gynecol Reprod Biol, 5: 203–207.

Beazley JM, Gillespie A (1971). Double-blind trial of prostaglandin E_2 and oxytocin in induction of labour. Lancet, 1: 152–155.

Blackburn MG, Mancusi-Unbaro HR, Orzalesi MM, Hobbins JC, Anderson GG (1973). Effects on the neonate of the induction of labor with prostaglandin $F_{2\alpha}$ and oxytocin. Am J Obstet Gynecol, 116: 847–853.

Bremme K, Bygdeman M (1980a). Induction of labor by

oxytocin or prostaglandin E₂. Acta Obstet Gynecol Scand, 11–21.

Bremme K, Bygdeman M (1980b). A comparative study of uterine activity and fetal heart rate pattern in labor induced with oral prostaglandin E₂ or oxytocin. Acta Obstet Gynecol Scand, 23–29.

Bremme K, Eneroth P (1980). Changes in serum hormone levels during labor induced by oral PGE₂ or oxytocin infusion. Acta Obstet Gynecol Scand, 31–43.

Bremme K, Eneroth P, Samuelson K (1984). Estriol and cholic acid in maternal serum in induced labor. Gynecol Obstet Invest, 17: 120–126.

Calder AA, Embrey MP (1975). Comparison of intravenous oxytocin and prostaglandin E₂ for induction of labour using automatic and non-automatic infusion techniques. Br J Obstet Gynaecol, 82: 728–733.

Egarter C, Schurz B, Wagner G, Grunberger W, Husslein P (1987). Comparison between prostaglandin E₂ gel and oxytocin in medically indicated labour induction. Geburtshilfe Frauenheilkd, 47: 337–340.

Ekman G, Granstrom L, Ulmsten U (1986). Induction of labor with intravenous oxytocin or vaginal PGE₂ suppositories. Acta Obstet Gynecol Scand, 65: 857–859.

Elliott JP, Flaherty JF (1984). The use of breast stimulation to prevent postdate pregnancy. Am J Obstet Gynecol, 149: 628–632.

Embrey MP (1969). The effect of prostaglandins on the human pregnant uterus. J Obstet Gynaecol Br Commnwlth, 76: 783–798.

Gowenlock AH, Taylor DS, Sanderson JH (1975). Biochemical and haematological changes during the induction of labour at term with oxytocin, prostaglandin E₂ and prostaglandin F₂α. Br J Obstet Gynaecol, 82: 215–220.

Haeri AD, Scher J, Davey DA, Leader M (1976). Comparison of oral prostaglandin E₂ and intravenous oxytocin for induction of labor. S Afr Med J, 50: 516–518.

Karim SMM, Trussell, RR, Patel, RC, Hillier, K (1968). Response of pregnant human uterus to prostaglandin F₂α-induction of labour. Br Med J, 4: 621–623.

Kennedy JH, Quinn MA, Howie PW, Calder AA (1978). Single shot prostaglandin gel for labor induction. Prostaglandins, 15: 169–173.

Le Maire WJ, Spellacy WN, Shevach AB, Gall SA (1972). Changes in plasma estriol and progesterone during labor induced with prostaglandin F₂α or oxytocin. Prostaglandins, 2: 93–101.

Lykkesfeldt G, Osler M (1979). A comparison of three methods for inducing labor: oral prostaglandin E₂, buccal desaminooxytocin, intravenous oxytocin. Acta Obstet Gynecol Scand, 58: 321–325.

Lykkesfeldt G, Osler M (1981). Induction of labor with oral prostaglandin E₂ and buccal demoxytocin without amniotomy. Acta Obstet Gynecol Scand, 60: 429–430.

Macer J, Buchanan D, Yonekura ML (1984). Induction of labor with prostaglandin E₂ vaginal suppositories. Obstet Gynecol, 63: 664–668.

MacLennan AH, Green RC (1980). The effect of intravaginal prostaglandin F₂α on labour after spontaneous and artificial rupture of the membranes. Austral NZ J Obstet Gynaecol, 20: 87–90.

Mathews DD, Hossain H, Bhargava S, D'Souza F (1976). A randomised controlled trial of an oral solution of prostaglandin E₂ and oral oxytocin used immediately after low amniotomy for induction of labour in the presence of a favourable cervix. Curr Med Res Opin, 4: 233–240.

Miller JF, Welply GA, Elstein M (1975). Prostaglandin E₂ tablets compared with intravenous oxytocin in induction of labour. Br Med J, 1: 14–16.

Naismith WCMK, Barr W, MacVicar J (1973). Comparison of intravenous prostaglandins F₂α and E₂ with intravenous oxytocin in the induction of labour. J Obstet Gynaecol Br Commnwlth, 80: 531–535.

Rangarajan NS, La Croix GE, Moghissi KS (1971). Induction of labor with prostaglandin. Obstet Gynecol, 38: 546–550.

Ratnam SS, Khew KS, Chen C, Lim TC (1974). Oral prostaglandin E₂ in induction of labour. Austral NZ J Obstet Gynaecol, 14: 26–30.

Read MD, Martin RH (1974). A comparison between intravenous oxytocin and oral prostaglandin E₂ for the induction of labour in parous patients. Curr Med Res Opin, 2: 236–239.

Scher J, Davey DA, Baillie P, Friend J, Friend DM (1972). A comparison of prostaglandin F₂α and oxytocin in the induction of labour. S Afr Med J, 46: 2009–2012.

Secher NJ, Lange AP, Hassing Nielsen F, Thomson Pedersen G, Westergaard JG (1981). Induction of labor with and without primary amniotomy. A randomized study of prostaglandin E₂ tablets and intravenous oxytocin. Acta Obstet Gynecol Scand, 60: 237–241.

Sivasuriya M, Tan KL, Salmon YM, Karim SMM (1978). Neonatal serum bilirubin levels in spontaneous and induced labour. Br J Obstet Gynaecol, 85: 619–623.

Somell C, Larsson B (1983). Priming and induction of labor with oral PGE₂ in patients with low Bishop score. Acta Obstet Gynecol Scand, 62: 315–320.

Spellacy WN, Gall SA, Shevach AB, Holsinger KK (1973). The induction of labor at term. Comparisons between prostaglandin F₂α and oxytocin infusion. Obstet Gynecol, 41: 14–21.

Ulmsten U, Wingerup L, Andersson KE (1979). Comparison of prostaglandin E₂ and intravenous oxytocin for induction of labor. Obstet Gynecol, 54: 581–584.

Ulstein M, Sagen N, Eikhom SN (1979). A comparative study of labor induced by prostaglandin E₂ and buccal tablets of demoxytocin. Int J Gynaecol Obstet, 17: 243–245.

Vakhariya VR, Sherman AI (1972). Prostaglandin F₂α for induction of labor. Am J Obstet Gynecol, 113: 212–222.

Vroman S, Thiery M, Yo Le Sian A, Depiere M, Vanderheyden C, Derom R, Van Kets H, Brouckaert J (1972). A double blind comparative study of prostaglandin F₂α and oxytocin for the elective induction of labor. Eur J Obstet Gynecol Reprod Biol, 4: 115–123.

Westergaard JG, Lange AP, Pedersen GT, Secher NJ (1983). Oral oxytocics for induction of labor. Acta Obstet Gynecol Scand, 62: 103–110.

Wildemeersch DA, Schellen AMCM (1976). Double-blind trial of prostaglandin F₂α and oxytocin in the induction of labour. Curr Med Res Opin, 4: 263–266.

64 Prelabour rupture of the membranes at term

John Grant and Marc J. N. C. Keirse

1 Introduction

Prelabour rupture of the membranes at term is defined as spontaneous rupture of the membranes after 37 weeks of gestation and before the onset of regular uterine contractions. In the literature it is often referred to as 'premature rupture of the membranes', but for reasons explained elsewhere (see Chapter 43) we believe 'prelabour rupture' to be a more appropriate expression than 'premature rupture', especially when it occurs at term. The incidence of the condition varies from 6 to 19 per cent of all term births, depending on three major determinants. The most important of these relates to whether the diagnostic criterion is rupture of the membranes before the onset of regular uterine contractions (no matter how long the latent period before contractions begin (Johnson *et al.* 1981; Kappy *et al.* 1979, 1982; Fayez *et al.* 1978; Morales and Lazar 1986), or whether a specified latent period (varying from 1 to 24 hours in different publications) before the onset of contractions has to occur (Lanier *et al.* 1965; Duff *et al.* 1984; Conway *et al.* 1984; Hauth *et al.* 1977; Magos *et al.* 1983; Westergaard *et al.* 1983; Lange *et al.* 1981; Ekman-Ordeberg *et al.* 1985; Schutte *et al.* 1983). Other variables relate to whether the incidences are population-based or hospital-based (most of the studies have been hospital-based), and to the cut-off point between term and preterm gestations, which in different studies varies from 36 to 38 weeks of gestation.

2 Diagnosis

There is no consensus regarding the method of diagnosis of prelabour rupture of membranes, and this subject has been addressed in the allied Chapter on preterm prelabour rupture of the membranes (see Chapter 43). Most authors require that a woman with a history suggestive of prelabour rupture of membranes undergo a speculum examination in which a sterile speculum is inserted into the vagina, avoiding contact with the cervix, to allow visualization of amniotic fluid either as a pool in the posterior vaginal fornix or coming through the cervix on fundal pressure (Johnson *et al.* 1981; Kappy *et al.* 1979, 1982; Fayez *et al.* 1978; Morales and Lazar, 1986; Duff *et al.* 1984; Conway *et al.* 1984; Magos *et al.* 1983; Ekman-Ordeberg *et al.* 1985). In most publications (Kappy *et al.* 1979, 1982; Fayez *et al.* 1978; Conway *et al.* 1984; Ekman-Ordeberg *et al.* 1985), a positive speculum examination is sufficient for the diagnosis to be made. Some authors accept a positive nitrazine test or positive fern test on vaginal fluid if no amniotic fluid is seen in the vagina (Kappy *et al.* 1979, 1982; Fayez *et al.* 1978; Ekman-Ordeberg *et al.* 1985). Others (Johnson *et al.* 1981) require fluid to be seen in the vagina and a positive nitrazine test. Others again (Duff *et al.* 1984) require positive nitrazine and positive fern test results, in addition to fluid being seen. To complete the picture of diversity, Lanier *et al.* (1985) and Schutte *et al.* (1983) performed nitrazine or fern tests on fluid escaping from the vagina without performing a speculum examination. False positive and false negative results can occur with all of these procedures (Friedman and McElin 1969; Smith 1976; Gorodeski *et al.* 1982; see also Chapter 43).

3 Prognosis

Most women with prelabour rupture of membranes at term will go into labour soon after the membranes rupture (Johnson *et al.* 1981; Kappy *et al.* 1979, 1982; Fayez *et al.* 1978; Morales and Lazar 1986; Duff *et al.* 1984; Conway *et al.* 1984). Considering only recent studies (and pooling the results) of the women allowed to go into spontaneous labour, 69 per cent (95 per cent confidence interval 65–73 per cent) will deliver within 24 hours (Kappy *et al.* 1979, 1982; Fayez *et al.* 1978; Morales and Lazar 1986; Duff *et al.* 1984, Conway *et al.* 1984), and 86 per cent (95 per cent confidence interval 82–90 per cent) will do so within 48 hours (Kappy *et al.* 1979, 1982; Morales and Lazar 1986). A remarkably constant 2 to 5 per cent of women will be undelivered after 72 hours (Johnson *et al.* 1981; Kappy *et al.* 1979, 1982; Morales and Lazar, 1986), and roughly the same proportion will remain undelivered after 7 days (Kappy *et al.* 1979, 1982). These women probably represent a high risk group, with serious underlying dystocia. It is possible that these women may have a deficiency in prostaglandin production or in their prostanoid biosynthesis pathway (Keirse *et al.* 1987), which is responsible not only for their failure to go into spontaneous labour, but also for the frequently observed poor progress in cervical dilatation with conventional means of inducing labour.

The main concerns related to prelabour rupture of membranes occurring at term are maternal and neonatal infection and an increased incidence of caesarean section, either because induction of labour fails to achieve sufficient progress in cervical dilatation, or because of decelerations of the fetal heart rate, possibly related to lack of liquor and cord compression, or because of underlying dystocia caused by or resulting from prelabour rupture of the membranes.

Maternal and neonatal infection has been the main complication to worry obstetricians. Indeed, in the early reports, maternal *mortality* was a frequent cause of concern (see reviews by Webb 1967; Gunn *et al.* 1970; Johnson *et al.* 1981; Daikoku *et al.* 1982). With latent periods of more than 24 hours, the incidence of maternal infection in various studies has been reported to range from 10 to 28 per cent (Johnson *et al.* 1981; Lanier *et al.* 1965; Gunn *et al.* 1970; Daikoku *et al.* 1982; Schutte *et al.* 1983). In a review of 6425 women with prelabour rupture of membranes at term delivered at Johns Hopkins Hospital in Baltimore in the United States between 1951 and 1964, Johnson *et al.* (1981) found a perinatal mortality rate of 15 per 1000 among white babies if intrapartum fever was absent, and of 119 per 1000 if it was present; the corresponding figures for non-white babies were 23 per 1000 and 144 per 1000. With intrapartum fever, 80 per cent of the perinatal deaths in whites and 93 per cent of the deaths in non-

whites were stillbirths. The perinatal mortality was greater with latent periods of more than 72 hours.

These studies produced persuasive evidence that prelabour rupture of the membranes at term was associated with maternal and fetal or neonatal infection which resulted in a significant risk of maternal and perinatal mortality. A controlled trial conducted in the 1950s showed that routine prescription of antibiotics in labour was associated with a statistically significant reduction in perinatal mortality (Smith *et al.* 1956). But in the 1960s, two controlled trials of prophylactic antibiotics conducted in both term and preterm pregnancies with prelabour rupture of the membranes (Lebherz *et al.* 1963; Brelje *et al.* 1966; see Chapter 43), which together involved more than 2000 women, failed to show any effect on perinatal mortality.

The changing prognosis of prelabour rupture of the membranes at term in the second half of this century is readily apparent. So are changes in the prognosis for both mother and baby even when intrauterine infection is diagnosed (Koh *et al.* 1979; Yoder *et al.* 1983). Data collected over long periods, some of which include women who delivered more than 20 years ago, are of questionable relevance to current obstetric practice. The maternal deaths mostly occurred in women with prolonged, severe intrauterine infection, who often had inadequate antibiotic therapy judged by today's standards, if they had received any care at all before becoming moribund. Uterine rupture was seen in many of them, either because of underlying, unrecognized dystocia, or because intrauterine infection may predispose to that complication. In more recently conducted studies of prelabour rupture of the membranes at term, maternal mortality is almost unknown, and even perinatal death from infection has become rare (Yoder *et al.* 1983).

4 Care of the woman with prelabour rupture of the membranes at term

4.1 Induction of labour or expectant care?

In the 1950s and 1960s, concern about maternal and fetal infection led to the widespread practice of immediate induction of labour when a diagnosis of prelabour rupture of membranes at term was made (Russell and Anderson 1962; Webster 1969; Gunn *et al.* 1970). Following adoption of this policy, however, concern arose that it led to high caesarean section rates (attributed to 'unreadiness' of the cervix and uterus for labour) and higher rates of infectious morbidity in women undergoing caesarean section than in those delivered vaginally (see Chapter 73). The view thus evolved that a more conservative policy (involving awaiting the spontaneous onset of labour) would result in a higher proportion of vaginal deliveries and a lower rate of infectious maternal morbidity (Kappy *et al.* 1979, 1982; Conway *et al.* 1984).

Although there have been 3 controlled trials comparing an active policy of uterine stimulation with a more conservative approach for the care of women with prelabour rupture of membranes at term, none of these has used formal randomization. In the trial by Duff *et al.* (1984) women were allocated to the different policies according to the day of the week on which they were admitted to hospital (two obstetric teams were responsible for the labour suite on alternate days of the week). Fayez *et al.* (1978) allocated the women under their care by hospital record numbers, and Morales and Lazar (1986) used both day of the week and hospital record number in their allocation to induction of labour or expectant care. In all three of the trials intravenous oxytocin was used for stimulation of uterine contractions. In none of the trials was there any indication that

observers were blinded to the group allocation when assessing maternal and neonatal infection rates.

The data from these trials (Table 64.1) suggest that active management with induction of labour after prelabour rupture of membranes at term leads to an increase in the use of caesarean section for delivery, and an increase in the rate of maternal pelvic infection. The increased incidence of maternal infection in the induced group may have been due to the larger number of caesarean sections and digital vaginal examinations in this group. Morales and Lazar (1986) reported a three-fold higher number of vaginal examinations in women in the induced group than in the control group, and the average interval between the first vaginal examination and delivery in the two groups was 17 hours and 4 hours respectively. The overall rate of serious neonatal infection in the trials was very low (less than 1 per cent), and no differential effects of the two policies were detected (Table 64.1).

Table 64.1 Effect of active management of prelabour rupture of membranes at term on caesarean section rates

Study	EXPT		CTRL		Odds ratio	Graph of odds ratios and confidence intervals						
	n	(%)	n	(%)	(95% CI)	0.01	0.1	0.5	1	2	10	100
Fayez *et al.* (1978)	3/53	(5.66)	2/59	(3.39)	1.69 (0.28–10.13)							
Duff *et al.* (1984)	12/59	(20.34)	5/75	(6.67)	3.40 (1.23–9.45)							
Morales and Lazar (1986)	31/150	(20.67)	11/167	(6.59)	3.39 (1.77–6.49)							
Typical odds ratio (95% confidence interval)					3.20 (1.89–5.40)							

Effect of active management of prelabour rupture of membranes at term on maternal infection

Fayez *et al.* (1978)	4/53	(7.55)	7/59	(11.86)	0.62 (0.18–2.13)							
Duff *et al.* (1984)	9/59	(15.25)	3/75	(4.00)	3.94 (1.20–12.94)							
Morales and Lazar (1986)	18/150	(12.00)	7/167	(4.19)	2.92 (1.29–6.61)							
Typical odds ratio (95% confidence interval)					2.21 (1.22–3.99)							

Effect of active management of prelabour rupture of membranes at term on serious neonatal infection

Fayez *et al.* (1978)	0/53	(0.00)	3/59	(5.08)	0.14 (0.01–1.42)							
Duff *et al.* (1984)	1/59	(1.69)	0/75	(0.00)	9.69 (0.19–99.99)							
Morales and Lazar (1986)	0/150	(0.00)	0/167	(0.00)	1.00 (1.00–1.00)							
Typical odds ratio (95% confidence interval)					0.42 (0.06–3.01)							

None of the trials specifically addressed the questions of the length of labour, analgesia, and the degree of discomfort experienced by the woman. Data on the intervals between rupture of the membranes and delivery in the 2 trials that provided these data for both groups (Duff *et al.* 1984; Morales and Lazar 1986) indicate that the interval was reduced from an average of about 30 hours to about 24 hours. This average gain of 6 hours appears to have been accompanied by a longer duration of labour in the induced group than in the control group. In the trial of Duff *et al.* (1984), women receiving expectant care had a mean (SD) length of labour of 9 (5) hours. The length of labour in the induced group is not stated, but these women delivered on average 25 (12) hours after rupture of the membranes compared with 30 (27) hours in the expectant group. Subtracting the mean intervals between rupture of the membranes and the onset of labour from the mean intervals between membrane rupture and delivery in the trial of Morales and Lazar (1986) provides a duration of labour of 15 hours in the induced group compared with only 6 hours in the group with expectant care.

There is thus some suggestive evidence that the active policy exposes the mother not only to a higher risk of caesarean section and infectious morbidity, but also to a longer and presumably less comfortable labour, without any demonstrated benefit.

4.2 The choice between induction policies

In the light of the evidence that induction of labour in these circumstances has harmful effects, it is ironic that no less than 5 controlled trials have addressed the question of which oxytocic drug should be used to achieve it. Furthermore, these trials leave a number of uncertainties about the extent to which bias was controlled. In 4, the method of random allocation was not stated (Hauth *et al.* 1977; Lange *et al.* 1981; Wester-

gaard *et al.* 1983; Ekman-Ordeberg *et al.* 1985); in the fifth it was based on the woman's hospital number (Magos *et al.* 1983).

As shown in Table 64.2, all 5 trials used the prostaglandin PGE_2. In three of the trials the drug was administered in the form of oral tablets; in 1 trial, as a 3 mg vaginal pessary, repeated after 4 hours if considered necessary; and in the last trial, in a dose of 4 mg administered vaginally in a starch gel. In the control groups of all but 1 of the 5 trials, oxytocin was administered intravenously; in the fifth, the buccal oxytocin derivative, desamino-oxytocin, was used (Table 64.2).

The available evidence, poor as it may be, suggests that, if uterine contractions are to be stimulated at all in the presence of prelabour rupture of membranes at term, the use of prostaglandins rather than oxytocin is less likely to increase the rate of caesarean section (Table 64.3). There was no difference in the incidence of infectious morbidity in either mother or baby across the trials that provided data on these outcomes (Table 64.3).

Differences in the length of labour, or the interval from uterine stimulation to delivery, cannot be adequately assessed from these trials. For example, one of the trials (Hauth *et al.* 1977) showed a statistically significantly shorter interval from membrane rupture to delivery in the prostaglandin group than in the oxytocin group, but prostaglandin treatment was started 3 hours and oxytocin 12 hours after rupture of the membranes.

4.3 Prophylactic antibiotics

The 2 controlled trials of prophylactic antibiotics conducted in the 1960s together involved more than 2000 women with prelabour rupture of the membranes at variable gestational ages, most of whom were at term (Lebherz *et al.* 1963; Brelje *et al.* 1966). These trials, which have been discussed elsewhere (see Chapter 43), utilized antibiotic treatments that would no longer be

Table 64.2 Characteristics of the trials comparing prostaglandin E_2 with oxytocin for induction of labour after prelabour rupture of the membranes

Author and years	Allocation	Number of women PGE₂	Oxytocin	PGE₂ dose and route	Oxytocin dose and route
Hauth *et al.* (1977)	random, not described	50	50	orally 0.5–1.0 mg/hr	intravenous dose?
Lange *et al.* (1981)	random, not described	99	102	orally 0.5–1.5 mg/hr	intravenous up to 45 mU
Westergaard *et al.* (1983)	random, not described	109	84	orally 0.5–1.5 mg/hr	buccal 50 U/30 min
Magos *et al.* (1983)	hospital number	15	21	vaginal 3 mg pessary	intravenous up to 32 mU
Ekman-Ordeberg *et al.* (1985)	random, not described	10	10	vaginal 4 mg in gel	intravenous up to 24 mU

Table 64.3 Effect of prostaglandins vs oxytocin for prelabour rupture of membranes at term on caesarean section

Study	EXPT n	EXPT (%)	CTRL n	CTRL (%)	Odds ratio (95% CI)	Graph of odds ratios and confidence intervals
Hauth et al. (1977)	7/50	(14.00)	11/50	(22.00)	0.58 (0.21–1.61)	
Lange et al. (1981)	0/99	(0.00)	3/102	(2.94)	0.14 (0.01–1.33)	
Westergaard et al. (1983)	6/109	(5.50)	4/84	(4.76)	1.16 (0.32–4.18)	
Magos et al. (1983)	0/15	(0.00)	1/21	(4.76)	0.18 (0.00–9.60)	
Ekman-Ordeberg et al. (1985)	0/10	(0.00)	4/10	(40.00)	0.09 (0.01–0.79)	
Typical odds ratio (95% confidence interval)					0.50 (0.25–1.00)	

Table 64.4 Effect of neonatal prophylactic antibiotics after prelabour ruptured membranes at term on neonatal infection

Study	EXPT n	EXPT (%)	CTRL n	CTRL (%)	Odds ratio (95% CI)	Graph of odds ratios and confidence intervals
Wolf and Olinsky (1976)	0/24	(0.00)	4/25	(16.00)	0.12 (0.02–0.94)	
Typical odds ratio (95% confidence interval)					0.12 (0.02–0.94)	

used. Although they failed to show any effect on the incidence of fetal and neonatal infection, a statistically significant reduction in the incidence of infectious maternal morbidity postpartum was observed after antibiotic prophylaxis. In some centres, this has led to the adoption of policies involving routine administration of antibiotics *after* delivery to women with prolonged rupture of the membranes. Although the utility of this approach has not been addressed in randomized comparisons, it would be worth assessing which women, without overt signs of infection, might benefit from postpartum antibiotic prophylaxis.

One randomized trial has addressed the question of whether prophylactic antibiotics should be given to the baby after birth in women with prolonged prelabour rupture of membranes, some of whom were at term (Table 64.4). Forty-nine infants whose mothers had ruptured membranes for more than 24 hours and who did not have clinical evidence of infection at birth were randomly allocated to a prophylactic antibiotic regime of penicillin and kanamycin, or to a control group. There was some support for the idea that prophylactic antibiotics reduced the risk of infection, but the trial requires replication on a larger sample, with blind assessment of infant outcomes.

5 Conclusions

Evidence from the only reasonably well-controlled studies suggests that stimulation of uterine contractions after prelabour rupture of membranes at term does more harm than good. This applies in particular when oxytocin, rather than prostaglandins, are used to stimulate contractions. These forms of care should not be used other than in the context of appropriately sized, properly randomized trials, in which maternal and infant morbidity is assessed by observers who are unaware of the allocated group. Until this prior question has been addressed satisfactorily, comparisons of different oxytocic treatment regimens are unwarranted unless they also involve comparison with a randomized group receiving no oxytocics.

There may be a role for prophylactic antibiotic administration to mothers, neonates, or both if delivery has occurred more than 24 hours after rupture of the membranes at term. It would be worth assessing in properly controlled trials what women and babies, without overt signs of infection, might benefit from postpartum antibiotic prophylaxis.

References

Brelje MC, Kaltreider DF, Kassir L (1966). The use of vaginal antibiotics in premature rupture of the membranes. Am J Obstet Gynecol, 94: 889–897.

Conway DI, Prendiville WJ, Morris A, Speller DCE, Stirrat GM (1984). Management of spontaneous rupture of the membranes in the absence of labor in primigravid women at term. Am J Obstet Gynecol, 150: 947–951.

Daikoku NH, Kaltreider F, Khouzami VA, Spence M, Johnson JWC (1982). Premature rupture of membranes and spontaneous preterm labour: Maternal endometritis risks. Obstet Gynecol, 59: 13–20.

Duff P, Huff RW, Gibbs RS (1984). Management of premature rupture of membranes and unfavorable cervix in term pregnancy. Obstet Gynecol, 63: 597–702.

Ekman-Ordeberg G, Uldbjerg N, Ulmsten U (1985). Comparison of intravenous oxytocin and vaginal prostaglandin E_2 gel in women with unripe cervixes and premature rupture of the membranes. Obstet Gynecol, 66: 307–310.

Fayez JA, Hasan AA, Jonas HS, Miller GL (1978). Management of premature rupture of the membranes. Obstet Gynecol, 52: 17–21.

Friedman ML, McElin TW (1969). Diagnosis of ruptured fetal membranes. Clinical study and review of literature. Am J Obstet Gynecol, 104: 544–550.

Gorodeski IG, Haimovitz L, Bahari CM (1982). Reevaluation of the pH, ferning and nile blue sulphate staining methods in pregnant women with premature rupture of the fetal membranes. J Perinat Med, 10: 286–292.

Gunn GC, Mishell DR, Morton DG (1970). Premature rupture of the membranes. Am J Obstet Gynecol, 106: 469–483.

Hauth JC, Cunningham FG, Whalley PJ (1977). Early labour initiation with oral PGE_2 after premature rupture of the membranes at term. Obstet Gynecol, 49: 523–526.

Johnson JWC, Daikoku NH, Niebyl JR, Johnson TRB, Khouzami VA, Witter RF (1981). Premature rupture of the membranes and prolonged latency. Obstet Gynecol, 57: 547–556.

Kappy KA, Cetrulo CL, Knuppel RA, Ingardia CJ, Sbarra AJ, Scerbo JC, Mitchell GW (1979). Premature rupture of the membranes: A conservative approach. Am J Obstet Gynecol, 134: 655–661.

Kappy KA, Cetrulo CL, Knuppel RA, Ingardia CJ, Sbarra AJ, Scerbo JC, Mitchell GW (1982). Premature rupture of the membranes at term: A comparison of induced and spontaneous labours. J Reprod Med, 27: 29–33.

Keirse MJNC, Noort W, Erwich JJHM (1987). The role of prostaglandins and prostaglandin synthesis in the pregnant uterus. In: Priming and Induction of Labour by Prostaglandins. 'A State of the Art'. Keirse MJNC, de Koning Gans HJ (eds). Leiden: Boerhaave Committee for Postacademic Medical Education, pp 1–25.

Koh KS, Chan FH, Monfared AH, Ledger WJ, Paul RH (1979). The changing perinatal and maternal outcome in chorioamnionitis. Obstet Gynecol, 53: 730–734.

Lange AP, Secher NJ, Nielsen FH, Pederson GT (1981). Stimulation of labor in cases of premature rupture of the membranes at or near term. Acta Obstet Gynecol Scand, 60: 207–210.

Lanier LR, Scarbrough RW, Fillingim DW, Baker RE (1965). Incidence of maternal and fetal complications with rupture of the membrane before onset of labour. Am J Obstet Gynecol, 93: 398–404.

Lebherz TB, Hellman LP, Madding R, Anctil A, Arje SL (1963). Double-blind study of premature rupture of the membranes. Am J Obstet Gynecol, 87: 218–225.

Magos AL, Noble MCB, Wong Ten Yuen A, Rodeck CH (1983). Controlled study comparing vaginal prostaglandin E_2 pessaries with intravenous oxytocin for the stimulation of labour after spontaneous rupture of the membranes. Br J Obstet Gynaecol, 90: 726–731.

Morales WJ, Lazar AJ (1986). Expectant management of rupture of the membrane at term. South Med J, 79: 955–958.

Russell KP, Anderson GV (1962). The aggressive management of ruptured membranes. Am J Obstet Gynecol, 83: 930–934.

Schutte MF, Treffers PE, Kloosterman GJ, Soepatmi S (1983). Management of premature rupture of membranes: The risk of vaginal examination to the infant. Am J Obstet Gynecol, 146: 395–400.

Smith JA, Jennison RF, Langley FA. (1956). Perinatal infection and perinatal death. Clinical aspects. Lancet, 2: 903–906.

Smith RP (1976). A technic for the detection of rupture of the membranes. A review and preliminary report. Obstet Gynecol, 48: 172–176.

Webb GA (1967). Maternal death associated with premature rupture of the membranes. Am J Obstet Gynecol, 98: 594–601.

Webster A (1969). Management of premature rupture of the fetal membranes. Obstet Gynecol Surv, 24: 485–496.

Westergaard JG, Lange AP, Pederson GT, Secher NJ (1983). Use of oral oxytocics for stimulation of labor in cases of premature rupture of the membranes at term. Acta Obstet Gynecol Scand, 62: 111–116.

Wolf RL, Olinsky A (1976). Prolonged rupture of fetal membranes and neonatal infections. S Afr Med J, 50: 574–576.

Yoder PR, Gibbs RS, Blanco JD, Castaneda YS, St Clair PJ (1983). A prospective, controlled study of maternal and perinatal outcome after intra-amniotic infection at term. Am J Obstet Gynecol, 145: 695–701.

65 Induction of labour after fetal death

Marc J. N. C. Keirse and Humphrey H. H. Kanhai

1 Introduction

The pattern of fetal death has changed dramatically during the past three decades. Thirty years ago, about half of all stillbirths resulted from fetal death during labour (Butler and Alberman 1969). Today, however, more than 80 per cent of the fetuses who die do so before the onset of labour (Macfarlane *et al.* 1986). In addition, although the overall rate of antepartum fetal deaths has declined, those deaths that do occur now tend to occur earlier in pregnancy than previously. In 1958, more than half of all stillbirths occurred after 37 weeks of gestation (Gruenwald 1969). Fetal deaths as late in pregnancy as this are now the exception rather than the rule, the majority now occurring in the preterm and very preterm periods (Rush *et al.* 1976; Kanhai 1981). In our own department, for example, more than 80 per cent of fetal deaths are now diagnosed before 37 weeks, and about half of these have been diagnosed by 28 weeks (Kanhai and Keirse 1986). This shift to a predominance of fetal deaths in earlier gestations has other consequences because the interval between fetal death and delivery is likely to be longer if death occurs earlier in pregnancy. In one series, for example, this interval was longer than 4 weeks in 20 per cent of cases when fetal death occurred between 28 and 32 weeks, but in only 3 per cent if the fetus had died after 38 weeks of gestation (Grandin and Hall 1960).

These shifts in the occurrence of fetal death from the intrapartum toward the antepartum period, and from late pregnancy toward midpregnancy have major consequences for care. Fetal death now occurs at a time when the expected end of pregnancy is still a long way off and the onset of spontaneous labour after fetal death (the timing of which was always difficult to predict with confidence in individual cases) is more likely to be delayed than in previous times.

2 Diagnosis

Because women are now more involved in their care during pregnancy, fetal death is suspected and brought to medical attention earlier than used to be the case. The means of confirming the diagnosis have also improved. In the past, confirmation of suspected fetal death depended on radiological signs and tests such as urinary oestrogen or gonadotrophin excretion, all of which had significant error rates and required an appropriate delay after fetal demise in order to be conclusive. Schulman *et al.* (1979), for example, reported that plasma progesterone levels in 65 women carrying a dead fetus for periods from 3 days to 8 weeks were within the normal range for gestation, averaging about 80 per cent of the mean observed in normal pregnancies.

In the past, those obstetricians who were sceptical about a test result suggesting that the baby was dead were sometimes rewarded by the birth of a live infant. Less prudent clinicians, who induced labour on the basis of test results, sometimes found themselves delivering live infants who subsequently died from immaturity or other complications of unwarranted elective delivery (Fawzy and Basiony 1979).

Accurate diagnosis of fetal death is obviously a fundamental prerequisite for effective care of the woman with suspected fetal death. This has been made considerably easier with the introduction of real time ultrasound. Ultrasound visualization of the pulsating fetal heart provides a secure basis for rejecting a tentative diagnosis of fetal death. Failure to observe such pulsation is not, however, an infallible way of confirming suspected fetal death. Failure to observe heart wall motion and valvular function on ultrasound is sometimes, albeit rarely, followed by 'reversion' to normal and the birth of a live infant which had been presumed to be dead (Pitkin 1987).

We have found it wise to insist that the diagnosis of fetal death should only be made if two experienced observers concur, either after a sufficiently long and careful single ultrasound examination, or after two separate examinations. Women readily accept the sometimes longer periods of uncertainty that result from this cautious approach if the reasons for these precautions have been explained to them. On the rare occasions when fetal death is suspected it is quite unacceptable to leave the examination to an inexperienced ultrasonographer, or one who has no mandate to communicate the diagnosis to the mother.

Once the diagnosis has been made, women should have the opportunity to adapt to it. Rushed decisions at this time are unnecessary. On the contrary, women should be given time to consider the options and to decide what they want. They must be allowed the time to grieve and make decisions within the environment in which they feel most secure. Most women will want to return home, even if only for a brief period. It is important to remember to ask the woman how she arrived at the hospital or clinic for the ultrasound examination. She should not have to drive at such a time, or go home unescorted. Allowing a woman to leave alone and unescorted after confirmation of an intrauterine fetal death amounts to negligent practice.

3 Choosing between active and expectant care

Ideally, the choice between active intervention to end pregnancy and the expectant approach (awaiting spontaneous labour) should be based on unbiased comparisons of the relative merits of these two approaches. Such data are not available, however. From a somatic point of view, and given appropriate means to induce labour after fetal death, there are no overwhelming benefits or hazards for either one of these two broad approaches to care. Both the advantages and the disadvantages of the active and the expectant policies relate almost exclusively to emotional and psychological aspects. As the woman herself is the best judge of these, she should be the one to make the choice. Her care-

givers should assist her by providing her with the information she needs in order to make an informed choice, and ensure that whatever option she chooses is implemented with as little psychological and physical discomfort as possible.

It is incorrect to assume that all women desire the most rapid method of delivery when intrauterine fetal death has occurred. For some, learning of the death is the worst moment; carrying the dead fetus *in utero* still permits a closeness of mother and baby that will be lost once delivery occurs. Many, on the other hand, are anxious to proceed at once to delivery of the baby. Some may even suggest that this should be done by caesarean section. A decision by the caregiver to induce labour, if made with little consultation or input by the woman and her partner, may be seen by the parents as a way of compensating for guilt, or as the search for a quick solution. Discussing the facts and alternatives with the woman and her partner conveys compassion and understanding. Often it will help to defuse initial feelings of anger, suspicion, inadequacy and guilt, which are typically felt by all, caregivers and women alike, after such a disastrous finding.

The main advantage of the expectant option is the absence of any need for intervention. The woman can stay at home, and she will avoid procedures that might turn out to be less effective and more risky than anticipated. Some women, although probably only a small minority, feel that a continuation of the closeness with the baby even after it has died is meaningful to them, and they prefer to let nature take its course.

Disadvantages of the expectant option are mainly emotional and relate to the unpredictable and usually long time during which the woman may have to carry the dead baby. Sometimes, she or her relatives may be under the impression that the baby may rot inside her and exude toxins that can poison her. It is obviously important to attempt to dispel such fears, but their emotional impact will not necessarily be lost. Other disadvantages of expectant care relate to the process of maceration that starts after fetal death. Not only may this result in the stillborn baby being more unsightly and therefore possibly more distressing to the parents, it may also render the autopsy findings and chromosome analysis less informative that they would otherwise have been. This latter consequence may be a handicap in trying to establish the cause of death to provide a basis for effective counselling for a subsequent pregnancy.

The only real somatic hazard of the expectant policy relates to a possible increase in the risk of disturbances in blood coagulation. These are most likely to occur when fetal death has been caused by placental abruption, and retention of the dead fetus virtually never occurs under these circumstances (Grandin and Hall 1960; Csapo 1977). Not only are disorders of coagulation rare in association with other causes of fetal death, the hypofibrinogenaemia that is held to be responsible for these disorders occurs very slowly and is rarely clinically significant in the first four to five weeks after fetal death (Pritchard 1959). By the time that clinically significant alterations in coagulation mechanisms have occurred, the chances are that delivery will have supervened (Tricomi and Kohl 1957; Grandin and Hall 1960).

The only advantage of an active policy to effect delivery in the care of women with a dead fetus is that they can be offered the option of ending a pregnancy that has lost its purpose. Its advantage is therefore entirely of a psychological and emotional nature. The disadvantages of an active policy relate to the means through which it is effected. If the policy is implemented by caesarean section, its hazards will largely outweigh its benefits (see Chapter 70). It is an option, however, that some women may request soon after the diagnosis of fetal death has been made as a quick way to resolve a terrible situation; it is not always readily apparent to them why this 'quick fix' is inappropriate. If induction of labour is considered, the efficacy and safety of the particular method selected will be the most influential factor in considering the relative merits of the policy. If the policy is effected by judicious use of an appropriate prostaglandin preparation, the risks are not likely to be greater than those associated with elective delivery in an otherwise uncomplicated pregnancy.

4 Choice of methods for inducing labour

Before prostaglandins became available, attempts to induce labour after fetal death sometimes turned into iatrogenic nightmares because of the unreliability and the risks of the available methods (Keirse 1982a). The older literature contains examples of women that failed to deliver in spite of repeated attempts over the course of anything up to two years (Donald 1969). The methods used included oestrogen administration (Martin and Menzies 1955), intra-amniotic injection of hypertonic solutions (Courtney *et al.* 1971), and high doses of oxytocin (Loudon 1959; Liggins 1962; Ursell 1972). Discouraged by oestrogen administration (which was aptly described as 'playing for time') and a number of maternal deaths attributed to hypertonic intrauterine instillations (Donald 1969), most obstetricians have tended to rely on high doses of oxytocin, if they were at all inclined to pursue elective delivery. Effective doses of oxytocin nearly always led to some degree of water retention (Liggins 1962), and the infusions often had to be stopped and then repeated after a suitable delay. Instead of diminishing emotional anguish, the procedure thus often aggravated it, leaving the woman exasperated and exhausted after every failed attempt to induce labour.

4.1 Natural prostaglandins

The availability of natural prostaglandins, first used for this indication by Karim in 1970, dramatically changed the prospects for inducing labour after intrauterine fetal death. Within a decade of their introduction, cumulative clinical experience with the administration of prostaglandins for this indication extended to more than 1500 women included in over 50 published reports (Karim *et al.* 1979; Keirse 1982a). Although all of these studies were reports of case series with no formal controls, they indicated the overwhelming superiority of prostaglandins compared with previously available methods to induce labour after fetal death.

A summary of these studies is presented in Table 65.1. This shows that successful induction (vaginal delivery following a single course of treatment) was achieved in 95 per cent of cases or more, irrespective of the prostaglandin used and the dose in which it was administered. The doses used have varied considerably, some authors reporting mean doses more than 10 times higher than those reported by others using the same

Table 65.1 Cumulative experience with the natural prostaglandins, PGE_2 and $PGF_{2\alpha}$, for induction of labour after intrauterine fetal death in the first decade of their introduction for that purpose (based on review of the literature from 1970 to 1979 after Keirse 1982b)

Prostaglandin and route of administration	Number of women	Success		Mean dose (mg)		Mean interval (hr:min)		
		No.	Percent	Lowest	Highest	Median	Lowest	Highest
Intravenous PGE_2	269	255	94.8	0.58 –	7.3	11:22	7:42 –	17:26
Intravenous $PGF_{2\alpha}$	174	166	95.4	8.7 –	52.3	9·20	7:00 –	19:15
Extra-amniotic PGE_2	115	112	97.4	0.45 –	3.8	8:48	7:06 –	17:12
Extra-amniotic $PGF_{2\alpha}$	41	40	97.6	3.5 –	120.0	12:00	10:12 –	15:44
Intra-amniotic $PGF_{2\alpha}$	86	85	98.8	5.6 –	78.3	10:50	8:22 –	10:57
Vaginal PGE_2	899	872	97.0	26.0 –	90.0	9:50	6:18 –	19.15
Total	1584	1530	96.6				6:18 –	19:15

route of administration (Table 65.1). The mean intervals between induction of labour and fetal death in all of the case series that included at least 6 women ranged from just over 6 hours to almost 20 hours (Table 65.1). The medians of these means, calculated for the two prostaglandins (PGE$_2$ and PGF$_{2\alpha}$) administered by the same route, showed no consistent differences (Table 65.1). In keeping with the higher uterotonic propensity of PGE$_2$ (see Chapter 62), the doses of PGE$_2$ and PGF$_{2\alpha}$ were, of course, markedly different. Nor do these data indicate that one route of administration is markedly inferior or superior to others in terms of achieving delivery, or in terms of the mean intervals between induction of labour and delivery reported in the various studies that have documented their use (Table 65.1).

The impression gained from these and other studies has been that labour is more readily induced by natural prostaglandins after the fetus has died, than when the fetus is alive at comparable gestational age (Luengo *et al.* 1977; Karim *et al.* 1979; Schulman *et al.* 1979; Wallenburg *et al.* 1980; Keirse 1982a). In the absence of controlled comparisons between the various dose regimens and routes of administration of prostaglandins for inducing labour after fetal death, conclusions need to be derived from a careful assessment of whatever other evidence is available.

Intravenous administration, although undoubtedly efficacious at infusion rates of 0.25 to 4 µg PGE$_2$ or 2.5 to 40 µg PGF$_{2\alpha}$ per minute, titrated according to the myometrial response, has now largely been superseded because of a relatively high incidence of side-effects in comparison with local routes of administration. Experience with intra-amniotic administration has been limited and was mostly gathered in the early days of clinical prostaglandin research. When the fetus has died it is often difficult to identify a clear amniotic pool in which to administer the drug, or impossible to obtain a sample of clear fluid to guarantee that the right compartment has been found. This and post-mortem changes in the fetal membranes (that render the degree of absorption of the drug into the myometrium and into the maternal circulation rather unpredictable) mean that intra-amniotic administration is probably one of the least suitable approaches.

Vaginal administration of PGE$_2$, usually in the form of 20 mg suppositories, is probably the most widely used approach nowadays because of its convenience and ease of administration. For it to have any effect on the uterus, absorption into the circulation is necessary. Consequently there is a high rate of the undesirable side-effects that are characteristic of all systemic administrations of large doses of prostaglandins. In one large multicentre survey (Southern *et al.* 1978), for example, of 709 women treated with PGE$_2$ suppositories after fetal death, 56 per cent reported vomiting, 43 per cent had diarrhoea, 22 per cent experienced chills

and shivering, and 40 per cent had a temperature rise above 38.1 °C. Fear of an infectious process may well lead to unwarranted antibiotic treatment in these cases of pyrexia, particularly since it is not universally known that prostaglandin administration also increases leucocytosis and effects differential cell counts, resulting in a relative increase in neutrophils and a relative decrease in lymphocytes (Keirse and Bennebroek Gravenhorst 1977; Wallenburg *et al.* 1980). The frequency of side-effects observed in the large survey reported by Southern and his colleagues (1978) cited above is reflected in the results of other, smaller surveys reporting on the use of vaginal PGE$_2$ suppositories for induction of labour after fetal death (Kent and Goldstein 1976; Lauersen and Wilson 1977; Scher *et al.* 1980; Kanhai and Keirse 1986). In addition to the high incidence of associated side-effects, vaginal PGE$_2$ administration has the additional disadvantage that rupture of the membranes or bleeding early during treatment may interfere with the administration and absorption of subsequent doses of the drug.

Extra-amniotic administration of natural prostaglandins, either by continuous infusion using 1- to 2-hourly injections through an indwelling (Foley type) catheter, or by administration in a viscous gel, appears to produce the lowest incidence of systemic, particularly gastrointestinal, side-effects (Karim *et al.* 1979; Scher *et al.* 1980). The method requires insertion of a catheter into the extra-amniotic space, however, which in addition to being bothersome for the woman and limiting her freedom of movement during labour, carries an undetermined risk of introducing infection, and requires some experience in order to avoid rupture of the membranes and premature expulsion of the catheter. These complications occur in a sizable minority of cases and may require administration of additional oxytocic agents, such as intravenous oxytocin or prostaglandins administered by another route, to ensure completion of the induction process.

When intrauterine fetal death occurs in late pregnancy, which applies to only a minority of all cases of fetal death before labour, it will usually be possible to induce labour with any one of the prostaglandin regimens that are employed for other inductions. This is an important consideration as the experience of individual clinicians with elective delivery of dead fetuses is likely to be limited. Methods with which one is thoroughly accustomed tend to perform better than those that are only rarely needed and require careful study before being applied. This is of little help, however, at the earlier gestational ages when the sensitivity of the uterus to prostaglandins is much lower than it is at term. At these stages of pregnancy the choice between the various routes for administering natural prostaglandins is not easy; despite their efficacy in inducing labour and delivery, they all have several drawbacks.

4.2 Prostaglandin analogues

Soon after the clinical use of prostaglandins became a practical proposition, great efforts were directed at the synthesis of structurally modified analogues, which might overcome some of the drawbacks of the natural compounds. A great variety of such compounds has been synthesized. Many of them have been clinically tested for termination of pregnancy (Amy 1982; Keirse 1982b); some of them have been applied to the induction of labour after intrauterine fetal death (Karim and Ratnam 1976; Ylikorkala *et al.* 1976; Karim *et al.* 1979; Fawzy and Basioni 1979). None of these or any subsequent studies have been formally controlled comparisons either between natural prostaglandins or prostaglandin analogues or between various prostaglandin analogues, although a few studies using historical or contemporary non-randomized controls within the same institution have been reported (Keirse and Bennebroek Gravenhorst 1977; Gruber and Baumgarten 1980; Keirse and Lobatto 1983).

These analogues are not suitable for induction of labour with a live fetus, first, because toxicity studies are inadequate to judge the possible effects of these synthetic substances and their metabolites on infant development and, second, because their longer half-life makes them more prone to cause uterine hyperstimulation that may be hazardous to a live fetus. For the induction of labour after fetal death, they offer a number of potential advantages, however. Their longer duration of action results in less need for continuous administration, thus permitting intermittent doses and alternative routes of administration. This does not necessarily mean that the incidence of side-effects will be reduced; for this to be achieved there needs to be a differential effect in potency on different organ systems. A general increase in potency merely implies, as demonstrated in practice (Wiqvist *et al.* 1972), that both effects and side-effects occur at a lower dose. However, some of these analogues, especially the multi-substituted prostaglandin E$_2$ analogue, 16-phenoxy-17,18,19,20-tetranor-methylsulphonylamide (sulprostone), exhibit greater utero-selectivity than the parent compound from which they have been derived (Hess *et al.* 1979).

Only two prostaglandin PGF$_{2\alpha}$ analogues have been reported to be used on a wider scale than that of small observational studies to explore their effects. Both, 15(S),15-methyl-PGF$_{2\alpha}$ and 2a,2b-dihomo-15(S),15-methyl-PGF$_{2\alpha}$ methyl ester, were found to have a high efficacy for inducing labour after fetal death with success rates of 98 per cent or more and mean induction to delivery intervals of less than 12 hours in series which involved at least 50 women each (Karim and Ratnam 1976; De Gezelle *et al.* 1980; Wallenburg *et al.* 1980; Karim *et al.* 1982). The incidence of gastrointestinal side-effects, on the other hand, has been very high,

particularly with 15(S),15-methyl-PGF$_{2\alpha}$. From the studies that have been conducted it is not clear, however, whether or not the drugs were used at optimal doses. Doses have usually been derived from experience gathered in 2nd-trimester abortions, and there is some evidence that the dose response relationships that apply in these circumstances may not be applicable to the induction of labour after fetal death. For instance, Wallenburg and his colleagues (1980) reported on a multicentre study conducted in The Netherlands in which two consecutive series of women had labour induced because of fetal death with either 250 μg or 125 μg 15(S),15-methyl-PGF$_{2\alpha}$ administered intramuscularly every 2 hours. The lower dose was as effective as the higher dose in inducing labour, and side-effects occurred with comparable frequency in association with the two regimens (of 52 women receiving the lower dose, 48 per cent experienced vomiting and 62 per cent diarrhoea; of the 45 women receiving the higher dose, 56 per cent vomited and 56 per cent had diarrhoea (Wallenburg *et al.* 1980).

Results obtained with the PGE$_2$ analogue, sulprostone, appear to be superior to those obtained with the PGF$_{2\alpha}$ analogues, although no formal comparisons between the drugs have been reported. Comparative studies that have been reported have used historical controls (Keirse and Lobatto 1983), and are therefore prone to bias. From the available literature, however, it is clear that the incidence of side-effects, most notably vomiting and diarrhoea, is considerably lower with sulprostone than with any of the PGF$_{2\alpha}$ analogues. This is likely to be due to the greater utero-selectivity of this compound (Hess *et al.* 1979), but may also to some extent reflect the fact that the parent compound PGE$_2$, when given in large equipotent doses (as required, for instance, in 2nd-trimester abortion) also produces less gastrointestinal side-effects than PGF$_{2\alpha}$.

Sulprostone, although suitable for both intravenous and intramuscular administration, is probably best administered intravenously. The optimal dose schedules for either intravenous or intramuscular administration after intrauterine fetal death have not been clearly established, however; as for the PGF$_{2\alpha}$ analogues discussed above, dose schedules have been constructed on the basis of experience with 2nd-trimester abortions.

In an attempt to provide more rationally based and formally evaluated treatment regimens for the induction of labour after fetal death, a multicentre trial was conducted in which women in the participating centres were assigned to two different treatment groups by centralized telephone randomization (Kanhai and Keirse 1989). One group was assigned to receive a continuous intravenous infusion of 1 μg sulprostone per minute; the other group was assigned to receive an infusion of 3 μg per minute for 8 hours, until the

Table 65.2 Effect of low dose vs. high dose sulprostone for induction of labour after fetal death on vomiting

Study	EXPT		CTRL		Odds ratio	Graph of odds ratios and confidence intervals						
	n	(%)	*n*	(%)	(95% CI)	0.01	0.1	0.5	1	2	10	100
Kanhai and Keirse (1989)	8/43	(18.60)	16/42	(38.10)	0.39 (0.15–0.99)							
Typical odds ratio (95% confidence interval)					0.39 (0.15–0.99)							

Effect of low dose vs. high dose sulprostone for induction of labour after fetal death on diarrhoea

Kanhai and Keirse (1989)	1/43	(2.33)	6/42	(14.29)	0.21 (0.04–0.97)							
Typical odds ratio (95% confidence interval)					0.21 (0.04–0.97)							

Effect of low dose vs. high dose sulprostone for induction of labour after fetal death on pyrexia

Kanhai and Keirse (1989)	2/43	(4.65)	7/42	(16.67)	0.29 (0.07–1.13)							
Typical odds ratio (95% confidence interval)					0.29 (0.07–1.13)							

Effect of low dose vs. high dose sulprostone for induction of labour after fetal death on use of epidural analgesia

Kanhai and Keirse (1989)	7/43	(16.28)	8/42	(19.05)	0.83 (0.27–2.51)							
Typical odds ratio (95% confidence interval)					0.83 (0.27–2.51)							

Effect of low dose vs. high dose sulprostone for induction of labour after fetal death on not delivered within 12 hours

Kanhai and Keirse (1989)	23/43	(53.49)	21/42	(50.00)	1.15 (0.49–2.68)							
Typical odds ratio (95% confidence interval)					1.15 (0.49–2.68)							

Effect of low dose vs. high dose sulprostone for induction of labour after fetal death on not delivered within 24 hours

Kanhai and Keirse (1989)	4/43	(9.30)	8/42	(19.05)	0.45 (0.13–1.52)							
Typical odds ratio (95% confidence interval)					0.45 (0.13–1.52)							

Effect of low dose vs. high dose sulprostone for induction of labour after fetal death on not delivered within 36 hours

Kanhai and Keirse (1989)	1/43	(2.33)	1/42	(2.38)	0.98 (0.06–15.88)							
Typical odds ratio (95% confidence interval)					0.98 (0.06–15.88)							

Effect of low dose vs. high dose sulprostone for induction of labour after fetal death on manual removal of the placenta

Kanhai and Keirse (1989)	14/43	(32.56)	16/42	(38.10)	0.79 (0.32–1.91)							
Typical odds ratio (95% confidence interval)					0.79 (0.32–1.91)							

Table 65.2—*continued* Effect of low dose vs. high dose sulprostone for induction of labour after fetal death on blood loss > 500 ml

Study	EXPT n	(%)	CTRL n	(%)	Odds ratio (95% CI)	Graph of odds ratios and confidence intervals
Kanhai and Keirse (1989)	5/43	(11.63)	3/42	(7.14)	1.68 (0.40–7.15)	
Typical odds ratio (95% confidence interval)					1.68 (0.40–7.15)	

maximum dose of 1500 µg per 24 hours was reached, which if necessary could be repeated the next day. The latter, higher dosage regimen had been the one recommended by the manufacturer and used in previous studies for inducing labour after fetal death. Both vomiting and diarrhoea were statistically significantly less frequent with the lower dose regimen, and the incidence of pyrexia followed a similar trend (Table 65.2). This reduction in side-effects was not achieved at the cost of any lengthening of the induction to delivery interval, or an increased incidence of placental retention or excessive bleeding (Table 65.2). The lower dose regimen also resulted in a reduction of costs: 32 of the 43 women (74 per cent) assigned to the low dose did not require more than 2 ampoules (500 µg each) and 39 (91 per cent) required less than 3 ampoules. In the high dose group these figures were respectively 4 (10 per cent) and 12 (29 per cent) of 42 women.

5 Care during labour and delivery

Care for the woman with a dead fetus does not stop once a decision to induce labour has been reached, nor with the choice of drugs to implement the policy. Irrespective of whether labour is induced or occurs spontaneously, several elements of care will require extra attention above and beyond that which applies to all labours and deliveries.

Although it should be possible to ensure that pain is controlled during labour, the side-effects of the drugs used to induce labour may be very distressing and exacerbate the psychological distress which will have resulted from confirmation of the fetal death. This makes the need for psychological support all the more crucial in these circumstances, and women with a dead fetus should never be left alone in labour (see Chapter 49).

The delivery of the stillborn baby should be conducted with all the care that is appropriate during the delivery of a living infant. For the mother, her baby has been a living person, and she will expect him or her to be treated with the dignity and respect that is accorded to other persons (see Chapter 85).

6 Conclusions

6.1 Implications for current practice

Ultrasound is the definitive method for diagnosing intrauterine fetal death, but the diagnosis should only be made if two experienced observers concur after a sufficiently intensive examination. The diagnosis, once confirmed, should be communicated to the woman at once. Women should be allowed time to adapt to the reality of the diagnosis and should then be offered the choice of induction of labour or expectant care. Neither form of care should expose her to somatic risks, and the decision should be made on the psychological and emotional grounds of which the woman herself is the best judge.

If induction of labour is chosen, this should be implemented with the use of a prostaglandin or a prostaglandin analogue. Thus far and regrettable as it may be, the choice of the particular compound and its route of administration will often depend, not on what is considered to be ideal, but on what is available in a particular country. In the later weeks of pregnancy the most effective method is likely to be the method of which the caregiver has adequate experience from inducing labour in other pregnancies. Earlier in gestation, prostaglandin analogues (sulprostone in particular) if available, constitute the treatment of choice. Where such compounds are not available, a natural prostaglandin can be used by any one of a variety of routes, none of which will be ideal. Our preference is for extra-amniotic administration, although there are no formal comparisons to justify this judgement.

6.2 Implications for future research

The introduction of natural prostaglandins and prostaglandin analogues for inducing labour after fetal death represented an important advance over the very unsatisfactory options that were previously available. Although this judgement could be made confidently without carefully controlled trials, it is necessary (and obviously feasible) to mount multicentre randomized trials to assess the relative merits of different prostaglandins and prostaglandin analogues in this situation. There is still considerable scope for developing preparations, routes of administration, and dosage schedules which minimize the unpleasantness for women of a labour which is destined to end with the birth of a dead

References

Amy JJ (1982). Termination of second trimester pregnancy with prostaglandin analogues. In: Second Trimester Pregnancy Termination. Keirse MJNC, Bennebroek Gravenhorst J, Van Lith DAF, Embrey MP (eds). The Hague: Leiden University Press, pp 115–131.

Butler NR, Alberman ED (1969). Perinatal Problems. Edinburgh: Churchill Livingstone.

Courtney LD, Boxall RR, Child P (1971). Permeability of membranes of dead fetus. Br Med J, 1: 492–493.

Csapo AI (1977). The 'see-saw' theory of parturition. In: The Fetus and Birth. Ciba Foundation Symposium No. 47. Amsterdam: Elsevier, pp 159–195.

De Gezelle H, Thiery M, Parewijck W, Decoster JM (1980). Prostaglandin F_{2a} for interrupting pregnancy, managing intrauterine death and molar pregnancy and induced labor. Int J Gynaecol Obstet, 17: 362–367.

Donald I (1969). Practical Obstetric Problems. London: Lloyd-Luke.

Fawzy A, Basioni BA (1979). The use of sulprostone in the management of death in utero and molar pregnancy. Singapore J Obstet Gynaecol, 10: 39–42.

Grandin DJ, Hall RE (1960). Fetal death before the onset of labor. An analysis of 407 cases. Am J Obstet Gynecol, 79: 237–243.

Gruber WS, Baumgarten K (1980). Intravenous prostaglandin E_2 methyl sulfonamide for induction of fetal death in utero. Am J Obstet Gynecol, 137: 8–14.

Gruenwald P (1969) Stillbirth and early neonatal death. In: Perinatal Problems. Butler NR, Alberman ED (eds). Edinburgh: Churchill Livingstone, pp 163–183.

Hess HJ, Schaaf TK, Bindra JS, Johnson MR, Constantine JW (1979). Structure-activity considerations leading to sulprostone. In: International Sulprostone Symposium. Friebel K, Schneider A, Wurfel H (eds). Berlin: Schering, pp 29–37.

Kanhai HHH (1981). Achtergronden en konsekwenties van vroeggeboorte. Leiden University: MD thesis.

Kanhai HHH, Keirse MJNC (1986). Beëindiging van de zwangerschap na foetale sterfte antepartum. In: Prostaglandines in de Verloskunde en Gynaecologie. Keirse MJNC (ed). Amsterdam: Excerpta Medica, pp 100–118.

Kanhai HHH, Keirse MJNC (1989). Induction of labour after fetal death: A randomized controlled trial of two prostaglandin regimens. Br J Obstet Gynaecol, 96: 1400–1404.

Karim SMM (1970). The use of prostaglandin E_2 in the management of missed abortion, missed labour and hydatiform mole. Br Med J, 3: 196–197.

Karim SMM, Ratnam SS (1976). Termination of abnormal intrauterine pregnancies with intramuscular administration of dihomo-15-methyl prostaglandin F_{2a}. Br J Obstet Gynaecol, 83: 885–889.

Karim SMM, Lim AL, Prasad RNV, Yeo KC, Ng SC, Salmon YM, Choo HT, Ratman SS (1979a). Termination of abnormal intrauterine pregnancy with intramuscular administration of sulprostone. Singapore J Obstet Gynaecol, 10: 33–37.

Karim SMM, Ng SC, Ratman SS (1979b). Termination of abnormal intrauterine pregnancy with prostaglandins. In: Practical Applications of Prostaglandins and their Synthesis Inhibitors. Karim SMM (ed). Lancaster: MTP Press, 319–374.

Karim SMM, Ratman SS, Hutabarat H, Hanafiah J, Simanjuntak P, Teoh SK, Ong SK, Sen DK, Sinathuray TA (1982). Termination of pregnancy in cases of intrauterine fetal death, missed abortion, molar and anencephalic pregnancy with intramuscular administration of 2a,2b-dihomo-15(S)-15-methyl-PGF_{2a}-methyl ester—a multicenter study. Ann Acad Med (Singapore), 11: 508–512.

Keirse MJNC (1979). Epidemiology of pre-term labour. In: Human Parturition. Keirse MJNC, Anderson ABM, Bennebroek Gravenhorst J (eds). The Hague: Leiden University Press, pp 219–234.

Keirse MJNC (1982a). Termination of pregnancy after intrauterine fetal death. In: Second Trimester Pregnancy Termination. Keirse MJNC, Bennebroek Gravenhorst J, Van Lith DAF, Embrey MP (eds). The Hague: Leiden University Press, pp 138–154.

Keirse MJNC (1982b) Current status of prostaglandins for termination of pregnancy. J Drug Res, 7: 1359–1366.

Keirse MJNC, Bennebroek Gravenhorst J (1977). Het inleiden van de baring bij intra-uteriene vruchtdood. Ned Tijdschr Geneeskd, 123: 1195–1199.

Keirse MJNC, Lobatto R (1983). Synthetische prostaglandine analoga voor het inleiden van de baring bij intrauteriene vruchtdood. J Drug Res, 8: 1561–1566.

Kent DR, Goldstein AI (1976). Prostaglandin E_2 induction of labor for fetal demise. Obstet Gynecol, 48: 475–478.

Lauersen NH, Wilson KH (1977). Induction of labor in patients with missed abortion and fetal death in utero with prostaglandin E_2 suppositories. Am J Obstet Gynecol, 127: 609–611.

Liggins GC (1962). The treatment of missed abortion by high dosage Syntocinon intravenous infusion. J Obstet Gynaecol Br Commnwlth, 69: 227–281.

Loudon JDO (1959). The use of high concentration oxytocin intravenous drips in the management of missed abortion. J Obstet Gynaecol Br Empire, 66: 277–281.

Luengo J, Keirse MJNC, Bennebroek Gravenhorst J (1977). Extra-amniotic prostaglandin F_{2a} for intra-uterine death and fetal abnormality. Eur J Obstet Gynecol Reprod Biol, 7: 325–329.

Macfarlane A, Cole S, Hey E (1986). Comparison of data from regional perinatal mortality surveys. Br J Obstet Gynaecol, 93: 1224–1232.

Martin RH, Menzies DN (1955). Oestrogen therapy in missed abortion and labour. J Obstet Gynaecol Br Empire, 62: 256–258.

Pitkin RM (1987) Fetal death: diagnosis and management. Am J Obstet Gynecol, 157: 583–589.

Pritchard JA (1959). Fetal death in utero. Obstet Gynecol, 14: 593–580.

Rush RW, Keirse MJNC, Howat P, Baum JD, Anderson ABM, Turnbull AC (1976). Contribution of preterm delivery to perinatal mortality. Br Med J, 2: 965–968.

Scher J, Jeng DY, Moshirpur J, Kerenyi TD (1980). A comparison between vaginal prostaglandin E₂ suppositories and intrauterine extra-amniotics prostaglandins in the management of fetal death in utero. Am J Obstet Gynecol, 137: 769–772.

Schulman H, Saldana L, Lin CC, Randolph G (1979). Mechanism of failed labor after fetal death and its treatment with prostglandin E₂. Am J Obstet Gynecol, 133: 742–752.

Southern EM, Gutknecht GD, Mohberg NR, Edelman DA (1978). Vaginal prostaglandin E₂ in the management of fetal intrauterine death. Br J Obstet Gynaecol, 85: 437–441.

Tricomi V, Kohl SG (1957). Fetal death in utero. Am J Obstet Gynecol, 74: 1092–1097.

Ursell W (1972). Induction of labour following fetal death. J Obstet Gynaecol Br Commnwlth, 79: 260–264.

Wallenburg HCS, Keirse MJNC, Freie HMP, Blacquiére JF (1980). Intramuscular administration of 15(S)-15-methyl prostaglandin F₂ₐ for induction of labour in patients with fetal death. Br J Obstet Gynaecol, 87: 203–209.

Wiqvist N, Béguin F, Bygdeman M, Toppozada M (1972). Recent aspects on systemic administration of prostaglandin. In: The Prostaglandins—Clinical Applications in Human Reproduction. Southern EM (ed). Mount Kisco: Futura, pp 295–306.

Ylikorkala O, Kirkinen P, Jarvinen PA (1976). Intramuscular administration of 15-methyl-prostaglandin F₂ₐ for induction of labour in patients with intrauterine fetal death or an anencephalic fetus. Br J Obstet Gynaecol, 83: 502–504.

Part VIII

Care during labour

66 Care during the second stage of labour

Jennifer Sleep, Joyce Roberts, and Iain Chalmers

1 Introduction

In some respects it is undesirable to separate consideration of care during delivery from care during the first stage of labour. The foundation for effective care during the second stage of labour—confidence of the mother in those providing care—should have been created earlier in labour, and preferably during pregnancy. Nevertheless, the second stage is a period during which the whole tempo and nature of activities surrounding labour tend to change. It is a time when women may become vulnerable and dependent on the influence of those who assist them. Discussion about aspects of care is not easy at this time, and this reality leaves the caregiver with even more than usual responsibility to safeguard the interests of the mother and baby.

2 Diagnosis of the onset of the second stage

By definition, the second stage of labour, which ends with the birth of the baby, begins when the cervix is fully dilated. This 'anatomical' onset may or may not coincide with the onset of the expulsion phase, when the mother begins to feel the urge to bear down. In up to two-thirds of women, the urge to bear down occurs before the cervix is fully dilated (Roberts *et al.* 1987).

The mother herself may signal the transition into the expulsive phase, sometimes in words, sometimes by action, sometimes by a change in the expression on her face, or in the way she may squeeze her companion's hand. If the presenting part is visible at the introitus, full dilatation is easily confirmed. If the mother feels that she wishes to start pushing when the progress of labour up to that point gives reason to believe that the cervix may not be fully dilated, it is often appropriate to check cervical dilatation. If, as is sometimes the case (particularly in nulliparae), the cervix is only 6 or 7 cm dilated, the woman should be asked to try to find the position in which she feels most comfortable and able to resist the urge to push. If there is only a rim of cervix left and the woman has an irresistible urge to push, however, she may feel better doing so, and it is unlikely that any harm will come from this spontaneous pushing as long as she does not exhaust herself (Roberts *et al.* 1987).

When an epidural anaesthetic has been administered for pain relief in labour, maternal bearing down efforts are reduced, delayed, or abolished (see Chapter 57). Because the woman is usually in a supine or semi-recumbent position, abdominal palpation is a satisfactory way of gauging descent of the presenting part, and full dilatation can be tentatively diagnosed in this way and confirmed either by the appearance of the presenting part at the vulva or by vaginal examination.

3 Pushing during the second stage

In a study of healthy nulliparous women who had received no formal childbirth education and were allowed to push spontaneously without any directions from those caring for them, three to five relatively brief (4 to 6 second) bearing down efforts were made with each contraction (Roberts *et al.* 1987). The number of bearing-down efforts per contraction increased as the second stage progressed and most were accompanied by the release of air. The minority that were not were accompanied by very brief periods of breath-holding (lasting less than 6 seconds). Despite this pattern of breathing, the average length of the second stage of labour was 45 minutes, and did not exceed 95 minutes for any of the 31 women studied.

The duration of breath holding (less than 6 seconds) in the minority of women who spontaneously used this technique contrasts with the 10–30-second duration which is widely advocated for sustained, directed bearing-down efforts. The practice of attempting to override the spontaneous pattern of expulsive efforts by encouraging sustained, directed bearing down efforts during the second stage of labour is very widespread, in spite of the fact that the wisdom of this practice has been challenged intermittently for at least 30 years (Beynon 1957). The available evidence from controlled trials suggests that sustained bearing down efforts involving the Valsalva manoeuvre result in shorter second stages of labour than bearing down efforts consisting of shorter 'pushes' accompanied by air-release or exhalation (Table 66.1). The wisdom of the common advice to women to make strenuous, bearing-down efforts accompanied by sustained breath-holding has been questioned, however, because of the potentially adverse haemodynamic consequences of the Valsalva manoeuvre (Bassell *et al.* 1980; Roberts 1980; Yeates and Roberts 1984; McKay and Roberts 1985). In addition to respiratory-induced alterations in cardiovascular haemodynamics, maternal bearing down efforts, particularly when the mother is in a supine position, have been shown to be associated with com-

pression of the distal aorta and reduced blood flow to the uterus and lower extremities (Bassell *et al.* 1980). In combination with sustained maternal breath-holding, this effect may compromise fetal oxygenation.

In all three of the published controlled trials comparing different approaches to bearing down in which cord umbilical arterial pH assessments were available, mean cord umbilical arterial pH was lower in the group in which sustained or early bearing down had been encouraged (Table 66.2). In a large study in which the method of allocation to the different bearing down policies is less clearly described (de la Fuente *et al.* 1984), these differences were statistically significant.

Sustained bearing-down efforts also appear to predispose to abnormalities of the fetal heart rate (Knauth and Haloburdo 1986) and depressed Apgar score (Martinez-Lopez *et al.* 1984). These findings are consistent with the observations made in the study of primiparac using only spontaneous expulsive efforts (Roberts *et al.* 1987): the restoration of the baby's heart rate to the baseline level which existed at the beginning of the second stage of labour was much faster than in other reports in the literature.

Despite the limitations of the available evidence, a fairly consistent pattern emerges. Although the widespread policy of directing women to use sustained and early bearing-down efforts may well result in a modest decrease in the duration of the second stage, this does not appear to confer any benefit; indeed it seems to compromise maternal–fetal gas exchange.

4 Position during the second stage

The use of upright positions such as standing, sitting on a specially designed chair, or squatting for delivery is

Table 66.1 The effect of sustained (Valsalva) vs. exhalatory bearing down efforts on the average length of the second stage of labour (in minutes)

Study	*n*	Sustained Mean (SD)	Exhalatory Mean (SD)	Diff.	*p*-value
Barnett and Humenick (1982)	10	25 (11)	44 (18)	− 19	< 0.05
Martinez-Lopez *et al.* (1984)	96	21 (NA)	33 (NA)	− 12	< 0.05
Knauth and Haloburdo (1986)	17	46 (NA)	46 (NA)	0	NS

Table 66.2 The effect of sustained bearing down efforts during the second stage of labour on mean umbilical arterial pH

Study	*n*	Sustained Mean (SD)	Control Mean (SD)	Diff.	*p*-value
Caldeyro-Barcia *et al.* (1985)	80	7.28 (NA)	7.32 (NA)	− 0.04	NS
Barnett and Humenick (1982)	10	7.28 (0.54)	7.32 (0.62)	− 0.06	NS
Martinez-Lopez *et al.* (1984)	96	7.26 (NA)	7.33 (NA)	− 0.07	NS

common in many cultures (see Chapter 6). During the past two decades, people have come to question the recumbent positions that women giving birth in institutions have been expected to adopt for delivery. As is the case with respect to position during the first stage of labour (see Chapter 55), constraining women to adopt positions for delivery which they find awkward or uncomfortable can only be justified if there is good evidence that such a policy has important advantages for the health of either the mother or her baby.

Several clinical trials have been reported in which the recumbent position has been compared with upright posture during delivery. In most of these, either specially designed obstetric chairs or a back rest or wedge were used to support the upright position. In one trial (Stewart *et al.* 1983), the women in the recumbent control group could be propped up to almost the same angle of elevation as the upright group (e.g. 15–20 degrees), so the nature of an 'upright position' was variable among as well as within some trials.

Three other controlled trials with somewhat different designs are relevant. Two of these compared the dorsal recumbent position with a 15-degree left tilt (Humphrey *et al.* 1973, 1974; Johnstone *et al.* 1987). The other trial (Van Lier 1984) involved studying fetal variables that were potentially related to uterine blood flow, in the lateral and supine positions: 30 women were asked to alternate between an upright (55-degree elevation) and recumbent (10-degree elevation) position for as many series of three contractions as possible before they indicated a preference to remain at a particular angle of elevation.

In only two of the nine trials for which the relevant information is available were upright positions associated with longer mean durations of the second stage of labour, and in these the mean duration only differed by 1–2 minutes (Table 66.3). There is no evidence, however, that posture during the second stage of labour affects the incidence of either operative delivery (Table 66.4) or perineal trauma/episiotomy (Table 66.5). The differences that have been observed in controlled trials could be a reflection of chance variation.

Women using birth chairs during the second stage of labour are at increased risk of postpartum haemorrhage (Table 66.6). This tendency is reflected in a higher incidence of low haemoglobin (Table 66.7) and an increased need for blood transfusion (Table 66.8). It seems unlikely that this tendency to postpartum haemorrhage is due to an increased risk of bleeding from the placental site; it is more likely to arise from perineal trauma exacerbated by obstructed venous return, particularly in the light of observations of excessive perineal oedema and haemorrhoids in women who are upright in birth chairs for extended periods of time (Goodlin and Frederick 1983; Cottrell and Shannahan 1986).

The effects of maternal position during the second stage of labour on the condition of the baby have been examined by several investigators. Abnormal fetal heart rate patterns have been less frequently observed in women who adopted upright postures for delivery (Table 66.9), possibly partly because the method or frequency of fetal heart rate monitoring has differed according to the mother's position. In the two trials for which data are available, however, mean umbilical arterial pH was higher in babies born to women who had used the upright position for delivery (Table 66.10). These effects have been attributed to the avoidance of the aortocaval compression that is associated with recumbency. Both the observations themselves and this interpretation are consistent with the results of a study in which women were asked to change from their sides to their backs late in the first stage and during the second stage of labour (Kurz *et al.* 1982): adoption of the supine position was found to be associated with a substantial decrease in fetal oxygenation. This alteration in fetal acid–base status was also observed in two trials comparing the effects of the supine position with a 15 degree left lateral tilt (Humphrey *et al.* 1973; 1974; Johnstone *et al.* 1987).

Table 66.3 The effect of upright vs. recumbent position on the average length of the second stage of labour (in minutes)

Study		Upright Mean (SD)	Recumbent Mean (SD)	Diff.	*p*-value
Chan (1963)		29 (NA)	33 NA	− 4	NS
Liu (1974)		34 (NA)	75 (NA)	−41	<0.01
Stewart *et al.* (1983)	*Primip*	81 (65)	94 (79)	− 13	NS
	Multip	18 (19)	26 (24)	− 8	NS
Marttila *et al.* (1983)	*Primip*	43 (34)	41 (24)	+ 2	NS
	Multip	20 (25)	20 (37)	0	NS
Liddell and Fisher (1985)		53 (31)	59 (41)	− 6	NS
Turner *et al.* (1986)	*Primip*	6 (NA)	55 (NA)	+ 1	NS
	Multip	19 (NA)	19 (NA)	0	NS

Table 66.4 Effect of upright vs. recumbent position in second stage of labour on instrumental vaginal delivery

Study	EXPT		CTRL		Odds ratio	Graph of odds ratios and confidence intervals
	n	(%)	*n*	(%)	(95% CI)	0.01 0.1 0.5 1 2 10 100
Crowley (unpub)	80/637	(12.56)	89/596	(14.93)	0.82 (0.59–1.13)	
Hemminki *et al.* (1986)	17/88	(19.32)	8/87	(9.20)	2.27 (0.98–5.29)	
Turner *et al.* (1986)	37/318	(11.64)	38/318	(11.95)	0.97 (0.60–1.57)	
Stewart *et al.* (1983)	10/94	(10.64)	12/90	(13.33)	0.78 (0.32–1.88)	
Liddell and Fisher (1985)	11/27	(40.74)	7/21	(33.33)	1.36 (0.42–4.37)	
Chan (1963)	23/93	(24.73)	25/95	(26.32)	0.92 (0.48–1.77)	
Marttila *et al.* (1983)	2/50	(4.00)	6/50	(12.00)	0.34 (0.08–1.44)	
McManus and Calder. (1978)	4/19	(21.05)	5/19	(26.32)	0.75 (0.17–3.30)	
Typical odds ratio (95% confidence interval)					0.92 (0.73–1.14)	

Table 66.5 Effect of upright vs. recumbent position in second stage of labour on perineal trauma/episiotomy

Study	EXPT		CTRL		Odds ratio	Graph of odds ratios and confidence intervals
	n	(%)	*n*	(%)	(95% CI)	0.01 0.1 0.5 1 2 10 100
Crowley (unpub)	501/637	(78.65)	485/596	(81.38)	0.84 (0.64–1.12)	
Turner *et al.* (1986)	249/318	(78.30)	226/318	(71.07)	1.47 (1.03–2.09)	
Stewart *et al.* (1983)	67/86	(77.91)	76/91	(83.52)	0.70 (0.33–1.47)	
Liddell and Fisher (1985)	20/27	(74.07)	16/21	(76.19)	0.90 (0.24–3.30)	
Typical odds ratio (95% confidence interval)					1.00 (0.82–1.24)	

Table 66.6 Effect of upright vs. recumbent position in second stage of labour on estimated blood loss > 500 ml

Study	EXPT		CTRL		Odds ratio	Graph of odds ratios and confidence intervals
Crowley (unpub)	32/637	(5.02)	22/596	(3.69)	1.37 (0.80–2.37)	
Turner *et al.* (1986)	28/318	(8.81)	19/318	(5.97)	1.51 (0.83–2.74)	
Stewart *et al.* (1983)	12/94	(12.77)	4/90	(4.44)	2.84 (1.02–7.89)	
Typical odds ratio (95% confidence interval)					1.57 (1.08–2.28)	

Table 66.7 Effect of upright vs. recumbent position in second stage of labour on haemoglobin <11 g postpartum

Study	EXPT		CTRL		Odds ratio	Graph of odds ratios and confidence intervals						
	n	(%)	n	(%)	(95% CI)	0.01	0.1	0.5	1	2	10	100
Crowley (unpub)	72/629	(11.45)	49/591	(8.29)	1.42 (0.98–2.07)							
Typical odds ratio (95% confidence interval)					1.42 (0.98–2.07)							

Table 66.8 Effect of upright vs. rcumbent position in second stage of labour on blood transfusion postpartum

Study	EXPT		CTRL		Odds ratio	Graph of odds ratios and confidence intervals						
	n	(%)	n	(%)	(95% CI)	0.01	0.1	0.5	1	2	10	100
Crowley (unpub)	12/637	(1.88)	7/596	(1.17)	1.60 (0.64–3.95)							
Typical odds ratio (95% confidence interval)					1.60 (0.64–3.95)							

Table 66.9 Effect of upright vs. recumbent position in second stage of labour on abnormal fetal heart rate patterns

Study	EXPT		CTRL		Odds ratio	Graph of odds ratios and confidence intervals						
	n	(%)	n	(%)	(95% CI)	0.01	0.1	0.5	1	2	10	100
Crowley (unpub)	19/637	(2.98)	36/596	(6.04)	0.49 (0.28–0.84)							
Marttila *et al.* (1983)	7/29	(24.14)	10/25	(40.00)	0.49 (0.16–1.52)							
McManus and Calder (1978)	1/20	(5.00)	1/20	(5.00)	1.00 (0.06–16.58)							
Typical odds ratio (95% confidence interval)					0.50 (0.31–0.81)							

Table 66.10 The effect of upright vs. recumbent position on mean umbilical artery pH

Study	Upright Mean (SD)	Recumbent Mean (SD)	Diff.	p-value
Schneider-Affeld and Martin (1982)	7.21 (NA)	7.17 (NA)	+0.04	NS
Caldeyro-Barcia *et al.* (1985)	7.32 (NA)	7.28 (NA)	+0.04	<0.05

Table 66.11 The effect of lateral tilt vs. dorsal position for birth on mean (SD) umbilical artery pH

Study	n	Lateral tilt Mean (SD)	Dorsal position Mean (SD)	Diff.	p-value
Humphrey *et al.* (1973)	40	7.251 (0.059)	7.247 (0.087)	+0.003	0.05
Johnstone *et al.* (1987)	58	7.24 (0.06)	7.19 (0.10)	+0.05	<0.05

Babies whose mothers had adopted the dorsal position had lower umbilical cord arterial pH values than those whose mothers had been placed in a left lateral tilt (Table 66.11). The available data also suggest that an upright position during the second stage of labour leads to a reduced incidence of depressed Apgar score (Table 66.12).

Without exception, the clinical trials that included an assessment of the position preferred by mothers during the second stage of labour elicited more frequent positive responses from the group that had used the upright position. The perceived advantages included less pain (Marttila *et al.* 1983; Schneider-Affeld and Martin 1982), less backache (Liddell and Fisher 1985; Stewart *et al.* 1983), and a desire to use a birth chair or upright position for a subsequent birth (Marttila *et al.* 1983; Hemminki *et al.* 1986). In the study by Van Lier (1984), who asked 30 women to experience a series of three contractions alternately in the upright and recumbent positions, 19 expressed a preference for the upright position because it was more comfortable and easier to bear down, four preferred being recumbent, and seven women had no preference. After trying each position at least two times, the women who indicated a preference for staying in an upright position preferred an angle of 48 degrees (range 32 to 62 degrees) elevation.

Only four of the clinical trials assessed or commented on the birth attendant's perceptions of the position adopted by the woman during the second stage of labour. In the trial by Chan (1963), 7 out of 100 obstetricians indicated that delivering parturients in the upright position was 'inconvenient'. Stewart and his colleagues (1983) reported that midwives had found the chair 'satisfactory'. The fourteen nurse midwives and three physicians in training interviewed by Van Lier

(1984) were generally positive about the chair, but expressed concern about some inconvenience in accessing the perineum for difficult procedures. The prior preferences of the midwives involved in the trial reported by Hemminki *et al.* (1986) persisted throughout the study.

Evidence that intra-abdominal pressure can be increased effectively in the squatting position, along with radiological reports of an increased sagittal diameter of the pelvic outlet in the squatting position (Davies and Renning 1964; Borell and Fernstrom 1967; Russell 1982), has resulted in renewed interest in the potential advantages of squatting for birth (McKay 1984; McKay and Roberts 1985; Romond and Baker 1985). Adoption of the squatting position for excretion, resting, and other reasons is not common in many industrialized societies, and many people find it uncomfortable. However, the relative merits and possible disadvantages of the squatting position for birth have not yet been systematically explored.

5 Duration of the second stage

The second stage of labour has been considered to be a time of particular risk to the fetus for well over a century (Hamilton 1861). More than a half a century ago De Lee (1920) emphasized it dramatically in his classic recommendation of 'prophylactic forceps' as soon as the cervix was fully dilated. Echoes of these views exist today in the widespread policies for imposing arbitrary limits on the length of the second stage. A national survey in England found that there tended to be limits of one hour for nulliparae and half an hour for multiparae (Garcia *et al.* 1986), but some obstetricians have proposed limits as low as 20 and 30 minutes for

Table 66.12 Effect of upright vs. recumbent position in second stage of labour on Apgar score <7 at 1 minute

Study	EXPT		CTRL		Odds ratio	Graph of odds ratios and confidence intervals
	n	(%)	n	(%)	(95% CI)	0.01 0.1 0.5 1 2 10 100
Crowley (unpub)	7/637	(1.10)	6/596	(1.01)	1.09 (0.37–3.26)	
Hemminki *et al.* (1986)	1/88	(1.14)	8/87	(9.20)	0.19 (0.05–0.74)	
Turner *et al.* (1986)	2/318	(0.63)	2/318	(0.63)	1.00 (0.14–7.13)	
Liddell and Fisher (1985)	4/27	(14.81)	2/21	(9.52)	1.61 (0.29–8.85)	
Carpenter (unpub)	0/20	(0.00)	2/20	(10.00)	0.13 (0.01–2.13)	
Marttila *et al.* (1983)	0/50	(0.00)	4/50	(8.00)	0.13 (0.02–0.93)	
Typical odds ratio (95% confidence interval)					0.54 (0.28–1.03)	

nulliparae and multiparae respectively (Roemer *et al.* 1976).

It is true that statistical associations have been demonstrated between prolonged second stage of labour and obviously undesirable outcomes such as infant mortality, postpartum haemorrhage, puerperal febrile morbidity (Hellman and Prystowski 1952), and neonatal seizures (Minchom *et al.* 1987), as well as with outcomes of less certain significance relating to the acid–base status of the baby at birth (Roemer *et al.* 1976; Katz *et al.* 1987). On their own, these associations are not sufficient justification, however, for concluding that the length of the second stage of labour, *per se*, is the crucial variable. After an analysis in which he failed to find any evidence of an association between the length of the second stage of labour and a variety of adverse outcomes, Cohen (1977) concluded that 'elective termination of labor simply because an arbitrary period of time has elapsed in the second stage is clearly not warranted'.

Two policies to curtail the second stage of labour in the absence of overt maternal or fetal problems have been examined in controlled trials. In the first of these (Wood *et al.* 1973), 11 women whose babies' heads had become visible at the vulva were actively encouraged to push and episiotomies (and, in one case, forceps) were used to expedite delivery. They were compared with a randomized control group of 11 women for whom a more conservative approach was adopted. Mean(SD) umbilical arterial pH values were statistically significantly higher (7.28(0.04)) in the expedited group than in the control group (7.23(0.06)). In the second of the two controlled trials (Katz *et al.* 1982), 25 nulliparae who had been in the second stage of labour for between 20 and 30 minutes were alternately allocated either to elective delivery with the vacuum extractor, or to continue labouring until spontaneous delivery had occurred. Mean umbilical cord arterial pH values were statistically significantly higher in the expedited group (7.25) than in the conservatively managed group (7.16). The results of both of these trials thus suggest that

curtailing the length of the second stage of labour can modify the decline in fetal pH that tends to occur during labour with the passage of time (Pearson and Davies 1974; Roemer *et al.* 1976). However, without some evidence that this policy has a beneficial effect on less ambiguous outcomes, the maternal trauma and occasional fetal trauma resulting from the increased surgical interference that the policy involves can hardly be justified (Alexander *et al.* 1987).

The effects of trying to reduce the length of the second stage in women with epidural anaesthesia by encouraging earlier pushing in these circumstances has also been evaluated in three randomized trials (McQueen and Mylrea 1977; Maresh *et al.* 1983; Buxton *et al.* 1988). There is a tendency for rotational forceps deliveries to be more common among those women who had been encouraged to bear down relatively early (Table 66.13). In none of the studies was there any evidence that a policy of early bearing down had any compensating advantages for either the mother or the baby.

Decisions about curtailing the second stage of labour should be based on the same principles of monitoring the well-being of mother and baby that apply during the first stage of labour (see Chapters 53 and 54). If the mother's condition is satisfactory, the baby's condition is satisfactory, and there is evidence that progress is occurring with descent of the presenting part, there are no grounds for intervention.

Maternal exhaustion can occur at any time during labour, but is more likely to occur during the second stage when the extra effort of pushing is added to the stress of the contractions. On the other hand, if the mother is not unduly distressed, and is not actively pushing (particularly when she has epidural analgesia), there is no reason to think that the second stage is any more likely to cause exhaustion than the first stage.

Unless there are good reasons for doing otherwise therefore, it is important that, throughout the second stage of labour, any sense of urgency felt by the mother or her partner is allayed.

Table 66.13 Effect of early vs. late pushing with epidural anaesthesia in second stage of labour on rotational forceps deliveries

Study	EXPT		CTRL		Odds ratio	Graph of odds ratios and confidence intervals						
	n	(%)	*n*	(%)	(95% CI)	0.01	0.1	0.5	1	2	10	100
McQueen and Mylrea (1977)	18/50	(36.00)	9/49	(18.37)	2.41 (1.00–5.81)							
Buxton *et al.* (1988)	3/19	(15.79)	4/22	(18.18)	0.85 (0.17–4.25)							
Maresh *et al.* (1983)	11/39	(28.21)	4/34	(11.76)	2.70 (0.87–8.36)							
Typical odds ratio (95% confidence interval)					2.12 (1.12–4.02)							

Monitoring the fetal heart using intermittent auscultation may on occasions pose difficulties, as it is sometimes hard to find the fetal heart when the baby moves down into the pelvis. It can be frustrating and uncomfortable for the woman to have people continually trying to listen to her baby's heart, or to have to change her position in order to facilitate fetal auscultation. In these circumstances, electronic fetal monitoring is often more comfortable and less disruptive for the woman.

Assessment of failure of progress in labour must be considered only in terms of descent of the presenting part, as dilatation of the cervix is, by definition, complete. Failure of the presenting part to descend may be due to inadequate or inco-ordinate uterine contractions, to malposition or malpresentation of the baby, or to cephalopelvic disproportion. The cause of this failure to progress must be diagnosed and appropriately treated. This may require as little as a change of posture. Malpresentation, or minor degrees of cephalopelvic disproportion, may also sometimes be overcome by encouraging the mother to vary her position. Intravenous oxytocin can be used if contractions are inadequate, although a decision to do so should be taken with particular caution in multiparae. Instrumental or manual manipulation, or sometimes caesarean section may be necessary (see Chapters 53, 71, and 72).

6 Care of the perineum

The importance of intervening to expedite delivery only on the basis of clear maternal or fetal indications and not 'because of the clock' will all tend to minimize perineal trauma during childbirth, as will selection of the vacuum extractor rather than forceps for instrumental delivery when this is indicated (see Chapter 71). Reducing the risk of perineal trauma is important because it can cause discomfort of a degree that can dominate the experience of early motherhood and because it sometimes results in significant disability during the months and years that follow (Kitzinger 1981).

Perineal damage may occur either from spontaneous laceration or because the accoucheur attempts to prevent more serious problems by performing an episiotomy. Whatever the cause, perineal damage is very common. Although some individual accoucheurs appear to be particularly skillful in assisting delivery in a way that minimizes perineal trauma, it is usual for at least two-thirds of all primigravidae to sustain trauma sufficient to require suturing.

6.1 Guarding and massaging the perineum

The practice of guarding the perineum, with the birth attendant's hand held against the perineum during contractions, is widespread. It is believed that this practice supports the tissues sufficiently to reduce the risk of spontaneous trauma. It is difficult to believe that fairly modest external pressure of this kind is likely to have much effect in the face of the very high internal pressures which are exerted during expulsive contractions. The practice might be more logical if combined with gentle pressure applied to the fetal head as a means of controlling the speed of crowning, as this is the time that the perineal tissues appear to be most at risk of spontaneous damage. Unfortunately, there have been no formal evaluations of the alternative strategies.

'Ironing out' or massaging the perineum as the second stage advances, sometimes with an emollient such as olive oil or the application of a hot pad, are also measures designed to stretch the tissues and reduce the risk of trauma. These techniques have enthusiastic advocates (see, for example, Davis 1981; Flint 1986), as well as detractors. The latter suggest that touch may be a disruptive distraction and that the increase in vascularity and oedema in tissues that are already at risk of trauma is counterproductive (Noble 1983). Neither of these diametrically opposed opinions can be supported with evidence from controlled comparisons. The only trial of perineal massage conducted so far refers to massage started six weeks prior to labour (Avery and Burket 1986). Unfortunately, the methodological weaknesses of the study are such that the results do not provide any basis for guiding clinical practice.

6.2 Episiotomy

As already noted (see Section 5, above), if monitoring during the second stage of labour suggests that either the fetus or the mother has become distressed during the second stage of labour, or that progress has ceased, it may be necessary to hasten delivery either by instrumental delivery (see Chapter 71) or by episiotomy.

Like any surgical procedure, episiotomy carries a number of risks. Indeed, the excessive blood loss, haematoma formation, and infection that sometimes follow episiotomy have sometimes been fatal (Golde and Ledger 1977; Shy and Eschenbach 1979; Ewing *et al.* 1979). Trauma involving the anal sphincter and rectal mucosa seems likely to predispose to these rare but serious problems and only rarely to occur spontaneously (Thorp *et al.* 1987). Complications of these third and fourth degree lacerations include rectovaginal fistulae, loss of rectal tone, and perineal abscess formation (Thorp *et al.* 1987).

All the case reports of serious complications of episiotomy cited above relate to clinical practice in North America, where midline incisions are preferred to the mediolateral approach used in the United Kingdom. The two operations have been compared in only one controlled trial (Coats *et al.* 1980). Unfortunately, interpretation of the results is compromised because selection bias may well have been operating during recruitment to the trial: allocation was based on the terminal digit of the woman's case record, and those who received the mediolateral operation were more likely to have had rotational or breech deliveries. Even with this likely bias against the mediolateral operation, third degree lacerations occurred in 39 of 163 women (24 per cent) in the midline episiotomy group and in only 22 of 193 (9 per cent) of those in the mediolateral group. The perineum was significantly less bruised in the women who had had the midline operation but the amount of pain experienced was similar in the two groups, as were the proportions of women requiring analgesics. Women in the midline episiotomy group began intercourse significantly earlier than those who had a mediolateral incision. At follow-up the investigators judged the cosmetic appearance and texture of the scar to be somewhat better following the midline operation. Well-controlled research to assess the short and long term advantages and disadvantages of midline and mediolateral episiotomies is long overdue.

Episiotomies are sometimes performed using scissors, sometimes with a scalpel. Those who favour scissors maintain that they are less likely to damage the presenting part of the baby and more likely to promote haemostasis in the wound edges because of their crushing as well as cutting action. Those who favour the scalpel say that it minimizes trauma and is thus followed by better healing of the perineal wound. There are no data on which to base any judgements about the validity of these claims. Whatever the line of incision of the episiotomy and the instrument used to perform the operation, it must be preceded by adequate infiltration of a local anaesthetic.

6.3 Liberal use of episiotomy

The most common cause of perineal damage is episiotomy. In a review of the English language literature from 1860 to 1980, Thacker and Banta (1983) stated that this procedure is carried out on between 50 and 90 per cent of women giving birth to their first child, thus making it the most commonly performed surgical procedure in the United States (Banta and Thacker 1982). Although this extensive use of episiotomy has been questioned (House 1980; Hofmeyr and Sonnendecker 1987), the prevailing view appears to be that the policy is justified. Put in the words of the author of one modern obstetric textbook: 'The modern accoucheur simply looks for reasons why an episiotomy should *not* be performed. There are few' (Dewhurst 1976).

Liberal use of an operation with the risks described above, however rare these may be, could only be justified by evidence that it confers worthwhile benefits if used frequently. There are three postulated benefits of a liberal use of episiotomy. These are first, prevention of damage to the anal sphincter and rectal mucosa (third and fourth degree lacerations) and easier repair and better healing than with a spontaneous tear;

second, prevention of trauma to the fetal head; and third, prevention of serious damage to the muscles of the pelvic floor (Banta and Thacker 1982). A substantial review of the English language literature was unable to uncover any evidence to support these postulated benefits of liberal use of episiotomy (Thacker and Banta 1983).

6.3.1 Prevention of severe perineal trauma

Liberal use of (mediolateral) episiotomy has been compared to restricted use in only two randomized controlled trials (Sleep *et al.* 1984; Harrison *et al.* 1984). The results of a third trial are uninterpretable because the randomization broke down (House *et al.* 1986). In addition, however, there are two other trials, one an evaluation of a birth chair (Stewart *et al.* 1983), the other an evaluation of team midwifery care (Flint and Poulengeris 1987), in which episiotomy was used more liberally in one of the two experimental groups than in the other. Data on perineal trauma from these trials have been incorporated in the analyses that follow because there is no evidence of a systematic effect of the principal independent variables studied in those trials on this particular outcome (see Section 4 above, and Chapter 10).

In the trial by Sleep and her colleagues (1984), women were allocated either to a policy in which the midwife was asked to 'try to prevent a perineal laceration' (by performing an episiotomy if considered necessary), or to a policy of trying to avoid an episiotomy (other than for 'fetal indications'); the resulting episiotomy rates in the two groups were 51 per cent and 10 per cent respectively. In the trial by Harrison *et al.* (1984) women were allocated either to routine episiotomy (100 per cent), or to restricted episiotomy (which resulted in a rate of 8 per cent). In the other two trials (Stewart *et al.* 1983; Flint and Poulengeris 1987) the episiotomy rates were 43 per cent versus 20 per cent, and 42 per cent versus 34 per cent, respectively.

Liberal use of episiotomy is associated with higher overall rates of perineal trauma (Table 66.14). There is no evidence that this policy reduces the risk of serious perineal or vaginal trauma (Table 66.15), but it seems to be protective against anterior trauma around the labia and urethra (Table 66.16).

In only one of the trials (Sleep *et al.* 1984) were analyses of the longer term experiences of the randomized cohorts reported. The two groups experienced a comparable amount of perineal pain assessed at 10 days and 3 months postpartum (Table 66.17). Although women allocated to liberal use of episiotomy resumed intercourse somewhat later than those who had experienced restricted use of the operation, the proportions of women experiencing pain on intercourse 3 months and 3 years after delivery was almost identical (Table 66.18).

Table 66.14 Effect of liberal use of episiotomy in spontaneous vaginal delivery on any posterior perineal trauma

Study	EXPT		CTRL		Odds ratio	Graph of odds ratios and confidence intervals
	n	(%)	n	(%)	(95% CI)	0.01 0.1 0.5 1 2 10 100
Sleep *et al.* (1984)	380/502	(75.70)	329/498	(66.06)	1.59 (1.21–2.09)	
Stewart *et al.* (1983)	76/90	(84.44)	68/94	(72.34)	2.03 (1.01–4.08)	
Flint and Poulengeris (1987)	334/438	(76.26)	336/443	(75.85)	1.02 (0.75–1.39)	
Harrison *et al.* (1984)	89/89	(100.0)	73/92	(79.35)	8.90 (3.45–22.97)	
Typical odds ratio (95% confidence interval)					1.47 (1.21–1.78)	

Table 66.15 Effect of liberal use of episiotomy in spontaneous vaginal delivery on any severe trauma (perineal or vaginal)

Study	EXPT		CTRL		Odds ratio	Graph of odds ratios and confidence intervals
	n	(%)	n	(%)	(95% CI)	0.01 0.1 0.5 1 2 10 100
Sleep *et al.* (1984)	1/502	(0.20)	4/498	(0.80)	0.30 (0.05–1.72)	
Flint and Poulengeris (1987)	0/438	(0.00)	2/443	(0.45)	0.14 (0.01–2.19)	
Harrison *et al.* (1984)	5/89	(5.62)	0/92	(0.00)	8.00 (1.36–47.14)	
Typical odds ratio (95% confidence interval)					1.01 (0.32–3.16)	

Table 66. 16 Effect of liberal use of episiotomy in spontaneous vaginal delivery on anterior trauma

Study	EXPT		CTRL		Odds ratio	Graph of odds ratios and confidence intervals
	n	(%)	n	(%)	(95% CI)	0.01 0.1 0.5 1 2 10 100
Sleep *et al.* (1984)	87/502	(17.33)	131/498	(26.31)	0.59 (0.44–0.80)	
Typical odds ratio (95% confidence interval)					0.59 (0.44–0.80)	

Table 66.17 Effect of liberal use of episiotomy in spontaneous vaginal delivery on perineal pain at 10 days

Study	EXPT		CTRL		Odds ratio	Graph of odds ratios and confidence intervals
	n	(%)	n	(%)	(95% CI)	0.01 0.1 0.5 1 2 10 100
Sleep *et al.* (1984)	101/446	(22.65)	99/439	(22.55)	1.01 (0.73–1.38)	
Typical odds ratio (95% confidence interval)					1.01 (0.73–1.38)	

Effect of liberal use of episiotomy in spontaneous vaginal delivery on perineal pain at 3 months

Study	EXPT		CTRL		Odds ratio	Graph
Sleep *et al.* (1984)	35/457	(7.66)	33/438	(7.53)	1.02 (0.62–1.67)	
Typical odds ratio (95% confidence interval)					1.02 (0.62–1.67)	

Table 66.18 Effect of liberal use of episiotomy in spontaneous vaginal delivery on dyspareunia at 3 months

Study	EXPT		CTRL		Odds ratio	Graph of odds ratios and confidence intervals						
	n	(%)	*n*	(%)	(95% CI)	0.01	0.1	0.5	1	2	10	100
Sleep *et al.* (1984)	74/457	(16.19)	86/438	(19.63)	0.79 (0.56–1.11)							
Typical odds ratio (95% confidence interval)					0.79 (0.56–1.11)							

Effect of liberal use of episiotomy in spontaneous vaginal delivery on dyspareunia ('ever') at 3 years

Sleep *et al.* (1987)	45/340	(13.24)	52/324	(16.05)	0.80 (0.52–1.23)							
Typical odds ratio (95% confidence interval)					0.80 (0.52–1.23)							

6.3.2 Prevention of fetal trauma

Neither of the two randomized trials (Sleep *et al.* 1984; Harrison *et al.* 1984) provides any evidence to support the suggestion that liberal use of episiotomy minimizes trauma to the fetal head. In the trial carried out by Sleep *et al.* (1984), the distribution of Apgar scores was similar in the two groups, as was the rate of admission to the special care nursery. In the group with liberal use of episiotomy, 7.6 per cent of the babies were admitted to a special care baby unit compared with 5.7 per cent in the group with restricted use of episiotomy. Harrison *et al.* (1984) commented only that 'the Apgar scores at one and 10 minutes for babies born to mothers in the two groups did not indicate a difference in rating'.

6.3.3 Prevention of urinary stress incontinence

The question of whether stress incontinence is caused or aggravated by vaginal delivery remains controversial. A long-held belief is that injury to the pelvic floor muscles or to their nerve supply or to the interconnecting fascia is an inevitable consequence of vaginal delivery, particularly if the delivery is difficult (Malpas *et al.* 1949). This in turn, it is argued, may cause genital prolapse and stress incontinence.

A frequent claim in support of liberal use of episiotomy is that it prevents pelvic relaxation during delivery and thereby prevents urinary incontinence and genital prolapse (e.g. Willson 1981; Flood 1982). If the intention really were to protect the pelvic floor, a much more extensive incision than is usual would almost certainly be required (Goodlin 1983). As noted above, however, liberal and restricted use of episiotomy are associated with contrasting patterns of trauma: liberal use is associated with a lower frequency of anterior vaginal and labial tears (Sleep *et al.* 1984; Stewart *et al.* 1983). This raises the possibility that episiotomy may have a more specific protective effect on the tissues around the bladder neck.

The findings in an observational study of two groups of women who were matched on some prognostic variables, but had different forms of perineal care, is consistent with this. Women with vaginal tears not only had more labial tears, but also more cystocoeles (Brendsel *et al.* 1981). A small matched-pair study, however, found no statistically significant differences in the rates of genital prolapse between women who had and did not have an episiotomy, and perineometer readings were similar in the two groups (Brendsel *et al.* 1979).

Childbirth itself is often blamed for long term, persistent stress incontinence, but many women already have stress incontinence during pregnancy. The prevalence of this symptom increases steadily to a rate of 40 to 70 per cent by the end of pregnancy (Francis 1960a,b; Stanton *et al.* 1980). For most women the symptom resolves in the first few weeks after birth, but in an important minority it persists. According to Stanton and his colleagues (1980), about 6 per cent of first time mothers still have stress incontinence at the six-week postnatal check-up, although few of them had the symptom before pregnancy. About 10 per cent of multiparous mothers, most of whom had this symptom prior to the pregnancy, also had stress incontinence at 6 weeks postpartum. In Francis's series (1960a,b) only 6 per cent of the women who had stress incontinence in pregnancy had persistent incontinence, but the symptom returned in a further 38 per cent when they developed a precipitating factor such as a cough. Francis (1960b) was emphatic that in none of the women in her series did stress incontinence appear for the first time postnatally. Others, however, have reported that the puerperium is the time of onset in anything between 4 per cent (Beck and Hsu 1965) and 19 per cent (Iosif 1981) of all women who have stress incontinence postnatally.

Suggestive evidence that both urinary and faecal incontinence result from damage to the nerves of the pelvic floor muscles has come from Snooks and Swash and their colleagues (Snooks and Swash 1984, Snooks *et al.* 1984, 1985). They found that in 75 per cent of women with faecal incontinence of no clear cause there is histological evidence of denervation of the pelvic floor muscles, especially the puborectalis and the external anal sphincter muscles. Women who also have stress urinary incontinence have slowed conduction in the perineal branch of the pudendal nerve which innervates the periurethral voluntary sphincter muscle (Snooks and Swash 1984). More recent studies in women with urinary stress incontinence only, have shown slowed conduction in the perineal branch of the pudendal nerve with normal conduction to the external anal sphincter muscle (Snooks *et al.* 1985).

Slowed conduction in the pudendal nerve is common immediately after vaginal delivery (but not following caesarean section), and it is usually transitory (Snooks *et al.* 1984). Delay in return to normal conduction is more common following instrumental delivery and in multiparae. Not all women with stress incontinence show abnormal conduction patterns, however, and stress incontinence associated with vaginal delivery is still most commonly attributed to stretching or damage to pelvic muscles and fascia, and in particular the perineal body.

Whatever the aetiology of postpartum stress incontinence may be, there is no good evidence that more liberal use of episiotomy is protective against this distressing condition. The hypothesis that liberal use of episiotomy protects against the subsequent development of urinary stress incontinence has been tested in a long term follow-up study (Sleep and Grant 1987) of a randomized trial (Sleep *et al.* 1984). In the 3-month follow-up described in the original report, 19 per cent of women reported urinary incontinence (15 per cent of primiparae and 22 per cent of multiparae); 6 per cent of them needed to wear a pad because of the incontinence. Participants have since been recontacted 3 years after delivery; 674 out of the original 1000 women responded (they were equally divided between the two groups). Rates and severity of incontinence were almost identical in the two trial groups (Table 66.19) and this similarity persisted when deliveries in the subsequent 3 years were taken into account. Thus, there is no support for the hypothesis that liberal use of episiotomy prevents long term urinary incontinence.

This conclusion is consistent with the finding of an observational study of postnatal perineal muscle function using a perineometer (Gordon and Logue 1985). There was association between pressure measurements and the form of perineal management (perineum intact, second degree tear, episiotomy) or delivery (spontaneous vaginal, instrumental vaginal, caesarean section). There was, however, striking variation in pressure measurements among women within groups categorized by these characteristics of the delivery.

Urinary stress incontinence is common, and causes embarrassment and discomfort to a large number of women. Even a relatively small reduction in its prevalence is therefore potentially important. There is no evidence, however, that alternative methods of perineal care during delivery make a difference to the risk of stress incontinence, and little evidence that the extent of perineal trauma is important. Even if neurological

Table 66.19 Effect of liberal use of episiotomy in spontaneous vaginal delivery on urinary incontinence at 3 months

Study	EXPT		CTRL		Odds ratio	Graph of odds ratios and confidence intervals						
	n	(%)	*n*	(%)	(95% CI)	0.01	0.1	0.5	1	2	10	100
Sleep *et al.* (1984)	85/457	(18.60)	83/438	(18.95)	0.98 (0.70–1.37)							
Typical odds ratio (95% confidence interval)					0.98 (0.70–1.37)							

Effect of liberal use of episiotomy in spontaneous vaginal delivery on urinary incontinence at 3 years

Sleep *et al.* (1987)	44/333	(13.21)	45/310	(14.52)	0.90 (0.57–1.40)							
Typical odds ratio (95% confidence interval)					0.90 (0.57–1.40)							

Effect of liberal use of episiotomy in spontaneous vaginal delivery on 'stress' urinary incontinence at 3 years

Sleep *et al.* (1987)	105/333	(31.53)	103/310	(33.23)	0.93 (0.67–1.29)							
Typical odds ratio (95% confidence interval)					0.93 (0.67–1.29)							

damage to the perineal branch of the pudendal nerve is sustained during delivery, it is hard to see how it could be prevented by a change in the current methods of management. Perhaps pelvic floor exercises during pregnancy or programmes after delivery may make a difference, but this remains to be confirmed (see Chapter 79).

7 Delivery

Women may choose a variety of positions for delivery if they are encouraged to discover for themselves which is most comfortable for them, and accoucheurs should be sensitive to these differences between women. In the light of the evidence already reviewed, there is no justification for requiring, or actively encouraging, a supine position during delivery. Women who choose to lie down for delivery often appear to find the (left or right) lateral position comfortable (Irwin 1978).

The woman will depend on the midwife's guidance to moderate her pushing effort to allow an unhurried, gentle delivery of the head. This can be achieved by interspersing short pushing efforts with periods of panting, so giving the tissues time to relax and stretch under pressure. Using this approach, several contractions may occur before the head crowns and is delivered. The mother may wish to look at and touch her baby at this point.

After delivery of the head, the shoulders rotate internally. It is expedient to check that the umbilical cord is not tightly wound around the baby's neck. If it is, it may be possible to loosen it, then loop it over the baby's head; if necessary, it can be clamped and severed. Once rotation is complete, the shoulders are delivered one at a time to reduced the risk of perineal trauma. When the mother is in the semi-recumbent position, the anterior shoulder may deliver first; in the squatting or kneeling position, the posterior shoulder may be released first. The mother may then grasp her baby and complete the rest of the delivery herself.

Difficulty with delivery of the shoulders is rare following spontaneous delivery of the head, but if the baby has felt large on abdominal palpation, the accoucheur should be alert for and prepared to deal with shoulder dystocia. It is important that delivery of the shoulders should not be attempted until they have rotated into the antero-posterior axis. Posterior traction on the head, combined with the mother's expulsive efforts, is usually sufficient to effect delivery of the anterior shoulder. The accoucheur should, however, be aware of techniques to overcome the problem of shoulder dystocia on the rare occasions on which it does occur. These include wide abduction of the mother's thighs and complete flexion of her hips; manual rotation of the posterior shoulder anteriorly; and, if necessary, sustained suprapubic pressure exerted by an assistant directly above the pubic bone.

8 Conclusions

8.1 Implications for current practice

There are no data to support a policy of directed pushing during the second stage of labour, and some evidence to suggest that it may be harmful. The practice should be abandoned. Similarly, there are no data to justify restricting women to a supine position during the second stage of labour. With some reservations, the data tend to support the use of upright positions. There is a tendency for recumbency to lengthen the second stage of labour, to reduce the incidence of spontaneous births, to increase the incidence of abnormal fetal heart rate patterns, and to reduce umbilical cord blood pH. Although some birth attendants report that upright positions sometimes caused them inconvenience, there has been a consistently positive response from the women who have used an upright position for birth.

On the other hand, at least some of the birthing chairs that have been introduced during recent years appear to predispose to perineal oedema and venous engorgement which, in conjunction with perineal trauma, can result in the loss of substantial amounts of blood. Use of a birthing chair is not, however, the only way of adopting an upright position during labour. The mother should be encouraged to use the position that she prefers.

There is no evidence to suggest that, when the second stage of labour is progressing and the condition of both mother and fetus is satisfactory, the imposition of any arbitrary upper limit on its duration is justified. Such limits should be discarded.

There is no evidence to support the practice of 'ironing out' or massaging the perineum, or claims that liberal use of episiotomy reduces the risk of severe perineal trauma, improves perineal healing, prevents fetal trauma, or reduces the risk of urinary stress incontinence after delivery. Episiotomy should be used only to relieve fetal or maternal distress, or to achieve adequate progress when it is the perineum that is responsible for lack of progress.

8.2 Implications for future research

Ways of adopting an upright position during the second stage of labour other than chairs, particularly squatting and semi-squatting positions, should be more systematically explored and their effects assessed.

Some individual practitioners appear to be particularly skilled in minimizing perineal trauma during delivery and their methods should be studied with a view to disseminating them more widely. Controlled trials should be mounted to assess the value of massaging the perineum, both during preparation for delivery and during delivery itself.

The relative merits of midline and mediolateral episiotomies require more systematic comparison than they have received so far. Trials could be mounted with a factorial design to enable comparison of scissors and scalpel for making the incision.

References

Alexander S, Cantraine F, Schwers J (1987). Apgar score and cord pH in relation to length of second stage. In: Fetal and Neonatal Physiological Measurements. Rolfe P (ed). London: Butterworths, pp 59–64.

Avery MD, Burket BA (1986). Effect of perineal massage on the incidence of episiotomy and perineal laceration in a nurse midwifery service. J Nurs Midwifery, 31: 128–134.

Banta D, Thacker SB (1982). The risks and benefits of episiotomy: a review. Birth, 9: 25–30.

Barnett MM, Humenick SS (1982). Infant outcome in relation to second stage labor pushing method. Birth, 9: 221–229.

Bassell GM, Humayun SG, Marx GF (1980). Maternal bearing down efforts—another fetal risk? Obstet Gynecol, 56: 39–41.

Beck RP, Hsu N (1965). Pregnancy, childbirth and the menopause related to the development of stress incontinence. Am J Obstet Gynecol, 91: 821–823.

Beynon CL (1957). The normal second stage of labour: a plea for reform in its conduct. J Obstet Gynaecol Br Empire, 64: 815–820.

Borell U, Fernstrom I (1967). The mechanisms of labor. Radiol Clin North Am, 5: 73–85.

Brendsel C, Peterson G, Mehl LE (1979). Episiotomy: facts, fictions, figures, and alternatives. In: Compulsory Hospitalization or Freedom of Choice in Childbirth. Stewart D, Stewart L (eds). National Association of Parents and Professionals for Safe Alternatives in Childbirth (NAPSAC), pp 139–144.

Brendsel C, Peterson G, Miehl C (1981). The role of episiotomy in pelvic symptomatology. In: Episiotomy—Physical and Emotional Aspects. Kitzinger S (ed). London: National Childbirth Trust, pp 36–44.

Buxton EJ, Redman CWE, Obhrai M (1988). Delayed pushing with lumbar epidural in labour—does it increase the incidence of spontaneous delivery? J Obstet Gynaecol, 8: 258–261.

Caldeyro-Barcia R (1984). Delivery in a sitting position. Paper presented at 2nd Symposium of Perinatal Medicine, Campinas, Brasil.

Caldeyro-Barcia R, Alonso JG, Sugo M, Barron R, Dellepiane M (1985). Fetal outcome of humanised labour (unpublished).

Carpenter ME (1977). The effect of maternal position during labor on fetal outcome. Masters thesis, University of Oregon, USA.

Chan DP (1963). Positions during labour. Br Med J, 1: 100–102.

Coats PM, Chan KK, Wilkins M, Beard RJ (1980). A comparison between midline and mediolateral episiotomies. Br J Obstet Gynaecol, 87: 408–412.

Cohen WR (1977). Influence of the duration of second stage labor on perinatal outcome and puerperal morbidity. Obstet Gynecol, 49: 266–269.

Cottrell BH, Shannahan MD (1986). Effect of the birth chair on duration of second stage labor and maternal outcome. Nurs Res, 35: 364–367.

Crowley P (unpublished). The Coombe Lying-In Hospital Birthing Chair Trial.

Davies JW, Renning EL (1964). The birth canal—practical applications. Medical Times, 92: 75–86.

Davis E (1981). Heart and Hands. New Mexico: John Muir Publications, pp 102–103.

De Lee JB (1920). The prophylactic forceps operation. Am J Obstet Gynecol, 1: 34–44.

de la Fuente P, Hernandez-Garcia JM, Martinez V (1984). Evolution de l'équilibre acido–basique selon le type d'expulsion. J Gynecol Obstet Biol Reprod (Paris), 13: 629–634.

Dewhurst CJ (1976). Integrated Obstetrics and Gynaecology for Postgraduates (2nd edn). Oxford: Blackwell Scientific Publications.

Ewing TL, Smale LE, Elliott FA (1979). Maternal deaths associated with postpartum vulvar edema. Am J Obstet Gynecol, 134: 173–179.

Flint C (1986). Sensitive Midwifery. London: Heinemann, pp 101–102.

Flint C, Poulengeris P (1987). The 'Know Your Midwife' Report. London: Heinemann.

Flood C (1982). The real reasons for performing episiotomies. World Med, 6 Feb: 51.

Francis WJA (1960a). Disturbances of bladder function in relation to pregnancy. J Obstet Gynaecol Br Empire, 67: 353–366.

Francis WJA (1960b). The onset of stress incontinence. J Obstet Gynaecol Br Empire, 67: 899–903.

Garcia J, Garforth S, Ayers S (1986). Midwives confined? Labour ward policies and routines. Research and the Midwife Conference, Manchester, 1985. University of Manchester: Research and the Midwife Conference Proceedings, pp 74–80.

Golde S, Ledger WJ (1977). Necrotizing fasciitis in postpartum patients. Obstet Gynecol, 50: 670–673.

Goodlin RC (1983). On protection of the maternal perineum during birth. Am J Obstet Gynecol, 62: 393–394.

Goodlin RC, Frederick IB (1983). Postpartum vulvar edema associated with the birthing chair. Am J Obstet Gynecol, 146: 334.

Gordon H, Logue M (1985). Perineal muscle function after childbirth. Lancet, 2: 123–125.

Hamilton G (1861). Classical observations and suggestions in obstetrics. Edinburgh Med J, 7: 313–321.

Harrison RF, Brennan M, North PM, Reed JV, Wickham EA (1984). Is routine episiotomy necessary? Br Med J, 288: 1971–1975.

Hellman LH, Prystowski H (1952). The duration of the second stage of labor. Am J Obstet Gynecol, 61: 1223–1233.

Hemminki E, Virkkunen A, Makela A, Hannikainen J, Pulkkis E, Moilanen K, Pasanen M (1986). A trial of delivery in a birth chair. J Obstet Gynaecol, 6: 162–165.

Hofmeyr GJ, Sonnendecker EWW (1987). Elective episiotomy in perspective. S Afr Med J, 71: 357–359.

House MJ (1980). Episiotomy—indications, technique and results. Midwife, Health Visitor and Community Nurse, 16: 6–9.

House MJ, Cario G, Jones MH (1986). Episiotomy and the perineum: a random controlled trial. J Obstet Gynaecol, 7: 107–110.

Humphrey M, Hounslow D, Morgan S, Wood C (1973). The influence of maternal posture at birth on the fetus. J Obstet Gynaecol Br Commnwlth, 80: 1075–1080.

Humphrey M, Chang A, Wood EC, Morgan S, Hounslow D (1974). A decrease in fetal pH during the second stage of labour, when conducted in the dorsal position. J Obstet Gynaecol Br Commnwlth, 81: 600–602.

Iosif S (1981). Stress incontinence during pregnancy and in the puerperium. Int J Gynaecol Obstet, 19: 13–20.

Irwin HW (1978). Practical considerations for the routine application of left lateral Sims' position for vaginal delivery. Am J Obstet Gynecol, 131: 129–133.

Johnstone FD, Aboelmagd MS, Harouny AK (1987). Maternal posture in second stage and fetal acid base status. Br J Obstet Gynaecol, 94: 753–757.

Katz M, Lunenfeld E, Meizner I, Bashan N, Gross J (1987). The effect of the duration of the second stage of labour on the acid–base status of the fetus. Br J Obstet Gynaecol, 94: 425–430.

Katz Z, Lancet M, Dgani R, Ben-Hur H, Zalel Y (1982). The beneficial effect of vacuum extraction on the fetus. Acta Obstet Gynecol Scand, 61: 337–340.

Kitzinger S (1981). Some Women's Experiences of Episiotomies. London: National Childbirth Trust.

Knauth DG, Haloburdo EP (1986). Effect of pushing techniques in birthing chair on length of second stage labor. Nurs Res, 35: 49–51.

Kurz CS, Schneider H, Huch R, Huch A (1982). The influence of the maternal position on the fetal transcutaneous oxygen pressure (tcpO$_2$). J Perinat Med, 10 (Suppl 2): 74–75.

Liddell HS, Fisher PR (1985). The birthing chair in the second stage of labour. Austral NZ J Obstet Gynaecol, 25: 65–68.

Liu YC (1974). Effects of an upright position during labor. Am J Nurs, 74: 2202–2205.

Malpas P, Jeffcoate TNA, Lister UM (1949). The displacement of the bladder and urethra during labour. J Obstet Gynaecol Br Empire, 56: 949–960.

Maresh M, Choong KH, Beard RW (1983). Delayed pushing with lumbar epidural analgesia in labour. Br J Obstet Gynaecol, 90: 623–627.

Martinez-Lopez V, de la Fuenta P, Iniguez A, Freese UE, Mendez-Bauer C (1984). Comparison of two methods of bearing down during second stage. Paper presented at the 31st Meeting of the Society for Gynecologic Investigation, 21–24 March.

Marttila M, Kajanoja P, Ylikorkala O (1983). Maternal half-sitting position in the second stage of labor. J Perinat Med, 11: 286–291.

McKay S (1984). Squatting: an alternate position for the second stage of labor. Matern Child Nurs, 9: 181–183.

McKay S, Roberts J (1985). Second stage labor: what is normal? J Obstet Gynecol Neonatal Nurs, 14: 101–106.

McManus TJ, Calder AA (1978). Upright posture and the efficiency of labour. Lancet, 1: 72–74.

McQueen J, Mylrea L (1977). Lumbar epidural analgesia in labour. Br Med J, 1: 640–641.

Minchom P, Niswander K, Chalmers I, Dauncey M, Newcombe R, Elbourne D, Mutch L, Andrews J, Williams G (1987). Antecedents and outcome of very early neoantal seizures in infants born at or after term. Br J Obstet Gynaecol, 94: 431–439.

Noble E (1983). Childbirth with Insight. Boston: Houghton Mifflin, p 88.

Pearson JF, Davies P (1974). The effect of continuous lumbar epidural analgesia upon fetal acid–base status during the second stage of labour. J Obstet Gynaecol Br Commnwlth, 80: 975–979.

Roberts J (1980). Alternative positions for childbirth. Part II: Second stage of labor. J Nurs Midwifery, 25: 13–19.

Roberts JE, Goldstein SA, Gruener JS, Maggio M, Mendez-Bauer C (1987). A descriptive analysis of involuntary bearing down efforts during the expulsive phase of labour. J Obstet Gynecol Neonatal Nurs, 16: 48–55.

Roemer VM, Harms K, Buess H, Horvath TJ (1976). Response of fetal acid–base balance to duration of second stage of labour. Int J Obstet Gynaecol, 14: 455–471.

Romond JL, Baker IT (1985). Squatting in childbirth: a new look at an old tradition. J Obstet Gynecol Neonatal Nurs, 14: 406–411.

Russell JG (1982). The rationale of primitive delivery positions. Br J Obstet Gynaecol, 89: 712–715.

Schneider-Affeld F, Martin K (1982). Delivery from a sitting position. J Perinat Med, 10 (Suppl 2): 70–71.

Shy KK, Eschenbach DA (1979). Fatal perineal cellulitis from an episiotomy site. Obstet Gynecol, 54: 292–298.

Sleep J, Grant A (1987). West Berkshire perineal management trial: three year follow up. Br Med J, 295: 749–751.

Sleep JM, Grant A, Garcia J, Elbourne D, Spencer J, Chalmers I (1984). West Berkshire perineal management trial. Br Med J, 289: 587–590.

Snooks SJ, Swash M (1984). Abnormalities of the innervation of the urethral striated musculature in incontinence. Br J Urol, 56: 401–405.

Snooks SJ, Setchell M, Swash M, Henry MM (1984). Injury to innervation of pelvic floor sphincter musculature in childbirth. Lancet, ii: 546–550.

Snooks SJ, Badenoch DF, Tiptaft RC, Swash M (1985). Perineal nerve damage in genuine stress incontinence—an electrophysiological study. Br J Urol, 57: 422–426.

Stanton SL, Kerr-Wilson R, Grant Harris V (1980). The incidence of urological symptoms in normal pregnancy. Br J Obstet Gynaecol, 87: 897–900.

Stewart P, Hillan E, Calder AA (1983). A randomised trial to evaluate the use of a birth chair for delivery. Lancet, 1: 1296–1298.

Thacker SE, Banta HD (1983). Benefits and risks of episiotomy: and interpretative review of the English language literature, 1860–1980. Obstet Gynecol Surv, 38: 322–338.

Thorp JM, Bowes WA, Brame RG, Cefalo R (1987). Selected use of midline episiotomy: effect on perineal trauma. Obstet Gynecol, 70: 260–262.

Turner MJ, Romney ML, Webb JB, Gordon H (1986). The birthing chair: an obstetric hazard? J Obstet Gynaecol, 6: 232–235.

Van Lier DJ (1984). Effect of maternal position on the second stage of labour (unpublished dissertation). Medical Center Graduate College, University of Illinois.

Willson J R (1981). Obstetrics—gynecology: a time for a change. Am J Obstet Gynecol, 141: 857–863.

Wood C, Ng KH, Hounslow D, Benning H (1973). Time—an important variable in normal delivery. J Obstet Gynaecol Br Commnwlth, 80: 295–300.

Yeates DA, Roberts JE (1984). A comparison of two bearing-down techniques during the second stage of labor. J Nurs Midwifery, 29: 3–11.

67 Care during the third stage of labour

Walter Prendiville and Diana Elbourne

1 Introduction

In the excitement of giving birth to a baby, the delivery of the placenta (the third stage of labour) is often considered to be of little importance to the new mother. However, one of the events associated with this stage—postpartum haemorrhage—remains an important cause of both maternal morbidity and mortality (Gilliat 1949; Greenhill 1951; Department of Health and Social Security 1982; Hall *et al.* 1985; Department of Health and Social Security 1986; Gilbert *et al.* 1987).

The introduction of oxytocic drugs for the treatment of postpartum haemorrhage has been regarded as 'one of the enduring achievements of modern science' (Moir 1964). It was the pioneering work of Moir (1932) that led to the discovery that ergometrine was the active principle on which the known oxytocic effect of ergot had depended (Dudley and Moir 1935). Following the introduction of ergometrine into obstetric practice half a century ago (Dudley and Moir 1935), this drug became widely accepted as a means of controlling postpartum haemorrhage. Reviewing the use of ergometrine in obstetric practice, Moir wrote in 1955, 'Few drugs can have become so firmly established in so short a time and few drugs can be so completely indispensable as ergometrine now is'. He described a fall in the death rate from postpartum haemorrhage from its previously static level of approximately 0.3 per 1000 births throughout the 1930s to 0.06 per 1000 births in 1952, coincident with the introduction of the use of oxytocics (Moir 1955). While ascribing this fall in death rate

primarily to the use of ergometrine, he acknowledged the possible confounding influence of such factors as the widespread introduction of blood transfusion services and the advent of sulphonamides and penicillin. This period was also a time of dramatic socioeconomic changes. The improved nutrition and the antenatal care women received may also have contributed to the reduced incidence of postpartum haemorrhage. Nevertheless, few would dispute the claim that the introduction of ergometrine as an effective oxytocic in obstetric practice has prevented death from postpartum haemorrhage in a substantial number of women.

Because the spectre of postpartum haemorrhage continues to dominate the management of the third stage of labour, particularly for the accoucheur who has actually been confronted with an unpredicted torrent of blood before or soon after the delivery of the placenta, we begin this chapter by giving consideration to how this serious complication of childbirth should be treated (without reiterating those aspects of the management of severe haemorrhage which have been covered in the earlier chapter on antepartum haemorrhage (Chapter 37)). We go on to discuss the management of retained placenta, a complication which predisposes to postpartum haemorrhage, and of inversion of the uterus.

The majority of the chapter, however, is given over to a consideration of the effects of active management of the third stage of labour and its various components—routine *prophylactic* use of oxytocic drugs, early clamping and division of the umbilical cord, and controlled cord traction for delivery of the placenta—because these obstetric practices were introduced with the intention of preventing both postpartum haemorrhage and retained placenta.

2 The management of third stage complications

2.1 Postpartum haemorrhage

Postpartum haemorrhage is usually defined as bleeding from the genital tract of 500 ml or more in the first 24 hours following delivery of the baby. Some people use 600 ml as the cut-off point (Beischer and Mckay 1986). Burchell (1980) estimates that the average blood loss in singleton vaginal deliveries is 600 ml (and nearly 1,000 ml for twins) and suggests that a more useful clinical diagnosis would include only cases where the estimated blood loss was 1000 ml or more. Whatever the actual cut-off point used, it is important to acknowledge that clinical estimates of the amount of blood lost tend to underestimate the actual volume of blood lost by between 34 and 50 per cent (Newton at al. 1961; Brant 1966, 1967; Quinlivan *et al.* 1970; Prendiville *et al.* (1988a). These problems in estimating the amount of blood lost are one reason that estimates of the incidence of postpartum haemorrhage vary from less than 5 per cent (Hall *et al.* 1985) to more than 10 per cent (Gilbert *et al.* 1987).

The care for the woman with postpartum haemorrhage obviously depends on assessment of the clinical situation and intends to achieve prompt arrest of the bleeding before the situation becomes critical. The source of the bleeding must be rapidly determined and corrected. If it is traumatic, this will require surgical repair; if it is due to uterine atony, contraction of the uterus must be achieved by ensuring that the uterus is empty and well contracted by 'rubbing up a contraction' and the use of oxytocics.

Oxytocin and ergometrine have been the traditional first line approach to achieve contraction of the uterus in these circumstances. Since numerous reports of the superior haemostatic effect of prostaglandins have appeared, it may well be that these agents should be the first line of approach in severe postpartum haemorrhage due to uterine atony (Tagaki 1976; Toppozada *et al.* 1981; Hyashi *et al.* 1984; Buttino and Garite 1986; Thiery 1986). Although the superiority of prostaglandins for this condition has not been demonstrated in controlled trials, their dramatic effect in the arrest of haemorrhage when all other measures have failed justify the conclusion that these drugs are indeed worth trying in these circumstances (Thiery 1986) and may negate the need for uterine packing, internal artery ligation or even hysterectomy.

2.2 Retained placenta

Retained placenta is the failure to deliver the placenta

before a certain time limit. The limit leading to the diagnosis is not consistently defined in the literature (Selinger *et al.* 1986). Beischer and Mckay (1986) allow 20 minutes; Whitfield (1981) on the other hand considers that no time limit need be exceeded before arriving at a diagnosis if active management has been employed. Few would dispute the diagnosis after an hour has elapsed.

The conventional treatment of retained placenta is manual removal following digital separation of the placenta from the uterine wall (Whitfield 1981) usually under either general anaesthesia or epidural block. Other methods, however, have been proposed. Jarcho (1928) postulated that distension of the chorionic villi by a saline infusion into the umbilical vein would promote placental separation and Golan (1983) reported a 100 per cent success rate in 10 cases treated with intraumbilical vein injection of oxytocin. Three studies have attempted to measure the effectiveness of intraumbilical view oxytocin vs. intraumbilical vein saline upon the incidence of retained placenta and prolonged third stage. Chestnut and Wilcox (1987) in a randomized controlled double-blind study assessed this intervention at 5 minutes after delivery (i.e. before a diagnosis of retained placenta had been made). Selinger *et al.* (1986) in an equally well controlled trial studied the same procedure in women at 20 minutes after delivery (ie after a diagnosis of retained placenta had been made). Similarly, Kristiansen *et al.* (1987) randomized women with retained placenta 20 minutes after delivery into one of three groups: in the first 10 international units of oxytocin diluted in 10 ml of sodium chloride (0.9 per cent) were injected into the umbilical vein; in the second, only sodium chloride was injected; the third group received no injection but manual removal of the placenta was planned. Table 67.1 details the results of these three studies. They did not reveal any benefit from use of intraumbilical vein oxytocin over intraumbilical vein saline. Kristiansen *et al.* (1987) compared the effect of intraumbilical vein injection (of oxytocin or saline) with no injection and found no advantage of the injection, but the sample size of the study was too small to exclude a clinically important effect. This trial needs to be undertaken using a far larger sample size than has been studied so far.

Selinger et al (1986) noted that waiting 60 minutes (before resorting to manual removal) will almost halve the number of women who will require manual removal with its attendant anaesthetic risks, and that umbilical vein infusion of oxytocin has nothing to offer in this condition.

2.3 Inversion of the uterus

Remarkably, inversion of the uterus has been reported in the non-pregnant uterus (Dapaah and Nel 1986) as well as the puerperium. It is now very rare (Beischer

Table 67.1 Effect of umbilical vein oxytocin vs. placebo for retained placenta on retained placenta

Study	EXPT n	(%)	CTRL n	(%)	Odds ratio (95% CI)	Graph of odds ratios and confidence intervals
Selinger *et al.* (1986)	9/15	(60.00)	8/15	(53.33)	1.30 (0.31–5.38)	
Kristiansen *et al.* (1987)	10/19	(52.63)	7/16	(43.75)	1.41 (0.38–5.24)	
Chestnut and Wilcox (1987)	1/37	(2.70)	2/41	(4.88)	0.56 (0.06–5.56)	
Frappell *et al.* (1988)	14/22	(63.64)	15/19	(78.95)	0.49 (0.13–1.84)	
Typical odds ratio (95% confidence interval)					0.90 (0.43–1.89)	

Graph scale: 0.01 0.1 0.5 1 2 10 100

and Mckay 1986). It may occur as a result of excessive cord traction in the presence of a relaxed uterus, vigorous fundal pressure or exceptionally high intra-abdominal pressure as a result of coughing or vomiting. Inappropriate cord traction without counter pressure to prevent fundal descent is said to result in the occasional case of uterine inversion (Fell 1966). Also, in unskilled domiciliary deliveries, uterine inversion and resultant death has been described (Massoudnia 1973). Treatment involves replacement of the inversion either manually (Dewhurst and Bevis 1951) or by O'Sullivan's hydrostatic method (1945).

3 Active management of the third stage

Active management of the third stage of labour, with its components of *prophylactic* use of oxytocic drugs, early clamping and division of the umbilical cord, and controlled cord traction for delivery of the placenta, has been widely adopted in an attempt to prevent both postpartum haemorrhage and retained placenta. This is reflected in the results of a survey of policies for the care of normal women in consultant and general practitioner maternity units in England in 1984 (Garcia *et al.* 1987), which showed that an active management policy with Syntometrine and controlled cord traction was universal in those units that had a policy for third stage management.

Some women using the maternity services have begun to question the routine use of an active approach for managing the third stage of labour (Chamberlain 1985; Milton 1985).

Dunn, a British paediatrician, has for many years claimed that it may interfere with physiological processes to the detriment of both mother and baby (Dunn 1966a, b, 1973, 1985; Dunn *et al.* 1966). More recently, Inch (1985) has offered evidence to suggest that routine active management of the third stage of labour promotes a 'cascade of intervention'.

3.1 Effects of routine, prophylactic use of oxytocics

While few would dispute the contribution of oxytocic drugs in the treatment of postpartum haemorrhage, the *routine, prophylactic* administration of oxytocic drugs to reduce the risk of postpartum haemorrhage has not been so universally accepted. During the 1940s several reports claimed a beneficial effect of routine administration of ergometrine for the management of the third stage of labour (see review by Dumoulin 1981). At this time the use of prophylactic oxytocic administration in the form of ergometrine (ergonovine in the United States) appeared to be popular in the United States (Martin and Dumoulin 1953) but was accepted less enthusiastically in the United Kingdom. Indeed, the practice was roundly condemned by Kerr and Moir (1949) in their textbook *Operative Obstetrics*.

In 1953, however, Du Vigneaud *et al.* synthesized oxytocin and Embrey and his colleagues (1963) subsequently reported advantages of combining this with ergometrine, as Syntometrine. The value of the combined preparation was claimed to lie in the rapid effect of the oxytocin and the sustained effect of ergometrine (Embrey *et al.* 1963). Within a few years of Syntometrine's introduction in the United Kingdom it became routine practice to administer this combined preparation prophylactically, usually in association with controlled cord traction to deliver the placenta (Kimbell 1958; Spencer 1962). In the United Kingdom and elsewhere it has now become standard teaching to advocate routine oxytocic administration for managing the third stage of labour (Fleigner and Hibbard 1966; Hibbard 1964; Llewellyn-Jones 1986; Myles 1985; Beischer and Mackay 1986; Turnbull 1976; Hickman 1978; Bender and Tindall 1980; Clayton *et al.* 1980; Marsh 1985).

We were able to identify nine trials (Prendiville *et al.* 1988b) published over a span of 34 years that compared women who did or did not receive oxytocic preparations (Daley 1951; McGinty 1956; Friedman 1957;

Table 67.2 Controlled trials of routine oxytocics in the third stage of labour

Study					Sample size				
No.	Author	Entry criteria	Drug	Route	Oxytocic	Control	Timing	Third stage management	Outcome data
1	Daley (1951)	Labour <48 hr; parity <5; spontaneous vertex delivery; singleton; no APH, hydramnios or traumatic haemorrhage	Ergometrine (0.5 mg)	IM into thigh	490	510	At crowning of head	Dorsal position; wait for signs of placental separation	Length of third stage (min); mean blood loss (oz); PPH (⩾20 oz); retained placenta (⩾1 hr); manual removal of placenta
2	McGinty (1956)	Delivered vaginally under Demerol or Scopolamine analgesia	Ergonovine (0.2 mg) Methergine (0.2 mg) Pitocin (5 units) (Control 1 ml saline)	IV IV IM IV	50 50 50	50	With birth of anterior shoulder	Not stated	Systolic and diastolic BP: significant elevation = 20 mg Hg rise in systolic since admission; severe elevation = systolic 170 mm Hg; PPH; headache, vertigo, dizziness, nausea and vomiting
3	Friedman (1975)	All vaginal deliveries except those for whom 'adequate observation was not obtained'	Pitocin (10 units) Ergonovine maleate (0.2 mg) Methergine tartrate (0.2 mg) Dihydroergotamine methane-sulfonate (1.0 mg)	IM IM or IV IM IM	214 210 167 126	177	After delivery of placenta	Not stated	Uterine atony; blood loss (ml); nausea and vomiting; BP: abnormal = systolic >140 mm Hg, diastolic >90 mm Hg; mild elevation = rise of 15 mm Hg systolic and/or 10 mm Hg diastolic; moderate = rise of 25 and/or 20; severe = rise of >20
4	Newton et al. (1961)	All term deliveries without antepartum complications and at low risk of intrapartum complications	Syntocinon (1 ml; 10 units)	IM	50	50	After delivery of placenta	Wait for placental separation, permit spontaneous expulsion by gentle fundal pressure and cord traction	Mean blood loss (ml) on delivery table and within 1 hr after leaving delivery table; need for further oxytocics; mean pulse rate; subjective feelings
5	Howard et al. (1964)	All vaginal deliveries	Oxytocin (3.0 IV) Methergine maleate (0.2 mg) (Control 0.9% sodium chloride)	IV IV IV	479 505	475	After delivery of placenta	Not stated	Need for further oxytocics; blood loss (ml); BP rises in diastolic and systolic <10 mm Hg, 10–20 mm Hg, >20 mm Hg

Table 67.2 Controlled trials of routine oxytocics in the third stage of labour—*continued*

No.	Author	Entry criteria	Drug	Route	Oxytocic	Control	Timing	Third stage management	Outcome data
6	Vaughan Williams *et al.* (1974)	All requiring IV infusion during labour, and expected to have spontaneous vaginal deliveries, except those with antenatal or labour complications	Ergometrine (0.5 mg) IV Ergometrine (0.5 mg) IV Oxytocin (10 units) IV Syntometrine (1 ml) IM and diazepam (10 mg) IM		5 10 7 9 10	10	After delivery of baby; with birth of anterior shoulder	Controlled cord traction	Central venous pressure (cm of water); blood loss (ml) in first postpartum hr
7	Hacker and Biggs (1979)	Spontaneous vaginal deliveries; no BP > 130/80 mg Hg in pregnancy or labour; postpartum blood loss < 200 ml	Syntometrine (oxytocin 5 IU + ergometrine maleate 0.5 mg) Ergometrine (0.5 mg) IV	IM	10 10	6	20 min after delivery (of baby or placenta?)	Not stated	Rise in systolic and/or diastolic BP
8	Kerekes and Domokos (1979)	Spontaneous vaginal deliveries	$PGF_{2\alpha}$ (1 mg) Ergometrine (0.2 mg) IV	Intra-myo-metrial	47 50	43	After cord Clamping	Not stated	Mean blood loss up to delivery of placenta and within subsequent 2 hr (ml); Hb 48 hr postpartum; mean length of third stage; uterine subinvolution; postpartum fertility
9	Rooney *et al.* (1985)	All spontaneous deliveries 'unless excluded by a doctor'	Syntometrine (1 ml)	IM	346	278	With birth of anterior shoulder	50% used controlled cord traction	Blood loss (ml); transfusions; Hb; length of third stage need for subsequent oxytocics; retained placenta; manual removal of placenta

Newton *et al.* 1961; Howard *et al.* 1964; Vaughan Williams *et al.* 1974; Hacker and Biggs 1979; Kerekes and Domokos 1979; Rooney *et al.* 1985). Overall, the trials included 4494 women of whom 1599 had been allocated to a 'no oxytocic' control group. The sample sizes of individual trials ranged from 26 to 1459 women (Table 67.2). The criteria for trial entry varied considerably between the studies, as did the drugs studied and their route and timing of administration. In most of the studies, the principal outcome of interest was blood loss, variously defined (Table 67.3).

The available data suggest that routine administration of oxytocics decreases the frequency of postpartum haemorrhage (Table 67.3). The results imply that routine use of oxytocics might reduce a 10 per cent risk of

postpartum haemorrhage to about 6 per cent. In the light of this finding it is not surprising that routine prophylaxis with oxytocics resulted in a reduced need to use these drugs therapeutically (Table 67.4).

The effect of the policy on retention of the placenta is far from clear. Information about retained placenta and manual removal of the placenta could be obtained from only two studies (Daley 1951; Rooney *et al.* 1985), and these cannot be assumed to be representative of all. Although there is some suggestion from these limited data that routine administration of oxytocics reduces the risk of retained placenta, this finding can easily reflect either selective presentation of outcome data or the play of chance. One other trial (Kerekes and Domokos 1979) provides evidence of possible rele-

Table 67.3 Effect of prophylactic oxytocics in third stage of labour on postpartum haemorrhage

Study	EXPT		CTRL		Odds ratio	Graph of odds ratios and confidence intervals						
	n	(%)	n	(%)	(95% CI)	0.01	0.1	0.5	1	2	10	100
Howard *et al.* (1964)	24/963	(2.49)	25/470	(5.32)	0.43 (0.23–0.78)							
McGinty (1956)	1/150	(0.67)	5/50	(10.00)	0.04 (0.01–0.27)							
Daley (1951)	45/490	(9.18)	80/510	(15.69)	0.55 (0.38–0.80)							
Rooney *et al.* (1985)	34/346	(9.83)	42/278	(15.11)	0.61 (0.38–0.99)							
Friedman (1957)	24/717	(3.35)	2/177	(1.13)	2.19 (0.82–5.83)							
Typical odds ratio (95% confidence interval)					0.57 (0.44–0.73)							

Table 67.4 Effect of prophylactic oxytocics in third stage of labour on need for further oxytocics

Study	EXPT		CTRL		Odds ratio	Graph of odds ratios and confidence intervals						
	n	(%)	n	(%)	(95% CI)	0.01	0.1	0.5	1	2	10	100
Howard *et al.* (1964)	46/984	(4.67)	58/475	(12.21)	0.32 (0.21–0.49)							
Newton *et al.* (1961)	1/50	(2.00)	11/50	(22.00)	0.15 (0.05–0.51)							
Friedman (1957)	100/717	(13.95)	36/177	(20.34)	0.61 (0.39–0.96)							
Typical odds ratio (95% confidence interval)					0.40 (0.30–0.55)							

vance, in that the mean duration of the third stage was longer in the control group (7.3 minutes) than in groups given ergometrine (5.7 minutes) or prostaglandin $F_{2\alpha}$ (3.9 minutes). The 99 per cent confidence limits of these estimates do not overlap.

Only two of the studies analysed (McGinty 1956; Friedman 1957) provided information about hypertension as a potential side-effect (defined as over 170 mm Hg systolic, or over both 140 mm Hg systolic and 90 mm Hg diastolic, respectively). In each of these studies a statistically significant hypertensive effect of oxytocics was demonstrated. More general data on blood pressure were available in four studies (Table 67.5). Analysis of these data suggests that the prophylactic use of oxytocics leads to a rise in blood pressure. These results support the suggestion that oxytocics increase the risk of hypertension, although part of the effect may be explained by reduction of the risk of hypotension caused by blood loss.

Our analysis supports the hypothesis that routine use of oxytocic drugs in the management of the third stage of labour reduces the risk of postpartum haemorrhage, but this policy appears to increase the risk of hypertension.

Older uncontrolled studies have suggested that the introduction of routine oxytocic prophylaxis resulted in up to a 90 per cent reduction in the rate of postpartum haemorrhage (Lister 1950; Martin and Dumoulin 1953). The evidence reviewed here suggests that this is an overestimate: the reduction seems more likely to be in the order of 30–40 per cent. This level of reduction in the incidence of a serious and not uncommon complication of childbirth remains of great importance.

The advantages of the prophylactic oxytocics must be considered together with the rare but serious morbidity which has sometimes been attributed to their administration. Maternal deaths from cardiac arrest (Department of Health and Social Security 1975) and intracerebral haemorrhage (Ringrose 1962) have been attributed to ergometrine, as have non-fatal instances of cardiac arrest and myocardial infarction (Browning 1974; Valentine *et al.* 1977; Taylor and Cohen 1985), postpartum eclampsia (Hofmeister and Brown 1953; McFadyen 1960; Abouleish 1976), and pulmonary oedema in cardiac patients (Casady *et al.* 1960; Dumoulin 1981) as a result of the venous vasoconstriction which is known to occur with ergometrine (Brooke and Robinson 1970; Greenhalf and Evans 1970; Vaughan Williams *et al.*

Table 67.5 Effect of prophylactic oxytocics in third stage of labour on blood pressure elevation

Study	EXPT		CTRL		Odds ratio	Graph of odds ratios and confidence intervals						
	n	(%)	n	(%)	(95% CI)	0.01	0.1	0.5	1	2	10	100
Howard *et al.* (1964)	158/983	(16.07)	50/475	(10.53)	1.57 (1.15–2.15)							
McGinty (1956)	43/150	(28.67)	6/50	(12.00)	2.45 (1.17–5.15)							
Hacker and Biggs (1979)	9/20	(45.00)	0/6	(0.00)	6.77 (1.03–44.35)							
Friedman (1957)	14/717	(1.95)	1/177	(0.56)	2.32 (0.64–8.33)							
Typical odds ratio (95% confidence interval)					1.76 (1.33–2.33)							

1974). Because these events are so rare, the available randomized trials cannot provide useful estimates of the extent to which they may be attributed to oxytocic administration.

Certain other rare but definite adverse consequences of routine oxytocic administration include intrauterine asphyxia of an undiagnosed second twin (Dunn 1966c), and neonatal convulsions in a baby mistakenly injected with an oxytocic instead of prophylactic vitamin K (Whitfield and Salfield 1980; Pandey and Haines 1982).

In principle, randomized trials should be able to provide useful information about adverse effects which are less serious but more prevalent. In fact, the nine studies reviewed here provided little usable information in this respect. Five of the trials made some mention of possible adverse effects, but apart from the investigation of hypertensive effects, there were few systematic attempts to quantify side-effects. Howard and colleagues (1964) merely reported a 'paucity of subjective side effects'. Daley (1951) stated that there were none. In answer to an enquiry, 'How do you feel?', half an hour after treatment, the proportion of women in Newton's study (Newton *et al.* 1961) who answered positively or negatively did not differ between the two trial arms. Only one woman in McGinty's trial (1956) complained of nausea, vomiting, and headache. Friedman (1957) reported no significant differences in nausea and vomiting between controls and the oxytocin and dihydroergotamine groups, but noted statistically significant increases in these symptoms in the ergonovine and methergine groups. In view of the fact that ergometrine is known to lower serum prolactin levels (Shane and Naftolin 1974; Weiss *et al.* 1975; Canales *et al.* 1976), it is unfortunate that none of the trials has investigated whether or not it interferes with breast-feeding.

On balance, the evidence suggests that the benefits of routine oxytocic administration outweigh the likely risks.

3.2 Comparisons of different oxytocics

The previous section has demonstrated the effects of oxytocics in general for the management of the third stage of labour. The present section extends this process by examining controlled trials in which different oxytocics are compared with each other (Elbourne *et al.* 1988).

Seventeen trials were identified in 16 published papers (McGinty 1956; Friedman 1957; Fugo and Dieckmann 1958; Barbaro and Smith 1961; Bonham 1963; Neiminen and Jarvinen 1963; Howard *et al.* 1964; Soiva and Koistinen 1964; Francis *et al.* 1965 (a,b); Vaughan Williams *et al.* 1974; Sorbe 1978; Hacker and Biggs 1979; Kerekes and Domokos 1979; Docherty and Hooper 1981; Dumoulin 1981; Symes 1984). These reports with sample sizes ranging from 11 to 2067 were published over a period of 24 years (from 1957 to 1984) (Table 67.6).

The oxytocic drugs evaluated can be divided into four categories: ergot alkaloids, oxytocin, prostaglandins, and a mixture of oxytocin and ergometrine (Syntometrine). The route of administration was usually intramuscular or intravenous (only one being intramyometrial). The oxytocics were administered at the crowning of the head, at delivery of the anterior shoulder, or at the end of the second stage, to at the end of the third stage.

Ergot alkaloids and oxytocin were compared in seven trials (McGinty 1956; Friedman 1957; Fugo and Dieckmann 1958; Nieminen and Jarvinen 1963; Howard *et al.* 1964; Vaughan Williams *et al.* 1974; and Sorbe 1978). Syntometrine was compared with ergot alkaloids in nine trials (Barbaro and Smith 1961; Bonham 1963; Nieminen and Jarvinen 1963; Soiva and Koistinen 1964; Francis *et al.* (one publication reporting two trials) 1965; Vaughan Williams *et al.* 1974; Hacker and Biggs 1979; and Docherty and Hooper 1981). Syntometrine was compared to oxytocin in five trials (Nieminen and Jarvinen 1963; Vaughan Williams *et al.* 1974;

Table 67.6 Controlled trials comparing different oxytocics in the third stage of labour

Trial	Entry criteria	Drug	Route	Timing	Sample size	Third stage management	Outcomes
McGinty (1956)	Delivered vaginally under Demerol or Scopolamine analgesia	Ergonovine 0.2 mg	IV	With delivery of anterior shoulder	50	Not stated	Systolic and diastolic BP significant elevation = 20 mm Hg rise in systolic since admission; severe elevation = systolic > 170 mm Hg; PPH; headache
		Methergine 0.2 mg	IV	With delivery of anterior shoulder	50		
		Pitocin 5 units	IM	With delivery of anterior shoulder			
		5 units	IV		50		
Friedman (1957)	All vaginal deliveries except those for whom 'adequate observation was not obtained'	Oxytocin (10 units)	IM	After delivery of placenta	214	Not stated	Uterine atony; blood loss (cc); nausea and vomiting; BP abnormal = systolic > 140 mm Hg, diastolic > 90 mm Hg; mild elevation = rise of 15 mm
		Ergonovine maleate (0.2 mg)	IM or IV	After delivery of placenta	210		
		Methergine tartrate (0.2 mg)	IM or IV	After delivery of placenta	167		Hg systolic and/or 10 mm Hg diastolic; moderate = rise of 25 and/or 20; severe = rise of > 20
		Dihydro-ergotamine methane-sulfonate (1.0 mg)	IM	After delivery of placenta	126		
Barbaro and Smith (1961)	All vaginal deliveries > 28 weeks	SE505 (5 units syntocin and 0.5 mg ergometrine maleate in 1 ml)	IM	Immediately after delivery of fetus	300	Not stated	Blood loss (clinical estimation); PPH (> 600 ml); mean length of 3rd stage (min)
		0.5 mg ergometrate maleate +	IV	Immediately after delivery of fetus.	300		
		0.5 mg ergometrine maleate	IM	After delivery of placenta			
Bonham (1963)	All vaginal deliveries except: multiple pregnancies, previous PPH or MRP, forceps, breech, parity ≥ 4, syntocinon infusions in 1st or 2nd stages	Ergometrine (0.5 mg)	IM	At crowning of head	217	Half controlled cord traction; half maternal effort, fundal pressure (classical pistoning technique)	Blood loss including loss on linen and swabs. Loss recorded in 20 ml steps above 100 ml; PPH (≥ 568 ml) mean loss; length of 3rd stage; manual removal of placenta
		Ergometrine (0.5 mg) + hyaluronidase (1500 units)	IM	At crowning of head	177		
		Ergometrine (0.5 mg) + oxytocin (5 units)	IM	At crowning of head	199		
Nieminen and Jarvinen (1963)	Not stated	OCM 505 (Methergin 0.5 mg + Syntocinon 5 IU)	IM	With delivery of anterior shoulder	689	Active	Duration of 3rd stage (minutes) haemorrhage (g), retained placenta

Table 67.6 Controlled trials comparing different oxytocics in the third stage of labour—*continued*

Trial	Entry criteria	Drug	Route	Timing	Sample size	Third stage management	Outcomes
Nieminen and Jarvinen (1963) —*continued*		Methergin 0.1–0.2 mg	IV	With delivery of anterior shoulder	689		
		Syntocinon 5 IU	IM	With delivery of anterior shoulder	689		
Howard et al. (1964)	All vaginal deliveries	Oxytocin 3.0 IU	IV	After delivery of placenta	479	Not stated	Need for further oxytocics; blood loss (ml) BP rises in diastolic and systolic <10 mm Hg, 10–20 mm Hg, 20+ mm Hg
		Methergine maleate 0.2 mg	IV	After delivery of placenta	505		
Soive and Koistinen (1964)	Spontaneous singleton cephalic deliveries	Syntometrine	IM	Immediately after birth of baby	560	No efforts to express placenta during 1st 3rd stage contraction	Blood loss (g); PPH (>500 g); length of 3rd stage retained placenta MRP; puerperal complications
		Methergin (0.12–0.2 mg)	IV	Immediately after birth of baby	280 (+280 historical controls)		
Francis et al. (1965)	All except: previous blood loss >2 oz; instrumental deliveries; breeches; twins; APH; severe anaemia; IV oxytocin in 1st and 2nd stages	Ergometrine (0.5 mg)	IM	After delivery of placenta	300	Brandt–Andrews after signs of descent	Blood loss (oz) including a swabs). Retained placenta (not delivered with 20 min)
		Syntometrine (0.5 ml)	IM	After baby born and cord divided	287		
		Syntometrine (1.0 ml)	IM	After baby born and cord divided	300		
Francis et al. (1965)	As above	Ergometrine (0.5 mg) + water (1.0 ml)	IM IM	End of 2nd stage End of 3rd stage	183	As above	As above
		Syntometrine (1.0 ml) + water (1.0 ml)	IM IM	End of 2nd stage End of 3rd stage	171		
		Water (1.0 ml) + Ergometrine (0.5 ml)	IM IM	End of 2nd stage End of 3rd stage	167		
Vaughan Williams et al. (1974)	All requiring intravenous infusion during labour, and to have spontaneous vaginal deliveries, except those with antenatal or labour complications	Ergometrine (0.5 mg)	IV	After delivery of baby	5	Controlled cord traction	Central venous pressure (cm of water); blood loss (ml) in first postpartum hr
		Ergometrine (0.5 mg)	IV	With delivery of anterior shoulder	10		

Table 67.6 Controlled trials comparing different oxytocics in the third stage of labour—*continued*

Trial	Entry criteria	Drug	Route	Timing	Sample size	Third stage management	Outcomes
		Oxytocin 10 units	IV	With delivery of anterior shoulder	7		
		Syntometrine 1 ml	IM	With delivery of anterior shoulder	9		
		Syntometrine 1 ml and diazepam 10 mg	IM	With delivery of anterior shoulder	10		
Sorbe (1978)	Not stated	Oxytocin (10 IU)	IV	With delivery of anterior shoulder	506	Not stated	Blood loss (ml); PPH (>600 ml) Crede's manoeuver; MRP; length of 3rd stage, placental retention, uterine
		Ergometrine (0.2 mg)	IV	With delivery of anterior shoulder	543		
Hacker and Biggs (1979)	Spontaneous vaginal deliveries; No BP >130/ 80 mm Hg in pregnancy or labour; postpartum blood loss <200 ml	Syntometrine (oxytocin 5 IU + ergometrine maleate 0.5 mg)	IM	20 min after delivery	10	Not stated	Rise in systolic and/or diastolic BP
		Ergometrine (0.5 mg)	IV	20 min after delivery	10		
Kerekes and Domokos (1979)	Spontaneous vaginal deliveries	Prostaglandin $F_{2\alpha}$ (1 mg)	Intra-myo-metrial	After cord clamping	47	Not stated	Mean blood loss up to delivery of placenta and within subsequent 2 hr (ml); Hb 48 hr postpartum; mean length of 3rd stage; uterine subinvolution; postpartum fever
		Ergometrine (0.2 mg)	IV	After cord clamping	50		
Docherty and Hooper (1981)	Normal patients. Spontaneous vertex deliveries without episiotomies, oxytocin infusions; if used in labour were stopped at delivery	Oxytocin (10 units)	IM	Not stated	25	Not stated	Mean blood loss (ml), nausea, vomiting
		Ergometrine maleate (0.5 mg) with oxytocin (5 units)	IM		25		
Dumoulin (1981)	Caesarian sections excluded. Otherwise not stated	Syntometrine	IM	After delivery of head	1000	Not stated	Primary PPH; mean blood loss (ml); Secondary PPH; manual removal of placenta
		Oxytocin (10 IU)	IM	After delivery of head	250		

Table 67.6 Controlled trials comparing different oxytocics in the third stage of labour—*continued*

Trial	Entry criteria	Drug	Route	Timing	Sample size	Third stage management	Outcomes
Dumoulin (1981)—*continued*		Oxytocin (10 IU)	IM	After delivery of head	500		
Symes (1984)	Primigravidae vaginal deliveries	Oxytocin (5 units + ergometrine (0.5 mg)	IM	With delivery of anterior shoulder	5	Not stated	Serum prolactin
		Oxytocin (5 units)	IM	With delivery of anterior shoulder	6	Active	
Fugo and Dieckmann (1985)	Not stated	U3772 (80 mg)	IV	When anterior shoulder visible	151	MRP if placenta undelivered in 10 min; 'shoehorn' if placenta protruding and traction	Time/ delivery of placenta after oxytocic; blood loss (cc/ml) BP; subjective side-effects
		Syntocinon (2 IU)	IV	When anterior shoulder visible	156		
		Ergonovine (4 mg)	IV	When anterior shoulder visible	149		
		Pitocin (2 IU)	IV	When anterior shoulder visible	168		

Docherty and Hooper 1981; Dumoulin 1981; Symes 1984). Only one study (Kerekes and Domokos 1979) compared an ergot alkaloid with a prostaglandin. There were no comparisons of prostaglandins with either oxytocin or Syntometrine.

3.2.1 Oxytocin vs. ergot alkaloids

The seven trials in which oxytocin was compared with ergot alkaloids provide no evidence that these two kinds of oxytocics differ greatly in their effects on the incidence of postpartum haemorrhage (Table 67.7). In the trial of Vaughan Williams and her colleagues (1974) there was no information on postpartum haemorrhage, although the mean blood loss was higher in the ergot alkaloid groups than in the oxytocin group. The typical odds ratio derived from the remaining six trials is 0.78 (95 per cent confidence interval 0.56–1.09) which tends to suggest that oxytocin is somewhat more effective. This estimate, however, is heavily influenced by the two trials (Friedman 1957; Sorbe 1978) in which bias is most likely to have been operating.

In only three papers was the oxytocic given before the end of the third stage and was placental delivery considered as an outcome. They did not use strictly comparable endpoints, but all three trials suggest that oxytocin is less likely than ergot alkaloids to lead to a delay in placental delivery. Nieminen and Jarvinen (1963) found a greater risk of prolonged third stage (>30 min) and retained placenta in the ergometrine group. Sorbe (1978) found that oxytocin was less likely than ergot alkaloids to be associated with a prolonged third stage, a trapped or partially retained placenta and a need for manual removal of the placenta. Fugo and Dieckmann (1958) found no statistically significant differences between the trial arms in terms of the interval to 'spontaneous' delivery of the placenta, over 60 per cent being delivered within three minutes of oxytocic administration. However, manual removal was performed in a very high proportion of women (24 per cent in the ergotrate group and 17 per cent in the oxytocin groups) 'to train residents in this procedure'!

Five of the seven papers provided information on pressor effects. Vaughan Williams and her colleagues

Table 67.7 Effect of prophylactic oxytocin vs. ergot derivatives in third stage of labour on postpartum haemorrhage

Study	EXPT		CTRL		Odds ratio	Graph of odds ratios and confidence intervals
	n	(%)	n	(%)	(95% CI)	0.01 0.1 0.5 1 2 10 100
Howard *et al.* (1964)	15/470	(3.19)	9/493	(1.83)	1.75 (0.78–3.94)	
Fugo and Dieckmann (1958)	0/324	(0.00)	0/149	(0.00)	1.00 (1.00–1.00)	
McGinty (1956)	0/50	(0.00)	1/100	(1.00)	0.22 (0.00–14.26)	
Nieminen and Jarvinen (1963)	9/689	(1.31)	10/689	(1.45)	0.90 (0.36–2.22)	
Sorbe (1978)	33/506	(6.52)	52/543	(9.58)	0.66 (0.43–1.03)	
Friedman (1957)	4/214	(1.87)	20/503	(3.98)	0.52 (0.21–1.27)	
Typical odds ratio (95% confidence interval)					0.78 (0.56–1.09)	

Table 67.8 Effect of prophylactic oxytocin vs. ergot derivatives in third stage of labour on blood pressure elevation

Study	EXPT		CTRL		Odds ratio	Graph of odds ratios and confidence intervals
	n	(%)	n	(%)	(95% CI)	0.01 0.1 0.5 1 2 10 100
Howard *et al.* (1964)	69/479	(14.41)	91/504	(18.06)	0.77 (0.55–1.07)	
McGinty (1956)	17/50	(34.00)	26/100	(26.00)	1.47 (0.70–3.12)	
Friedman (1957)	0/214	(0.00)	14/503	(2.78)	0.23 (0.07–0.74)	
Typical odds ratio (95% confidence interval)					0.78 (0.58–1.06)	

(1974) showed that oxytocin was less likely than ergometrine to cause a rise in central venous pressure. Fugo and Dieckmann (1958) merely stated that there were no significant differences in blood pressure between the groups. A typical odds ratio of 0.78 (with 95 per cent confidence limits at 0.58 and 1.06) for blood pressure elevation was derived from the only three trials that provided data suitable for meta-analysis (Table 67.8). Thus, the available evidence suggests that oxytocin is less likely to cause hypertension than are ergot alkaloids.

These three studies also commented on side-effects such as headache, nausea, and vomiting. Howard and his colleagues (1964) and McGinty (1956) reported no differences in this respect between women given oxytocin and ergot alkaloids, but in Friedman's trial (1957) these effects were stated to be significantly worse in the ergot alkaloid than in the oxytocin group.

3.2.2 Syntometrine vs ergot alkaloids alone

There was no statistically significant difference in the rate of postpartum haemorrhage between Syntometrine

and ergot alkaloids in the six trials for which data were available (Table 67.9). The available data suggest that Syntometrine is somewhat less likely than ergot alkaloids to be associated with a prolonged third stage (Table 67.10).

Only Hacker and Biggs (1979) considered blood pressure and they found that Syntometrine was less likely than ergometrine to be associated with a 20 mm Hg elevation of diastolic blood pressure.

3.2.3 Syntometrine vs oxytocin

The two trials with data on postpartum haemorrhage which compared Syntometrine with oxytocin alone suggested that Syntometrine is superior for reducing the risk of postpartum haemorrhage (Table 67.11). This was reflected in Docherty and Hooper's (1981) and in Dumoulin's (1981) findings of a lower mean blood loss in the Syntometrine group (383 ml vs. 278 ml; 264 ml vs. 230 ml respectively). In contrast, Vaughan Williams and her colleagues (1974), who presented no data on postpartum haemorrhage as such, reported that there had been a higher mean blood loss in the

Table 67.9 Effect of prophylactic syntometrine vs. ergot derivatives in third stage of labour on postpartum haemorrhage

Study	EXPT		CTRL		Odds ratio	Graph of odds ratios and confidence intervals
	n	(%)	*n*	(%)	(95% CI)	0.01 0.1 0.5 1 2 10 100
Francis *et al.* (1965)	4/171	(2.34)	17/150	(11.33)	0.23 (0.10–0.56)	
Barbaro and Smith (1961)	39/300	(13.00)	10/300	(3.33)	3.62 (2.02–6.49)	
Francis *et al.* (1965)	18/587	(3.07)	10/300	(3.33)	0.92 (0.41–2.03)	
Nieminen and Jarvinen (1963)	5/689	(0.73)	10/689	(1.45)	0.51 (0.18–1.41)	
Bonham (1963)	5/391	(1.28)	19/792	(2.40)	0.57 (0.24–1.34)	
Soiva and Koistinen (1964)	18/560	(3.21)	19/560	(3.39)	0.95 (0.49–1.82)	
Typical odds ratio (95% confidence interval)					1.02 (0.75–1.39)	

Table 67.10 Effect of prophylactic oxytocin vs. ergot derivatives in third stage of labour on prolonged third stage

Study	EXPT		CTRL		Odds ratio	Graph of odds ratios and confidence intervals
	n	(%)	*n*	(%)	(95% CI)	0.01 0.1 0.5 1 2 10 100
Nieminen and Jarvinen (1963)	10/689	(1.45)	19/689	(2.76)	0.53 (0.25–1.11)	
Typical odds ratio (95% confidence interval)					0.53 (0.25–1.11)	

Table 67.11 Effect of prophylactic syntometrine vs. oxytocin in third stage of labour on postpartum haemorrhage

Study	EXPT		CTRL		Odds ratio	Graph of odds ratios and confidence intervals
	n	(%)	*n*	(%)	(95% CI)	0.01 0.1 0.5 1 2 10 100
Nieminen and Jarvenin (1963)	5/689	(0.73)	9/689	(1.31)	0.56 (0.20–1.61)	
Dumoulin (1981)	52/1000	(5.20)	74/750	(9.87)	0.50 (0.35–0.72)	
Typical odds ratio (95% confidence interval)					0.50 (0.36–0.71)	

Syntometrine groups (with or without diazepam) than in the oxytocin group (184 ml vs. 99 ml).

The length of the third stage was reported explicitly in only one of the trials (Nieminen and Jarvinen 1963). The odds of a prolonged third stage (> 30 min) were reduced with Syntometrine, but retained placenta was more common after using this drug, although neither difference was statistically significant. Dumoulin (1981) merely noted that the incidence of manual removal of the placenta was not significantly different between the two treatment groups.

None of these trials examined blood pressure eleva-tion as an outcome, but Vaughan Williams and her colleagues (1974) considered the effects of oxytocics on mean central venous pressure and showed that it was more likely to rise after Syntometrine than after oxyto-cin used alone. This effect was not detected if women had been given diazepam late in the first stage of labour.

Symes (1984) showed that Syntometrine suppresses serum prolactin levels and that it may therefore have an adverse effect on breastfeeding. As there was no evi-dence for a comparable effect of oxytocin, he concluded that this was due to the ergot alkaloid part of Synto-metrine.

Table 67.12 Controlled trials of umbilical cord management in the third stage of labour—*continued*

	Study population	Cord management	Sample size	Outcomes studied
Siddal and Richardson (1953)	Not documented	A) Prompt cord clamping B) Cord milked before ligation	100 100	Neonatal Hgb and haematocrit; maternal Hgb, neonatal red cell count
Colozzi (1954)	Uncomplicated, vaginal deliveries 'without incident'	A) Immediate cord clamping B) Late cord clamping, baby held on mother's abdomen C) Late cord clamping, baby held below level of placenta D) Cord milked before clamping	25 25 25 25	Neonatal Hgb, neonatal red cell count
Whipple *et al.* (1957)	Healthy women, full term spontaneous vaginal deliveries	A) Cord clamped <10 sec postpartum B) Cord clamped at 3 min, baby held below placenta C) Cord clamped at 3 min, baby held above placenta D) Cord milked before clamping	10 11 8 9	Neonatal blood volume, Hgb, haematocrit and bilirubin
Pao-Chen and Tsu-Shan (1960)	Singleton, full term, vaginal; mothers without infection	A) Immediate cord clamping B) Cord clamped after pulsation ceased	73 55	Hgb, infant body weight changes; body length changes, jaundice, infant morbidity, PPH, MRP
Newton and Moody (1961)	Normal women delivered at term	A) Immediate cord clamping B) Cord clamped after pulsation ceased C) Cord clamped after pulsation ceased and after it had been milked	20 19 9	Placental weight and blood volume
Taylor *et al.* (1963)	Premature vaginal deliveries, diabetics excluded	A) Cord clamped before 1 min B) Cord clamped after 1 min	199 141	Neonatal mortality from RDS, birthweight
Buckels and Usher (1965)	Uncomplicated, fullterm vaginal deliveries	A) Cord clamped within 5 sec B) Cord clamped after 5 min	15 17	Neonatal haematocrit, pH, pCO_2, HCO_3, bilirubin, blood pressure and cardiac diameter, respiratory grunting
Dunn *et al.* (1966)	Rh+ve women in normal labour at term following uncomplicated pregnancy	A) Immediate clamping B) Cord clamped after 3 min	11 11	Feto–maternal transfusion haematocrit
Spears *et al.* (1966)	Vaginal delivery, cord cases were excluded	A) Cord clamped before 1 min B) Cord clamped before 3 min	222 202	Respiratory distress, birthweight, Apgar score
Frank and Gabriel (1967)	Premature infants 1000–1500 g	A) Cord clamped before 2 breaths B) Cord clamped after 2 breaths	61 129	Respiratory distress syndrome; mortality from respiratory distress syndrome
Botha (1968)	'Normal' vaginal deliveries	A) Cord clamped B) Cord not clamped	30 30	Duration of 3rd stage, maternal blood loss
Daily *et al.* (1970)	Full term, vaginal, spontaneously delivered; uneventful perinatal course	A) Cord clamped within 10 sec and before first breath B) Cord clamped after 5 min, with placenta held 20 cm above baby; no 'milking'	7 7	Transthoracic impedance (TTI); birthweight, neonatal Hb and haematocrit

Table 67.12 Controlled trials of umbilical cord management in the third stage of labour—*continued*

	Study population	Cord management	Sample size	Outcomes studied
Terry (1970)	Uncomplicated pregnancy, spontaneous onset of labour, spontaneous vaginal delivery	A) Immediate cord clamping but placental end left unclamped B) Controlled cord traction; no clamping	58 67	Feto–maternal transfusion
Johansen *et al.* (1971)	Normal women in labour, compatible blood groups	A) After cessation of pulsation, cord clamped ×2 and cut B) After cessation of pulsation, cord clamped and cut, placental end free to drain	 110 90	Feto–maternal transfusion
Yao *et al.* (1971)	Spontaneous vaginal deliveries with no perinatal complications	A) Cord clamped at 5–10 sec B) Cord clamped at 3–5 min	24 33	Expiratory grunting, birthweight, respiratory rate, heart rate
Saigal *et al.* (1972)	Vaginal deliveries; exclusions: IUGR, diabetes, infection, erythroblastosis	A) Immediate clamping B) Clamping at 1 min, baby held below placenta C) Clamping at 5 min, baby held below placenta D) Clamping at 1 min, baby held above placenta	51 48 48 23	Cord haematocrit, neonatal venous haematocrit, blood volume, plasma volume, RBC volume, bilirubin, RDS
Philip (1973)	Caucasian mothers, uncomplicated pregnancies, no blood group incompatibility	A) Cord clamping before regular respirations B) Cord clamping after regular respirations	28 29	Residual placental blood volume, neonatal bilirubin, haematocrit, reticulocyte count, and fluid intake and output
Nelson *et al.* (1980)	Low obstetric risk, <37 weeks interested in Leboyer, would attend prenatal classes	A) Cord clamped and cut, before 60 sec B) Cord clamped and cut after pulsation ceased	26 28	PPH, complications, puerperal infections, perinatal asphyxia and hypothermia, respiratory rate >60, polycythaemia, birthweight, hyperbilirubinaemia, residual placental blood volume
Moncrieff *et al.* (1986)	Consecutive primiparae, vaginal delivery	A) Cord clamped, controlled cord traction B) Cord clamped and cut, placental end let free then controlled cord traction	72 69	Feto–maternal transfusion
Hofmeyer *et al.* (1986)	Singleton cephalic presentation <35/40	A) Cord clamped immediately baby delivered B) Cord clamped at 1 min after baby delivered + Syntometrine	14 24	Periventricular and intraventricular haemorrhage, birthweight, Apgar scores

Table 67.13 Effect of early cord clamping on the duration of the third stage of labour

Study	Early cord clamping	Control
Pao-Chen and Tsu-Shan (1960)	average duration 8.4 min $n = 73$	average duration 10.2 min $n = 55$
Botha (1968)	mean duration 3.5 min ± 2.0 $n = 30$	mean duration 10.5 min ± 4.0 $n = 30$

3.3 Timing and route of oxytocic administration

Although, as Table 67.6 demonstrates, there was considerable variation between trials in terms of the timing of oxytocic administration, only in Vaughan Williams' trial (1974) and in Francis and colleagues' second trial (1965) was timing of a particular drug—ergometrine—explicitly compared. Neither trial could identify any differential effect ascribable to the timing of administration.

Similarly, while a number of trials (Hacker and Biggs 1979; Kerekes and Domokos 1979; Nieminen and Jarvinen 1963; Soiva and Koistinen 1963; and Vaughan Williams *et al.* 1974) compared intravenous ergot alkaloids with other oxytocics given intramuscularly, none have compared the effect of using different routes of administration for the same drug.

3.4 Early clamping and division of the umbilical cord

Precisely when the umbilical cord should be ligated and divided has been a controversial matter for many years. By the end of the nineteenth century, Kostlin (1898, cited in *Lancet* 1962) had already collected over 50 references on the subject. Active management of the third stage of labour usually entails clamping and dividing the umbilical cord relatively early, prior to beginning controlled cord traction. It has been suggested that pre-empting physiological equilibration of the blood volume within the feto–placental unit in this way predisposes to retained placenta, postpartum haemorrhage, feto–maternal transfusion, and a variety of unwanted effects in the neonate, respiratory distress in particular (Usher 1959; Bound *et al.* 1962; Dunn *et al.* 1966; Dunn 1966a,b, 1973, 1985; Botha 1968; Inch 1985).

There appears to be general agreement that delayed cord clamping is associated with a placental transfusion to the baby varying between 20 per cent and 50 per cent of neonatal blood volume depending on when the cord is clamped and at what level the baby is held prior to

clamping (De Marsh *et al.* 1942; Ballantine 1947; Gunther 1957; Usher *et al.* 1963; Oh *et al.* 1966; Yao *et al.* 1968; McCue 1968; Yao and Lind 1974; Peltonen 1981; Linderkamp 1982).

Several randomized trials have addressed various aspects of cord care: the timing of cord clamping, milking the cord, and the relative heights of baby and placenta. Details of these trials are presented in Table 67.12. The way in which the cord was managed varied from one trial to the next. For example, 'early cord clamping' means clamping the cord before 10 seconds in the study of Yao et al (1971) but means clamping the cord before one minute in the trials done by Spears *et al.* (1966), Buckels and Usher (1965), Taylor *et al.* (1963) and Nelson *et al.* (1980). Similarly, the endpoints studied varied from trial to trial. In spite of these difficulties we have attempted to synthesize the data generated by this body of research.

3.4.1 Maternal effects

The results of two trials confirm that early cord clamping leads to heavier placentae and a higher mean residual placental blood volume, but neither of these studies discussed the clinical relevance of these observations (Newton and Moody, 1961; Phillip 1973). The available data (Pao-Chen and Tsu-Shan 1960; Botha 1968) concerning the effect of early cord clamping on the duration of the third stage are presented in Table 67.13. These two trials are not strictly comparable because the timing of cord clamping differed. Also allocation to cord clamping or not was not random and the numbers studied were small. However, they arrived at the same conclusion: that early cord clamping reduces the length of the third stage. In a further trial (Dunn *et al.* 1966), manual removal of the placenta was not required in any of the 11 women in whom the cord was clamped immediately after delivery of the baby and in 2 of 11 women who had the cord clamped between 3 and 10 minutes after delivery.

Three trial reports provide data on maternal blood loss (Pao-Chen and Tsu-Shan 1960; Botha 1968; Nel-

Table 67.14 Effect of early umbilical cord clamping in third stage of labour on postpartum haemorrhage

Study	EXPT		CTRL		Odds ratio	Graph of odds ratios and confidence intervals						
	n	(%)	*n*	(%)	(95% CI)	0.01	0.1	0.5	1	2	10	1
Nelson *et al.* (1980)	1/26	(3.85)	1/28	(3.57)	1.08 (0.07–17.74)							
Pao-Chen and Tsu-Shan (1960)	7/73	(9.59)	5/55	(9.09)	1.06 (0.32–3.50)							
Botha (1968)	1/30	(3.33)	0/30	(0.00)	7.39 (0.15–99.99)							
Typical odds ratio (95% confidence interval)					1.22 (0.42–3.53)							

son *et al.* 1980). The effect of early cord clamping on blood loss after delivery are shown in Table 67.14. True random allocation was employed in only one (Nelson *et al.* 1980) of these three trials. Neither the individual nor the typical odds ratios show a statistically significant effect of the timing of cord clamping on the postpartum haemorrhage rate.

Four controlled trials have addressed the question of feto–maternal transfusion (Dunn *et al.* 1966; Terry 1970; Johansen *et al.* 1971; Moncrieff *et al.* 1986). The study by Dunn *et al.* (1966) did not suggest any effect of early cord clamping. The other three trials assessed the effect of allowing free bleeding from the placental end of the cord, and the results are shown in Table 67.15. The methodological quality of these four trials is similar. None of them used strictly random allocation. A further controlled trial by Ladipo (1972), where the method of allocation was not reported, supports the findings of the three trials in Table 67.15. These are that free placental drainage after early cord clamping is associated with a reduced risk of feto–maternal transfusion. Furthermore Lapido estimated that 30 per cent (*n* = 100) of patients denied placental drainage had a sufficiently large feto–maternal transfusion (0.25 ml) to be associated with a high incidence of rhesus immunization 6 months after delivery. Women whose third stage was managed by placental drainage immediately postpartum or after cessation of cord pulsation had 0.25 ml placental transfusions in 7.9 per cent (*n* = 62) and 10.2 per cent (*n* = 38) respectively.

3.4.2 Neonatal effects

Fifteen controlled trials compared the effect of different cord management practices on the neonate (Siddal and Richardson 1953; Colozzi 1954; Whipple *et al.* 1957; Pao-Chen and Tsu-Shan 1960; Taylor *et al.* 1963; Buckels and Usher 1965; Dunn and Fraser 1966; Spears *et al.* 1966; Frank and Gabriel 1967; Daily *et al.* 1970; Yao *et al.* 1971, Saigal *et al.* 1972, Phillip 1973, Nelson *et al.* 1980; Hofmeyr *et al.* 1986). Haematological indices were studied in some of these and the results

confirm that early cord clamping reduces the extent of placental transfusion to the baby. Babies born after early cord clamping have lower haemoglobin values (Siddall and Richardson 1953; Colozzi 1954; Whipple *et al.* 1957; Pao-Chen and Tsu-Shan 1960; Daily *et al.* 1970) and haematocrits (Whipple *et al.* 1957; Buckels and Usher 1965; Dunn and Fraser 1966; Daily *et al.* 1970; Saigal *et al.* 1972; and Phillip 1973). In all three trials which included sequential assessment of haemoglobin, differences between the two experimental groups diminished over time (Siddall and Richardson 1953; Colozzi 1954; Pao-Chen and Tsu-Shan 1960). In the study with the longest follow-up (Pao-Chen and Tsu-Shan 1960) the difference in haemoglobin levels had virtually disappeared by 6 weeks of age and was undetectable at 6 months after birth.

3.4.2.1 Neonatal respiratory maladaptation One of the problems confounding assessment of the relative frequency of 'respiratory distress' is the difficulty of finding a universally acceptable definition. As can be seen from Table 67.12 the study populations and method of cord management varied between these studies.

The effects of early cord clamping on the incidence of a variety of forms of neonatal respiratory maladaptation are shown in Table 67.16. (Taylor *et al.* 1963; Buckels and Usher 1965; Spears *et al.* 1966; Frank and Gabriel 1967; Yao *et al.* 1971).

Respiratory grunting was investigated by two authors (Buckels and Usher 1965; Yao *et al.* 1971) These authors' study populations were similar. Entry bias was not considered optimum by us in either study but cord management was similar in both studies. The results from these two trials were inconsistent (Table 67.17).

Two trials (Spears *et al.* 1966 and Frank and Gabriel 1967) separately and together both suggest that late cord clamping results in less neonatal 'respiratory distress' but the effect is not statistically significant (Table 67.18).

Table 67.15 Effect of free bleeding from placental end of umbilical cord on feto-maternal transfusion

Study	EXPT		CTRL		Odds ratio	Graph of odds ratios and confidence intervals						
	n	(%)	*n*	(%)	(95% CI)	0.01	0.1	0.5	1	2	10	100
Terry (1970)	27/58	(46.55)	45/67	(67.16)	0.43 (0.21–0.88)							
Moncrieff *et al.* (1986)	32/68	(47.06)	61/72	(84.72)	0.19 (0.09–0.38)							
Johansen *et al.* (1971)	28/90	(31.11)	34/110	(30.91)	1.01 (0.55–1.84)							
Typical odds ratio (95% confidence interval)					0.47 (0.32–0.70)							

Table 67.16 Effect of early cord clamping on neonatal respiratory maladaptation

Study	Early cord clamping group	Control	Outcome studied
	Table 67.12 study group A	Table 67.12 study group B	
Taylor *et al.** (1963)	15.5% 22.9% 19/199	14.4% 25% 25/141	Tachypnoea Dyspnoea Death
Buckels and Usher (1965)	42 2/15 2/15 3/15 2/15	43 6/17 0/17 9/17 6/17	Mean respiration rate Chest retraction Grunting Decreased at entry Rates
Spears *et al.* (1966) Term infants	8/12 2/192 25/192	5/187 1/187 22/187	Respiration rate >60 Air exchange at 3 hr 'Poor' 'Respiratory distress' at first breath
Spears *et al.* (1966) Premature infants	4/30 1/30 13/30	2/15 2/15 6/15	Respiration rate >60 Air exchange at 3 hr 'Poor' 'Respiratory distress' at first breath
Frank and Gabriel (1967)	19/61 5/19	35/129 0/14	'Respiratory distress' Mortality in infants with hyaline membrane disease
Yao *et al.* (1971)	0/24	13/33	Expiratory grunting

*Percentage adjusted to allow for differences in birthweight distribution of early and late clamped infants

Table 67.17 Effect of early umbilical cord clamping in third stage of labour on neonatal grunting

Study	EXPT n	(%)	CTRL n	(%)	Odds ratio (95% CI)	Graph of odds ratios and confidence intervals 0.01 0.1 0.5 1 2 10 100
Yao *et al.* (1971)	0/24	(0.00)	13/33	(39.39)	0.11 (0.03–0.38)	
Buckels and Usher (1965)	2/15	(13.33)	0/17	(0.00)	9.07 (0.54–99.99)	
Typical odds ratio (95% confidence interval)					0.23 (0.07–0.71)	

Table 67.18 Effect of early umbilical cord clamping in third stage of labour on neonatal respiratory distress

Study	EXPT n	(%)	CTRL n	(%)	Odds ratio (95% CI)	Graph of odds ratios and confidence intervals 0.01 0.1 0.5 1 2 10 100
Spears *et al.* (1966)	38/222	(17.12)	28/202	(13.86)	1.28 (0.76–2.16)	
Frank and Gabriel (1967)	19/61	(31.15)	35/129	(27.13)	1.22 (0.62–2.39)	
Typical odds ratio (95% confidence interval)					1.26 (0.83–1.90)	

Table 67.19 Effect of early cord clamping on neonatal plasma bilirubin levels

Study	Early cord clamping				Control group				Difference of means
	Study group Table 67.12	Mean sample time	Bilirubin value (mean) mg %	Sample size (n)	Study group Table 67.12	Mean sample time	Bilirubin value (mean) mg %	Sample size (n)	
Whipple et al. (1957)	A	77.7 hr	2.8	9	B	83 hr	5.5	11	−2.7
Buckels and Usher (1965)	A	72 hr	3.77	15	B	72 hr	3.87	17	−0.1
Saigal et al. (1972)	A (full term babies)	72 hr	3.2	15	C (full term babies)	72 hr	7.7	15	−4.5
	A (premature babies)	72 hr	9.8	36	C (premature babies)	72 hr	14.4	33	−4.6
Phillip* (1973)	A	72 hr	3.9	14	B	72 hr	3.6	13	+0.3
Nelson et al.† (1980)	A	72 hr	5 babies had bilirubin value ⩾ 12	26	B	72 hr	12 babies had bilirubin value ⩾ 12		

* Cord clamped relative to onset of respirations
† In both groups the cord was clamped after pulsation ceased

Table 67.20 Effect of early umbilical cord clamping in third stage of labour on neonatal jaundice

Study	EXPT		CTRL		Odds ratio	Graph of odds ratios and confidence intervals						
	n	(%)	n	(%)	(95% CI)	0.01	0.1	0.5	1	2	10	100
Nelson et al. (1980)	5/26	(19.23)	12/28	(42.86)	0.34 (0.11–1.07)							
Pao-Chen and Tsu-Shan (1960)	16/55	(29.09)	9/38	(23.68)	1.31 (0.52–3.32)							
Typical odds ratio (95% confidence interval)					0.77 (0.37–1.57)							

3.4.2.2 Neonatal bilirubin and jaundice In four out of the five trials in which neonatal bilirubin levels were measured they were lower in the babies born after early cord clamping (Whipple et al. 1957; Buckels and Usher 1965; Saigal et al. 1972; Phillip 1973; and Nelson et al. 1980) (Table 67.19). The effects of early cord clamping on the incidence of clinical jaundice are shown in Table 67.20 (Pao-Chen and Tsu-Shan 1960; Nelson et al. 1980). It is difficult to draw clinically relevant information from this table. The trials differ in that the diagnostic criteria for clinical jaundice was based on visual assessment in Pao-Chen and Tsu-Shan's study, and was only performed on two trials of each study group. It was not related to morbidity. In Nelson et al.'s study the median time of cord clamping was 45 seconds in the early clamping group. By this time most placental blood would already have been transferred to the infant. Taken together these two trials do not provide conclusive evidence about the effect of early cord clamping on neonatal jaundice.

3.5 Controlled cord traction

Aristotle appears to have been the first person to advocate cord traction as a means of expediting delivery of the placenta (Aristotle, reprinted 1786). Similar advice was given by a number of authors of textbooks in the eighteenth and nineteenth centuries including Mauriceau (1694) and Ould (1741). Levy and Moore

(1985) reckoned that it was likely that 'cord traction as a method of third stage management was continued during the late nineteenth and early twentieth century but, paradoxically, its use was not advocated in the standard textbooks of midwifery and obstetrics, perhaps partially due to the possibility of introducing infection by handling the cord and partially due to the widespread acceptance of Crede's method of fundal pressure to expel the placenta'.

Brandt (1933) and Andrews (1940, revived academic interest in this approach to third stage management. Further modification of the technique by Spencer (1962), who also advocated prophylactic oxytocic therapy, produced the technique today known as controlled cord traction. In this, controlled traction on the cord is maintained while being countered with upward pressure on the lower segment of the uterus by a hand placed on the lower abdomen.

There have been two controlled trials in which controlled cord traction has been compared with a less active approach, albeit one which sometimes entailed use of fundal pressure (Bonham 1963; Kemp 1971) (Table 67.21). Controlled cord traction was associated with a lower mean blood loss and shorter third stages, but the trials provide insufficient data to warrant any firm conclusions about its effects on either postpartum haemorrhage (Table 67.22) or manual removal of the placenta (Table 67.23). One of the two investigators (Kemp 1971) noted that the umbilical cord had ruptured in 3 per cent of the women managed with controlled cord traction, but that women were more likely to find fundal pressure uncomfortable.

3.6 Active vs. expectant management of the third stage

When a particular element has been the focus of the experiment, it is often difficult or impossible to assess from the research reports that we have reviewed above, which other elements of active management of the third stage of labour have also been used.

In a recent randomized controlled trial in the third stage of labour (Prendiville *et al.* 1988b), 846 women were allocated to active management (prophylactic oxytocic, early cord clamping and controlled cord traction) and 849 to expectant or 'physiological' management (no prophylactic oxytocic, cord clamping after placental

Table 67.21 Details of trials of controlled cord traction

Study	Entry criteria	Third stage management		Sample size		
		CCT	Control	CCT	Control	
Bonham (1963)	Spontaneous vaginal deliveries, singletons Cephalic presentation No 3rd stage complications No 1st/2nd stage oxytocins used	IM oxytocic (ergometrine or ergometrine + hyaluronidase or ergometrine + oxytocin) maternal effort and abdominal, i.e. fundal pressure	IM oxytocic (ergometrine or ergometrine + hyaluronidase or ergometrine + oxytocin) maternal effort and abdominal, i.e. fundal pressure	593	590	Length of 3rd stage; postpartum haemorrhage; manual removal of placenta
Kemp (1971)	Not documented	IM syntometrine with anterior shoulder, immediate cord clamping controlled cord traction	IM syntometrine with anterior shoulder, i.e. fundal pressure after signs of separation	379	334	Length of 3rd stage; postpartum haemorrhage; secondary postpartum haemorrhage; cord rupture; manual removal of placenta

Table 67.22 Effect of cord traction vs. fundal pressure in third stage of labour on postpartum haemorrhage

Study	EXPT		CTRL		Odds ratio	Graph of odds ratios and confidence intervals						
	n	(%)	n	(%)	(95% CI)	0.01	0.1	0.5	1	2	10	10
Bonham (1963)	7/593	(1.18)	17/590	(2.88)	0.43 (0.19–0.95)							
Kemp (1971)	6/379	(1.58)	5/334	(1.50)	1.06 (0.32–3.49)							
Typical odds ratio (95% confidence interval)					0.57 (0.29–1.11)							

Table 67.23 Effect of cord traction vs. fundal pressure in third stage of labour on manual removal of placenta

Study	EXPT		CTRL		Odds ratio	Graph of odds ratios and confidence intervals
	n	(%)	n	(%)	(95% CI)	0.01 0.1 0.5 1 2 10 100
Bonham (1963)	5/593	(0.84)	6/590	(1.02)	0.83 (0.25–2.71)	
Kemp (1971)	3/379	(0.79)	6/334	(1.80)	0.45 (0.12–1.67)	
Typical odds ratio (95% confidence interval)					0.63 (0.26–1.52)	

delivery, no controlled cord traction, and maternal effort aided by gravity). The two groups were comparable at entry. Virtually all the women in the active group received their allocated management compared to about half in the 'physiological' group. Women allocated to active management had less blood loss, fewer blood transfusions, shorter third stages and less need for therapeutic oxytocics, but were more likely to vomit than those allocated to 'physiological' management.

In terms of neonatal effects the increased placental transfusion associated with expectant management resulted in a higher mean birthweight and a higher neonatal haematocrit as well as an increase in the incidence of jaundice and the need for phototherapy.

These results held true for a 'low risk' subset of women (spontaneous onset of labour without augmentation, epidurals or prolonged first or second stages of labour) and their babies.

4 Conclusions

4. Implications for current practice

The evidence from controlled trials supports the routine use of oxytocic drugs in the third stage of labour because of a reduced risk of postpartum haemorrhage. The reduction in risk is likely to be in the order of 30 to 40 per cent. This advantage must be weighed against the relatively small risk of hypertension and the disadvantages attending the routine use of injections.

The evidence available provides no support for the continued prophylactic use of ergometrine. This drug offers no advantage over oxytocin in reducing blood loss and it is associated with a greater risk of hypertension and vomiting.

Early cord clamping reduces the length of the third stage of labour. The available evidence does not reveal any effect upon blood loss or postpartum haemorrhage. In rhesus negative women it should be avoided because it increases the risk of feto–maternal transfusion. As a package, the active management of labour is superior to 'physiological' or expectant management by virtue of its significant protective effect with respect to postpartum haemorrhage.

In the presence of severe intractable postpartum haemorrhage it is worth trying prostaglandin therapy, but which preparation, dose, or route of administration is unclear.

4.2 Implications for future research

Active management is made up of many interlocking and interdependent variables. There is a need to scrutinize the following components of active management by large randomized controlled trials, using factorial designs where possible.

(i) choice of oxytocic
(ii) route of oxytocic
(iii) timing of oxytocic
(iv) timing of cord clamping
(v) value of signs of placental separation
(vi) effects of controlled cord traction

Some aspects of the 'physiological' package may also need further investigation. For instance, the role of early suckling is currently the subject of a trial in Malawi (Bullough, personal communication). The influence of maternal posture and maternal effort also need investigation.

Where 'physiological' or expectant management is the usual practice it would be justifiable to mount a large, randomized controlled trial comparing it with active management. If this were to be tried in some 'Third World' countries, then as oxytocics are unstable at high ambient temperatures (Longland and Roebottom 1987), it may be necessary either to consider the feasibility of using existing oxytocics or to synthesize new forms of the drugs able to withstand high temperatures. This topic is being considered by the World Health Organization, Maternal and Child Health Division in Geneva (Guidotti, personal communication).

In the context of a trial of active versus 'physiological' management, there is also a need to investigate whether it is preferable to resort to the full complement of active management (rather than a piecemeal approach) when there is a need to interrupt the process of physiological management.

Turning to the treatment of third stage problems,

because the 'optimal management' of retained placenta is unknown, the effect of intraumbilical vein injection of oxytocin or saline (compared to no injection) should be evaluated.

In the presence of severe postpartum haemorrhage the urgency of the clinical situation precludes the implementation of a controlled trial where the individual patient is the unit. However, a trial of management

protocol using various prostaglandins administered by different routes versus other oxytocics would be feasible when an obstetric department was the unit for randomization. In this way it should be possible to discover the most effective way of treating postpartum haemorrhage which remains a potent cause of maternal morbidity and mortality.

References

Abouleish E (1976). Postpartum hypertension and convulsion after oxytocic drugs. Anaesth Analg, 55: 813–815.

Andrews CJ (1940). Sth Med Surg, 102: 605.

Aristotle (1786). The Complete Works. London: E Wilson.

Ballantine GN (1947). Delayed ligation of the umbilical cord. Penn Med J, 50: 726–728.

Barbaro CA, Smith GO (1961). Clinical trial of SE 505—a new oxytocic mixture. Austral NZ J Obstet Gynaecol, 1: 147–150.

Beischer NA, Mackay EV (1986). Obstetrics and the Newborn. Eastbourne: Ballière Tindall, pp 360 and 375.

Bender S, Tindall VR (1980). Practical Student Obstetrics. London: Heinemann, p 209.

Bonham DG (1963). Intramuscular oxytocics and cord traction in the third stage of labour. Br Med J, 2: 1620–1623.

Botha MC (1968). The management of the umbilical cord in labour. S Afr J Obstet Gynaecol, 6: 30–33.

Bound JP, Harvey PW, Bagshaw HB (1962). Prevention of pulmonary syndrome of the newborn. Lancet, 1: 1200.

Brandt ML (1933). The mechanism and management of the third stage of labour. Am J Obstet Gynecol, 25: 662–666.

Brant HA (1966). Blood loss at caesarean section. J Obstet Gynaecol Br Commwlth, 73: 456–457.

Brant HA (1967). Precise estimation of post partum haemorrhage: difficulties and importance. Br Med J, 1: 398–400.

Brooke OG, Robinson BF (1970). Effect of ergotamine and ergometrine in forearm venous compliance in man. Br Med J, 1: 139–142.

Browning DJ (1974). Serious side effects of ergometrine and its use in routine obstetric practice. Med J Austral, 1: 957–959.

Buckels LJ, Usher R (1965). Cardiopulmonary effects of placental transfusion. J Pediatr, 67: 239–46.

Burchell RC (1980). Postpartum haemorrhage. In: Current Therapy in Obstetrics and Gynecology. Quilligan ES (ed). Philadelphia: W B Saunders, p 69.

Buttino L, Garite TJ (1986). The use of 15 methyl F2 alpha prostaglandin for the control of postpartum haemorrhage. Am J Perinatol, 3: 241–243.

Canales ES, Garrido JT, Zarate A, Mason M, Soria J (1976). Effect of ergonovine on prolactin secretion and milk let down. Obstet Gynecol, 48: 228–229.

Casady GN, Moore DC, Brindenbaugh LD (1960). Postpartum hypertension after use of vasoconstrictor and oxytocic drugs. JAMA, 172: 101–105.

Chamberlain GVP (1985). Discussion. In: Litigation and obstetrics and gynaecology. Chamberlain GVP, Orr CJB,

Sharp F (eds). London: Royal College of Obstetricians and Gynaecologists, p 272.

Chestnut DH, Wilcox LL (1987). Influence of umbilical vein administration of oxytocin on the third stage of labor: A randomized, double-blind placebo-controlled trial. Am J Obstet Gynaecol, 157: 160–162.

Clayton SG, Lewis TLT, Pinker G (1980). Obstetrics by Ten Teachers. London: Arnold, p 124.

Colozzi AE (1954). Placental transfusion. New Engl J Med, 250: 629–632.

Daily W, Olsson T, Victorin L (1970). Transthoracic impedance. V. Effects of early and late cord clamping of the umbilical cord with special reference to the ratio air to blood during respiration. Acta Paediatr Scand (Suppl 207): 57–72.

Daley D (1951). The use of intramuscular ergometrine at the end of the second stage of normal labour. J Obstet Gynaecol, 57: 388–97.

Dapaah V, Nel J (1986). Spontaneous inversion of an adolescent non-pregnant uterus. J Obstet Gynaecol, 7: 146.

Department of Health and Social Security (1975). Report on confidential enquiries into maternal deaths 1970-1972. London: Her Majesty's Stationery Office.

Department of Health and Social Security (1982). Report on confidential enquiries into maternal deaths 1976–1978. London: Her Majesty's Stationery Office.

Department of Health and Social Security (1986). Report on confidential enquiries into maternal deaths 1979–1981. London: Her Majesty's Stationery Office.

De Marsh QB, Windle WF, Alt HL (1942). Blood volume of newborn infant in relation to early and late clamping of umbilical cord. Am J Dis Child, 63: 1123–1129.

Dewhurst CJ, Bevis DCA (1951). Acute puerperal inversion of the uterus. Lancet, 2: 452.

Docherty PW, Hooper M (1981). Choice of an oxytocic agent for routine use at delivery. J Obstet Gynaecol, 2: 60.

Dudley HW, Moir JC (1935). The substance responsible for the traditional clinical effect of ergot. Br Med J, 1: 520–523.

Dumoulin JG (1981). A reappraisal of the use of ergometrine. J Obstet Gynaecol, 1: 178–181.

Dunn PM (1966a). The placental venous pressure during and after the third stage of labour following early cord ligation. J Obstet Gynaecol Br Commwlth, 73: 747–756.

Dunn PM (1966b). Postnatal placental respiration. Dev Med Child Neurol, 8: 607.

Dunn PM (1966c). Ergometrine and the undiagnosed twin. Br Med J, 2: 1535.

Dunn PM (1973). Caesarean section and the prevention of

respiratory distress syndrome of the newborn. In: Perinatal Medicine. Bossart H *et al.* (eds). Berne: Hans Huber, pp 138–145.

Dunn PM (1985). Management of childbirth in normal women: the third stage and fetal adaptation. In: Perinatal Medicine; Report of the IX European Congress Perinatal Medicine, Dublin. Lancaster: MTP Press.

Dunn PM, Fraser ID, Raper AB (1966). Influence of early cord ligation on the transplacental passage of foetal cells. J Obstet Gynaecol Br Commwlth, 73: 757–760.

Du Vigneaud V, Ressler C, Tippet S (1953). The sequence of amino acids in oxytocin with a proposal for the structure of oxytocin. J Biol Chem, 205: 949.

Elbourne D, Prendiville W, Chalmers I (1988). Choice of oxytocic preparation for routine use in the management of the third stage of labour: an overview of the evidence from controlled trials. Br J Obstet Gynaecol, 95: 17–30.

Embrey MP, Barber DTC, Scudamore JH (1963). Use of syntometrine in prevention of post partum haemorrhage. Br Med J, 1: 1387–1389.

Fell MR (1966). Management of the third stage. Br Med J, 2: 764.

Fleigner JR, Hibbard BM (1966). Active management of the third stage of labour. Br Med J, 2: 622–623.

Francis HH, Miller JM, Porteous CR (1965). Clinical trial of an oxytocin–ergometrine mixture. Austral NZ J Obstet Gynaecol 5: 47–51.

Frank DJ, Gabriel M (1967). Timing of cord ligation and newborn respiratory distress. Am J Obstet Gynecol, 97: 1142–1144.

Friedman EA (1957). Comparative clinical evaluation of post-partum oxytocics. Am J Obstet Gynecol, 73: 1306–1313.

Fugo NW, Dieckmann WJ (1958). A comparison of oxytocic drugs in the management of the placental stage. Am J Obstet Gynecol, 76: 141–146.

Garcia J, Garforth S, Ayers S (1987). The policy and practice of midwifery study: introduction and methods. Midwifery, 3: 2–9.

Gilbert L, Porter W, Brown V (1987). Postpartum haemorrhage a continuing problem. Br J Obstet Gynaecol, 94: 67–71.

Gilliat W (1949). Transactions of the 12th Congress of Obstetrics and Gynaecology, Canada, p 271.

Golan A, Lider ALB, Wexler S, David MP (1983). A new method for the management of retained placenta. Am J Obstet Gynecol, 146: 708.

Greenhalf JO, Evans DJE (1970). Effect of ergometrine on the central venous pressure in the third stage of labour. J Obstet Gynaecol Br Commwlth, 77: 1066–1069.

Greenhill JP (1951). Year Book of Obstetrics and Gynaecology. Chicago: Year Book Publishers, p 230.

Gunther M (1957). The transfer of blood between baby and placenta in the minutes after birth. Lancet, 1: 1277–1280.

Hacker NF, Biggs JSG (1979). Blood pressure changes when uterine stimulants are used after normal delivery. Br J Obstet Gynaecol, 86: 633–636.

Hall MH, Halliwell R, Carr-Hill R (1985). Concomitant and repeated happenings of complications of the third stage of labour. Br J Obstet Gynaecol, 92: 732–738.

Hibbard BM (1964). The third stage of labour. Br Med J, 2: 1485–1488.

Hickman MA (1978). An Introduction to Midwifery. Oxford: Blackwell, p 166.

Hofmeister FJ, Brown RC (1953). Postpartum convulsions. Am J Obstet Gynecol, 65: 498–504.

Hofmeyr GJ, Bolton KD, Bowen DC, Govan JJ (1986). Periventricular/intraventricular haemorrhage and umbilical cord clamping: findings and hypothesis. S Afr Med J, 73: 104–106.

Howard WF, McFadden PR, Keettel WC (1964). Oxytocic drugs in fourth stage of labor. JAMA, 189: 411–413.

Hyashi RH, Castillo MS, Noah ML (1984). Management of severe postpartum haemorrhage due to uterine atony using an analogue of prostaglandin F$_2$alpha. Obstet Gynecol, 63: 806.

Inch S (1985). Management of the third stage of labour—Another cascade of intervention? Midwifery, 1: 114–122.

Jarcho B (1928). Management of retained placenta. Surg Gynecol Obstet, 46: 265.

Johansen JK, Schache E, Stürup AG (1971). Feto–maternal transfusion and free bleeding from the umbilical cord. Acta Obstet Gynecol Scand, 50: 193–195.

Kemp J (1971). A review of cord traction in the third stage of labour from 1963 to 1969. Med J Austral, 1: 899–903.

Kerekes L, Domokos N (1979). The effect of prostaglandin F$_2$alpha on third stage labour. Prostaglandins, 18: 161–166.

Kerr JMM, Moir JC (1949). Operative Obstetrics. London: Ballière, Tindall & Cox, pp 54 and 810.

Kimbell N (1958). Brandt–Andrews technique of delivery of the placenta. Br Med J, 1: 203–204.

Kristiansen FV, Frost L, Kaspersen P, Moller BR (1987). The effect of oxytocin injection into the umbilical vein for the management of the retained placenta. Am J Obstet Gynecol, 156: 979–980.

Ladipo OA (1972). Management of the third stage of labour, with particular reference to reduction of feto–maternal transfusion. Br Med J, 1: 721–723.

Lancet (1962). Placental transfusion. Lancet, 1: 1222–1223.

Levy V, Moore J (1985). The midwife's management of the third stage of labour. Nursing Times, 81: 47–50.

Linderkamp O (1982). Placental transfusion: determinants and effects. Clin Perinatol, 9: 559–593.

Lister UM (1950). The use of intravenous oxytocics in the second stage of labour. J Obstet Gynaecol Br Empire, 57: 210.

Longland P, Roebottom PC (1987). Stability at room temperature of medicines normally recommended for cold storage. Pharmaceut J, 288: 147–51.

Llewellyn-Jones D (1986). Fundamentals of Obstetrics and Gynaecology (4th edn), Vol. 1. London: Faber & Faber, p 135.

Marsh GN (1985). Modern Obstetrics in General Practice. Oxford: Oxford University Press.

Martin JD, Dumoulin JG (1953). Use of intravenous ergometrine to prevent post partum haemorrhage. Br Med J, 1: 643–646.

Massoudnia N (1973). Inversion of the uterus in Iran. Gerburtshilfe Frauenheilk, 33: 901.

Mauriceau F (1694). Traite des maladies des femmes grosses. Vol 1, Ed 4, Paris.

McCue CM, Garner FB, Hurt WG, Schelin EC, Sharpe AE (1968). Placental transfusion. J Pediatr 72: 15–21.

McFadyen IR (1960). Postpartum pre-eclampsia. Lancet, 2: 1009–1010.

McGinty LB (1956). A study of the vasopressor effects of oxytocics when used intravenously in the third stage of labour. West J Surg, 64: 22–28.

Milton PJD (1985). Natural childbirth and home deliveries—clinical aspects. In: Litigation and obstetrics and gynaecology. Chamberlain GVP (ed). London: Royal College of Obstetricians and Gynaecologists, pp 279–299.

Moir JC (1932). The action of ergot preparation on the puerperal uterus. Br Med J: 1119–1122.

Moir JC (1955). The history of present day use of ergot. Can Med Assoc J, 72: 727–734.

Moir JC (1964). The obstetrician bids and the uterus contracts. Br Med J, 2: 1025–1029.

Moncrieff D, Parker Williams J, Chamberlain G (1986). Placental drainage and feto–maternal transfusion. Lancet, 2: 453.

Myles MF (1985). Textbook for Midwives (10th Edn). Edinburgh: Churchill Livingstone, pp 331–336.

Nelson NM, Enkin MW, Saigal S, Bennett KJ, Milner R, Sackett DL (1980). A randomized clinical trial of the Leboyer approach to childbirth. New Engl J Med, 302: 655–660.

Newton M, Mosey LM, Egli GE, Gifford WB, Hull CT (1961). Blood loss during and immediately after delivery. Obstet Gynecol, 17: 9–18.

Nieminen U, Jarvinen PA (1963). A comparative study of different medical treatments of the third stage of labour. Ann Chir Gynaecol Fenn, 53: 424–429.

Oh W, Blankenship W, Lind J (1966). Further study of neonatal blood volume in relation to placental transfusion. Ann Paediatr, 20: 147–159.

O'Sullivan JV (1945). Acute inversion of the uterus. Br Med J, 2: 282.

Ould F (1741). A Treatise of Midwifery in Three Parts. Dublin: Nelson, pp 57–67.

Pandey SK, Haines CI (1982). Accidental administration of ergometrine to a newborn infant. Br Med J, 285: 693.

Pao-Chen W, Tsu-Shan K (1960). Early clamping of the umbilical cord. A study of its effect on the infant. Chin Med J, 80: 351–355.

Peltonen T (1981). Placental transfusion advantage and disadvantage. Eur J Pediatr, 137: 141–146.

Phillip AGS (1973). Further observations on placental transfusion. Obstet Gynecol, 47: 334–343.

Prendiville WJ, Elbourne DR, Chalmers I (1988a). The Bristol third stage trial: active versus physiological management of the third stage of labour. Br Med J, 297: 1295–1300.

Prendiville WJ, Elbourne DR, Chalmers I (1988b). The effects of routine oxytocic administration in the management of the third stage of labour: An overview of the evidence from controlled trials. Br J Obstet Gynaecol, 95: 3–16.

Quinlivan WLG, Brock JA, Sullivan H (1970). Blood volume changes, blood loss associated with labour. 1 Correlation of changes in blood volume measured by I^{131} albumin and Evans blue dye, with measured blood loss. Am J Obstet Gynecol, 106: 843–849.

Ringrose CAD (1962). The obstetrical use of ergot. Can Med Assoc J, 87: 712–714.

Rooney I, Hughes P, Calder A (1985). Is routine administration of syntometrine still justified in the management of the third stage of labour? Health Bull, 43: 99–101.

Saigal S, O'Neill A, Surainder Y, Chua LB, Usher R (1972). Placental transfusion and hyperbilirubinemia in the premature. Pediatrics, 49: 406–419.

Selinger M, MacKenzie I, Dunlop P, James D (1986). Intra-umbilical vein oxytocin in the management of retained placenta. A double blind controlled study. J Obstet Gynaecol, 7: 115–117.

Shane JM, Naftolin F (1974). Effect of ergonovine maleate on puerperal prolactin. Am J Obstet Gynecol, 120: 129–131.

Siddall RS, Richardson RP (1953). Milking or stripping the umbilical cord. Effect on vaginally delivered babies. Obstet Gynaecol, 1: 230–233.

Soiva K, Koistinen U (1964). Clinical experience with simultaneous intramuscular injection of oxytocin and methyl–ergometrine. Ann Chir Gynaecol, 53: 173–186.

Sorbe B (1978). Active pharmacologic management of the third stage of labor. Obstet Gynecol, 52: 694–697.

Spears RL, Anderson GV, Brotman S, Farrier J, Kwan J, Masto A, Perrin L, Stebbins R (1966). The effect of early versus late cord clamping on signs of respiratory distress. Am J Obstet Gynecol, 95: 564–568.

Spencer PM (1962). Controlled cord traction in management of the third stage of labour. Br Med J, 1: 1728–1732.

Symes JB (1984). A study on the effect of ergometrine on serum prolactin levels following delivery. J Obstet Gynaecol, 5: 36–38.

Tagaki S, Yoshida T, Togo Y (1976). The effects of intramyometrial injections of prostaglandin PGF_2 on severe postpartum haemorrhage. Prostaglandins, 12: 565–579.

Taylor GJ, Cohen B (1985). Ergonovine-induced coronary artery spasm and myocardial infarction after normal delivery. Obstet Gynecol, 66: 821–822.

Taylor PM, Bright NH, Birchard EL (1963). Effect of early versus delayed clamping of the umbilical cord on the clinical condition of the newborn infant. Am J Obstet Gynecol, 86: 893–898.

Terry MF (1970). A management of the third stage to reduce feto–maternal transfusion. J Obstet Gynaecol Br Commwlth, 77: 129–132.

Thiery M (1986). Prostaglandins for the treatment of hypotonic postpartum haemorrhage. In: Prostaglandin Perspectives 2: 10.

Toppozada M, El-Bossati M, El Rahman HA, Shams El-Din AH (1981). Control of intractable atonic postpartum haemorrhage by 15-methyl prostaglandin F_{2a}. Obstet Gynecol, 58: 327–330.

Turnbull AC (1976). Obstetrics—traditional use of ergot compounds. Postgrad Med J, 52 (Suppl 1): 15–16.

Usher R, Shepherd M, Lind J (1963). The blood volume of the newborn infant and placental transfusion. Acta Paediatr Scand, 52: 497–512.

Usher R (1959). The respiratory distress syndrome of prematurity: a preliminary report. Paediatr Int, 9: 141.

Valentine BH, Martin MA, Phillips NV (1977). Collapse during operation following intravenous ergometrine. Br J Anaesth, 49: 81–82.

Vaughan Williams C, Johnson A, Ledward R (1974). A comparison of central venous pressure changes in the third stage of labour following oxytocic drugs and diazepam. J Obstet Gynaecol Br Commwlth, 81: 596–599.

Weiss G, Klein S, Shenkman L, Katooka K, Hollander CS (1975). Effect of methylergonovine on puerperal prolactin secretion. Obstet Gynecol, 46: 209–210.

Whipple GA, Sisson TRC, Lund CJ (1957). Delayed ligation of the umbilical cord. Obstet Gynecol, 10: 603–610.

Whitfield CR (1981). Complications of the third stage of labour. In: Integrated Obstetrics and Gynaecology for Postgraduates. Dewhurst J, (ed). Oxford: Blackwell, p 437.

Whitfield MF, Salfield SAW (1980). Accidental administration of syntometrine in adult dosage to the newborn. Arch Dis Child, 55: 68–70.

Yao AC, Hirvensalo M, Lind J (1968). Placental transfusion rate and uterine contraction. Lancet, 1: 380-384.

Yao AC, Link J and Vourenkoski V (1971). Expiratory grunting in the late cord clamped normal neonate. Pediatrics, 48: 865–70.

Yao AC, Lind J (1974). Placental transfusion. Am J Dis Child, 127: 128–141.

68 Repair of perineal trauma after childbirth

1 Introduction	1170
2 Technique of perineal repair	1171
3 Subcuticular or interrupted sutures for perineal skin closure?	1171
4 The choice of absorbable suture materials for perineal repair	1173
5 Comparisons of 'absorbable' materials with non-absorbable materials removed during the puerperium	1177
6 Who should perform the repair?	1179
7 Conclusions	
7.1 Implications for current practice	1180
7.2 Implications for future research	1180

1 Introduction

In the developed world as many as 70 per cent of women are likely to require repair of perineal trauma following childbirth (Sleep et al. 1984). As might be expected, the majority of these women experience some perineal pain or discomfort in the immediate postpartum period (see Chapter 79), but even 3 months later, as many as 20 per cent still have problems (such as dyspareunia) likely to be related to perineal trauma and its repair.

Given the magnitude of the problem it is surprising that perineal repair following childbirth has been the subject of so little scientifically sound research. The underlying reason for this apparent lack of interest is most likely the clinical perspective on the morbidity which can result. The symptoms caused by perineal trauma usually remain unrecognized by the operator who performed the repair, they are believed to resolve with time in nearly all cases and thus they are not rated as particularly serious. The lack of interest amongst both those who sponsor and those who conduct research in obstetrics possibly also reflects an attitude that considers study of such problems unglamorous, and not really 'true science'. The technique of repair and the choice of suture material, in addition to the nature and extent of the trauma, are likely to have a bearing on the extent of morbidity associated with perineal trauma. A telephone survey conducted in 1986 of a random sample of 50 English maternity units (34 specialist units and 16 general practitioner units) revealed a wide variation in the 'most popular' materials for perineal repair of the deep tissues and the skin (Grant 1986). The results are summarized in Table 68.1.

The variation in clinical practice is, in fact, even wider than this simple tabulation suggests. Thirteen different combinations of materials for the deeper tissue and skin were mentioned. As many as a quarter of the

Table 68.1 Suture materials used for perineal repair in a random sample of 50 English maternity units (Grant 1986)

Material	Deep tissues (% units)	Skin (% units)
Plain catgut	13	8
Chromic catgut	63	49
Polyglycolic acid (Dexon)	12	12
Polyglycolic acid plus lactic acid (Vicryl)	5	5
Glycerol-impregnated catgut (Softgut)	7	8
Silk	—	15
Nylon	—	2

Note: some units used two materials equally; this is the reason for the non-even percentages.

units surveyed used two or more combinations equally frequently, the most extreme example of this being a hospital in which the four obstetricians all had individual and markedly different policies. With one exception, glycerol-impregnated catgut was only used in specialist consultant units, whereas plain catgut for the deeper tissues with silk to the skin was a combination popular with general practitioners. Chromic catgut for all layers was clearly most popular, being the choice in 50 per cent of those units with a consistent policy. Polyglycolic acid sutures (either the homopolymer (Dexon; Davis and Geck Ltd) or the copolymer with lactide, (Vicryl; Ethicon Ltd)) used for both deeper tissues and the skin was the choice in 17 per cent of units. Other reported combinations included glycerol-impregnated catgut (Softgut; Davis & Geck Ltd) throughout (8 per cent), and chromic catgut for the deep tissue with silk to the skin (6 per cent).

The technique of skin closure also varied considerably. When absorbable materials were chosen for skin closure 59 per cent of units predominantly used interrupted sutures, and only 7 per cent predominantly used continuous subcuticular suturing; 34 used the two techniques equally often.

Clearly, there is no clinical consensus within England as to which materials and which technique of skin closure should be used. Can the few controlled studies which have been conducted help to make an informed choice?

2 Technique of perineal repair

Perineal trauma is most commonly repaired in 'layers'. The three stages are repair of the vagina, repair of the deeper perineal tissues, and closure of the skin. The vaginal trauma may be repaired with a continuous suture or (less commonly) with interrupted sutures. In theory a continuous stitch might 'concertina' the vagina and for this reason a continuous, locking stitch is sometimes recommended. No controlled studies have compared these techniques. The vaginal stitch is started at the apex of the vaginal trauma and continued down to about the level of the fourchette. The deeper perineal injuries are usually closed with interrupted sutures in one or two stages depending on the extent of the trauma, but sometimes continuous 'running' sutures are used. Some operators 'bury' the knots of these stitches believing that this makes wound breakdown less likely. Again, there are no relevant controlled studies. The skin is commonly closed with interrupted transcutaneous sutures. Alternatively, a continuous subcuticular suture using an absorbable material may be used. Details of these techniques are available elsewhere (for example, Isager-Sally *et al.* 1986).

An alternative approach has been advocated by Pretorius (1982). His technique is simply to appose the deeper tissues with 'a few catgut sutures'. Although Pretorius claims that perineal trauma managed in this way heals satisfactorily with minimal discomfort, the evidence unfortunately remains anecdotal and no formal evaluative studies have been reported.

3 Subcuticular or interrupted sutures for perineal skin closure?

Four controlled studies (Banninger *et al.* 1978; Detlefson *et al.* 1980; Isager-Sally *et al.* 1986; Mahomed *et al.* 1989) have compared continuous subcuticular with interrupted transcutaneous suturing techniques for closure of the perineal skin. All four trials used similar materials and techniques for repair of the deeper tissues in their two trial groups. In the first three, polyglycolic acid (Dexon) sutures were used throughout. Mahomed *et al.* (1989) Southmead Perineal Suture Study had a balanced factorial design and approximately 50 per cent were repaired with polyglycolic acid and 50 per cent with chromic catgut in each trial group. The four trials are described in summary in Table 68.2.

The three earlier (but smaller) trials (Banninger *et al.* 1978; Detlefson 1980; Isager-Sally *et al.* 1986) all suggested that the continuous, subcuticular technique was associated with fewer short term problems. Although women in the Southmead trial reported somewhat more pain on the second postpartum day after subcuticular repair, by the tenth day this trend was reversed. Thus the overview strongly suggests that continuous, subcuticular sutures are associated with

Table 68.2 Randomized trials comparing continuous with interrupted suturing techniques for closure of the perineal skin following perineal trauma—description of the studies

Study	Entry criteria	'Continuous' group (*n*)	'Interrupted' group (*n*)
Banninger *et al.* (1978)	Episiotomy Primigravidae Normal delivery	Subcuticular PGA (80) PGA to deeper tissue	Interrupted PGA (80) PGA to deeper tissue
Detlefson *et al.* (1980)	Mediolateral and median episiotomies	Subcuticular PGA (52) PGA to deeper tissue	Interrupted PGA (65) PGA to deeper tissue
Isager-Sally *et al.* (1986)	Mediolateral episiotomy	Subcuticular PGA (267) PGA to deeper tissue	Interrupted PGA (263) PGA to deeper tissue
Mahomed and Grant (1989)	Perineal trauma requiring repair following vaginal delivery	Subcuticular (533) 50% chromic catgut 50% PGA Similar materials to deeper tissues	Interrupted (524) 50% chromic catgut 50% PGA Similar materials to deeper tissues

PGA = polyglycolic acid

Table 68.3 Effect of continuous vs. interrupted sutures for perineal repair on short-term pain

Study	EXPT		CTRL		Odds ratio	Graph of odds ratios and confidence intervals						
	n	(%)	n	(%)	(95% CI)	0.01	0.1	0.5	1	2	10	100
Mahomed et al. (1989)	130/447	(29.08)	148/461	(32.10)	0.87 (0.65–1.15)							
Isager-Sally et al. (1986)	24/262	(9.16)	60/261	(22.99)	0.36 (0.23–0.57)							
Banninger et al. (1978)	7/80	(8.75)	8/80	(10.00)	0.86 (0.30–2.49)							
Typical odds ratio (95% confidence interval)					0.69 (0.55–0.88)							

Table 68.4 Effect of continuous vs. interrupted sutures for perineal repair on long-term pain

Study	EXPT		CTRL		Odds ratio	Graph of odds ratios and confidence intervals						
	n	(%)	n	(%)	(95% CI)	0.01	0.1	0.5	1	2	10	100
Isager-Sally et al. (1986)	77/265	(29.06)	96/250	(38.40)	0.66 (0.46–0.95)							
Mahomed et al. (1989)	57/465	(12.26)	51/451	(11.31)	1.10 (0.73–1.64)							
Typical odds ratio (95% confidence interval)					0.83 (0.63–1.09)							

Table 68.5 Effect of continuous vs. interrupted sutures for perineal repair on dyspareunia

Study	EXPT		CTRL		Odds ratio	Graph of odds ratios and confidence intervals						
	n	(%)	n	(%)	(95% CI)	0.01	0.1	0.5	1	2	10	100
Mahomed et al. (1989)	116/459	(25.27)	94/443	(21.22)	1.25 (0.92–1.71)							
Isager-Sally et al. (1986)	45/265	(16.98)	58/250	(23.20)	0.68 (0.44–1.04)							
Detlefsen et al. (1980)	20/52	(38.46)	44/65	(67.69)	0.31 (0.15–0.64)							
Typical odds ratio (95% confidence interval)					0.90 (0.71–1.14)							

less pain than interrupted transcutaneous sutures in the immediate postpartum period (Table 68.3). The three trials which provided the relevant data are also consistent in that women repaired with a subcuticular suture reported less analgesic use in the puerperium. Both Detlefson and Isager-Sally reported less long term pain and dyspareunia associated with subcuticular suturing. Mohamed et al., on the other hand, found little if any difference in pain at 3 months' postpartum, but somewhat more dyspareunia in the continuous suture group. Putting the results from these three trials together suggests that there are no substantial differences between the two techniques in respect of long term pain

(Table 68.4) and dyspareunia (Table 68.5).

The need for resuturing is a rarer adverse outcome. None of the women in either of Banninger's groups was resutured, but resuturing was required by three women in each group in the Southmead trial. As will be discussed later, it is common for absorbable suture materials (which in theory should not need removal) to be removed during the puerperium. In the Southmead trial, 18 per cent of women who had a continuous suture and 29 per cent of the women who had interrupted sutures had sutures removed during the first 10 days postpartum, a further 26 per cent and 37 per cent respectively had to have sutures removed during the 3 months after delivery. Despite this, a similar proportion (7 per cent) complained of 'still feeling stitches' at the 3-month follow-up.

The lack of consistency between the results of the Southmead trial and the other three trials may reflect the skills and preferences of the operators. Thirty per cent of the repairs in the Southmead trial were performed by midwives. This was a relatively new development in the hospital. There is clear evidence that some of the midwives disliked the technically more difficult subcuticular technique: when a woman was allocated to subcuticular suturing the repair was more likely to be performed by a junior doctor; and as many as 18 per cent of women allocated to subcuticular suturing were repaired with interrupted transcutaneous sutures. It should be noted, however, that most of the repairs in the trial reported by Isager-Sally and his colleagues were performed by midwives. One interpretation of this review could be that interrupted, transcutaneous sutures should be used by those who are relatively inexperienced in perineal repair whereas more experienced operators should use a continuous subcuticular stitch. Another interpretation is that the inconsistency may reflect a publication bias. The three published trials all suggest that subcuticular suturing is superior.

4 The choice of absorbable suture materials for perineal repair

The absorbable materials most commonly used for perineal skin closure are polyglycolic acid and chromic catgut. One attraction of absorbable materials is that the same materials can be used for all layers. Seven controlled studies (Tompkins and Lea 1972; Beard *et al.* 1974; Livingstone *et al.* 1974; Rogers 1974; Banninger *et al.* 1978; Roberts and McKay Hart 1983; Mahomed *et al.* 1989) have compared polyglycolic acid and catgut (mostly chromic catgut) when used for all layers with a similar technique used in each trial for the two groups. These trials are summarized in Table 68.6. Three used interrupted skin sutures, two continuous sutures, one half interrupted and a half continuous. Details of the suturing technique used in the seventh trial are not known.

Data for four principal measures of outcome—short term perineal pain, short-term analgesia use, longer term pain, and dyspareunia—where available, have been considered. The Tompkins and Lea paper provides no useful data and no extra information has been supplied by the authors. The report in this paper of less pain in the early puerperium associated with polyglycolic acid sutures is, however, consistent with all the other

Table 68.6 Randomized trials comparing polyglycolic acid and catgut for repair of perineal trauma—description of the studies

Study	Entry criteria	Polyglycolic acid group (*n*)	Catgut group (*n*)
Tompkins and Lea (1972)	Episiotomy	PGA to all layers (25) Subcuticular to skin	Chromic catgut to all layers (25) Subcuticular to skin
Beard *et al.* (1974)	Mediolateral episiotomy Normal delivery	PGA to all layers (100) Subcuticular to skin	Chromic catgut to all layers (100) Subcuticular to skin
Livingstone *et al.* (1974)	Mediolateral episiotomy Primigravidae Instrumental or normal delivery	PGA to all layers (50) Interrupted to skin	Plain catgut (50) Interrupted to skin
Rogers (1974)	Episiotomy— median and mediolateral	PGA to all layers (299) Type of skin suture not stated	Chromic catgut to all layers (301) Type of skin suture not stated
Banninger *et al.* (1978)	Episiotomy Primigravidae Normal delivery	PGA to all layers (80) Interrupted to skin	Chromic catgut to all layers (73) Interrupted to skin
Roberts and McKay Hart (1983)	Mediolateral episiotomy Instrumental or normal delivery	PGA to all layers (88) Interrupted to skin	Catgut to all layers (84) Interrupted to skin
Mahomed *et al.* (1989)	Perineal trauma requiring repair	PGA to all Layers (275) Interrupted and subcuticular to skin	Chromic catgut to all layers (263) Interrupted and subcuticular to skin

published trials (Table 68.7). The results for analgesia use during the immediate puerperium also suggest that women whose perineal trauma was repaired with poly-glycolic sutures suffer less pain during the early puer-perium than those repaired with either chromic or plain catgut (Table 68.8).

Unfortunately, only one of the seven trials, all of which suggest such clear-cut short term advantages for polyglycolic sutures, includes adequate follow-up after discharge from hospital. Only 46 (30 per cent) of the 160 women in the Swiss trial (Banninger *et al.* 1978) returned for reassessment 3 months after delivery: four women in each group complained of persistent dyspar-eunia. More complete longer term follow-up data are only available for the Southmead Suture Study (Mahomed *et al.* 1989). The available data suggest that both perineal pain (Table 68.9) and dyspareunia (Table 68.10) were equally common in the trial's two groups 3 months after delivery.

A striking finding in the Southmead study was that the reported removal of some suture material was far more common in the polyglycolic acid group. This was particularly marked in the first 10 days (77/230 vs. 27/232) but persisted up to 3 months (94/232 vs. 48/233). The commonest reasons given were 'irritation' and 'tightness'. Anecdotes of stitch abscess associated with polyglycolic sutures were not supported in the trial findings.

Only two trials (Banninger *et al.* 1978; Mahomed *et al.* 1989) reported cases which were judged to require resuturing. The 2 cases in the Swiss trial and 3 cases in the British trial were all in the catgut groups. This is consistent with the finding of Livingstone and col-leagues of only 1 case of major dehiscence in their polyglycolic acid group as opposed to 3 in the catgut group.

The comparisons between catgut and polyglycolic acid which have been discussed so far have all been between the materials when used to repair all layers. In the analysis of the Southmead trial comparing the two

Table 68.7 Effect of polyglycolic acid vs. catgut for perineal repair on short-term pain

Study	EXPT		CTRL		Odds ratio	Graph of odds ratios and confidence intervals
	n	(%)	*n*	(%)	(95% CI)	0.01 0.1 0.5 1 2 10 100
Roberts and McKay Hart (1983)	23/88	(26.14)	29/84	(34.52)	0.67 (0.35–1.29)	
Livingstone *et al.* (1974)	39/50	(78.00)	48/50	(96.00)	0.21 (0.06–0.66)	
Beard *et al.* (1974)	64/100	(64.00)	72/100	(72.00)	0.69 (0.38–1.25)	
Rogers (1974)	155/299	(51.84)	225/301	(74.75)	0.37 (0.27–0.52)	
Mahomed *et al.* (1989)	130/270	(48.15)	134/253	(52.96)	0.83 (0.59–1.16)	
Banninger *et al.* (1978)	14/80	(17.50)	29/73	(39.73)	0.34 (0.17–0.68)	
Typical odds ratio (95% confidence interval)					0.54 (0.44–0.65)	

Table 68.8 Effect of polyglycolic acid vs. catgut for perineal repair on analgesia use

Study	EXPT		CTRL		Odds ratio	Graph of odds ratios and confidence intervals
	n	(%)	*n*	(%)	(95% CI)	0.01 0.1 0.5 1 2 10 100
Roberts *et al.* (1983)	32/88	(36.36)	49/84	(58.33)	0.42 (0.23–0.76)	
Beard *et al.* (1974)	21/100	(21.00)	36/100	(36.00)	0.48 (0.26–0.89)	
Mahomed *et al.* (1989)	129/270	(47.78)	135/254	(53.15)	0.81 (0.57–1.14)	
Typical odds ratio (95% confidence interval)					0.64 (0.49–0.84)	

Table 68.9 Effect of polyglycolic acid vs. catgut for perineal repair on long term pain

Study	EXPT		CTRL		Odds ratio	Graph of odds ratios and confidence intervals						
	n	(%)	*n*	(%)	(95% CI)	0.01	0.1	0.5	1	2	10	100
Mahomed *et al.* (1989)	25/232	(10.78)	28/233	(12.02)	0.88 (0.50–1.57)							
Typical odds ratio (95% confidence interval)					0.88 (0.50–1.57)							

Table 68.10 Effect of polyglycolic acid vs. catgut for perineal repair on dyspareunia 3 months postpartum

Study	EXPT		CTRL		Odds ratio	Graph of odds ratios and confidence intervals						
	n	(%)	*n*	(%)	(95% CI)	0.01	0.1	0.5	1	2	10	100
Mahomed *et al.* (1989)	56/227	(24.67)	56/228	(24.56)	1.01 (0.66–1.54)							
Banninger *et al.* (1978)	4/25	(16.00)	4/21	(19.05)	0.81 (0.18–3.69)							
Typical odds ratio (95% confidence interval)					0.99 (0.66–1.49)							

materials for repair of the perineal skin (the materials for the deeper tissues were balanced to be the same in the groups), there was no evidence of a difference in short term pain. Polyglycolic acid sutures were much more likely to be removed, particularly in the first ten days postpartum (148/451 vs. 69/454), again because of 'irritation' and 'tightness'. But resuturing was less common in the polyglycolic acid group (1/458 vs. 5/458).

In the analysis comparing the two materials when used to repair the vagina and deeper perineal tissues, the use of polyglycolic acid sutures was associated with a lower use of analgesia (48 per cent vs. 54 per cent, $p = 0.03$) and a suggestion of less pain in the immediate postpartum period. More women reported removal of dissolvable material in this group, however (19 per cent vs. 15 per cent), although not to the extent seen when these materials were used for all layers or for the skin alone (see above). This last analysis will be referred to again later during discussion of the choice of absorbable material to use for the deeper tissues.

Most of the evidence thus points to polyglycolic acid sutures causing less pain in the immediate postpartum period, albeit with a tendency to cause irritation sufficient to lead to the removal of some sutures in an important minority of cases. The limited evidence available suggests no major difference in the long term with the possible exception of a greater risk of dehiscence leading to resuturing associated with catgut. If the choice is in respect of the deep tissues only (for example, in combination with a removable skin suture) polyglycolic acid again appears superior.

Polyglycolic acid sutures cause minimal tissue reaction (Craig *et al.* 1975), and this contrasts with chromic catgut and silk (see below), both of which elicit a polymorphonuclear reaction (Lawrie *et al.* 1959; Capperauld 1975). This may explain why the use of polyglycolic acid sutures is associated with less pain in the immediate postpartum period. The knotting properties of polyglycolic acid and chromic catgut are also different. First throws of polyglycolic sutures hold better; double throws are needed with catgut but the stitch can be tightened with the second throw. Another suggested explanation for the trial findings is that they reflect differences in the tightness of the stitches rather than differences in the materials *per se*.

Two polyglycolic acid suture materials are commercially available: the homopolymer, 'polyglycolide' (Dexon; Davis and Geck Ltd) and the copolymer with lactide, 'polyglactide' (Vicryl; Ethicon Ltd). All seven trials discussed above have evaluated polyglycolide (Dexon). There are no direct comparisons between the two formulations in this context. It seems likely that they will behave similarly. The manufacturing method used for braiding the filaments does appear different and for this reason polyglycolide (Dexon) is somewhat rougher in texture. Passage through the tissues may be more traumatic but knots are more secure (Trimbos and Klopper 1985). First throws of polyglycolide (Dexon) hold better; polyglactide (Vicryl) behaves more like catgut and double or triple throws are needed to prevent knot slippage. The implications of this are that different knotting techniques are required for the two materials (Rahman and Way 1972). The first throw of polyglycolide (Dexon) must be positioned correctly whereas the positioning of the knot can be decided at the second throw with polyglactide (Vicryl). Teflon coating of Dexon (marketed as Dexon plus) produces a smoother surface. Much of the coating may come off during passage through tissues so Dexon plus is likely to behave like untreated Dexon in other respects. Both polyglycolide (Dexon) and polyglactide (Vicryl) cause minimal tissue reaction (Craig *et al.* 1975). The two materials also lose their tensile strength at very similar rates: about 50 per cent loss in 20 days and 100 per cent loss in 30 days (Capperauld 1984). The 10 per cent lactide component of polyglactide (Vicryl) may explain its slightly speedier resorption pattern: 70 days compared with 90 days (Capperauld 1984).

The only other published trial of two absorbable materials (Spencer *et al.* 1986) compared glycerol-impregnated catgut (soft catgut—Braun) with chromic catgut, both materials being used for all layers. The trial is summarized in Table 68.11.

The use of glycerol-impregnated catgut was associated with statistically significantly more pain 10 days after delivery and an increased prevalence of dyspareunia 3 months' postpartum. A further follow-up 3 years after delivery has recently been completed (Grant *et al.*, 1989). This has revealed that the increased prevalence of dyspareunia has persisted, reports of pain during sexual intercourse being nearly twice as common in the glycerol-impregnated catgut group (Table 68.11). On the basis of this trial there appears to be no place for glycerol-impregnated catgut sutures for repair of perineal trauma. Another finding in the trial by Spencer *et al.* (1986) was that untreated catgut stitches were much more likely to be removed in the puerperium than were glycerol-treated sutures (11.5 per cent vs. 2.4 per cent in the first 10 days; and 16.4 per cent vs.

Table 68.11 Effect of glycerol-impregnated catgut vs. chromic catgut for perineal repair on perineal pain at 10 days

Study	EXPT		CTRL		Odds ratio	Graph of odds ratios and confidence intervals						
	n	(%)	*n*	(%)	(95% CI)	0.01	0.1	0.5	1	2	10	100
Spencer *et al.* (1986)	107/335	(31.94)	75/321	(23.36)	1.53 (1.09–2.16)							
Typical odds ratio (95% confidence interval)					1.53 (1.09–2.16)							

Effect of glycerol-impregnated catgut vs. chromic catgut for perineal repair on analgesia at 10 days

Spencer *et al.* (1986)	12/335	(3.58)	6/321	(1.87)	1.90 (0.74–4.84)							
Typical odds ratio (95% confidence interval)					1.90 (0.74–4.84)							

Effect of glycerol-impregnated catgut vs. chromic catgut for perineal repair on perineal pain at 3 months

Spencer *et al.* (1986)	30/339	(8.85)	24/332	(7.23)	1.24 (0.71–2.17)							
Typical odds ratio (95% confidence interval)					1.24 (0.71–2.17)							

Effect of glycerol-impregnated catgut vs. chromic catgut for perineal repair on dyspareunia at 3 months

Spencer *et al.* (1986)	78/300	(26.00)	57/292	(19.52)	1.44 (0.98–2.12)							
Typical odds ratio (95% confidence interval)					1.44 (0.98–2.12)							

Effect of glycerol-impregnated catgut vs. chromic catgut for perineal repair on dyspareunia at 3 years

Grant *et al.* (1989)	51/263	(19.39)	29/253	(11.46)	1.83 (1.14–2.95)							
Typical odds ratio (95% confidence interval)					1.83 (1.14–2.95)							

6.9 per cent in the first 3 months). 'Maternal discomfort' was the most common reason given for this. Glycerol-impregnated catgut was reported by the operators in this trial to be easier to straighten out and less likely to dry out. Drying out is one possible explanation for this difference in the rates of suture removal. It is noteworthy that, as discussed above, polyglycolic acid sutures were more likely to be removed than untreated chromic catgut when these two materials were compared. Spencer and his colleagues were confident that the higher rate of suture removal in the group sutured with chromic catgut than in the group sutured with glycerol impregnated catgut explained only a relatively small amount of the difference in both the extent of perineal pain at 10 days and the dyspareunia rates at 3 months experienced by the two groups. Nevertheless, this does raise questions about the practice of leaving materials such as catgut and polyglycolic acid to dissolve.

5 Comparisons of 'absorbable' materials with non-absorbable materials removed during the puerperium

Six controlled studies have compared absorbable with non-absorbable skin sutures (Table 68.12). Four (Hansen *et al.* 1975; Bendsen and Madsen 1980; Buchan and Nicholls 1980; Mahomed *et al.* 1989) compared polyglycolic acid sutures with interrupted silk. In two of these the polyglycolic acid sutures were subcuticular, in one interrupted, and in the fourth 50 per cent interrupted and 50 per cent continuous. All except the study conducted by Hansen and colleagues used similar materials for the deeper tissues in the two trial groups. The groups repaired with polyglycolic acid sutures left to dissolve generally had less pain (Table 68.13) and used less analgesia in the first 5 days after delivery.

The situation in respect of longer term morbidity is less clear. Buchan and Nicholls reported more long term pain and dyspareunia in the polyglycolic acid group but do not provide the data in a form which would allow them to be pooled with those from the other trials. The results of the other trials tend to support this but taken on their own, provide no clear evidence of a difference in long term pain (Table 68.14) or dyspareunia (Table 68.15).

The other two trials which compared absorbable with non-absorbable skin sutures compared polyglycolic acid with the polyamide nylon (Isager-Sally *et al.* 1986) and chromic catgut with the polyamide Supramid (Gaasemyr *et al.* 1977). Their results are consistent

Table 68.12 Randomized trials comparing absorbable with non-absorbable skin sutures for repair of perineal trauma—description of the studies

Study	Entry characteristics	Absorbable group (n)	Non-absorbable group (n)
PGA vs. silk Hansen *et al.* (1975)	Mediolateral episiotomy	Interrupted PGA to skin (136) PGA to deeper tissues	Interrupted silk to skin (145) Chromic catgut to deeper tissues
Bendsen and Madsen (1980)	Episiotomy	Subcuticular PGA to skin (108) PGA to deeper tissues	Interrupted silk to skin (103) PGA to deeper tissues
Buchan and Nicholls (1980)	Mediolateral episiotomy Primigravidae Normal delivery	Subcuticular PGA to skin (70) Chromic catgut to deeper tissues	Interrupted silk to skin (70) Chromic catgut to deeper tissues
Mahomed *et al.* (1989)	Perineal trauma requiring repair following vaginal delivery	45% subcuticular and 55% interrupted PGA to skin (535) 50% PGA and 50% chromic catgut to deeper tissues	Interrupted silk to skin (517) 50% PGA and 50% chromic catgut to deeper tissues
PGA vs. nylon Isager-Sally *et al.* (1986)	Mediolateral episiotomy	50% subcuticular (535) and 50% interrupted PGA to skin PGA to deeper tissues	Interrupted nylon to skin (267) Plain catgut to deeper tissues
Catgut vs. Supramid Gaasemyr *et al.* (1977)	Mediolateral episiotomy Normal delivery	Chromic catgut to skin (40) (? interrupted) Chromic catgut to deeper tissues	Interrupted Supramid (60) Chromic catgut to deeper tissues

Table 68.13 Effect of polyglycolic acid vs. silk for perineal repair on short term pain

Study	EXPT		CTRL		Odds ratio	Graph of odds ratios and confidence intervals						
	n	(%)	n	(%)	(95% CI)	0.01	0.1	0.5	1	2	10	100
Mahomed et al. (1989)	142/450	(31.56)	140/444	(31.53)	1.00 (0.76–1.33)							
Bendsen and Modsen (1980)	24/108	(22.22)	62/103	(60.19)	0.21 (0.12–0.36)							
Hansen et al. (1975)	16/136	(11.76)	22/145	(15.17)	0.75 (0.38–1.48)							
Typical odds ratio (95% confidence interval)					0.72 (0.57–0.92)							

Effect of polyglycolic acid vs. nylon for perineal repair on short term pain

Study	EXPT		CTRL		Odds ratio	Graph
Isager-Sally I et al. (1986)	370/523	(70.75)	236/269	(87.73)	0.39 (0.28–0.55)	
Typical odds ratio (95% confidence interval)					0.39 (0.28–0.55)	

Effect of chromic catgut vs. Supramid for perineal repair on short term pain

Study	EXPT		CTRL		Odds ratio	Graph
Gaasemyr et al. (1977)	29/40	(72.50)	43/60	(71.67)	1.04 (0.43–2.53)	
Typical odds ratio (95% confidence interval)					1.04 (0.43–2.53)	

Table 68.14 Effect of polyglycolic acid vs. silk for perineal repair on long term pain (3 months)

Study	EXPT		CTRL		Odds ratio	Graph of odds ratios and confidence intervals						
	n	(%)	n	(%)	(95% CI)	0.01	0.1	0.5	1	2	10	100
Mahomed et al. (1989)	54/458	(11.79)	54/450	(12.00)	0.98 (0.66–1.46)							
Hansen et al. (1975)	15/124	(12.10)	12/135	(8.89)	1.41 (0.64–3.12)							
Typical odds ratio (95% confidence interval)					1.05 (0.74–1.51)							

Effect of chromic catgut vs. Supramid for perineal repair on longer term pain (6 weeks)

Study	EXPT		CTRL		Odds ratio	Graph
Gaasemyr et al. (1977)	3/40	(7.50)	5/60	(8.33)	0.89 (0.21–3.88)	
Typical odds ratio (95% confidence interval)					0.89 (0.21–3.88)	

Effect of polyglycolic acid vs. nylon for perineal repair on longer term pain (3 months)

Study	EXPT		CTRL		Odds ratio	Graph of odds ratios and confidence intervals						
	n	(%)	*n*	(%)	(95% CI)	0.01	0.1	0.5	1	2	10	100
Isager-Sally *et al.* (1986)	173/515	(33.59)	87/266	(32.71)	1.04 (0.76–1.42)							
Typical odds ratio (95% confidence interval)					1.04 (0.76–1.42)							

Table 68.15 Effect of polyglycolic acid vs. silk for perineal repair on dyspareunia

Study	EXPT		CTRL		Odds ratio	Graph of odds ratios and confidence intervals						
	n	(%)	*n*	(%)	(95% CI)	0.01	0.1	0.5	1	2	10	100
Mahomed *et al.* (1989)	105/400	(26.25)	94/379	(24.80)	1.08 (0.78–1.49)							
Hansen *et al.* (1975)	5/124	(4.03)	5/135	(3.70)	1.09 (0.31–3.86)							
Typical odds ratio (95% confidence interval)					1.08 (0.79–1.48)							

Effect of polyglycolic acid vs. nylon for perineal repair on dyspareunia (3 months)

Isager-Sally *et al.* (1986)	103/515	(20.00)	57/266	(21.43)	0.92 (0.64–1.32)							
Typical odds ratio (95% confidence interval)					0.92 (0.64–1.32)							

with the polyglycolic acid vs. silk trials: less pain and analgesia in the polyglycolic acid group in the short term, no clear difference in the longer term (Tables 68.13 and 68.14). Polyamides would be expected to cause less pain than silk because they cause less tissue reaction and pass easily through the tissues. Handling and knotting polyamides, however, is less easy. They tend to be stiff and have a 'memory', and they thus require three or four throws in a knot. The handling properties of silk on the other hand, are probably the best of all suture materials, and it knots easily and securely (Capperauld 1975). These latter characteristics almost certainly explain silk's continuing popularity for perineal repair (see Table 68.1), despite its unsuitability in terms of increased discomfort.

6 Who should perform the repair?

As already hinted, it seems likely that the skills of the operator are as important, if not more important, than the materials and techniques used. There is, however, little research evidence on the effects of skill on symptoms associated with perineal repair. Experience does not necessarily result in a better outcome—the same mistakes may be made with increasing confidence. There is an urgent need for this to be clarified in respect of the repair of perineal trauma.

Because perineal repairs are performed in such large numbers they are often delegated to a junior obstetrician or a medical student. There are signs, however, that in the United Kingdom this situation is changing. A resolution passed at the British Royal College of Midwives' Representatives meeting in 1985 'deplored the fact that repair of episiotomy is still undertaken by medical students'. Perineal repair is now an integral part of midwifery training and a survey conducted in 1984 revealed that midwives were suturing the perineum in over 60 per cent of consultant units and it was planned that they would do so in a further 10 per cent in the near future (Garcia *et al.* 1986). Training is likely to have an important effect on the outcome of perineal repair but has been a neglected area for research. The usual approach is still 'see three, do three, and now you are on your own!' Video recordings have been introduced in some places to supplement this, and apparatuses on which to practice suturing are becoming available. Ideally, the usefulness of these developments should also be carefully assessed before they are introduced widely.

7 Conclusions

7.1 Implications for current practice

On the basis of currently available research evidence, polyglycolic acid sutures (Dexon or Vicryl) should be chosen for both the deep layers and the skin. Questions still remain about the long term implications of this policy, but generally speaking, the available evidence is reassuring. The very frequent need to remove polyglycolic acid material in the puerperium because of irritation indicates either that this material is not ideal, or that the stitches were tied too tightly.

A continuous subcuticular stitch appears to be preferable to interrupted transcutaneous sutures, particularly for the experienced operator; but the easier, interrupted technique may well cause fewer problems in the hands of the inexperienced or novice operator. If worries about the long term effects of using absorbable material (or some other reason) lead to a choice of a material which must be removed in the puerperium there is no clear evidence from clinical research on which to base the choice. Silk is easiest to handle and knot, whereas a polyamide such as nylon appears preferable in terms of the tissue reaction. Whichever

material is chosen for the skin, polyglycolic acid appears to be the material of choice for the deeper tissues.

7.2 Implications for future research

An 'absorbable' material (polyglycolic acid) which requires (some) removal from as many as 40 per cent of women cannot be wholly satisfactory. Given these concerns a useful development would seem to be a continuous, subcuticular, synthetic, 'non-absorbable' skin suture which could be removed easily in the early puerperium. Unfortunately, the methods currently used for fixing the ends in other sites, such as beads or clips or multiple-throw knots, may not be suitable for the perineum. Once these problems are overcome this approach should be compared with subcuticular polyglycolic acid skin suturing.

Pretorius's (1982) claims for his technique of leaving the vaginal mucosa and perineal skin unsutured should also be taken seriously and tested formally in a sufficiently large randomized trial.

Other areas needing research are the training of operators and the implications for both mothers and midwives of the extension of the midwifery role to include perineal suturing.

Research into the repair of episiotomies and perineal tears remains surprisingly neglected. There can be no doubt about its relevance for improving the comfort of literally millions of women throughout the world.

References

Banninger V, Buhrig H, Schreiner WE (1978). A comparison between chromic catgut and polyglycolic acid sutures in episiotomy repair. Geburtshilfe Frauenheilkd, 30: 30–33.

Beard R, Boyd I, Sims C (1974). A trial of polyglycolic acid and chromic catgut sutures in episiotomy repair. Br J Clin Pract, 28: 409–410.

Bendsen J, Madsen H (1980). Intracutaneous suturing of episiotomy wounds. Comparison between polyglycolic acid (Dexon) intracutaneously and silk sutures in the skin. Ugeskr Laeger, 142: 3120–3122.

Buchan PC, Nicholls JAJ (1980). Pain after episiotomy—a comparison of two methods of repair. J R Coll Gen Pract, 30: 297–300.

Capperauld I (1975). Sutures in wound repair. Postgraduate Surgery Lectures, Vol 3. McFarland J (ed). London: Butterworths, pp 9–24.

Capperauld I (1984). Sutures and dressings. In: Wound Healing for Surgeons. Bucknall TE, Ellis H (eds). London: Ballière Tindall, pp 75–93.

Craig PH, Williams JA, Davis KW, Magoun AD, Levy AJ, Bogdansky S, Jones JP (1975). A biologic comparison of polyglactin 910 and polyglycolic acid synthetic absorbable sutures. Surg Gynecol Obstet, 141: 1–10.

Detlefson A, Vinther S, Larsen P, Schroeder E (1980). Intradermal suturing of episiotomy wounds compared with interrupted sutures. Ugeskr Laeger, 142: 3117–3120.

Gaasemyr M, Hovland E, Bergsjo P (1977). Suturaterialets betydning for tilheling etter episiotomi—sammenlikning mellom cromcatgut og supramid. Fra Medisinske Publikasjoner, 2: 1–5.

Garcia J, Garforth S, Ayers S (1986). Midwives confined? Labour ward policies and routines. Research and the Midwife Conference, Manchester 1985. Research and the Midwife Conference Proceedings 1986: 2–30.

Grant A (1986). Repair of episiotomy and perineal tears. Br J Obstet Gynaecol, 93: 417–419.

Grant A, Sleep J, Ashurst H, Spencer JAD (1989). Dyspareunia associated with the use of glycerol-impregnated catgut to repair perineal trauma – report of a three-year follow-up study. Br J Obstet Gynaecol, 96: 741–3.

Hansen MK, Selnes A, Simonsen E, Sorensen KM, Pederson GT (1975). Polyglycolic acid (Dexon) used as suture material for the repair of episiotomies. Ugeskr Laeger, 137: 617–620.

Isager-Sally L, Legarth J, Jacobson B, Bustofte E (1986). Episiotomy repair—immediate and long-term sequelae. A prospective randomized study of three different methods of repair. Br J Obstet Gynaecol, 93: 420–425.

Lawrie P, Angus GE, Reese AJ (1959). The absorption of surgical catgut. Br J Surg, 46: 638–642.

Livingstone E, Simpson D, Naismith WCMK (1974). A comparison between catgut and polyglycolic acid sutures in episiotomy repair. J Obstet Gynaecol Br Commnwlth, 81: 245–247.

Mahomed K, Grant A, Ashurst H, James D (1989). South-mead perineal suture trial. Br J Obstet Gynaecol, 96: 1272–80.

Pretorius GP (1982). Episiotomy. Br Med J, 284: 1332.

Rahman MS, Way S (1972). Polyglycolic acid surgical sutures in gynaecological surgery. J Obstet Gynaecol Br Commnwlth, 79: 849–851.

Roberts ADG, McKay Hart D (1983). Polyglycolic acid and catgut sutures with and without oral proteolytic enzymes, in the healing of episiotomies. Br J Obstet Gynaecol, 90: 650–653.

Rogers RE (1974). Evaluation of post-episiorrhaphy pain: polyglycolic acid vs. catgut sutures. Milit Med, 139: 102–104.

Sleep J, Grant A, Garcia J, Elbourne D, Spencer J, Chalmers I (1984). West Berkshire perineal management trial. Br Med J, 289: 587–590.

Spencer JAD, Grant A, Elbourne D, Garcia J, Sleep J (1986). A randomized comparison of glycerol-impregnated chromic catgut with untreated chromic catgut for the repair of perineal trauma. Br J Obstet Gynaecol, 93: 426–430.

Tompkins MG, Lea RH (1972). The use of polyglycolic acid sutures in obstetrics and gynecology. Can Med Assoc J, 106: 675–677.

Trimbos JB, Klopper PJ (1985). Knot security of synthetic absorbable suture material: a comparison of polyglycolic acid and polyglactin 910. Eur J Obstet Gynecol Reprod Biol, 19: 183–190.

69 Variations in operative delivery rates

Jonathan Lomas and Murray Enkin

1 Introduction

A baby can be born in only a limited number of ways. He or she may enter the world spontaneously through the mother's vagina with, perhaps, only some guidance or non-operative assistance from attendants; a vaginal birth may be effected by operative means, with the use of forceps or vacuum extraction; finally, birth may be accomplished abdominally by caesarean section. All of these modes of birth have been used since antiquity, with varying success. Two thousand years of experience and observation have resulted in neither evidence nor consensus as to the best approach in many circumstances.

It might seem reasonable to assume that for each baby, and for each birth one of these ways to be born would be the best; that is, would be the most likely to result in the best health outcomes for mother, baby, or both. While this assumption may be plausible, it is not a useful guide to practice for at least two reasons. First, although the needs and values of the mother, baby, and caregiver are often similar, they are not always congruent. The definition of 'best outcomes' may vary from time to time, from place to place, and from person to person. Second, even when there is agreement about what would constitute the most desirable outcomes, there is little data on which to base the decisions as to the best way to achieve them.

Until less than three centuries ago choices in the means of childbirth were severely restricted. The maternal and infant mortality associated with operative delivery was appalling. Operative intervention in birth was undertaken as a measure of desperation, when all other means failed. Although a variety of instruments (hooks, knives, trocars, craniotribes, cranioclasts, and other prehensile instruments) were available to facilitate delivery when progress was obstructed by malposition, contracted pelvis, or ineffective uterine action, the mutilating and destructive operations carried out on the fetus often resulted in serious damage to the mother as well.

The use of obstetric forceps for the delivery of a living child was probably known as early as the second or third century AD. Forceps were clearly shown in a birth room scene on a marble bas-relief believed to be from this era, recently discovered near Rome (Speert 1973). Ignored or forgotten, however, the forceps fell into disuse until discovered or rediscovered by a member of the famous (or infamous) Chamberlen family toward the close of the sixteenth century. The invention remained a closely guarded family secret for nearly a hundred years, passing from one Chamberlen to another through three generations.

In 1710 Hugh Chamberlen translated into English the textbook of obstetrics by the great French obstetrician, Francois Mauriceau, in which Mauriceau had described the then current techniques of embryotomy in minute detail. In notes from 'the translator to the reader', Chamberlen laments 'I can (not) approve of that practice because my father, my brothers and myself (tho none else in Europe as I know) have, by God's blessing and our industry, attained to and long practiced a way to deliver women in this case without any prejudice to them or their infants; tho all others (being obliged, for want of such an expedient, to use the common way) do, and much endanger if not destroy one or both with hooks. I will now take leave to offer an apology for not publishing the secret I mention we have to extract children without hooks; viz. there being my father and two brothers living that practice this art, I cannot esteem it my own to dispose of nor publish it without injury to them.' One must view with amazement the contrast between Chamberlen's sensitivity to avoid injury to his family, and his callousness toward the injury that might occur to those women or babies who were 'endangered or destroyed by the hooks', as well as the power of the entrepreneurial spirit that allowed this life-preserving invention to remain the secret of one family for almost a century.

The 'expedient' did not remain a family monopoly for long after Hugh Chamberlen's apology. A contemporary commented 'He who keeps secret so beneficial an instrument deserves to have a worm devour his vitals for all eternity' (de la Motte, quoted in Graham 1951). Hugh's son, Hugh Junior, perhaps because he had no sons to hand it on to, sold the family secret a short time later. In his 1733 book in which the first detailed design of the instrument was published, Edmund Chapman stated that the forceps are 'now well known by all the principal men of the profession, both in town and country'.

Caesarean section, the delivery of a child by cutting through the walls of the abdomen and uterus, and perhaps the most dramatic of all surgical operations, has a much longer history than does the use of obstetrical forceps. Various myths and legends from different regions suggest that abdominal birth was widely believed to be the godly way to enter the world. A person who had been cut out of his mother's body was still considered as 'unborn' as late as the eighteenth century. Macbeth who bore a 'charmed life, which must not yield to one of woman born' was slain by Macduff who was 'from his mother's womb untimely ripped' (Shakespeare 1605).

The operation was known in biblical times. Although it may originally have been intended to be undertaken only after the death of the mother, it was at times also carried out on living, (usually moribund) women. Maternal survival, although rare, did occur. The talmudic expounders of Jewish law (about AD 500) prescribed different ritual observances for 40 days after the birth for women who 'bears through the belly wall', thus at least implicitly suggesting that sometimes the mother lived (Boss 1961).

Medical opinion on the caesarean operation has long been divided. A number of obstetricians (cited in Trolle 1982) recommended caesareans in cases of contracted pelvis, but Mauriceau in 1668 (translated by Chamber-

len 1710) stated 'I do not know if there was ever any law, Christian or Civil, which doth ordain the martyring and killing the mother to save the child'. Indications became more liberal with the passage of time. In the third edition of his book, issued in 1681, Mauriceau acknowledged that 'if it is preferable to save the life of the child instead of that of the mother, a caesarean section must be performed; as, for instance, in case of an heir presumptive, because the welfare of the public is more important than that of the individual' (quoted in Trolle 1982).

Despite the occasional survivor, the caesarean operation was fraught with enormous danger to the mother. Aitken (1785) reported with masterful understatement that 'this formidable operation, intended to save mother and child, has been performed during many centuries with various success. In Britain it has never fully had the desired effect, all the mothers having died.' In Paris not a single successful Caesarean section was performed between the years 1787 and 1876 (Budin 1901, cited in Williams 1903). Matters were only slightly better in America: Harris (1887, quoted in Williams 1903) pointed out that the operation was much more successful when the abdomen was ripped open by the horns of an infuriated bull. He collected 9 such cases with 5 recoveries, and compared this with the experience in New York, where 11 Caesarean sections had been performed with only 1 patient surviving.

Fortunately the picture is considerably different today. Operative delivery, both vaginal and abdominal, can be carried out with a high degree of safety, and at times with great advantage to both mother and baby. Few would agree with the seriously recommended extreme positions of recommending forceps delivery for all babies as did DeLee in 1921, or of offering elective caesarean section to all pregnant women (Feldman and Freiman 1985). Nevertheless, operative delivery, appropriately and effectively used, possesses an enormous potential for the preservation of life and health, greater perhaps than that of any other surgical procedure. Used inappropriately or improperly, however, it is still capable of great harm.

In this chapter we will first report the available data on operative delivery rates across different countries and at different times, noting the extent to which the different rates vary. As the variability noted is far greater than can be reasonably explained by differences in the populations served or the facilities available, we will explore possible non-medical reasons for operative delivery and discuss the relative roles of these and the medical indications.

2 International comparisons of overall operative delivery rates

Table 69.1 shows operative delivery rates across a large

Table 69.1 Rates of operative delivery, cross-national comparisons, comparable year

Country, year	a Caesarean	b Forceps	c Vacuum	b+c Instrum.	a+b+c total op.
Canada 1980	16.1	17.8	0.5	18.3	34.4
USA 1980	16.5	18.4	0.5	18.9	35.4
England/Wales 1980	8.8			12.5	21.3
Netherlands 1980	4.7	1.7		6.3	11.0
Sweden 1979	12.0	0.3	3.6	7.1	18.1
Scotland 1979	10.7	13.0	6.8	13.3	24.0
Denmark 1979	10.7	0.7	—	9.3	20.0
Norway 1979	8.3	3.2	8.6	6.6	14.9
France 1981	10.7		3.4		
Finland 1979	11.9	0.3	3.4	3.7	15.6
Czechoslovakia 1981	4.0	1.3	1.0	2.3	6.3

Sources:
Canada—Statistics Canada, Institutional care statistics (Dr Nair). Data are for fiscal year 1980–81. Adjustments for under reporting in the province of Quebec are absent for this year and result in an underestimate of the caesarean section rate for Canada of about 1.5 percentage points.
USA—National Center for Health Statistics (Dr Placek): National hospital discharge survey for caesarean section rates and for instrumental vaginal delivery.
England and Wales—Macfarlane and Mugford (1984) Birth counts: statistics of pregnancy and childbirth. London: HMSO.
The Netherlands—Office of the Medical Registrar (Dr Hoogendoorn), The Netherlands.
Sweden, Scotland, Denmark, Norway, Czechoslovakia—Bergsjø *et al.* (1983).
Switzerland—Federal Office of Statistics (Dr Paccaud), Switzerland.

selection of countries in or around 1980. These varied from highs of nearly 35 per cent in the United States and Canada to lows of 10.3 per cent in The Netherlands and 6.3 per cent in Czechoslovakia. High rates of one form of operative delivery are generally associated with high rates of the other. The only situation in which substitution occurs is between the two forms of instrumental vaginal delivery—vacuum extraction and forceps—which appear to be considered alternate means of achieving the same ends.

A number of studies (Bergsjø *et al.* 1983; Hemminki 1983; Macfarlane and Mugford 1984; Olshan *et al.* 1984; Thiery and Derom 1986) have failed to detect any relation between crude perinatal mortality rates and the level of operative deliveries. This is not surprising, because the main determinants of perinatal death are not likely to be influenced by the method of delivery. It should be noted, however, that the variations in the countries listed, with the exception of The Netherlands and Czechoslovakia, occur mainly at relatively high rates of operative intervention. It is quite possible that perinatal outcomes may be compromised below some minimum level of surgical delivery. Data to support this suggestion is available from Czechoslovakia (Fig. 69.1), where the overall caesarean section rate in 1986 was 6.51 per cent, and the crude perinatal mortality 10.9 per thousand. Although there were no statistically significant differences in crude perinatal mortality rates

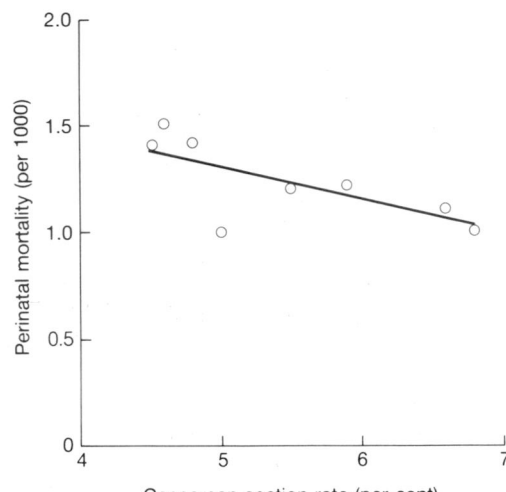

Fig. 69.1 Relation of perinatal mortality rate for babies over 3000 g (excluding non-viable malformations) to caesarean section rates, Czechoslovakian provinces, 1986 (data from Stembera 1987).

between provinces with different caesarean section rates, there was a statistically significantly lower perinatal mortality in infants over 3000 g with no lethal congenital abnormalities associated with higher rates of caesarean section, within a range of 4 to 7 per cent. (Fig. 69.1) (Stembera 1987).

In Table 69.2 the annual rates of caesarean delivery since 1965 are displayed for Canada, United States, England and Wales, and The Netherlands. Irrespective of the initial rate of caesarean section, which varied somewhat across the four countries, they have all increased over this time period. These increases have not, however, brought their caesarean section rates closer together. Rather, the rates in the four countries have diverged because of their different rates of increase in the use of caesarean section. From 1968 to 1983 the caesarean section rate increased 2.5-fold in England and Wales, 3-fold in The Netherlands, 3.7-fold in Canada, and 3.8-fold in the United States.

The instrumental vaginal delivery rates presented in Table 69.3 show more marked variation between countries in the earlier years than the later; thus there has been, in this case, some convergence of rates over time. In 1980 there was still, however, a threefold difference between the instrumental vaginal delivery rates of the lowest rate country (The Netherlands, 6 per cent) and the highest (Canada, 18.3 per cent).

Figures 69.2 to 69.5 show instrumental vaginal delivery and caesarean section rates for each of the four countries, and suggest that as higher rates of caesarean section are reached these may finally have some moderating influence on the instrumental vaginal delivery rate. Particularly in the United States in the early 1970s, and to a lesser extent in Canada and in England and Wales in the late 1970s, the instrumental vaginal delivery rate started to edge down. The United States had a decline of 53 per cent in the instrumental vaginal delivery rate in the 1970s, while the caesarean rate was climbing; the latter, however, climbed at 5 times the pace that the former declined. Because the indications for caesarean section and instrumental vaginal delivery, while at times overlapping, are sometimes quite distinct, the extent of any substitution effect is difficult to determine.

What is not difficult to determine from all these data is that there are marked international variations in almost every aspect of operative delivery utilization: the rates of total operative delivery, the relative proportions of instrumental vaginal and caesarean delivery, the type of instrumental vaginal delivery, and the rates of change in all of these over time. These high levels of variation are, not surprisingly, also found for the indication-specific rates of caesarean section both between and within countries or regions.

Table 69.2 Caesarean section rates 1965–84: Canada, USA, England and Wales, and The Netherlands

Country	1965	1966	1967	1968	1969	1970	1971	1972	1973	1974	1975	1976	1977	1978	1979	1980	1981
Canada	—	—		4.8	5.2	6.0	6.4	7.2	8.0	9.0	9.6	10.8	12.1	13.9	14.7	15.2	15.8
USA	4.5	4.7	5.1	5.3	—	5.5	5.8	7.0	8.0	9.2	10.4	12.1	13.7	15.2	16.5	16.5	17.9
Eng./Wales	3.5	3.4	3.8	4.0	4.3	4.3	4.6	4.9	5.0	5.3	5.7	6.3	7.1	7.3	8.2	8.8	9.1
Netherlands	—	—	—	1.8	2.0	2.0	2.1	2.3	2.5	2.7	2.8	2.9	3.5	3.9	3.9	4.3	4.7

Sources:
Canada—See Table 69.1
Notes: 1) Caesarean data: Quebec adjustments absent after 1978, hence rates are understatement by up to 1.5 pe.
USA—See Table 69.1, and Taffel *et al.* (1987)
England and Wales—See Table 69.1
The Netherlands—See Table 69.1

Table 69.3 Instrumental vaginal delivery rates 1965–84: Canada, USA, England and Wales, and The Netherlands

Country	1965	1966	1967	1968	1969	1970	1971	1972	1973	1974	1975	1976	1977	1978	1979	1980	1981
Canada	—	—	—	10.2	11.8	13.4	16.9	16.5	17.2	17.5	17.6	16.3	15.7	20.4	18.8	18.3	17.2
USA	—	—	—	37.6	40.6	38.6	38.2	37.3	36.3	35.1	—	—	—	—	—	17.8	—
Eng./Wales	5.8	6.0	7.5	7.9	8.2	8.8	9.4	10.5	11.0	12.0	12.4	13.0	13.4	13.3	13.1	12.9	12.5
Netherlands	—	—	—	2.3	2.4	2.7	3.7	3.7	4.0	4.3	4.7	5.0	5.4	5.7	6.1	6.0	—

Sources:
Canada—Statistics Canada, except: instrumental vaginal delivery 1968–70; Chalmers and Richards (1978)
Notes: 1) ICD 8 to ICD 9 change in 1978–79 results in spurious change in rate for subsequent years
USA—National natality survey 1972, 1980 (includes only forceps delivery) National Centre for Health Statistics
England and Wales—Macfarlane and Mugford, 1984
The Netherlands —1968–70—Chalmers and Richards
       —1971–80—Office of the Registrar, Dr Hoogendoorn

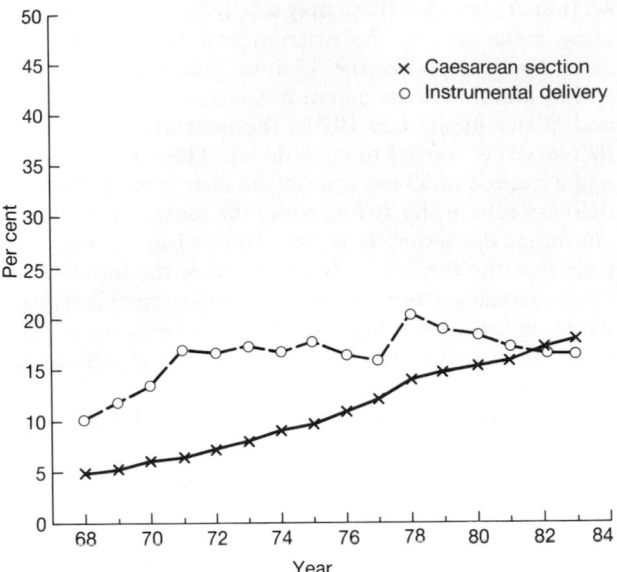

Fig. 69.2 Operative delivery rates, Canada, 1968–83.

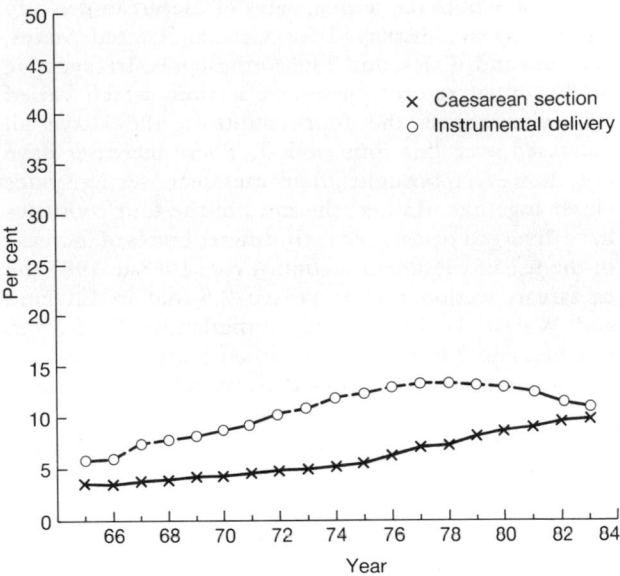

Fig. 69.4 Operative delivery rates, England and Wales, 1965–83.

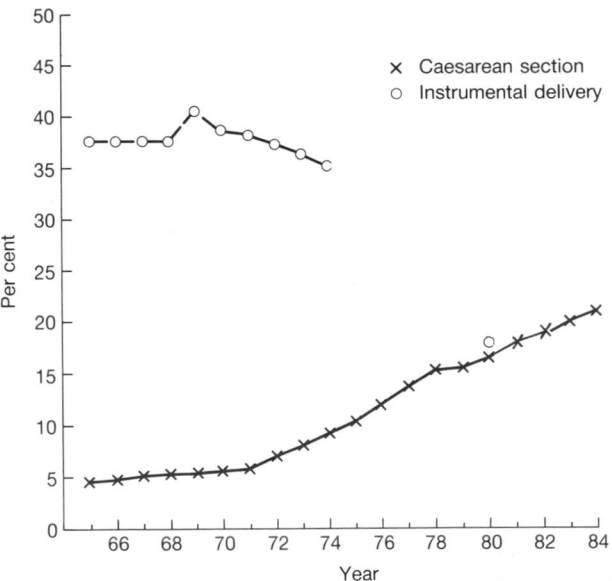

Fig. 69.3 Operative delivery rates, United States, 1965–84.

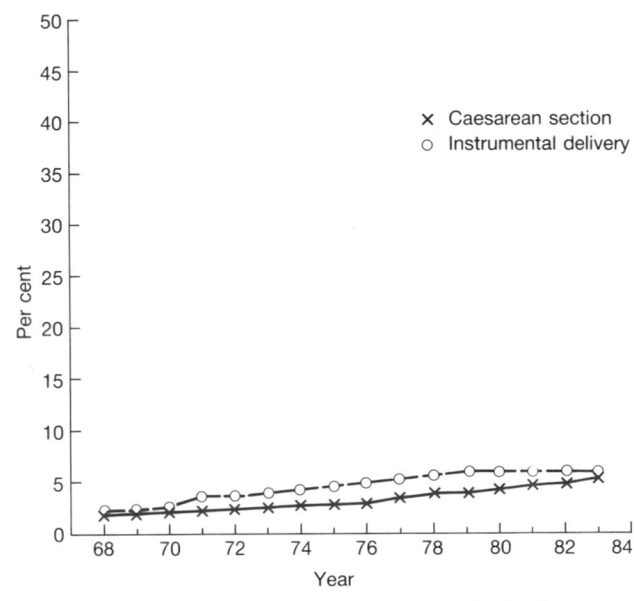

Fig. 69.5 Operative delivery rates, The Netherlands, 1968–82.

3 Obstetrical indications for caesarean section

3.1 International comparisons

Without more specific knowledge about the actual indications being used for operative delivery it is difficult to make judgments about how appropriate the various overall rates of intervention described above actually are. Given the wide variability, it is highly unlikely that the rate in every country is appropriate. The availability of such indication-specific data is limited in the case of caesarean section and non-existent in the case of instrumental vaginal delivery.

Table 69.4 shows the data that we could locate for the rates of caesarean section by indication in selected countries. Previous caesarean section, and breech pre-

Table 69.4 Rates of caesarean section by indication, crossnational comparisons, about 1980 caesarean rate for each indication (per hundred cases with that diagnosis)

Country (total CS rate)	Previous CS	Breech
Canada (15.2)	96	55
United States (16.5)	97	66
England and Wales (8.8)		76
Sweden (12.3) (1981)		93
Scotland (12.5) (1982)	97	67
Norway (8.3)	57	45

Data sources:
Canada—Statistics Canada, Institutional care statistics (Dr Nair)
USA—National Center for Health Statistics, National hospital discharge survey (Dr Placek)
　　—Taffel *et al.* (1987)
England and Wales, Sweden, Scotland, Norway—Notzon *et al.* (1987)

sentation were the only important indications for which we could find comparable and reliable data. While data on dystocia would have been welcomed, we could not reconcile the differences in use of the term. In some cases it included both cephalopelvic disproportion and prolonged labour, while in others it was restricted to cephalopelvic disproportion, rendering comparison of indication-specific rates meaningless. The variations for such imprecise diagnostic categories as dystocia and fetal distress could be partly attributable to the use of more or less liberal diagnostic criteria, which would result in higher or lower proportions of 'true' candidates for caesarean section being allowed into the diagnostic group.

Nevertheless, these limited data once again provide the now familiar picture of wide variations in practice. In countries of apparently similar demographic, cultural, and economic characteristics (Sweden and Norway, for example) one sees twofold differences in the rate of caesarean section for breech presentation.

Unfortunately, the diagnosis-specific data required

to address this area of variability is not widely reported. Such an analysis of variations in both diagnosis of potential caesarean indications and variations in the actual rates of caesarean intervention for those diagnoses is possible only where reasonably comprehensive reporting of this data exists. One such location is the Canadian province of Ontario.

3.2 A case study—Ontario

Anderson and Lomas (1985), using hospital discharge data that captured all hospital births in the province of Ontario for 1982, analysed diagnostic and procedure data for variations in both diagnostic class and use of caesarean section in the teaching and community hospitals of the four southern regions of the province. The area covered includes 90 per cent of the provincial population of 8.5 million people, and had 109 112 births in 1982. The regions are roughly comparable on demographic and obstetric variables (Table 69.5).

Table 69.6 displays the indication-specific caesarean section rates for four major indications—previous caesarean section, breech presentation, dystocia (including prolonged labour), and fetal distress. The figures in the table are for the percentage of women in whom a diagnosis of the particular indication was made who received a caesarean section for that indication. Women who had previous caesareans consistently received a repeat caesarean in the community hospitals of all regions; among the teaching hospitals as few as 77 per cent or as many as 94 per cent of these women received repeat caesareans. These data suggest that most obstetricians in community hospitals routinely perform repeat caesareans, whereas within some regions obstetricians in some teaching hospitals are bringing some trials of labour to successful vaginal delivery.

In both teaching and community hospitals there appears to be uncertainty as to the proportion of breech presentations that should be delivered by caesarean. As few as 55 per cent of babies presenting as a breech may be delivered by caesarean (community hospitals in region 2), or as many as 75 per cent (teaching hospitals

Table 69.5 Comparability of the four regions of Southern Ontario on obstetric and demographic factors (1981)

Demographic factors	Region 1	2	3	4
Population (thousands)	1273	1694	3694	1185
Mean age of mothers at birth (years)	26.3	26.8	27.6	26.9
% of primiparous mothers	43.3	43.9	46.9	46.4
median birthweight (g)	3401	3420	3369	3417
% births <2500 g	5.8	5.6	5.9	6.0
% births <1500 g	0.85	0.89	0.88	0.80
% births <1000 g	0.37	0.38	0.38	0.29

Table 69.6 Variations in indication-specific caesarean section rates across the four regions of Southern Ontario, 1982

Hospital type	(percentage of cases with this diagnosis treated by caesarean section)							
	Teaching Hospitals				Community Hospitals			
Region	1	2	3	4	1	2	3	4
Indications								
Previous caesarean	77.2%	84.6%	93.6%	91.6%	98.5%	96.8%	98.8%	97.0%
Breech presentation	55.1	65.0	71.5	74.7	57.2	54.8	67.4	61.4
Dystocia	70.6	22.1	33.3	30.7	43.1	28.7	32.4	25.3
Fetal distress	35.6	36.6	23.2	22.1	76.6	22.2	49.0	30.1

in region 4). There is as much variability within the two hospital types as there is between them.

The use of caesarean in cases of dystocia is extremely variable. As few as 22 per cent (teaching hospitals in region 2), or as many as 70 per cent (teaching hospitals in region 1) with this diagnosis receive a caesarean. Given the equivocal nature of the diagnosis of dystocia (see Chapter 53), this variability presumably reflects not only a differential use of caesarean for dystocia, but also more liberal or conservative use of the diagnostic label of dystocia.

The use of caesarean section for fetal distress shows similarly large variation, from as low as 22 per cent (teaching hospitals in regions 3 and 4 and community hospitals in region 2) to as high as 76 per cent (community hospitals in region 1). Again, this variability may be related more to the differential use of the diagnostic label than to differential likelihood of using caesarean for a (theoretical) objective and replicable definition of fetal distress.

The effect of different uses of the diagnostic label is unlikely to be the case for previous caesarean or breech presentation, because these are clear-cut and well defined conditions. The figures in Table 69.7 are the percentages of deliveries in which particular diagnoses are made. These data do indeed show greater variability in the frequency with which a diagnosis of dystocia or fetal distress is made than is the case for previous caesarean and breech presentation.

Comparing the data in Table 69.7 to those in Table 69.6, it is clear that regions with high rates of diagnosis for dystocia or fetal distress have a commensurately low proportion of patients in these categories going on to caesarean section (see, for instance, dystocia in the community hospitals in region 4). This implies a more liberal use of the diagnostic label in these hospitals—a use that may not be closely related to the need for caesarean intervention. Conversely, hospitals with low rates of diagnosis for dystocia or fetal distress have commensurately high proportions of patients in these categories going on to caesarean section (see, for instance, fetal distress in the community hospitals of region 1). This implies a conservative use of the diagnostic label, which is presumably more closely tied to the need for caesarean intervention.

Variation therefore occurs not only in the rate of application of caesarean section to a particular diagnosis, but also in the frequency of the initial diagnosis itself. These variations are not explained by any major differences in the nature of the women giving birth in the different regions (see Table 69.5). While the observation that variations exist in the diagnosis of some indications may explain part of the variable rate of caesarean section, this cannot explain all of the variation. Breech presentation is not an equivocal diagnosis open to differing rates of identification, and yet we still see major differences in the use of caesarean for this indication. Furthermore, with such elastic boundaries

Table 69.7 Variations in frequency of diagnosis of caesarean section indications across the four regions of Southern Ontario, 1982

Hospital type	(percentage of all births with this diagnosis)							
	Teaching Hospitals				Community Hospitals			
Region	1	2	3	4	1	2	3	4
Indications								
Previous caesarean	8.4%	8.3%	8.7%	7.7%	7.5%	6.3%	8.0%	6.9%
Breech presentation	5.2	4.1	3.8	4.0	2.3	2.8	2.7	3.2
Dystocia	4.1	11.2	8.9	13.6	7.2	12.4	11.3	14.0
Fetal distress	3.6	7.3	9.4	8.8	1.4	5.6	3.2	3.0

around the diagnostic classes of fetal distress and dystocia there is likely to be some substantial slippage from a policy of applying caesarean intervention to only those women for whom true benefit is likely to accrue to mother or baby (see Chapters 53 and 54).

3.3 Reasons for variation in rates

There are, no doubt, differences in the obstetrical characteristics of the population served, and in the amount and sophistication of the equipment available in the different regions described in these studies of variation in overall and indication-specific caesarean section rates. The differences in population and equipment are, however, unlikely to be of a magnitude capable of explaining away the two- and threefold differences in rates of intervention observed. Thus the observed differences in operative delivery rates suggest that collectively the obstetrical community is uncertain as to when caesarean section is indicated, and represent substantive differences in clinical policy adopted by the obstetric communities of the various areas studied.

The ultimate determinants of this clinical policy should be the available evidence in the research literature on the appropriate use of caesareans. The variation in intervention rates outlined above could be symptomatic of either a paucity of such research evidence, or of so much conflicting evidence that the appropriate clinical policy is far from clear, with the result that any number of policies can be justified. The nature of the obstetrical research literature is not sufficient to explain the degree of variation observed, for a number of reasons.

First, one might reasonably expect that, in the absence of evidence or in a climate of conflicting evidence, the most judicious strategy would be to make changes in policy slowly. This has not been the case. The caesarean section rate has increased rapidly in the recent past.

Second, the obstetrical communities in different areas seem to be consistent in moving toward more frequent use of operative intervention in birth, even if the rate of this response and the particular indications used are not consistent. This trend has, if anything, been despite rather than because of the research evidence.

Third, the indication-specific caesarean section rates are far from being supported by the research evidence. This is true even when existing clinical practice is consistent or near consistent, as in the case of repeat sections for women with a previous caesarean section. Five prospective studies of women with previous caesarean section have shown that the current repeat section rate of 90 per cent or more in this population cannot be justified on the grounds of increased safety or improved outcomes (Gibbs 1980; Benedetti *et al.* 1982; Meier and Porreco 1982; Martin *et al.* 1983; Paul *et al.*

1985) (see Chapter 70). A similar situation holds for the increasing use of caesarean section in women with uncomplicated breech presentations at term: randomized trials have failed to demonstrate any advantage for elective over selective caesarean birth (Gimovsky *et al.* 1983; Collea *et al.* 1978) (see Chapter 42).

Thus, far from there being either no research evidence or conflicting research evidence, there is some consistent evidence that is being ignored by obstetricians. Relative risks and benefits to mother, baby, or both, do not appear to be the major determining factors in the decisions to utilize operative delivery. If the research evidence on the risks, benefits, and costs of operative delivery does not determine clinical practice, then what does?

The clinical policies adopted by physicians are frequently influenced by far more than the research evidence (Eddy 1982). A review of the potential role of some of these 'non-medical' indications for operative delivery may help to explain some of the large variations observed in the use (and abuse) of interventions during labour and delivery.

Medical and non-medical indications for operative delivery cannot be neatly divided into tidy self-contained categories. Many factors, such as the age or previous reproductive history of the mother, have clear associations with potential medical reasons for operative delivery, but may also precipitate courses of action not based on medical requirement.

There are, however, other factors that do not obviously relate to any medical indication for intervention, yet which have been shown to be influential on the clinician's decision to undertake an operative delivery; some of these will be discussed in the following section of this chapter.

4 Non-medical patient-related determinants

4.1 Socioeconomic status

Porreco (1985), in a non-randomized comparative study, claimed to have shown that the introduction of a formal protocol for public 'clinic' patients in Denver resulted in a far lower caesarean section rate than in the private 'office practice' patients where no such protocol was used. An alternative, and possibly more plausible, explanation of the findings is that they merely reflected an existing tendency for clinicians to perform fewer operative deliveries on 'public' than on 'private' patients.

The relation between socioeconomic class and health status is well-recognized and acknowledged (Townsend and Davidson 1982; Oakley *et al.* 1982). Less well-recognized and acknowledged is the relationship between social class and medical care. This relationship is not a new phenomenon; it predates current practice by hundreds of years. In the nineteenth century practitioners believed that different obstetrical practices were suitable for a prostitute, a 'worthy' poor woman, a middle class housewife, or an upper class society woman (Bogden 1978). In 1958, Erhardt and Gold showed caesarean rates of 3.5 per cent in New York Municipal hospitals (which looked after only the indigent population), 4.2 per cent among the general service patients of voluntary hospitals, and 6.3 per cent for the private patients in the voluntary hospitals. A quarter of a century later, in 1980, the rates in these hospitals had increased, as they had in the country as a whole, but the differential remained: 15 per cent caesareans in the municipal hospitals, 16.4 per cent for general service patients in the voluntary hospitals, and 22.5 per cent for the private patients (Hurst and Summey 1984).

Goldfarb (1984) used national survey data in the United States to show, among other things, that the caesarean section rate in 1977 was 11.9 per cent in government hospitals, but 13.1 per cent in for-profit hospitals. She also noted that the type of insurance coverage held by the mother was related to the caesarean section rate. In 1977 those without insurance (likely among the poorest in the population) had a caesarean section rate of 10.7 per cent, whereas those with commercial or Blue Cross insurance had rates of 13.2 per cent and 13.9 per cent respectively.

Similar findings have been reported in a more recent survey in the United States (Haynes de Regt et al. 1986). After adjusting for other differences between the groups these authors showed that low risk primiparous women had a caesarean section rate of 15.2 per cent in private care, but only 11.2 per cent in public care. For some specific indications the difference was even more marked. Seventy-one per cent of primiparous women with malpresentations in private care received caesarean section, compared to 45 per cent in clinic care. Using Apgar scores, birth injuries and neonatal death as outcomes studied, the authors could not attribute any unfavorable outcome difference in the clinic group to the difference in caesarean section rates. In fact, in private care there were statistically significantly more patients with low Apgar scores and birth injuries. These United States data strongly suggest that, independent of medical necessity, the socioeconomic status of the patient, or the location of care influences the probability of a woman having a caesarean section.

This observation is not restricted to the United States. Janowitz et al. (1984) reported even more marked differences in caesarean section rates for women of differing socioeconomic status in a large maternity hospital in Brazil. In a sample of nearly 6000 women the caesarean section rate in 1980–81 was 7.5 per cent among the indigent, 9.5 per cent among publicly insured patients, and 49.6 per cent among private

patients. In England and Wales in 1980 the caesarean rate among women using pay beds in NHS hospitals was 19.6 per cent, compared with 9 per cent for ordinary NHS patients; also, an estimated 24.2 per cent of women using pay beds had instrumental vaginal deliveries, compared to an instrumental vaginal delivery rate of 13.1 per cent under the NHS (Macfarlane and Mugford 1986)

Haynes de Regt et al. (1986) noted that while 3.6 per cent of the clinic patients in her study had babies with a birthweight below 2000 g, only 1.9 per cent of the private patients' babies were below this weight. Janowitz's Brazilian data show that the incidence of noncephalic presentation among private patients was 4.2 per cent, but among the publicly insured and indigent was 5.5 per cent and 6.2 per cent respectively. Thus, a variant of the 'inverse care law' (Hart 1971) seems clearly to apply in obstetrical practice, with those most likely to be ill (the poor) being the least likely to receive medical intervention. (Whether or not they would have been better off to have received it is, of course, quite another question).

4.2 Influence of malpractice litigation

One explanation offered for the clinic/private difference in caesarean section rates is the clinicians' increased fear of a malpractice suit brought by the more educated and potentially more demanding private patients who, in an era of a low birth rate, have high expectations for healthy babies. In the United States malpractice suits can be brought directly against a physician by a private patient, but a general service patient is obliged to sue the hospital, and it is the hospital that pays if an award is made to the patient (Hurst and Summey 1984). This fear, it is said, leads to more defensive medicine including a lower threshold for resorting to caesarean section.

The intangible spectre of the malpractice suit threat has become integral to the culture of obstetrical care, and seems to loom ever-larger as a major factor in the rising caesarean section rate. Clinicians increasingly claim it to be a prime influence over their decisions to perform caesareans. Fear of malpractice suits was 'the most frequent reason for the increase in the caesarean section rate' given by physicians during interviews in both the United States (Marieskind 1979) and United Kingdom (Maternity Alliance 1983).

The reality of the threat will vary according to the particular legal system in a country and the population's propensity to resort to the courts for redress. More important as an influence on practice than the reality of the threat will be the clinician's *perception* of the seriousness and frequency of malpractice claims. But the fact that the public/private differences long predated the 'malpractice crisis', and the fact that we see both the rise over time in the caesarean rate and the public/private differences in caesarean rates in countries that are much less litigious than the United States, suggests that many factors in addition to fear of a malpractice suit are influencing the inappropriate use of caesarean section.

4.3 Women's expectations

Even outside the issue of the fear of malpractice litigation, women's expectations or demands are cited by obstetricians as part of the upward pressure on caesarean section rates—'the patient made me do it' is not unheard of as a reason for undertaking a caesarean section. The extent to which women's demands actually influences practice is undocumented. However, one recent paper reports the results of polling obstetricians on whether or not they would accede to a woman's demand for a caesarean section in four hypothetical situations where there were clearly no medical grounds for the procedure. Over 90 per cent at least stated that they would not acquiese (Johnson *et al.* 1986).

The expectations and demands of women undoubtedly have some influence on decisions for or against operative delivery. Demands and expectations *for* an operative delivery, however, are more easily satisfied than are those for less interventive approaches. McClain (1985), in a survey of reasons given by pregnant women with a previous caesarean section (and eligible for a trial of labour) for choosing trial of labour or repeat caesarean section, stated that 'three characteristics of women's strategies for childbirth care after a previous caesarean section were especially noteworthy. First, childbirth care plans were based on social expectations and goals as well as on medical information and advice supplied by physicians. Second, reasons supporting a plan of action were multiple and reinforcing, not single dimensional and unconnected. Third, although information about medical risk influenced decisions, safety considerations were neither the sole nor even the primary reasons for respondent's choices. Furthermore, women did not seek out actual probabilities of complications. Rather, they evaluated benefits and hazards as a package and projected mental images of themselves participating in scenarios of likely consequences depending upon which option they selected'.

By establishing such scenarios women are presumably setting up powerful expectations for the events that may occur during labour and delivery. The influence of this expectation on actual events will obviously be related in part to the extent to which the scenario is grounded in real possibilities, but will also be related to the extent to which it coincides or conflicts with the counterpart scenario that the obstetrician brings to the labour and delivery. A woman with a desire or expectation for a caesarean is more likely than one with the converse to have that desire fulfilled in the current North American, and some European, obstetrical environments.

5 Non-medical professional-related determinants

5.1 Financial incentives

The different rates of caesarean section noted earlier for women of different socioeconomic status may also be interpreted as related to the different financial incentives that accompany patients with different types of insurance coverage (or no insurance coverage). Indeed, a principal conclusion of the Janowitz *et al.* (1984) study was that 'it appears likely that financial incentives did play a role in physician decisions on whether to perform caesarean deliveries'. The care of indigent or publicly insured women, or clinic care in general, will frequently be paid for on the basis of salary remuneration, whereas private care is usually on a fee-for-service basis. Often there is a larger fee for caesarean than for vaginal delivery.

The influence of this type of financial incentive for surgical intervention is by no means restricted to obstetrical procedures. It has been implicated for large numbers of elective surgical procedures in studies that compare elective surgery rates across countries with different remuneration mechanisms for their physicians (Vayda 1973; McPherson *et al.* 1981). Countries with a fee-for-service remuneration system generally appear to demonstrate higher intervention rates than those with physicians on salary. Similarly, elective surgery rates are at least 20 per cent lower in American Health Maintenance Organizations, which are paid a lump sum per month for all patients' care, than in fee-for-service practices (Manning *et al.* 1984). One study has specifically shown a lower rate of caesarean section in these Health Maintenence Organizations than in fee-for-service practice (Williams and Hawes 1979). Most important, these differences in surgery rates have never been shown to have any effect on the health status of the different populations (Gaus *et al.* 1976).

However, while financial incentives are no doubt a factor in decisions regarding operative delivery, their influence should not be overestimated. In many countries operating under a fee-for-service system the difference between the fees for caesarean and vaginal delivery is not large or, in more recent times, has actually been removed (Barros *et al.* 1986). Furthermore, the proportion of an obstetrician's income accounted for by these fees is small enough that any explicit influence is likely to be negligible. Finally, the influence of direct financial incentives will be far less than the indirect financial incentive represented by the ability to control the time and duration of the obstetrician's involvement when a caesarean section is performed, in contrast to the absence of such control with a spontaneous labour and delivery.

5.2 Convenience

A number of studies have looked at the convenience factor for obstetricians by comparing the proportion of births that occur on weekdays versus weekends and during the day versus at night (Macfarlane 1978, 1979, 1984; Phillips *et al.* 1982; Evans *et al.* 1984; Hurst and Summey 1984; Macfarlane and Mugford 1984; Paccaud *et al.* 1984).

The studies all find a large difference in the incidence of caesarean sections between night and day or weekend and weekday. For instance, Phillips *et al.* (1982) found in 1979—1980 that only 9.6 per cent of repeat sections in their hospital occurred on the weekend. (A random distribution would have resulted in 28.5 per cent on the weekend.) Most of the elective caesarean sections done today, at least in North America, are for previous caesarean section and are therefore mostly discretionary (see Chapter 70). Despite the consistent finding that the incidence of respiratory distress syndrome is less among infants whose mothers were allowed to go into labour prior to their section than in those of mothers who were sectioned without the benefit of labour (Cohen and Carson 1985; Bowers *et al.* 1982; Callen *et al.* 1979; Toffle *et al.* 1978), elective caesarean section without the benefit of a period of spontaneous labour persists as the norm. This adds support to the interpretation that the repeat caesarean section rate is influenced by the convenience, to both the woman and the obstetrician, of scheduled operations.

Turning to the above mentioned studies on the time distribution of the non-elective caesarean sections we find that all but one (Phillips *et al.* 1982) demonstrate a preference factor for either one or both of weekdays and daytime. For instance, data from one New York voluntary hospital in 1980 revealed that between 60 and 65 per cent of primary caesarean sections were done during daytime hours (7 a.m. to 6 p.m.) (Hurst and Summey 1984).

While it is not possible to give an exact assessment of the extent to which the convenience factor influences the caesarean section rate, the above data leave little doubt that it is important. Of particular concern is the extent to which this factor influences the decision to perform an elective repeat caesarean section for women with a previous section.

5.3 Professional discipline

Each professional group develops its own set of norms and accepted practices that are perpetuated by numerous subtle and not-so-subtle mechanisms, including peer pressure, educational programmes, and formal standards. These norms will affect the practice patterns of the discipline's members and therefore, in obstetrical care, potentially affect the operative delivery rate. Obstetricians, general practitioners, and midwives do not share identical norms and values (see Chapter 9).

Operative delivery rates tend to be lower when women of equivalent risk status are cared for by midwives or general practitioners (see Chapters 10, 11). One general practitioner has been moved to declare obstetricians as a 'risk factor for caesarean delivery' (Klein 1986).

Different characteristics *within* a professional group, as well as between such groups are associated with the proneness of a practitioner to intervene. While no data is available on the influence of the obstetrican's sex on the caesarean section rate, Domenighetti *et al.* (1985) showed that male gynaecologists were about twice as likely to perform hysterectomies as were female gynaecologists.

Practitioner training programmes constitute a major influence on patterns of practice. Among many obstetrical training programmes it has become accepted practice to teach that the delivery of a breech should be performed by caesarean section. Clearly this has implications for the ability to make changes to the policy once graduates of such programmes are out in independent practice. When, as at present, the research evidence tilts toward an alternative course of action—in this case, the vaginal delivery of the uncomplicated term breech—these graduates do not have the skill to undertake such action and they will therefore unnecessarily perpetuate an inappropriate intervention. Precepts taught during training can become self-perpetuating.

The influences of authority do not, however, cease upon graduation to independent practice. A substantial body of evidence is now accumulating on the existence of 'educational influentials' in local communities (Hiss *et al.* 1978; Parboosingh and Lockyer 1984). These are individuals who, by dint of their personality, status, and past history come to be regarded as an exemplar for practice in a community; interestingly enough they will not always be in a position of formal authority. The basis upon which these individuals develop their practice norms is not clear; what is clear is that they can have a substantial impact on the practice patterns in a community, and that changes in a community's practice patterns will often be mediated through their activities.

5.4 Availability of technology

At an aggregate level, the teaching or referral status of a hospital will often be a proxy for the availability of technology. The regional neonatal intensive care units, high risk antenatal monitoring equipment, and sophisticated labour and delivery monitoring facilities found at this type of hospital often coincides with high intervention rates in labour and delivery. Goldfarb (1984) showed that in the United States in 1977 the caesarean section rate in large (500 or more beds) teaching hospitals with neonatal intensive care units was 15.5 per cent, whereas in small (less than 100 beds) or medium-sized (100 to 300 beds) community hospitals without neonatal intensive care units the caesarean section rates were 10.2 per cent and 11.8 per cent respectively.

While some of this association is to be expected because of the referral bias toward more high risk patients, there are studies to suggest that the introduction of the technology itself results in higher intervention rates regardless of the case-mix effect. In all of the randomized trials of electronic fetal monitoring there was a higher rate of caesarean section in the electronically monitored group (see Chapter 54). In another study the introduction of a perinatology service to one US hospital resulted in a rise in the caesarean section rate over a twelve month period (1980 to 1981) from 14.3 per cent to 18.5 per cent (Gleicher *et al.* 1985). Although some of the increase could be attributed to a 'marginal shift in admitting pattern' toward higher risk patients, a substantial portion of the increase was due to staff obstetricians' 'shock response' to the service's introduction. By implementing some utilization review procedures the caesarean section rate was returned to its former level in the subsequent year. The study showed that, in the absence of careful monitoring of a department's activities, the introduction of technology can unduly increase the intervention rate.

6 Conclusions

The operative delivery rates of a country, region, district or hospital are not important in and of themselves. They are important because they represent the aggregation of each practitioner's individual clinical policy to their regional or national level. They are the result of many thousands of individual decisions, made on a day-to-day basis by different practitioners, in varying circumstances. An optimal and rational view of obstetrical practice would be that, despite the variable nature of the circumstances under which each of these decisions is made, a common and powerful determinant of each one would be the existing evidence on the risks, benefits, and costs of the action to be undertaken. If this were the case, while there would be a great variation in the decisions made in different situations, one would expect to see little variability in the overall rates of operative delivery, other than that which could be explained by differences in the nature of the women giving birth, the available facilities, or by absent or conflicting research evidence.

The data presented in this chapter show that this is not the case. The variations observed are far too great to be explained by differences in the population served, the facilities available, or the weakness of the evidence. In some situations where consistency does exist, as in the use of repeat caesareans to women with a previous caesarean section, the research evidence not only does

not support the nature of the policy but actually refutes it.

Thus we are left to search in directions other than the research evidence to explain the determinants of the observed operative delivery rates. Non-medical determinants of operative delivery include the socioeconomic status of the woman, the influence of malpractice litigation, financial incentives and convenience for the clinician, the educational background and professional discipline of the clinician, and the increased availability of technology. The extent to which these non-medical determinants influence the observed operative delivery rates cannot be exactly calculated, but it is likely to be as great or greater than the influence of medical indications.

More research on this area of influence on operative delivery rates is clearly called for. While it is a difficult area to research, the studies reviewed above show that such research is possible. There is an urgent need for quantitative research on the effects of women's expectations and demand, fear of malpractice, increased use of technology, different remuneration mechanisms, the 'deskilling' of practitioners in techniques such as vaginal breech delivery, and the training of the practitioner. In a more general sense we need to do research to improve our understanding of the determinants of clinical policies—how they come about, what influences them, how they can be changed and the relative contributions of their various determinants.

In trying to understand and influence current obstetric practice we must utilize our existing limited knowledge on the determinants of clinical policies. It is clearly not good enough to assume that the publication of research results will automatically change practice patterns to match the new evidence. If inappropriate and wildly variable practice patterns are to be made more appropriate and more uniform we must pay attention to the non-medical factors that appear to have such a powerful influence over practice patterns.

Our own work (Anderson and Lomas 1984, 1985; Panel 1986; Lomas 1986) is trying to move in this direction. We are currently engaged in a series of studies designed to glean from the research evidence the appropriate practice policies for caesarean section, to acknowledge this appropriate practice using consensus conference techniques, and to do randomized trials on the effectiveness of different strategies for disseminating the conclusion and for promoting appropriate practice.

Identification of inappropriate and inconsistent practice patterns in obstetrics will become increasingly important in the next decade, as an emerging cost-consciousness makes it less and less acceptable to spend resources on interventions that are being used at rates far in excess of what can be considered appropriate, or even 'good medicine'. It has recently been estimated that in 1982 the United States spent, in direct costs only, $1,251,000,000 on caesarean sections and the care associated with them (Fuchs and Perrault 1986). Such enormous expenditures cannot, and likely will not, escape significant scrutiny for much longer. The most

appropriate future course of events will see the obstetrical community itself addressing this important issue to reduce the caesarean section rate and to attenuate the existing degree of variation seen in that rate.

References

Aitken J (1785). Principles of midwifery or puerperal medicine. Edinburgh: Edinburgh Lying-in Hospital.

Anderson GM, Lomas J (1984). Determinants of the increasing cesarean birth rate: Ontario Data 1979–1982. New Engl J Med, 311: 887–892.

Anderson GM, Lomas J (1985). Explaining variations in cesarean section rates: patients, facilities, or policies? Can Med Assoc J, 132: 253–259.

Barros FC, Vaughan JP, Victora CG (1986). Why so many cesarean sections? The need for a further policy change in Brazil. Health Policy and Planning, 1: 19–29.

Benedetti TJ, Platt L, Druzin M (1982). Vaginal delivery after previous cesarean section for a non-recurrent cause. Am J Obstet Gynecol, 142: 358–359.

Bergsjø P, Schmidt E, Pusch D (1983). Differences in the reported frequencies of some obstetrical interventions in Europe. Br J Obstet Gynaecol, 90: 629–632.

Bogden JD (1978). Care or Cure? Childbirth practices in 19th century America. Feminist Studies, 4: 92–103.

Boss J (1961). The antiquity of caesarean section with maternal survival: the Jewish tradition. Med Hist, 5: 117–131.

Bowers SK, MacDonald HM, Shario ED (1982). Prevention of iatrogenic neonatal respiratory distress syndrome: elective repeat cesarean section and spontaneous labour. Am J Obstet Gynecol, 143: 186–188.

Callen P, Goldsworty S, Graves L, Harvey D, Mellows H, Parkinson C (1979). Mode of delivery and the Lecithin/Sphingomyelin Ratio. Br J Obstet Gynaecol, 86: 965–968.

Chalmers I, Richards M (1978). Intervention and causal inference. In: Benefits and Hazards of the New Obstetrics. Chard T, Richards M (eds). London: Spastics International Medical Publications.

Chapman E (1733). An essay for the improvement of midwifery. Quoted in Graham H (1951): Eternal Eve, the History of Gynaecology and Obstetrics. New York: Doubleday.

Cohen M, Carson BS (1985). Respiratory morbidity benefit of awaiting onset of labour after elective cesarean section. Obstet Gynecol, 65: 818–824.

Collea JV, Rabin SC, Weghorst G, Quilligan EJ (1978). The randomized management of term frank breech presentation: vaginal delivery versus cesarean section. Am J Obstet Gynecol, 131: 186–195.

DeLee JB (1921). The prophylactic forceps operation. Am J Obstet Gynecol, 1: 34–44.

Domenighetti G, Luraschsi P, Marazzi A (1985). Hysterectomy and sex of the gynecologist. New Engl J Med, 313: 1482.

Eddy DM (1982). Clinical policies and the quality of clinical practice. New Engl J Med, 307: 343–347.

Erhardt CL, Gold EM (1958). Cesarean section in New York City: incidence and mortality during 1954–55. Obstet Gynecol, 11: 241–49.

Evans MI, Richardson DA, Sholl JS, Johnson BA (1984). Cesarean section: assessment of the convenience factor. J Reprod Med, 29: 670–673.

Feldman GB, Freiman JA (1985). Prophylactic cesarean section at term? New Engl J Med, 312: 1264–1267.

Fuchs VR, Perreault L (1986). Expenditures for reproduction-related health care. JAMA, 255: 76–81.

Gaus CR, Cooper BS, Hirschman CJ (1976). Contrasts in HMO and fee-for-service performance. Soc Secur Bull, 39: 3–4.

Gibbs CE (1980). Planned vaginal delivery following cesarean section. Clin Obstet Gynecol, 2: 507–515.

Gimovsky ML, Wallace R, Schifrin BS, Paul RH (1983). Randomized management of the nonfrank breech presentation at term: a preliminary report. Am J Obstet Gynecol, 146: 34–40.

Gleicher N, Vermesh M, Rotmensch Z, Thornton J, Elrod H, (1985). Cesarean section patterns: influence of a perinatology service. Mt Sinai J Med, 52: 100–105.

Goldfarb (1984). Who received cesareans: patient and hospital characteristics hospital cost and utilization project, research note No. 4. The United States Department of Health and Human Services, DHHS Publication No. (PHS) 84–3345.

Graham H (1951). Eternal Eve, the History of Gynaecology and Obstetrics. Garden City, New York: Doubleday.

Hart J T (1971). The inverse care law. Lancet i: 405–412.

Haynes de Regt R, Minkoff HL, Feldman J, Schwarz RH (1986). Relation of private or clinic care to the cesarean birth rate. New Engl J Med, 315: 619–624.

Hemminki E (1983). Obstetric practice in Finland, 1950–1980: changes in technology and its relation to health. Medical Care, 21: 1131–1141.

Hiss RG, MacDonald R, David WR (1978). Identification of physician educational influentials in small community hospitals. Proceedings Annual Conference on Research in Medical Education, 17: 283–288.

Hoogendorn D. Personal communication.

Hospital In-Patient Enquiry (1986). Maternity Tables (1977–1981) Series MB4. Quoted in News and Notes, Lancet i: 569–570.

Hurst M, Summey PS (1984). Childbirth and social class: the case of cesarean delivery. Soc Sci Med, 18: 621–631.

Janowitz B, Wallace S, Araujo G, Araujo L (1984. Method of payment and the cesarean birth rate in a hospital in Northeast Brazil. J Health Politics, Policy and Law, 9: 515–526.

Johnson SR, Elkins TE, Strong C, Phelan JP (1986). Obstetric decision-making: responses to patients who request cesarean delivery. Obstet Gynecol, 67: 847–850.

Klein MC (1986). Do family doctors prevent cesarean sections? (Are obstetricians a risk factor for cesarean section?) Mimeo, Department of Family Practice, McGill University, Montreal, Canada.

Lomas J (1986). The consensus process and evidence dissemination. Can Med Assoc J, 134: 1340–1341.

Macfarlane A, Mugford M (1984). Birth counts: statistics of pregnancy and childbirth. London: Her Majestys' Stationery Office.

Macfarlane A, Mugford M (1986). An epidemic of caesareans? J Matern Child Health, 11: 38–42.

Macfarlane A (1978). Variations in numbers of births and perinatal mortality by day of the week in England and Wales. Br Med J, 2: 1670–1673.

Macfarlane A (1979). Day of the week variations in numbers of births and perinatal mortality rates. J Matern Child Health, 4: 415–416.

Macfarlane A (1984). Day of birth. Lancet, 2: 695.

Manning WG, Leibowitz A, Goldberg GA, Rogers WH, Newhouse JP (1984). A controlled trial of the effect of a prepaid group practice on use of services. New Engl J Med, 310: 1505–1510.

Marieskind HI (1979). An evaluation of cesarean section in the United States. Report to the Office of the Secretary, Department of Health Education and Welfare, Washington, DC.

Martin JN, Harris BA, Huddleston JF, Morrison JC (1983). Vaginal delivery following previous caesarean birth. Am J Obstet Gynecol, 146: 255–263.

Maternity Alliance (1983). One Birth in Nine—Caesarean Section trends since 1978. London: Maternity Alliance.

Mauriceau F (1668), translated by Chamberlen H (1710). The Diseases of Women with Child, and in Childbed, as also, the Best Means of Helping Them in Natural and Unnatural Labours. London: Andrew Bell.

McClain CS (1985). Why women choose trial of labour for repeat cesarean section. J Family Pract, 21: 210–216.

McPherson K, Strong PM, Epstein A, Jones L (1981). Regional variations in the use of common surgical procedures: within and between England and Wales, Canada and the United States of America. Soc Sci Med, 15A: 273–88.

Meier PR, Porreco RP (1982). Trial of labour following cesarean section: the two year experience. Am J Obstet Gynecol, 144: 671–678.

Notzon FG, Placek PJ, Taffel SM (1987). Comparisons of national caesarean section rates. New Engl J Med, 316: 386–389.

Oakley A, Macfarlane AJ, Chalmers I (1982). Social class, stress and reproduction. In: Disaease and the environment. Rees AR, Purcell H (eds). Chichester: John Wiley, pp 11–50.

Olshan AF, Shy KK, Luthy DA, Hickock D, Weiss NS, Daling JR (1984). Cesarean birth and neonatal mortality in very low birth weight infants. Obstet Gynecol, 64: 267–270.

Paccaud F, Neury JE, Ackermann-Liebrich U (1984). Weekend births. Lancet, 2: 470.

Panel (1986). Indications for cesarean section: final statement of the panel of The National Consensus Conference on aspects of cesarean birth. Can Med Assoc J, 134: 1348–1352.

Parboosingh J, Lockyer J (1984). How physicians make changes in their clinical practice: a study of physicians that facilitate this process. Annals of the Royal College of Physicians and Surgeons of Canada, 17: 429–435.

Paul RH, Phelan JP, Yeh S (1985). Trial of labour in the patient with a prior cesarean birth. Am J Obstet Gynecol, 151: 297–304.

Phillips RN, Thornton J, Gleicher N (1982). Physician bias in cesarean sections. JAMA, 248: 1082–1084.

Porreco RP (1985). High cesarean section rate: a new perspective. Obstet Gynecol, 65: 307–311.

Shakespeare W (1605). Macbeth.

Speert H (1973). Iconographia Gyniatrica: a Pictorial History of Gynecology and Obstetrics. Philadelphia: F A Davis.

Stembera Z (1987). Unpublished data, in preparation for J Cs. Gynacologie.

Taffel SM, Placek PJ, Liss T (1987). Trends in the United States cesarean section rates and reasons for the 1980–85 rise. Am J Public Health, 77: 955–959.

Thiery M, Derom R (1986). Review of evaluation studies on caesarean section Part I: Trends in caesarean section and perinatal mortality. In: Perinatal Care Delivery Systems: Description and Evaluation in European Community Countries. Kaminski M, Breart G, Buekens P, Huisjes H, McIlwaine G, Selbman HK (eds). Oxford: Oxford University Press.

Toffle R, MacFee M, Porreco RP (1978). The management of elective repeat cesarean section. J Reprod Med, 21: 277–281.

Townsend P, Davidson N (1982). Inequalities in Health: The Black Report. Harmondsworth: Penguin Books.

Trolle D (1982). The history of caesarean section. Acta Historica Scientiarum Naturalium et Medicinalium, Vol 33. Copenhagen: C A Reitzel.

Vayda E (1973). A comparison of surgical rates in canada and in England and Wales. New Engl J Med, 289: 1224–1229.

Williams JW (1903). Obstetrics. New York and London: Appleton.

Williams RL, Hawes WE (1979). Cesarean section, fetal monitoring and perinatal mortality in California. Am J Public Health, 69: 864–874.

70 Labour and delivery following previous caesarean section

Murray Enkin

1 Introduction

In the year 1500 Jacob Nufer, a swine gelder, delivered his wife of a living child by caesarean section after thirteen midwives and two lithotomists had given both up for lost. Mrs Nufer, who eventually lived to the ripe old age of 77, subsequently gave birth naturally to five more children, including one set of twins (Graham 1951). Apparently the question of repeat caesarean section was not raised.

Indeed, the issue was not seriously addressed during the ensuing four centuries. So few mothers survived the original operation that the question of whether or not to repeat a caesarean section in subsequent pregnancies was irrelevant (see Chapter 69). The late nineteenth century, however, saw a number of breakthroughs, including the advent of antiseptic surgical technique and the concept of suturing the uterine wound, which had previously been left open to drain (Sänger 1882; Kehrer 1882; cited in Trolle 1982). (Kehrer also advocated making the incision in the thin lower segment. Various modifications of Sänger's fundal incision were proposed soon after his original contribution, but Kehrer's important suggestion of the lower segment operation was forgotten until revived by Kerr almost 40 years later (see Chapter 72).

As maternal mortality fell with improved operative technique, however, the question of how best to care for the woman in her next pregnancy became real and pressing. That vaginal delivery after caesarean section was possible had already been demonstrated by Mrs Nufer (although some historians have suggested that in reality she had an abdominal pregnancy rather than a caesarean section). Repeated caesarean section was also compatible with maternal survival. Playfair (1885) stated 'there are authenticated cases in which it has been performed twice, thrice, or even in one instance four times on the same patient. A second operation on the same patient affords a better prognosis than a first, probably because peritoneal adhesions resulting from the first operation have shut off the general abdominal cavity from the uterine wound.' Williams (1903), while agreeing that a subsequent operation was 'even better borne than the first', admonished that 'the occurrence of pregnancy after a caesarean section is not always devoid of danger, as cases have been reported in which the cicatrix ruptured in the latter part of the subsequent gestation. This, however,' he stated 'is a very unusual occurrence'.

As time went on this 'unusual occurrence' became less unusual. In 1921 Kerr drew attention to the hazards of the classical operation: 'The weakness in caesarean section at the present time is that it leaves behind a uterus permanently injured and liable to rupture should another pregnancy occur. Until we can secure an absolutely sound cicatrix the operation of caesarean section cannot be extended as far as many of us desire. It is no use shutting our eyes to the fact that caesarean section performed in the manner generally favoured (vertical incision in the uterine fundus) leaves the uterine wall very decidedly weakened.' Kerr's plea in this paper was not for repeat caesarean section, but for more widespread utilization of the Kehrer transverse lower segment incision, which he had recently reintroduced. Holland (1921a) estimated that the frequency of rupture of the classical scar in subsequent pregnancy or labour was 4 per cent. With the lower segment operation the risk was much less. 'So far', Holland claimed, 'only one case of ruptured scar has been reported, and this is not a fair case as the upper end of the incision had to be extended upwards onto the body of the uterus. At the same time it must be remembered that very few of the lower segment operations have been done compared to the many thousands by the classical method.' (By 1921 Kerr himself had performed only 22 lower segment caesarean sections and Holland only nine (Holland 1921b).) Much later, with vastly more experience behind them, Kerr and Moir (1949) were still able to report that 'neither of us personally has ever witnessed a rupture of a transverse lower segment wound, and at a repeat operation only very occasionally found it to be thinned out'.

Dewhurst (1957) summarized the British experience and position clearly. Collecting and synthesizing the six recently published series of pregnancy and labour following caesarean section in the United Kingdom, he reaffirmed and emphasized the large differences in risk between the classical and the lower segment operation. He further raised the question as to whether an apparent uterine defect seen at caesarean section before the onset of labour is evidence that extension of the 'tear' is certain, or whether such a uterus would not often withstand the forces of labour without apparent effect. He concluded that 'whether we view rupture of the uterine scar from the point of view of its incidence or its severity, these figures seem to justify the view that, other things being equal, an attempt at vaginal delivery after a previous lower segment caesarean section can be made with a considerable degree of safety.'

It is not surprising, given these testimonials by the doyens of British obstetrics, that rupture of the lower segment scar was little feared by their confrères. Opinion in America was distinctly at variance with that in Britain. In its earlier years the caesarean operation appeared to be less often fatal there than in the United Kingdom, and this may at least in part explain the greater readiness of American obstetricians to resort to repeat surgery. The risks of uterine rupture received far greater attention than did the other risks attendant upon caesarean section.

In 1916 Edwin Cragin presented a paper entitled 'Conservatism in obstetrics' to the Eastern Medical Society of the city of New York. In that paper he acknowledged the 'brilliant results' of 'radical surgical obstetrics', but posed the question 'Are we, in our enthusiasm over radical obstetric surgery, neglecting the fundamentals of obstetrics, the routine precautionary methods which may make the resort to radical obstetric surgery unnecessary?'. His eloquent plea to avoid the primary caesarean section unless it was absolutely essential has been largely forgotten; his dictum that the usual rule should be 'once a caesarean always a caesarean' became the watchword of American obstetrics.

'Once a caesarean always a caesarean' was a reasonable recommendation under the circumstances prevailing at the time. Primary caesarean sections for reasons other than a major degree of pelvic contraction were 'exceptional and infrequent' (Cragin 1916). Only classical caesarean sections were performed at that time. These left scars more liable to catastrophic rupture in subsequent pregnancies than would be the scars from the lower segment caesarean sections usually performed today. Even the lower segment operations performed in North America at the time frequently utilized a vertical incision, which often tended to encroach upon the upper segment.

Routine performance of elective repeat caesarean section became established practice in America during the ensuing decades. An editorial opinion in the 1950 *Year Book of Obstetrics and Gynecology* (Greenhill 1950) stated: 'It is far safer to perform repeat cesarean sections in nearly all cases than to permit vaginal delivery. There is practically no mortality connected with elective cesarean section. The only disadvantage from repeat cesarean sections is limitation of the size of the family—but few couples desire more than three or four children anyway.'

In 1953 Riva and Teich (1961) embarked upon a policy that allowed women scheduled for repeat caesarean section to go into labour in order to develop an adequate lower uterine segment. In many of these women they found that labour was progressing rapidly, and it was sometimes not possible to accomplish the planned surgery before vaginal delivery occurred. As examination of the uterus following delivery revealed few defects from previous caesarean sections, they decided to permit planned trials of labour. From 1953 to 1960 there were 214 women who had had a previous caesarean section, and 158 of these (74 per cent) gave birth vaginally. This change in policy resulted in a fall in the total caesarean section rate in their hospital from 2.9 per cent to 1.5 per cent. There were no uterine ruptures, and no maternal deaths among the women delivered vaginally. Among the women delivered surgically one death occurred postpartum in a patient who had had 3 consecutive caesarean sections for cephalopelvic disproportion. The 5 fetal deaths in the entire series were all associated with other conditions (3 abruptions in early pregnancy, 1 Rhesus and 1 ABO sensitization).

The discussion following Riva and Teich's paper illustrated the tenor of obstetrical thinking of the time. Reis (1961) started the discussion by asking 'So what? I cannot understand what is to be gained by permitting vaginal delivery after previous caesarean section. I certainly know what is to be lost.' Greenhill (1961) said 'There is little justification for subjecting a woman to the hazards of possible rupture and the sequelae of severe haemorrhage, especially when the (maternal) mortality associated with cesarean section is only 0.1 or 0.2 per cent'.

Riva did get some support. Ware (1961) pointed out that 'The high incidence of successful vaginal deliveries after cesarean sections proves that many first cesareans are unnecessary', and Robert Douglas (1961) admitted to performing 80 per cent repeat sections on the private service, compared to 50 per cent on the ward service. 'In common with Riva's experience' he said, 'there was one (maternal) death in the entire group, a women delivered by repeat section'. There was a 'slightly higher perinatal mortality on our private service where a large number of repeat sections were performed. This may be accounted for by a higher incidence of prematurity. Also, there appears to be slightly more problems with pulmonary ventilation in the infant delivered by elective repeat section'.

The general adoption of the transverse lower segment incision revolutionized the management of labour and delivery. Today over 90 per cent of caesarean operations are of this type (Lowe *et al.* 1976). Despite these operative changes that have dramatically minimized the risks of vaginal delivery subsequent to caesarean section, the doctrine of 'once a caesarean always a caesarean' has continued as stated policy in many institutions.

In 1978, 98.9 per cent of all pregnant women with a previous caesarean section were delivered surgically in the United States. Previous caesarean birth accounted for over 30 per cent of all caesarean deliveries, and repeat caesarean has been estimated to have contributed 27 per cent of the overall rise in caesarean delivery between 1970 and 1978 (US Department of Health and Human Services 1981). The Ontario data for 1982 (Anderson and Lomas 1984) show that an increasing proportion of caesarean sections are attributed to this indication, and previous caesarean section accounts for 68 per cent of the increase in the caesarean section rate between 1979 and 1982. The National Institute of Health consensus conference in the United States (US Department of Health and Human Services 1981) and

the Canadian National Consensus Conference on Aspects of Cesarean Birth (Panel 1986) have helped to focus public and professional attention on these data (see Chapter 69).

Two general propositions underlie the current widespread practice of repeat caesarean section: that trial of labour, with its inherent risk of uterine rupture, represents a significant hazard to the well-being of mother and baby, and that planned repeat caesarean operations is virtually free of risk. It is important to examine the validity of both these propositions, and to consider the relative hazards associated with each.

2 Results of a trial of labour

2.1 Delivery outcome

No randomized or systematically controlled trials have been carried out to compare the results of elective caesarean section vs. trial of labour for women who have had a previous caesarean section. In the absence of such trials, the best available data on the relative safety of trial of labour comes from the prospective cohort comparative studies that have been reported (Table 70.1). As can be seen from this table, of a total of 8899 pregnant women with a history of one caesarean section, 6097 (68.5 per cent) were allowed a trial of labour. Of 7131 women allowed a trial of labour, 5683 (79.9 per cent) gave birth vaginally. Thus, for the series for which total data are available 54.7 per cent of all women with a previous caesarean section gave birth vaginally.

A number of retrospective studies have also compared the effects of elective caesarean section versus trial of labour in women who have had one previous caesarean section. There is far greater potential for bias in these retrospective studies than is the case in the prospective studies, and one should be cautious in drawing conclusions from them. Nevertheless, it is interesting to note that by and large they are similar to and support the conclusions from the prospective studies. Data from these studies are presented in Table 70.2.

2.2 Uterine dehiscence or rupture

Uterine dehiscence or rupture (the data available do not allow these two conditions to be quantified separately) occurred in 0.5 to 2.0 per cent of the women who had elective caesarean sections, and in 0.5 to 3.3 per cent of the women in the trial of labour groups in the prospective cohort studies (Table 70.3(a)). Dehiscences or ruptures occurred in 31 of the 2027 women who had elective caesarean sections (1.5 per cent) and in 33 of the 4153 women allowed a trial of labour (0.8 per cent). Most of these were minor in nature, and had no sequelae. At least four of them were in women who had

Table 70.1 Delivery outcomes in women with a previous caesarean section—prospective studies

Series	Total number *n*	Elective caesarean *n* (%)	Trial of labour TOL *n* (%)	Vag. Del. *n* (%)	Caesarean *n* (%)	Dehiscence/ rupture *n* (%)
Duff *et al.* (1988)	281	54 (19.2)	227 (80.3)	167 (59.4)	60 (21.4)	1 (0.4)
Gibbs (1980)	1558	366 (23.6)	1192 (76.5)	746 (62.5)	446 (37.4)	6 (0.5)
Martin *et al.* (1983)	698	555 (79.5)	143 (20.5)	89 (62.2)	54 (37.8)	4 (2.8)
Meier and Porreco (1982)	269	62 (23.0)	207 (77.0)	175 (84.5)	32 (15.4)	1 (0.4)
Molloy *et al.* (1987)	2176	395 (18.2)	1781 (81.8)	1618 (74.4)	163 (9.2)	8 (0.4)
Paul *et al.* (1985)	1209	458 (37.9)	751 (62.1)	614 (81.8)	137 (18.2)	11 (1.5)
Phelan *et al.* (1987)	2708	912 (33.7)	1796 (66.3)	1465 (81.6)	331 (18.4)	39 (2.2)
Subtotal	8899	2802 (31.5)	6097 (68.5)	4874 (79.9)	1223 (20.1)	70 (1.1)
Benedetti *et al.* (1982)			89	71 (79.8)	18 (20.2)	3 (3.4)
Davey *et al.* (1987)			70	35 (50.0)	35 (50.0)	6 (0.6)
Horenstein and Phelan (1985)			732	595 (81.3)	137 (18.7)	15 (2.0)
MacKenzie *et al.* (1984)			143	108 (75.5)	35 (24.5)	0 (0.0)
Total			7131	5683 (79.7)	1448 (20.3)	94 (1.3)

Note: 1. Merrill and Gibbs (1978) was excluded, as these patients were included in Gibbs (1980)
2. Martin *et al.* (1983) includes 8 unplanned vaginal deliveries in the elective CS group

Table 70.2 Delivery outcomes in women with a previous caesarean section—retrospective studies

Series	Total number *n*	Elective caesarean *n* (%)	Trial of labour TOL *n* (%)	Vag. Del. *n* (%)	Caesarean *n* (%)	Dehiscence/ rupture *n* (%)
Baker (1955)	100	17 (17.0)	83 (83.0)	74 (89.2)	9 (10.8)	1 (1.2)
Beall *et al.* (1984)	857	556 (64.9)	301 (35.1)	233 (77.4)	68 (22.6)	6 (2.0)
Boucher *et al.* (1984)	852	544 (63.8)	308 (36.2)	240 (77.9)	68 (22.1)	4 (1.3)
Case *et al.* (1971)	1513	570 (37.7)	943 (62.3)	817 (86.6)	126 (13.4)	19 (2.0)
Clark *et al.* (1984)	852	544 (63.8)	308 (36.2)	240 (77.9)	68 (22.1)	7 (2.2)
Eglinton *et al.* (1984)	803	495 (61.6)	308 (38.4)	240 (77.9)	68 (22.1)	6 (1.9)
Gellman *et al.* (1984)	220	135 (51.4)	85 (38.6)	76 (89.4)	9 (10.6)	0 (0.0)
Graham (1984)	1551	1309 (84.4)	242 (15.6)	166 (69.0)	76 (31.4)	0 (0.0)
Hadley *et al.* (1986)	171	131 (76.6)	40 (23.4)	32 (80.0)	8 (20.0)	0 (0.0)
Jarrell *et al.* (1985)	799	583 (73.0)	216 (27.0)	142 (65.7)	74 (34.3)	12 (5.6)
Koppenol and Westerink (1980)	438	264 (60.3)	174 (39.7)	111 (63.8)	63 (36.2)	1 (0.6)
McGarry (1969)	415	81 (19.5)	334 (80.5)	242 (72.5)	92 (27.5)	1 (0.3)
Mootabar *et al.* (1984)	778	476 (61.2)	302 (38.8)	165 (54.6)	137 (45.5)	5 (1.6)
Morewood *et al.* (1973)	423	180 (42.6)	243 (57.4)	171 (70.4)	72 (29.6)	3 (1.2)
Ngu and Quinn (1985)	1029	566 (55.0)	463 (45.0)	276 (59.6)	187 (40.4)	0 (0.0)

Table 70.2 Delivery outcomes in women with a previous caesarean section—retrospective studies—*continued*

Series	Total number n	Elective caesarean n (%)	Trial of labour TOL n (%)	Trial of labour Vag. Del. n (%)	Trial of labour Caesarean n (%)	Dehiscence/ rupture n (%)
Nielsen and Hokegard (1984)	224	81 (36.2)	143 (63.8)	91 (63.6)	52 (36.4)	1 (0.7)
Riva and Teich (1961)	214	20 (9.4)	194 (90.6)	158 (81.4)	36 (18.6)	1 (0.5)
Saldana *et al.* (1979)	226	81 (45.8)	145 (64.2)	56 (38.6)	89 (61.4)	0 (0.0)
Tahilramaney *et al.* (1984)	836	528 (63.2)	308 (36.8)	238 (77.9)	68 (22.1)	6 (1.9)
Vlies and Dewhurst (1975)	48	9 (17.3)	39 (81.2)	35 (89.8)	4 (10.2)	1 (2.5)
Wadhawan and Narone (1983)	451	132 (29.3)	319 (70.7)	201 (63.0)	118 (37.0)	1 (0.3)
Whiteside *et al.* (1983)	579	385 (66.5)	194 (33.5)	148 (76.3)	46 (23.7)	1 (0.5)
Yeh *et al.* (1984)	112	34 (30.4)	78 (69.6)	57 (73.1)	21 (26.9)	1 (1.3)
Demianczuk *et al.* (1982)	92			50 (54.3)	42 (45.7)	4 (4.4)
Finley and Gibbs (1986)	1156			745 (64.4)	411 (35.6)	5 (0.4)
Horenstein *et al.* (1984)	282			217 (77.0)	65 (23.0)	6 (2.1)
O'Connor (1983)	243			191 (78.6)	52 (21.4)	0 (0.0)
Pauerstein *et al.* (1969)	43			22 (51.2)	21 (48.8)	3 (7.0)
Rudick *et al.* (1984)	115			102 (88.7)	13 (11.3)	1 (0.9)
Van Gelderen *et al.* (1986)	52			31 (59.6)	21 (40.4)	3 (5.8)

Table 70.3(a) Maternal morbidity in women with a previous caesarean section—prospective studies

Series	Elective caesarean n	Dehiscence/ rupture n (%)	Fever/ infection n (%)	Other morbidity n (%)	Trial of labour n	Dehiscence) rupture n (%)	Fever/ infection n (%)	Other morbidity n (%)
Benedetti *et al.* (1982)					89	3 (3.3)		
Gibbs (1980)	366	3 (0.1)	138 (37.7)	18 (4.9)	1192	6 (0.5)	275 (23.1)	43 (3.6)
Martin *et al.* (1983)	555	3 (0.05)	54 (9.8)	91 (16.6)	143	4 (2.8)	1 (1.1)	38 (25.2)
Meier and Porreco (1982)	62	1 (1.6)	21 (33.9)	6 (9.6)	207	1 (0.5)	5 (2.4)	2 (0.1)
Paul *et al.*(1985)	197	4 (2.0)	23 (11.7)		726	16 (2.2)	51 (7.0)	
Phelan *et al.* (1987)	847	20 (2.4)	163 (19.2)	14 (1.7	1796	3 (2.2)	159 (8.9)	5 (0.3)

Table 70.3(b) Maternal morbidity in women with a previous caesarean section—prospective studies

Series	Trial of labour, vaginal delivery n	Dehiscence/ rupture n (%)	Fever/ infection n (%)	Other morbidity n (%)	Trial of labour, caesarean section n	Dehiscence) rupture n (%)	Fever/ infection n (%)	Other morbidity n (%)
Benedetti *et al.* (1982)	71	3 (4.2)			18	0 (0.0)		
Gibbs (1980)	746	3 (0.04)	34 (4.6)	15 (2.0)	446	3 (0.7)	241 (54.0)	28 (6.2)
Martin *et al.* (1983)	89	1 (1.1)	1 (1.1)	17 (19.1)	54	3 (5.5)	10 (18.5)	21 (38.9)
Meier and Porreco (1982)	175	0 (0.0)	2 (1.1)	0 (0.0)	32	1 (3.1)	3 (9.4)	2 (6.3)
Paul *et al.* (1985)	596	11 (1.8)	14 (2.3)		130	5 (3.8)	37 (27.0)	
Phelan *et al.* (1987)	1465	22 (1.5)	53 (3.6)		331	17 (5.1)	106 (32.0)	

previously had vertical incisions. Three women required a hysterectomy for uterine rupture, one in the elective caesarean group and two after trial of labour. No mother in these studies died.

2.3 Maternal morbidity

Data from the prospective comparative cohort studies (Table 70.3(a)) show that febrile morbidity rates were consistently and substantially higher in the groups of women who underwent elective caesarean section (range 9.8 to 37.7 per cent) than in the groups of women who had a trial of labour, including both those who had an emergency caesarean section and those who had a vaginal delivery (range 2.4 to 23.1 per cent). Although the febrile morbidity rates were highest among the women who underwent caesarean section after a trial of labour (range 9.4 to 54.0 per cent), these were more than counterbalanced by the lower rate (range 1.1 to 4.6 per cent) in the two-thirds of women who give birth vaginally after a trial of labour (Table 70.3(b)).

Blood transfusions, endometritis, abdominal wound infections, thromboembolic phenomena, anaesthetic complications, pyelonephritis, pneumonia, and septicemia are also less common in women who have a vaginal delivery following low transverse caesarean section than in women who undergo a repeat caesarean section (Case *et al.* 1971; Merrill and Gibbs 1978; Gibbs 1980; Minkoff and Schwarz 1980).

2.4 Perinatal morbidity and mortality

Perinatal mortality and morbidity rates are similar with trial of labour and elective caesarean section in the reported series in which it is possible to determine them. Such comparisons, however, are of little value, because the groups compared are not equivalent. The decision to perform a repeat caesarean section or to permit a trial of labour may be made on the basis of whether or not the fetus is living or dead, anomalous, or immature.

3 Risks of caesarean section to the mother

3.1 Maternal mortality

Based on in-hospital maternal mortality data derived from the Professional Activities Study of the Commission on Professional and Hospital Activities, Petitti *et al.* (1982) found that the rate of maternal death associated with caesarean section (40.9 per 100 000 births) was four times that associated with all vaginal deliveries (9.8 per 100 000 births). The maternal death rate associated with elective repeat caesarean section (17.9 per 100 000 births), although lower than that associated with caesarean sections overall, was still twice the rate associated with all vaginal deliveries, and nearly four

times the mortality rate associated with uncomplicated vaginal deliveries (4.9 per 100 000 births).

Maternal mortality from caesarean section *per se* is difficult to estimate, as inevitably some of the deaths observed are caused by the condition which necessitated the caesarean section in the first place. Evrard and Gold (1977), reviewing maternal deaths that had occurred in Rhode Island during the period 1965–75 found, that the risk of death associated with caesarean section was 26 times greater than that for vaginal delivery. Frigoletto *et al.* (1980a), on the other hand, reported 10 231 consecutive caesarean sections at the Boston Hospital for women, with no maternal mortality whatsoever. Rubin and his colleagues (1981) found, by linking live birth certificates to death certificates, 16 maternal deaths after caesarean section in Georgia during the period 1975–76, five more than the 11 deaths reported through vital records alone. They concluded that caesarean deaths were seriously under-reported. Nine of these 16 deaths were attributed by the authors to the caesarean section *per se*. With these 9 attributable deaths as numerator, and 15 188 caesarean deliveries as denominator (9/15 188), the caesarean-attributed maternal mortality rate was 59.3 per 100 000 caesarean deliveries. In the same period of time, the maternal mortality rate for all vaginal births (14/144 045) was 9.7 per 100 000 deliveries—a sixth of the rates associated with caesarean birth.

In summary, while it is not possible to quantitate exactly the extent of increased risk of death to the mother from elective caesarean section, the data available suggest that it is at least twice, and probably not more than four times that to be expected from vaginal delivery (Petitti *et al.* 1982).

3.2 Maternal morbidity

Most forms of maternal morbidity are higher with caesarean section than with vaginal delivery. The extent of infectious morbidity is documented in the chapter on antibiotics and caesarean section (see Chapter 73). In addition to the risks of anaesthesia attendant to all surgery, there are risks of operative injury (Eisenkop *et al.* 1982; Nielsen and Hokegard 1984), effects on subsequent fertility (Hurry *et al.* 1984; Hemminki *et al.* 1985) and of psychological morbidity as well (Garel *et al.* 1987). The relative risk of morbidity with trial of labour or elective caesarean section was discussed in Section 2.3.

4 Risks of caesarean section to the child

The major hazards to the child relate to the risks of respiratory distress contingent on either the caesarean delivery or on iatrogenic preterm birth. The incidence of death due to hyaline membrane disease was higher in babies born by elective caesarean section during the 1958 British Perinatal Mortality Survey (4 per 1000 live births) than in babies born by caesarean section after labour had commenced (3 per 1000), or by the vaginal route (2 per 1000) (Fedrick and Butler 1970). This higher incidence associated with elective caesarean section remained after correcting for differences in gestational age (Butler and Alberman 1969). Pharyngeal aspirate lecithin/sphingomyelin ratios are significantly lower in babies born by elective section than in those born following elective induction of labour (Callen *et al.* 1979). Lung gas volumes are significantly lower, and midvolume total pulmonary resistance significantly higher in babies born by elective caesarean section than in those born vaginally; babies born by emergency caesarean have intermediate values (Boon *et al.* 1981). Benson *et al.* (1969) noted an increased proportion of babies weighing less than 2500 g in his 'elective caesarean at term' group compared to a matched group of vaginal deliveries (8.4 per cent v. 5.7 per cent). Both 1 and 5 minute Apgar scores were significantly lower in the caesarean section group.

Using a rigid protocol of early bimanual examination and midpregnancy ultrasonography, Frigoletto and his colleagues (1980b) managed to decrease their use of amniocentesis to 10–20 per cent of cases. Among 1497 repeat caesarean deliveries, 23 babies (1.5 per cent) developed respiratory distress syndrome. Four of these infants were delivered electively, and had been believed by the obstetrician to be at term. The availability of more accurate and readily available dating with ultra-

sound (see Chapter 27) may decrease the risk of iatrogenic preterm delivery. Nevertheless, it is unlikely that this risk can ever be completely eliminated.

5 Balance of risks and benefits

Shy *et al.* (1981) used the technique of decision analysis in an attempt to determine the optimal delivery policy after previous caesarean section. Using data derived from a review of the English language literature since 1950, the authors estimated the probabilities of various outcomes (Figs 70.1 to 70.4). Maternal mortality data were obtained from two large Professional Activity Study reports (Lowe *et al.* 1976; Commission on Professional and Hospital Activities 1977). For repeat caesarean section, cohort data were available to estimate the probabilities of iatrogenic 'prematurity' associated with elective repeat caesarean section prior to labour, and of non-iatrogenic 'prematurity' associated with spontaneous labour prior to the scheduled date for elective caesarean section. Data were also available to estimate the probability of perinatal mortality for both of these sources of 'prematurity'.

The decision analysis predicted 4.6 maternal deaths and 158 perinatal deaths in a hypothetical cohort of 10 000 planned elective caesarean sections (Figs 70.1 and 70.3), compared to 3.6 maternal deaths and 119 perinatal deaths in a hypothetical cohort of the same size who had planned trial of labour (Figs 70.2 and 70.4). While the validity of these predictions is, of course, dependent on the accuracy of the data on which they were based, and no sensitivity analysis was per-

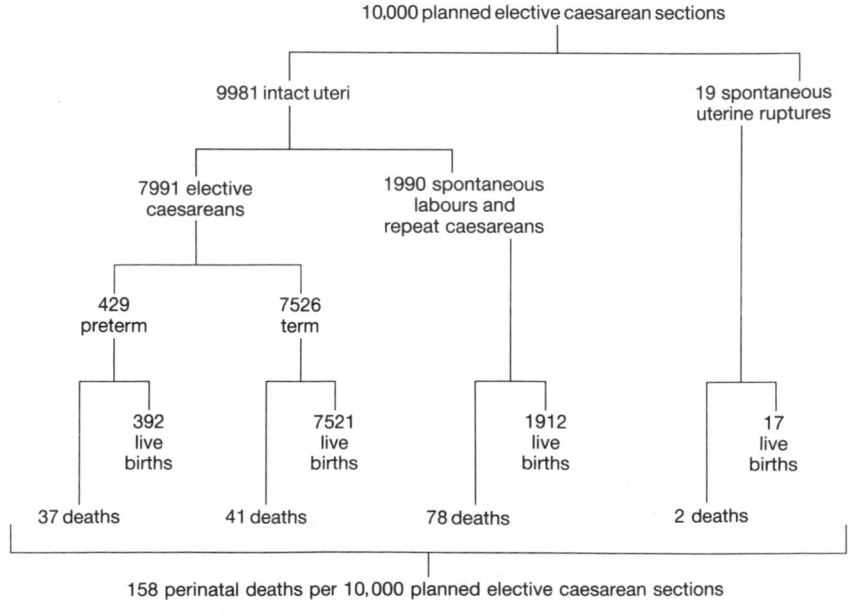

Fig. 70.1 Perinatal mortality for planned elective caesarean section (after Shy 1981)

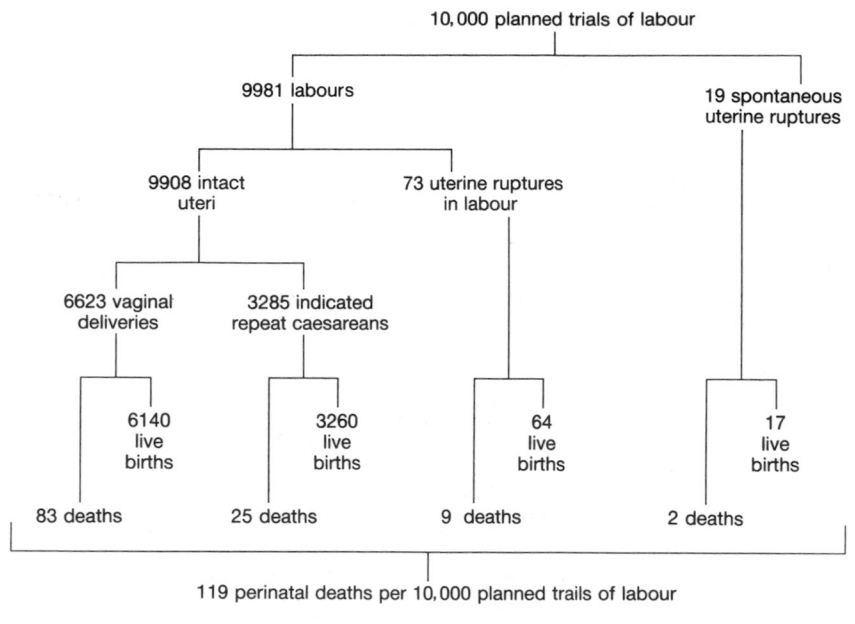

Fig. 70.2 Perinatal mortality for planned trial of labour (after Shy 1981)

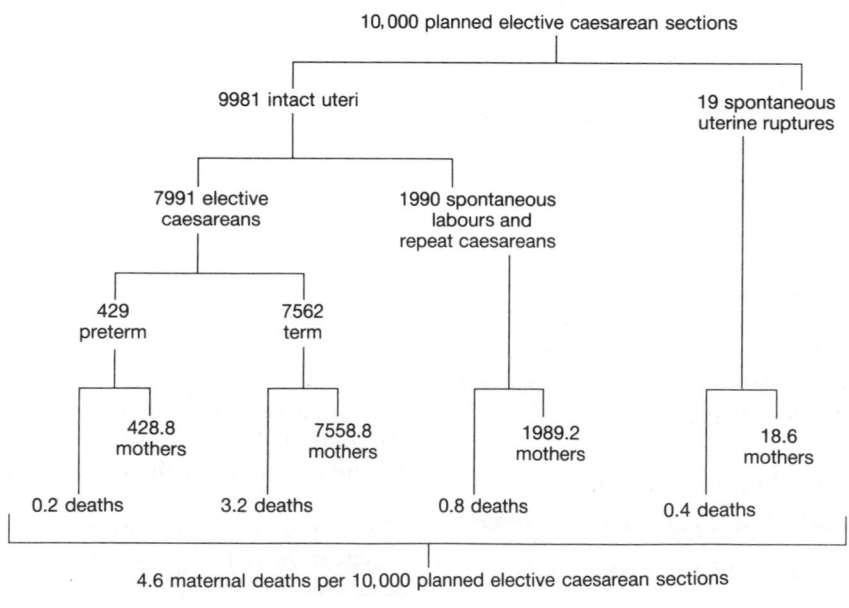

Fig. 70.3 Maternal mortality for planned elective caesarean section (after Shy 1981)

formed, their results support the impression from a variety of clinical reports, that a trial of labour is not associated with greater risk of death for either the infant or the mother. This is true both because uterine rupture makes only an insignificant contribution to the overall incidence of perinatal and maternal mortality for women undergoing a trial of labour, and because the use of routine elective caesarean section may be associated with other risks of mortality to both mother and baby which more than counterbalance the risks of uterine rupture.

Silver and Minogue (1987) carried the decision analysis comparing trial of labour and elective repeat caesarean section considerably further. They con-

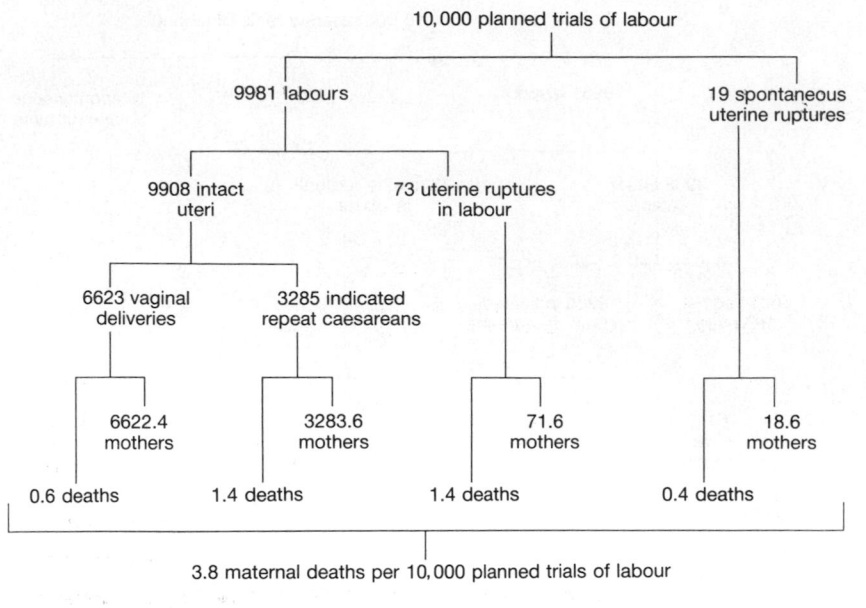

Fig. 70.4 Maternal mortality for planned trial of labour (after Shy 1981)

sidered the probabilities and utilities of a number of other possible outcomes, including the need for hysterectomy, uterine rupture, iatrogenic 'prematurity', need for future repeat caesarean sections, prolonged hospitalization and recovery, additional cost, failed trial of labour, discomfort of labour, and inconvenience of awaiting labour. Over a wide range of probabilities and utilities, which included all reasonable values, trial of labour proved to be the logical choice.

A mathematical, utilitarian approach comparing the balance of risks and benefits of trial of labour with those of planned caesarean section will not always be the best way to choose a course of action. Such an approach can, however, provide important data which will be helpful in arriving at the best decision.

6 Factors to consider in the decision about a trial of labour

6.1 More than one previous caesarean section

Data on the results of trials of labour in women who have had more than one previous caesarean section tend to be buried in studies of trial of labour after previous caesarean section as a whole. Two studies have specifically looked at women with more than one previous caesarean section (Porreco and Meier 1983; Farmakides *et al.* 1987), but give comparative data only on the indications for the initial caesarean section, rather than on the cohorts with more than one previous caesarean section who had elective repeat caesarean section or

trial of labour. The available data on delivery outcome for trial of labour in women who have had more than one previous caesarean section are presented in Table 70.4. The overall vaginal delivery rate of (range 58.0 to 81.0 per cent) is little different from that seen in women who have had one previous caesarean section. Phelan *et al.* (1987) included 8 women with three or more previous caesarean sections in his series, with 7 vaginal deliveries (88 per cent). Lawson (1987) also reported a successful vaginal delivery after 3 previous caesarean sections.

The rate of uterine dehiscence in these women who have had more than one previous caesarean section (range 0 to 3.8 per cent) is slightly higher than the dehiscence rate for women with only 1 previous caesarean (range 0.4 to 2.8 per cent), but all dehiscences were asymptomatic and without serious sequelae. There was no maternal or perinatal mortality associated with any of the trials of labour after more than one previous caesarean section reported in these series. No data has been reported on other maternal or infant morbidity specifically associated with multiple previous caesarean sections.

While the number of cases reported is still small, the available evidence does not suggest that the woman who has had more than one previous caesarean section should be treated any differently from the woman who has had only one caesarean section.

6.2 Reason for the primary caesarean section

Delivery outcomes as they relate to the indication

Table 70.4 Delivery outcomes in women with more than one previous caesarean section

| Series | Total number n | Elective caesarean n (%) | Trial of labour | | | |
			TOL n (%)	Vag. Del. n (%)	Caesarean n (%)	Dehiscence/ rupture n (%)
Case *et al.* (1971)	353					8 (2.2)
Farmakides *et al.* (1987)	121	64 (52.9)	57 (47.1)	44 (77.2)	13 (22.8)	1 (1.8)
Martin *et al.* (1983)	192	173 (90.1)	19 (9.9)	12 (63.2)	7 (36.8)	0 (0.0)
Paul *et al.* (1985)	286	261 (91.3)	25 (8.7)	18 (72.5)	7 (28.0)	—
Phelan *et al.* (1987)	322	188 (58.4)	134 (41.6)	98 (73.1)	36 (36.7)	—
Porreco and Meier (1983)			21	17 (81.0)	4 (19.0)	0 (0.0)
Riva and Teich (1961)	84	8 (9.5)	76 (90.6)	50 (66.0)	26 (34.0)	0 (0.0)
Saldana *et al.* (1979)	59	21 (35.8)	38 (64.4)	22 (58.0)	16 (42.0)	—
Tahilramaney *et al.* (1984)			185			7 (3.8)

Table 70.5 Vaginal deliveries with a trial of labour in women with a previous caesarean section by indication for primary caesarean section

| Series | Dystocia/CPD | | Breech/Malpres | | Fetal distress | | Other | |
	n	Vag. (%)	n	Vag. (%)	n	Vag. (%)	n	Vag. (%)
Benedetti *et al.* (1982)	—	—	51	40; (80.0)	10	6 (60.0)	28	26 (92.8)
Clark *et al.* (1984)	61	39 (63.9)	94	81 (86.2)	38	31 (81.6)	115	89 (77.4)
Demianczuk *et al.* (1982)	33	13 (39.4)	—	— —	—	— —	59	37 (66.1)
Duff *et al.* (1988)	131	89 (67.9)	—	— —	—	— —	96	78 (81.3)
Eglinton *et al.* (1984)	61	39 (63.9)	94	84 (89.3)	38	31 (81.6)	92	69 (75.0)
Farmakides *et al.* (1987)	23	16 (69.6)	11	10 (90.9)	8	6 (75.0)	15	12 (80.0)
Gellman *et al.* (1983)	7	5 (71.4)	13	12 (92.3)	10	8 (80.0)	22	18 (81.8)
Graham (1984, 1987)	48	30 (62.5)	90	67 (74.4)	25	13 (52.0)	38	31 (81.6)
Hadley *et al.* (1986)	14	9 (64.3)	—	— —	—	— —	25	22 (88.0)
Jarrell *et al.* (1987)	78	42 (54.0)	72	54 (75.0)	—	— —	66	46 (70.0)
MacKenzie *et al.* (1984)	25	15 (60.0)	—	— —	—	— —	118	93 (78.8)
Martin *et al.* (1987)	48	30 (62.5)	31	19 (61.3)	31	20 (64.5)	30	16 (53.3)
McGarry (1969)	146	90 (61.6)	36	28 (77.8)	45	36 (80.0)	107	88 (82.2)
Meier and Porreco (1982)	83	65 (78.3)	74	65 (87.8)	27	25 (92.6)	23	20 (87.0)
Morewood *et al.* (1973)	106	71 (67.0)	—	— —	56	44 (78.6)	81	56 (69.1)
Mootabar *et al.* (1984)	163	77 (47.2)	—	— —	—	— —	133	84 (63.1)
Ngu and Quinn (1985)	169	75 (44.4)	80	55 (68.8)	110	72 (65.5)	104	74 (71.2)
Paul *et al.* (1985)	319	245 (76.8)	135	123 (91.1)	67	56 (83.6)	230	190 (82.6)
Phelan *et al.* (1987)	812	622 (76.6)	332	294 (88.6)	168	140 (83.3)	484	409 (84.5)
Saldana *et al.* (1979)	90	25 (27.7)	3	3 (100.0)	16	9 (56.0)	28	15 (53.5)
Seitchik and Rao (1982)	58	40 (69.0)	13	12 (92.3)	10	8 (80.0)	22	18 (81.8)
Whiteside *et al.* (1983)	53	30 (56.6)	60	53 (82.0)	—	— —	29	22 (75.8)

for the primary caesarean section are presented in Table 70.5. The greatest likelihood of vaginal delivery is seen when the first caesarean section was done because of breech presentation (range 66.1 to 100 per cent), and vaginal delivery rates are lowest when the initial indication was failure to progress in labour, dystocia, or cephalopelvic disproportion (range 39.4 to 78.3 per cent). Even when the indication for the first caesarean section was disproportion, dystocia, or failure to progress, however, successful vaginal delivery occurred over 50 per cent of the time in most published series, and the rate was over 75 per cent in the largest series reported (Phelan *et al.* 1987). It is clear that a history of caesarean section for dystocia is not a contraindication to a trial of labour, and has only a small effect on the likelihood of vaginal birth when a trial of labour is permitted.

Reviewing the 13 cases of rupture of lower segment scars which occurred in 110 000 deliveries over a 12-year period, Salzmann (1964) found only one case in which the primary caesarean section was done for disproportion, the others having been indicated by placenta praevia, abruptio, toxaemia, transverse lie, prolapsed cord, and diabetes. The one case of uterine rupture in which the primary procedure was carried out for 'cephalopelvic disproportion' was actually an elective caesarean section performed on an elderly primigravida after 13 hours of ineffective mild contractions with intact membranes, and an uneffaced and undilated cervix. Thus it appears that in this series there were no ruptures when the primary operation was performed after a thorough test of labour had thinned out the lower uterine segment. Other reports also confirm the safety of trial of labour even when the first caesarean section was done for cephalopelvic disproportion (Pauerstein 1966; Pauerstein *et al.* 1969; Demianczuk *et al.* 1982). This should not be surprising. Caesarean sections for dystocia or disproportion are usually performed after many hours of labour, and through a thin, well-developed lower segment. Operations for haemorrhage and other non-repetitive indications are often performed before the onset of labour or during the early first stage, when the lower segment of the uterus is not yet well-developed.

6.3 Previous vaginal delivery

Mothers who have had a previous vaginal delivery in addition to their previous caesarean sections are more likely to deliver vaginally after trial of labour than mothers with no previous vaginal deliveries (Table 70.6). This advantage is increased even further in those mothers whose previous vaginal delivery was subsequent to rather than prior to the primary caesarean section (Paul *et al.* 1985).

While higher rates of vaginal delivery were seen in women who had previously given birth vaginally as well as by caesarean section, vaginal delivery still occurred in 50 to 80 per cent of the women who had not previously given birth vaginally.

6.4 Type of previous incision in the uterus

Modern experience with other than lower segment caesarean sections is limited. There is, however, a growing trend towards the use of vertical incisions in preterm caesarean sections (Keeping *et al.* 1980). This, and the unfortunately not rare 'inverted T' incision sometimes necessary to allow delivery, show that consideration of the type of uterine scar is still relevant.

The potential dangers of uterine rupture are related to the rapid 'explosive' rupture which is most likely to be seen in women who have had a classical midline scar. The majority of dehiscences found following lower

Table 70.6 Vaginal delivery after trial of labour according to whether or not a previous vaginal delivery had occurred

Series	*n*	Previous vaginal delivery		No previous vaginal delivery	
		n	Vag. (%)	*n*	Vag. (:%)
Benedetti *et al.* (1982)	89	45	38 (84.4)	44	35 (79.5)
Demianczuk *et al.* (1982)	90	16	13 (81.2)	74	37 (50.0)
Graham (1984)	242	50	41 (82.0)	192	125 (64.1)
Koppenol and Westerink (1980)	174	31	24 (77.4)	143	118 (82.5)
Martin *et al.* (1983)	162	33	29 (87.9)	129	72 (55.8)
Mgu and Quinn (1985)	465	160	128 (80.0)	296	154 (52.0)
Pauerstein *et al.* (1969)	43	13	6 (45.2)	30	16 (53.3)
Riva and Teich (1961)	138	58	52 (89.6)	80	57 (71.2)
Whiteside *et al.* (1983)	191	63	55 (87.3)	128	93 (72.6)

Table 70.7 Relative risk of uterine rupture in labour with classical and lower segment caesarean scars (after Dewhurst 1957)

Series		Classical					Lower segment			
	n	Elective caesarean n (%)	Trial of labour n (%)	Vaginal delivery n (% TOL)	Rupture n (% TOL)	n	Elective caesarean n (%)	Trial of labour n (%)	Vaginal delivery n (% TOL)	Rupture n (% TOL)
Lawrence (1953)*	400	222 (55.5)	178 (44.5)	74 (41.6)	4 (2.2)	449	139 (30.9)	310 (69.0)	121 (39.0)	2 (0.6)
Brown (1951)*	16	16	16	16 (100.0)	0 (0.0)	76		76	76 (100.0)	1 (1.3)
Baker (1955)						100	17 (17.0)	83 (83.0)	74 (89.16)	1 (1.2)
Dewhurst (1956)*	84	44 (52.4)	40 (47.6)	31 (77.5)	7 (17.5)	635	283 (44.6)	352 (55.4)	235 (66.8)	3 (0.3)
Bruce (1953)*						41		41	34 (82.9)	0 (0.0)
Winchester and Brown (1954)*				69	6 (8.7)	229			112	1 (0.9)

*Cited in Dewhurst (1957)

segment transverse incisions are 'silent', 'incomplete', or incidentally discovered at the time of repeat caesarean section. While scars found at repeat caesarean section can be described as 'dangerous' (meaning thin or 'windowed'), only a small proportion of them actually demonstrated a rupture (Case *et al.* 1971). What the fate of these 'dangerous' scars would actually have been, had labour been permitted, can only be surmised.

Following a classical caesarean section, rupture of the scar is not only more serious than rupture of a lower segment scar, it is also more likely to occur. Rupture may occur suddenly during the course of pregnancy, prior to labour, and before a repeat caesarean section could be scheduled. Dewhurst (1957), combined the results of six series of pregnancy and labour following caesarean section published from the British Isles (Table 70.7). There were 762 viable pregnancies following classical caesarean section, with 17 ruptures (2.2 per cent) and 1530 viable pregnancies following lower segment caesarean sections, with 8 ruptures (0.5 per cent); that is, the scar of the classical operation was more than four times as likely to rupture in a subsequent pregnancy as was that of the lower segment incision.

Dewhurst (1957) was able to collect from the literature 100 cases of rupture of a classical scar and 55 of a lower segment scar. There were 5 maternal deaths among the women with ruptured classical scar, while all 55 mothers survived the rupture of a lower segment scar. While women with rupture of the classical scar presented with the typical features of rupture—severe abdominal pain, and collapse—the majority of women with lower segment rupture did not present with such serious clinical signs. Pain was present in 9 of the 55 cases of rupture of a lower segment scar, and tenderness in eleven. In only 3 cases did collapse occur. A serious clinical picture appeared only in those few cases where the early signs were not recognized.

Well over half (49/86) of the ruptured classical scars and almost a quarter (11/45) of the lower segment scars in Dewhurst's series (1957) occurred prior to the onset of labour. Of 19 classical scar ruptures before labour, 16 had clinical signs of rupture calling for urgent treatment; in 11 cases of lower segment scar rupture only 2 gave rise to clinical features suggesting that rupture had occurred, and 9 were accidental findings at caesarean section.

Unfortunately, even in the older literature, there are very few data on the risk of uterine rupture of a vertical scar in the lower segment (US Department of Health and Human Services 1981). Donnelly and Franzoni (1964) reported on 30 years' experience of trial labour at the Margaret Hague Maternity Hospital in New Jersey. Of the (unstated number of) women who had had a previous caesarean section, many of which had been with a vertical incision in the lower segment, 51 per cent delivered vaginally. There were 26 caesarean scar ruptures between 1931 and 1961, in 219 755 deliveries; 10 (38.5 per cent) of these occurred before the onset of labour, and 6 of them were in women who had a previous classical or low-vertical uterine incision.

Palerme and Friedman (1966) found an incidence of rupture of 2.2 per cent in classical incision scars, 1.3 per cent in vertical incision lower segment scars and 0.7 per cent in transverse incision lower segment scars. The distinction between the risk of rupture of vertical and transverse lower segment scars may be related to extension of the lower segment vertical incision into the upper segment of the uterus. In many reports, lower segment vertical and transverse scar ruptures are not considered separately (US Department of Health and Human Services 1981).

There is a similar dearth of data regarding the prognosis for pregnancy after a previous hysterotomy. Clow and Crompton (1973) found two 'dangerous' scars, one of which was ruptured, in 46 patients who reached third trimester after a previous hysterotomy. Vlies and Dewhurst (1975) reported one rupture in 52 consecutive cases. The child lived and the uterus was repaired without complication. Thirteen of the 52 patients had caesarean sections, and in 2 the scars were described as 'thin' and were reinforced at operation; the remainder delivered vaginally and uneventfully.

The uncertain denominators in the reported series make it difficult to quantitate the risk of rupture with a previous classical or vertical incision lower segment scar. It is clear, however, that the risk that such a rupture may occur, that it may occur prior to the onset of labour, and that it may have serious sequelae, are considerably greater with such scars than with transverse incision lower segment scars. It would seem reasonable that women who have had a hysterotomy, a vertical uterine incision, or an 'inverted T' incision be treated in subsequent pregnancies in the same manner as women who have had a classical caesarean section, and that trial of labour, if permitted at all, should be carried out with great caution, and with acute awareness of the increased risks entailed.

6.5 Gestational age at previous caesarean section

During the past decade improved neonatal care has increased the survival rate of preterm babies, and this in turn has led to a reduction in the stage of gestation at which obstetricians are prepared to perform primary caesarean sections for fetal indications. This has resulted in caesarean sections being used to deliver babies as early as 26–28 weeks. At these early gestations the lower segment is poorly formed, and so-called 'lower segment' operations at this period of gestation are in reality transverse incisions in the body of the uterus. Whether or not such an incision confers any advantage over a classical incision remains in doubt. Indeed, some authors now recommend performing a classical incision under these circumstances (Keeping *et al.* 1980).

In a retrospective chart review of women who underwent a primary caesarean section for delivery of a preterm fetus between 24 and 35 weeks gestation, 163 women who had undergone a classical uterine incision were matched for gestational age and year of delivery with controls who had undergone a lower segment transverse uterine incision. Postpartum fever was more frequently seen (16 per cent) in the women who had had the classical caesarean section than in the control group (6 per cent, $p < 0.01$). Other post-operative maternal complications were not significantly different in the two groups, and there were no differences in uncorrected perinatal mortality (Halperin *et al.* 1988). Over 50 per cent of the women in both groups had no subsequent pregnancies. Of those who did become pregnant, four of the 70 women with previous classical scars had scar dehiscences or silent ruptures, as compared with none of the 71 women who had transverse incisions (Halperin *et al.* 1988).

While this small retrospective series suggests an increased hazard for the vertical incision, and does suggest the relative safety of the lower segment transverse incision for the preterm caesarean section, it is not sufficiently large to give great reassurance. Whichever of these incisions is used at these early gestational ages, their consequences for subsequent pregnancies are currently unknown. It is quite possible, in theory at least, that they may result in a greater morbidity in future pregnancies than that associated with the lower segment operation at term.

6.6 Integrity of the scar

The decision to advise for or against a trial of labour may be influenced by an assessment of the integrity of the scar. This assessment may be helped by knowledge of the operative technique used at the previous caesarean section, of the operative findings at the time of surgery, of whether an extension of the operative incision had occurred, and of the nature of the post-operative course.

Attempts have been made since 1955 to assess the integrity of the uterine scar directly, by means of hysterography (Baker 1955). Numerous articles have been published describing the hysterographic appearance of scars and suggesting their implications for subsequent pregnancies (Poidevin and Bockner 1958; Poidevin 1961; Ruiz-Velasco *et al.* 1964). Minor deformities appeared commonly or universally, and are taken to indicate a normal process of scar formation. Larger defects are interpreted to imply a weak scar, and believed to necessitate repeat caesarean section.

Lepage *et al.* (1959) found no relationship between the hysterographic appearance of the scar and other variables such as the length of labour, parity, age, indication for section, duration of labour, or suture technique used, although others (Poidevin 1961; Waniorek 1967) relate large defects to intra-operative or post-operative complications. It seems well-established (Keirse and Mingeot 1974) that the pouching effects seen hysterographically actually represent an escape of radiopaque substance through a sinus tract, and indicates a true defect in the myometrium.

The shape of the X-ray image alone does not predict the condition of the scar, or how it will behave in subsequent pregnancies (Ruiz-Velasco and Gamiz 1966). Most defective scars found on hysterography are clinically benign (Zilberman *et al.* 1968). The large proportion of small defects noted, combined with the low incidence of clinical rupture of the uterus in subsequent labours, has tended to dampen enthusiasm for hysterography in Europe. In North America, largely due to the policy of 'once a caesarean always a caesarean', the procedure was never widely practised. It enjoyed a wave of popularity, but is seldom performed today.

7 Care during a trial of labour

7.1 Use of oxytocics

The use of oxytocin for induction or augmentation of labour in women who have had a previous caesarean section has remained controversial, because of speculation that there might be an increased risk of uterine rupture or dehiscence. This view is not universally held, nor is it strongly supported by the available data.

Ryan (1960), who included 10 women with previous caesarean sections in his series of oxytocin inductions, did not consider a uterine scar to be a contraindication to oxytocin induction of labour, although 'every member of the medical and nursing staff regarded oxytocin in the presence of a section scar with anxiety'. McGarry (1969) used oxytocin in 81 women with a previous caesarean section, commenting that 'if the uterus could be expected to withstand normal labour, then initiation of labour by oxytocin is justified'. MacKenzie *et al.* (1984) reported a series of 143 women previously delivered by caesarean section in whom labour was induced with vaginal instillation of prostaglandin E$_2$, followed by oxytocin when necessary. One hundred and eight of these women (76 per cent) gave birth vaginally, and no uterine dehiscences or ruptures occurred. Many current authors (e.g. Duff *et al.* 1988) have, in their reported series, used oxytocin as indicated for induction or augmentation of labour.

Others have suggested that the use of oxytocin is associated with greater risk (Demianczuk *et al.* 1982),

and that its use be avoided (Gellman *et al.* 1983). Review of the reported case series (Table 70.8), however, shows that the increased risk of uterine rupture, if any, with the use of oxytocin is extremely small.

Such comparisons, of course, are rendered invalid by the fact that the cohorts of women who received, or did not receive oxytocin, may have differed in many other respects in addition to the use of oxytocin. Nevertheless, the high vaginal delivery rates and low dehiscence rates noted in these women suggest that oxytocin should be used for induction or augmentation of labour whenever indicated in women who have had a previous caesarean section, using the same precautions that should always attend its use.

7.2 Regional analgesia and anaesthesia

The use of regional (caudal or epidural) analgesia in labour for the woman with a previous caesarean section has been questioned because of fears that it might mask pain or tenderness, considered to be early signs of rupture of the scar (Gibbs 1980; Plauche *et al.* 1984). Pearce and Ravi (1976) report a case of rupture of a uterine scar in a women given epidural analgesia. Although the woman had no discomfort, and her blood pressure and pulse and the fetal heart rate remained normal, abdominal examination revealed an irregular uterine outline. At laparotomy, the baby was found to be lying outside the uterus, having been extruded through a large tear extending across the whole length of the previous lower segment incision.

The extent of the risk of masking a catastrophic uterine rupture is difficult to quantitate. It must be minuscule; no other case reports were found. In a number of reported series (e.g. Martin *et al.* 1983; Flamm *et al.* 1984; Graham 1984; Hadley *et al.* 1986; Duff *et al.* 1988) regional block is used whenever requested by the woman for pain relief, and no difficulties were encountered with this policy. Pain and tenderness of the scar are neither sensitive nor specific signs of impending uterine rupture. Case *et al.* (1971) reported that of 20 caesarean sections performed because of pain and tenderness in labour, in only one was a dehiscence noted. Dehiscences of the scar are usually asymptomatic, and even frank rupture may not be associated with any of the classical signs or symptoms, including pain, even in the absence of regional analgesia (Phelan *et al.* 1987). Meehan *et al.* (1972) recommended the use of caudal analgesia, not only for the patient's comfort, but because it makes it possible to assess the lower segment scar directly during labour. The value, if any, of such assessments has not, however, been established.

There does not appear to be any increased hazard of or from uterine rupture associated with the use of regional anaesthesia for women who have had a previous caesarean section. It is sensible, safe, and justified to use analgesia for the woman with a lower segment

Table 70.8 Vaginal delivery and dehiscence/rupture after trial of labour with and without the use of oxytocin

Series	n	No oxytocin			Oxytocin		
		n (%)	Vag. (%)	D/R (%)	n (%)	Vag. (%)	D/R (%)
Benedetti *et al.* (1982)	89	73 (82.0)	59 (80.8)	2 (2.7)	16 (18.0)	12 (75.0)	1 (6.3)
Carlsson *et al.* (1980)	119	43 (36.1)	41 (95.3)	0 (0.0)	76 (63.9)	64 (84.2)	0 (0.0)
Demianczuk *et al.* (1980)	92	69 (75.0)	40 (58.0)	1 (1.4)	23 (25.0)	10 (43.5)	2 (8.7)
Flamm *et al.* (1984)	230	136 (59.1)	120 (88.2)	0 (0.0)	94 (40.9)	61 (64.9)	0 (0.0)
Flamm *et al.* (1987)	1776	1291 (72.7)	1005 (77.8)	6 (0.5)	485 (27.3)	309 (63.7)	5 (1.0)
Horenstein *et al.* (1984)	292	234 (80.1)	168 (71.8)	3 (1.3)	58 (19.9)	31 (53.4)	3 (5.2)
Horenstein and Phelan (1985)	732	443 (60.5)	395 (89.2)	6 (1.4)	289 (39.5)	200 (69.2)	9 (3.1)
MacKenzie *et al.* (1984)*	143	48 (33.6)		0 (0.0)	95 (66.4)		0 (0.0)
McGarry (1969)	334	251 (75.1)	191 (76.1)	0 (0.0)	83 (24.9)	51 (61.4)	1 (1.2)
Martin *et al.* (1983)	162	137 (84.6)	84 (61.3)	10 (7.3)	25 (15.4)	17 (68.0)	1 (4.0)
Meehan *et al.* (1972)	75	50 (66.7)		2 (4.0)	25 (33.3)		0 (0.0)
Meier and Porreco (1982)	207	165 (79.7)	141 (85.5)	0 (0.0)	42 (20.3)	34 (81.0)	1 (2.4)
Molloy *et al.* (1987)	1781	1062 (59.5)	984 (92.7)	2 (0.2)	719 (40.4)	634 (88.2)	6 (0.8)
Morewood *et al.* (1973)	243	198 (81.5)	143 (72.2)	3 (1.5)	45 (18.5)	28 (62.2)	0 (0.0)
Ngu and Quinn (1985)	463	386 (83.4)	220 (57.0)	0 (0.0)	77 (16.6)	56 (72.7)	0 (0.0)
O'Connor (1983)	243	211 (86.8)	169 (80.1)	0 (0.0)	32 (13.2)	22 (68.7)	0 (0.0)
Paul *et al.* (1985)	732	443 (60.5)	395 (89.2)	no dif	289 (39.5)	200 (69.2)	no dif
Phelan *et al.* (1987)	1796	1003 (55.8)	908 (90.5)	18 (2.0)	793 (44.2)	557 (70.2)	24 (3.0)
Riva and Teich (1961)	214	207 (96.7)	151 (72.9)	2 (1.0)	7 (3.3)	7 (100.0)	0 (0.0)
Saldana *et al.* (1979)	145	142 (97.9)	53 (37.3)	0 (0.0)	3 (2.1)	3 (100.0)	0 (0.0)
Van Gelderen *et al.* (1984)	52	30 (57.7)	17 (56.7)	2 (6.7)	32 (61.5)	14 (43.6)	1 (3.1)

* All women in this series received prostaglandin for cervical ripening

scar in the same manner as for the woman whose uterus is intact.

7.3 Manual exploration of the uterus

In many reports of series of vaginal births after previous caesarean section, (e.g. MacKenzie *et al.* 1984; Phelan *et al.* 1987) mention is made of the fact that the uterus was explored postpartum in all cases, in a search for asymptomatic uterine rupture or dehiscence. In an editorial commentary in the 1970 *Year Book of Obstetrics and Gynecology*, Greenhill (1970) recommended that every patient who has previously had a caesarean section should have a vaginal examination to detect any defect in the anterior lower segment. (He also recommended manual exploration of the uterus after every delivery, regardless of whether or not the woman has had a previous caesarean section.) He did not give any evidence to support his recommendation.

Manual exploration of a scarred uterus immediately following a vaginal delivery is often inconclusive (Poi-

devin and Bockner 1958). It is difficult to be sure whether or not the thin, soft lower segment is intact. In any case, in the absence of bleeding or systemic signs, an asymptomatic rupture discovered postpartum does not require any treatment, so the question of diagnosis would be academic. Baxter (1958) reports two cases in which this diagnosis was made, and no repair or other intervention was undertaken; both patients made uneventful recoveries.

No studies have shown any benefit from routine manual exploration of the uterus in women who have had a previous caesarean section. There is always a risk of introducing infection by the manual exploration, or of converting a dehiscence into a larger rupture. Browne and McGrath (1965) suggest that a reasonable compromise would consist of increased vigilance in the hour after delivery of the placenta, reserving internal palpation of the lower segment for women with signs of abnormal bleeding. Based on the available data, this would seem to be a practical and feasible approach.

8 Rupture of the scarred uterus during pregnancy and labour

Complete rupture of the uterus can be a life-threatening emergency. Fortunately the condition is rare in modern obstetrics, despite the increase in caesarean section rates, and serious sequelae are even more rare. Fedorkow *et al.* (1987) reported the experience over 20 years in a major Canadian teaching hospital and referral centre. From 1966 to 1985 there were 15 cases of uterine rupture encountered in 52 854 deliveries, an overall incidence of 0.3 per 1000 deliveries. There was no change in the incidence over time, with 4 to 5 cases in each quinquennium. Of the 15 women who suffered a uterine rupture, only 7 had previously had a caesarean section, including one with a vertical scar. Suggested causes in the other 8 women were uterine trauma from previous dilatation and curettage or laparoscopy (3), forceps delivery (2), bicornuate uterus (1), precipitous delivery (1), and oxytocin (1). Ten of the 15 women were in labour. Two gave birth vaginally, the remaining 13 underwent caesarean section. Four of the ruptures were incidentally found at caesarean section. The rupture site was repaired in 11, and 4 women underwent hysterectomy. None of the women, and none of the babies died.

Thus, although previous caesarean section is often considered to be the most common cause of uterine rupture, in this large (for the developed world) series, it was involved in less than half the cases.

The rate of uterine rupture (excluding asymptomatic dehiscence) for women with a singleton vertex presentation who underwent a trial of labour after a previous lower segment transverse incision caesarean section was 5/2268, or 0.22 per cent in the prospective series reviewed by the panel for the Canadian National Consensus Conference on Aspects of Caesarean Section (Panel 1986). The incidence of complete rupture was 1 in 1156 trials of labour (0.09 per cent) in the series reported by Finley and Gibbs (1986). To put these rates into perspective, on the basis of 11 819 births at a Canadian teaching centre (Cohen *et al.* 1985), the probability of requiring an emergency caesarean section for reasons other than uterine rupture (fetal distress, cord prolapse, or antepartum haemorrhage) was 2.7 per cent (confidence interval 2.4 to 2.9 per cent), or 30 times as high as the risk of uterine rupture with a trial of labour. In Finley and Gibbs' series (1986) the likelihood that a woman undergoing a trial of labour would require an emergency caesarean delivery for reasons unrelated to the scar (abruptio, cord prolapse, or fetal distress) was 15 in 1156 (1.3 per cent) or 14 times as high as the risk of uterine rupture.

Rupture of a lower segment scar does not produce a catastrophic picture requiring extraordinary facilities. Hospitals whose capabilities are so limited that they cannot deal promptly with problems associated with a trial of labour are also incapable of dealing appropriately with other obstetrical emergencies (Shearer 1981). Any obstetrical department that is prepared to look after patients with much more frequently encountered conditions such as placenta praevia, abruptio placentae, prolapsed cord, and acute fetal distress should be able to manage a trial of labour safely after a previous lower segment caesarean section.

9 Gap between evidence and practice

Obstetric practice has been slow to reflect the scientific evidence confirming the safety of trial of labour after previous caesarean section. The degree of opposition to vaginal birth after caesarean section, in North America in particular, is difficult to explain, considering the strength of the available evidence that trials of labour are, under proper circumstances, both safe and effective.

Sloan (1968) interviewed a number of obstetricians in private practice in New York, asking them the following question: 'Assuming you could be shown documentation and overwhelming evidence of the safety of permitting labour following caesarean section, would you allow this to alter your management?' Eighty per cent of his respondents answered in the negative! Sloan found this difficult to explain. He postulated that many clinicians who are today's teachers are expressing the dictum to which they were exposed as students. 'We are', he said, 'presented on the one hand with evidence pointing out what may well be an archaic practice and on the other the strength of the convictions of those who practice our specialty and are the teachers of our future clinicians.'

If policies of routine repeat caesarean section could be considered an archaic practice in 1968, they must be even more so today. Two national consensus statements (US Department of Health and Human Services 1981; Panel 1986), and two national professional bodies (American College of Obstetrics and Gynecology 1982, 1985; Society of Obstetricians and Gynecologists of Canada 1982) have recommended policies of trial of labour after previous caesarean section.

Increasing numbers of pregnant women, as well as professionals, are vehemently protesting the status quo. For a variety of reasons many women prefer to attempt a vaginal birth after a caesarean section. Their earlier caesarean experience may have been emotionally or physically difficult. They may be unhappy because they were separated from their partners or from their babies. They may well wonder if it was all necessary in the first place. They may be aware of the accumulated evidence on the relative safety and advantages of trial of labour, and simply be looking for a better experience this time. According to Keolker (1981), there is another, less obvious benefit from vaginal birth after caesarean section. Because an informed decision on this subject requires knowledge and study on the part of the woman, her sense of control and participation are greatly enhanced.

In recent years a number of consumer 'shared predicament' groups have appeared, with the expressed purposes of demythologizing caesarean section, of combatting misinformation, and of disseminating both accurate information and their own point of view: 'Although some doctors are informed and supportive many still adhere to "Once a caesarean always a caesarean", and I'm not sure they will change until we women who've been sectioned inform ourselves, search for support, work for changes in our local hospital, and refuse to take "no" for an answer' (Ryder 1982). Special prenatal classes are available for many parents who elect to attempt a vaginal birth after caesarean (Shearer 1982).

Current incidence data on repeat caesarean section, and consideration of the factors that may be involved in the continuing North American practice are discussed in the chapter on variations in operative delivery rates (see Chapter 69).

10 Conclusions

10.1 Implications for current practice

The recommendations of the panel of the Canadian Consensus Conference on Aspects of Caesarean Birth (Panel 1986) are in accord with the available evidence. They state that 'A trial of labour after a previous caesarean section should be recommended for women who meet all the following criteria: one low transverse incision caesarean section, a singleton vertex presentation, and no absolute indication for caesarean section (such as a placenta praevia) in the present pregnancy. The likelihood of vaginal birth after caesarean section appears to be independent of the indication for the first cesarean section (including "cephalopelvic disproportion" and "failure to progress"). Suspected fetal macrosomia (birth weight over 4000 g) is not in itself a contraindication to a trial of labour.'

'A history of classical, low vertical or unknown uterine incision or hysterotomy remains a contraindication to a trial of labour.'

References

American College of Obstetrics and Gynecology Committee on Obstetrics: Maternal and Fetal Medicine (1982). Guidelines for vaginal delivery after a cesarean childbirth. Statement.
American College of Obstetrics and Gynecology (1985).

'Epidural anaesthesia may be used for the usual obstetric indications.'

'Hospitals providing obstetric care should ensure the availability of blood, operating rooms, neonatal resuscitation, and nursing, anaesthetic and surgical personnel so that a caesarean section can be started within approximately 30 minutes for any women in labour, including a woman undergoing a trial of labour.'

The panel further recommended, for women undergoing a trial of labour after previous caesarean section '(a) antenatal evaluation by a qualified obstetrician, (b) intrapartum notification of and/or consultation with the obstetrician or surgeon and the anaesthetist to be involved in an emergency and (c) skilled evaluation of labour and routine maternal and fetal surveillance.

'In addition, the panel feels that the continuous presence of the physician during labour is not necessary. Continuous electronic monitoring of the fetal heart rate is not routinely indicated; however minimum standards for recording the fetal heart rate in labour should be followed (i.e. auscultation after a contraction every 15 minutes in the active phase of the first stage of labour and every 5 minutes in the second stage).

'Adequate information should be provided so that a woman can make an informed decision on the choice between repeat elective caesarean section and trial of labour. Every effort should be made to accommodate this decision. Physicians working in hospitals that are unable to fulfil the woman's wishes should so inform the patient and advise her of the nearest facility that can.'

10.2 Implications for future research

The panel also noted that '(a) a trial of labour after more than one caesarean section may be a reasonable alternative to repeat elective caesarean section, but to date there are not sufficient data to confirm or refute this; (b) there is insufficient evidence to make a recommendation regarding a trial of labour with twins or with breech presentation; (c) although the data on oxytocin stimulation are reassuring, more information is necessary, and in the meantime oxytocin should be used with caution; and (d) there are insufficient data in the literature to allow comment on induction of labour' (Panel 1986).

In view of the rarity of adverse outcomes from a trial of labour, randomized trials to determine the safety of such trials in the situations noted would not be feasible. Prospective cohort data should, however, be maintained and published, to guide future policy.

Guidelines for vaginal delivery after a previous cesarean birth. ACOG Newsletter, February 1985, p 8.
Anderson GM, Lomas J (1984). Determinants of the increasing cesarean birth rate. Ontario data 1979 to 1982. New Engl J Med, 311: 887–892.
Baker K (1955). Vaginal delivery after lower segment caesarean section. Surg Gynecol Obstet, 100: 690–696.

Baxter J (1958). Vaginal delivery after caesarean section. Rupture of the lower segment scar. J Obstet Gynaecol Br Empire, 65: 87–88.

Beall M, Eglinton GJ, Clark SL, Phelan JP (1984). Vaginal delivery after previous cesarean section in women with unknown types of uterine scar. J Reprod Med, 29: 31–35.

Benedetti TJ, Platt L, Druzin M (1982). Vaginal delivery after cesarean section for a nonrecurrent cause. Am J Obstet Gynecol, 142: 358–359.

Benson RG, Berendes H, Weiss W (1969). Fetal compromise during elective cesarean section. Am J Obstet Gynecol, 105: 579–588.

Boon AW, Milner AD, Hopkin IE (1981). Lung volumes and lung mechanics in babies born vaginally and by elective and emergency lower segmental cesarean section. J Pediatr, 98: 812–814.

Boucher M, Tahilramaney MR, Eglinton GS, Phelan JP (1984). Maternal morbidity as related to trial of labor after a previous cesarean delivery—a quantitative analysis. J Reprod Med, 29: 12–16.

Browne ADH, McGrath J (1965). Vaginal delivery after previous caesarean section. J Obstet Gynaecol Br Commnwlth, 72: 557–563.

Browne O'D (1951). A summary of 100 vaginal deliveries in the Rotunda Hospital following previous caesarean section. J Obstet Gynaecol Br Empire, 58: 555–557.

Bruce DF (1953). Labour following caesarean section. Glasgow Med J, 34: 354–364.

Butler NR, Alberman ED (1969). Perinatal Problems: The Second Report of the 1958 British Perinatal Mortality Survey. Edinburgh: Churchill Livingstone.

Callen P, Goldsworthy S, Graves L, Harvey D, Mellows H (1979). Mode of delivery and the lecithin/sphingomyelin ratio. Br J Obstet Gynaecol, 86: 965–968.

Carlsson C, Nybell-Lindahl G, Ingemarsson I (1980). Epidural block in patients who have previously undergone caesarean section. Br J Anaesth, 52: 827–829.

Case BD, Jeffcoate N, Randle GH (1971). Caesarean section and its place in modern obstetric practice. J Obstet Gynaecol, 78: 203–214.

Clark S, Eglinton GS, Beall MD, Phelan JP (1984). Effect of indication for previous cesarean section on subsequent delivery outcome in patients undergoing a trial of labor. J Reprod Med, 29: 22–25.

Clow WM, Crompton AC (1973). The wounded uterus: Pregnancy after hysterotomy. Br Med J, 1: 321–323.

Cohen MS, Ong G, Palahniuk R, Cumming M (1985). Obstetrical anesthesia and cesarean section. Presented at the National Consensus Conference on Aspects of Cesarean Birth, Niagara-on-the-Lake, Ontario, 24–26 October, 1985.

Commission on Professional and Hospital Activities (1977). Hospital mortality in PAS hospitals US, 1974–1975. Ann Arbor: CPHA, p 128. (cited in Shy *et al.* 1981)

Cragin EB (1916). Conservatism in obstetrics. New York Med J, 104: 1–3.

Davey MR, Moodley J, Hofmeyr GJ (1987). Labour after caesarean section – the problem of scar dehiscence. S Afr Med J, 71: 766–768.

Demianczuk NN, Hunter DJS, Taylor DW (1982). Trial of labour after previous cesarean section: Prognostic indicators of outcome. Am J Obstet Gynecol, 142: 640–642.

Dewhurst CJ (1956). Reports of societies. J Obstet Gynaecol Br Empire, 63: 125–129.

Dewhurst CJ (1957). The ruptured caesarean section scar. J Obstet Gynaecol Br Empire, 64: 113–118.

Donnelly JP, Franzoni KT (1964). Uterine ruptures: a 30 year survey. Obstet Gynecol, 23: 774–777.

Douglas R (1961). Discussion of Riva and Teich (1961). Am J Obstet Gynecol, 81: 508–509.

Duff P, Southmayd K, Read JA (1988). Outcome of trial of labor in patients with a single previous low transverse cesarean section for dystocia. Obstet Gynecol, 71: 380–384.

Eisenkop SM, Richman R, Platt LD, Paul RH (1982). Urinary tract injury during cesarean section. Obstet Gynecol, 60: 591–596.

Eglinton GS, Phelan JP, Yeh S, Diaz F, Wallace TM, Paul RH (1984). Outcome of a trial of labor after prior cesarean delivery. J Reprod Med, 29: 3–8.

Evrard JR, Gold EM (1977). Cesarean section and maternal mortality in Rhode Island. Obstet Gynecol, 50: 594–597.

Farmakides G, Duvivier R, Schulman H, Schneider E, Biordi J (1987). Vaginal birth after two or more previous cesarean sections. Am J Obstet Gynecol, 156: 565–566.

Fedorkow DM, Nimrod CA, Taylor PJ (1987). Ruptured uterus in pregnancy: a Canadian hospital's experience. Can Med Assoc J, 137: 27–29.

Fedrick J, Butler NR (1970). Certain causes of neonatal death. I: Hyaline membranes. Biol Neonate, 15: 229–255.

Finley BE, Gibbs CE (1986). Emergent cesarean delivery in patients undergoing a trial of labor with a transverse lower-segment scar. Am J Obstet Gynecol, 155: 936–939.

Flamm BL, Dunnett C, Fischermann E, Quilligan EJ (1984). Vaginal delivery following cesarean section: Use of oxytocin augmentation and epidural anaesthesia with internal tocodynamic and internal fetal monitoring. Am J Obstet Gynecol, 148: 759–763.

Flamm BL, Goings JR, Fuelberth NJ, Fischermann E, Jones C, Hersh E (1987). Oxytocin during labor after previous cesarean section: Results of a multicenter study. Obstet Gynecol, 70: 709–712.

Frigoletto FD, Ryan KJ, Phillippe M (1980a). Maternal mortality rate associated with cesarean section: An appraisal. Am J Obstet Gynecol, 136: 969–970.

Frigoletto FD, Phillippe M, Davies IJ, Ryan KJ (1980b). Avoiding iatrogenic prematurity with elective repeat cesarean section without the routine use of amniocentesis. Am J Obstet Gynecol, 137: 521–524.

Garel M, Lelong N, Kaminski M (1987). Psychological consequences of caesarean childbirth in primiparas. J Psychosom Obstet Gynaecol, 6: 197–209.

Gellman E, Goldstein MS, Kaplan S, Shapiro WJ (1983). Vaginal delivery after caesarean section. Experience in private practice. JAMA, 249: 2935–2937.

Gibbs CE (1980). Planned vaginal delivery following cesarean section. Clin Obstet Gynecol, 23: 507–515.

Graham H. (1951). Eternal Eve: The History of Gynecology and Obstetrics. Garden City, New York: Doubleday, p 138.

Graham RA (1984). Trial labor following previous cesarean section. Am J Obstet Gynecol, 149: 35–45.

Greenhill JP (1950). Editorial. Year Book of Obstetrics and Gynecology. Chicago: Year Book Publishers, pp 203–204.

Greenhill JP (1961). Discussion of Riva and Teich, 1961. Am J Obstet Gynecol, 81: 509–510.

Greenhill JP (1970). Editorial. Year Book of Obstetrics and Gynecology. Chicago: Year Book Publishers, pp 202–203.

Hadley CB, Mennuti MT, Gabbe SG (1986). An evaluation of the relative risks of a trial of labor versus elective repeat cesarean section. Am J Perinatol, 3: 107–114.

Halperin ME, Moore DC, Hannah WJ (1988). Classical versus low segment transverse incision for preterm caesarean section. Maternal complications and outcome of subsequent pregnancies. Br J Obstet Gynaecol, 95: 990–996.

Hemminki E, Graubard BI, Hoffman HJ, Mosher WD, Fetterly K. (1985). Cesarean section and subsequent fertility: Results from the 1982 national survey of family growth. Fertil Steril, 43: 520–528.

Holland E (1921a). Rupture of the caesarean section scar in subsequent pregnancy or labour. J Obstet Gynaecol Br Empire, 28: 488–522.

Holland E (1921b). Methods of performing caesarean section. J Obstet Gynaecol Br Empire, 28: 349–357.

Horenstein JM, Eglinton GS, Tahilramaney MP, Boucher M, Phelan JP (1984). Oxytocin use during a trial of labor in patients with previous cesarean section. J Reprod Med, 29: 26–30.

Horenstein JM, Phelan JP (1985). Previous cesarean section: The risks and benefits of oxytocin usage in a trial of labor. Am J Obstet Gynecol, 151: 564–569.

Hurry DJ, Larsen B, Charles D (1984). Effects of postcesarean section febrile morbidity on subsequent fertility. Obstet Gynecol, 64: 256–260.

Jarrell MA, Ashmead GG, Mann LI (1985). Vaginal delivery after cesarean section: a five-year study. Obstet Gynecol, 65: 629–632.

Keeping JD, Morrison J, Chang AM (1980). Classical caesarean section in preterm deliveries. Austral NZ J Obstet Gynaecol, 20: 103–105.

Kehrer FA (1882). Über ein Modificirtes Verfahren beim Kaiserschnitte. Arch Gynaek, 19: 177–209.

Keirse MJNC, Mingeot RA (1974). Dehiscent caesarean section scar on hysterography. Br J Radiol, 47: 191–192.

Keolker K (1981). Vaginal birth after cesarean. Simkin P (ed). Seattle: The Pennypress.

Kerr, JMM (1921). Indications for caesarean section. J Obstet Gynaecol Br Empire, 28: 338–348.

Kerr JM, Moir C (1949). Operative Obstetrics (5th edn). London: Baillière, Tindall & Cox.

Koppenol W, Westerink M (unpublished data) (1980). Management of previous caesarean section. Glasgow Royal Maternity Hospital, Glasgow.

Lawrence RF (1953). Vaginal delivery after caesarean section. J Obstet Gynaecol Br Empire, 60: 237–243.

Lawson GW (1987). Vaginal delivery after 3 previous caesarean sections. Austral NZ J Obstet Gynaecol, 27: 115–116.

Lepage F, Noel B, Lemerre L, Schramm B (1959). Étude hystérographique des césariennes segmentaires. Gynécologie et Obstétrique, 58: 506–517.

Lowe JA, Klassen DE, Loup RJ (1976). Caesarean section in US PAS Hospitals. PAS Report, 14: 1.

MacKenzie IZ, Bradley S, Embree MP (1984). Vaginal prostaglandin and labour induction for patients previously delivered by caesarean section. Br J Obstet Gynaecol, 91: 7–10.

McGarry JA (1969). The management of patients previously delivered by caesarean section. J Obstet Gynaecol Br Empire, 76: 137–143.

Martin JN, Harris BA, Huddleston JF, Morrison JC, Propst MG, Wiser WL, Perlis HW, Davidson JT (1983). Vaginal delivery following previous cesarean birth. Am J Obstet Gynecol, 146: 255–263.

Meehan FP, Moolgaoker AS, Stallworthy J (1972). Vaginal delivery under caudal analgesia after caesarean section and other major uterine surgery. Br Med J, ii: 740–747.

Meier PR, Porreco RP (1982). Trial of labor following cesarean section: a two-year experience. Am J Obstet Gynecol, 144: 671–678.

Merrill BS, Gibbs CE (1978). Planned vaginal delivery after cesarean section. Obstet Gynecol, 52: 50–52.

Minkoff HL, Schwarz RH (1980). The rising cesarean section rate: Can it safely be reversed? Obstet Gynecol, 56: 135–143.

Molloy BG, Sheil O, Duignan NM (1987). Delivery after caesarean section: Review of 2176 consecutive cases. Br Med J, 294: 1645–1647.

Morewood GA, O'Sullivan MJ, McConney J (1973). Vaginal delivery after cesarean section. Obstet Gynecol, 42: 589–595.

Mootabar H, Dwyer JF, Surur F, Dillon TF (1984). Vaginal delivery following previous cesarean in 1983. Int J Gynecol Obstet, 22: 155–160.

Ngu A, Quinn MA (1985). Vaginal delivery following cesarean section. Austral NZ J Obstet Gynaecol, 25: 41–43.

Nielson TF, Hokegard K-H (1984). Cesarean section and intraoperative surgical complications. Acta Obstet Gynecol Scand, 63: 103–108.

O'Connor KM (1983). How safe is induction of labour following a previous caesarean section? J Obstet Gynaecol, 4: 86–87.

Palerme GR, Friedman EA, (1966). Rupture of the gravid uterus in the third trimester. Am J Obstet Gynecol, 94: 571.

Panel (1986). Indications for cesarean section: Final statement of the panel of the National Consensus Conference on Aspects of Cesarean Birth. Can Med Assoc J, 134: 1348–1352.

Pauerstein CJ (1966). Once a section, always a trial of labor? Obstet Gynecol, 28: 273.

Pauerstein CJ, Karp L, Muher S (1969). Trial of labour after low segment caesarean section. South Med J, 62: 925–928.

Paul RH, Phelan JP, Yeh S (1985). Trial of labor in a patient with a prior cesarean birth. Am J Obstet Gynecol, 151: 297–304.

Pearce DJ, Ravi P (1976). Rupture of uterine scar in a patient given epidural analgesia. Lancet, i: 1177–1178.

Petitti DB, Cefalo RC, Shapiro S, Whalley P (1982). In-hospital maternal mortality in the United States: Time trends and relation to method of delivery. Obstet Gynecol, 59: 6–11.

Phelan JP, Clark SL, Diaz F, Paul RH (1987). Vaginal birth after cesarean. Am J Obstet Gynecol, 157: 1510–1515.

Plauche WC, Von Almen W, Muller R (1984). Catastrophic uterine rupture. Obstet Gynecol, 64: 792–797.

Playfair WS (1885). A Treatise on the Science and Practice of Midwifery. Philadelphia: Lea Brothers, p 513.

Poidevin LO, Bockner VY (1958). A hysterographic study of

uteri after caesarean section. J Obstet Gynaecol Br Empire, 65: 278–283.

Poidevin LO (1961). The value of hysterography in the prediction of cesarean section wound defects. Am J Obstet Gynecol, 81: 67–71.

Porreco RP, Meier PR (1983). Trial of labor in patients with multiple previous sections. J Reprod Med, 28: 770–772.

Reis R (1961). Discussion of Riva and Teich (1961). Am J Obstet Gynecol, 81: 508.

Riva HL, Teich JC (1961). Vaginal delivery after cesarean section. Am J Obstet Gynecol, 81: 501–510.

Rubin GL, Peterson HB, Rochat RW, McCarthy BJ, Terry JS (1981). Maternal death after cesarean section in Georgia. Am J Obstet Gynecol, 139: 681–685.

Rudick V, Niv D, Helman-Peri M, Geller E, Ovni A, Golan A (1984). Epidural analgesia for planned vaginal delivery following previous cesarean section. Obstet Gynecol, 64: 621–623.

Ruiz-Velasco V, Guerrero R, Morales A, Gamiz R (1964). Post-cesarean section hysterographic control. Am J Obstet Gynecol, 90: 222–226.

Ruiz-Velasco V, Gamiz R, (1966). Prognosis of the caesarean section scar. Am J Obstet Gynecol, 95: 1119–1121.

Ryan TJ (1960). Further observations on the safety of the pitocin drip. J Obstet Gynaecol Br Empire, 67: 962–965.

Ryder F (1982). The cesarean section. Maternal Health News 7(2): 14.

Sänger (1882). Zur Rehabilitirung des Classischen Kaiserschnittes. Arch Gynaek, 19: 370–399.

Saldana LR, Schulman H, Reuss L (1979). Management of pregnancy after cesarean section. Am J Obstet Gynecol, 135: 555–561.

Salzmann B (1964). Rupture of low segment cesarean section scars. Obstet Gynecol, 23: 460–466.

Seitchik J, Rao VRR (1982). Cesarean delivery in nulliparous women for failed oxytocin augmented labor: route of delivery in subsequent pregnancy. Am J Obstet Gynecol, 143: 393–397.

Shearer E (1982). Education for vaginal birth after cesarean. Birth 9: 31–34.

Shearer E (1981). NIH consensus development task force on cesarean childbirth: the process and the result. Birth Family J, 8(1): 25–30.

Shy KK, LoGerfo JP, Karp LE (1981). Evaluation of elective repeat cesarean section as a standard of care: an application of decision analysis. Am J Obstet Gynecol, 139: 123–129.

Silver RK, Minogue J (1987). When does a statistical fact become an ethical imperative? Am J Obstet Gynecol, 157: 229–233.

Sloan D (1968). Inconclusive conclusion. Am J Obstet Gynecol, 101: 133–136.

Society of Obstetricians and Gynecologists (1982). The increasing cesarean section rate. SOGC Bulletin III (3).

Tahilramaney MP, Boucher M, Eglinton GS, Beall M, Phelan JP (1984). Previous cesarean section and trial of labor: factors related to uterine dehiscence. J Reprod Med, 29: 17–21.

Trolle D (1982). The history of caesarean section. Acta Hist Sci Nat Med, 33: 1–109.

US Department of Health and Human Services (1981). Cesarean childbirth. NIH Publication No. 82-2067.

Van Gelderen CJ, England MJ, Naylor GA, Katzeff TC (1986). Labour in patients with a caesarean section scar. The place of oxytocin augmentation. S Afr Med J, 70: 529–532.

Vlies PR, Dewhurst CJ (1975). Pregnancy and labour following hysterotomy. Int J Gynaecol Obstet, 13: 162–164.

Wadhawan S, Narone JN (1983). Outcome of labor following previous cesarean section. Int J Gynaecol Obstet, 21: 7–10.

Waniorek A (1967). Hysterography after caesarean section for evaluation of suturing technic. Obstet Gynecol, 29: 192–199.

Ware HH (1961). Discussion of Riva and Teich (1961). Am J Obstet Gynecol, 81: 510.

Whiteside DC, Mahan CS, Cook JC (1983). Factors associated with successful vaginal delivery after cesarean section. J Reprod Med, 28: 785–788.

Williams JW (1903). Obstetrics. New York: Appleton.

Winchester G, Brown R (1954). Symposium on caesarean section. IV. Caesarean section, with special reference to subsequent childbearing. Transactions of the Edinburgh Obst. Soc. Session 106, 1953–54. Edinburgh Med J, 61(Tr): 63–70.

Yeh S, Huang X, Phelan JP (1984). Post term pregnancy after previous cesarean section. J Reprod Med, 29: 41–44.

Zilberman A, Sharf M, Polishuk WZ (1968). Evaluation of caesarean section scar by hysterography. Obstet Gynecol 32: 153–157.

71 Instrumental vaginal delivery

Aldo Vacca and Marc J. N. C. Keirse

1 Introduction

When a valid indication for expediting the birth of the baby exists, instrumental vaginal delivery may be selected on the basis of a number of factors. These include the condition of the fetus and mother; progress in labour; dilatation of the cervix; the station of the presenting part; position and moulding of the fetal head; comfort, morale, and co-operation of the mother; experience and attitudes of the operator; and the availability of correct equipment.

Few indications for instrumental delivery are absolute, and there are considerable regional and international differences in the rate of instrumental deliveries (Chalmers and Richards 1977) (see Chapter 69). It may be helpful, therefore, to categorize indications for instrumental delivery as either 'standard' or 'special' indications (Table 72.1). A higher level of judgement and skill is required to use instruments for special indications.

2 Conditions for instrumental delivery

2.1 Condition of the fetus and mother

The state of both the fetus and the mother are important in selecting the most appropriate method for operative vaginal delivery. Severe fetal distress is often quoted as an indication for using forceps rather than vacuum extraction because many operators believe that vacuum extraction is too slow. This belief has largely

Table 71.1 Standard and special indications for instrumental vaginal delivery

A *Standard indications for operative delivery*: (the fetal head is engaged and the cervix is fully dilated).

- Delay in the second stage of labour with the fetal head stationed at the outlet of the pelvis, on the pelvic floor or in the midpelvis
- Fetal distress
- Elective shortening of the second stage of labour for fetal or maternal benefit.

B *Special indications for operative delivery*:

- Delay in the second stage of labour associated with malposition of the fetal head where borderline disproportion is suspected
- Prolapse of the umbilical cord when the cervix is fully dilated.

C *Special indications for forceps only*:

- Face presentation
- Delivery of the head in breech presentation

D *Special indications for vacuum extraction only*:

- Fetal distress or delay associated with fetal malposition in a multipara after the cervix is widely but not fully dilated
- Delivery of the second twin when the head is not quite engaged or still high
- After symphysiotomy (Bird and Bal 1967; Gebbie 1982)

resulted from the recommendation that time should be allowed for the development of an adequate caput succedaneum (chignon) before traction is applied (Chalmers JA 1971). However, Wider *et al.* (1967) and Svenningsen (1987) showed that the desired level of negative pressure could be attained in one step once the vacuum cup had been correctly applied, and that gradual and stepwise increases in negative pressure are not necessary. In experienced hands, application-to-delivery interval is no slower for vacuum extraction than for forceps (see below).

A number of maternal medical conditions, such as severe pre-eclampsia, cardiac disease, cerebral aneurysm, and increased risk of retinal detachment may indicate instrumental delivery to avoid excessive maternal exertion during the expulsion phase of the second stage of labour. Forceps are usually preferred in such circumstances since they are less dependent on maternal expulsive effort than vacuum extraction. The need for maternal pushing can be reduced, however, if normal uterine action is maintained throughout the second stage of labour, using oxytocin if necessary, and if time is allowed for the head to descend to the pelvic floor, using epidural analgesia if necessary to alleviate bearing down sensations. Application of the vacuum cup to promote flexion of the head, and traction during contractions to cause steady progress will nearly always result in easy delivery without undue effort on the part of the mother.

2.2 Progress in labour

A conceptual division of the second stage of labour into two distinct phases (O'Driscoll and Meagher 1980) is useful in relation to instrumental delivery. The first phase extends from the time of full dilatation of the cervix until the fetal head reaches the pelvic floor, and it may be regarded as an extension of the first stage of labour. The second phase extends from the time the head reaches the pelvic floor until the baby is born. Liberal use of oxytocin may be better than premature instrumental delivery for the treatment of delay in the first phase of the second stage of labour. If the baby must be delivered by forceps or vacuum extraction and there is evidence of hypotonic uterine action, oxytocin should be administered to enhance contractions during the procedure. This is especially important if vacuum extraction is the method chosen.

2.3 Dilatation of the cervix

Although it is generally agreed (albeit with some exceptions, e.g. Moolgaoker 1970) that forceps should not be applied to the fetal head unless the cervix is fully dilated, there is still some controversy about the use of the vacuum extractor in such circumstances (Chalmers JA 1975). Bird (1982) advised caution when using the

instrument before the cervix was fully dilated. He regarded this as one of its 'special uses' and listed strict conditions that should be fulfilled before such procedures were attempted.

2.4 Station, position, and moulding of the fetal head

Station of the head has been traditionally assessed by relating the lowest part of the fetal head to the ischial spines. By this method, engagement is defined as having occurred when the lowest point is at or below the ischial spines, for at this stage the biparietal diameter of the head is assumed to have passed through the plane of the brim of the pelvis. In normal labours such an assumption is usually correct, but in difficult situations where pronounced moulding causes elongation of the head, or where a prominent caput succedaneum obscures a clear definition of the lowest cranial point, the head may appear to be lower in the pelvis than is actually the case. Crichton (1974) emphasized the potential dangers of misjudging the station of the fetal head when performing instrumental delivery, and devised a practical and reliable method of establishing the level by estimating the proportion of the head, expressed in fifths, palpable abdominally. The pitfall of making a wrong diagnosis of engagement can be reduced by considering both the number of fifths of head palpable abdominally and the findings obtained by vaginal examination (see Chapter 53).

Moulding may be used as an indicator of the extent of compression to which the fetal head has been subjected during labour. When considered together with the number of fifths of head above the pelvic brim, it provides useful evidence for the diagnosis of cephalopelvic disproportion (Philpott 1982) (see Chapter 31). Stewart (1982) proposed a system for assessing moulding that allowed comparison of results from one vaginal examination to another (Fig. 71.1). In slight moulding the parietal bones are touching but not overlapping at the sagittal suture line; in moderate moulding, one parietal bone is overlapping the other, but it can be reduced to the normal position by finger pressure; and in severe moulding the overlapping of the bones cannot easily be reduced.

The degree of moulding should always be assessed before attempting operative vaginal delivery. If severe moulding is present, as is often found with the deflexed and asynclitic heads in occipitoposterior and lateral positions, additional force created by applying forceps or vacuum extractor without first correcting the position and thus relieving compression of the head may increase the risk of intracranial injury. Correction of the malposition and asynclitism, on the other hand, may often allow safe vaginal delivery.

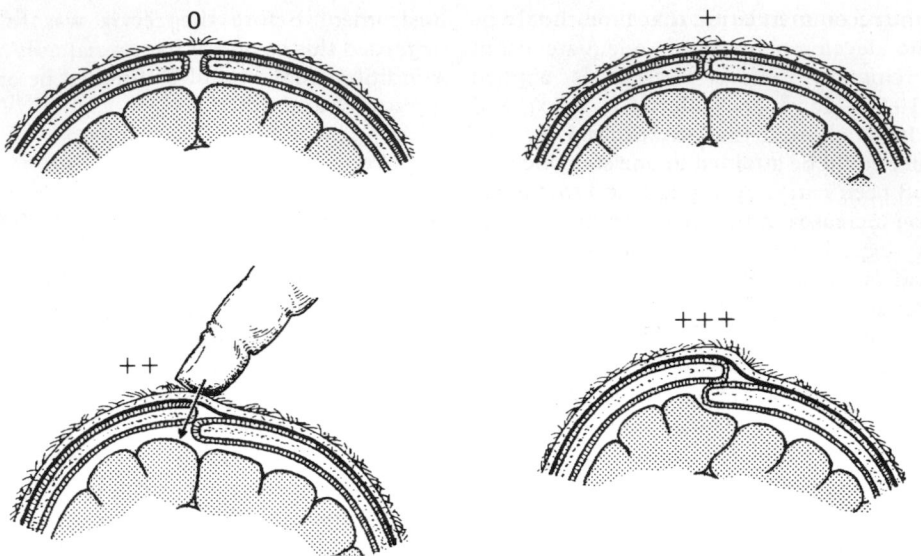

Fig. 71.1 Degrees of moulding according to Stewart (1982).

2.5 Comfort, morale, and co-operation of the mother

Certain aspects of pain relief should be considered in relation to instrumental delivery. Epidural analgesia can predispose to instrumental delivery and malposition of the fetal head (Hoult et al. 1977). On the other hand, Doughty (1969) reported a decrease in the forceps delivery rate despite increasing use of epidural analgesia. Bailey and Howard (1983) analysed the outcomes of labours of women who delivered before and after introduction of an epidural service and found that although initially there was an increase in the forceps rate it subsequently fell to pre-epidural levels. Jouppila *et al.* (1979) concluded that segmental epidural analgesia did not seem to disturb the normal progress of labour nor increase the frequency of fetal malpositions and instrumental deliveries. At the Mater Mothers Hospital in Brisbane, the instrumental delivery rate in nulliparae has decreased despite increasing use of epidural block.

It is clear that effective epidural analgesia will modify or abolish the mother's urge and ability to push, and hence will result in altered mechanisms during the second stage of labour (see Chapter 57). The effect of the use of instrumental delivery will depend on the way that the second stage is managed in the light of these altered mechanisms (see Chapter 66).

Fetal distress and delay in the second stage of labour are common indications for instrumental delivery and under such circumstances it is hardly surprising that maternal anxiety is increased. Some of that anxiety may be relieved if the expectant mother and her partner are fully informed of the reasons for operative delivery and if they receive continuous support. If instrumental delivery is required, the attendant should explain the reasons for the procedure and emphasize the need for the mother's active involvement in the delivery. The greater the maternal co-operation and expulsive effort, the less the need for traction by the operator.

2.6 Analgesia for instrumental delivery

Effective and appropriate analgesia should be provided before instrumental delivery is undertaken. In general, less pain relief is needed for vacuum extraction than for forceps delivery (Vacca *et al.* 1983). Forceps procedures at the pelvic outlet and most non-rotational midpelvic procedures are usually managed satisfactorily with infiltration of the perineum or pudendal nerve block. Outlet vacuum extractions require no analgesia unless episiotomy is performed.

Procedures that require forceps rotation of the fetal head should virtually always be performed under epidural or spinal block. With few exceptions, perineal infiltration alone suffices for rotational and non-rotational vacuum extractions from the midpelvis.

Epidural analgesia and general anaesthesia should not be implemented for the purpose of vacuum extraction, because they impair maternal expulsive powers. If the mother has already received epidural analgesia and vacuum extraction is undertaken, the operator should help her to compensate for the loss of pushing sensation by telling her when she is bearing down effectively. Injury to the fetus is more likely to occur if the operator relies entirely on increased traction to overcome decreased maternal expulsive effort.

2.7 Traction and compression forces acting on the fetal head

In order for the fetal head to pass through the birth canal, the powers exerted on it must be greater than the sum of the resisting forces in the pelvis. Such powers may be enhanced by increasing the propulsive forces (uterine contractions, voluntary maternal expulsive effort); by applying traction to the fetal head (forceps or vacuum extraction); or by reducing the resisting forces so that the existing powers are rendered more effective (ensuring optimum presenting diameters of the fetal head). In normal labour, compression force acting on the fetal head depends on friction of the maternal tissues, the presenting diameters of the head in relation to the pelvis, and the strength of the expulsive powers. Force is modified by the pliable nature of the scalp bones, which allows the head to reduce its dimensions in one plane and increase them in another, and by rotation and flexion of the fetal head as an adaptation to the sigmoid birth tract.

Many investigators have tried to define what forces constitute safe levels for traction and compression. During the expulsive phase of the second stage of labour, forces acting on the fetal head have been calculated to be between 8.4 kg (Pearse 1966) and 15 kg (Lindgren 1960). Estimates of average traction forces with forceps have ranged from 16 kg (Wylie 1935) to 23 kg (Moolgaoker *et al.* 1979), although investigators have pointed out that normal babies have been delivered using measured pulls well in excess of these averages. With crossed forceps, the proportion of the traction force that is transmitted to the fetal head as compression force has been estimated to be between 25 per cent (Laufe 1971) and 50 per cent (Kelly and Sines 1966).

The vacuum extractor accepts pulls of between 15 kg (Chamberlain 1980) and 20 kg or more (Saling and Hartung 1973) before the cup becomes detached. The maximal traction force increases with increasing vacuum and with increasing cup size (Duchon *et al.* 1988). Some authors regard cup detachment as an inherent safety mechanism of the vacuum extractor, but Issel (1977) warns that sudden changes when the cup is pulled off may lead to brain injury from compression–decompression effects. Duchon *et al.* (1988) recently compared the forces exerted by different vacuum cups on the fetal scalps in a laboratory setting. They found that the Bird modified Malmström cup exerted greater force ($0.79 \, \text{kg/cm}^2$) than the more recent Mity-Vac and Soft Cup devices which exerted forces of, respectively, 0.68 and $0.63 \, \text{kg/cm}^2$. These devices will therefore accept less traction before detachment occurs than the classical cups.

Pearse (1966) has shown that traction and compression forces exerted on the fetal head are greater when delivery occurs in the occipito-posterior position.

Resistance to delivery is least when the largest diameters of the head meet the widest dimensions of the pelvis at any given level in the birth canal. Biparietal applications of the forceps blades and flexing median applications of the vacuum cup to the fetal head, followed by traction in the line of the axis of the pelvis, will result in optimum presenting diameters that require the least additional force to effect delivery.

Ultimately, it is the operator who decides how much extra force in addition to the compression forces of labour, will be exerted on the fetal head as a result of instrumental delivery. The total force exerted on the fetal head during instrumental delivery will depend on the duration of the procedure and on the number and strength of pulls. Some descent of the head should occur with each pull. No descent with traction should be regarded by the operator as a reason to abandon the procedure in favour of caesarean section.

2.8 The operator and the attitudes of the attendants

The operator is a major determinant of the success or failure of instrumental delivery. Unfavourable results are almost invariably caused by the user's unfamiliarity with either the instrument or the basic rules governing its use (Aguero and Alvarez 1962). In the English-speaking world in general, forceps is the preferred instrument, and adequate familiarity with the vacuum extractor is less common. The situation is the reverse in many European countries where the use of forceps is uncommon (Bergsjø *et al.* 1983; Ryden 1986). Bowes and Bowes (1980) expressed concern that obstetricians in training in the United States have little opportunity to acquire adequate experience in the correct use of midcavity forceps, and Iffy *et al.* (1984) pointed out that the majority of specialist obstetricians in the United States have been trained only in the use of forceps and have had little or no opportunity to become familiar with the vacuum extractor. Familiarity with both vacuum extraction and forceps is thus rare.

Operators, whatever their seniority, who are unfamiliar with one or other method should acquire experience of the technique in question by commencing with outlet procedures, graduating to midpelvic operations under supervision, and only after mastering the technique in these circumstances, attempt such procedures as are listed in the special groups. It is inadvisable and potentially dangerous to use one instrument for routine work and to reserve the other for specially challenging situations.

The extent to which a mother will accept the appearance of her baby after forceps or vacuum extraction will be influenced by the attitudes and reassurances of the staff, not only of those who perform the procedures, but also, of the paediatricians, midwives, and nurses who care for mothers and babies after birth. It is important to reassure mothers that bruising with forceps or vacuum extractor is transient, that a chignon will disappear in a matter of hours, and that markings from the vacuum cup or forceps blades will leave no traces after a few days. A careless remark, however well-intentioned, may lead to unnecessary anxiety for the mother.

3 Equipment and techniques

Although injury to mother and baby from operative delivery with either forceps or vacuum extractor has been widely documented, it can be difficult to ascertain to what extent this is caused by the instrument itself and to what extent it is due to the circumstances surrounding its use (Ryden 1986). Every procedure has a potential for injury to mother or baby. When a clear-cut indication for expediting delivery exists, the relative benefits of operative vaginal and abdominal delivery must be weighed against their risks. When the choice is made in favour of operative vaginal delivery, knowledge of the instrument and its proper use and limitations become of paramount importance.

3.1 Forceps

Since the introduction of forceps numerous modifications have been devised in attempts to improve the efficiency and safety of the instrument for specific obstetric situations. Changes have been made to the blades, shanks, locking and traction devices, pelvic and cephalic curves, and in the relation between the two branches from crossed, to divergent and parallel designs (Laufe 1985). Forceps can be grouped on a functional basis into non-rotational and rotational types, depending on whether the primary function is to exert traction or to correct malposition prior to exerting traction.

Forceps operations can be categorized into outlet procedures (when the fetal head is on view and the sagittal suture is in the antero-posterior diameter of the pelvis), midpelvic non-rotational procedures (when the head is in an oblique occipito-anterior position but not on view), and midpelvic rotational procedures (when the occiput is in occipito-lateral or posterior positions). For outlet and midpelvic non-rotational procedures, one of the classical (non-rotational) forceps such as the Simpson, Neville Barnes, Haig Ferguson, and Elliott varieties are usually employed. Forceps with parallel shanks (Shute 1958) or divergent blades (Laufe 1968) are preferred by some operators because it is claimed that a reduced compression force is applied to the fetal head (Seidenschnur and Koepcke 1979; Laufe 1971).

Specialized forceps have been developed for midpelvic rotation of the fetal head in occipito-lateral and posterior positions. Kielland's forceps have remained the most popular of the rotational forceps in common use. Instrumental procedures in transverse arrest are among the most difficult of all forceps operations, because marked asynclitism may render correct application difficult. The Barton forceps with a hinged anterior blade and markedly curved posterior blade were designed specifically for use in such occipito-lateral positions. Parry-Jones (1972) recommended that Barton's forceps be used for lateral positions of the occiput and Keilland's forceps for occipito-posterior positions. Laufe (1956) discussed the relative advantages and disadvantages of the Kielland and Barton forceps, and outlined the reasons for introducing his new design the Kielland–Barton–Laufe forceps, which also incorporated a hinged anterior blade. Similarly, Moolgaoker (1962) listed some of the mechanical drawbacks of the Kielland forceps and described advantages of a forceps of his own design.

Three main methods have been described for the application of the Kielland forceps: the classical (or inversion), the wandering, and the direct (Parry-Jones 1952). The inversion method is rarely used in modern obstetric practice. When the occiput is latero-posterior or lateral the wandering technique for applying the anterior blade is usually the method of choice; when the occiput is sacral, the direct method is preferable. More recently, Parry-Jones (1972) detailed the method of using Barton's forceps in occipito-lateral and occipito-posterior positions. He believed Barton's forceps had one great advantage over other rotational forceps in that they allow spontaneous rotation of the head during traction, provided the axis traction handle is used. He warned that, without the traction bar, a small amount of rotational force applied to the end of the handles of the forceps imparted a considerable amount of force to the fetal head due to the overall length of the forceps and the angle at which the blades lie to the shanks. Dennen (1964) regarded the shape of the Barton forceps as a disadvantage for traction when the axis traction handle was used. No controlled trials to assess the relative merits and hazards of these different types of forceps have been reported.

Rotation with forceps should not be forceful, and it should be undertaken as a separate procedure from traction. Rotation should usually precede traction. Sometimes it is necessary to displace the head somewhat upwards in order to accomplish rotation. At times rotation can be better accomplished after slight descent of the head to a lower station. Rotation and traction performed simultaneously may place undue strain on the spinal column of the fetus and result in serious injury to the cervical cord (Pridmore 1974).

Forceps are correctly applied to the side of the head when the blades are located symmetrically between the orbits and the ears, reaching from the parietal eminences to the malar areas and cheeks (Fig. 71.2). With such applications, described as biparietal or cephalic, pressure is evenly distributed over the least vulnerable

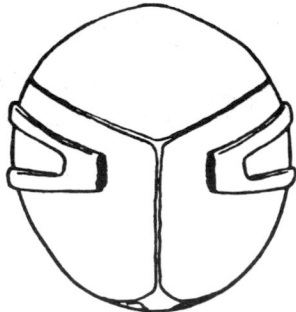

Fig. 71.2 Correct application of forceps to the fetal head.

areas, and the head is maintained in an attitude of flexion, resulting in optimum diameters presenting for delivery. In this position the forceps correspond to the 'pivot point' of the head which is the midpoint of the biparietal diameter (Dennen 1964). If the pivot point is not in the centre of the blades, traction causes the head to become either overextended or overflexed.

In practice, correct application can be diagnosed by relating the position of the posterior fontanelle and sagittal suture to the position of the forceps. The posterior fontanelle should be about one finger's breadth in front of the plane of the shanks and equidistant from the blades; the sagittal suture should be perpendicular to the middle of the plane of the shanks. If the posterior fontanelle is more than one finger's breadth above the plane of the shanks, the pivot point of the head will be above the centre of the blades and traction will cause the head to extend. If the sagittal suture is closer to one or other of the shanks, the application will be asynclitic.

When the head is deflexed and asynclitic, the diameters that are offered for delivery are larger than optimum; unless corrected, more forceful traction will be necessary to achieve delivery. Forceps can only minimally correct a deflexion attitude, and significant degrees of deflexion should be corrected before forceps are applied. Because deflexion and asynclitism are nearly always associated with the malpositioned head, rotation to the occipito-anterior position should be performed before exerting traction with forceps. If the head is arrested with the occiput lying directly posterior and distending the perineum, it is probably wiser to accomplish delivery in the face-to-pubis position.

Forceps are sometimes used to assist delivery in face presentations provided the head is well down in the pelvic cavity and the chin is anterior. Mento-posterior presentations should be managed by caesarean section (Myerscough 1982).

With a breech presentation it is important that the aftercoming head be delivered gently. In some cases this can be better accomplished with forceps (Milner 1975). Traction with the forceps is exerted directly on the head and not through the vertebral column, thereby reducing the risk of injury to the spinal cord. Although any of the classical varieties of forceps may be used, the Piper forceps were specifically designed for use on the aftercoming head. For details of technique of forceps the reader is referred to standard texts such as Dennen (1964), Myerscough (1982), and Pritchard *et al.* (1985). Scalp and facial injuries following instrumental delivery are related to the ease with which operative vaginal delivery is accomplished. Herbertson *et al.* (1985) studied the use of pads slipped over the forceps blades in a randomized controlled trial. They showed that markings and abrasions on the face and scalp were significantly reduced with the use of padded forceps compared with unpadded forceps.

3.2 Vacuum extraction

Although early attempts at vacuum extraction for delivery were described by Yonge (1706) and Simpson (1848), these procedures had little impact on obstetric practice. Interest in vacuum extraction as a method of assisting vaginal delivery was revived by Malmström (1954). The method is practised extensively in some parts of the world (Bergsjø *et al.* 1983) although its use in English-speaking countries is sporadic (Chalmers and Richards 1977). Malmström's (1954) original design is still the most popular form of the instrument and is usually employed as described by Chalmers (1971).

An important modification to Malmström's vacuum extractor was introduced by Bird (1976) who recognized that difficult vacuum extractions, failure of the procedure, and injuries to the neonate were sometimes the result of failing to correct deflexion of the fetal head. In order to increase manoeuvrability of the cup to achieve a more correct application on the fetal head, Bird altered the attachment of the suction tube from the central position of the dome (as found in the Malmström version) to the lateral wall of the cup. This design was called the 'posterior cup' and Bird recommended its use specifically for posterior and lateral positions of the occiput. Earlier, Bird (1969) had introduced his first modification, the 'anterior cup' for use in anterior positions of the occiput. More recently, he (1982) altered the traction system from a chain on the dome of the cup to a cord (string) attached to the rim. This latest design has been called the 'New Generation' cup and is available in anterior and posterior varieties (Bird 1982).

For malpositions of the fetal head, the new generation Bird posterior cup is more manoeuvrable than the Malmström cup because of the lateral attachment of the suction tube and the smooth dome of the cup. Carmody *et al.* (1986) compared the 'New Generation' cup with the original Bird cup in a randomized controlled trial and could find no evidence that the newer designs improved outcome compared with the original cups (Table 71.2). Bird's claims that his cups offer advan-

Table 71.2 Effect of New Generation vs. original Bird vacuum extraction on failure to deliver (selected instrument)

Study	EXPT		CTRL		Odds ratio	Graph of odds ratios and confidence intervals						
	n	(%)	n	(%)	(95% CI)	0.01	0.1	0.5	1	2	10	100
Carmody *et al.* (1986)	9/60	(15.00)	7/63	(11.11)	1.41 (0.49–4.01)							
Typical odds ratio (95% confidence interval)					1.41 (0.49–4.01)							

Effect of new generation vs. original Bird vacuum extraction on cup detachment

| Carmody *et al.* (1986) | 9/60 | (15.00) | 4/60 | (6.67) | 2.35 (0.75–7.40) | | | | | | | |
| Typical odds ratio (95% confidence interval) | | | | | 2.35 (0.75–7.40) | | | | | | | |

Effect of new generation vs. original Bird vacuum extraction on Apgar score <7 at 1 min

| Carmody *et al.* (1986) | 10/60 | (16.67) | 8/63 | (12.70) | 1.37 (0.51–3.71) | | | | | | | |
| Typical odds ratio (95% confidence interval) | | | | | 1.37 (0.51–3.71) | | | | | | | |

Effect of new generation vs. original Bird vacuum extraction on Apgar score <7 at 5 mins

| Carmody *et al.* (1986) | 2/60 | (3.33) | 0/63 | (0.00) | 7.90 (0.49–99.99) | | | | | | | |
| Typical odds ratio (95% confidence interval) | | | | | 7.90 (0.49–99.99) | | | | | | | |

Effect of new generation vs. original Bird vacuum extraction on endotracheal intubation

| Carmody *et al.* (1986) | 4/60 | (6.67) | 7/63 | (11.11) | 0.58 (0.17–2.00) | | | | | | | |
| Typical odds ratio (95% confidence interval) | | | | | 0.58 (0.17–2.00) | | | | | | | |

Effect of new generation vs. original Bird vacuum extraction on scalp injuries

| Carmody *et al.* (1986) | 17/60 | (28.33) | 19/63 | (30.16) | 0.92 (0.42–1.99) | | | | | | | |
| Typical odds ratio (95% confidence interval) | | | | | 0.92 (0.42–1.99) | | | | | | | |

Effect of new generation vs. original Bird vacuum extraction on admission to special care nursery

| Carmody *et al.* (1986) | 3/60 | (5.00) | 4/63 | (6.35) | 0.78 (0.17–3.56) | | | | | | | |
| Typical odds ratio (95% confidence interval) | | | | | 0.78 (0.17–3.56) | | | | | | | |

Effect of new generation vs. original Bird vacuum extraction on use of phototherapy

| Carmody *et al.* (1986) | 14/60 | (23.33) | 7/63 | (11.11) | 2.35 (0.92–6.00) | | | | | | | |
| Typical odds ratio (95% confidence interval) | | | | | 2.35 (0.92–6.00) | | | | | | | |

tages over the original Malmström design for positions that require rotation received support from the data of an observational study in Portsmouth (Table 71.3).

O'Neil *et al.* (1981) devised a method of traction which he adapted to the Bird cup patterns and claimed that the cups withstood greater oblique traction force than either the Malmström or Bird cups, a claim that was not substantiated in a randomized comparison made by Thiery *et al.* (1987). In a randomized trial, which involved 410 women at term with a healthy singleton fetus, no differences were found between the two type of cups except that failure to deliver was more frequent in women allocated to the O'Neil cup (3 per cent) than in women allocated to the Malmström cup (0.5 per cent; Table 71.4). Both instruments had a high success rate, which probably relates to the fact that vacuum extraction was usually conducted as an elective rather than as an indicated procedure (Thiery, personal communication).

Table 71.3 Difference between the Bird and Malmström cups for rotational vacuum extraction (data from an observational study in Portsmouth, England)

Type of cup	No. of women	Per cent flexing applications	Failure rate (%)	Neonatal injury (%)
Bird	176	72	13	15
Malmström	68	37	28	29
Total	244	62	17	19

Randomized comparisons of the soft, bell-shaped cups such as the Silastic (Ottolini, 1980) and Silc models (Wiqvist 1984) with rigid cups have not yet been reported. In theory at least, such cups would appear to be inferior to the cups described earlier because their design and size often does not allow the attainment of a correct application on the fetal head. They are rather inefficient instruments when the fetal head is midpelvic (Berkus *et al.* 1986) or malpositioned (Hastie and MacLean 1986). On the basis of current evidence their use should probably be restricted to easy or to outlet procedures.

A randomized trial has compared two models of the soft cups, Silastic and Mity-Vac (Dell *et al.* 1985) (Table 71.5). Although the Mity-Vac cups resulted in fewer scalp injuries other than cephalhaematoma and appeared to be more effective in achieving delivery, the number of women involved was small.

All the vacuum cups are satisfactory for outlet and non-rotational midpelvic operations provided the operator is familiar with the vacuum extractor. The posterior cup is preferable when the occiput is lateral or posterior. Operators would be well advised to develop confidence in the use of the rigid anterior cup for outlet

and non-rotational midpelvic procedures because the basic technique of vacuum extraction is similar in all positions of the occiput, and experience gained with the anterior cup will prove invaluable when the more difficult rotational operations are attempted using the posterior cup.

The vacuum extractor must be maintained in good working order. An airtight seal within the pump and tubing is essential for the success of the procedure. The equipment should be serviced regularly and any defective parts replaced. Operators should test the instrument for leakage immediately before applying the cup to the baby's head. For details of technique and care of the equipment the reader is referred to Bird (1976; 1982) and Thiery (1985).

A correct application of the vacuum cup on the fetal head is one of the most important determinants of outcome. Bird (1976) emphasized the importance of flexion in vacuum extraction. He showed that traction applied to a vacuum cup in the axis of the pelvis maintains or promotes complete flexion and synclitism of the fetal head if the centre of the cup is either on or directly behind the posterior end of the mento-vertical diameter. If it is in front of this point it causes deflexion. In practical terms this 'flexing point' is located on the sagittal suture 3 cm in front of the posterior fontanelle. For vacuum extraction the flexing point is the most important landmark on the fetal head. It corresponds to the pivot point described by Dennen (1964) for forceps. The ideal application for vacuum extraction is achieved when the centre of the cup is superimposed on the flexing point. Correct and incorrect applications of the 50 mm cup are shown diagrammatically in Fig. 71.3.

It should be appreciated that the 50 mm cup has a maximum diameter of 60 mm due to the curved edges of the cup. Assuming that the length of the sagittal suture is approximately 9 cm in the average term baby, when the centre of the cup is over the flexing point the leading edge of the cup will be at least 3 cm behind the anterior fontanelle. The operator can confirm that the cup is correctly positioned when there is 3 cm or more between the leading edge of the cup and the anterior fontanelle, with the cup placed symmetrically over the sagittal suture. This application is called 'flexing median' and operators should strive to achieve it with every vacuum extraction whatever the position of the fetal head. If the distance between anterior fontanelle and cup is less than 3 cm, the application is deflexing. When the centre of the cup is situated more than 1 cm to one or other side of the midline, the application is described as paramedian and will cause asynclitism.

Thus there are four possible applications of the cup: (a) flexing median; (b) flexing paramedian; (c) deflexing median; and (d) deflexing paramedian (Fig. 71.3). The effect of application of the cup on the outcome of the

Table 71.4 Effects of O'Neil vs. Malmström vacuum extraction on failure to deliver with selected instrument

Study	EXPT		CTRL		Odds ratio	Graph of odds ratios and confidence intervals
	n	(%)	*n*	(%)	(95% CI)	0.01　0.1　0.5　1　2　10　1
Thiery *et al.* (1987)	6/200	(3.00)	1/210	(0.48)	4.48 (1.01–19.95)	
Typical odds ratio (95% confidence interval)					4.48 (1.01–19.95)	

Effect of O'Neil vs. Malmström vacuum extraction on cup detachment/leakage

Thiery *et al.* (1987)	17/200	(8.50)	28/210	(13.33)	0.61 (0.33–1.13)	
Typical odds ratio (95% confidence interval)					0.61 (0.33–1.13)	

Effect of O'Neil vs. Malmström vacuum extraction on low Apgar score at 1 min

Thiery *et al.* (1987)	7/200	(3.50)	6/210	(2.86)	1.23 (0.41–3.72)	
Typical odds ratio (95% confidence interval)					1.23 (0.41–3.72)	

Effect of O'Neil vs. Malmström vacuum extraction on low Apgar score (<7) at 5 min

Thiery *et al.* (1987)	3/200	(1.50)	5/210	(2.38)	0.63 (0.16–2.56)	
Typical odds ratio (95% confidence interval)					0.63 (0.16–2.56)	

Effect of O'Neil vs. Malmström vacuum extraction on endotracheal intubation

Thiery *et al.* (1987)	4/200	(2.00)	3/210	(1.43)	1.40 (0.32–6.25)	
Typical odds ratio (95% confidence interval)					1.40 (0.32–6.25)	

Effect of O'Neil vs. Malmström vacuum extraction on scalp injuries

Thiery *et al.* (1987)	10/200	(5.00)	11/210	(5.24)	0.95 (0.40–2.29)	
Typical odds ratio (95% confidence interval)					0.95 (0.40–2.29)	

Effect of O'Neil vs. Malmström vacuum extraction on hyperbilirubinaemia (>12 mg/100 ml)

Thiery *et al.* (1987)	38/200	(19.00)	43/210	(20.48)	0.91 (0.56–1.48)	
Typical odds ratio (95% confidence interval)					0.91 (0.56–1.48)	

Table 71.5 Effects of Silastic vs. Mityvac vacuum extraction on failure to deliver with the selected instrument

Study	EXPT		CTRL		Odds ratio	Graph of odds ratios and confidence intervals						
	n	(%)	n	(%)	(95% CI)	0.01	0.1	0.5	1	2	10	100
Dell *et al.* (1985)	10/36	(27.78)	4/37	(10.81)	2.94 (0.93–9.37)							
Typical odds ratio (95% confidence interval)					2.94 (0.93–9.37)							

Effect of Silastic vs. Mityvac vacuum extraction on Apgar score <7 at 1 min

| Dell *et al.* (1985) | 4/36 | (11.11) | 2/37 | (5.41) | 2.11 (0.40–11.08) | | | | | | | |
| Typical odds ratio (95% confidence interval) | | | | | 2.11 (0.40–11.08) | | | | | | | |

Effect of Silastic vs. Mityvac vacuum extraction on Apgar score <7 at 5 min

| Dell *et al.* (1985) | 0/36 | (0.00) | 0/37 | (0.00) | 1.00 (1.00–1.00) | | | | | | | |
| Typical odds ratio (95% confidence interval) | | | | | 1.00 (1.00–1.00) | | | | | | | |

Effect of Silastic vs. Mityvac vacuum extraction on cephalhaematoma

| Dell *et al.* (1985) | 5/36 | (13.89) | 6/37 | (16.22) | 0.84 (0.23–2.99) | | | | | | | |
| Typical odds ratio (95% confidence interval) | | | | | 0.84 (0.23–2.99) | | | | | | | |

Effect of Silastic vs. Mityvac vacuum extraction on scalp injuries other than cephalhaematoma

| Dell *et al.* (1985) | 16/36 | (44.44) | 6/37 | (16.22) | 3.75 (1.39–10.13) | | | | | | | |
| Typical odds ratio (95% confidence interval) | | | | | 3.75 (1.39–10.13) | | | | | | | |

Effect of Silastic vs. Mityvac vacuum extraction on use of phototherapy

| Dell *et al.* (1985) | 2/36 | (5.56) | 0/37 | (0.00) | 7.82 (0.48–99.99) | | | | | | | |
| Typical odds ratio (95% confidence interval) | | | | | 7.82 (0.48–99.99) | | | | | | | |

procedure in malpositions of the fetal head is shown in Table 71.6. In the series from which these data were derived (Vacca, unpublished observations) high failure and neonatal injury rates were associated with deflexing applications, and outcome was worse still when cup applications were also paramedian. All four major injuries were associated with deflexing applications of the cup, and all but one of these also had paramedian applications. The most favourable outcome is obtained with flexing, median applications of the cup. Deflexing

applications of the cup are far less likely to result in anterior rotation of the occiput (Table 71.6).

Lasbrey *et al.* (1964) showed that the risk of injury to the infant was directly related to the number of pulls with the vacuum extractor. The effect of application of the vacuum cup on neonatal injury has been considered in other sections of this chapter and is shown in Table 71.6. Sudden cup detachments are often associated with injury to the scalp of the infant.

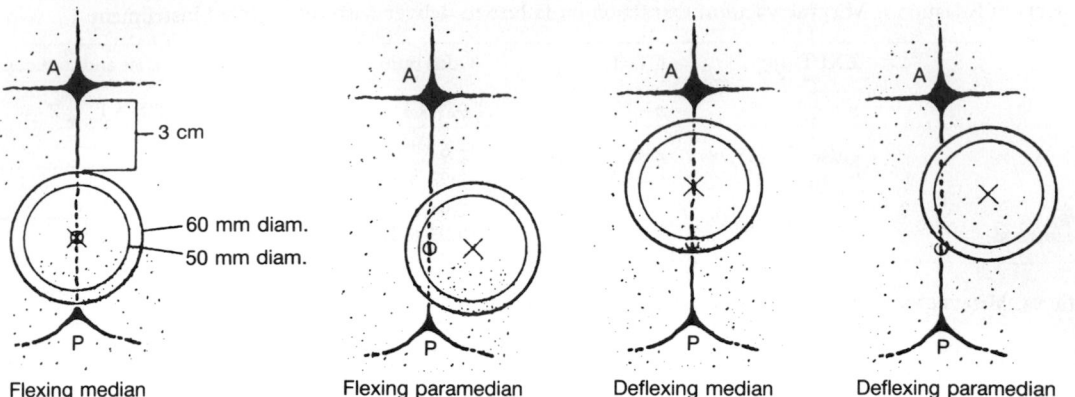

Fig. 71.3 Applications of a 50-mm vacuum cup: the 'flexing median' application should be used in order to avoid deflexion and/or asynclitism.

Table 71.6 The effect of different applications of the cup on the outcome of rotational vacuum extractions

Cup application	No. of women	Successful rotation (%)	Failure rate (%)	Neonatal injury (%)
Flexing	151	94	8	9
median	103	96	4	5
paramedian	48	90	17	17
Deflexing	93	27	32	35
median	38	24	29	21
paramedian	55	29	35	45
Total	244	68	17	19

4 Vacuum extraction or forceps?

4.1 General uses

Forceps delivery and vacuum extraction have been compared in five controlled trials (Dell *et al.* 1985; Ehlers *et al.* 1974; Fall et al. 1986; Lasbrey *et al.* 1964; Vacca *et al.* 1983) (Tables 71.7 to 71.18). One other study (Nyirjesy *et al.* 1963) contained a randomized series but the data derived from these unbiased comparisons were aggregated with those derived from a non-randomized series. The senior author has confirmed that disaggregation of the results relating to the randomized series is no longer possible (Nyirjesy, personal communication).

4.1.1 Efficiency of the method

Data on the duration of the procedure from the time the instrument was applied to the actual time of delivery was available in three of the six studies. The mean time between the decision to deliver and delivery was similar for both forceps and vacuum extraction. The range of

the decision-to-delivery interval was much greater for forceps than for vacuum extraction (Vacca *et al.* 1983). The more frequent longer time intervals with forceps were probably partly due to the time needed to institute the more complex forms of analgesia required for forceps delivery than for vacuum extraction.

4.1.2 Effects on the mother

Information about failure of the instrumental procedure was available in four of the nine studies. All four studies consistently showed a higher failure rate for vacuum extraction than for forceps; the cumulative data and typical odds showed this to be statistically significant (Table 71.7).

Only two of the studies (Lasbrey *et al.* 1964; Vacca *et al.* 1983) provided information about analgesia and anaesthesia. Table 71.8 shows that general and regional anaesthesia were more likely to be used if instrumental vaginal delivery was attempted with forceps than if it was attempted with vacuum extraction, which also explains the wider variation in the time to delivery with forceps delivery noted above. In spite of the use of these more powerful forms of pain relief, in the only study in which their views were sought, mothers were more likely to report having experienced moderate or severe pain if they had been allocated to forceps delivery (Table 71.9).

Significant maternal injuries were reported in three of the five controlled comparisons of forceps delivery and vacuum extraction and were statistically significantly more common in women allocated to forceps delivery (Table 71.10).

4.1.3 Effects on the infant

There is no evidence that choice of instrument has an effect on the proportion of infants with an Apgar score of less than 7 at 1 minute (Table 71.11). The available evidence suggests a tendency for the Apgar score of

Table 71.7 Effect of vacuum extraction vs. forceps delivery on failure to deliver with the selected instrument

Study	EXPT		CTRL		Odds ratio	Graph of odds ratios and confidence intervals						
	n	(%)	n	(%)	(95% CI)	0.01	0.1	0.5	1	2	10	100
Dell *et al.* (1985)	14/73	(19.18)	3/42	(7.14)	2.58 (0.89–7.48)							
Lasbrey *et al.* (1964)	12/121	(9.92)	3/131	(2.29)	3.88 (1.37–11.02)							
Vacca *et al.* (1983)	19/142	(13.38)	15/144	(10.42)	1.33 (0.65–2.71)							
Ehlers *et al.* (1974)	13/107	(12.15)	0/99	(0.00)	7.73 (2.52–23.72)							
Typical odds ratio (95% confidence interval)					2.55 (1.60–4.07)							

Table 71.8 Effect of vacuum extraction vs. forceps delivery on use of regional or general anesthesia

Study	EXPT		CTRL		Odds ratio	Graph of odds ratios and confidence intervals						
	n	(%)	n	(%)	(95% CI)	0.01	0.1	0.5	1	2	10	100
Lasbrey *et al.* (1964)	3/121	(2.48)	25/131	(19.08)	0.19 (0.09–0.41)							
Vacca *et al.* (1983)	70/152	(46.05)	105/152	(69.08)	0.39 (0.25–0.62)							
Typical odds ratio (95% confidence interval)					0.33 (0.22–0.48)							

Table 71.9 Effect of vacuum extraction vs. forceps delivery on moderate to severe pain at delivery

Study	EXPT		CTRL		Odds ratio	Graph of odds ratios and confidence intervals						
	n	(%)	n	(%)	(95% CI)	0.01	0.1	0.5	1	2	10	100
Garcia *et al.* (1985)	7/33	(21.21)	12/32	(37.50)	0.46 (0.16–1.33)							
Typical odds ratio (95% confidence interval)					0.46 (0.16–1.33)							

Table 71.10 Effect of vacuum extraction vs. forceps delivery on significant maternal injury

Study	EXPT		CTRL		Odds ratio	Graph of odds ratios and confidence intervals						
	n	(%)	n	(%)	(95% CI)	0.01	0.1	0.5	1	2	10	100
Dell *et al.* (1985)	21/73	(28.77)	22/45	(48.89)	0.42 (0.20–0.91)							
Lasbrey *et al.* (1964)	2/121	(1.65)	10/131	(7.63)	0.27 (0.08–0.86)							
Vacca *et al.* (1983)	17/152	(11.18)	39/152	(25.66)	0.38 (0.21–0.68)							
Typical odds ratio (95% confidence interval)					0.38 (0.24–0.58)							

Table 71.11 Effect of vacuum extraction vs. forceps delivery on Apgar score <7 at 1 min

Study	EXPT		CTRL		Odds ratio	Graph of odds ratios and confidence intervals						
	n	(%)	*n*	(%)	(95% CI)	0.01	0.1	0.5	1	2	10	100
Dell *et al.* (1985)	6/73	(8.22)	2/45	(4.44)	1.81 (0.42–7.87)							
Vacca *et al.* (1983)	42/152	(27.63)	46/152	(30.26)	0.88 (0.54–1.44)							
Typical odds ratio (95% confidence interval)					0.95 (0.59–1.51)							

Table 71.12 Effect of vacuum extraction vs. forceps delivery on Apgar score <7 at 5 min

Study	EXPT		CTRL		Odds ratio	Graph of odds ratios and confidence intervals						
	n	(%)	*n*	(%)	(95% CI)	0.01	0.1	0.5	1	2	10	100
Dell *et al.* (1985)	0/73	(0.00)	0/45	(0.00)	1.00 (1.00–1.00)							
Lasbrey *et al.* (1964)	19/121	(15.70)	11/131	(8.40)	2.00 (0.93–4.29)							
Vacca *et al.* (1983)	10/152	(6.58)	7/152	(4.61)	1.45 (0.55–3.86)							
Typical odds ratio (95% confidence interval)					1.77 (0.97–3.23)							

Table 71.13 Effect of vacuum extraction vs. forceps delivery on cephalhaematoma

Study	EXPT		CTRL		Odds ratio	Graph of odds ratios and confidence intervals						
	n	(%)	*n*	(%)	(95% CI)	0.01	0.1	0.5	1	2	10	100
Dell DL *et al.* (1985)	11/73	(15.07)	1/45	(2.22)	4.03 (1.19–13.71)							
Fall *et al.* (1986)	7/20	(35.00)	2/16	(12.50)	3.21 (0.72–14.35)							
Vacca *et al.* (1983)	14/152	(9.21)	8/152	(5.26)	1.80 (0.76–4.27)							
Typical odds ratio (95% confidence interval)					2.49 (1.31–4.72)							

Table 71.14 Effect of vacuum extraction vs. forceps delivery on scalp injuries other than cephalhaematoma

Study	EXPT		CTRL		Odds ratio	Graph of odds ratios and confidence intervals						
	n	(%)	*n*	(%)	(95% CI)	0.01	0.1	0.5	1	2	10	100
Dell *et al.* (1985)	22/73	(30.14)	23/45	(51.11)	0.41 (0.19–0.89)							
Vacca *et al.* (1983)	7/152	(4.61)	14/152	(9.21)	0.49 (0.20–1.19)							
Typical odds ratio (95% confidence interval)					0.44 (0.25–0.79)							

Table 71.15 Effect of vacuum extraction vs. forceps delivery on use of phototherapy

Study	EXPT		CTRL		Odds ratio	Graph of odds ratios and confidence intervals						
	n	(%)	*n*	(%)	(95% CI)	0.01	0.1	0.5	1	2	10	100
Dell *et al.* (1985)	2/73	(2.74)	0/45	(0.00)	5.11 (0.29–89.66)							
Vacca *et al.* (1983)	10/152	(6.58)	8/152	(5.26)	1.27 (0.49–3.28)							
Typical odds ratio (95% confidence interval)					1.45 (0.59–3.58)							

Table 71.16 Effect of vacuum extraction vs. forceps delivery on retinal haemorrhage

Study	EXPT		CTRL		Odds ratio	Graph of odds ratios and confidence intervals						
	n	(%)	*n*	(%)	(95% CI)	0.01	0.1	0.5	1	2	10	100
Fall *et al.* (1986)	4/20	(20.00)	3/16	(18.75)	1.08 (0.21–5.56)							
Ehlers *et al.* (1974)	69/107	(64.49)	47/112	(41.96)	2.46 (1.45–4.18)							
Typical odds ratio (95% confidence interval)					2.28 (1.37–3.77)							

infants allocated to vacuum extraction to be lower 5 minutes after delivery than those allocated to forceps delivery (Table 71.12).

Vacuum extraction is more likely to cause cephalhaematoma than forceps (Table 71.13), but forceps are more likely to cause other kinds of scalp injuries (Table 71.14). In the trial by Vacca and his colleagues (1983), neonatal jaundice was found to be statistically significantly more common in babies for whom vacuum extraction was chosen as the method of delivery. This was usually mild, but there is not enough evidence available to assess whether vacuum extraction is more likely than forceps delivery to be followed by jaundice of a degree to give rise to medical (Table 71.15) or maternal concern (Garcia *et al.* 1985).

It is unclear whether vacuum extraction predisposes to retinal haemorrhage compared with forceps delivery (Table 71.16). The methodologically sounder of the two trials for which data on retinal haemorrhages are available (Fall *et al.* 1986) showed similar rates in babies delivered by vacuum and in babies delivered with forceps, but the number of affected babies was very small and so the confidence limits surrounding this 'no difference' estimate are very wide. The other published report of a comparison of the two instruments (Ehlers *et al.* 1974) found more babies with retinal haemorrhages in the vacuum extraction group. However, the method of allocation and the analysis may well have led to important selection bias, and there was no evidence that any attempt had been made to blind the

observers to the group assignment of the babies they were examining. In a recently published observational study (Van Zundert *et al.* 1986), the rate of retinal haemorrhage in babies born to women who had epidural anaesthesia was similar to those whose mothers had either narcotic analgesia or no analgesia, even though twice as many mothers in the epidural group had been delivered by vacuum extraction.

Predictably, there is not enough information available to judge the relative effects of the two instruments on the risk of perinatal death (Table 71.17), or the long term condition of the infants (Table 71.18). In the only follow-up study of cohorts randomized to the two instruments, the incidence of problems was similar in the vacuum and forceps groups, but the numbers of infants studied was too small to exclude anything other than very dramatic differential effects of the two instruments (Carmody *et al.* 1986).

McBride *et al.* (1979) examined the effect of various methods of operative delivery on developmental outcome at 5 years of age and could find no deleterious effect attributable to the method of delivery. Varner (1983) reviewed the literature on neuropsychiatric sequelae of midforceps deliveries and pointed out that because of the retrospective nature of the studies few valid conclusions could be drawn from the results. Bjerre and Dahlin (1974) and Blennow *et al.* (1977) studied the long term development of infants born by vacuum extraction and found no differences between them and infants born spontaneously. Carmody *et al.*

Table 71.17 Effect of vacuum extraction vs. forceps delivery on perinatal death

Study	EXPT		CTRL		Odds ratio	Graph of odds ratios and confidence intervals
	n	(%)	n	(%)	(95% CI)	0.01 0.1 0.5 1 2 10 100
Dell *et al.* (1985)	0/73	(0.00)	0/45	(0.00)	1.00 (1.00–1.00)	
Fall *et al.* (1986)	0/20	(0.00)	0/16	(0.00)	1.00 (1.00–1.00)	
Lasbrey *et al.* (1964)	1/121	(0.83)	3/121	(2.48)	0.36 (0.05–2.61)	
Vacca *et al.* (1983)	1/152	(0.66)	0/152	(0.00)	7.39 (0.15–99.99)	
Ehlers *et al.* (1974)	0/107	(0.00)	0/112	(0.00)	1.00 (1.00–1.00)	
Typical odds ratio (95% confidence interval)					0.67 (0.11–3.89)	

Table 71.18 Effect of vacuum extraction vs. forceps delivery on readmission by hospital

Study	EXPT		CTRL		Odds ratio	Graph of odds ratios and confidence intervals
	n	(%)	n	(%)	(95% CI)	0.01 0.1 0.5 1 2 10 100
Carmody *et al.* (1986)	14/152	(9.21)	11/152	(7.24)	1.30 (0.57–2.94)	
Typical odds ratio (95% confidence interval)					1.30 (0.57–2.94)	

Effect of vacuum extraction vs. forceps delivery on confirmed or suspected hearing abnormalities

Carmody *et al.* (1986)	8/152	(5.26)	5/152	(3.29)	1.62 (0.53–4.90)	
Typical odds ratio (95% confidence interval)					1.62 (0.53–4.90)	

Effect of vacuum extraction vs. forceps delivery on suspected strabismus/vision abnormality

Carmody *et al.* (1986)	8/152	(5.26)	6/152	(3.95)	1.35 (0.46–3.93)	
Typical odds ratio (95% confidence interval)					1.35 (0.46–3.93)	

(1986) reassessed at 9 months of age babies who were born during the Portsmouth randomized trial comparing forceps and vacuum extraction (Vacca *et al.* 1983) and found no significant differences in the babies.

4.1.4 Views of the staff

The opinions of staff about forceps and vacuum extraction were sought in one randomized trial (Vacca *et al.* 1983). When the main trial was completed, but before results were available, the attitudes of operators, paediatric and midwifery staff of the hospital were surveyed by questionnaire (Garcia *et al.* 1985). Replies made it clear that many of the staff had very little prior knowledge of the vacuum extractor, but that the experience of the trial and working with an advocate of the method had influenced their views. Most said that their attitudes about the methods of instrumental delivery had changed since the trial started and that they had a new familiarity with the vacuum extractor and a willingness to consider its use in a wider range of circumstances. In general the staff were confident that maternal trauma and pain were reduced with vacuum extraction compared with forceps delivery. Obstetricians and paediatricians were divided in their predictions about which instrument caused less infant injury but were cautious about infant well-being following delivery. Forceps delivery was thought to be quicker by the majority of obstetricians and paediatricians and half of the midwives.

While reduction in maternal trauma was seen as the most significant advantage of the vacuum extractor, the perceived disadvantages of the instrument were the general lack of experience in its use, its greater complexity and poor maintenance of the equipment. Staff also referred to problems of the newborn that they felt were associated with the use of the vacuum extractor such as chignon, markings, and an increase in jaundice (Garcia *et al.* 1985).

4.2 Specific uses

In addition to the general indications for which the choice between vacuum extraction and forceps delivery is largely dictated by the preferences of the accoucheur and the mother, each of these instruments has a number of specific indications. These are not so much specific indications for the use of one instrument, as contraindications to the use of the other instrument.

Specific uses for forceps thus relate to fetal presentations for which vacuum extraction would clearly be inappropriate (face presentation) or not feasible (aftercoming head in breech delivery).

Specific uses for vacuum extraction, on the other hand, do not relate to fetal presentation but rather to the likelihood of severe maternal injury if forceps were to be used. Thus, vacuum extraction can, if necessary, be more readily applied than forceps when the cervix is not fully dilated, although delivery by caesarean section will usually be more appropriate in these circumstances. In general, the use of vacuum extraction before full dilatation should be undertaken with great caution (Bird 1982), and only when prompt delivery is mandatory and when it is likely that the cervix will readily recede. Similarly, to avoid maternal injury, vacuum extraction is the procedure of choice if instrumental delivery is required after symphysiotomy.

A particularly valuable specific indication for vacuum extraction relates to delivery of the second infant in twin pregnancy. Since full dilatation has already been achieved and resistance in the birth canal is minimal after delivery of the first infant, vacuum extraction can be valuable for expediting delivery of a non-engaged or poorly engaged second infant in the event of fetal distress. All of these specific indications, however, require familiarity and expertise with the instrument used.

5 Conclusions

5.1 Implications for current practice

Apart from the specific uses that apply to either forceps or vacuum extraction these instruments are to a large extent interchangeable. The available evidence indicates, however, that the use of forceps is more likely to result in severe maternal injury and is more dependent on the use of adequate analgesia or anaesthesia than is vacuum extraction in order to avoid serious maternal discomfort.

With adequate experience and proper placement of the vacuum cup most deliveries that require instrumental rotation of the head can be accomplished by vacuum extraction. This experience should not be difficult to obtain and should form part of all residency training programmes in obstetrics.

The widely held belief that vacuum extraction is too slow to be useful when rapid delivery is required for fetal distress can now firmly be laid to rest. With proper technique the interval between deciding on the need for instrumental delivery and delivery itself is no longer with vacuum extraction than with forceps.

Although there is no adequate evidence on which to judge the difference between these instruments on long term outcomes of neonatal morbidity, there is a distinct difference in short term outcomes. Cephalhaematoma and subgaleal haematoma occur more frequently with vacuum extraction, but other types of injuries of the head and face are more frequently observed after forceps delivery.

On balance, it would appear that for instrumental rotational deliveries vacuum extraction should be preferred over forceps. The same may hold, albeit to a lesser extent, for most other operative vaginal deliveries as well. Reserving one instrument for routine applications and the other for especially difficult situations would be ill-advised, however. Difficult extractions, whether by forceps or by vacuum extraction, should not be undertaken unless the operator has considerable expertise with the instrument chosen. Delivery by caesarean section should be considered as an alternative.

5.2 Implications for future research

The few randomized comparisons of vacuum versus forceps delivery that have been conducted thus far have tended to concentrate on short term measures of delivery outcome, maternal discomfort, and neonatal morbidity. Suggestions of an increase in retinal haemorrhages in the neonate after vacuum extraction in particular have given rise to concern. There is an urgent need to determine whether these are observed more frequently after vacuum extraction than after forceps delivery, when observers are blinded to the mode of delivery of the babies that they are examining, and what influence, if any, they have on long term infant outcomes. The important question is whether the two methods of delivery show differences in terms of sensory and intellectual functions of the infant.

References

Aguero O, Alvarez H (1962). Fetal injuries due to the vacuum extractor. Obstet Gynecol, 19: 212–217.

Bailey PW, Howard FA (1983). Epidural analgesia and forceps delivery: laying a bogey. Anaesthesia, 38: 282–285.

Bergsjø P, Schmidt E, Pusch D (1983). Differences in the reported frequencies of some obstetrical interventions in Europe. Br J Obstet Gynaecol, 90: 628–632.

Berkus MD, Ramamurthy RS, O'Connor PS, Brown K, Hayashi RH (1985). Cohort study of Silastic obstetric vacuum cup deliveries: 1, Safety of the instrument. Obstet Gynecol, 66: 503–509.

Berkus MD, Ramamurthy RS, O'Connor PS, Brown K, Hayashi RH (1986). Cohort study of Silastic obstetric vacuum cup deliveries: II. Unsuccessful vacuum extraction. Obstet Gynecol, 68: 662–666.

Bird GC (1969). Modification of Malmström's Vacuum Extractor. Br Med J, 3: 526.

Bird GC (1976). The importance of flexion in vacuum extractor delivery. Br J Obstet Gynaecol, 83: 194–200.

Bird GC (1982). The 'New Generation' Vacuum Extractor. In: Vacuum Extractor Manual. Gothenburg: A B Vacuum Extractor.

Bird GC, Bal JS (1967). Subcutaneous symphysiotomy in association with the vacuum extractor. J Obstet Gynaecol Br Commwlth, 74: 266–269.

Bjerre I, Dahlin K (1974). The long term development of children delivered by vacuum extraction. Dev Med Child Neurol, 16: 378–381.

Blennow G, Svenningsen MW, Gustafson B, Sunden B, Cronquist S (1977). Neonatal and prospective follow up study of infants delivered by vacuum extraction (VE). Acta Obstet Gynecol Scand, 56: 189–194.

Bowes WA, Bowes C (1980). Current role of the midforceps operation. Clin Obstet Gynecol, 23: 549–557.

Carmody F, Grant A, Somchiwong M (1986). A randomized comparison of the 'New Generation' cup with the original Bird cup. J Perinat Med, 14: 95–100.

Carmody F, Grant A, Mutch M, Vacca A, Chalmers I (1986). Follow-up of babies delivered in a randomized comparison of vacuum extraction and forceps delivery. Acta Obstet Gynecol Scand, 65: 763–766.

Chalmers I, Richards M (1977). Intervention and causal inference in obstetric practice. In: Benefits and Hazards of the New Obstetrics. Chard T, Richards M (eds). London: Heinemann, p 34.

Chalmers JA (1971). The Ventouse. London: Lloyd-Luke.

Chalmers JA (1975). The use of the vacuum extractor to accelerate the first and second stages of labour. Clinics Obstet Gynaecol, 2: 203–220.

Chamberlain G (1980). Forceps and vacuum extraction. Clin Obstet Gynaecol, 7: 511–527.

Chukudebelu WO (1978). Vacuum extraction before full cervical dilation. Int Surg, 63: 89–90.

Crichton D (1974). A reliable method of establishing the level of the fetal head in obstetrics. S Afr Med J, 48: 784–787.

Dell DL, Sightler SE, Plauche WC (1985). Soft cup vacuum extractor: a comparison of outlet delivery. Obstet Gynecol, 66: 624–628.

Dennen EH (1964). Forceps Deliveries (2nd edn). Philadelphia: F A Davis.

Doughty A (1969). Selective epidural analgesia and the forceps rate. Br J Anaesth, 41: 1058–1062.

Duchon MA, DeMund MA, Brown RH (1988). Laboratory comparison of modern vacuum extractors. Obstet Gynecol, 71: 155–158

Ehlers N, Jensen IK, Hansen KB (1974). Retinal haemorrhages in the newborn—a comparison of delivery by forceps and by vacuum extractor. Acta Ophthalmol, 52: 73–82.

Fall O, Ryden G, Finnstrom K, Finnstrom O, Leijon I (1986). Forceps or vacuum extraction? A comparison of effects on the newborn infant. Acta Obstet Gynecol Scand, 65: 75–80.

Garcia J, Anderson J, Vacca A, Elbourne D, Grant A, Chalmers I (1985). Views of women and their medical and midwifery attendants about instrumental delivery using vacuum extraction and forceps. J Psychosom Obstet Gynaecol, 4: 1–9.

Gebbie D (1982). Symphysiotomy. Clin Obstet Gynaecol, 9: 663–683.

Hastie SJ, MacLean AB (1986). Comparison of the use of the Silastic Obstetric Vacuum Extractor to Kielland's Forceps. Asia-Oceania J Obstet Gynaecol, 12: 63–68.

Hebertson RM, Sanders MS, Warenski JC, Heywood ER, Larkin RM, Bryson MJ (1985). Obstetric forceps pad designed to reduce infant trauma. Obstet Gynecol, 65: 275–278.

Hoult IJ, MacLennan AH, Carrie LES (1977). Lumbar epidural analgesia in labour: relation to fetal malposition and instrumental delivery. Br Med J, 1: 14–16.

Iffy L, Lancet M, Kessler I (1984). The vacuum extractor. In: Operative Perinatology, (1st edn). Iffy L, Charles D (eds). New York: Macmillan, Chapter 14, p 582.

Issel EP (1977). Zur mechanischen einwirkung der geburtshilflichen Zange auf den fetalen Schädel. Zbl Gynäkol, 9: 487–497.

Jouppila R, Jouppila P, Karinen JM, Hollmen A (1979). Segmental epidural and analgesia in labour: related to the progress of labour, fetal malposition and instrumental delivery. Acta Obstet Gynecol Scand, 58: 135–139.

Kelly JV, Sines G (1966). An assessment of the compression and traction forces. Am J Obstet Gynecol, 96: 521–537.

Lasbrey AH, Orchard CD, Crichton D (1964). A study of the relative merits and scope for vacuum extraction as opposed to forceps delivery. S Afr J Obstet Gynaecol, 2: 1–3.

Laufe LE (1956). New obstetric forceps. Obstet Gynecol, 7: 91–96.

Laufe LE (1968). A new divergent outlet forceps. Am J Obstet Gynecol, 101: 509–512.

Laufe LE (1971). Divergent and crossed obstetrics forceps. Comparative study of compression and traction forces. Obstet Gynecol, 38: 885–887.

Laufe LE (1985). Obstetric Forceps in Gynaecology and Obstetrics, Vol 2. Sciarra (ed). Philadelphia: Harper & Row, 99: 1 20.

Lindgren L (1960). The causes of foetal head moulding in labour. Acta Obstet Gynecol Scand, 39: 46–62.

Malmström T (1954). Vacuum extraction—an obstetrical instrument. Acta Obstet Gynecol Scand, 3: Suppl 4.

Maltau JM, Egge K, Moe N (1984). Retinal hemorrhages in the preterm neonate. Acta Obstet Gynecol Scand, 63: 219–221.

McBride WG, Black BP, Brown CJ, Dolby RM, Murray AD,

Thomas DB (1979). Method of delivery and developmental outcome at 5 years of age. Med J Austral, 1: 301–304.

Milner RD (1975). Neonatal mortality of breech deliveries with and without forceps to the aftercoming head. J Obstet Gynaecol Br Commwlth, 82: 783–785.

Moolgaoker A (1962). A new design of obstetric forceps. J Obstet Gynaecol Br Commwlth, 69: 450-457.

Moolgaoker A (1970). A safe alternative to caesarean section? J Obstet Gynaecol Br Commwlth, 77: 1077–1087.

Moolgaoker AS, Ahamed SOS, Payne PR (1979). A comparison of different methods of instrumental delivery based on electronic measurements of compression and traction. Obstet Gynecol, 54: 299–309.

Myerscough PR (1982). The obstetric forceps and the ventouse. In: Munro Kerr's Operative Obstetrics (10th edn). London: Baillière Tindall, pp 276–294.

Nyirjesy I, Hawks DL, Falls HC, Munsat TL, Pierce WE. (1963). A comparative clinical study of the vacuum extractor and forceps. Am J Obstet Gynecol, 65: 1071–1082.

O'Driscoll K, Meagher D (1980). Progress of labour: second stage. In: Active Management of Labour. Eastbourne: W B Saunders, p 35.

O'Driscoll K, Jackson RJA, Gallagher JT (1970). Active management of labour and cephalopelvic disproportion. J Obstet Gynaecol Br Commwlth, 77: 385–389.

O'Neil AGB, Skull E, Michael C (1981). A new method of traction for the vacuum cup. Austral NZ J Obstet Gynaecol, 21: 24–25.

Ottolini JL (1980). Instructions for the Silastic Obstetrical Vacuum Cup. Midland, Michigan: Dow Corning Corporation.

Parry-Jones E (1952). Kielland's Forceps. London: Butterworth.

Parry-Jones E (1972). Barton's Forceps. London: Sector Publishing.

Pearse WH (1965). Forceps versus spontaneous delivery. Clin Obstet Gynecol, 8: 813–821.

Philpott RH (1982). The recognition of cephalopelvic disproportion. Clin Obstet Gynaecol, 9: 609–624.

Pridmore BR, Hey EN, Aherne WA (1974). Spinal cord injury of the fetus during delivery with Kielland's forceps. J Obstet Gynaecol Br Commwlth, 81: 168–172.

Pritchard JA, MacDonald PC, Gant NF (eds) (1985). Forceps delivery and related techniques. In: Williams Obstetrics (17th edn). Norwalk: Appleton-Century-Crofts, pp 837–850.

Ryden G (1986). Vacuum extraction or forceps. Br Med J, 292: 75–6.

Saling E, Hartung M (1973). Analyses of tractive forces during the application of vacuum extracion. J Perinat Med, 1: 245–251.

Seidenschnur G, Koepcke E (1979). Fetal risk in delivery with Shute parallel forceps: analysis of 1,503 forceps deliveries. Am J Obstet Gynecol, 135: 312–317.

Shute W B (1958). An obstetrical forceps using a new principle of parallelism. Proceedings of the Second International Congress of Obstet and Gynecol, 11: 645.

Simpson JY (1848). Cited in: Chalmers JA (1971). The Ventouse. London: Lloyd-Luke, pp 2–3.

Stewart KS (1982). In: Munro Kerr's Operative Obstetrics (10th edn). Myerscough PR (ed). London: Baillière Tindall, p 32.

Svenningsen L (1987). Birth progression and traction forces developed under vacuum extraction after slow or rapid application of suction. Eur J Obstet Gynecol Reprod Biol, 26: 105–12.

Thiery M (1985). Obstetric vacuum extraction. In: Obstet Gynecol Annual. Wynn RM (ed). Norwalk: Appleton-Century-Crofts, pp 73–111.

Thiery M, Van Den Broeke R, Kermans G, Parewijck W, Dhont M, Vanlancker M, Van Kets H, Defoort P, Derom R, Vanhaesebrouck P (1987). A randomized study of two cups for vacuum extraction. J Perinat Med, 15: 129–136.

Vacca A, Grant A, Wyatt G, Chalmers I (1983). Portsmouth Operative Delivery trial: a comparison of vacuum extraction and forceps delivery. Br J Obstet Gynaecol, 90: 1107–1112.

Van Zundert A, Jansen J, Vaes L, Soetens M, de Vel M, Van der Aa P (1986). Extradural anaesthesia and retinal haemorrhage in the newborn. Br J Anaesth, 58: 1017–1021.

Varner MW (1983). Neuropsychiatric sequelae of midforceps deliveries. Clin Perinatol, 10: 455–460.

Wider JA, Erez S, Steer CM (1967). An evaluation of the vacuum extractor in a series of 201 cases. Am J Obstet Gynecol, 98: 24–31.

Wiqvist N (1984). The Silc Cup—An Obstetrical Instrument. Gothenburg: Menox AB.

Wylie B (1935). Traction in forceps deliveries. Am J Obstet Gynecol, 2: 425–435.

Yonge J (1706). Cited in: Chalmers JA (1971). The Ventouse. London: Lloyd-Luke, 1.

72 Technique of caesarean section

Jim Pearson and Gareth Rees

1 Introduction

The term caesarean section, contrary to popular belief, is derived neither from the fabulous story of the birth of Julius Caesar in 100 BC, nor from the Roman Law which prescribed the operation when a mother died near term with a fetus still alive. In fact it arose during the middle ages from the Latin verb *caedere*—to cut. As 'section' also means 'to cut' the term caesarean section is a pleonasm.

The first serious work on the subject was by Rousset in 1581, but from the sixteenth century to the middle of the nineteenth century the mortality rate was so high as to almost prohibit the operation; Lepage (1878) stated that not a single woman operated upon in Paris between 1799 and 1877 recovered. Measures such as symphysiotomy, craniotomy, and other forms of embriotomy were employed in its place (see Chapters 70, 71).

In early times the midline uterine 'classical' incision was used. The uterine incision was usually left unsutured because it was widely believed that the suture material thus buried encouraged suppuration, and that the alternating contractions and relaxations of the uterus forbade the employment of a suture.

An alternative approach was introduced by Porro (1876) who, after extracting the fetus, amputated the body of the uterus, removed the ovaries and fixed the cervical stump to the lower end of the abdominal wound where the bleeding was controlled by means of a noose. This radical procedure reduced the maternal mortality by about half.

The first satisfactory method of suturing the classical incision was popularized by Sänger in 1882 and consisted of deep and superficial rows of sutures. With the addition of antiseptic techniques, this was the method of operating still strongly supported by T Watts Eden in 1915, in whose hands the maternal mortality rate had fallen to 3 per cent and the fetal mortality rate to 6 per cent, a rate lower than that for symphysiotomy.

Sänger's operation gave good results in 'clean' cases, but was disappointing in infected cases. Various extraperitoneal approaches to the uterine cavity were therefore devised in the hope of avoiding general peritonitis. Two approaches were employed, lateral and median. The lateral approach consisted of a left lateral incision down to the peritoneum, which with the bladder, was dissected off the lower segment. The vagina was incised transversely and the child removed via the cervix (Thomas 1870). The median approach was via a midline incision. The peritoneum and bladder were separated, and the child removed through the part of the lower segment beneath the loose peritoneum of the uterovesical pouch. These procedures were difficult, and accidental ingress to the bladder or the peritoneal cavity largely nullified their benefits.

Although previously described by Kehrer (1882,

cited in Trolle 1982), the name which is most closely associated with the struggle for acceptance of the now universally performed lower segment caesarean section is that of Munro Kerr. He first used the transverse lower segment incision in 1911, but it was slow to be accepted because it was perceived to have greater technical difficulties than the classical operation. Support for its use gradually grew in the 1930s and 1940s despite much opposition. Munro Kerr contended that the scar was stronger and thus less liable to rupture, and that it should result in a lower maternal mortality if widely adopted. His vindication came at the 12th British Congress of Obstetrics and Gynaecology in 1949, where several papers were read demonstrating that the adoption of this approach was a major contributing factor to the rapidly falling maternal death rate. Munro Kerr, already some years retired, was invited to the platform. After making generous reference to the speakers, he pointed out the lower segment operation had, perhaps for the first time, been referred to in nothing but words of praise. Breaking from his theme, he threw his arms above his head and exclaimed in exultation, 'Alleluia! The strife is o'er, the battle done.' (Kerr 1949).

Despite Munro Kerr's understandable gratification with the results of the technique that Kehrer had introduced and championed, caesarean section is still not always as safe an operation as it is often thought to be. Potentially avoidable deaths still occur. The main causes of death associated with caesarean section are haemorrhage, sepsis, pulmonary embolism, and, of increasing importance, anaesthesia. Because the majority of anaesthetic deaths are potentially avoidable, this aspect of care for caesarean section will be considered first in this chapter.

2 Anaesthesia for caesarean section

The anaesthesia necessary for caesarean section poses the greatest risks of the procedure for both mother and child. The aim of good obstetric anaesthesia is to maximize the safety and comfort of the mother and to minimize depression of the baby.

Next to associated maternal disease, anaesthesia is the largest single cause of maternal death associated with caesarean section, accounting for over a fifth of the mortality (Department of Health and Social Security 1986) (Table 72.1). Similar findings were reported by the Confidential Enquiries into Maternal Deaths in Scotland (Scottish Home and Health Department 1978). Pulmonary aspiration of gastric contents and difficult intubation were the major factors involved (Table 72.2). The conclusion drawn in these reports was that the deaths were due to substandard care, and

Table 72.1 Causes of maternal mortality associated with caesarean section, England and Wales 1979–81

Cause	Number	Per cent
Anaesthesia	19	21.9
Hypertensive disease	13	14.9
Pulmonary embolus	7	8.0
Haemorrhage	7	8.0
Sepsis	4	4.6
Other direct causes	9	10.4
Associated diseases	28	32.2
Total	87	100.0

From: Report on confidential enquiries into maternal deaths in England and Wales, 1979–81.

Table 72.2 Causes of maternal mortality associated with anaesthesia for caesarian section, England and Wales 1967–81

Year	Pulmonary aspiration	Difficult intubation	Total deaths
1978–81	8	8	22
1976–78	11	16	30
1973–75	13	7	31
1970–72	16	5	37
1967–69	26	10	50
1967–81	74	46	170

recommendations were made for the procurement of better obstetric anaesthetic services, including more trained anaesthetists, provision of skilled anaesthetic assistance, better monitoring equipment and improved administrative practices (see Chapter 52). Nationally collected data on neonatal outcome are not available. The effects of anaesthesia on newborn morbidity and neurobehavioural patterns has been extensively studied (Palahniuk et al. 1977; Hollmen et al. 1978).

The obstetric anaesthetist is concerned to reduce to the minimum the likelihood that the infant delivered by caesarean section will be depressed, either by drugs given to the mother before delivery, or by biochemical changes caused by the anaesthetic technique. A major cause of biochemical depression is the effects upon maternal cardiovascular dynamics imposed by the pregnant uterus when the patient is supine (Crawford *et al.* 1972). Three controlled trials (Crawford *et al.* 1972; Clemetson *et al.* 1973; Downing *et al.* 1974) have examined the effect of lateral tilt of the patient to relieve the pressure of the uterus on the vena cava. All showed trends in the direction of improvements in most or all parameters of the biochemical status of the umbilical cord blood with the use of lateral tilt. Statistically significant improvements were noted in umbilical artery and vein pH, pCO_2, and oxygen saturation (Tables 72.3 and 72.4). These improved biochemical indices were reflected in a trend towards higher Apgar scores in the babies delivered in the lateral tilt groups.

Anatomically the inferior vena cava lies anterior and to the right of the spinal column, so that tilting the mother towards her left side should prove more effective than a rightward tilt. This hypothesis was tested and confirmed by Brock-Utne *et al.* (1978), who randomly allocated 75 women to left or right tilt. A significant decrease (> 20 mm Hg) in blood pressure occurred in 4/38 (10.5 per cent) of women with a left tilt compared to 11/37 (29.7 per cent) of women with a right tilt. Apgar scores of the infants in the two groups were similar, but the average time to spontaneous

respiration was lower with the left tilt (17.6 ± 3.8 seconds vs. 27.5 ± 4.8 seconds). The umbilical cord blood gases showed a statistically significantly less fetal respiratory acidaemia in the left tilt group (Table 72.5).

These findings, although perhaps of little consequence to the healthy mother and her uncompromised fetus, could be of vital importance when fetal compromise is either present or imminent.

2.1 Types of anaesthesia

Four methods of anaesthesia are in current use for caesarean section: general anaesthesia, epidural anaesthesia, spinal anaesthesia, and less commonly, local infiltration. Selection of the method to be used depends on whether the operation is an emergency or elective, the experience of the anaesthetist, whether maternal disease is present, and the preference of the mother. After consideration of safety, the preference of the mother should be of paramount importance (De Vore 1979).

The selection of the safest method is sometimes clear cut. For example, the method of choice in the mother who is bleeding profusely is general anaesthesia: epidural or spinal anaesthesia would be inappropriate and dangerous because of the autonomic blockade associated with their use. On the other hand, there is still

Table 72.3 Effect of lateral tilt vs. supine position for caesarean section on umbilical artery blood gases

	Tilt			No tilt			Difference between means	Statistical significance
	No.	Mean	± SD	No.	Mean	± SD		
pH								
Crawford *et al.* (1972)	63	7.31	0.04	87	7.27	0.09	0.39	$p < 0.001$
Clemetson *et al.* (1973)								
Spinal	10	7.31	0.05	10	7.27	0.09	0.04	NS
General	12	7.30	0.06	11	7.28	0.08	0.02	NS
Downing *et al.* (1974)	50	7.26	0.04	50	7.24	0.04	0.02	$p < 0.05$
pCO_2								
Crawford *et al.* (1972)	63	54.65	7.23	87	60.37	12.24	5.72	$p < 0.001$
Clemetson *et al.* (1973)								
Spinal	10	48.7	8.11	10	50.9	9.68	2.2	NS
General	12	55.5	9.82	11	51.3	10.84	4.2	NS
Downing *et al.* (1974)	50	51.7	7.78	50	51.3	7.78	0.4	NS
Base excess								
Crawford *et al.* (1972)	63	−4.3	2.4	87	−4.8	3.5	0.56	NS
Clemetson *et al.* (1973)								
Spinal	10	−2.0	1.9	10	−4.2	3.8	2.2	NS
General	12	−0.5	5.2	11	−2.7	4.5	2.2	NS
Downing *et al.* (1974)	50	5.9	2.8	50	6.6	3.5	0.7	NS
Oxygen saturation								
Clemetson *et al.* (1973)								
Spinal	10	26.7	14.8	10	16.7	7.3	10	NS
General	12	26.8	12.9	11	23.7	18.3	3.1	NS
Downing *et al.* (1974)	50	34.9	15.5	50	28.5	15.5	6.4	$p < 0.05$

Table 72.4 Effect of lateral tilt vs. supine position for caesarean section on umbilical vein blood gases

	Tilt			No tilt			Difference between means	Statistical significance
	No.	Mean	± SD	No.	Mean	± SD		
pH								
Crawford *et al.* (1972)	63	7.31	0.04	87	7.34	0.09	0.029	$p<0.02$
Clemetson *et al.* (1973)								
Spinal	10	7.37	0.56	10	7.33	0.11	0.04	NS
General	12	7.33	0.13	11	7.30	0.07	0.03	NS
Downing *et al.* (1974)	50	7.31	0.04	50	7.30	0.04	0.14	NS
pCO_2								
Crawford *et al.* (1972)	63	41.2	6.5	87	46.7	10.3	5.57	$p<0.001$
Clemetson *et al.* (1973)								
Spinal	10	37.8	7.3	10	42.0	10.1	4.2	NS
General	12	48.9	10.7	11	46.4	11.0	−2.5	NS
Downing *et al.* (1974)	50	42.5	5.7	50	44.3	5.7	1.8	NS
Base excess								
Crawford *et al.* (1972)	63	−3.47	2.34	87	−3.66	3.53	0.19	NS
Clemetson *et al.* (1973)								
Spinal	10	−4.2	3.0	10	−4.3	5.5	0.10	NS
General	12	−0.7	5.1	11	−3.8	3.1	3.1	NS
Downing *et al.* (1974)	50	−5.9	2.8	50	−6.6	3.5	0.7	NS
Oxygen saturation								
Clemetson *et al.* (1973)								
Spinal	10	65.2	13.4	10	45.2	10.9	20.0	$p<0.002$
General	12	55.3	18.6	11	50.0	17.9	5.3	NS
Downing *et al.* (1974)	50	71.7	12.7	50	63.3	14.1	8.4	$p<0.005$

Table 72.5 Effect of left lateral tilt vs. right lateral tilt for caesarean section on umbilical blood gases (after Brock-Utne *et al.* 1978)

	Left tilt		Right tilt		Difference between means	Statistical significant
	$n = 37$		$n = 38$			
	Mean	± SD	Mean	± SD		
Umbilical artery						
pH [H^+ mmol/l]	52.3	(1.4)	55.2	(1.1)		NS
pCO_2	48.6	(1.0)	51.2	(0.8)	2.6	$p<0.05$
Base excess	−7.1	(0.7)	−7.5	(0.6)	0.4	NS
PO_2	32.3	(1.4)	30.2	(1.4)	2.1	NS
Umbilical vein						
pH [H^+ mmol/l]	45.9	(0.9)	47.7	(0.9)		NS
pCO_2	40.2	(0.7)	43.2	(1.7)	3.0	$p<0.005$
Base excess	−5.5	(0.5)	−5.1	(0.7)	0.4	NS
pO_2	30.2	(1.4)	32.3	(1.4)	2.1	NS

controversy about the choice between epidural and general anaesthesia for a woman with severe pre-eclampsia. The anaesthetist must take all the relevant factors into consideration.

Anaesthesia for caesarean section can usually be managed equally successfully with either general or regional anaesthesia. Mothers are increasingly requesting epidural anaesthesia as it enables them to enjoy and share the moment of birth with their family, and offers them an alert and pain-free period after the operation.

In addition, medical and midwifery staff gain satisfaction from sharing in the pleasure of the mother.

2.2 General anaesthesia

The principal advantages of general anaesthesia are speed of induction, particularly important in an emergency situation, control of the airway following endotracheal intubation, and predictability of effect.

The disadvantages are related to major problems associated with the technique, such as pulmonary aspiration, inadequate airway control, maternal awareness, and neonatal depression, which if improperly managed can lead to maternal and fetal morbidity and mortality.

2.2.1 Pulmonary aspiration

Pulmonary aspiration of gastric contents is a major cause of maternal death associated with general anaesthesia. In the last 5 reports of confidential enquiries into maternal deaths in England and Wales, 74 of the 170 deaths (43.5 per cent) were due to pulmonary aspiration (Table 72.2). The available information suggests that the vast majority of these were due to liquid aspiration leading to Mendelson's syndrome and only a few due to aspiration of particulate material.

Anaesthetists have given considerable attention to preventing these tragedies. Approaches such as increasing the tone of the cardio-oesophageal (cardiac) sphincter or emptying the stomach are ineffective: first, because the gastro-oesophageal sphincter is incompetent in most mothers (Hart 1978) so that attempts to increase its tone with drugs will fail (Hey 1978), and secondly because none of the methods described completely empties the stomach (Holdsworth *et al.* 1974) (see Chapter 52).

Mendelson's syndrome is an acid pneumonitis, the severity of which depends on the pH of the aspirate. The practice of administering antacids to mothers in labour, first recommended by Taylor and Pryse-Davies in 1966, is now widespread. This practice is not without hazard. Particulate antacids such as aluminium hydroxide when aspirated in animals (Gibbs *et al.* 1979) and humans (Bond *et al.* 1979) lead to aggravation of the pulmonary lesion and it is for this reason that their replacement with aqueous antacids is recommended (Gibbs *et al.* 1981).

A variety of medications have been recommended to reduce the acidity of the gastric contents, including antacids and H2-receptor antagonists such as ranitidine or cimetidine (Thornburn and Moir 1987). Limited studies suggest that these drugs are free of adverse effects on the neonate (McAuley *et al.* 1985). (The effectiveness of all these methods is more completely discussed in Chapter 52.)

The most important measure in preventing pulmonary aspiration is occlusion of the oesophagus by cricoid pressure (Sellick 1961). It is the linchpin on which management should be based. The advantage of this method is its simplicity and effectiveness. It will prevent passive regurgitation of gastric contents against a hydrostatic pressure of 100 cm H_2O, which far exceeds that required to prevent pulmonary aspiration.

If this measure is so simple and effective, why is it that the cases of regurgitation and pulmonary aspiration continue to be reported? The most likely explanation is that the manoeuvre requires an assistant who is knowledgeable and capable. This is a *sine qua non*,

and the published enquiries report that, of the deaths due to Mendelson's syndrome, cricoid pressure has either not been applied, has been relaxed before intubation, or that it has been inefficiently performed. The method loses its effectiveness unless skilled help is available. The Wales Perinatal Mortality Initiative (1984–86) (Health Policy Division of the Welsh Office 1986) showed that 10 per cent of maternity units were not able to provide any skilled help, and in 33 per cent, trained assistance was not continuously available.

The next and equally important problem associated with general anaesthesia is the inability of the anaesthetist to intubate the trachea (Table 72.2). If the anaesthetist persists, death will result either from pulmonary aspiration or cardiac arrest subsequent to hypoxia.

Deaths due to Mendelson's syndrome or failed intubation are preventable and can be eradicated by improvements in clinical care, administrative arrangements and provision of drills for 'failed intubation'.

2.2.2 Awareness

Women expect to be asleep during general anaesthesia, and an anaesthetist's failure to produce unconsciousness is recognized in some circumstances to be negligent. A high inspired oxygen concentration of at least 50 per cent is required for the neonate to be delivered in optimal condition (Marx and Mateo 1971). An anaesthetic mixture of 50 per cent oxygen and 50 per cent nitrous oxide, unless supplemented with an inhalation agent such as 0.5 per cent halothane, 1 per cent enflurane or 0.75 per cent isoflurane, will lead to 25 to 30 per cent of patients being aware (Warren *et al.* 1983).

2.2.3 Neonatal depression

The possibility of depression of the neonate following general anaesthesia remains an important consideration, but if the fetus has not been previously compromised, well-conducted general anaesthesia will have minimal side-effects on the neonate. The use of intravenous induction agents such as thiopentone (Morgan *et al.* 1981) and supplementation with standard inhalation agents appear to have little or no effect on neonatal well-being (Palahniuk *et al.* 1977).

2.3 Epidural anaesthesia

Epidural anaesthesia for caesarean section is becoming increasingly popular with women, anaesthetists, and obstetricians. In some centres in Britain, more than 70 per cent of all elective caesarean sections are carried out with this technique (Moir and Thornburn 1986).

The main advantages are that the threat of pulmonary aspiration is reduced and the risk of 'failed endotracheal' intubation is eliminated. Other advantages are that regional anaesthesia allows the mother to see the infant at delivery, and the father to be present and interact with the mother at the birth. Breastfeeding can be started without delay.

The main problems associated with the use of regional anaesthesia, whether spinal or epidural, are related to the extensive block that is required for the surgical procedure. The extensive sympathetic blockade will be accompanied by a profound fall in blood pressure if there is any interference with the compensatory vasoconstrictive mechanisms that follow the block. The most common cause is compression of the inferior vena cava, which is easily averted by placing the woman on her side. Maternal hypotension must be treated immediately and aggressively, otherwise neonatal depression and maternal morbidity and mortality may ensue. The recent introduction of automatic non-invasive blood pressure monitors add to the safety of the method.

Another problem associated with an excessively high block is that the mother will not be able to protect her airway, with consequent risk of pulmonary aspiration of gastric contents. It should be noted that deaths from Mendelson's syndrome, although rare, have occurred in women receiving epidural or spinal anaesthesia (Department of Health and Social Security 1982).

What might be termed minor problems such as dural tap, intra-operative discomfort and backache, are balanced by the sore throat, the pains that sometimes follow the use of suxamethonium, and other minor sequelae associated with general anaesthesia. Nevertheless, these minor complications can cause considerable discomfort to the patient.

2.4 Spinal anaesthesia

Spinal anaesthesia is similar in many ways to epidural anaesthesia, except that less local anaesthetic drug is used and the speed of onset is much more rapid. The latter of these two qualities can be advantageous in circumstances where there is great urgency to perform surgery. On the other hand, the compensatory mechanisms can more readily be overwhelmed, and dangerous hypotension may develop. These problems are generally managed with prophylactic fluid loading and vasopressor administration. Ephedrine is the vasopressor most commonly recommended (Ralston *et al.* 1974).

The main disadvantage associated with spinal anaesthesia (or an inadvertent dural tap with epidural anaesthesia) is the development of severe headache. The incidence can be reduced to 1 or 2 per cent by the use of a 25- or 26-gauge spinal needle. Spinal headache that does not respond to bed rest and simple analgesia can be treated with an epidural infusion or with an epidural blood patch (Di Giovanni *et al.* 1972).

2.5 Local infiltration

Local infiltration is indicated in desperate situations, when the life of the mother would be at serious risk from the use of either regional or general anaesthesia. Typical examples of this would be severe maternal disease in regions of the world where there is a shortage of skilled anaesthetic personnel, medical and midwifery staff, or equipment. The trade off is between acceptance of discomfort by the mother and risk to her of mortality or serious morbidity. The technique was described by Ranney and Stanage (1975).

3 Technique of lower segment caesarean section

No two operators perform this operation in exactly the same way. Each surgeon during his or her apprenticeship gathers details of technique from their seniors, adopting and rejecting operative details as they progress, finally achieving a style of operating which gives the best results in their own hands. They will have found these methods adaptable to different problems that they meet in their surgical practice, and will normally serve them well, with little further change through the remainder of their professional careers.

(The account which follows is based on the personal experience of one of us (JFP) although reference is made to the findings of randomized trials wherever these are available.)

3.1 Preparation

With the suitably anaesthetized patient placed on the table with a left lateral tilt, the bladder is emptied with a catheter. Occasionally surgeons leave a catheter indwelling throughout the operation, draining into a gauze pad. The writer can recognize no logic in this practice and does not recommend it. The abdominal wall is painted with a suitable antiseptic agent such as povidone iodine from xiphisternum to mid-thigh, and sterile towelling draped around the area of the incision according to custom. The only point here that evokes strong feelings in the writer's mind is the unnecessary habit of fixing the towel clips to the skin.

3.2 The incision

The possible incisions are vertical or transverse. A randomized trial comparing transverse and vertical skin incisions for lower segment caesarean section (Haeri 1976) showed that more patients required blood transfusions with the transverse incision than the vertical (17/100 vs. 13/100), but there were fewer women with a post-operative haemoglobin less than 10 g/100 ml (28/100 vs. 36/100). Average operating time was longer with the transverse incision (53 minutes vs. 45 minutes). Febrile morbidity was seen less frequently with the transverse incision (30/100 vs. 48/100). None of these differences were statistically significant.

3.2.1 The midline suprapubic incision

The midline suprapubic incision, hallowed by tradition, has much to commend it, because it ensures even and adequate exposure of the pelvic viscera. A disadvantage is that upward extension requires that one either traverses the umbilicus, a site difficult to sterilize and finicky to repair, or one cuts obliquely to one side of the umbilicus leaving a less pleasing scar. Upward extension is, however, rarely necessary at caesarean section because the distance between the symphysis and umbilicus is much increased by the abdominal wall distension intrinsic to pregnancy. This incision formerly had a bad reputation among general surgeons who were called upon to repair the ventral hernias resulting from its use. Nowadays, the use of a nylon suture for the fascia has largely eliminated this troublesome complication. This incision is preferred in the delivery of high order multiple pregnancies (triplets and more), because there may be much oedema in the lower abdomen which restricts access.

3.2.2 The paramedian incision

With the operator standing to the patient's right, this is normally a right paramedian incision. The advantage of this approach in the lower abdomen is not as great as in the upper abdomen, because the posterior fascial layer of the rectus sheath is limited at the linea semilunaris, and at caesarean section divarication of the recti may further limit its value in protecting against dehiscence. On the other hand it extends upwards quite nicely if necessary, and as such is useful for the classical operation.

3.2.3 The Pfannenstiel incision

The popular Pfannenstiel incision (Pfannenstiel 1900) is cosmetically more acceptable than either of the vertical incisions, and less liable to result in wound disruption or incisional hernia. The down-curved skin incision however, is not truly along Langer's lines and careful repair is required to avoid subsequent unsightly guttering when the patient stands erect. The up and down subaponeurotic dissection of the rectus sheath may lead to troublesome bleeding from perforating vessels. Post-operative haematoma and abscess formation at this site is sufficiently common for some surgeons to drain this incision routinely. Because the peritoneal incision is vertical between the recti, considerable subaponeurotic dissection may be necessary if the infant is large.

3.2.4 The Cohen incision

The Cohen incision (Cohen 1972) is preferred by the writer for most obstetric and gynaecological work. Of relatively recent origin (1954) this incision is made straight, not curved, between two points 1 inch below and medial to the anterior superior iliac spines. Only the skin is cut, the subcutaneous tissue being incised transversely over a distance of 2 inches in the midline where few vessels exist, to the rectus sheath. The same incision can usefully divide the sheath for about an inch on either side of the midline. The subcutaneous fat is then separated along the line of incision from the rectus sheath by pushing a pair of closed curved scissors in the plane of cleavage, opening the blades and withdrawing them opened. The small rectus sheath incisions are now extended transversely with scissors and the space between the recti opened with the same instrument.

This space is stretched with fingers up and down, then two fingers of the operator pull the rectus muscle laterally and at the same time the assistant does likewise. The underlying peritoneum is opened as usual, but the peritoneum is cut transversely. To avoid the bladder it is better to enter the peritoneal cavity relatively high and to one side if in doubt.

This incision is rapid, virtually bloodless, and cosmetically acceptable. In ten years of routine use the writer has never seen a burst abdomen, but has seen one small midline ventral hernia. The Cohen incision can be used whatever other scars are present. The operator merely cuts through a previous Cohen incision but does not excise the previous scar, as this does not improve the end result. The incision through a previous Cohen incision often ends up a bit like a Pfannenstiel. Lateral separation of the recti may be difficult because of adhesions, and upward and downward subaponeurotic dissection of the fascia is often necessary. As the bladder may also be drawn up, the peritoneum is best entered at the highest extremity of the upper subaponeurotic flap, where it is often possible to cut the peritoneum transversely. Adhesions, however, may dictate a vertical peritoneal incision.

3.3 Abdominal packing

Traditionally, large damp gauze packs of a 3-foot length of 9-inch gauze were placed around the uterus to shield the rest of the abdominal cavity from soiling by the fluid contents of the uterus and this step is mentioned in almost every work on this subject. For many years the writer has omitted this step and no harm has been done thereby. There are two reasons for this. First, that if one does not put packs in, one cannot forget to remove them. Second, the gravid uterus and broad ligaments themselves act as good obturators before incision of the uterus, and following removal of the fetus and placenta, the uterus has shrunk so much that any pack inserted earlier is by that time performing no useful function. The more logical thing is to operate with a head down tilt and to use an efficient sucker, or better still, to have an efficient assistant to wield it.

3.4 The uterine incision

Having excluded uterine torsion or dextrorotation and

confirmed the presentation, a Doyen's retractor is introduced. The inch or so of loose uterovesical fold is identified, picked up with artery forceps above and below the midline, snipped through with scissors, which are then passed closed laterally to free the plane of cleavage, and withdrawn opened. The uterovesical fold is then divided transversely across the full width of the lower segment. The upper forceps is removed, the lower held up by the assistant, and the upper end of the bladder gently separated by two fingers. Pushing the bladder down with swabs may cause much oozing and is not recommended. The Doyen's retractor is then slipped into the retrovesical space thus formed.

A 2-inch transverse incision is then made in the lower segment using several gentle strokes of the scalpel, keeping the scalpel at right angles to the uterine wall until the membranes are seen shining through. The incision is extended to 3 inches using 7-inch curved Mayo's scissors (the membranes should now be bulging through nicely). Scissors are preferred to fingers as with their use the incision has cleaner edges, which facilitates repair. The fingers are finally used to stretch the incision to its full extent, thus minimizing the risk of damage to the uterine vessels at the angles.

3.5 The delivery

In a singleton pregnancy the mode of delivery depends on the presentation. At elective lower segment caesarean section the membranes are usually intact, therefore disimpaction is seldom required or is easy, as indeed is any other form of intrauterine manipulation, unless oligohydramnios is extreme. On the other hand the lower segment may be quite thick which may partly nullify the above advantages.

When the presentation is cephalic, the membranes are usually ruptured in non-elective operations and the hand is used to 'shoehorn' the head out of the brim and through the incision, the assistant exerting judicious fundal pressure to aid expulsion of the head. Manual delivery is less easy at elective section when the head is high and the lower segment thick. Under these conditions obstetric forceps are preferred. Although the Wrigley's forceps are popular, the writer uses Simpson's short straight forceps—although of some antiquity (1816) they can still be purchased and have the advantage of enabling the operator to get a good cephalic application whatever the attitude of the head. Thereafter the delivery incorporating the appropriate rotation is easily accomplished.

If the head is unexpectedly large and a Pfannenstiel or Cohen's incision has been made, it has been known for difficulty to be experienced in delivery of the head from between the recti. This is nearly always because the operator has made the fundamental error of performing an inadequate initial incision. The only way out of this unfortunate situation is to promptly divide

each rectus muscle transversely for about half its width. The recti are left unsutured. Should the breech present, the membranes are ruptured and a gentle breech extraction is performed using the same manoeuvres as in vaginal delivery. The aftercoming head is conveniently delivered by jaw-flexion and shoulder traction. If the aftercoming head is large, Wrigley's forceps are preferred to ensure controlled delivery.

The infant, having been delivered, is maintained in the head down position. The cord is then clamped and divided, and the baby is handed head down to the paediatrician.

In some cases of placenta praevia, the placental bed may lie directly beneath the uterine incision. The diagnosis has usually been made beforehand and careful ultrasonic examination should already have been made with a view to delineating the limits of the placenta. Armed with this information the surgeon should know the shortest route to the placental margin. The placenta is quickly separated along its natural plane of cleavage from the uterine wall in the direction of its nearest margin, the presenting part (usually the breech) is identified, a foot is grasped *through* the membranes and the presenting leg is delivered past the placenta and into the incision. The membranes rupture *en route*. The infant is then delivered as a breech. Should the head present, it is usually oblique and floating. The head is displaced upwards through the intact membranes and the external hand brings the breech and thus the foot, within reach. There is no place whatsoever for cutting or tearing through the substance of the placenta. This manoeuvre is no quicker, and can rapidly lead to fetal exsanguination.

3.6 The third stage

Oxytocin (5 international units) is injected intravenously by the anaesthetist following delivery, and the placenta delivered using cord traction once the uterus has contracted. At this point some operators eventrate the uterus to facilitate the repair. This technique seems harmless and indeed useful under general anaesthesia, but may cause pain when epidural block is used, and in these circumstances is not recommended.

There has been one randomized trial comparing extra-abdominal eventration of the uterus after delivery of the placenta to facilitate repair of the incision with intraperitoneal repair (Hershey and Quilligan 1978). Although there was no statistically significant difference in the overall morbidity rates between the two groups (71/159 vs. 75/149), women whose uteri were externalized had a lower rate of more serious morbidity (with fevers lasting more than 3 days) (7/159) than did women who underwent intra-abdominal repair (16/149). Blood loss was also somewhat lower in the eventration group, with a mean decrease in haematocrit of $6.2 \pm .35$ vs. 7.0 ± 0.43 $(0.05 < p < .1)$. Eventration was, however, accompanied by more intra-operative nausea and vomiting (5/159) vs. 1/149. These data suggest that exteriorization decreases the technical difficulty of the repair, reduces blood loss and the risk of subsequent prolonged morbidity, but may cause nausea or vomiting, presumably related to a vagal response, in women under regional anaesthesia.

3.7 Repair of the uterine incision

The writer prefers the two needle technique. Using a mounted atraumatic needle carrying No. 1 plain catgut, the angle suture is inserted through full thickness just beyond the lateral margin of the incision. The short end is clipped and the other end uncut. The same procedure is adopted on the other side. Starting at the far side a continuous running suture closes the incision, tied to the short end of the other angle suture, which is then held and retracted medially along the line of the incision to facilitate the commencement of the second layer. (No special attempt is made to exclude the decidua, although some surgeons believe that this is important.) Using the second suture the second layer invaginates the lower segment and consists of a continuous Lembert stitch which is tied into the short end of the other side.

The pelvic peritoneum should be sutured such as to leave a scar as small as possible, and is usually a continuous suture drawn together quite tightly so as to bunch up the peritoneum before being tied. The abdomen is then closed in the customary manner.

3.8 Complications

Surgical accidental damage at this operation may be minimized by ensuring correct initial orientation. It is important to take into account the effects of lateral tilt and uterine rotation before making the first incision.

3.8.1 Damage to the uterine vessels

Damage to the uterine vessels may be minor or major. The usual site is at the lateral angles of the lower segment incision, and usually involves branches of the uterine artery as they cross in a medial direction. The usual solution to this problem is to ensure that the angle suture is sufficiently laterally placed to ensure ligation, remembering of course to allow for vessel retraction.

If the main vessels are divided, the uterus is first eventrated and ligaturing sutures are placed about 1.5 cm above and below the site of damage. Because the suture is passed through the broad ligament from before backwards eventration of the uterus enables these sutures to be passed under direct vision (Fig. 72.1). The suture is then passed around the vessels and through the adjacent uterine wall. It is best to use a fairly large, half circle, round bodied, atraumatic needle carrying No. 2 chromic catgut. When placing the lower

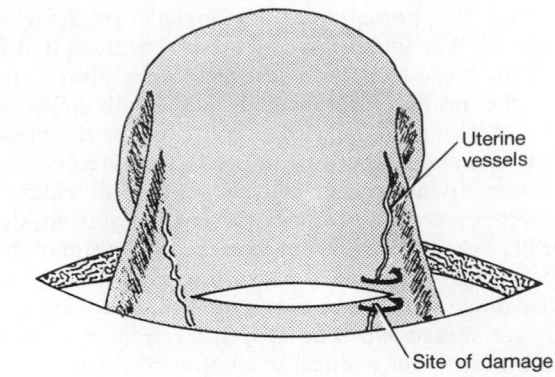

Fig. 72.1 Ligation of a damaged uterine blood vessel.

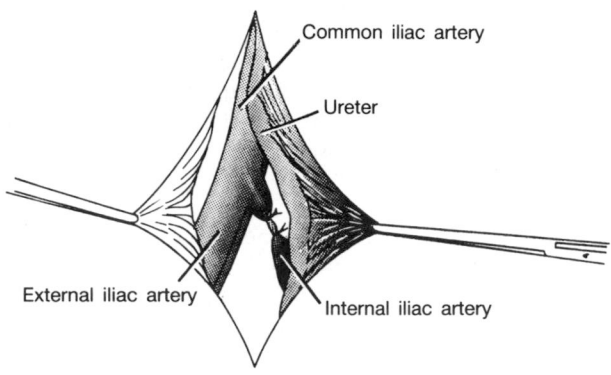

Fig. 72.2 Ligation of the internal iliac artery.

ligature, great care is required to avoid the ureter and the bladder.

Rarely the bleeding may not be so easily controlled, the edges of the uterine vessels might retract out of sight, or cause a rapidly enlarging broad ligament haematoma. In these circumstances ligature of the ipsilateral internal iliac artery may be required. This is not difficult and is achieved thus. With the uterus eventrated, the bowel is packed out of the pelvis, the ureter is identified as it passes forwards and medially at the bifurcation of the common iliac artery. The peritoneum is divided lateral and parallel to, and well clear of the ureter, along the line of the internal iliac artery. The ureter is retracted medially and a ligature of No. 1 silk is passed around the artery with a blunt aneurysm needle taking care not to damage the subjacent internal iliac vein. A second reinforcing suture is then passed 1.5 cm distal to the first and tied (Fig. 72.2). The broad ligament haematoma can then be evacuated and drained with a vacuum drain.

Ligature of the internal iliac artery is also useful in

severe uncontrollable bleeding from the lower segment that does not respond to treatment with oxytocics or prostaglandins, as may occur in cases of placenta praevia. It is quite permissible to ligate both internal iliac arteries in desperate situations. This latter measure has occasionally prevented recourse to total hysterectomy. Should the bleeding remain profuse despite these measures, then there should be no hesitation in resorting to total hysterectomy as a life-saving measure.

3.8.2 Accidental extension of the uterine incision

This complication occurs most frequently at repeat caesarean section. The lower segment is often very thin and fibrous, and, following removal of the baby, a fenestration or dehiscence in the lower segment is sometimes revealed. These are nearly always in the inferior flap and usually in the midline, extending downwards below the bladder towards the cervix. Before embarking on its repair the edges of the tear must be clearly demarcated and separated from the bladder (which is inspected for damage) and then repaired from below upwards with two rows of interrupted sutures. The lower segment incision is then repaired in the usual way.

3.8.3 Damage to the bladder

There are three main circumstances leading to damage to the bladder. First, the bladder may be entered during the process of opening the parietal peritoneum. This is unlikely during primary caesarean section, but may be a problem with a repeat procedure. This particular injury is most likely to occur when the woman has been in labour for some time, and the bladder has been drawn up along with the lower segment.

Second, the bladder may be drawn up and adherent to the anterior uterine wall because of previous surgery, and may be incised by mistake, or the bladder may be densely adherent and thus liable to damage during attempts to dissect it from the lower segment.

Third, the adherent bladder may be injured as part of a lower segment tear.

The edges of the hole in the bladder are first clearly demarcated and held with Allis tissue forceps. The surrounding bladder is mobilized from surrounding structures when necessary, so as to guarantee apposition without tension. Repair depends entirely on the shape and size of the hole. The ureters are scarcely ever involved, but the ureterovesical junction may be close. The torn edges of the bladder mucosa are brought together using a continuous Lembert invagination suture of fine chromic catgut. This suture line is reinforced by a second similar layer. On completion of the operation an indwelling Foley catheter or suprapubic drain is introduced and continuous bladder drainage is instituted. The bladder usually heals well, and if infection is avoided, convalescence is uneventful.

4 Technique of classical caesarean section

Conditions where classical caesarean section would be planned are unusual. Indications would include large fibroids which occupy the lower segment and conditions where the very size of the conceptus precludes delivery through the more limited lower segment—these would include such curiosities as conjoined twins. There is, however, an increasing ground-swell of opinion within the profession (unsupported by good evidence) that the elective preterm delivery of a breech may more safely be accomplished by this route. The lower segment at the beginning of the third trimester can be very much thicker than one thinks, and it is debatable as to whether it even exist as an anatomical entity at this time.

Even today the technique of this operation differs little from Sänger's operation of 1882. The preferred skin incision is a right paramedian incision extending about two inches above the level of the umbilicus. The peritoneum is opened in the midline and the uterus is carefully examined to determine the true longitudinal axis. This step is important, because to minimize blood loss the uterine incision should be made vertically in the midline of the uterus where the blood supply is generally poorest. The uterus is opened longitudinally with a scalpel over a distance of about 6 inches. If the placenta is encountered it is circumvented as previously described for the lower segment operation, and the fetus delivered either by the breech or the vertex, whichever is most convenient. Frequently an arm may prolapse through this incision. This should be promptly put back and replaced by one of the lower limbs.

Closure of the uterine incision is best carried out using strong (No. 2, for example) chromic catgut. There is no merit in attempting to bury the knots. Using a large curved needle, 'through-and-through' sutures are passed at one inch intervals for the length of the uterine incision and held at either end with haemostat forceps. The mass of uterine muscle is then closed with two layers of interrupted No. 2 chromic catgut, the most superficial layer of muscle being excluded. This latter layer is closed with a running suture of fine 2.0 chromic catgut. The 'through-and-through' sutures are tied next. These 'tension' sutures are inserted in order to minimize the tension put upon the uterine incision during the healing process. The abdomen is then closed in the usual way.

Whilst there may be a limited place for classical caesarean section, the trend towards its renaissance is partly based upon the fact that many of the statistics regarding the integrity of the scar stem from the pre-blood-transfusion—pre-antibiotic era. The fact remains that as the clinical circumstances for all patients in a given epoch were broadly similar, there is no doubt that fewer lower segment than classical scars rupture in subsequent pregnancies. This is so whether the patients have an elective section, go into labour or deliver vaginally. Furthermore, maternal and fetal mortality is considerably greater following a ruptured classical scar (Dewhurst 1957) (see Chapter 70).

5 Conclusions

Caesarean section, while still more hazardous than vaginal delivery, can be made a safer operation by meticulous attention to careful and correct technique, for both the anaesthesia and for the surgery.

References

Bond VK, Stoelting RK, Gupta CD (1979). Pulmonary aspiration syndrome after inhalation of gastric fluid containing antacids. Anesthesiology, 51: 452–453.

Brock-Utne JG, Buley RJR, Downing JW, Cuerden C (1978). S Afr Med, 54: 489–492.

Clemetson LAB, Hassan R, Mallikaryuneswara VR, Wallace G (1973). Tilt-bend caesarean section. Obstet Gynecol, 42: 290–296.

Cohen SJ (1972) Abdominal and Vaginal Hysterectomy. Oxford: Allen & Mowbray, pp 19–30.

Crawford JS, Burton M, Davies P (1972). Time and lateral tilt at caesarean section. Br J Anaesth, 44: 477–483.

Department of Health and Social Security (1982). Report on Confidential Enquiries in Maternal Deaths in England and Wales 1976–78. London: Her Majesty's Stationery Office.

Department of Health and Social Security (1986). Report on Confidential Enquiries in Maternal Deaths in England and Wales 1979–81. London: Her Majesty's Stationery Office.

DeVore JS (1979). Psychological anaesthesia for obstetrics. In: Anesthesia for obstetrics. Shnider SM, Levison G (eds). Baltimore: Williams & Williams, pp 65–74.

Dewhurst CJ (1957). The ruptured caesarean section scar. J Obstet Gynaecol Br Empire, 64: 113–118.

Di Giovanni AJ, Galbent MW, Wahle WM (1972). Epidural injection of autologans blood for post lumbar-puncture headache. Anesth Analg, 51: 226–232.

Downing JW, Coleman AJ, Mahomedymc MC, Jeal DE, Mahomedy YH (1974). Anaesthesia, 29: 696–703.

Gibbs CP, Sophr L, Schmidt D (1981). *In vitro* and *in vivo* evaluation of sodium citrate as an antacid. Anesthesiology, 55: A31.

Gibbs CP, Schwartz DJ, Wynne JW, Hood CI, Kuck EJ (1979). Antacid pulmonary aspiration in the dog. Anesthesiology, 51: 380–385.

Haeri AD (1976). Comparison of transverse and vertical skin incisions for caesarean section. S Afr Med J, 52: 33–34.

Hart DM (1978) Heartburn in pregnancy. J Int Med Res, 6: Suppl 1,1.

Health Policy Division of the Welsh Office (1986). Wales Perinatal Mortality Initiative, 1984–1986. Cardiff: Her Majesty's Stationery Office.

Hershey DW, Quilligan EJ (1978). Extraabdominal uterine exteriorization at cesarean section. Obstet Gynecol, 52: 189–192.

Hey VMF (1978). Gastro-oesophageal reflux in pregnancy: a review article. J Int Med Res, 6: Suppl 1,18.

Holdsworth JD, Furness RMB, Roulston RG (1974). A comparison of apomorphine and stomach tubes for emptying the stomach before general anaesthesia in obstetrics. Br J Anaesth, 46: 526–529.

Hollmen AI, Jouppila R, Koivisto M, Maata L, Pihlajaniemi R, Puukka M, Rantakyla P (1978). Neurologic activity of infants following anaesthesia for caesarean section. Anesthesiology, 48: 350–356.

Kerr M (1949). Quoted by Myerscough RP. In: Munro Kerr's Operative Obstetrics (9th edn). London: Baillière Tindall, p 519.

Lepage (*c.* 1878). Quoted by Watts Eden T. In: A Manual of Midwifery, (4th edn, 1915). London: J & A Churchill, p 719.

Marx GF, Mateo CV (1971). Effects of different oxygen concentration during general anaesthesia for elective caesarean section. Can Anaesth Soc J, 18: 587–593.

McAuley DM, Halliday HL, Johnston JR, Dundee JW (1985). Cimetidine in labour: absence of adverse effect on the high risk fetus. Br J Obstet Gynaecol, 92: 350–355.

Moir DD, Thornburn J (1986). Obstetric anaesthesia and analgesia (3rd edn). London: Baillière Tindall.

Morgan DJ, Blackman GL, Paul JD, Wolf LH (1981). Pharmokinetics and plasma binding of thiopental. Studies at caesarean section. Anesthesiology, 54: 474–480.

Palahniuk RJ, Scarliff J, Biehl D, Wiebe H, Sankaran K (1977). Maternal and neonatal effects of methoxyflurane, nitrous oxide and lumbar epidural anaesthesia for caesarean section. Can Anaesth Soc J, 34: 586–596.

Pfannensiel J (1900). Über die Vorteile des suprasymphysaren Fascienquerschnitts fur die gynäkologischen Koiliotomien, zugleich ein Beitrag zu der Indikations—stellung der Operations wege. Samml Klin Vortr (Neue Folge), Gynäk. No 68–98, 1897–1900 (Klin Votr, NF No 268, Gynäk, No 97, Feb).

Porro E (1876). Della amputazione utero-ovarica come complemento di Faglio cesario. Ann Univ Med Chir, 237: 289–350.

Ralston DH, Shnider SM, de Lorimes AA (1974). Effects of equipotent ephedrine, metaraminol, mephentermine and methoxamine on uterine blood flow in the pregnant ewe. Anesthesiology, 40: 354–370.

Ranney B, Stanage WF (1975). Advantages of local anaesthesia for caesarean section. Obstet Gynecol, 45: 163–167.

Rousset F (1581). Traitte nouveau de l'hystérotomotokie, ou enfantement césarien. Paris: Denys du Val.

Sänger M (1882). Sänger's operation—the so-called 'classical caesarean section'. Arch Gynecol, 19: 370.

Scottish Home and Health Department (1978). A report on an enquiry in maternal deaths in Scotland 1976–80. Edinburgh: HMSO.

Sellick BA (1961). Cricoid pressure to control regurgitation of stomach contents during induction of anaesthesia: preliminary communication. Lancet, 11: 404–406.

Taylor G, Pryse-Davies J (1966). Prophylactic use of antacids in the prevention of the acid-pulmonary aspiration syndrome (Mendelson's Syndrome). Lancet, 1: 288–291.

Thomas TG (1870). Gastro-elytrotomy; a substitute for the caesarean section. Am J Obstet Dis Wom, 3: 125–139.

Thornburn J, Moir DD (1987). Antacid therapy for emergency caesarean section. Anaesthesia, 42: 352–355.

Trolle D (1982). The history of caesarean section. Acta Historica Scientarium Naturalium et Medicinalium, 33: 1–109.

Warren TM, Datta S, Ostheimer GW, Naulty JS, Weiss JB, Morrison JA (1983). Comparison of the maternal and neonatal effects of halothane, enflurane and isoflurane for caesarean section. Anaesth Analg, 62: 516–520.

Watts Eden T (1915). A Manual of Midwifery (4th edn). London: J & A Churchill, pp 719–720.

73 Prophylactic antibiotics in association with caesarean section

Murray Enkin, Eleanor Enkin, Iain Chalmers, and Elina Hemminki

1 Introduction

Maternal morbidity after caesarean section has not been studied as systematically as has the maternal mortality associated with the operation (see Chapters 69 and 70). In part, this is due to differences of opinion about the criteria that should be used to define morbidity. 'Febrile morbidity', for example, has been variously defined as an oral temperature greater than 100.4 °F (38.0 °C) on any two of the first ten days postpartum excluding the first 24 hours (Hughes 1972); a temperature of 101.5 °F or greater in the first 24 hours post-operatively or of 101 °F or higher thereafter (Cunningham *et al.* 1978); or in terms of a 'fever index', computed as the number of degree-hours a patient accumulates when her temperature exceeds 99 °F during the postpartum period (Ledger and Kriewall 1973). 'Endometritis' is variably diagnosed on the basis of fever, uterine tenderness, and abnormal lochia—alone or in combination (Swartz and Grolle 1981). Before making a diagnosis of 'wound infection' some investigators have required a positive bacteriological culture in material taken from an inflamed or purulent wound (Moir-Bussy *et al.* 1984); others have required pus visible to the naked eye but not bacteriological confirmation (Pelle *et al.* 1986).

No doubt partly as a result of these varying defining criteria, the estimated incidence of maternal morbidity following caesarean section varies. The problem of post-operative infection can undoubtedly be substantial, however. Although some of the control groups in the trials reviewed below had no cases of endometritis, wound infection, or other serious infections (including such conditions as pelvic abscess, septic shock, and septic pelvic vein thrombophlebitis), the incidence of these conditions was sometimes as high as 85 per cent, 25 per cent, and 25 per cent respectively. Febrile morbidity, a proportion of which is likely to be caused by factors other than infection, appears to be an inevitable sequel to caesarean section for at least one in five women.

There have been a number of attempts to identify markers of an increased risk of infectious morbidity following caesarean section. Factors that have been shown in at least one investigation to be associated with an increased risk of post-operative infection include emergency caesarean section; labour and its duration; ruptured membranes and the duration of rupture; the socioeconomic status of the patient; vaginal examinations during labour and internal fetal monitoring; anaemia; obesity; general anaesthesia; and the skill of the operator (Swartz and Grolle 1981; Moir-Bussy *et al.* 1984; Pelle *et al.* 1986; Galask 1987; Ford *et al.* 1987). Unfortunately, interpretation of the available evidence is complicated by the fact that so many of these factors of putative aetiological importance are interrelated. The weight of evidence points to labour and ruptured membranes being the most important factors, the risk rising with increased duration of each. Obesity appears to be a risk factor of particular importance for wound infection (Moir-Bussy *et al.* 1984; Pelle *et al.* 1986).

Interest in the potential for reducing maternal morbidity following caesarean section by administering antibiotics prophylactically has existed since the time that these drugs first became available (Richards 1943; Hesseltine and Thelen 1946; Keettel and Plass 1950; Galask 1987). It was really not until 1968, however, when Miller and Crichton published a report based on a controlled trial conducted in South Africa, that the potential of this policy began to be investigated systematically. When Mead reviewed the subject in 1977 he referred to a total of 9 reports of relevant investigations; by 1981, Swartz and Grolle were able to draw on the results of 26 reports; in this chapter we have reviewed the results of over 90 reports of controlled trials (see Tables 73.1, 73.2 and 73. 3).

Table 73.1 Placebo-controlled trials of prophylactic antibiotic use in caesarean section

Trial	Manoeuvre	Exptl	Control
Apuzzio *et al.* (1982)	tigarcillin 6 g IV 1 dose after cord + 3 g IV 6–8 hr post-op	44/139	66/120
Bourgeois *et al.* (1985)	cefamandole 2 g irrigation	5/73	21/75
Conover and Moore (1984)	cefoxitin 2 g peritoneal irrigation	9/37	6/23
Conover and Moore (1984)	cefoxitin 2 g IV, 3 doses after cord clamped, 8 and 16 hr	1/31	8/33
Dashow *et al.* (1986)	cephapirin 2 g irrigation or cefamandole 2 g irrigation or moxalactam 2 g irrigation or ampicillin 2 g irrigation	54/283	22/77
Dillon *et al.* (1981)	cefoxitin 2 g IV, 3 doses after cord clamped, 4 and 10 hr	5/46	22/55
Duff and Park (1980)	ampicillin 1 g IV, 3 doses pre-op, 6 and 12 hr post-op	7/26	13/31
Duff *et al.* (1982)	ampicillin 1 g, 3 doses pre-op, 4 and 8 hr post-op	4/42	13/40
Elliott *et al.* (1982)	ampicillin, different doses (1 and 3 days)	18/83	10/20
Fugere *et al.* (1983)	cefoxitin 2 g 3 doses or cefazolin 1 g 3 doses after cord clamp, 6 and 12 hr	4/60	7/29
Gall (1979)	cefazolin 1 g IM pre-op + cefalothin 2 g 6, 12, 24 hr post-op	8/46	20/49

Table 73.1 Placebo-controlled trials of prophylactic antibiotic use in caesarean section – *continued*

Trial	Manoeuvre	Exptl	Control
Ganesh *et al.* (1986)	trimethoprin 240 + sulfamethoxazole IV 1 dose after cord clamped	6/29	13/28
Gibbs *et al.* (1972)	ampicillin 1 g, methacillin 1 g, kanamycin 0.5 g, 3 doses, pre-op, 2 and 8 hr post-op	9/33	17/28
Gibbs *et al.* (1981)	cefamandole 2 g 3 doses after cord clamp, 4 and 8 hr post-op	9/50	27/50
Gibbs *et al.* (1973)	ampicillin 1 g, kanamycin 0.5 g 3 doses, pre-op, 2 and 8 hr post-op	8/34	22/34
Gummerus (1984)	metronidazole 0.5 g IV, 1 dose 20 min after cord clamped	16/109	16/110
Hager and Williamson (1983)	cefamandole 0.5 g IV, 4 doses after cord clamp, 1, 6, 12 hr post-op	4/43	13/47
Harger and English (1981)	cefoxitin 2 g IV, 3 doses after cord clamp, 6 and 12 hr	26/196	68/190
Hawrylyshyn *et al.* (1983)	cefoxitin 2 g IV 1 dose after cord clamped, or 3 doses (+4 and 8 hr)	17/124	23/58
Karhunen *et al.* (1985)	tinadazole 0.5 g IV 1 dose after cord clamped	11/75	23/77
Kellum *et al.* (1985)	cefamandole 2 g irrigation	16/84	62/86
Kreutner *et al.* (1979)	cefalothin 1 g or cefamandole 1 g IV 3 doses, pre-op, 2 and 8 hr post-op	30/91	19/29
Kreutner *et al.* (1978)	cefazoline 1 g IV, 3 doses pre-op and 2 and 8 hr post-op	13/48	17/49
Levin *et al.* (1983)	cefoxitin 2 g, or cephapirin 2 g irrigation	8/85	11/43
Long *et al.* (1980) Rudd *et al.* (1981)	cefamandole 2 g irrigation	0/30	8/30
McCowan and Jackson (1980)	metrodnidazole 0.5 g IV pre-op + 2 g rectal suppository post-op	18/35	16/38
Miller and Crichton (1968)	ampicillin 0.5 g IM pre-op + 0.5 g q.i.d. × 6 days	39/150	70/150

Table 73.1 Placebo-controlled trials of prophylactic antibiotic use in caesarean section – *continued*

Trial	Prevalence of febrile morbidity or overall infection		
	Manoeuvre	Exprtl	Control
Moodley and Zeeman (1981)	lincomycin 0.6 g or metronidazole 0.5 g IV pre-op + t.i.d. × 2 days	7/40	4/20
Moro and Andrews (1974)	cephalothin 2 g IV pre-op + 1 g q.i.d. × 3 days + Cephalexin 0.50 q.i.d. × 5 days	6/74	20/74
Padilla *et al.* (1983)	ampicillin 2 g intra-operative, 1 dose	5/34	22/37
Phelan and Pruyn (1979)	cefazolin, 3 doses: 0.5 g pre-op and 2 hr post-op, + 1 g 8 hr post-op	11/61	18/61
Polk *et al.* (1982)	cefoxitin 2 g 3 doses after cord clamped, 4 and 8 hr post-op	23/138	49/128
Rehu and Jahkola (1980)	penicillin 10 mil U IV periop or clindamycin 500 mg IV periop + gentamycin 80 mg pre-op	7/88	13/40
Roex *et al.* (1986)	cefoxitin 2 g IV after cord clamped + 1 g IV 6 and 12 hr post-op	15/64	29/65
Ross *et al.* (1984)	metronidazole 500 mg IV pre-op + 500 mg suppository b.i.d. × 5 days	6/57	9/58
Saltzman *et al.* (1985)	ceftizoxime 2 g IV, 1 dose after cord clamped	7/50	16/49
Stage *et al.* (1982)	cephradine 1 g 2 doses pre-op and 4 hr post-op	29/133	25/66
Stiver *et al.* (1983)	cefoxitin 2 g or cefazolin 1 g IV 3 doses, after cord clamped, 4 and 8 hr post-op	30/243	40/111
Tully *et al.* (1983)	cefoxitin 2 g IV 3 doses after cord clamped, 4 and 8 hr post-op	16/45	17/54
Tzingounis *et al.* (1982)	cefuroxime 2 g IV, 10 doses pre-op + t.i.d. × 3 days	12/46	27/50
Wong *et al.* (1978)	cefazoline 1 g IV, 3 doses after cord clamped, 6 and 12 hr post-op pre-op and 4 and 8 hr post-op	22/48	30/48
Work (1977)	cephalothin 2 g IV, 3 doses pre-op and 4 and 8 hr post-op	14/40	27/40

Table 73.1 Placebo-controlled trials of prophylactic antibiotic use in caesarean section – *continued*

Trial	Prevalence of febrile morbidity or overall infection		
	Manoeuvre	Exprtl	Control
Young *et al.* (1983)	cefoxitin 1 g IV, 3 doses after cord clamped, 4 and 8 hr post-op	12/50	34/50

Table 73.2 No-treatment controlled trials of prophylactic antibiotic use in caesarean section

Trial	Prevalence of febrile morbidity or overall infection		
	Manoeuvre	Exprtl	Control
Adeleye and Osinusi (1981)	ampicillin 0.5 g pre-op + 0.25 g q.i.d. × 7 days	12/58	26/48
Bourgeois *et al.* (1985)	cefamandole 2 g irrigation	5/73	26/75
D'Angelo and Sokol (1980)	kefzol 1 g, 4 doses or keflex 0.5 g q6h × 5 days	12/49	20/31
De Palma *et al.* (1980)	cefamandole 2 g IV 72 hr or penicillin + gentamycin 72 hr	25/209	109/128
Elliott and Flaherty (1986)	cefoxitin 2 g, q.i.d. × 2 days or cefoxitin irrigation or cefoxitin 2 g q.i.d. × 2 days + irrigation	7/119	14/39
Gerstner *et al.* (1980)	metronidazole 500 mg IV t.i.d. × 4 days + 1 g suppository b.i.d. × 4 days	16/53	30/50
Gordon *et al.* (1979)	ampicillin 1 g pre-op + 2 doses or ampicillin 1 g at cord clamp + 2 doses	7/78	14/36
Itskovitz *et al.* (1979)	ampicillin 500 mg q.i.d. × 5 days or cephalothin 1 g q.i.d. × 1 day + cephalexin 0.5 g q.i.d. × 4 days	23/100	25/50
Kellum *et al.* (1985)	cefamandole 2 g irrigation	16/84	79/92
Long *et al.* (1980) Rudd *et al.* (1981)	cefamandole 2 g irrigation	0/30	7/30
Morrison *et al.* (1973)	penicillin 10 mil U pre-op + t.i.d. × 3 days + kanamycin 0.5 g IM b.i.d. × 2 days	25/115	59/115

Table 73.2 No-treatment controlled trials of prophylactic antibiotic use in caesarean section – *continued*

Trial	Prevalence of febrile morbidity or overall infection Manoeuvre	Exptl	Control
Oestreicher et al. (1987)	mezlocillin 4 g 1 dose	8/30	5/30
Rothbard et al. (1975)	cephalothin 2 g pre-op + q.i.d. × 2 days + kanamycin 1 g pre-op + 0.5 g b.i.d. × 2 days	6/47	23/53
Scarpignato et al. (1982) Mansani et al. (1984)	cefuroxime 0.75 g pre-op + 8, 16 hr or cefuroxime 0.75 g post-op 15 doses in 3 days	2/39	7/20
Schedvins and Moberg (1986)	cefuroxim 1.5 g q8h 3 doses plus cefadroxil 0.5 g b.i.d. 6 days	4/26	13/27

Table 73.3 Controlled trials of different regimens of prophylactic antibiotic use in caesarean section

Trial	Prevalence of febrile morbidity or overall infection Manoeuvre	A	B	C
Benigno et al. (1986)	A. piperacillin 2 g IV, 3 doses after cord clamped, 4 and 8 hr B. cefoxitin 2 g IV, 3 doses after cord clamped, 4 and 8 hr	35/136	37/147	
Boothby et al. (1984)	A. cefoxitin 2 g IV 4 doses B. cefoxitin 2 g by irrigation	2/50	2/53	
Conover and Moore (1984)	A. cefoxitin 2 g, 3 doses after cord clamped, 8 and 16 hr B. cefoxitin 2 g irrigation	1/31	9/37	
Crombleholme et al. (1987)	A mezlocillin 4 g 2 doses B. mezlocillin 4 g 3 doses	10/61	3/46	
D'Angelo and Sokol (1980)	A. kefzol 1 g, 4 doses, 1 day B. keflex 0.5 g q6h × 5 days	7/24	5/25	
Dashow et al. (1986)	A. cephapirin 2 g irrigation B. cefamandole 2 g irrigation C. moxalactam 2 g irrigation D. ampicillin 2 g irrigation	17/70	8/64	19/79 D: 10/ 70

Table 73.3 Controlled trials of different regimens of prophylactic antibiotic use in caesarean section – *continued*

Trial	Prevalence of febrile morbidity or overall infection Manoeuvre	A	B	C
De Palma et al. (1982)	A. penicillin 5 mil U + gentamyc 1 mg/kg 3 doses post-op B. cefamandole 2 g × 1, 1 g × 2 post-op C. cefamandole 2 g × 3 post-op	23/115	24/82	27/108
Donnenfeld et al. (1986)	A. cefazoline 1 g, 3 doses after cord clamped, 8 and 16 hr B. cefazoline 1 g irrigation	15/51	18/49	
Duff et al. (1987)	A. cefazolin 1 g 1 dose B. cefonicid 1 g 1 dose	18/96	15/103	
Elliott and Flaherty (1986)	A. cefoxitin 2 g, q.i.d. × 2 days B. cefoxitin irrigation C. cefoxitin 2 g q.i.d. × 2 days + irrigation	2/39	3/42	2/38
Elliott et al. (1982)	A. ampicillin 2 g at cord clamping + 1 g × 12 doses B. ampicillin 2 g at cord clamping + 1 g × 2 doses	3/37	15/46	
Ford (1986)	A. piperacillin 2 g 3 doses B. cefoxitin 2 g 3 doses	3/132	12/131	
Fugere et al. (1983)	A. cefoxitin 2 g 3 doses B. cefazolin 1 g 3 doses	1/30	3/30	
Gall and Hill (1987)	A. piperacillin 4 g 1 dose B. piperacillin 2 g 3 doses	8/60	3/56	
Gonen et al. (1986)	A. cefamandole 1 g 6 doses after cord clamped, then q6h B. cefamandole 2 g irrigation	18/107	15/101	
Gonik (1985)	A. cefotaxime 1 g after cord clamped B. cefoxatime 1 g IV, 3 doses after cord clamped, 6 and 12 hr	7/50	10/50	
Gordon et al. (1979)	A. ampicillin 1 g pre-op + 2 doses B. ampicillin 1 g at cord clamp + 2 doses	4/38	3/40	

Table 73.3 Controlled trials of different regimens of prophylactic antibiotic use in caesarean section – *continued*

Trial	Manoeuvre	Prevalence of febrile morbidity or overall infection		
		A	B	C
Hartert et al. (1987)	A. cefonicid 1 g 1 dose IV B. cefoxitin 2 g 4 doses	19/81	9/58	
Hawrylyshyn et al. (1983)	A. cefoxitin 2 g IV, 1 dose B. cefoxitin 2 g IV, 3 doses	8/64	5/60	
Itskovitz et al. (1979)	A. ampicillin 500 mg q.i.d. × 5 days B. cephalothin 1 g q.i.d. × 1 day + C. cephalexin 0.5 g q.i.d. × 4 days	15/50	15/50	8/50
Kreutner et al. (1979)	A. cefalothin 1 g 3 doses B. cefamandole 1 g 3 doses	18/48	12/43	
Levin et al. (1983)	A. cefoxitin 2 g irrigation B. cephapirin 2 g irrigation	3/41	5/44	
McGregor et al. (1986)	A. cefotan 2 g 1 dose at cord clamp B. cefoxatin 2 g IV, 3 doses after cord clamped, 4 and 8 hr	12/46	6/24	
Moodley and Zeeman (1981)	A. lincomycin 0.6 g 7 doses B. metronidazole 0.5 g 7 doses	2/20	5/20	
O'Leary et al. (1986)	A. ampicillin 2 g IV, 8 doses B. ampicillin 2 g IV, 8 doses + gentamycin 1 mg/kg 8 doses	19/61	12/62	
Parsons et al. (1985)	A. cefonamid 1 g 1 dose B. cefoxitin 2 g 5 doses	9/90	9/62	
Rehu and Jahkola (1980)	A. penicillin 10 mil U IV periop B. clindamycin 500 mg IV periop + gentamycin 80 mg pre-op	3/46	4/42	
Roex et al. (1987)	A. cefoxitin 2 g 1 dose B. cefoxitin 2 g + 1 g + 1 g, 3 doses	19/66	11/72	
Saltzman et al. (1986)	A. mezlocillin 4 g 1 dose	3/51	1/51	3/49

Table 73.3 Controlled trials of different regimens of prophylactic antibiotic use in caesarean section – *continued*

Trial	Manoeuvre	Prevalence of febrile morbidity or overall infection		
		A	B	C
	B. mezlocillin 4 g 3 doses C. cefoxitin 2 g 3 doses			
Saravolatz et al. (1985)	A. ceforanide 2 g at cord clamping B. ceforanide 2 g by irrigation	7/34	6/27	
Scarpignato et al. (1982) Mansani et al. (1984)	A. cefuroxime 0.75 g pre-op + 8, 16 hr B. cefuroxime 0.75 g post-op 15 doses in 3 days	0/19	2/20	
Stiver et al. (1983)	A. cefoxitin 2 g 3 doses B. cefazolin 1 g 3 doses	15/124	15/119	
Varner et al. (1986)	A. cefotetan 2 g IV 1 dose after clamp B. cefoxitin 2 g IV 3 doses after cord clamp, 4 and 8 hr	4/20	1/9	

The fact that this body of research is now so large is partly because of the undoubted importance of finding effective means of reducing maternal morbidity after caesarean section; partly due to the relative ease with which trials in this field can be mounted; and partly because of the undoubted commercial interest that exists in encouraging the routine use of antibiotics in association with an operation which continues to be used with increasing frequency (see Chapter 69).

In addition to evaluating the effects of antibiotics versus no antibiotics (Tables 73.1 and 73.2), the reports of relevant controlled trials have involved comparisons of alternative routes of antibiotic administration, different antibiotic drugs, and a variety of dosage schedules (Table 73.3). A majority of the studies has involved only women having unplanned caesarean sections; in a smaller number, the inclusion of women having elective operations has been specified; but in many papers the relation of morbidity to the indications for the operation have not been made clear. The outcome that has been studied most consistently has been 'post-operative febrile morbidity', variously defined by the authors (see above). Useful data is also available on the effect of antibiotic prophylaxis on the rate of serious clinical infections. As used in this chapter 'serious infection' refers to cases of septicaemia, pelvic abscess, general peritonitis, or cases specified by the authors as serious wound infections.

There is very little in the way of usuable information to allow an assessment of the extent to which toxic or allergic effects of antibiotics cause maternal morbidity. Similarly, information on the effects (good or bad) of policies of antibiotic prophylaxis at caesarean section on infants is scant. In the more recent trials, this may be because prophylaxis has been started after the umbilical cord has been clamped. In spite of these limitations, we believe that the information that is available can provide useful guidelines for current practice and future research.

2 Effects of antibiotic prophylaxis

2.1 Effect on risk of serious infection

Although there may be dispute about the clinical relevance of 'post-operative febrile morbidity' as an indicator of the effects of antibiotic prophylaxis in association with caesarean section, any effects on the incidence of serious post-operative infection should be taken seriously. As shown in Table 73.4, there is now overwhelming evidence that antibiotic prophylaxis reduces the risk of such infections (Odds ratio 0.24; CI 0.18–0.32). Not surprisingly, a protective effect of the same order of magnitude is seen when data are tabulated from trials in which endometritis has been specified as an outcome (Table 73.5). Although the size of the reduction in the risk of wound infection may be somewhat less, it is still substantial (Table 73.6). In summary, these protective effects of prophylactic antibiotics on important causes of maternal morbidity are of a degree and consistency across trials which are unlikely to be explained by biases within the studies conducted,

Table 73.4 Effect of prophylactic antibiotics in caesarean section (emergency and elective) on serious infection

Study	EXPT		CTRL		Odds ratio	Graph of odds ratios and confidence intervals
	n	(%)	*n*	(%)	(95% CI)	0.01 0.1 0.5 1 2 10 100
Apuzzio *et al.* (1982)	0/139	(0.00)	0/120	(0.00)	1.00 (1.00–1.00)	
Padilla *et al.* (1983)	1/34	(2.94)	2/37	(5.41)	0.55 (0.06–5.46)	
Gall (1979)	0/46	(0.00)	5/49	(10.20)	0.13 (0.02–0.79)	
Young *et al.* (1983)	2/50	(4.00)	8/50	(16.00)	0.27 (0.07–0.98)	
Stage *et al.* (1982)	0/133	(0.00)	0/66	(0.00)	1.00 (1.00–1.00)	
Ross *et al.* (1984)	0/57	(0.00)	1/58	(1.72)	0.14 (0.00–6.94)	
McCowan and Jackson (1980)	0/35	(0.00)	0/38	(0.00)	1.00 (1.00–1.00)	
Hager and Williamson (1983)	0/43	(0.00)	1/47	(2.13)	0.15 (0.00–7.46)	
Gibbs *et al.* (1981)	1/50	(2.00)	3/50	(6.00)	0.36 (0.05–2.61)	
Duff *et al.* (1982)	0/42	(0.00)	0/40	(0.00)	1.00 (1.00–1.00)	
Fugere *et al.* (1983)	0/60	(0.00)	0/29	(0.00)	1.00 (1.00–1.00)	
Gibbs *et al.* (1973)	0/34	(0.00)	1/34	(2.94)	0.14 (0.00–6.82)	
Gummerus (1984)	3/109	(2.75)	4/110	(3.64)	0.75 (0.17–3.38)	
Moodley and Zeeman (1981)	0/40	(0.00)	0/20	(0.00)	1.00 (1.00–1.00)	
Moro and Andrews (1974)	0/74	(0.00)	0/74	(0.00)	1.00 (1.00–1.00)	
Stiver *et al.* (1983)	1/243	(0.41)	1/111	(0.90)	0.42 (0.02–8.36)	
Work (1977)	0/40	(0.00)	0/40	(0.00)	1.00 (1.00–1.00)	

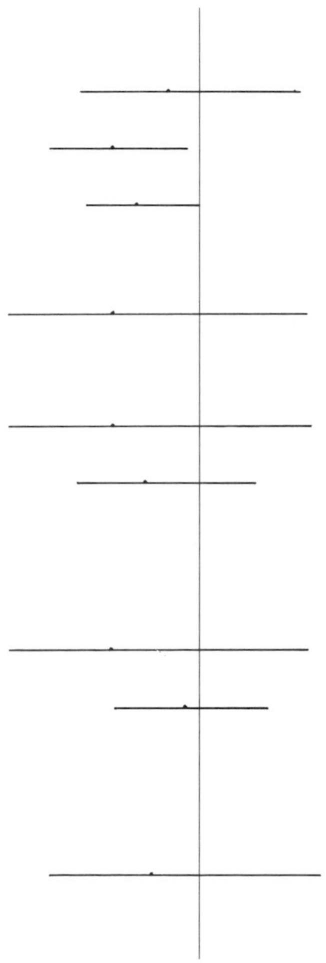

Table 73.4 Effect of prophylactic antibiotics in caesarean section (emergency and elective) on serious infection—*continued*

Study	EXPT n	(%)	CTRL n	(%)	Odds ratio (95% CI)	Graph of odds ratios and confidence intervals
Wong et al. (1978)	1/48	(2.08)	1/45	(2.22)	0.94 (0.06–15.23)	
Rehu and Jahkola (1980)	0/88	(0.00)	0/40	(0.00)	1.00 (1.00–1.00)	
Polk et al. (1982)	3/138	(2.17)	16/128	(12.50)	0.21 (0.08–0.54)	
Phelan and Pruyn (1979)	1/61	(1.64)	1/61	(1.64)	1.00 (0.06–16.17)	
Kreutner et al. (1978)	0/48	(0.00)	2/49	(4.08)	0.14 (0.01–2.19)	
Hawrylyshyn et al. (1983)	0/124	(0.00)	4/58	(6.90)	0.04 (0.00–0.34)	
Harger and English (1981)	0/196	(0.00)	0/190	(0.00)	1.00 (1.00–1.00)	
Saltzman et al. (1985)	0/50	(0.00)	0/49	(0.00)	1.00 (1.00–1.00)	
Karhunen et al. (1985)	2/75	(2.67)	5/77	(6.49)	0.42 (0.09–1.91)	
Gibbs et al. (1972)	1/33	(3.03)	1/28	(3.57)	0.85 (0.05–13.97)	
Tully et al. (1983)	0/45	(0.00)	2/54	(3.70)	0.16 (0.01–2.57)	
Roex et al. (1986)	0/64	(0.00)	0/65	(0.00)	1.00 (1.00–1.00)	
Duff and Park (1980)	0/26	(0.00)	0/31	(0.00)	1.00 (1.00–1.00)	
Kreutner et al. (1979)	3/91	(3.30)	3/29	(10.34)	0.23 (0.03–1.55)	
Elliott et al. (1982)	1/83	(1.20)	0/20	(0.00)	3.46 (0.02–99.99)	
De Palma et al. (1980)	14/209	(6.70)	37/128	(28.91)	0.18 (0.10–0.33)	
Miller and Crichton (1968)	1/150	(0.67)	8/150	(5.33)	0.20 (0.05–0.76)	
D'Angelo and Sokol (1980)	0/49	(0.00)	1/31	(3.23)	0.08 (0.00–4.23)	
Gerstner et al. (1980)	0/53	(0.00)	0/50	(0.00)	1.00 (1.00–1.00)	
Gordon et al. (1979)	0/78	(0.00)	0/36	(0.00)	1.00 (1.00–1.00)	
Scarpignato et al. (1982)	0/39	(0.00)	0/20	(0.00)	1.00 (1.00–1.00)	
Schedvins and Moberg (1986)	0/26	(0.00)	0/27	(0.00)	1.00 (1.00–1.00)	
Morrison et al. (1973)	8/115	(6.96)	31/115	(26.96)	0.24 (0.12–0.48)	
Itskovitz et al. (1979)	1/100	(1.00)	2/50	(4.00)	0.22 (0.02–2.45)	
Adeleye and Osinusi (1981)	5/58	(8.62)	15/48	(31.25)	0.23 (0.09–0.61)	
Rothbard et al. (1975)	0/47	(0.00)	0/53	(0.00)	1.00 (1.00–1.00)	
Typical odds ratio (95% confidence interval)					0.24 (0.18–0.32)	

Graph scale: 0.01 0.1 0.5 1 2 10 100

Table 73.5 Effect of prophylactic antibiotics in caesarean section (emergency and elective) on endometritis

Study	EXPT		CTRL		Odds ratio	Graph of odds ratios and confidence intervals
	n	(%)	*n*	(%)	(95% CI)	0.01 0.1 0.5 1 2 10 100
Apuzzio *et al.* (1982)	28/139	(20.14)	46/120	(38.33)	0.41 (0.24–0.71)	
Padilla *et al.* (1983)	5/34	(14.71)	21/37	(56.76)	0.17 (0.06–0.44)	
Gall (1979)	5/46	(10.87)	7/49	(14.29)	0.74 (0.22–2.46)	
Young *et al.* (1983)	10/50	(20.00)	30/50	(60.00)	0.19 (0.09–0.43)	
Stage *et al.* (1982)	1/133	(0.75)	9/66	(13.64)	0.07 (0.02–0.26)	
Ross *et al.* (1984)	0/57	(0.00)	4/58	(6.90)	0.13 (0.02–0.95)	
McCowan and Jackson (1980)	4/35	(11.43)	5/38	(13.16)	0.85 (0.21–3.42)	
Hager and Williamson (1983)	3/43	(6.98)	10/47	(21.28)	0.32 (0.10–1.03)	
Gibbs *et al.* (1981)	8/50	(16.00)	24/50	(48.00)	0.23 (0.10–0.54)	
Duff *et al.* (1982)	1/42	(2.38)	6/40	(15.00)	0.20 (0.04–0.95)	
Fugere *et al.* (1983)	2/60	(3.33)	2/29	(6.90)	0.44 (0.05–3.69)	
Ganesh *et al.* (1986)	6/29	(20.69)	13/28	(46.43)	0.32 (0.11–0.96)	
Gibbs *et al.* (1973)	6/34	(17.65)	20/34	(58.82)	0.18 (0.07–0.47)	
Gummerus (1984)	7/109	(6.42)	5/110	(4.55)	1.43 (0.45–4.58)	
Moodley and Zeeman (1981)	7/40	(17.50)	4/20	(20.00)	0.85 (0.21–3.36)	
Moro and Andrews (1974)	2/74	(2.70)	12/74	(16.22)	0.21 (0.07–0.63)	
Stiver *et al.* (1983)	8/243	(3.29)	10/111	(9.01)	0.31 (0.11–0.85)	
Tzingounis *et al.* (1982)	4/46	(8.70)	8/50	(16.00)	0.52 (0.15–1.72)	
Work (1977)	8/40	(20.00)	17/40	(42.50)	0.36 (0.14–0.91)	
Wong *et al.* (1978)	14/48	(29.17)	23/45	(51.11)	0.40 (0.18–0.92)	
Rehu and Jahkola (1980)	7/88	(7.95)	13/40	(32.50)	0.16 (0.06–0.44)	
Polk *et al.* (1982)	3/138	(2.17)	12/128	(9.38)	0.26 (0.09–0.74)	
Phelan *et al.* (1979)	5/61	(8.20)	7/61	(11.48)	0.69 (0.21–2.27)	
Kreutner *et al.* (1978)	6/48	(12.50)	11/49	(22.45)	0.51 (0.18–1.43)	
Mawrylyshyn *et al.* (1983)	9/124	(7.26)	17/58	(29.31)	0.17 (0.07–0.41)	
Harger and English (1981)	20/196	(10.20)	38/190	(20.00)	0.47 (0.27–0.81)	
Saltzman *et al.* (1985)	3/50	(6.00)	12/49	(24.49)	0.24 (0.08–0.72)	

Table 73.5 Effect of prophylactic antibiotics in caesarean section (emergency and elective) on endometritis—*continued*

Study	EXPT n	(%)	CTRL n	(%)	Odds ratio (95% CI)	Graph of odds ratios and confidence intervals
					(0.15–0.77)	
Gibbs *et al.* (1972)	7/33	(21.21)	8/28	(28.57)	0.68 (0.21–2.16)	
Tully *et al.* (1983)	3/45	(6.67)	11/54	(20.37)	0.33 (0.11–1.01)	
Roex *et al.* (1986)	2/64	(3.13)	9/65	(13.85)	0.26 (0.07–0.88)	
Dillon *et al.* (1981)	2/46	(4.35)	16/55	(29.09)	0.19 (0.07–0.52)	
Duff and Park (1980)	2/26	(7.69)	13/31	(41.94)	0.18 (0.05–0.57)	
Kreutner *et al.* (1979)	22/91	(24.18)	13/29	(44.83)	0.37 (0.15–0.93)	
Elliott *et al.* (1982)	16/83	(19.28)	10/20	(50.00)	0.20 (0.07–0.61)	
De Palma *et al.* (1980)	25/209	(11.96)	109/128	(85.16)	0.05 (0.03–0.07)	
Miller and Crichton (1968)	1/150	(0.67)	8/150	(5.33)	0.20 (0.05–0.76)	
Gerstner *et al.* (1980)	7/53	(13.21)	15/50	(30.00)	0.37 (0.15–0.95)	
Gordon *et al.* (1979)	6/78	(7.69)	12/36	(33.33)	0.15 (0.05–0.43)	
Scarpignato *et al.* (1982)	2/39	(5.13)	6/20	(30.00)	0.12 (0.03–0.59)	
Schedvins and Moberg (1986)	2/26	(7.69)	9/27	(33.33)	0.22 (0.06–0.81)	
Itskovitz *et al.* (1979)	13/100	(13.00)	14/50	(28.00)	0.36 (0.15–0.88)	
Adeleye and Osinusi (1981)	5/58	(8.62)	15/48	(31.25)	0.23 (0.09–0.61)	
Rothbard *et al.* (1975)	1/47	(2.13)	8/53	(15.09)	0.21 (0.05–0.82)	
Oestreicher *et al.* (1987)	6/30	(20.00)	10/30	(33.33)	0.51 (0.16–1.59)	
Typical odds ratio (95% confidence interval)					0.25 (0.22–0.29)	

Table 73.6 Effect of prophylactic antibiotics in caesarean section (emergency and elective) on wound infection

Study	EXPT		CTRL		Odds ratio	Graph of odds ratios and confidence intervals
	n	(%)	*n*	(%)	(95% CI)	
Apuzzio *et al.* (1982)	2/139	(1.44)	5/120	(4.17)	0.36 (0.08–1.60)	
Padilla *et al.* (1983)	0/34	(0.00)	5/37	(13.51)	0.13 (0.02–0.80)	
Gall (1979)	1/46	(2.17)	4/49	(8.16)	0.30 (0.05–1.83)	
Young *et al.* (1983)	1/50	(2.00)	4/50	(8.00)	0.29 (0.05–1.71)	
Stage *et al.* (1982)	3/133	(2.26)	12/66	(18.18)	0.10 (0.03–0.31)	
Ross *et al.* (1984)	7/57	(12.28)	7/58	(12.07)	1.02 (0.34–3.10)	
McCowan and Jackson. (1980)	9/35	(25.71)	7/38	(18.42)	1.52 (0.51–4.58)	
Hager and Williamson (1983)	1/43	(2.33)	1/47	(2.13)	1.09 (0.07–17.82)	
Gibbs *et al.* (1981)	0/50	(0.00)	2/50	(4.00)	0.13 (0.01–2.15)	
Duff *et al.* (1982)	0/42	(0.00)	0/40	(0.00)	1.00 (1.00–1.00)	
Fugere *et al.* (1983)	1/60	(1.67)	3/29	(10.34)	0.14 (0.02–1.14)	
Gibbs *et al.* (1973)	0/34	(0.00)	5/34	(14.71)	0.12 (0.02–0.73)	
Gummerus (1984)	3/109	(2.75)	5/110	(4.55)	0.60 (0.15–2.46)	
Moodley and Zeeman (1981)	2/40	(5.00)	4/20	(20.00)	0.19 (0.03–1.14)	
Moro and Williamson (1974)	0/74	(0.00)	2/74	(2.70)	0.13 (0.01–2.15)	
Stiver *et al.* (1983)	6/243	(2.47)	17/111	(15.32)	0.12 (0.05–0.30)	
Tzingounis *et al.* (1982)	2/56	(3.57)	4/50	(8.00)	0.44 (0.09–2.27)	
Work (1977)	3/40	(7.50)	1/40	(2.50)	2.83 (0.38–20.86)	
Wong *et al.* (1978)	2/48	(4.17)	3/45	(6.67)	0.61 (0.10–3.70)	
Rehu and Jahkola (1980)	4/88	(4.55)	4/40	(10.00)	0.40 (0.09–1.85)	
Polk *et al.* (1982)	3/138	(2.17)	9/128	(7.03)	0.33 (0.10–1.03)	
Phelan and Pruyn (1979)	2/61	(3.28)	1/61	(1.64)	1.97 (0.20–19.30)	
Kreutner *et al.* (1978)	0/48	(0.00)	2/49	(4.08)	0.14 (0.01–2.19)	
Hawrylyshyn *et al.* (1983)	2/124	(1.61)	2/58	(3.45)	0.43 (0.05–3.57)	
Harger and English (1981)	2/196	(1.02)	14/190	(7.37)	0.20 (0.07–0.55)	
Saltzman *et al.* (1985)	1/50	(2.00)	2/49	(4.08)	0.50 (0.05–4.88)	
Larhunen *et al.* (1985)	9/75	(12.00)	23/77	(29.87)	0.34 (0.16–0.75)	

Graph of odds ratios and confidence intervals scale: 0.01 0.1 0.5 1 2 10 100

Table 73.6 Effect of prophylactic antibiotics in caesarean section (emergency and elective) on wound infection—*continued*

Study	EXPT		CTRL		Odds ratio	Graph of odds ratios and confidence intervals
	n	(%)	n	(%)	(95% CI)	0.01 0.1 0.5 1 2 10 100
Gibbs et al. (1972)	0/33	(0.00)	0/28	(0.00)	1.00 (1.00–1.00)	
Tully et al. (1983)	1/45	(2.22)	2/54	(3.70)	0.61 (0.06–6.03)	
Roex et al. (1986)	1/64	(1.56)	7/65	(10.77)	0.21 (0.05–0.87)	
Duff and Park (1980)	0/26	(0.00)	1/31	(3.23)	0.16 (0.00–8.14)	
Kreutner et al. (1979)	3/91	(3.30)	0/29	(0.00)	3.82 (0.27–54.99)	
Elliott et al. (1982)	1/83	(1.20)	1/20	(5.00)	0.14 (0.00–4.70)	
Miller and Crichton (1968)	13/150	(8.67)	23/150	(15.33)	0.53 (0.27–1.07)	
Gerstner et al. (1980)	3/53	(5.66)	9/50	(18.00)	0.31 (0.09–1.01)	
Gordon et al. (1979)	0/78	(0.00)	1/36	(2.78)	0.04 (0.00–2.86)	
Scarpignato et al. (1982)	0/39	(0.00)	0/20	(0.00)	1.00 (1.00–1.00)	
Schedvins et al. (1986)	2/26	(7.69)	1/27	(3.70)	2.08 (0.21–20.93)	
Itskovitz et al. (1979)	1/100	(1.00)	2/50	(4.00)	0.22 (0.02–2.45)	
Adeleye and Osinusi (1981)	11/58	(18.97)	14/48	(29.17)	0.57 (0.23–1.40)	
Rothbard et al. (1975)	2/47	(4.26)	7/53	(13.21)	0.34 (0.09–1.33)	
Oestreicher et al. (1987)	4/30	(13.33)	17/30	(56.67)	0.15 (0.05–0.44)	
Typical odds ratio (95% confidence interval)					0.35 (0.28–0.44)	

or selective publication of only those studies that have suggested protective effects.

Because the rates of infection associated with unplanned caesarean sections are higher than those following elective operations, the absolute numbers of serious infections avoided by prophylactic administration of antibiotics in association with the former will be greater than those avoided by a similar policy implemented in the latter circumstances. The evidence that is available suggests that prophylactic antibiotics may achieve an order of risk reduction for both endometritis (Table 73.7) and wound infection (Table 73.8) which is at least as great among women having planned operations as that among women having emergency procedures. This conclusion is strengthened by analysis of the larger amount of data that are available in respect of the effects of antibiotic prophylaxis on the risk of post-operative febrile morbidity in women who have had planned caesarean sections (Table 73.9).

2.2 Effect on post–operative febrile morbidity

Although there may be more dispute about the clinical significance of post-operative febrile morbidity than about the importance of the clinical infections discussed above, its higher incidence as an outcome means that it is possible to distinguish effects of antibiotic prophylaxis in smaller, more homogeneous groups of trials.

Tables 73.10 and 73.11 show that the risk of post-operative febrile morbidity is reduced (by a comparable amount) by both broad spectrum penicillins (Odds ratio 0.33; CI 0.26–0.42) and cephalosporins (Odds ratio 0.33; CI 0.29–0.39). The only trial to have assessed the prophylactic effect of trimethoprim and sulphamethoxazole in these circumstances (Ganesh *et al.* 1986) also found a statistically significantly reduced risk of post-operative febrile morbidity, but the confidence interval is wide (Odds ratio 0.32; CI 0.11–0.96).

The most striking risk reduction in post-operative

Table 73.7 Effect of prophylactic antibiotics for elective caesarean section on endometritis

Study	EXPT		CTRL		Odds ratio	Graph of odds ratios and confidence intervals
	n	(%)	*n*	(%)	(95% CI)	0.01 0.1 0.5 1 2 10 100
Gibbs *et al.* (1973)	2/17	(11.76)	3/10	(30.00)	0.31 (0.04–2.25)	
Duff *et al.* (1982)	1/42	(2.38)	6/40	(15.00)	0.20 (0.04–0.95)	
Padilla *et al.* (1983)	4/18	(22.22)	9/17	(52.94)	0.28 (0.07–1.08)	
Phelan and Pruyn (1979)	1/24	(4.17)	2/22	(9.09)	0.45 (0.04–4.61)	
Levin *et al.* (1983)	0/21	(0.00)	2/18	(11.11)	0.11 (0.01–1.81)	
Karhunen *et al.* (1985)	1/26	(3.85)	0/24	(0.00)	6.84 (0.14–99.99)	
Gibbs *et al.* (1972)	0/11	(0.00)	2/13	(15.38)	0.15 (0.01–2.49)	
Duff and Park (1980)	0/15	(0.00)	6/17	(35.29)	0.11 (0.02–0.61)	
Dillon *et al.* (1981)	0/18	(0.00)	4/20	(20.00)	0.13 (0.02–0.98)	
Rothbard *et al.* (1975)	0/16	(0.00)	0/16	(0.00)	1.00 (1.00–1.00)	
Itskovitz *et al.* (1979)	9/33	(27.27)	10/17	(58.82)	0.27 (0.08–0.89)	
Typical odds ratio (95% confidence interval)					0.23 (0.13–0.42)	

Table 73.8 Effect of prophylactic antibiotics for elective caesarean section on wound infection

Study	EXPT		CTRL		Odds ratio	Graph of odds ratios and confidence intervals
	n	(%)	*n*	(%)	(95% CI)	0.01 0.1 0.5 1 2 10 100
Gibbs *et al.* (1973)	0/17	(0.00)	3/10	(30.00)	0.05 (0.00–0.62)	
Padilla *et al.* (1983)	0/18	(0.00)	3/17	(17.65)	0.11 (0.01–1.16)	
Phelan and Pruyn (1979)	0/24	(0.00)	1/22	(4.55)	0.12 (0.00–6.25)	
Gibbs *et al.* (1972)	0/11	(0.00)	2/13	(15.38)	0.15 (0.01–2.49)	
Rothbard *et al.* (1975)	0/16	(0.00)	1/16	(6.25)	0.14 (0.00–6.82)	
Typical odds ratio (95% confidence interval)					0.10 (0.03–0.36)	

Table 73.9 Effect of prophylactic antibiotics for elective caesarean section on febrile morbidity

Study	EXPT		CTRL		Odds ratio	Graph of odds ratios and confidence intervals
	n	(%)	*n*	(%)	(95% CI)	0.01 0.1 0.5 1 2 10 100
Gall (1979)	4/21	(19.05)	7/19	(36.84)	0.42 (0.11–1.65)	
Gibbs *et al.* (1973)	4/17	(23.53)	4/10	(40.00)	0.47 (0.09–2.50)	
Duff *et al.* (1982)	4/42	(9.52)	13/40	(32.50)	0.25 (0.09–0.73)	
Padilla *et al.* (1983)	4/18	(22.22)	9/17	(52.94)	0.28 (0.07–1.08)	
Phelan and Pruyn (1979)	5/24	(20.83)	3/22	(13.64)	1.63 (0.36–7.39)	
Kreutner *et al.* (1978)	2/18	(11.11)	6/23	(26.09)	0.39 (0.08–1.83)	
Levin *et al.* (1983)	0/21	(0.00)	2/18	(11.11)	0.11 (0.01–1.81)	
Karhunen *et al.* (1985)	1/26	(3.85)	1/24	(4.17)	0.92 (0.06–15.20)	
Gibbs *et al.* (1972)	0/11	(0.00)	8/13	(61.54)	0.07 (0.01–0.37)	
Duff and Park (1980)	0/15	(0.00)	6/17	(35.29)	0.11 (0.02–0.61)	
Dillon *et al.* (1981)	1/18	(5.56)	6/20	(30.00)	0.21 (0.04–1.04)	
Parsons *et al.* (1985)	5/47	(10.64)	0/22	(0.00)	4.76 (0.68–33.07)	
Rothbard *et al.* (1975)	0/16	(0.00)	4/16	(25.00)	0.11 (0.01–0.86)	
Itskovitz *et al.* (1979)	9/33	(27.27)	10/17	(58.82)	0.27 (0.08–0.89)	
Typical odds ratio (95% confidence interval)					0.32 (0.21–0.49)	

Table 73.10 Effect of broad spectrum penicillin vs. placebo for caesarean section on post-operative febrile morbidity

Study	EXPT		CTRL		Odds ratio	Graph of odds ratios and confidence intervals
	n	(%)	*n*	(%)	(95% CI)	0.01 0.1 0.5 1 2 10 100
Duff *et al.* (1982)	4/42	(9.52)	13/40	(32.50)	0.25 (0.09–0.73)	
Padilla *et al.* (1983)	5/34	(14.71)	22/37	(59.46)	0.15 (0.06–0.40)	
Apuzzio *et al.* (1982)	44/139	(31.65)	66/120	(55.00)	0.39 (0.24–0.63)	
Duff *et al.* (1980)	7/26	(26.92)	13/31	(41.94)	0.52 (0.18–1.54)	
Elliott *et al.* (1982)	18/83	(21.69)	10/20	(50.00)	0.24 (0.08–0.72)	
Miller *et al.* (1968)	39/150	(26.00)	70/150	(46.67)	0.41 (0.26–0.66)	
Gordon *et al.* (1979)	7/78	(8.97)	14/36	(38.89)	0.14 (0.05–0.38)	

Table 73.10 Effect of broad spectrum penicillin vs. placebo for caesarean section on post-operative febrile morbidity—*continued*

Study	EXPT		CTRL		Odds ratio	Graph of odds ratios and confidence intervals
	n	(%)	*n*	(%)	(95% CI)	0.01 0.1 0.5 1 2 10 100
Adeleye and Osinusi (1981)	12/58	(20.69)	26/48	(54.17)	0.24 (0.11–0.52)	
Itskovitz *et al.* (1979)	15/50	(30.00)	25/50	(50.00)	0.44 (0.20–0.97)	
Oestreicher *et al.* (1987)	6/30	(20.00)	10/30	(33.33)	0.51 (0.16–1.59)	
Typical odds ratio (95% confidence interval)					0.33 (0.26–0.42)	

Table 73.11 Effect of cephalosporins vs. placebo for caesarean section on post-operative febrile morbidity

Study	EXPT		CTRL		Odds ratio	Graph of odds ratios and confidence intervals
	n	(%)	*n*	(%)	(95% CI)	0.01 0.1 0.5 1 2 10 100
Fugere *et al.* (1983)	4/60	(6.67)	7/29	(24.14)	0.20 (0.05–0.77)	
Gall (1979)	8/46	(17.39)	20/49	(40.82)	0.33 (0.14–0.79)	
Gibbs *et al.* (1981)	9/50	(18.00)	27/50	(54.00)	0.21 (0.09–0.48)	
Hager and Williamson (1983)	4/43	(9.30)	13/47	(27.66)	0.31 (0.11–0.87)	
Moro and Andrews (1974)	6/74	(8.11)	20/74	(27.03)	0.27 (0.12–0.64)	
Stage *et al.* (1982)	29/133	(21.80)	25/66	(37.88)	0.45 (0.23–0.86)	
Stiver *et al.* (1983)	30/243	(12.35)	40/111	(36.04)	0.23 (0.13–0.40)	
Tzingounis V *et al.* (1982)	12/46	(26.09)	27/50	(54.00)	0.32 (0.14–0.72)	
Wong *et al.* (1978)	22/48	(45.83)	30/48	(62.50)	0.51 (0.23–1.14)	
Work (1977)	14/40	(35.00)	27/40	(67.50)	0.28 (0.12–0.66)	
Young *et al.* (1983)	12/50	(24.00)	34/50	(68.00)	0.17 (0.08–0.38)	
Conover and Moore (1984)	1/31	(3.23)	8/33	(24.24)	0.18 (0.04–0.73)	
Elliott *et al.* (1986)	2/39	(5.13)	14/39	(35.90)	0.16 (0.05–0.46)	
Harger and English (1981)	26/196	(13.27)	68/190	(35.79)	0.30 (0.19–0.47)	
Hawrylyshyn *et al.* (1983)	17/124	(13.71)	23/58	(39.66)	0.22 (0.10–0.47)	
Creutner *et al.* (1978)	13/48	(27.08)	17/49	(34.69)	0.70 (0.30–1.66)	
Phelan and Pruyn (1979)	11/61	(18.03)	18/61	(29.51)	0.53 (0.23–1.22)	
Polk *et al.* (1982)	23/138	(16.67)	49/128	(38.28)	0.34 (0.20–0.58)	
Saltzman *et al.* (1985)	7/50	(14.00)	16/49	(32.65)	0.36 (0.14–0.90)	

Table 73.11 Effect of cephalosporins vs. placebo for caesarean section on post-operative febrile morbidity—*continued*

Study	EXPT		CTRL		Odds ratio	Graph of odds ratios and confidence intervals						
	n	(%)	n	(%)	(95% CI)	0.01	0.1	0.5	1	2	10	100
Karhunen *et al.* (1985)	11/75	(14.67)	23/77	(29.87)	0.42 (0.20–0.90)							
Dillon *et al.* (1981)	5/46	(10.87)	22/55	(40.00)	0.23 (0.10–0.55)							
Roex *et al.* (1986)	15/64	(23.44)	29/65	(44.62)	0.39 (0.19–0.81)							
Tully *et al.* (1983)	16/45	(35.56)	17/54	(31.48)	1.20 (0.52–2.76)							
Kreutner *et al.* (1979)	30/91	(32.97)	19/29	(65.52)	0.26 (0.11–0.61)							
D'Angelo and Sokol (1980)	12/49	(24.49)	20/31	(64.52)	0.19 (0.08–0.48)							
Scarpignato *et al.* (1982)	2/39	(5.13)	7/20	(35.00)	0.10 (0.02–0.46)							
Schedvins and Moberg (1986)	4/26	(15.38)	13/27	(48.15)	0.23 (0.07–0.72)							
Itskovitz *et al.* (1979)	8/50	(16.00)	25/50	(50.00)	0.22 (0.10–0.50)							
Typical odds ratio (95% confidence interval)					0.31 (0.27–0.36)							

Table 73.12 Effect of broad spectrum penicillin + aminoglycoside vs. placebo for caesarean section on post-operative febrile morbidity

Study	EXPT		CTRL		Odds ratio	Graph of odds ratios and confidence intervals						
	n	(%)	n	(%)	(95% CI)	0.01	0.1	0.5	1	2	10	100
Gibbs *et al.* (1973)	8/34	(23.53)	22/34	(64.71)	0.19 (0.07–0.50)							
Rehu and Jahkola (1980)	7/88	(7.95)	13/40	(32.50)	0.16 (0.06–0.44)							
Gibbs *et al.* (1972)	9/33	(27.27)	17/28	(60.71)	0.26 (0.09–0.72)							
De Palma *et al.* (1980)	25/209	(11.96)	109/128	(85.16)	0.05 (0.03–0.07)							
Morrison *et al.* (1973)	25/115	(21.74)	59/115	(51.30)	0.28 (0.16–0.48)							
Rothbard *et al.* (1975)	6/47	(12.77)	23/53	(43.40)	0.23 (0.10–0.54)							
Typical odds ratio (95% confidence interval)					0.13 (0.10–0.17)							

febrile morbidity (Odds ratio 0.13; CI 0.10–0.17) was achieved when a combination of broad spectrum penicillins and aminoglycosides were used for prophylaxis (Table 73.12). The magnitude of the difference in effectiveness suggested by these indirect comparisons is not seen in direct comparisons however (see below).

There is currently no good evidence that the antiprotozoal drug metronidazole reduces the risk of post-operative febrile morbidity following caesarean section (Table 73.13). Even if the drug reduced the risk by as much as the lower boundary of the 95 per cent Confidence interval associated with the typical Odds ratio (0.48), it would still not be as effective as the antibiotics discussed above.

Table 73.13 Effect of metronidazole vs. placebo for caesarean section on post-operative febrile morbidity

Study	EXPT n	(%)	CTRL n	(%)	Odds ratio (95% CI)	Graph of odds ratios and confidence intervals
Ross *et al.* (1984)	6/57	(10.53)	9/58	(15.52)	0.65 (0.22–1.91)	
Gummerus (1984)	16/109	(14.68)	16/110	(14.55)	1.01 (0.48–2.14)	
McCowan and Jackson (1980)	18/35	(51.43)	16/38	(42.11)	1.45 (0.58–3.61)	
Moodley and Zeeman (1981)	7/40	(17.50)	4/20	(20.00)	0.85 (0.21–3.36)	
Gerstner *et al.* (1980)	16/53	(30.19)	30/50	(60.00)	0.30 (0.14–0.66)	
Typical odds ratio (95% confidence interval)					0.72 (0.48–1.08)	

3 Choice of antibiotic preparation

Studies comparing different antibiotic preparations can be divided into two groups: those comparing broad spectrum penicillins with cephalosporins, and those comparing a combination of broad spectrum penicillins and aminoglycosides with broad spectrum penicillins used alone. The evidence from trials in which broad spectrum penicillins and cephalosporins have been compared directly suggest that they have similar effects (Odds ratio 0.93; CI 0.62–1.39) on the risk of post-operative febrile morbidity (Table 73.14), a finding which supports the inferences based on the indirect comparisons derived from the placebo-controlled trials of the two classes of antibiotic (Tables 73.10 and 73.11).

The indirect comparisons of the placebo-controlled trials comparing a combination of broad spectrum antibiotics and aminoglycosides with broad spectrum antibiotics used alone suggested that the combination might be a more effective prophylactic (Tables 73.10 and 73.12). The results of trials in which direct compar-isons between the two regimens were made pointed in the same direction (Table 73.15), but the evidence is not sufficiently strong to warrant adoption of a regimen that is more complicated (and costly) and associated with increased risks of ototoxicity and nephrotoxicity caused by the aminoglycosides (Goodman *et al.* 1980).

4 Timing, dose, and frequency of administration

Although there is no suggestion from the available data that larger doses of antibiotics achieve prophylaxis more successfully than smaller doses (Table 73.16), the confidence interval surrounding the point estimate of 0.78 is wide and may mask a clinically important difference. The data do, however, suggest that relatively short courses of antibiotics are less effective than longer courses (Table 73.17), and that single-dose regimens are less effective than multiple-dose regimens (Table 73.18).

Table 73.14 Effect of broad spectrum penicillin vs. cephalosporins for caesarean section on post-operative febrile morbidity

Study	EXPT n	(%)	CTRL n	(%)	Odds ratio (95% CI)	Graph of odds ratios and confidence intervals
Saltzman *et al.* (1986)	1/51	(1.96)	3/49	(6.12)	0.34 (0.05–2.50)	
Benigno *et al.* (1986)	35/136	(25.74)	37/147	(25.17)	1.03 (0.60–1.76)	
Ford (1986)	3/132	(2.27)	12/131	(9.16)	0.28 (0.10–0.79)	
Itskovitz *et al.* (1979)	15/50	(30.00)	23/100	(23.00)	1.44 (0.66–3.14)	
Typical odds ratio (95% confidence interval)					0.89 (0.60–1.32)	

Table 73.15 Effect of aminoglycoside + broad spectrum penicillin vs. broad spectrum penicillin alone for caesarean section on post-operative febrile morbidity

Study	EXPT		CTRL		Odds ratio	Graph of odds ratios and confidence intervals
	n	(%)	n	(%)	(95% CI)	0.01 0.1 0.5 1 2 10 100
Rehu and Jahkola (1980)	4/42	(9.52)	3/46	(6.52)	1.50 (0.32–6.98)	
De Palma *et al.* (1982)	23/115	(20.00)	51/190	(26.84)	0.69 (0.40–1.18)	
O'Leary *et al.* (1986)	12/62	(19.35)	19/61	(31.15)	0.54 (0.24–1.21)	
Typical odds ratio (95% confidence interval)					0.68 (0.44–1.05)	

Table 73.16 Effect of smaller vs larger doses of prophylactic antibiotics for caesarean section on post-operative febrile morbidity

Study	EXPT		CTRL		Odds ratio	Graph of odds ratios and confidence intervals
	n	(%)	n	(%)	(95% CI)	0.01 0.1 0.5 1 2 10 100
Fugere *et al.* (1983)	3/30	(10.00)	1/30	(3.33)	2.87 (0.38–21.44)	
Stiver *et al.* (1983)	15/119	(12.61)	15/124	(12.10)	1.05 (0.49–2.25)	
De Palma *et al.* (1982)	24/82	(29.27)	27/108	(25.00)	1.24 (0.65–2.37)	
Typical odds ratio (95% confidence interval)					1.22 (0.75–1.97)	

Table 73.17 Effect of shorter vs. longer courses of prophylactic antibiotics for caesarean section on post-operative febrile morbidity

Study	EXPT		CTRL		Odds ratio	Graph of odds ratios and confidence intervals
	n	(%)	n	(%)	(95% CI)	0.01 0.1 0.5 1 2 10 100
Crombleholme *et al.* (1987)	10/61	(16.39)	3/46	(6.52)	2.50 (0.78–8.02)	
Elliott *et al.* (1982)	15/46	(32.61)	3/37	(8.11)	4.16 (1.46–11.81)	
D'Angelo *et al.* (1980)	7/24	(29.17)	5/25	(20.00)	1.63 (0.45–5.90)	
Scarpignato *et al.* (1982)	0/19	(0.00)	2/20	(10.00)	0.13 (0.01–2.24)	
Itskovitz *et al.* (1979)	15/50	(30.00)	8/50	(16.00)	2.19 (0.87–5.53)	
Typical odds ratio (95% confidence interval)					2.29 (1.34–3.89)	

Table 73.18 Effect of single vs. multiple doses of antibiotics for caesarean section on post-operative febrile morbidity

Study	EXPT		CTRL		Odds ratio	Graph of odds ratios and confidence intervals
	n	(%)	*n*	(%)	(95% CI)	0.01　0.1　0.5　1　2　10　100
McGregor *et al.* (1986)	12/46	(26.09)	6/24	(25.00)	1.06 (0.34–3.25)	
Saltzman *et al.* (1986)	3/51	(5.88)	4/100	(4.00)	1.53 (0.31–7.55)	
Hawrylyshyn *et al.* (1983)	8/64	(12.50)	5/60	(8.33)	1.55 (0.49–4.88)	
Roex *et al.* (1987)	19/66	(28.79)	11/72	(15.28)	2.20 (0.98–4.93)	
Gall and hill (1987)	8/60	(13.33)	3/56	(5.36)	2.51 (0.73–8.66)	
Gonik (1985)	7/50	(14.00)	10/50	(20.00)	0.66 (0.23–1.85)	
Varner *et al.* (1986)	4/20	(20.00)	1/9	(11.11)	1.82 (0.24–14.13)	
Hartert *et al.* (1987)	19/81	(23.46)	9/58	(15.52)	1.63 (0.71–3.77)	
Parsons *et al.* (1985)	9/90	(10.00)	9/62	(14.52)	0.65 (0.24–1.76)	
Typical odds ratio (95% confidence interval)					1.36 (0.95–1.95)	

Table 73.19 Effect of antibiotic irrigation vs. placebo at caesarean section on post-operative febrile morbidity

Study	EXPT		CTRL		Odds ratio	Graph of odds ratios and confidence intervals
	n	(%)	*n*	(%)	(95% CI)	0.01　0.1　0.5　1　2　10　100
Bourgeois *et al.* (1985)	5/73	(6.85)	48/150	(32.00)	0.25 (0.13–0.48)	
Dashow *et al.* (1986)	54/283	(19.08)	22/77	(28.57)	0.57 (0.31–1.05)	
Long *et al.* (1980)	0/30	(0.00)	15/60	(25.00)	0.17 (0.05–0.54)	
Conover *et al.* (1984)	9/37	(24.32)	6/23	(26.09)	0.91 (0.28–3.00)	
Elliott *et al.* (1986)	3/42	(7.14)	14/39	(35.90)	0.18 (0.06–0.52)	
Levin *et al.* (1983)	8/85	(9.41)	11/43	(25.58)	0.28 (0.10–0.79)	
Kellum *et al.* (1985)	16/84	(19.05)	141/178	(79.21)	0.08 (0.05–0.14)	
Typical odds ratio (95% confidence interval)					0.22 (0.17–0.30)	

Table 73.20 Effect of systemic antibiotics vs. antibiotic peritoneal irrigation for caesarean section on post-operative febrile morbidity

Study	EXPT		CTRL		Odds ratio	Graph of odds ratios and confidence intervals
	n	(%)	*n*	(%)	(95% CI)	0.01 0.1 0.5 1 2 10 100
Boothby *et al.* (1984)	2/50	(4.00)	2/53	(3.77)	1.06 (0.15–7.77)	
Conover and Moore (1984)	1/31	(3.23)	9/37	(24.32)	0.19 (0.05–0.73)	
Elliott *et al.* (1986)	2/39	(5.13)	3/42	(7.14)	0.71 (0.12–4.29)	
Saravolatz *et al.* (1985)	7/34	(20.59)	6/27	(22.22)	0.91 (0.27–3.09)	
Gonen *et al.* (1986)	18/107	(16.82)	15/101	(14.85)	1.16 (0.55–2.43)	
Donnenfeld *et al.* (1986)	15/51	(29.41)	18/49	(36.73)	0.72 (0.31–1.65)	
Typical odds ratio (95% confidence interval)					0.77 (0.50–1.21)	

5 Route of administration

Intra-operative irrigation with antibiotics is known to be more effective than irrigation with placebo in reducing the risk of post-operative febrile morbidity (Odds ratio 0.22; CI 0.17–0.30) (Table 73.19), and indirect comparisons suggest that this route of administration may be as effective (and possibly more effective) than systemic administration. Evidence from direct comparisons of the two routes of administration, however, provides no strong evidence that one route of administration is superior to the other (Table 73.20).

6 Potential adverse consequences of antibiotic prophylaxis

The evidence reviewed above suggests that the ambivalence that has been expressed in the past about the efficacy of antibiotic prophylaxis for caesarean section (*British Medical Journal* 1973; Mead 1977) is no longer appropriate. It is clear that effective means of reducing important post-operative morbidity are available, morbidity that can be very distressing to the women involved (National Childbirth Trust 1988). Our impression is that prophylactic use of antibiotics in association with caesarean section has been adopted more widely in North America than in many other parts of the world: the results of two fairly recent surveys conducted in England and Wales and Denmark, for example, suggest that antibiotic prophylaxis is used in only a small minority of women undergoing caesarean section in those countries (Moir-Bussy *et al.* 1984; Pelle *et al.* 1986). This reluctance to adopt antibiotic prophylaxis for caesarean section may reflect a lack of aware-

ness of the strength of the accumulated evidence that this policy can lead to a substantial reduction in the incidence of post-operative morbidity. It may also reflect concerns about possible adverse effects of antibiotic prophylaxis on the mother, the baby, or ecologically, by altering commensal bacterial flora or by promoting the emergence of drug resistant pathogens.

As we noted earlier, only a minority of the reports included information about adverse effects of the prophylactic agents used, and even in these reports the reference was usually rather casual, for example, that 'no adverse reactions were noted'. In those reports in which there was some sort of allusion to adverse reactions, there was generally no description of how they were sought, by whom and for how long. It is perhaps not surprising, therefore, that when it was estimated at all, the reported incidence of adverse reactions was very low—1 per cent or less. This is well below the rate of adverse reactions that one would expect of antibiotics, especially broad spectrum antibiotics given intravenously (Hemminki 1981). Like Duff (1987), we have not encountered any reports of serious maternal side-effects of antibiotic prophylaxis for caesarean section although there are case reports of at least two deaths from anaphylaxis in patients who received intra-operative injections of cephalothin during non-obstetric surgical procedures (Spruill *et al.* 1974). It is worth recalling that, in the 1950s, Posner *et al.* (1956) wrote that 'the ease of administration and the paucity of side reactions make tetracycline an ideal agent for the management of certain obstetric complications'. Now that the hepatotoxicity of tetracycline during pregnancy and its effects on the development of fetal teeth have been recognized it is easy to condemn the recommendation. To what extent is the apparent safety of the antibiotics used in more recent studies simply an indication of similar lack of knowledge?

Drug effects on the infant (which might include protective as well as unwanted effects) have not been studied systematically by the majority of investigators. In 1979, Gordon and his colleagues noted that, prior to their investigation, 'none of the reports had studied immediate or delayed neonatal infections, length of nursery stay, or even whether the antibiotics were continued in the nursery'. The study conducted by Gordon *et al.* (1979) was important because, although other evidence suggests that antibiotic prophylaxis for surgery should begin before the skin is incised (Pollock 1988), they were unable to detect any loss of effectiveness of ampicillin prophylaxis when administration of the drug was delayed until after the umbilical cord had been clamped. Although their trial was not large enough to exclude the possibility of an important decline in efficacy as a result of delaying administration of the drug in this way, their conclusions were subsequently supported by the results of a large non-randomized cohort study (Cunningham *et al.* 1983).

Preventing exposure of the baby to antibiotics by starting them after the umbilical cord has been clamped would seem to be a sensible precaution, even if there is some slight, as yet undetected, loss of prophylactic efficacy. Not only will babies be spared any unwanted effects of drugs that have crossed the placenta; they will also be spared the intensive investigations and neonatal administration of antibiotics which many paediatricians feel are mandatory because they are concerned that intrapartum fetal exposure to antibiotics may suppress microbial growth and thus mask neonatal sepsis (Cunningham *et al.* 1983).

Antibiotics received by the mother can also reach the baby through breast milk. The drug levels involved seem likely to be very low, particularly if the course of prophylactic antibiotics has been relatively short (Roex *et al.* 1987).

An important argument of those who have objected to routine antibiotic prophylaxis has been their concern about the effects of this practice on the bacterial flora: eradication of non-pathogenic bacteria giving way to pathogenic ones and a rise in resistance of bacteria in treated patients and in the hospital environment generally (Mead 1977; Chodak and Plant 1977; 1978). At least some antibiotics appear to cause these changes with relatively few doses (see Gibbs and Weinstein 1976; Gibbs *et al.* 1981; Stiver *et al.* 1984). Galask (1987), for example, showed in a placebo-controlled trial of a cephalosporin that although drug treatment was associated with a reduction in cultures positive for anaerobic gram-negative rods overall, there was an increase in the subgroup of cephalosporin-resistant organisms. There is some suggestion that certain prophylactic regimens—for example, trimethoprim and sulfamethoxazole (Ganesh *et al.* 1986)—may be less disruptive of flora yet remain effective.

7 Conclusions

7.1 Implications for current practice

The first step that should be taken to reduce the infectious morbidity that is so common following caesarean section is to minimise the numbers of unnecessary operations (see Chapters 69 and 70). The second step requires attention to the variety of factors that reduce the risk of infection following justified use of the operation. These include minimizing the length of hospital admission prior to surgery; delaying shaving of the operation site until immediately before the operation; sterilizing swabs and instruments, the hands of the operating team, the skin of the patient, and the air of the operating theatre (Pollock 1988); and paying attention to good surgical technique (see Chapter 72).

Decisions about whether or not to institute a policy of antibiotic prophylaxis should no longer depend on uncertainties about whether reductions in the risks of serious infections can be achieved in this way: they can. If the level of post-caesarean infectious morbidity is very low without a policy of antibiotic prophylaxis, the ratio of benefits to costs, in absolute terms, might argue against instituting such a policy. We think that such circumstances are rare and that the evidence we have reviewed justifies far wider adoption of antibiotic prophylaxis than currently exists. Although the incidence of adverse drug effects among women receiving prophylactic antibiotics seems very likely to have been underestimated in the body of literature we have reviewed, it is inconceivable that it could outweigh the reduction in serious maternal morbidity which can be achieved by a policy of antibiotic prophylaxis. Adverse drug effects in the baby can be lessened by beginning prophylaxis after the umbilical cord has been divided.

Adverse ecological effects on bacterial flora are more difficult to quantify and predict, but are potentially of greater concern than adverse drug reactions in individual mothers and babies. If prophylactic antibiotics are used routinely, genital tract cultures and drug sensitivity studies should be performed in all the women who become infected despite receiving prophylaxis, and the hospital bacteriology laboratory should conduct a periodic review of the susceptibility patterns of commonly isolated organisms to detect gradual changes in antibiotic resistance (Duff 1987).

The risk of these adverse ecological effects is likely to be reduced if the total load of antibiotics is reduced. Had our analysis suggested that single dose or short regimens were as effective as multiple dose or longer regimens, we would have been able to endorse the recommendations of others that the simpler regimens should be adopted. Their conclusions, however, seem likely to have been based on samples of insufficient size to exclude a clinically important advantage of the multiple dose and the longer regimens. Even so, the disadvantages of longer courses of antibiotics in terms of the resulting increase in the total antibiotic load, the numbers of women experiencing side effects, and the additional cost in financial terms may actually outweigh the advantages of their greater prophylactic efficacy relative to shorter or single-dose regimens (Freire *et al.* in press).

As far as choice of antibiotic is concerned, the broad spectrum penicillins are as effective as the cephalosporins. No strong case for adding aminoglycosides to broad spectrum penicillins can be made; on the basis of current evidence any increase in effectiveness which may result is likely to be marginal and would add the risk of otoxicity and nephrotoxicity associated with these drugs. Metronidazole currently has no place in antibiotic prophylaxis for caesarean section because there is no convincing evidence that it is effective.

7.2 Implications for future research

It is clear that withholding prophylactic antibiotics from women having caesarean section will increase the chances that they will experience serious morbidity, albeit rarely. The available evidence thus argues against inclusion of no-treatment controls in controlled trials of antibiotic prophylaxis associated with caesarean section, as it does in respect of antibiotic prophylaxis for other kinds of surgery (Baum *et al.* 1981). Those who wish to mount further trials with no-treatment controls, to quantify adverse effects more satisfactorily than is possible using the available data, will need to ensure that the women participating in such trials are aware of the evidence supporting the use of prophylactic antibiotics in association with caesarean section.

There is considerable scope for mounting very large trials to assess how long antibiotics must be administered to achieve worthwhile reductions in postpartum morbidity, while at the same time minimizing total antibiotic load and side-effects. The identification of prophylactic regimens that decrease morbidity without altering commensal bacterial flora would represent an important advance. Such trials should conduct longer term follow-up than has been usual in the research conducted in this field.

Concern continues to exist that the known beneficial effects of prophylactic antibiotics may be outweighed either by adverse ecological effects, or by unwanted long term effects on either mothers or breastfed babies, or both. These postulated disadvantages could be sought either by using non-experimental, epidemiological studies, or controlled trials using hospitals or hospital departments as the experimental units.

References

Adeleye JA, Osinusi BO (1981). The use of prophylactic antibiotics in caesarean sections. Singapore J Obstet Gynaecol, 12: 29–34.

Apuzzio JJ, Reyelt C, Pelosi M, Sen P, Louria DB (1982). Prophylactic antibiotics for cesarean section: comparison of high- and low-risk patients for endomyometritis. Obstet Gynecol, 59: 693–698.

Baum ML, Anish DS, Chalmers TC, Sacks HS, Smith H, Fagerstrom RM (1981). A survey of clinical trials of antibiotic prophylaxis in colon surgery: evidence against further use of no-treatment controls. New Engl J Med, 305: 795–799.

Benigno BB, Ford LC, Lawrence WD, Ledger WJ, Ling FW, McNeeley SG (1986). A double-blind, controlled comparison of piperacillin and cefoxitin in the prevention of postoperative infection in patients undergoing cesarean section. Surg Gynecol Obstet, 162: 1–7.

Boothby R, Benrubi G, Ferrell E (1984). Comparison of intravenous cefoxitin prophylaxis with intraoperative cefoxitin irrigation for the prevention of post-cesarean-section endometritis. J Reprod Med, 29: 830–2.

Bourgeois FJ, Pinkerton JA, Andersen W, Thiagarajah S (1985). Antibiotic irrigation prophylaxis in the high-risk cesarean section patient. Am J Obstet Gynecol, 153: 197–201.

Chodak GW, Plant ME (1977). Use of systemic antibiotics for prophylaxis in surgery. Arch Surg, 112: 326–334.

Chodak GW, Plant ME (1978). Wound infections and systemic antibiotic prophylaxis in gynecologic surgery: a review. Obstet Gynecol, 51: 123–127.

Conover WB, Moore TR (1984). Comparison of irrigation and intravenous antibiotic prophylaxis at cesarean section. Obstet Gynecol, 63: 787–791.

Crombleholme WR, Green JR, Ohm-Smith M, Dahrouge D, De Kay V, Rideout A, Sweet RL (1987). Cesarean section prophylaxis: comparison of two doses with three doses of mezlocillin. Am J Reprod Immunol Microbiol, 13: 71–75.

Cunningham FG, Hauth JC, Strong JD, Kappus SS (1978). Infectious morbidity following cesarean section. Obstet Gynecol, 52: 656–661.

Cunningham FG, Leveno KJ, DePalma RT, Roark M, Rosenfeld CR (1983). Perioperative antimicrobials for cesarean delivery: before or after cord clamping? Obstet Gynecol, 62: 151–154.

D'Angelo LJ, Sokol RJ (1980). Short- vs long-course prophylactic antibiotic treatment in cesarean section patients. Obstet Gynecol, 55: 583–586.

Dashow EE, Read JA, Coleman FH (1986). Randomized comparison of five irrigation solutions at cesarean section. Obstet Gynccol, 68: 473–478.

De Palma RT, Leveno KJ, Cunningham FG, Pope T, Kappus SS, Roark ML, Nobles BJ (1980). Identification and management of women at high risk for pelvic infection following cesarean section. Obstet Gynecol, 55: 185S–192S.

De Palma RT, Cunningham FG, Leveno KJ, Roark ML (1982). Continuing investigation of women at high risk for infection following cesarean delivery. Obstet Gynecol, 60: 53–59.

Dillon WP, Seigel MS, Lele AS, O'Leary JA (1981). Evaluation of cefoxitin prophylaxis for cesarean section. Int J Gynaecol Obstet, 19: 133–139.

Donnenfeld AE, Otis C, Weiner S (1986). Antibiotic prophylaxis in cesarean section. Comparison of intrauterine lavage and intravenous administration. J Reprod Med, 31: 15–18.

Duff P (1987). Prophylactic antibiotics for cesarean delivery: a simple cost-effective strategy for prevention of postoperative morbidity. Am J Obstet Gynecol, 157: 794–798.

Duff P, Park RC (1980). Antibiotic prophylaxis for cesarean section in a military population. Milit Med, 145: 377–381.

Duff P, Smith PN, Keiser JF (1982). Antibiotic prophylaxis in low-risk cesarean section. J Reprod Med, 27: 133–138.

Duff P, Robertson AW, Read JA (1987). Single-dose cefazolin vs cefonicid for antibiotic prophylaxis in cesarean delivery. Obstet Gynecol, 70: 718–721.

Editorial (1973). Prophylactic antibiotics in cesarean section. Br Med J, 2: 675–676.

Elliott JP, Flaherty JF (1986). Comparison of lavage or intravenous antibiotics at cesarean section. Obstet Gynecol, 67: 29–32.

Elliott JP, Freeman RK, Dorchester W (1982). Short vs long course of prophylactic antibiotics in cesarean section. Am J Obstet Gynecol, 143: 740–724.

Ford LC (1986). Cost of antibiotic prophylaxis in cesarean section. Drug Intell Clin Pharm, 20: 592–593.

Ford LC, Hammil HA, Lebherz TB (1987). Cost-effective use of antibiotic prophylaxis for cesarean section. Am J Obstet Gynecol, 157: 506–510.

Freire JM, Stachenko S, Fonberg E, Berlin J, Chalmers TC (in press). Meta-analysis of the evidence comparing single versus conventional treatment in lower urinary tract infections in adult women using amoxicillin and trimethoprim-sulfamethoxazole.

Fugere P, Turgeon P, Boucher M, Verschelden G, Lemay M (1983). Use of cephalosporins in antibiotic prophylaxis in women undergoing non-elective caesarean section. Can Med Assoc J, 129: 132–135.

Galask RP (1987). Changing concepts in obstetric antibiotic prophylaxis. Am J Obstet Gynecol, 157: 491–497.

Gall SA (1979). The efficacy of prophylactic antibiotics in caesarean section. Am J Obstet Gynecol, 134: 506–511.

Gall SA, Hill GB (1987). Single-dose vs multiple-dose piperacillin prophylaxis in primary cesarean operation. Am J Obstet Gynecol, 157: 502–506.

Ganesh V, Apuzzio JJ, Dispenziere B, Patel K, Bergen B, Louria DB (1986). Single-dose trimethoprim-sulfamethoxazole prophylaxis for cesarean section. Am J Obstet Gynecol, 154: 1113–1114.

Gerstner G, Kofler E, Huber J (1980). Perioperative metronidazol-prophylaxis for cesarean section. Z Geburtsh Perinatol, 184: 418–423.

Gibbs RS, Weinstein AJ (1976). Bacteriologic effects of prophylactic antibiotics in cesarean section. Am J Obstet Gynecol, 126: 226–229.

Gibbs RS, De Cherney AH, Schwarz RH (1972). Prophylactic antibiotics in cesarean section: a double-blind study. Am J Obstet Gynecol, 114: 1048–1053.

Gibbs RS, Hunt JE, Schwarz RH (1973). A follow-up study on prophylactic antibiotics in cesarean section. Am J Obstet Gynecol, 117: 419–422.

Gibbs RS, St Clair PJ, Castillo MS, Castaneda YS (1981).

Bacteriologic effects of antibiotic prophylaxis in high-risk cesarean section. Obstet Gynecol, 57: 277–282.

Gonen R, Samberg I, Levinski R, Levitan Z, Sharf M (1986). Effect of irrigation or intravenous antibiotic prophylaxis on infectious morbidity at cesarean section. Obstet Gynecol, 67: 545–548.

Gonik B (1985). Single- vs three-dose cefotaxime prophylaxis for cesarean section. Obstet Gynecol, 65: 189–193.

Goodman AG, Goodman LS, Gilman A (1980). The Pharmacological Basis of Therapeutics (6th edn). New York: Macmillan.

Gordon HR, Phelps D, Blanchard K (1979). Prophylactic cesarean section antibiotics: maternal and neonatal morbidity before or after cord clamping. Obstet Gynecol, 53: 151–156.

Gummerus M (1984). Perioperative short-term prophylaxis of puerperal infections following caesarean section with metronidazol. Geburtshilfe Frauenheilkd, 44: 570–572.

Hager WD, Williamson MM (1983). Effects of antibiotic prophylaxis on women undergoing non-elective cesarean section in a community hospital. J Reprod Med, 28: 687–690.

Harger JH, English DH (1981). Selection of patients for antibiotic prophylaxis in cesarean sections. Am J Obstet Gynecol, 141: 752–758.

Hartert RA, Benrubi G, Thompson RJ, Nuss RC (1987). Cefonicid vs cefoxitin for cesarean section prophylaxis. J Reprod Med, 32: 907–910.

Hawrylyshyn PA, Bernstein EP, Papsin FR (1983). Short-term antibiotic prophylaxis in high-risk patients following cesarean section. Am J Obstet Gynecol, 145: 285–289.

Hemminki E (1981). Adverse reactions to antibiotic drugs—the present scope of the problem in outpatient care and possibilities for improvement. Int J Health Serv, 11: 282–301.

Hesseltine HC, Thelen C (1946). Sulfonamides as a prophylactic agent in conjunction with cesarean section. Am J Obstet Gynecol, 52: 813–816.

Hughes EC (1972). Obstetric–Gynecoligic Terminology. Philadelphia: F A Davis, p 402.

Itskovitz J, Paldi E, Katz M (1979). The effect of prophylactic antibiotics on febrile morbidity following cesarean section. Obstet Gynecol, 53: 162–165.

Karhunen M, Koskela O, Teisala K, Suikkari AM, Mattila J (1985). Prophylaxis and treatment of anaerobic infections following caesarean section with tinidazole. Chemotherapy, 31: 228–236.

Keettel WC, Plass ED (1950). Prophylactic administration of penicillin to obstetric patients. JAMA, 142: 324–328.

Kellum RB, Roberts WE, Harris JB, Khansur N, Morrison JC (1985). Effect of intrauterine antibiotic lavage after cesarean birth on postoperative morbidity. J Reprod Med, 30: 527–529.

Kreutner AK, Del Bene VE, Delamar D, Huguley V, Harmon PM, Mitchell KS (1978). Perioperative antibiotic prophylaxis in cesarean section. Obstet Gynecol, 52: 279–284.

Kreutner AK, Del Bene VE, Delamar D, Bodden JL, Loadholt CB (1979). Perioperative cephalosporin prophylaxis in cesarean section: effect on endometritis in the high-risk patient. Am J Obstet Gynecol, 134: 925–935.

Ledger WJ, Kriewall TJ (1973). The fever index: a quantitative indirect measure of hospital acquired infections in obstetrics and gynecology. Am J Obstet Gynecol, 115: 514–520.

Levin DK, Gorchels C, Andersen R (1983). Reduction of post-cesarean section infectious morbidity by means of antibiotic irrigation. Am J Obstet Gynecol, 147: 273–277.

Long WH, Rudd EG Dillon MB (1980). Intrauterine irrigation with cefamandole nafate solution at cesarean section: a preliminary report. Am J Obstet Gynecol, 138: 755–758.

Mansani FE, Caltabiano M, Condemi V, Scarpignato C (1984). Short- or long-term antibiotic prophylaxis in obstetrical and gynecological surgery? Acta Biomed Ateneo Parmense, 55: 147–151.

McCowan L, Jackson P (1980). The prophylactic use of metronidazole in caesarean section. NZ Med J, 92: 153–155.

McGregor JA, French JI, Makowski E (1986). Single-dose cefotetan versus multidose cefoxitin for prophylaxis in cesarean section in high-risk patients. Am J Obstet Gynecol, 154: 955–960.

Mead PB (1977). Prophylactic antibiotics and antibiotic resistance. Seminars Perinatol, 1: 101–111.

Miller RD, Crichton D (1968). Ampicillin prophylaxis in caesarean section. S Afr J Obstet Gynaecol, 6: 69–70.

Moir-Bussy BR, Hutton RM, Thompson JR (1984). Wound infection after caesarean section. J Hosp Infect, 5: 359–370.

Moodley J, Zeeman DJ (1981). Prophylactic and antimicrobial therapy using lincomycin in patients undergoing emergency caesarean section. S Afr Med J, 59: 911–913.

Moro M, Andrews M (1974). Prophylactic antibiotics in cesarean section. Obstet Gynecol, 44: 688–692.

Morrison JC, Coxwell WL, Kennedy BS, Schreier PC, Wiser WL, Fish SA (1973). The use of prophylactic antibiotics in patients undergoing cesarean section. Surg Gynecol Obstet, 136: 425–428.

National Childbirth Trust (1988). Postnatal Infection. London: National Childbirth Trust.

O'Leary JA, Mullins JH, Andrinopoulos GC (1986). Ampicillin vs ampicillin–gentamicin prophylaxis in high-risk primary cesarean section. J Reprod Med, 31: 27–30.

Oestreicher M, Oestreicher S, Dudenhausen JW (1987). Prospective study on the question of single-dose antibiotic prophylaxis for primarily indicated abdominal cesarean section. Z Geburtsh Perinatol, 191: 12–14.

Padilla SL, Spence MR, Beauchamp PJ (1983). Single-dose ampicillin for cesarean section prophylaxis. Obstet Gynecol, 61: 463–466.

Parsons MT, Gibson R, Rimando-Ramos J, Spellacy WN (1985). Comparison of single-dose cefonicid and multiple-dose cefoxitin for surgical prophylaxis in women undergoing cesarean section. Adv Therapy, 2: 233–239.

Pelle H, Jepsen OB, Larsen SO, Bo J, Christensen F, Dreisler A, Jorgensen PJ, Kirstein A, Kjoller M, Lange A, Laursen K, Nickelsen CNA, Osler M, Rasmussen H (1986). Wound infection after cesarean section. Infect Control, 7: 456–461.

Phelan JP, Pruyn SC (1979). Prophylactic antibiotics in cesarean section: a double-blind study of cefalozin. Am J Obstet Gynecol, 133: 474–478.

Polk BF, Krache M, Phillippe M, Munoz A, Hutchinson D, Miao L, Schoenbaum SC (1982). Randomized clinical trial of perioperative cefoxitin in preventing maternal infection after primary cesarean section. Am J Obstet Gynecol, 142: 983–987.

Pollock AV (1988). Surgical prophylaxis the emerging picture. Lancet, 1: 225–230.

Posner AC, Konicoff NG, Prigot A (1955–1956). Tetracycline in obstetric infections. Antibiotics Annual, pp 345–348.

Rehu M, Jahkola M (1980). Prophylactic antibiotics in caesarean section: effect of a short preoperative course of benzyl penicillin or clindamycin plus gentamicin on postoperative infectious morbidity. Ann Clin Res, 12: 45–48.

Richards WR (1943). An evaluation of the local use of sulfonamide drugs in certain gynecological operations. Am J Obstet Gynecol, 46: 541–545.

Roex AJM, Puyenbroek JI, MacLaren DM, Van Geijn HP, Arts NFT (1986). A randomized clinical trial of antibiotic prophylaxis in cesarean section: maternal morbidity, risk factors and bacteriological changes. Eur J Obstet Gynecol Reprod Biol, 22: 117–124.

Roex AJM, Puyenbroek JI, Van Loenen AC, Arts NFT (1987). Single- vs three-dose cefoxitin prophylaxis in caesarean section: a randomized clinical trial. Eur J Obstet Gynecol Reprod Biol 25: 293–298.

Roex AJM, van Loenen AC, Puyenbroek JI, Arts NFT (1987). Secretion of cefotoxin in breast milk following short-term prophylactic administration in caesarean section. Eur J Obstet Gynecol Reprod Biol 25: 299–302.

Ross L, Mason P, Barnet-Lamb M, Robinson RE, Warren R (1984). Prophylactic metronidazole in patients with ruptured membranes undergoing emergency caesarean section. J Obstet Gynaecol, 5: 32–35.

Rothbard MJ, Mayer W, Wystepek A, Gordon M (1975). Prophylactic antibiotics in cesarean section. Obstet Gynecol, 45: 421–424.

Rudd EG, Long WH, Dillon MB (1981). Febrile morbidity following cefamandole nafate intrauterine irrigation during cesarean section. Am J Obstet Gynecol, 141: 12–16.

Saltzman DH, Eron LJ, Kay HH, Sites JG (1985). Single-dose antibiotic prophylaxis in high-risk patients undergoing cesarean section. Obstet Gynecol, 65: 655–657.

Saltzman DH, Eron LJ, Tuomala RE, Protomastro LJ, Sites JG (1986). Single-dose antibiotic prophylaxis in high-risk patients undergoing cesarean section: a comparative trial. J Reprod Med, 31: 709–712.

Saravolatz LD, Lee C, Drukker B (1985). Comparison of intravenous administration with intrauterine irrigation with ceforanide for non-elective cesarean section. Obstet Gynecol, 66: 513–516.

Scarpignato C, Caltabiano M, Condemi V, Mansani FE (1982). Short-term vs long-term cefuroxime prophylaxis in patients undergoing emergency cesarean section. Clin Ther, 5: 186–192.

Schedvins K, Moberg PJ (1986). Prevention of postoperative infection in cesarean section after rupture of the membranes. Int J Gynaecol Obstet, 24: 165–168.

Spruill FG, Mincttte LJ, Sturner WQ (1974). Two surgical deaths associated with cephalothin. JAMA, 229: 440–441.

Stage AH, Glover DD, Vaughan JE (1982). Low-dose cephradine prophylaxis in obstetric and gynecologic surgery. J Reprod Med, 27: 113–119.

Stiver HG, Forward KR, Livingstone RA, Fugere P, Lemay

M, Verschelden G, Hunter JDW, Carson GD, Beresford P, Tyrrell DL (1983). Multicenter comparison of cefoxitin vs cefazolin for prevention of infectious morbidity after non-elective cesarean section. Am J Obstet Gynecol, 145: 158–163.

Stiver HG, Tyrrell DL, Livingstone RA, Lemay M, Hunter JDW, Beresford P (1984). Comparative cervical microflora shifts after cefoxitin or cefazolin prophylaxis against infection following cesarean section. Am J Obstet Gynecol, 149: 718–721.

Swartz WH, Grolle K (1981). The use of prophylactic antibiotics in cesarean section. J Reprod Med, 26: 595–609.

Tully JL, Klapholz H, Baldini LM, Friedland GH (1983). Perioperative use of cefoxitin in primary cesarean section. J Reprod Med, 28: 827–832.

Tzingounis V, Makris N, Zolotas J, Michalas S, Aravantinos D (1982). Cefuroxime prophylaxis in caesarean section. Pharmatherapeutica, 3: 140–143.

Varner MW, Weiner CP, Petzold R, Galask RP (1986). Comparison of cefotetan and cefoxitin as prophylaxis in cesarean section. Am J Obstet Gynecol, 154: 951–954.

Wong R, Gee CL, Ledger WJ (1978). Prophylactic use of cefazolin in monitored obstetric patients undergoing cesarean section. Obstet Gynecol, 51: 407–411.

Work BA Jr (1977). Role of preventive antibiotics in patients undergoing cesarean section. S Afr Med J, 70: 44–45.

Young R, Platt L, Ledger W (1983). Prophylactic cefoxitin in cesarean section. Surg Gynecol Obstet, 157: 11–14.

74 Preterm delivery

Marc J. N. C. Keirse

1 Introduction

'Interest in the survival of the small baby has rattled the chains of conventional thinking in obstetrics today'.

Zuspan and Christian 1983

'When I see heroic efforts, including cesarean section, performed for fetal distress when a fetus is less than 26 weeks of gestation, I think obstetricians should visit schools and homes for blind children and children with other handicaps secondary to excessive prematurity. We have over-sold the public on medical miracles'.

Editorial commentary 1988

For a normally formed infant there is no risk greater than to be born too early. The transition from fetus to newborn is a hurdle to survival more than 100 times higher for the preterm infant than it is for the infant born at term (Rush *et al.* 1976; Keirse and Kanhai 1981). As preterm birth is the most important single determinant of adverse outcome of pregnancy, in terms of both the chances (Rush *et al.* 1976; Keirse and Kanhai 1981), and the quality (Keirse and Kanhai 1981; Yu *et al.* 1984b; Lefebvre *et al.* 1988) of survival, the main objectives of care should be to improve both the probability of living for the infant and the quality of life for the survivor.

Preterm delivery, while readily defined as the birth of an infant with a gestational age of less than 37 completed weeks, i.e. less than 259 days (FIGO News 1976; World Health Organization 1977), is not a single, homogeneous entity. Its incidence and the risk of adverse outcome in terms of mortality and morbidity is not equally distributed among the different gestational ages that are all defined as being preterm. Nor would all the risk of adverse outcome be abolished if, by some magical means, delivery could be postponed until term (Chng 1981). On the contrary, in the institutions where the matter has been documented, more than 20 per cent of preterm deliveries are the result of deliberate obstetric intervention to end a pregnancy because the obstetrician believes that the risks of a continuing pregnancy to mother or fetus have become unacceptably high (Rush *et al.* 1976; Rush *et al.* 1978; Chng 1981; Keirse and Kanhai 1981).

In comparison to birth at term, preterm birth is associated with a much higher incidence of inadequate fetal growth (Tamura *et al.* 1984), prelabour rupture of the membranes (see Chapter 43), multiple pregnancy (McKeown and Record 1952), placenta praevia (Kaltreider and Kohl 1980), placental abruption (Kaltreider and Kohl 1980), fetal congenital malformations (Rush *et al.* 1976), abnormal fetal lie (Scheer and Nubar 1976) and severe maternal disease (Kaltreider and Kohl 1980), all of which add their own problems to the care required during childbirth. Thus, care for preterm labour and delivery encompasses the whole spectrum of care for almost all major problems in obstetrics.

Only a few decades ago the prognosis for the survival of very preterm infants was so poor that obstetricians were not inclined to consider special care for their delivery. The philosophy of the time was 'survival of the fittest', often in a cold delivery room and with minimal attention at birth. The prevailing belief was that any measures taken to increase the survival rate would only result in increasing numbers of handicapped children who would be a burden to their families and society (Drillien 1958).

In the last two decades the pendulum has swung full circle. Statements such as 'the smaller the fetus, the larger should be the episiotomy' (Bieniarz *et al.* 1983) or 'evidence has accumulated that cesarean section may be preferable to vaginal delivery for all singleton infants of very low birthweight' (Ross and Stubblefield 1984), now suggest that it is the mothers, not the infants, who are a burden to their family. The evidence in support of these statements is no greater than that for the earlier beliefs.

The swing of the pendulum from therapeutic nihilism to zealous intervention has been prompted by enthusiastic reports from neonatologists who claim a much better outlook for preterm infants graduating from intensive neonatal care. These claims are unquestionably justified (Kitchen and Campbell 1971), but too many unwarranted conclusions have been drawn from such observational data. Too many uncontrolled comparisons have been presented as if they provided evidence rather than hypotheses. As an example, Stewart and her colleagues (Stewart and Reynolds 1974; Stewart 1977; Stewart *et al.* 1977; Fairweather and Stewart 1983) have repeatedly reported that infants of very low weight delivered by caesarean section have statistically significantly better outcomes than infants delivered vaginally. These data, which are frequently cited in support of abdominal delivery for most, if not all, very preterm infants are heavily biased by the inclusion of infants born outside the referral hospital. The authors themselves appear to be quite convinced that their observational and uncontrolled data provide sufficient 'evidence' to warrant routine caesarean section for all non-vertex presentations (Fairweather and Stewart 1983).

In fact, it is only recently that the pendulum has begun to return to the middle, and that zealous interventionism is being replaced by active care for delivery, which need not necessarily be (Nwaesei *et al.* 1987) nor be labelled (Dillon and Egan 1981) as aggressive. Paradoxically, this has occurred for the same reasons that earlier prompted more aggressive management and more surgical delivery of the preterm infant. The more recent trend appears to have been brought about by the realization that, with appropriate care and attention during and after labour and delivery, outcomes are also improving in infants whose gestational age is too low for obstetricians to resort to caesarean section with confidence (Herschel *et al.* 1982; Kitchen *et al.* 1985; Yu *et al.* 1986b; Nwaesei *et al.* 1987).

2 Nature and range of preterm delivery

'It should be recognised that mothers and babies delivered before 37 weeks of gestation are a heterogeneous group. Data collection should ensure that analysis by individual week of gestation is possible'.

Thirteenth Study Group of the Royal College of Obstetricians and Gynaecologists 1985.

2.1 Types of preterm delivery

Although it has long been known that preterm delivery encompasses a bewildering variety of different conditions which influence outcome, Rush *et al.* (1976) in Oxford were the first to distinguish various forms of preterm birth clearly. They pointed out that preterm delivery, as it presents itself to the obstetrician during pregnancy, is a distinctly different entity from preterm delivery as seen after pregnancy, by the neonatologist. There are substantial differences in the outcome of preterm delivery, according to the perspective of those who accumulate the data. Many reported data do not include stillbirths or grossly malformed infants, and they rarely contain reference to the significant pathology that may be present in mother or fetus before delivery. This is particularly relevant to the provision of care for preterm delivery, since many of the characteristics of that care have been and still are dictated by the reported outcomes of liveborn infants who have received modern intensive neonatal care.

2.1.1 Antepartum death and lethal malformations

Rush *et al.* (1976) found that in as many as 12 per cent of all preterm deliveries, none of the different forms of care available would have had any influence on the outcome, since all of these infants had either died before the onset of labour or before admission, or had malformations that were incompatible with life. These 12 per cent of births, however, accounted for 63 per cent of the total perinatal mortality associated with preterm delivery. There have been surprisingly few other attempts at distinguishing what can and what cannot be achieved by the kind of care that can be offered for preterm delivery, and those that have been made have not been representative of geographically defined populations. The conclusions of such studies conducted in widely different settings are remarkably similar (Table 74.1). They show that, because the baby

Table 74.1 Stillbirths and lethal congenital malformations among preterm deliveries in singleton and in all pregnancies

Source of data and authors	Singleton pregnancies			Multiple + singleton pregnancies		
	Number of births	Stillborn or malformed		Number of births	Stillborn or malformed	
		Per cent of infants	Per cent of deaths		Per cent of infants	Per cent of deaths
Oxford 1973–74 (Rush *et al.* 1976)	446	11.9	67.9	486	11.7	62.6
Cape Town 1974–75 (Rush *et al.* 1978)	– data not available –			2329	15.0	65.2
Aberdeen 1975 (Chng 1981)	99	9.1	56.3	– data not available –		
Leiden 1974–78 (Kanhai 1981)	476	15.0	65.1	578	13.7	62.7
Leiden 1979–83 (Van Kamp *et al.* 1989)	544	13.6	66.0	674	12.7	60.2

is either already dead or has lethal congenital malformations, in about 10 to 15 per cent of preterm deliveries the objectives of care should be directed entirely at maternal rather than at fetal or neonatal interests. More than half of the perinatal mortality associated with preterm birth (Table 74.1) will thus not be affected by any form of care that can be provided during labour and delivery. On the other hand, the type of care may markedly affect maternal morbidity and well-being. For example, caesarean section undertaken to deliver a lethally malformed infant will expose the mother to considerable morbidity with no possible hope of benefit to the infant. It may leave her to face an obstetric future with a uterine scar in the body rather than in the lower segment of the uterus, and thus increase her risk of uterine rupture in subsequent pregnancies (see Chapter 70). The frequency with which preterm delivery occurs in the presence of a dead or malformed fetus is ample justification for a careful ultrasound examination before any form of care that carries a substantial risk of maternal morbidity is undertaken.

2.1.2 Multiple pregnancy

About 10 per cent of Caucasian women who give birth preterm have a multiple pregnancy. Multiple births are 15 times more frequent among preterm births than among births at term, and preterm multiple births constitute nearly half of all multiple births (Keirse 1979). This is an important point to consider since it has been shown that these infants, 20 per cent of all liveborn preterm infants, have a higher rate of mortality (Rush *et al.* 1976; Keirse and Kanhai 1981) and a higher incidence of respiratory distress syndrome than singleton infants, even after correcting for differences in gestational age (Keirse and Kanhai 1981; Verloove-

Vanhorick and Verwey 1987). The neonatal mortality of all very preterm infants born alive at less than 32 weeks' gestation in The Netherlands in 1983 (Verloove-Vanhorick *et al.* 1986) was 10 per cent higher after a multiple than after a singleton birth (30 vs. 20 per cent). Also, the in-hospital mortality was higher after a multiple than after a singleton birth (33 vs. 23 per cent; Verloove-Vanhorick and Verwey 1987). Infants from multiple pregnancies, when born alive, have gestational age-specific mortality rates which are comparable to singleton infants who are at least 1 to 2 weeks less mature.

Increasing reliance on ultrasound examination in pregnancy (see Chapter 27) has made it extremely rare to be confronted at delivery with one more infant than was accounted for. However, if this occurs at preterm delivery it is likely to be distressing to the mother and the caregivers and risky for the unexpected infant. Given the frequency of multiple pregnancy in preterm deliveries, a firm diagnosis of the number of fetuses, if not already available, should be obtained by ultrasound examination before delivery is undertaken.

2.1.3 Elective delivery

Subtracting the 25 per cent of preterm pregnancies (representing 35 per cent of preterm infants) with either antepartum fetal death, lethal malformations, or multiple pregnancy does not reduce the remaining 75 per cent of preterm deliveries to a homogeneous group. About one-third of the remainder do not result from the spontaneous onset of labour, but from deliberate obstetric intervention to end pregnancy, either by induction of labour or by elective caesarean section (Rush *et al.* 1976; Chng 1981; Keirse and Kanhai 1981; Van Kamp *et al.* 1989). Even at gestational ages below 32 weeks, this category is becoming increasingly important (Table 74.2), and it constitutes an entirely different obstetric problem from that of delivery following the spontaneous onset of labour.

The issue of how best to achieve delivery is of secondary importance to that of whether one should even attempt to achieve delivery at that time. Unfortunately, such decisions are often made on very flimsy, albeit well-intentioned, grounds. Not only are patterns of fetal and maternal disease extremely variable in respect of their prognostic significance, but current tests of fetal well-being lack precision (see Chapters 29 and 30). Neonatal prognosis, if elective delivery is to be undertaken, cannot be assumed to be similar to that after preterm delivery following the spontaneous onset of labour. While there is a wealth of data on survival, morbidity, and follow-up of low birthweight, very low birthweight (<1500 g) and less than 1000 g infants, there is a dearth of information on how relevant these data are to the outcome of electively delivered infants, as opposed to infants born after the spontaneous onset

Table 74.2 Characteristics of birth and in-hospital mortality and morbidity in infants born alive before 32 weeks (224 days) of gestation in The Netherlands in 1983 (data from Verloove-Vanhorick and Verwey 1987)

Characteristics	No. of infants	Per cent
Characteristics of birth		
After prelabour rupture of membranes	453	44.8
More than 24 hours after rupture of membranes	226	22.4
After use of tocolytic drugs (any time)	533	52.8
After corticosteroid administration	173	17.1
Part of a multiple pregnancy	263	26.0
Breech presentation	293	29.0
Elective delivery*	155	15.3
Caesarean section	321	31.8
Characteristics and morbidity (confirmed diagnoses only) of newborn		
Congenital malformations	96	9.5
Weight below 10th centile for gestation	171	16.9
Respiratory distress syndrome	417	41.2
Intracranial haemorrhage	251	24.8
Convulsions	66	6.5
Septicaemia	133	13.2
In-hospital mortality of liveborn infants		
Neonatal deaths (28 days)	285	28.2
In-hospital deaths	310	30.7
Total	1010	100

*Defined as any delivery following any obstetrical intervention aimed at bringing pregnancy to an end before the onset of spontaneous labour and/or spontaneous rupture of the membranes.

of labour. The very few studies that have addressed this issue have all been hospital-based and have limited their attention either to first week mortality (Rush *et al.* 1976, 1978; Chng 1981) or to mortality and morbidity during the neonatal period (Keirse and Kanhai 1981; Kanhai and Keirse 1982). The difficulties of drawing generalizable conclusions are apparent when the indications for elective preterm delivery are compared for the three studies that provide relevant data (Table 74.3).

Table 74.3 Indications for elective preterm delivery of singleton infants born alive without lethal malformations

Indications for elective delivery	Per cent of elective preterm deliveries		
	Rush *et al.* 1976	Rush *et al.* 1978	Keirse and Kanhai 1981
Hypertension	40	39	6
Antepartum haemorrhage	14	22	13
Diabetes	10	7	12
Fetal growth retardation	7	18	29
Rhesus isoimmunization	7	3	36
Others	22	11	4
Total	100	100	100

2.1.4 Maternal and fetal pathology

The above has indicated that for more than half of the infants delivered preterm the issue of preterm delivery is rather different from what is intuitively understood by that term. In these circumstances, the perspectives of care for delivery are dominated by issues such as the absence of any chance of infant survival, the complexities of multiple pregnancy, and the question of whether and how to put an end to a pregnancy that is at no risk of imminent delivery.

The remaining infants and mothers, once again, still do not form a homogeneous group. For about half of them preterm labour and delivery ensue, causally or incidentally, from pathological processes in the mother, such as hypertension (see Chapter 24) or antepartum haemorrhage (see Chapter 37), or in the baby, such as stagnation of fetal growth (see Chapter 26). These disease processes are often the same, though not necessarily of similar severity, as those that prompt elective preterm delivery in other women (Table 74.3). Not surprisingly, the occurrence of preterm labour in these circumstances is often interpreted as an indication that nature itself has indicated the need to remove the fetus from a hostile intrauterine environment. Whether that interpretation is correct or not may be difficult to ascertain, but it is apparent that it can influence the type of care provided.

The fact that half of the preterm deliveries that result from spontaneous preterm labour in singleton pregnancies are complicated by maternal or fetal pathology (Keirse and Kanhai 1981), has major implications for the care for preterm labour and delivery. While such pathology occurs far more frequently in association with preterm delivery than with term delivery, the specific requirements with regard to care will be similar to those that are needed at term (see Chapters 53 and 54).

Purely obstetrical problems also occur more frequently when labour starts preterm rather than at term. These too have consequences for care during delivery. Among these are fetal malpresentation (see Chapter 42) and prolonged rupture of the membranes, especially following prelabour rupture of the membranes which occurs in nearly half of all otherwise uncomplicated preterm deliveries of singleton infants (see Chapter 43).

2.2 Gestational age

'Given that follow-up of some form should be done for the sake of the patients, it is then important, for the sake of hypothetical patients in the future, to subject the results to careful scrutiny'.

Scott 1987

2.2.1 Range of gestation

Although preterm delivery is internationally defined as delivery at less than 37 completed weeks (259 days) of gestation (FIGO News 1976; World Health Organization 1977; World Health Organization 1979), preterm delivery at 36 weeks is not very different from delivery at 37 weeks. Cut-off points drawn for demographic and public health reasons, particularly when they need to be arrived at by international consensus, have a tendency to follow the reality of clinical practice at a safe distance rather than to light the way. Thus, the expression 'prematurity', which had been defined first as a birthweight of 2500 g or less (World Health Organization 1950) and later as a gestational age of less than 37 weeks (World Health Organization 1961), was abolished and replaced by 'preterm' (World Health Organization 1969) long after it had become obvious that 'born too early' does not mean the same as 'born too small', and that two different definitions of the same word are not very helpful in distinguishing these two situations.

Preterm delivery rates in developed countries, as a proportion of all births, range from 5 to 8 per cent, with a few exceptions. In the United States rates of preterm delivery are 7.2 per cent for whites and 15.7 per cent for blacks (Paneth 1986). In Western Europe, data from

geographically defined areas show preterm delivery rates of between 5 and 8 per cent of all births (Alberman 1977; Bakketeig and Hoffman 1981; Ericson *et al.* 1984; Hall 1985; Piekkala *et al.* 1986; Rumeau-Rouquette 1986). Similar rates have been reported from Australia (Bryce and Stanley 1985). Data on the incidence of preterm delivery in some countries are incomplete or not reliable, because several countries do not routinely register gestational age at birth (Macfarlane and Mugford 1984; Keirse 1987).

The incidence of preterm delivery increases with increasing gestational age up to the cut-off point at 37 weeks. From the few data that are available on geographically defined populations, less than a quarter of preterm deliveries occur below 32 weeks. In the United States, in 1983, 1.8 per cent of liveborn infants had a gestational age of less than 32 weeks (National Center for Health Statistics 1985). The incidence of very preterm birth in that country is, like the incidence of all preterm births, markedly higher among the black than among the white population (Paneth 1986). The incidence of very preterm birth for singleton infants in Britain, in 1970, was 1.2 per cent (Chamberlain 1975). In The Netherlands, in 1983, 0.6 per cent of liveborn infants had a gestational age of less than 32 weeks (Verloove-Vanhorick *et al.* 1986). Data from Norway and Finland, which include infants born in the 32nd week, show incidences of 1.5 per cent of all singleton births in Norway (Hoffman and Bakketeig 1984) and of 1.1 per cent of live births in Finland (Heinonen *et al.* 1988).

The fact that preterm delivery at 35 and 36 weeks is not seen to be clinically very different from delivery at 37 weeks does not imply that the risks associated with delivery at these times in gestation are the same as they are at term. Preterm infants with a birthweight above the low birthweight threshold of 2500 g still have a neonatal mortality risk that is well above that of infants born at term (Battaglia *et al.* 1966; Keirse and Kanhai 1981). Part of this increased risk is undoubtedly attributable to the greater likelihood of maternal and fetal pathology in pregnancies that end outside the range of statistical normality (Kanhai 1981; see also Chapter 47). Care for preterm delivery will need to take account of this increased risk even with apparently 'normal' birthweight. Paneth *et al.* (1986) recently suggested that the reliance on birthweight rather than on gestational age as the major screening criterion for morbidity may explain some of the excess mortality that occurs in infants with 'mature' weight and preterm gestation in hospitals without neonatal intensive care units.

It is particularly the delivery of the very preterm infant that presents the greatest challenge. The notion 'very preterm' has not acquired the same general recognition as has 'preterm', but it is commonly used to denote infants with a gestational age of less than 32 completed weeks, i.e. less than 224 days. Although this cut-off point is of great epidemiological value, with respect to individual care the challenge of very preterm delivery cannot start or stop at an arbitrarily chosen cut-off point in gestation. The lower the gestational age, the greater the risk to the infant and the greater the challenge for care. Opinions on the assumed viability of infants readily influence care for delivery and, by pre-ordaining outcome they can easily become self-fulfilling prophesies.

There is no specific gestational age or estimated fetal weight at which a 'hands-off approach', as it was named by Nwaesei *et al.* (1987), suddenly changes from being negligent to being appropriate. Nor is there a specified gestational age or estimated fetal weight above or below which a 'hands-on approach' should automatically result in the use of surgical procedures to effect delivery. Too frequently the term 'active intervention on behalf of the infant' in reality is a euphemism for considering the fetus as the patient, and the mother as a type of envelope from which the patient needs to be extracted in order to receive all the 'benefits' of modern perinatal care. On the other hand, 'passive management for maternal considerations' sometimes conveys merely therapeutic nihilism and quiescent neglect of both the fetus and the mother. Nearly always, care for preterm delivery will have to steer in between these two undesirable courses, guided by the balance between potential benefit and potential harm to both mother and infant.

Advances in perinatology and improvements in the survival rate of tiny babies continue to lead to re-evaluation of, and adjustments in, the care for delivery of the very preterm infant. Such adjustments usually are not based on evidence, but on hopes that the next frontier will be won as readily as the previous ones. There is every need to ensure that these frontiers are not won at the expense of massive areas of waste land (Kirkley 1980).

It is not practical to suggest that controlled experimentation should determine from what gestational age onwards active management in the interest of the infant should determine the pattern of care. It is practical, however, to suggest that individual elements of care should be demonstrated to provide more benefit than harm before they are widely applied at ever lowering gestational ages. Clearly, measures which have been demonstrated to be beneficial for the infant and produce little harm for the mother, such as corticosteroid administration (see Chapter 45), may be applied with far greater confidence at very low gestational ages than other measures, such as non-selective caesarean section, which confer far more dubious benefits, if any, to the infant and substantial hazards to the mother (see Chapter 70).

2.2.2 *Estimated weight or gestational age as a basis for care options*

Care for preterm delivery is largely governed, as it should be, by the anticipated outcome of delivery and the anticipated effects of care. Unfortunately, most data on outcome have limited utility, as they rarely relate to gestational age categories. Postnatal measurement of birthweight has been the framework for the presentation of survival data for decades. Birthweight was readily available to neonatologists. It is reasonably objective; it circumvented the difficulties of adequate determination of gestational age; and it required no ascertainment on the part of the neonatologist of any (un)reliable data that the mother or the obstetrician might have to offer.

A wealth of information is thus available on short- and long-term outcomes of infants weighing less than 1000 g, less than 1500 g, less than 2000 g or less than 2500 g. The majority of these infants are, of course, born preterm and this applies in particular to the lower weight categories. For instance, only 27 of 1338 infants (2 per cent) born in The Netherlands in 1983 with a weight less than 1500 g had a gestational age of 37 weeks or more (Verloove-Vanhorick and Verwey 1987). Nevertheless, when data on infant outcome relate mainly to postnatal weight, it implies that care before birth for these infants and their mothers will be based on the opinion of a clinician as to how much the baby is likely to weigh after he or she has been delivered.

Experienced clinicians will usually take into account that the birthweight-specific data on which they have to base their care options include infants whose intrauterine growth was restrained, and who were therefore born at a more mature gestational age than would be expected from birthweight alone. Usually, they will also take into account that most of the data refer to infants delivered not from their mothers, but to neonatal units after all of the selection processes that occurred between the delivery and transfer to a neonatal unit. What they cannot take into account, however, is what the actual weight of the baby will be at delivery. This must be estimated either by a well-educated, but notoriously inaccurate guess (see Chapter 26), based on clinical examination; by extrapolating ultrasound measurements of dimension to weight; or on the basis of what the average baby will weigh at any given gestational age. The (in)accuracy of weight estimations at gestations of 26 to 32 weeks is exemplified in a recent study of Luthy *et al.* (1987). They conducted a randomized controlled trial of electronic monitoring in preterm labour at two North American university centres, using an estimated fetal weight of 700 to 1750 g at 26 to 32 weeks of gestation as the entry criterion. As many as 130 of the 376 women (35 per cent) enrolled in the study subsequently needed to be excluded because their infants weighed more than the 1750 g cut-off point at birth.

Great advances have been made in the accuracy of estimation of fetal weight by ultrasound examination (see Chapter 27). In most hands, however, its accuracy is still far from perfect. This applies in particular to the low weight ranges and, as is often the case for preterm delivery, when the measurements need to be made with some urgency and by whoever happens to be available. The accuracy claimed by experienced research fellows with ample time to obtain the best measurements possible in a non-labouring woman is hardly representative of what can predictably be obtained in the care for preterm delivery.

There is no evidence that estimation of fetal weight prior to preterm delivery improves either the provision of care for delivery or the outcome for the infant. No controlled clinical experimentation has been conducted to answer the question as to whether the prediction of birthweight and its use in selecting alternative forms of care confers more benefit than harm. This would certainly be necessary, as it can be inferred from some studies that determining patterns of care on the basis of weight estimations carries great hazards.

Wallace et al. (1984), for instance, found that 75 per cent of infants estimated to weigh less than 1500 g and admitted to a trial of caesarean section vs. vaginal delivery, actually weighed more than 1500 g at birth. As many as 24 per cent weighed even more than 2000 g. This, according to Wallace et al. (1984) led to 16 per cent of all women entered in their trial being subjected to caesarean section while no probable benefit for the infant could be anticipated. Paul et al. (1979), in a study designed to evaluate the merits of fetal monitoring and caesarean section for the very low birthweight infant, reported an opposite hazard of fetal weight estimations. In infants with a birthweight between 1000 and 1500 g they found that infants whose weight had been correctly estimated to be more than 1000 g had a mortality rate of 20 per cent, while those who had been incorrectly estimated to weigh less than 1000 g had a more than doubled mortality rate of 49 per cent. Underestimation of fetal weight, which appears to be quite common in the preterm infant (Luthy et al. 1987), may lead to the infant being denied the level of care for delivery that would have been given if the weight had been correctly estimated.

Erroneous judgements that a baby is too small to be salvageable have a strong tendency to become self-fulfilling prophesies. On the other hand, if the general rules include 'the presence of an experienced staff obstetrician and neonatologist at the delivery of every infant whose expected birthweight is less than 1500 g' (Bowes 1983), as they do in some places, an estimated weight of 1600 g may be the most dangerous hazard that an infant of 1250 g will ever have to overcome.

Even if birthweight could be determined with a 100 per cent accuracy before birth, the available evidence still suggests that this information would be inferior to gestational age as a determinant of infant outcome and care options. Epidemiological studies have demonstrated that birthweight is a better predictor of mortality than is gestational age when the whole range of gestation from 20 to over 40 weeks is considered (Abernathy et al. 1966; Susser et al. 1972; Hellier and Goldstein 1979). This does not apply to neonatal mortality and morbidity in the very preterm infant, where maturity is more important than organ weight. Population-based data from two countries showed that for these infants estimated gestational age is a better predictor of both neonatal mortality (Verloove-Vanhorick et al. 1986; Heinonen et al. 1988) and risk of intraventricular haemorrhage (Van de Bor et al. 1987) than is known birthweight. This does not imply that birthweight is unimportant, as very preterm infants with low weight for gestation have an even higher mortality than infants of the same gestational age with appropriate weights for gestation (Heinonen et al. 1985, 1988).

Very low birthweight infants with a low birthweight for gestation are sometimes believed to have a lower mortality risk than infants with an appropriate weight for gestation (Hoskins et al. 1983; Goldenberg et al. 1985a; Yu et al. 1986a). This is true, but only within birthweight-defined populations. An infant of low weight for gestation will automatically be born later in gestation than an infant of the same weight who is of appropriate weight for gestation. This does not mean, as is sometimes inferred, that an infant of low weight for gestation has a better chance of survival than an infant born at the same gestational age with an appropriate weight for gestation.

In conclusion, decisions on care for preterm delivery should be based primarily on gestational age and should only be refined, but not replaced by estimates of birthweight. A carefully taken menstrual history and ascertainment of any prior assessment of gestational age during pregnancy will be far more useful for the woman in preterm labour than attempts to determine fetal weight. In the absence of any evidence that estimation of fetal weight improves outcome, it is not justified to substitute weight estimation for a careful assessment of the menstrual history and gestational age as the basis for care decisions.

3 Place of and preparations for delivery

'Obstetricians have a predilection for delivering their patients in a sub-arctic environment'.

Roberton 1977

3.1 Place of delivery

The most dangerous place for a preterm baby to be delivered is in a hospital with caregivers who believe that they have, but do not in reality have, the equipment and skills necessary to effectively care for these tiny babies before and after birth. Misplaced self-confidence cannot make up for lack of facilities and equipment; for lack of persons capable of managing and handling that equipment; for lack of manpower to ensure around the clock utilization of these resources; nor for lack of collaboration among professionals in and across various disciplines. It can, and often does, result in failure of timely referral to institutions where such facilities are available.

Whenever possible, delivery of the very young and very small fetus should be referred to a centre with adequate facilities and personnel to cope with the intensive perinatal care that these mothers and babies require. It is clearly inappropriate to electively deliver such infants in institutions where these facilities are less than optimal. Population-based studies in which the risk of mortality of very preterm and very low birth-weight babies is related to the hospital at which birth took place, regardless of antenatal or neonatal trans-port, provide strong arguments for concentrating these deliveries in centres with adequate perinatal facilities (Paneth *et al*. 1982, 1987; Verloove-Vanhorick *et al*. 1988).

In the absence of controlled trials between antenatal and neonatal referral, such data provide the best evidence available on the effects of concentrating early preterm deliveries in intensive perinatal care centres. These studies have demonstrated that gestational age-specific and birthweight-specific mortalities are much lower for infants delivered in perinatal care centres than in other obstetric departments. Paneth *et al*. (1987) in New York for instance, found no difference in the mortality risk of normal birthweight infants delivered at term between different levels of hospital care. Infants of low weight and preterm gestation, however, showed marked differences in mortality according to the level of hospital care. Paneth *et al*. (1987) concluded that, in their population, intrauterine referral of preterm and growth-retarded infants to tertiary care settings had the potential to reduce mortality by almost 12 per cent. The preference for antenatal, as opposed to neonatal, refer-ral of very preterm infants is supported by a wealth of other information on the effects of regionalization of perinatal care (Harris *et al*. 1978; Bowes 1981; Hor-wood *et al*. 1982; Saigal *et al*. 1982; Goldenberg *et al*. 1983; Scott *et al*. 1984; see also Chapter 12).

How large the effect is of referring preterm deliveries to centres with intensive perinatal care units, is difficult to judge from the data that are thus far available. This is due to the absence of controlled trials and to the confounding effect of using birthweight instead of gestational age cut-offs as mentioned earlier. A conser-vative estimate is that moving the mother from the average obstetrical unit to a unit with intensive perina-tal care facilities is roughly equivalent to a gain of at least one week in the duration of gestation. It is unfor-tunate that such estimates cannot be made with greater precision, as they would be very helpful as guidelines in the provision of care for a large number of preterm deliveries. Indeed, most obstetrical teams will readily be able to appreciate the difference that, for instance, a 10 days' gain in gestation would make for delivery at, say, 26 or 36 weeks of gestation. Obviously, these caregivers would still need to consider the influence of maternal or fetal pathology, as they do at term (see Chapter 12).

Unfortunately, it is not uncommon for small preterm infants to be delivered in hospitals that lack the facilities to provide the special level of care that is necessary. Verloove-Vanhorick and her colleagues (Verloove-Vanhorick and Verwey 1987; Verloove-Vanhorick *et al*. 1988), for instance, found that 37 per cent of all infants with a weight of less than 1500 g, who were born in The Netherlands in 1983, were delivered in hospitals with little or no facilities for special perinatal care. Yet 70 per cent of the mothers had been hospitalized before deli-very, which would indicate that many of them could have been transported to a perinatal centre well before delivery could have occurred. A questionnaire survey conducted among Australian obstetricians by Trud-inger and Boshell (1987) indicated that as many as 25 per cent of the respondents considered it reasonable to deliver an infant of 32 weeks' gestation in a hospital without neonatal intensive care facilities. There were large differences by state, in that 32 per cent of obstetri-cians in some states as opposed to only 2 per cent in another state, felt that delivery at 32 weeks could be cared for at a hospital without an intensive neonatal care unit (Trudinger and Boshell 1987). It is inconceiv-able that differences of this magnitude could result from differences in the characteristics of preterm in-fants from one state to another. They indicate that there is a wide difference of opinion among obstetricians as to what constitutes appropriate care for preterm delivery, and that some of these opinions are out of touch with the reality of preterm birth.

3.2 Preparations for delivery

The woman at imminent risk of preterm delivery re-quires an immediate assessment as to the appropriate-ness of transfer to a perinatal centre. This will depend on gestational age, on the facilities that are available (which may be sufficient for delivery at 36 but not at 31 weeks), and on the imminence of the expected delivery.

If the woman is in labour, it is wise to administer tocolytic drugs in order to postpone delivery at least until after arrival at the perinatal centre (see Chapter

44). Administration of corticosteroids should be commenced before transfer, unless delivery is likely to be delayed for more than 48 hours, or gestational age has advanced beyond the stage at which respiratory distress syndrome is likely to be a problem (see Chapter 45).

Given the frequency with which preterm delivery occurs in the presence of maternal disease (Keirse and Kanhai 1981), the institutions where preterm delivery is undertaken should be able to draw not only on the expertise of neonatologists or perinatologists, but on that of a host of other professionals who may be needed to provide counselling or advice. Ultrasound equipment should be available for every preterm labour or delivery, along with persons who can handle that equipment and correctly interpret its findings. Full laboratory facilities should be available at all times. Resuscitation equipment (see Chapter 75) should be available on the spot and the presence and proper working order of this equipment should be verified before each delivery.

Fetal assessment prior to delivery should identify multiple pregnancy; ensure whether the fetus is alive and well; differentiate the normally formed from the congenitally malformed fetus; and correctly establish fetal presentation. As mentioned earlier, ascertainment of gestational age, and careful review of the gestational data and evidence established during antenatal care is mandatory.

All of these are prerequisites for proper care for preterm delivery and a policy of caesarean section for all is definitely not an adequate substitute.

A professional who is skilled in resuscitation and who can devote all his or her attention to the infant should be in attendance at all preterm deliveries. This is readily achieved where labour and neonatal wards are adjacent (as they should be). Where distances present a problem, every effort should be made, first, to ensure that these distances are phased out in the foreseeable future and, second, to increase staffing levels so that no preterm baby in the meantime will be delivered without appropriate neonatal attention. It has been suggested that decisions to effect abdominal rather than vaginal delivery, are sometimes guided by the need to ensure the presence of a skilled resuscitator at birth (Westgren 1985), but it is surely wrong to inflict major surgery on the mother simply to ensure that a qualified professional will be present to take care of the baby.

3.3 Prevention of intraventricular haemorrhage

Intraventricular haemorrhage is an important cause of mortality and morbidity in the very preterm infant (Thorburn *et al.* 1981; see also Tables 74.2 and 74.4). Most of these haemorrhages originate from the subependymal germinal matrix (Hambleton and Wigglesworth 1976; Ment *et al.* 1987), which dissipates grad-

Table 74.4 Recorded causes of in-hospital mortality of infants born alive before 32 weeks (224 days) of gestation in The Netherlands in 1983 (data from Verloove-Vanhorick and Verwey 1987)

Recorded causes of death	No. of infants	Per cent
Congenital malformation	21	6.8
Respiratory distress syndrome	127	41.8
Intracranial haemorrhage	105	33.9
Congenital infection	18	5.8
Septicaemia	50	16.1
Necrotizing enterocolitis	9	2.9
Others	134	43.2
Total	310	100

ually as gestational age increases (Pape and Wigglesworth 1979). The risk of haemorrhage is inversely related to gestational age, ranging from more than 70 per cent under 26 weeks' gestation to less than 10 per cent after 33 weeks' gestation (Allan and Philip 1985; Szymonowicz 1987). More than 90 per cent of the haemorrhages occur in infants below 35 weeks' gestation (Garcia-Prats *et al.* 1982).

Since the large majority of these haemorrhages occur within 24 hours of birth, and mostly in the first few hours of life (Beverley *et al.* 1984; Mcidcll *et al.* 1985; Szymonowicz 1987), there have been numerous attempts to correlate their occurrence with characteristics of labour and delivery. In some reports, higher incidences have been described in babies delivered vaginally than in those delivered by caesarean section (Kosmetatos *et al.* 1980; Greisen and Block-Petersen 1983; Beverley *et al.* 1984), while in others it was found that this applied only to elective caesarean sections done before the onset of labour (Tejani *et al.* 1984; Anderson *et al.* 1988). Still others found no difference between babies delivered vaginally and abdominally (Levene *et al.* 1982; Bada *et al.* 1984; Kitchen *et al.* 1985; Van de Bor *et al.* 1987). Relationships have been described with labour (Anderson *et al.* 1988), the length of labour (Meidell *et al.* 1985), fetal heart rate abnormalities in labour (Strauss *et al.* 1985), 'intrauterine asphyxia' (Westgren *et al.* 1986), fetal presentation at birth (Lamont 1985), low Apgar score at delivery (Tejani *et al.* 1984) and so forth. For each of these studies, others can be quoted that found no such effects, and in general it is impossible to establish to what extent the findings reflect the type of cases involved rather than potential cause and effect relationships. The largest study to date, derived from a national cohort of infants born before 32 weeks of gestation in The Netherlands in 1983 (Verloove-Vanhorick *et al.* 1986), found only one delivery-related event (rupture of the membranes for more than 24 hours before delivery) to be statistically significantly associated with the incidence of intraventricular haemorrhage. This was associated with a lower incidence of intracranial haemorrhage than that in the total group of 484 infants (Van de Bor *et al.* 1987), but this study too suffers all the drawbacks of observational data discussed elsewhere (see Chapter 1).

Two trials have addressed the possibility of reducing the incidence of intraventricular haemorrhage in preterm infants by administration of phenobarbitone to the mother before delivery (Morales and Koerten 1986; Shankaran *et al.* 1984, 1986). Earlier investigations had examined whether administration of phenobarbitone to preterm infants after delivery could reduce the incidence of intraventricular haemorrhage. The controlled studies (Ruth 1985; Kuban *et al.* 1986; Anwar *et al.* 1986; Donn *et al.* 1981; Morgan *et al.* 1982; Whitelaw *et al.* 1983; Bedard *et al.* 1984; Porter *et al.* 1985) overall failed to show a beneficial effect of the administration of phenobarbitone to the neonate.

The two trials in which phenobarbitone was administered to the mother provided data that are far more encouraging than those obtained with administration to the neonate. In these two trials phenobarbitone was administered before elective or spontaneous delivery at less than 32 weeks (Morales and Koerten 1986) or during spontaneous labour with intact or ruptured membranes before 35 weeks (Shankaran *et al.* 1984, 1986). Both trials indicate that this treatment has considerable potential for reducing the incidence of intraventricular haemorrhage (Tables 74.5 and 74.6) and of neonatal mortality in preterm infants (Table 74.7).

Unfortunately, neither of the two trials used methodology of sufficient rigour to exclude the possibility of selection bias. In one of them randomization was based on the hospital chart number (Morales and Koerten 1986) and in the other it was by means of a card deck (Shankaran *et al.* 1986), but in both trials the diagnosis of intraventricular haemorrhage was made without knowledge of the type of treatment received. The reduction in the incidence of both intraventricular haemorrhage and neonatal death in these two trials (Morales and Koerten 1986; Shankaran *et al.* 1984, 1986) is such that strong confirmation or denial of the benefits of this treatment is urgently required. Fortunately, further trials are currently under way (Hanson 1988; Molina 1988).

Table 74.5 Effect of maternal phenobarbital for the prevention of intraventricular haemorrhage in preterm infants on intraventricular haemorrhage

Study	EXPT		CTRL		Odds ratio	Graph of odds ratios and confidence intervals						
	n	(%)	*n*	(%)	(95% CI)	0.01	0.1	0.5	1	2	10	100
Morales and Koerten (1986)	16/75	(21.33)	35/75	(46.67)	0.33 (0.17–0.64)							
Shankaran *et al.* (1986)	8/25	(32.00)	13/23	(56.52)	0.38 (0.12–1.17)							
Typical odds ratio (95% confidence interval)					0.34 (0.19–0.60)							

Table 74.6 Effect of maternal phenobarbital for the prevention of intraventricular haemorrhage in preterm infants on severe intraventricular haemorrhage

Study	EXPT		CTRL		Odds ratio	Graph of odds ratios and confidence intervals						
	n	(%)	*n*	(%)	(95% CI)	0.01	0.1	0.5	1	2	10	100
Morales and Koerten (1986)	4/75	(5.33)	15/75	(20.00)	0.27 (0.10–0.70)							
Shankaran *et al.* (1986)	0/25	(0.00)	5/23	(21.74)	0.10 (0.02–0.64)							
Typical odds ratio 95% confidence interval)					0.22 (0.09–0.51)							

Table 74.7 Effect of maternal phenobarbital for the prevention of intraventricular haemorrhage in preterm infants on mortality

Study	EXPT		CTRL		Odds ratio	Graph of odds ratios and confidence intervals						
	n	(%)	n	(%)	(95% CI)	0.01	0.1	0.5	1	2	10	100
Morales and Koerten (1986)	3/75	(4.00)	10/75	(13.33)	0.31 (0.10–0.96)							
Shankaran *et al.* (1986)	2/25	(8.00)	8/23	(34.78)	0.20 (0.05–0.81)							
Typical odds ratio (95% confidence interval)					0.26 (0.11–0.63)							

4 Route of delivery

'Without some randomized method of selection I do not believe that it is possible to come to a really honest answer as to the best route of delivery'.

Beard 1977

One of the main decisions in the care for preterm delivery, and certainly the most controversial one, is the choice between vaginal delivery and caesarean section. One would expect a wealth of evidence to be available for selecting the best of these approaches from the volume of literature that has been published on this issue. This is not the case. Calls for clinical trials to provide unbiased comparisons between vaginal and abdominal routes of delivery have been published for more than a decade (Beard 1977; Crowley 1981; Grant 1986). Yet, there have been very few attempts to put these recommendations into practice, and those that were attempted were abandoned before, or soon after they started.

4.1 Randomized trials

Wallace *et al.* (1984) attempted to determine the best route of delivery for infants with a vertex presentation at 26 to 33 weeks' gestation. The trial was abandoned after 40 women had been enrolled because of 'an unacceptably high frequency of infants subsequently found to weigh in excess of 1500 g (Wallace *et al.* 1984). A high frequency of babies weighing more than 1500 g should have been anticipated. Brenner *et al.* (1976), in the United States where the trial was conducted, found 1500 g to be the 50th centile of weight for gestation at 31 weeks, and it is thus logical that the majority of infants delivered up to 33 weeks will weigh more than 1500 g.

Unfortunately, the data of Wallace *et al.* (1984) as presented are uninterpretable. Of the 40 women entered, 25 were assigned to attempted caesarean section and only 15 to attempted vaginal delivery. Results are not presented according to whether women were assigned to receive caesarean section or vaginal deli-very. Instead, the data relate to 18 caesarean sections and 20 vaginal deliveries, which included 5 women allocated to attempted caesarean section who delivered before that policy could be implemented. The two remaining women, apparently both in the caesarean section group, were excluded because of 'inadvertent entry' with non-vertex presentation.

Another trial, designed to determine the best route of delivery for singleton live infants between 26 and 31 weeks of gestation, was cancelled within 6 months after it started (Lumley *et al.* 1985). The trial envisaged to include infants in vertex and in breech presentation, provided that there were no fetal abnormalities on ultrasound examination. Only 4 of 33 women who actually delivered between 26 and 31 weeks of gestation in that period had been entered into the trial. Nearly half of all women who were eligible for participation in the trial had been withdrawn at the discretion of obstetricians, who had already become 'irrevocably convinced that most very low birthweight infants benefit from caesarean section' (Lumley *et al.* 1985).

At least three additional trials have been instigated to examine the best route of delivery for preterm infants presenting by the breech. Only one of these, started at the University of Iowa in 1978, actually recruited women for participation in the trial. 'Because of slow patient accrual, possible changing care practices, and increasing medico-legal concerns, the study of premature breeches pretty much fizzled out' (FJ Zlatnik, personal communication 1984) after only 38 women had been entered out of a total of 114 women who met the eligibility criteria and were delivered during that period. The other two trials, in Canada (S Effer, personal communication 1980) and in The Netherlands (PE Treffers and M Van Pel, personal communication 1987), were not commenced, apparently for lack of funding.

4.2 Breech presentation

'We are greatly concerned about authors who in recent publications admit to deficiencies in the evidence that they present and yet conclude that cesarean section is the method of choice for delivery of the very low-birth weight breech infant.

Effer *et al.* 1983

Most of the discussion regarding route of delivery has centred on the preterm breech. Breech presentation is far more common in preterm infants than it is in term infants, and for a variety of reasons breech presentation at delivery carries a higher risk than cephalic presentation does (see Chapter 42). Breech presentation has also paved the way for instituting so-named 'prophylactic caesarean section' as a safer method of delivery, and for extending the assumed benefits of that approach to the remainder of the population without adequate evidence that the assumed gain in safety is indeed a gain and not a loss.

A large number of studies have compared the outcome of vaginal breech delivery with that following caesarean section (Bowes 1977; Cruikshank and Pitkin 1977; Goldenberg and Nelson 1977; Ingemarsson *et al.* 1978; Lyons and Papsin 1978; Bowes *et al.* 1979; De Crespigny and Pepperell 1979; Duenhoelter *et al.* 1979; Haesslein and Goodlin 1979; Karp *et al.* 1979; Lewis and Seneviratne 1979; Mann and Gallant 1979; Paul *et al.* 1979; Woods 1979; Crowley and Hawkins 1980; Miller *et al.* 1980; Smith *et al.* 1980; Hochuli and Käch 1981; Kaupilla *et al.* 1981; Nisell *et al.* 1981; Cox *et al.* 1982; Geirsson *et al.* 1982; Gimovski and Paul 1982; Effer *et al.* 1983; Fairweather and Stewart 1983; Greisen *et al.* 1983; Lamont *et al.* 1983; Main *et al.* 1983; Bada *et al.* 1984; Frenzel *et al.* 1984; Kariniemi *et al.* 1984; Olshan *et al.* 1984; Petitti and Golditch 1984; Rosen and Chick 1984; Tejani *et al.* 1984; Wulf *et al.* 1984; Yu *et al.* 1984a; Goldenberg *et al.* 1985b; Van Eyck and Huisjes 1983; Westgren *et al.* 1985; Bodmer *et al.* 1986; Hielscher *et al.* 1986; Weisbach *et al.* 1986; Myers and Gleicher 1987; Verloove-Vanhorick and Verwey 1987; Doring and De Sousa 1988).

Most of these studies have been retrospective and most found higher survival rates after caesarean section than after vaginal delivery. Some of them also reported a lower frequency of morbidity following caesarean section than that observed after vaginal delivery. Some of these studies unquestionably compared apples with oranges. Smith *et al.* (1980), for instance, concluded that 'preterm infants of 26–34 weeks' gestation, presenting by breech, should have the benefit of caesarean section', on the basis of a comparison which, as Crowley (1981) pointed out, ignored the fact that the infants in the caesarean section group weighed substantially more than those delivered vaginally and included both vertex and breech presentations. In other studies genuine attempts were made to control as much as possible for confounding factors. Nevertheless, it is impossible to conclude that any of these studies have compared like with like.

It is impossible to assess the circumstances surrounding the choice between abdominal and vaginal delivery accurately enough to make valid and unbiased comparisons between caesarean section and vaginal delivery. In few fields is the question of selection bias (see Chapter 1) as strong as it is with regard to delivery of the preterm breech, and it is precisely in recognition thereof that so many calls have been made for a randomized trial between vaginal and abdominal delivery (Beard 1977; Crowley 1981; Grant 1986).

If the general policy is in favour of caesarean section for most, if not all, infants presenting by the breech at a certain gestational age, the comparisons will be biased in a number of ways. Infants delivered vaginally are more likely to be those who are rightly or wrongly considered to be too small, of too low gestational age, or too sick to receive sufficient benefit from caesarean section. These same infants are also likely to receive less dedicated care at vaginal delivery. Indeed, if their prognosis is too poor to warrant what is perceived to be the best form of care, it would seem illogical to invest a maximum of energy in what is perceived to be the inferior form of care. Infants delivered vaginally are more likely to be those whose mothers arrived too late in second stage labour to have a caesarean section. The care that these mothers and babies then receive may also be one of (sub)conscious despair because these mothers 'have selected themselves for vaginal delivery, and yet at the same time have denied themselves the benefits of expert management during the course of their labour' (Smith *et al.* 1981).

Infants who are delivered vaginally are also more likely to be those who have foregone the benefits of antenatal corticosteroid treatment (see Chapter 45), because delivery occurred too quickly for these drugs to be administered or to have their full effect. Infants delivered vaginally are certainly more likely to have been born in the absence of a senior obstetrician and neonatologist. If the general policy favours caesarean section, vaginal delivery by virtue of being unannounced and a rare occurrence, is likely to be assisted by a person whose technical skills and experience at breech delivery of tiny infants is virtually non-existent.

In contrast, infants delivered by caesarean section are more likely to be those for whom delivery could be planned in advance. They are more likely to be born as the result of elective obstetric intervention to end pregnancy. Delivery is more likely to have been preceded by thorough assessment of the fetal condition, possibly including ascertainment of lung maturation, and after full preparations were made for whatever special neonatal care was required. As is apparent from many comparative studies, these infants are more likely to be born later in gestation and to have birthweights that are higher than those of infants born vaginally. Commitment to survival of the infant on the part of the caregiver is both consciously and subconsciously likely to be much greater for infants delivered abdominally than for those delivered vaginally, if only to compensate for the risk and morbidity inflicted on the infant's mother.

5 Abdominal delivery

'Statements such as … "if in doubt, cut it out" are questionable at best'.

O'Leary and Pasley 1983

Although caesarean section is considered to be one of the safest of the major surgical procedures, it still carries considerable risk of mortality and morbidity (see Chapter 70). The technique of caesarean section has been fully described by Pearson and Rees (see Chapter 72), but some conditions should be met before it is applied to preterm delivery.

There is nothing worse than to open the peritoneal cavity and encounter a non-pregnant uterus, because the infant quietly slipped out of the vagina while everyone was preoccupied with the preparations for getting the infant delivered as quickly as possible. Both to avoid such rare disasters and to ensure an atraumatic delivery, it is essential to know what proportion of the infant is in or above the pelvic inlet. A vaginal or ultrasound examination will provide that information.

A careful ultrasound examination is essential before caesarean delivery of a preterm infant. There are several reasons for this. First, as mentioned earlier, it is important to differentiate the normally formed from the congenitally malformed fetus. Inflicting major surgery upon the mother to deliver an infant with lethal malformations cannot be described as effective care. Second, an exact diagnosis of the fetal presentation may allow correction of malpresentation before the uterus is incised. This may make all the difference between an easy caesarean delivery and a traumatic extraction of a malpositioned infant through a poorly formed and thick uterine segment. Third, when an infant needs to be delivered atraumatically through the type of lower segment incision that a preterm uterus will permit, it is unquestionably useful to know whether or not the placenta will be in the way. Little gain can be made in avoiding trauma to the aftercoming head, for instance, when this relatively large head needs to be delivered through a small incision in a thick uterine segment, which has the placenta as well as the body of the baby bulging through it.

At caesarean section, particularly when it is performed for breech presentation, it is important to assess whether the lower uterine segment possesses sufficient width to permit easy delivery of the head. Beginning with too small an incision, which then needs to be enlarged while the body of the baby is in the incision, is likely to lead to a more traumatic delivery than would have occurred during delivery via the vaginal route. Often, and particularly in elective preterm delivery, there will be little lower uterine segment, and whatever incision is made will be cut through the body of the uterus. Some authors therefore recommend a vertical rather than a transverse incision, but no controlled experiments have been conducted to evaluate the relative merits of the alternative policies (see Chapter 70). If the presentation is not longitudinal it is advisable to correct it to a longitudinal and preferably vertex presentation before the uterine incision is made. This is usually not too difficult, especially when there is no shortage of amniotic fluid, and the uterine relaxant effect of betamimetic treatment can be maintained up to the moment of delivery with that specific aim in mind.

At caesarean delivery it is just as important to strive for easy and gentle delivery of the fetal head as it is at vaginal delivery.

6 Vaginal delivery

'The smaller the fetus, the larger should be the episiotomy'.

Bieniarz *et al.* 1983

The head of the preterm baby, with its soft bones and wide skull sutures, is more vulnerable than that of the term baby to compression by the maternal pelvic tissues (particularly in nulliparae), and to sudden decompression when the baby emerges from the birth canal. Several measures have therefore been proposed to minimize the occurrence of these changes in intracranial pressure. They include liberal use of epidural analgesia to lower resistance in the birth canal; routine use of early episiotomy to remove the resistance of rigid perineal tissues; and routine use of 'prophylactic forceps' delivery in an attempt to counteract both compression before and decompression after birth.

6.1 Epidural and other analgesia

Adequate analgesia for labour and delivery is just as important for the mother delivering preterm as it is for women delivering at term. There have been few controlled studies on the provision of analgesia for preterm delivery, but those that have been reported (Kaltreider 1967) do not suggest that the issue is very different from that at term (see Chapter 57). The main difference may well be that mothers generally are less prepared for birth and more likely to be overcome by the suddenness of it all and by the large risks involved. Temptations to respond to that anxiety with heavy sedation must be resisted, particularly when they involve the use of drugs, such as diazepam, that induce retrograde amnesia. Too many mothers have a recall of being rushed into hospital pregnant and leaving it some days later without a baby and without any knowledge, other than hearsay, as to how they evolved from the pregnant to the non-pregnant state. Pain relief should be given when necessary; it is unkind and inappropriate to substitute sedation for analgesia.

Narcotics are bound to be more depressant for the preterm infant than they are for the term infant (see Chapter 57). The likelihood that the infant will require expert resuscitation increases with increasing use and increasing doses of narcotic drugs. It is probably wise to rely as much as possible on alternative forms of analgesia, including epidural analgesia, although there are no data from controlled observations that can substantiate that view. Some have suggested that liberal use of epidural analgesia improves infant outcome in preterm delivery, particularly when the infant is presenting by the breech (Crawford 1975). It is logical to assume that abolishing the urge to push before the cervix is fully dilated will reduce the risk of vaginal breech delivery. It is also reasonable to think that abolishing the urge to push against a partially dilated cervix and that relaxation of the pelvic musculature can offer protection against compression of the fetal head. There is no evidence, however, to show that what is logical in theory also occurs in practice. Consequently, there is as yet no place for routine use of epidural anaesthesia in order to protect the baby against supposed mechanical trauma at birth. Similar or even greater protection might be achieved by close communication with the woman and careful guidance.

6.2 Elective forceps delivery

In many places, prophylactic forceps have become accepted practice, but there have been few attempts to assess whether their assumed benefits exist. Some of the assumed benefits may be questioned on theoretical grounds. For instance, Healy and Laufe (1985) reported that the forceps designed by Simpson, Tucker–McLean and Luikart are the most commonly used instruments for outlet forceps deliveries in North America. These crossed instruments are effective levers and any compression applied at the handles is transmitted directly to the blades and hence to the fetal head. Crossed forceps transmit a substantial part of the traction force during delivery as compression force to the fetal head (see Chapter 71) which, especially when utilized by less experienced doctors, may be particularly damaging to the preterm baby with its soft bones and wide skull sutures (Wigglesworth and Pape 1980).

Only one trial has been reported comparing elective forceps with spontaneous delivery for the preterm infant (Maltau *et al.* 1984). The outcomes addressed were limited to retinal haemorrhages, which may or may not be an indicator of (traumatic) intracranial haemorrhages in the preterm neonate. In this trial 'a randomized selection into spontaneous birth versus forceps delivery was performed' (Maltau *et al.* 1984) for infants between 28 and 35 weeks' gestation, and data are reported on 23 babies in each group. The authors also reported, however, that 'additionally 4 infants randomized to spontaneous birth were excluded from the study due to their critical clinical condition which prohibited ophthalmological examination during the first 48 hours of life'. This statement casts some doubt on the nature of the 'randomized selection' that was applied.

Retinal haemorrhages were observed in 2 of 23 infants in the forceps group (which in this study consisted of 'gentle traction' with a small Simpson forceps) and in 1 of 23 infants in the spontaneous group. Extensive haemorrhage occurred in one infant in each group. The incidence of retinal haemorrhages (3 of 46; 6.5 per cent) was much lower in this small series of preterm infants than that observed by the same ophthalmologist in term infants born spontaneously (41 per cent) or by forceps (16 per cent) at the same institution (Egge *et al.* 1981).

Early observational studies reported a lower incidence of mortality (Russell and Betts 1952; Briscoe 1964) and of neurological morbidity at follow-up (Bishop *et al.* 1965) in preterm infants after elective outlet forceps delivery than after spontaneous delivery. More recently, Beverley *et al.* (1984) observed intraventricular haemorrhage in 12 of 30 infants (40 per cent) after spontaneous vertex delivery, and in 11 of 58 (19 per cent) delivered by forceps before 35 weeks' gestation. They concluded that '. . . protection of the head with forceps during vaginal vertex delivery in some part prevent the development of subsequent intraventricular haemorrhage'. Like the authors of earlier reports, they assumed that association and causation are synonymous, without addressing the question of selection bias and without correcting for gestational age differences in the two groups.

Other uncontrolled studies have arrived at entirely different conclusions. Haesslein and Goodlin (1979), for instance, found the incidence of intraventricular haemorrhage among infants born in vertex position with weights between 800 and 1350 g to be twice as high after elective low forceps delivery than after spontaneous delivery. Fairweather and Stewart (1983) found no statistical difference in neonatal outcome between the two methods of delivery in infants between 500 and 1500 g, though mortality was slightly higher in infants delivered by forceps. Schwartz *et al.* (1983) found no difference in mortality or in short term neonatal morbidity between 394 infants of 1000 to 2500 g delivered by low forceps and 671 delivered spontaneously; they reported that infants of 1000 to 2000 g delivered by forceps had a higher incidence of jaundice and sepsis than those delivered spontaneously. Looking more specifically at haemorrhages of traumatic origin, O'Driscoll *et al.* (1981) observed that, in a period of 17 years in which they dealt with a total of 110 344 births, the only preterm infants who died from traumatic intracranial haemorrhage, were those who were delivered by forceps. They suggested that 'this form of prophylaxis actually causes the lesion which it is meant to prevent' (O'Driscoll *et al.* 1981).

In conclusion, there is currently no evidence that routine use of forceps to deliver the preterm baby confers more benefit than harm. The theoretical considerations on which the policy is based are counterbalanced by the equally theoretical disadvantages of the types of instrument that are most commonly used. The old and uncontrolled observational data which are frequently cited in support of 'prophylactic' forceps delivery, must be offset against more recent, but equally uncontrolled, data demonstrating greater harm in infants so delivered than in those delivered spontaneously. Given the lack of evidence for any neonatal benefits and the clear potential for maternal injury and morbidity (see Chapter 71), recommendations for routine use of forceps to deliver the preterm baby in vertex presentation should be regarded as well-intentioned, but ill-conceived.

6.3 Routine use of early episiotomy

Apparently only one trial has addressed the question as to whether routine use of episiotomy for delivery of the preterm baby improves neonatal outcome (Lobb and Cooke 1986). Some attendant staff at the institution where the trial was conducted routinely performed an episiotomy, while others did not. Women whose babies were expected to weigh less than 1500 g at birth were randomly allocated to one or other of these two groups of staff. The staff apparently also differed in their use of forceps for delivery since 18 of 43 women (42 per cent) allocated to the practice of routine episiotomy had a forceps delivery compared with 4 of 51 (8 per cent) women in the other group. Furthermore, the process of randomization, details of which were not reported, failed to provide comparable groups. Infants whose mothers had been allocated to a policy of no episiotomy had a mean gestational age which was 2 weeks less and a mean birthweight which was 150 g less than the infants whose mothers had been allocated to the policy of routine episiotomy.

There were no traumatic intracranial haemorrhages among the 94 babies, but 22 had periventricular haemorrhages. Nine of these were born to the 43 mothers allocated to routine episiotomy and 13 were born to the 51 mothers assigned to the alternative policy. Conclusions as to whether a policy of routine episiotomy confers any benefit cannot be reached from this trial. To circumvent the discrepancies in gestational age, birthweight, and use of forceps between the two groups, the authors performed a sub-analysis on infants born without the use of forceps between 25 and 28 weeks of gestation; 8 of 15 (53 per cent) in the episiotomy group and 19 of 33 (57 per cent) in the no-episiotomy group had intraventricular haemorrhages. The authors concluded that their results 'do not support the use of episiotomy in preterm delivery' (Lobb and Cooke 1986).

The lack of controlled experimentation to obtain evidence that routine mutilation of the perineum and its short and long term sequelae (see Chapter 68) are counterbalanced by improvements in infant outcome, need not be surprising. What is surprising is that statements such as 'the smaller the fetus, the larger should be the episiotomy' have become a time-honoured policy (Kubli 1977) and are reiterated throughout the literature on preterm delivery in the absence of such evidence. The editors of a major text dealing with the controversies in providing care for delivery of the infant under 1500 g summarized it as follows: 'all authors re-emphasize the significance of . . . utilizing a generous episiotomy' (Zuspan and Christian 1983).

Some have suggested that 'large retractors which are introduced in the vagina and by which the perineum may be stretched sufficiently without being cut' may be equally effective (Kubli 1977), but again there are no controlled data to substantiate such claims. It certainly is incumbent upon those who advocate routine use of episiotomy, to familiarize themselves with the significant maternal morbidity and discomfort that result from episiotomy (see Chapter 68), and to provide evidence that there is at least some neonatal gain that can be offset against it.

6.4 Immediate care at birth

6.4.1 Cord clamping

Opinions as to when the cord should be clamped after preterm delivery vary as much as they do for term delivery (see Chapter 67). The physiological consequences of early versus late cord clamping have not been studied as well in the preterm infant as they have been at term. In the preterm infant, delayed cord clamping is associated with a 50 per cent increase in red cell volume and 56 per cent of this placental transfusion occurs within the first minute after birth (Saigal *et al.* 1972). Proponents of delayed clamping have suggested that the placental transfusion may expand the pulmonary bed and prevent respiratory distress; prevent hypovolaemia and hypotension; and increase haemoglobin concentrations and total body iron stores (see Chapter 67). Critics argue that the large transfusion may encourage pulmonary oedema and increase the risk of intracranial haemorrhage and hyperbilirubinaemia. From the available evidence, admittedly gathered predominantly in infants who were not born preterm, there does not seem to be any justification, at present, for rushing to clamp the cord on the basis of any of these postulated effects (see Chapter 67). In fact, some (Dunn PM, personal communication) have argued for many years that the preterm infant born at caesarean section should be delivered and handed to the neonatologist with the placenta still attached. Controlled experiments to assess the benefits of this approach are thus far not available.

At vaginal delivery, when delivery of the placenta cannot be as readily controlled as it can at caesarean section, the timing of cord clamping is likely to be largely influenced by the urgency of the need for specialist neonatal care.

Extrapolation of the data available on term delivery (see Chapter 67) to the preterm infant suggests that it may be worthwhile to observe a 1-minute delay between delivery and cord clamping. Hofmeyr *et al.* (1988) recently proposed that early cord clamping before the establishment of the pulmonary circulation may cause surges in arterial pressure sufficient to contribute to the development of intraventricular haemorrhage, and that a 1-minute delay between delivery and cord clamping may protect the preterm infant against haemorrhage. Hofmeyr *et al.* (1988) randomly assigned 38 infants born before 35 weeks of gestation to a policy of cord clamping either immediately at birth or after a delay of 1 minute. Ten of 13 (77 per cent) infants in the early, but only 8 of 23 infants (35 per cent) in the delayed clamping group developed signs of peri- or intraventricular haemorrhage on ultrasonography performed between 6 and 72 hours of birth. Nevertheless, conclusive interpretation of these results is difficult for three reasons. First, despite strict adherence to the randomization protocol, the two groups differed markedly in their incidence of low Apgar score, low arterial pH and very low birthweight. All of these, which could not have been influenced by the cord clamping policy, were more unfavourable in the early clamping group. Second, all five neonatal deaths occurred in the group with delayed clamping; this may have been due to the disproportionally larger number of very small and asphyxiated babies in this group, but it may also be related to the late clamping policy. Third, no ultrasonography was performed after 72 hours, and it is possible that the policy of delayed clamping may have postponed rather than prevented the occurrence of intraventricular haemorrhage. Indirect evidence that policies implemented at delivery can postpone the development of intraventricular haemorrhage was recently presented by Anderson *et al.* (1988). These authors observed that infants delivered by caesarean section had a lower incidence of intraventricular haemorrhage in the first few days after birth, but that the incidence at 7 days of age was the same as that observed after vaginal delivery. It remains therefore unknown whether alternative policies of cord clamping have a significant impact on neonatal outcome.

6.4.2 *Resuscitation*

As mentioned earlier, a paediatrician should be present at all preterm deliveries. For the very preterm and very small infant, that paediatrician should be an experienced neonatologist and decisions with regard to resuscitation and suctioning (see Chapter 75) should be his or her prerogative, taken in harmony with the parents and the obstetrician.

Some authors have recommended immediate intubation of all very small or very preterm infants at birth. There has been only one clinical trial comparing a policy of elective tracheal intubation with a policy of selective intubation (Drew 1982); it was conducted in infants weighing 1500 g or less, regardless of whether they showed signs of asphyxia at birth and this has been discussed elsewhere (see Chapter 75). As Tyson *et al.* (see Chapter 75) point out, the evidence that is available does not support elective intubation of preterm infants by persons who are not eminently proficient in the necessary skills. It is not justified to assume that the results of intubation by very experienced resuscitators can be reproduced by others with a lesser degree of skill; and in these circumstances the hazards are likely to be greater than the gain (see Chapter 75).

If an experienced obstetrician is a key issue at delivery of the very preterm baby, so is the presence of an experienced neonatologist. The major contribution of the obstetrician at this particular time is to ensure that the baby is not born into a 'comfortably' cool environment (Silverman *et al.* 1958). The simple measure of providing adequate heat in the delivery room can contribute more to subsequent neonatal well-being than any of the other measures that, in many places, are routinely applied to effect delivery of the preterm infant.

7 Conclusions

'There is a great temptation to take the simple path, uncritically follow the precepts of leaders in the field, or succumb to the seduction of the uncontrolled studies'.
Milner *et al.* 1984

Preterm delivery is an ordeal for both mother and baby. In addition, both may suffer its consequences for a lifetime. This is a matter that cannot be taken lightly by anyone who provides care for mother and baby at that time. This chapter has not dealt with the need to provide empathetic understanding and emotional support at and around preterm delivery. These essential elements are discussed in detail in other chapters in this book; it must be realized though that they are indispensable ingredients of effective care for preterm delivery.

7.1 Implications for current practice

Preterm delivery encompasses a variety of different clinical situations. In some the risk is little different from that of delivery at term; in others the utmost sophistication of facilities and skills is necessary if the infant is to have even a remote hope of intact survival. Many fetuses are already compromised by factors, such as congenital malformations, fetal disorders or complicating maternal illness, in addition to being preterm. Care for preterm delivery must, therefore be carefully individualized, taking all these factors into consideration.

The plan of care for preterm delivery should be governed by consideration of gestational age rather than of estimated weight, because gestational age is a better indicator of prognosis.

The baby should be delivered in an institution that has all the necessary facilities and skilled personnel readily available both before and after birth. It is clearly inappropriate to contemplate caesarean section for the very preterm infant where adequate facilities for intensive neonatal care do not exist. Transfer of the baby after birth is not as likely to be effective as birth in a centre that is adequately equipped and staffed to assess the fetus prior to delivery, ensure that the fetus is alive and well, rule out congenital malformations, accurately establish fetal presentation before delivery, and perform the skilled resuscitation that may be necessary at the moment of birth. Even for the woman in active labour, tocolytics may be an effective means of delaying delivery long enough to permit transfer of the mother to such a centre.

The choice of the best route of delivery, caesarean section or vaginal delivery, is by no means easy. The observational data on the differential effects of abdominal and vaginal delivery are all subject to such major biases, comparing unlike cohorts, that their results should be totally ignored. In the absence of guidance from controlled trials, caesarean section with its known risks to the mother should be the exception rather than the rule. This applies to the fetus presenting as a breech as well as to that presenting as a vertex.

A careful ultrasound examination is essential before caesarean delivery of a preterm infant, to ensure that the baby is free of lethal congenital malformations, to precisely determine the fetal presentation and allow correction if necessary before the uterus is incised, and to determine the position of the placenta, which may interfere with extraction of the baby. It is important that the incision be adequate in size, sometimes difficult with the poorly developed lower segment characteristic of the preterm uterus. Extraction of the baby through an inadequate incision may be at least as traumatic as the most difficult vaginal delivery.

The head of the preterm baby is more vulnerable to injury, either from compression or sudden expansion, than that of the baby at term. There is no evidence to suggest, however, that either elective forceps delivery or routine use of episiotomy will in any way reduce that risk. Indeed, there are strong theoretical reasons to believe that forceps delivery will actually increase the risk to the baby. The routine use of both of these procedures should be abandoned, unless they can be shown in controlled trials to confer more benefit than harm.

As the evidence in favour of early or late clamping of the umbilical cord is conflicting, the most reasonable recommendation would be to base the decision on when to perform this on the urgency of the need for resuscitation.

A paediatrician should be in attendance at all preterm deliveries. For the very preterm or very small infant, this should be an experienced neonatologist capable of making the decisions and performing the skilled resuscitation that may be necessary.

Prevention of asphyxia, avoidance of trauma and protection from cold stress at birth are main elements of care for preterm delivery. Meticulous attention to the features that should be present for all births, such as a warm environment and empathetic consideration, is even more important in preterm birth than it is for birth at term.

7.2 Implications for future research

The prognosis for the preterm baby needs to be better quantified, as a guide to individualization of care. For this, geographically rather than institutionally based data are required, and these data must be based on gestational age, rather than on birthweight alone.

When (and if) caesarean section has a place in the care for preterm delivery, either for the infant presenting as a breech or a vertex, are inherently answerable questions, if the repeated calls for randomized controlled trials are eventually heeded. They will not be answered until that time. The experience from unsuccessfully mounted trials in several countries suggests that randomization of practitioners or units to the two alternative forms of care may be a more successful avenue to pursue than the random assignment of individual women and babies to alternative policies within the same institution. The place, if any, for routine forceps delivery or episiotomy for delivery of the preterm baby can also be answered only in the context of randomized controlled trials of sufficient size. All of these would require multicentre collaboration for a definitive answer, but even small, single centre trials, if properly conducted and reported, could start to fill the enormous gaps in knowledge on the effects of procedures which have been advocated for decades without any evidence that they do more good than harm.

The small trials of phenobarbital administration to the mother to prevent intraventricular haemorrhage are promising. They deserve replication in trials that are more carefully controlled for allocation bias, so that their positive findings can be either confirmed or refuted.

The frequency with which very preterm infants continue to be delivered in institutions that do not possess an infrastructure capable of providing effective care for these fetuses and infants constitutes a major problem. More research should therefore be conducted into effective means to ensure that the mothers and babies who are in need of this very special care do indeed gain access to that care.

References

Abernathy JR, Greenberg BG, Donnelly JF (1966). Application of discriminant functions in perinatal death and survival. Am J Obstet Gynecol, 95: 860–867.

Alberman E (1977). Sociobiologic factors and birth weight in Great Britain. In: The Epidemiology of Prematurity. Reed DM, Stanley FJ (eds). Baltimore: Urban & Schwarzenberg, pp 145–156.

Allan WC, Philip AGS (1985). Neonatal cerebral pathology diagnosed by ultrasound. Clin Perinatol, 12: 195–218.

Anderson GD, Bada HS, Sibai BM, Harvey C, Korones SB, Magill HL, Wong SP, Tullis K (1988). The relationship between labor and route of delivery in the preterm infant. Am J Obstet Gynecol, 158: 1382–1390.

Anwar M, Kadam S, Hiatt IM, Hegyi T (1986). Phenobarbitone prophylaxis of intraventricular haemorrhage. Arch Dis Child, 61: 196–197.

Bada HS, Korones SB, Anderson GD, Magill HL, Wong SP (1984). Obstetric factors and relative risk of neonatal germinal layer/intraventricular hemorrhage. Am J Obstet Gynecol, 148: 798–804.

Bakketeig LS, Hoffman HJ (1981). Epidemiology of preterm birth: Results from a longitudinal study of births in Norway. In: Preterm Labour. Elder MG, Hendricks CH (eds). London: Butterworths, pp 17–46.

Battaglia FC, Frazier TM, Hellegers AE (1966). Birthweight, gestational age, and pregnancy outcome, with special reference to high birthweight-low gestational age infant. Pediatrics, 37: 417–422.

Beard R (1977). Discussion remark. In: Pre-term Labour. Proceedings of the Fifth Study Group of the Royal College of Obstetricians and Gynaecologists. Anderson A, Beard R, Brudenell JM, Dunn PM (eds). London: Royal College of Obstetricians and Gynaecologists, pp 361–362.

Bedard MP, Shankaran S, Slovis TL, Pantoja A, Dayal B, Poland RL (1984). Effect of prophylactic phenobarbital on intraventricular hemorrhage in high-risk infants. Pediatrics, 73: 435–439.

Beverley DW, Chance GW, Coates CF (1984). Intraventricular haemorrhage: Timing of occurrence and relationship to perinatal events. Br J Obstet Gynaecol, 91: 1007–1013.

Bieniarz J, Burd L, Scommegna A (1983). Management of preterm labor. In: Reid's Controversies in Obstetrics and Gynecology III. Zuspan FP, Christian CD (eds). Philadelphia: WB Saunders, pp 80–91.

Bishop EH, Israel SL, Briscoe CC (1965). Obstetric influences on the premature infant's first year of development: A report from the collaborative study of cerebral palsy. Obstet Gynecol, 26: 628–635.

Bodmer B, Benjamin A, McLean FH, Usher RH (1986). Has use of cesarean section reduced the risks of delivery in the preterm breech presentation? Am J Obstet Gynecol, 154: 244–250.

Bowes WA (1977). Results of the intensive perinatal management of very low birth weight infants (501–1500 g). In: Preterm Labour. Proceedings of the Fifth Study Group of the Royal College of Obstetricians and Gynaecologists. Anderson A, Beard R, Brudenell JM, Dunn PM (eds). London: Royal College of Obstetricians and Gynaecologists, pp 331–355.

Bowes WA (1981). A review of perinatal mortality in Colorado, 1971 to 1978, and its relationship to the regionalization of perinatal services. Am J Obstet Gynecol, 141: 1045–1052.

Bowes W (1983). Intensive obstetric management of the very low birth weight infant. In: Reid's Controversies in Obstetrics and Gynecology III. Zuspan FP, Christian CD (eds). Philadelphia: WB Saunders, pp 137–148.

Bowes WA, Taylor ES, O'Brien M, Bowes C (1979). Breech delivery: Evaluation of the method of delivery on perinatal results and maternal morbidity. Am J Obstet Gynecol, 135: 965–973.

Brenner WE, Edelman DA, Hendricks CH (1976). A standard of fetal growth for the United States of America. Am J Obstet Gynecol, 124: 555–564.

Briscoe CC (1964). Delivery of the premature infant. Clin Obstet Gynecol, 7: 695–706.

Bryce R, Stanley FJ (1985). Can prematurity be prevented? New Doctor, 36: 9–10.

Chamberlain R (1975). Birthweight and length of gestation. In: British Births 1970. Vol 1: The First Week of Life. London: Heinemann, pp 50–88.

Chng PK (1981). An analysis of preterm singleton deliveries and associated perinatal deaths in a total population. Br J Obstet Gynaecol, 88: 814–818.

Cox C, Kendall AC, Hommes H (1982). Changed prognosis of breech-presenting low birth weight infants. Br J Obstet Gynaecol, 89: 881–886.

Crawford JS (1975). Lumbar epidural analgesia for the singleton breech presentation. Anaesthesia, 30: 119–120.

Crowley P (1981). Mode of delivery and survival in babies weighing less than 2000 g at birth. Br Med J, 282: 71–72.

Crowley P, Hawkins DF (1980). Premature breech delivery: The caesarean section debate. J Obstet Gynaecol, 1: 2–6.

Cruikshank DP, Pitkin RM (1977). Delivery of the premature breech. Obstet Gynecol, 50: 367–369.

De Crespigny LJC, Pepperell RJ (1979). Perinatal mortality and morbidity in breech presentation. Obstet Gynecol, 53: 141–145.

Dillon WP, Egan EA (1981). Aggressive obstetric management in late second-trimester deliveries. Obstet Gynecol, 58: 685–690.

Donn SM, Roloff DW, Goldstein GW (1981). Prevention of intraventricular haemorrhage in pre-term infants by phenobarbitone: A controlled trial. Lancet, 2: 215–217.

Doring GK, De Sousa GAI (1988). Zum Wandel der Beckenendlagenentbindung. Geburtshilfe Frauenheilkd, 48: 150–154.

Drew JH (1982). Immediate intubation at birth of the very-low-birth-weight infant: Effect on survival. Am J Dis Child, 136: 207–210.

Drillien CM (1958). Growth and development in a group of children of very low birth weight. Pediatrics, 27: 452–464.

Duenhoelter JH, Wells CE, Reisch JS, Santos-Ramos R, Jimenez JM (1979). A paired controlled study of vaginal and abdominal delivery of the low birth weight breech fetus. Obstet Gynecol, 54: 310–313.

Editorial commentary (1988). Prognosis for infants born at 23 to 28 weeks' gestation. Obstet Gynecol Surv, 43: 445–447.

Effer SB, Saigal S, Rand C, Hunter DJS, Stoskopf B, Harder AC, Nimrod C, Milner R (1983). Effect of delivery mode on outcomes in the very low birth weight breech infant: Is the improved survival rate related to caesarean section or other perinatal care maneuvers? Am J Obstet Gynecol, 145: 123–128.

Egge K, Lyng G, Maltau J (1981). Effect of instrumental delivery on the frequency and severity of retinal hemorrhages in the newborn. Acta Obstet Gynecol Scand, 60: 153–155.

Ericson A, Eriksson M, Westerholm P, Zetterstrom R (1984). Pregnancy outcome and social indicators in Sweden. Acta Pediatr Scand, 73: 69–74.

Fairweather DVI, Stewart AL (1983). How to deliver the under 1500-gram infant. In: Reid's Controversies in Obstetrics and Gynecology III. Zuspan FP, Christian CD (eds). Philadelphia: WB Saunders, pp 154–164.

FIGO News (1976). Lists of gynecologic and obstetrical terms and definitions. Int J Gynaecol Obstet, 14: 570–576.

Frenzel J, Krause W, Sander I, Michels W (1984). Zur Früh- und Spätmorbidität mindergewichtiger Neugeborener (LBWI) nach Beckenendlagen in Abhängigkeit vom Entbindungsmodus. Z Geburtshilfe Perinatol, 188: 261–268.

Garcia-Prats JA, Procianoy RS, Adams JM, Rudolph AJ (1982). The hyaline membrane disease–intraventricular hemorrhage relationship in the very low birth weight infant: Perinatal aspects. Acta Paediatr Scand, 71: 79–84.

Geirsson RT, Namunkangula R, Calder AA, Lunan CB (1982). Preterm singleton breech presentation: The impact of traumatic intracranial haemorrhage on neonatal mortality. J Obstet Gynaecol, 2: 219–223.

Gimovski ML, Paul RH (1982). Singleton breech presentation in labor: Experience in 1980. Am J Obstet Gynecol, 143: 733–739.

Goldenberg RL, Nelson KG (1977). The premature breech. Am J Obstet Gynecol, 127: 240–244.

Goldenberg RL, Humphrey JL, Hake CB, Boyd BW, Wayne JB (1983). Neonatal deaths in Alabama. II: Policy and research implications derived from a comparison of birth-weight specific state and medical center neonatal mortality rates. Am J Obstet Gynecol, 145: 545–552.

Goldenberg RL, Nelson KG, Koski JF, Cutter GR (1985a).

Low birthweight, intrauterine growth retardation, and preterm delivery. Am J Obstet Gynecol, 152: 980–984.

Goldenberg RL, Nelson KG, Koski JF (1985b). Neonatal mortality in infants weighing 501–1000 g. Am J Obstet Gynecol, 151: 608–611.

Grant A (1986). Randomized trial of preterm breech delivery. Br Med J, 293: 562–563.

Greisen G, Block-Petersen M (1983). Intraventricular haemorrhage and method of delivery of very low birth weight infants. J Perinat Med, 11: 67–73.

Greisen G, Jacobsen JC, Ulrichsen H, Wyboe J (1983). Method of delivery of low birthweight infants. A retrospective analysis. J Perinat Med, 11: 162–168.

Haesslein HC, Goodlin RC (1979). Delivery of the tiny newborn. Am J Obstet Gynecol, 134: 192–200.

Hall MH (1985). Incidence and distribution of preterm labour. In: Pre-term Labour and its Consequences. Proceedings of the Thirteenth Study Group of the Royal College of Obstetricians and Gynaecologists. Beard RW, Sharp F (eds). London: Royal College of Obstetricians and Gynaecologists, pp 5–13.

Hambleton G, Wigglesworth JS (1976). Origin of intraventricular haemorrhage in the preterm infant. Arch Dis Child, 51: 651–659.

Hanson LM (1988). Antenatal phenobarbitone for prevention of intracranial haemorrhage. In: Oxford Database of Perinatal Trials. Oxford: Oxford University Press.

Harris TR, Isaman J, Giles HR (1978). Improved neonatal survival through maternal transport. Obstet Gynecol, 52: 294–300.

Healy DL, Laufe LE (1985). A survey of obstetric forceps residency training in North America. Am J Obstet Gynecol, 151: 54–58.

Heinonen K, Matilainen R, Ksoki H, Launiala K (1985). Intrauterine growth retardation (IUGR) in pre-term infants. J Perinat Med, 13: 171–178.

Heinonen K, Hakulinen A, Jokela V (1988). Survival of the smallest. Time trends and determinants of mortality in a very preterm population during the 1980s. Lancet, 2: 204–207.

Hellier JL, Goldstein H (1979). The use of birthweight and gestation to assess perinatal mortality risk. J Epidemiol Community Health, 33: 183–185.

Herschel M, Kennedy JL, Kayne HL, Henry M, Cetrulo CL (1982). Survival of infants born at 24 to 28 weeks' gestation. Obstet Gynecol, 60: 154–158.

Hielscher K, Renziehausen K, Muller K (1986). Der Einfluss des Entbindungsverfahrens auf die perinatale Mortalität und neonatale Morbidität untergewichtiger Beckenendlagen. Zbl Gynäkol, 108: 1465–1472.

Hochuli E, Käch O (1981). Die Beckenendlage. Geburtshilfe Frauenheilkd, 41: 23–31.

Hoffman HJ, Bakketeig LS (1984). Risk factors associated with the occurrence of preterm birth. Clin Obstet Gynecol, 27: 539–552.

Hofmeyr GJ, Bolton KD, Bowen DC, Govan JJ (1988). Periventricular/intraventricular haemorrhage and umbilical cord clamping. S Afr Med J, 73: 104–106.

Horwood SP, Boyle MH, Torrance GW, Sinclair JC (1982). Mortality and morbidity of 500 to 1499 gram birthweight infants liveborn to residents of a defined geographic region before and after neonatal intensive care. Pediatrics, 69: 613–620.

Hoskins EM, Elliot E, Shennan AT, Skidmore MB, Keith E (1983). Outcome of very low-birth weight infants born at a perinatal center. Am J Obstet Gynecol, 145: 135–140.

Ingemarsson I, Westgren M, Svenningsens NW (1978). Long-term follow-up of preterm infants in breech presentation delivered by caesarean section. Lancet, 2: 172–175.

Kaltreider DF (1967). Premature labor and meperidine analgesia. Am J Obstet Gynecol, 99: 989–993.

Kaltreider DF, Kohl S (1980). Epidemiology of preterm delivery. Clin Obstet Gynecol, 23: 17–31.

Kanhai HHH (1981). Achtergronden en konsekwenties van vroeggeboorte. Leiden University: MD thesis.

Kanhai HH, Keirse MJNC (1982). Perinatal hazards of elective versus spontaneous preterm birth. In: Proceedings of the Eighth European Congress of Perinatal Medicine. Thiery M, Senterre J, Derom R (eds). Angleur: Nelissen, p 8.

Kariniemi V, Jarvenpaa AL, Teramo K (1984). Fetal heart rate patterns and perinatal outcome of very low birthweight infants. Br J Obstet Gynaecol, 91: 18–22.

Karp LE, Doney JR, McCarthy T, Meiss PJ, Hall M (1979). The premature breech: Trial of labour or cesarean section. Obstet Gynecol, 53: 88–92.

Kaupilla O, Grönroos M, Aro P, Aittoniemi P, Kuoppala M (1981). Management of low birthweight breech delivery: Should caesarean section be routine? Obstet Gynecol, 57: 289–294.

Keirse MJNC (1979). Epidemiology of pre-term labour. In: Human Parturition. New Concepts and Developments. Keirse MJNC, Anderson ABM, Bennebroek Gravenhorst J (eds). The Hague: Leiden University Press, pp 219–234.

Keirse MJNC (1987). De Nederlandse perinatale sterfte in internationaal perspectief. Ned Tijdschr Geneeskd, 131: 905–909.

Keirse MJNC, Kanhai HHH (1981). An obstetrical viewpoint on preterm birth with particular reference to perinatal morbidity and mortality. In: Aspects of Perinatal Morbidity. Huisjes HJ (ed). Groningen: Universitaire Boekhandel Nederland, pp 1–35.

Kirkley WH (1980). Fetal survival: What price? Presidential address. Am J Obstet Gynecol, 137: 873–875.

Kitchen WH, Campbell DG (1971). Controlled trial of intensive care for very low birth weight infants. Pediatrics, 48: 711–714.

Kitchen W, Ford GW, Doyle LW, Rickards AL, Lissenden JV, Peperell RJ, Duke JE (1985). Caesarean section or vaginal delivery at 24 to 28 weeks' gestation: Comparison of survival and neonatal and two-year morbidity. Obstet Gynecol, 66: 149–157.

Kosmetatos N, Dinter C, Williams ML, Lourie H, Berne AS (1980). Intracranial hemorrhage in the premature: Its predictive features and outcome. Am J Dis Child, 134: 855–859.

Kuban KCK, Krishnamoorthy KS, Brown ER, Teele RL, Baglivo JA, Sullivan KF, Huff KR, White S, Cleveland RH, Allred EN, Spritzer KL, Skouteli HN, Cayea P, Epstein MF (1986). Neonatal intracranial hemorrhage and phenobarbital. Pediatrics, 77: 443–450.

Kubli F (1977). Discussion opener. In: Pre-term Labour.

Proceedings of the Fifth Study Group of the Royal College of Obstetricians and Gynaecologists. Anderson A, Beard R, Brudenell JM, Dunn PM (eds). London: Royal College of Obstetricians and Gynaecologists, pp 356–359.

Lamont RF (1985). Factors influencing the route of delivery of the preterm infant. In: Pre-term Labour and its Consequences. Proceedings of the Thirteenth Study Group of the Royal College of Obstetricians and Gynaecologists. Beard RW, Sharp F (eds). London: Royal College of Obstetricians and Gynaecologists, pp 263–271.

Lamont RF, Dunlop PDM, Crowley P, Elder MG (1983). Spontaneous preterm labour and delivery at under 34 weeks' gestation. Br Med J, 286: 454–457.

Lefebvre F, Bard H, Veilleux A, Martel C (1988). Outcome at school age of children with birthweight of 1000 g or less. Dev Med Child Neurol, 30: 170–180.

Levene MI, Fawer CL, Lamont RF (1982). Risk factors in the development of intraventricular haemorrhage in the preterm neonate. Arch Dis Child, 57: 410–417.

Lewis BV, Seneviratne HR (1979). Vaginal breech delivery or cesarean section. Am J Obstet Gynecol, 134: 615–618.

Lobb MO, Cooke RWI (1986). The influence of episiotomy on the neonatal survival and incidence of periventricular haemorrhage in very-low-birth-weight infants. Eur J Obstet Gynecol Reprod Biol, 22: 17–21.

Lumley J, Lester A, Renou P, Wood C (1985). A failed RCT to determine the best method of delivery for very low birth weight infants. Controlled Clin Trials, 6: 120–127.

Luthy DA, Shy KK, Van Belle G, Larson EB, Hughes JP, Benedetti TJ, Brown ZA, Effer S, King JF, Stenchever MA (1987). A randomized trial of electronic fetal monitoring in preterm labor. Obstet Gynecol, 69: 687–695.

Lyons ER, Papsin FR (1978). Caesarean section in the management of breech presentation. Am J Obstet Gynecol, 130: 558–561.

Macfarlane A, Mugford M (1984). Birth Counts. Statistics of Pregnancy and Childbirth. London: Her Majesty's Stationery Office.

Main DM, Main BK, Maurer MM (1983). Caesarean section versus vaginal delivery for the breech fetus weighing less than 1500 g. Am J Obstet Gynecol, 146: 580–584.

Maltau JM, Egge K, Moe N (1984). Retinal hemorrhages in the preterm neonate. A prospective randomized study comparing the occurrence of hemorrhages after spontaneous vs forceps delivery. Acta Obstet Gynecol Scand, 63: 219–221.

Mann LI, Gallant JM (1979). Modern management of the breech delivery. Am J Obstet Gynecol, 134: 611–614.

McKeown T, Record R (1952). Observations of fetal growth in multiple pregnancies in man. J Endocrinol, 8: 386–394.

Meidell R, Marinelli P, Pettett G (1985). Perinatal factors associated with early-onset intracranial hemorrhage in premature infants. Am J Dis Child, 139: 160–163.

Ment LR, Duncan CC, Ehrenkranz RA (1987). Intraventricular hemorrhage of the preterm neonate. Seminars Perinatol, 11: 132–141.

Miller EC, Kouam L, Schwientek S (1980). Zum problem des perinatalen Mortalität bei der Frühgeburt aus Beckenenddlage im Vergleich zur Schädellage. Geburtshilfe Frauenheilkd, 40: 1013–1021.

Milner RA, Enkin MW, Mohide PT (1984). The importance

of clinical trials in preterm labor. Clin Obstet Gynecol, 27: 606–613.

Molina RD (1988). Antenatal phenobarbital for the prevention of intracerebral hemorrhage in the premature infant. In: Oxford Database of Perinatal Trials. Oxford: Oxford University Press.

Morales WJ, Koerten J (1986). Prevention of intraventricular hemorrhage in very low birth weight infants by maternally administered phenobarbital. Obstet Gynecol, 68: 295–299.

Morgan MEI, Massey RF, Cooke RWI (1982). Does phenobarbitone prevent periventricular hemorrhage in very low-birth-weight babies? A controlled trial. Pediatrics, 70: 186–189.

Myers SA, Gleicher N (1987). Breech delivery: Why the dilemma? Am J Obstet Gynecol, 156: 6–10.

National Center for Health Statistics (1985). Monthly Vital Statistics Report, Vol. 34, No. 6, Suppl.

Nisell H, Bistoletti P, Palme C (1981). Preterm breech delivery. Early and late complications. Acta Obstet Gynecol Scand, 60: 363–366.

Nwaesei CG, Young DC, Byrne JM, Vincer MJ, Sampson D, Evans JR, Allen A, Stinson DA (1987). Preterm birth at 23 to 26 weeks' gestation: Is active obstetric management justified? Am J Obstet Gynecol, 157: 890–897.

O'Driscoll K, Meagher D, MacDonald D, Geoghegan F (1981). Traumatic intracranial haemorrhage in firstborn infants and delivery with obstetric forceps. Br J Obstet Gynaecol, 88: 577–581.

O'Leary JA, Pasley WW (1983). Once a breech, always a cesarean section. In: Reid's Controversies in Obstetrics and Gynecology III. Zuspan FP, Christian CD (eds). Philadelphia: WB Saunders, pp 235–239.

Olshan AF, Shy KK, Luthy DA, Hickok D, Weiss NS, Daling JR (1984). Cesarean birth and neonatal mortality in very low birthweight infants. Obstet Gynecol, 64: 267–270.

Paneth N (1986). Recent trends in preterm delivery rates in the United States. In: Prévention de la Naissance Prématurée. Papiernik E, Bréart G, Spira N (eds). Paris: INSERM, pp 15–30.

Paneth N, Kiely JL, Wallenstein S, Marcus M, Pakter J, Susser M (1982). Newborn intensive care and neonatal mortality in low-birth-weight infants. Population study. New Engl J Med, 307: 149–155.

Paneth N, Wallenstein S, Kiely JL, Snook CP, Susser M (1986). Medical care and preterm infants of normal birth weight. Pediatrics, 77: 158–166.

Paneth N, Kiely JL, Wallenstein S, Susser M (1987). The choice of place of delivery. Effect of hospital level on mortality in all singleton births in New York City. Am J Dis Child, 141: 60–64.

Pape KE, Wigglesworth JS (1979). Haemorrhage, Ischaemia and the Perinatal Brain. London: Heinemann.

Paul RH, Koh KS, Monfared AH (1979). Obstetric factors influencing outcome in infants weighing from 1001 to 1500 grams. Am J Obstet Gynecol, 133: 503–508.

Petitti DB, Golditch IM (1984). Mortality in relation to method of delivery in breech infants. Int J Gynaecol Obstet, 22: 189–193.

Piekkala MM, Kero P, Erkkola R, Sillanpää M (1986). Perinatal events and neonatal morbidity: An analysis of 5380 cases. Early Hum Dev, 13: 249–268.

Porter FL, Marshall RE, Moore J, Miller RH (1985). Effect of phenobarbital on motor activity and intraventicular hemorrhage in preterm infants with respiratory disease weighing less than 1500 g. Am J Perinatol, 2: 63–66.

Roberton NRC (1977). Immediate management of the preterm new-born infant. In: Pre-term Labour. Proceedings of the Fifth Study Group of the Royal College of Obstetricians and Gynaecologists. Anderson A, Beard RW, Brudenell JM, Dunn PM (eds). London: Royal College of Obstetricians and Gynaecologists, pp 315–330.

Rosen MG, Chick L (1984). The effect of delivery route on outcome in breech presentation. Am J Obstet Gynecol, 148: 909–914.

Ross MG, Stubblefield PG (1984). Clinical management of preterm birth. In: Preterm Birth: Causes, Prevention and Management. Fuchs F, Stubblefield PG (eds). New York: Macmillan, pp 279–287.

Rumeau-Rouquette C (1986). Evolution de la prématurité et de sa prévention en France. In: Prévention de la Naissance Prématurée. Papiernik E, Bréart G, Spira N (eds). Paris INSERM, pp 425–442.

Rush RW, Keirse MJNC, Howat P, Baum JD, Anderson ABM, Turnbull AC (1976). Contribution of preterm delivery to perinatal mortality. Br Med J, 2: 965–968.

Rush RW, Davey DA, Segall ML (1978). The effect of preterm delivery on perinatal mortality. Br J Obstet Gynaecol, 85: 806–811.

Russell GR, Betts WA (1952). Natal and neonatal factors in premature infant mortality. J Pediatr, 40: 727–732.

Ruth V (1985). Gehirnschutz mittels Phenobarbital bei Frühgeborenen mit sehr niedrigem Geburtsgewicht (VLBW)—Eine Studie unter kontrollierten Bedingungen. Klin Pädiatr, 197: 170–171.

Saigal S, O'Neill A, Surainder Y, Chua L, Usher R (1972). Placental transfusion and hyperbilirubinemia in the premature. Pediatrics, 49: 406–419.

Saigal S, Rosenbaum P, Stoskopf B, Milner R (1982). Follow-up of infants 501–1500 g birthweight delivered to residents of a geographically defined region with perinatal intensive care facilities. J Pediatr, 100: 606–613.

Scheer K, Nubar J (1976). Variation of fetal presentation with gestational age. Am J Obstet Gynecol, 125: 269–270.

Schwartz DB, Miodovnik M, Lavin JP (1983). Neonatal outcome among low birth weight infants delivered spontaneously or by low forceps. Obstet Gynecol, 62: 283–286.

Scott DT (1987). Premature infants in later childhood: Some recent follow-up results. Seminars Perinatol, 11: 191–199.

Scott KE, Peddle LJ, Rees EP (1984). Impact of regional organization and planned services to reduce perinatal mortality. In: Preterm Birth: Causes, Prevention and Management. Fuchs F, Stubblefield PG (eds). New York: Macmillan, pp 348–376.

Shankaran S, Ilagan N, Cepeda E, Moriana F, Bedard P, Poland RL, Ostrea EM (1984). Antenatal phenobarbital for prevention of neonatal intraventricular hemorrhage: Preliminary observations. Pediatr Res, 18: 346.

Shankaran S, Cepeda EE, Ilagan N, Mariona F, Hassan M, Bhatia R, Ostrea E, Bedard MP, Poland RL (1986). Antenatal phenobarbital for the prevention of neonatal intracerebral hemorrhage. Am J Obstet Gynecol, 154: 53–57.

Silverman WA, Fertig JW, Berger AP (1958). The influence

of the thermal environment upon survival of newly born premature infants. Pediatrics, 22: 876–886.

Smith ML, Spencer SA, Hull D (1980). Mode of delivery and survival in babies weighing less than 2000 g at birth. Br Med J 281: 1118–1119.

Smith ML, Spencer SA, Hull D (1981). Mode of delivery and survival in babies weighing less than 2000 g at birth. Br Med J 282: 72.

Stewart A (1977). Follow-up of pre-term infants. In: Preterm Labour. Proceedings of the Fifth Study Group of the Royal College of Obstetricians and Gynaecologists. Anderson A, Beard RW, Brudenell JM, Dunn PM (eds). London: Royal College of Obstetricians and Gynaecologists, pp 372–384.

Stewart AL, Reynolds EOR (1974). Improved prognosis for infants of very low birth weight. Pediatrics, 54: 724–735.

Stewart AL, Turcan DM, Rawlings G, Reynolds EOR (1977). Prognosis of infants weighing 1000 g or less at birth. Arch Dis Child, 52: 97–104.

Strauss AD, Kirz D, Modanlou HD, Freeman RK (1985). Perinatal events and intraventricular/subependymal hemmorhage in the very-low birthweight infant. Am J Obstet Gynecol, 151: 1022–1027.

Susser MW, Marolla FA, Fleiss J (1972). Birthweight, fetal age and perinatal mortality. Am J Epidemiol, 96: 197–204.

Szymonowicz W (1987). Periventricular haemorrhage and ischaemia in preterm infants. In: Prematurity. Yu VYH, Wood EC (eds). Edinburgh: Churchill Livingstone, pp 198–222.

Tamura RK, Sabbagha RE, Depp R, Vaisrub N, Dooley SL, Socol ML (1984). Diminished growth in fetuses born preterm after spontaneous labor or rupture of membranes. Am J Obstet Gynecol, 148: 1105–1110.

Tejani N, Rebold B, Tuck S, Ditroia D, Sutro W, Verma U (1984). Obstetric factors in the causation of early periventricular-intraventricular hemorrhage. Obstet Gynecol, 64: 510–515.

Thirteenth Study Group of The Royal College of Obstetricians and Gynaecologists (1985). Conclusions. In: Pre-term Labour and its Consequences. Proceedings of the Thirteenth Study Group of the Royal College of Obstetricians and Gynaecologists. Beard RW, Sharp F PM (eds). London: Royal College of Obstetricians and Gynaecologists, pp 401–402.

Thorburn RJ, Stewart AL, Hope PL, Lipscomb AP, Reynolds EOR, Pape KE (1981). Prediction of death and major handicap in very preterm infants by brain ultrasound. Lancet, 2: 1119–1121.

Trudinger BJ, Boshell L (1987). A survey of the management of premature labour by Australian obstetricians. Austral NZ J Obstet Gynaecol, 27: 188–195.

Van de Bor M, Verloove-Vanhorick SP, Brand R, Keirse MJNC, Ruys JH (1987). Incidence and prediction of periventricular-intraventricular hemorrhage in very preterm infants. J Perinat Med, 15: 333–339.

Van Eyck EA, Huisjes HJ (1983). Neonatal mortality and morbidity associated with preterm breech presentation. Eur J Obstet Gynecol Reprod Biol, 15: 17–23.

Van Kamp I, Kanhai HH, Keirse MJNC (1989). The changing pattern of preterm birth (in preparation).

Verloove-Vanhorick SP, Verwey RA (1987). Project on Pre-term and Small for Gestational Age Infants in The Netherlands 1983: A collaborative survey. Leiden University: MD thesis.

Verloove-Vanhorick SP, Verwey RA, Brand R, Bennebroek Gravenhorst J, Keirse MJNC, Ruys JH (1986). Neonatal mortality risk in relation to gestational age and birthweight. Results of a national survey of preterm and very-low-birthweight infants in The Netherlands. Lancet, 1: 55–57.

Verloove-Vanhorick SP, Verwey RA, Ebeling MCA, Brand R, Ruys JH (1988). Mortality in very preterm and very low birth weight infants according to place of birth and level of care: Results of a national collaborative survey of preterm and very low birth weight infants in the Netherlands. Pediatrics, 81: 404–411.

Wallace RL, Schifrin BS, Paul RH (1984). The delivery route for very-low-birth-weight infants. J Reprod Med, 29: 736–740.

Weisbach W, Menzel K, Wagner F (1986). Zur Morbidität und Mortalität in den Jahren 1984–85 aus Beckenendlage geborener Prämaturer mit einem Geburtsgewicht ≤ 1500 g. Eine propspektive Studie zur Fragestellung vaginaler oder abdominaler Entbindungsweg. Zbl Gynäkol, 108: 424–434.

Westgren M (1985). Discussion opener. In: Pre-term Labour and its Consequences. Proceedings of the Thirteenth Study Group of the Royal College of Obstetricians and Gynaecologists. Beard RW, Sharp F PM (eds). London: Royal College of Obstetricians and Gynaecologists, pp 273–276.

Westgren LMR, Songster G, Paul RH (1985). Preterm breech delivery: Another retrospective study. Obstet Gynecol, 66: 481–484.

Westgren LM, Malcus P, Svenningsen NW (1986). Intrauterine asphyxia and long-term outcome in preterm fetuses. Obstet Gynecol, 67: 512–516.

Whitelaw A, Placzek M, Dubowitz L, Lary S, Levene M (1983). Phenobarbitone for prevention of periventricular haemorrhage in very low birth-weight infants. Lancet, 2: 1168–1170.

Wigglesworth JS, Pape KE (1980). Pathophysiology of intracranial hemorrhage in the newborn. J Perinat Med, 8: 119–133.

Woods JR (1979). Effects of low birth weight breech delivery on neonatal morbidity. Obstet Gynecol, 53: 735–740.

World Health Organization (1950). Expert Group on Prematurity: Final Report. Geneva: World Health Organization, Technical Report Series No. 27.

World Health Organization (1961). Public Health Aspects of Low Birthweight. Geneva: World Health Organization, Technical Report Series No. 217.

World Health Organization (1969). Prevention of Perinatal Morbidity and Mortality. Geneva: World Health Organization, Public Health Papers No. 42.

World Health Organization (1977). Recommended definitions, terminology and format for statistical tables related to the perinatal period and use of a new certificate for cause of perinatal deaths. Acta Obstet Gynecol Scand, 56: 247–253.

World Health Organization (1979). Definitions and recommendations. International Statistical Classification of Diseases (9th Revision). Geneva: World Health Organization, vol 1: pp 763–768.

Wulf KH, Kastendieck E, Seelbach-Göbel B (1984). Zum

Geburtsmodus bei Frühgeborenen abdominal oder vaginal? Z Geburtshilfe Perinatol, 188: 249–255.

Yu VYH, Bajuk B, Cutting D, Orgill AA, Astbury J (1984a). Effect of mode of delivery on outcome of very-low-birth-weight infants. Br J Obstet Gynaecol, 91: 633–639.

Yu VYH, Orgill AA, Bajuk B, Astbury J (1984b). Survival and 2-year outcome of extremely preterm infants. Br J Obstet Gynaecol, 91: 640–646.

Yu VYH, Wong PY, Bajuk B, Orgill AA, Astbury J (1986a). Outcome of extremely-low-birthweight infants. Br J Obstet Gynaecol, 93: 162–170.

Yu VYH, Loke HL, Bajuk B, Szymonowicz W, Orgill AA, Astbury J (1986b). Prognosis for infants born at 23 to 28 weeks' gestation. Br Med J, 293: pp 1200–1203.

Zuspan FP, Christian CD (1983). Editorial comment. In: Reid's Controversies in Obstetrics and Gynecology III. Zuspan FP, Christian CD (eds). Philadelphia: WB Saunders, 171–173.

75 Immediate care of the newborn infant

Jon Tyson, William Silverman, and Joan Reisch

1 Introduction

Given the success of human evolution and the exceptionally high survival rate of human infants, it would seem clear that little more than a clear airway and adequate warmth are required to support the first few minutes of neonatal adaptation to extrauterine life for the vast majority of newborns. Despite this, there are striking variations from place to place in the patterns of care and interventions that newborns receive in the immediate post-delivery period. This variety reflects both the inherent resilience and adaptability of the newborn infant and the lack of consensus among caregivers as to the best approach.

This chapter on the immediate postnatal care of the newborn infant is divided into three sections. In the first, we discuss the immediate postnatal care of the apparently healthy normal newborn infant, and some prophylactic measures that have been proposed or recommended for all infants. The second section deals with a number of prophylactic measures that have been proposed for certain subgroups of infants who are considered to be at increased risk of subsequent morbidity. The final section of our chapter discusses some of the measures used for immediate resuscitation of ill newborn infants.

We have used two basic approaches in reviewing our subject. First, to provide information about the scope and variability of recommendations for the immediate postnatal care of newborn infants, we conducted a survey of thirteen major textbooks of obstetrics, maternal–fetal medicine, neonatology, and paediatrics (Tyson, unpublished data). Our survey revealed that some topics, such as tracheal suctioning of infants born after passage of meconium *in utero*, were almost always addressed with specific but highly variable recommendations. Others, for example the use of blood volume expanders in resuscitation, were dealt with by offering rather vague advice. Some important but difficult topics, such as the evaluation of resuscitation services, or the perplexing indications for withholding resuscitative measures, tend not to be addressed at all.

Second, using widely accepted methodological standards for research, we reviewed the information that was available from controlled trials, and we have presented and emphasized the results of those trials that we judged, independently, to have been methodologically adequate (Tyson *et al.* 1983).

2 Immediate care of the normal newborn

2.1 Welcoming the newborn

In his book, *Birth without Violence* (1975), Frederick Leboyer painted a graphic picture of the slapping, sucking out, and cacophony which so often seemed to characterize the immediate care of normal newborn infants. He went on to describe a number of measures to minimize 'the shock of the newborn's first separation experiences'—the use of a dark delivery room, delayed clamping of the umbilical cord, gentle massage, and a warm bath for the infant. Leboyer claimed that infants so treated would grow up to be healthier and free of conflict. Superior development was reported in an uncontrolled follow-up study (Rappoport 1976).

Nelson and colleagues (1980) conducted a randomized trial assessing the effect of Leboyer deliveries on infant neurobehavioural status in the first hour of life, at 24 and 72 hours after birth, and at 8 months of age. No statistically significant effects, either beneficial or harmful, were found in this study or in a clinical trial conducted by Kliot and Silverstein (1984). In a third and as yet unpublished study (Sorrells-Jones 1983), Leboyer deliveries were associated with increased infant alertness in the delivery room and changes in maternal–infant interaction (increased maternal smiling and talking to the infant) on the second postpartum day. No effect on subsequent infant development was identified.

The fact that no specific advantages of the specific measures advocated by Leboyer have been demonstrated should not, however, be taken to mean that the newborn should not be treated with the regard and respect due to any sentient human being.

2.2 Ensuring a clear airway

Although a routine of suctioning to remove secretions from the newborn's oral and nasal passages has been widely recommended, a need for this practice has never been established, and it is by no means universally carried out. The practice is not without potential hazards, including cardiac arrhythmias, laryngospasm, and pulmonary artery vasospasm. Possible benefits include improved air exchange, reduced likelihood of aspiration of secretions, and perhaps reduced acquisition of any pathogens present in the amniotic fluid or birth canal. Controlled trials would be required to evaluate the balance between the potential hazards and the potential benefits of airway suctioning. In the absence of evidence from such trials, the practice cannot be recommended with confidence.

If nasal and pharyngeal suctioning is to be used, care should be taken to minimize pharyngeal stimulation. Suction bulbs, rather than catheters should be used, based on the evidence that suction bulbs are less likely to induce cardiac arrhythmias (Cordero and Hon 1971).

The practice of routine gastric suctioning appears to be even more tenuously based. It seems to have been introduced into practice following the poorly tested suggestion that the respiratory distress of infants of diabetic women often resulted from aspiration that might be prevented by gastric suctioning (Gellis *et al.* 1949). As the passage of the tube during the immediate neonatal period may produce bradycardia or laryngospasm (Cordero and Hon 1971) and disruption of prefeeding behaviour (Widstrom *et al.* 1987), there is no justification for routine gastric suctioning in the delivery room.

2.3 Maintaining body temperature

The recommendation that all babies be kept warm immediately after birth is based on extrapolation from an extensive body of evidence about thermal physiology of both newborn animals and human neonates (Sinclair 1978). With the possible exception of extremely small infants (those weighing less than 750 g), there is solid observational evidence that neonates maintain their body temperature in a cool environment at the metabolic cost of increased energy expenditure. A randomized clinical trial conducted in a delivery room compared acid–base homeostasis in healthy full term infants who were thermally protected with a radiant warmer with control infants who were left uncovered for 2 hours after delivery (Gandy *et al.* 1964). Vigorous neonates exposed in cold delivery rooms experienced marked drops in body temperature and metabolic acidosis. Blood pH in these infants was maintained by respiratory compensation and a reduced $PaCO_2$.

A variety of studies have demonstrated that the postnatal fall in infant temperature can be reduced by skin-to-skin contact between the infant and mother. Gardner (1979) reported that rectal temperature 15 minutes after delivery was the same for infants given skin-to-skin contact as for infants kept in heated beds. Fardig (1980) noted that skin and rectal temperature during the first 45 minutes after birth was higher among infants given immediate skin-to-skin contact than among infants given delayed skin-to-skin contact after a period under a radiant warmer or infants kept under a radiant warmer from birth.

The postnatal fall in temperature can also be reduced by the use of an incubator (Miller and Oliver 1966), or a radiant warmer (Dahm and Jones 1972; Stephenson *et al.* 1970), by drying the infant (Dahm and Jones 1972), or by covering the infant's body or head with insulated material (Baum and Scopes 1968; Besch *et al.* 1971; Holzman 1985; de Saintonge *et al.* 1979).

Despite the contributions of the above studies, many unanswered questions remain about the effects of the early thermal environment on individual babies. The limits of the vague advice to 'reduce initial heat loss and warm to compensate for relatively large losses' have not been explored in depth. Little attention has been given to the findings of Perlstein *et al.* (1974) who reported that short periods of cold stress during the first two postnatal days enhanced the ability of newborns to withstand subsequent cold stress. The effects of different methods of supplying heat to newborns also deserve further evaluation (Marks *et al.* 1986).

2.4 Prophylactic administration of vitamin K to prevent haemorrhagic disease

Most of the textbooks we reviewed recommend routine parenteral administration of vitamin K to all newborn infants and the 'official' guideline in the United States is unequivocal (American Academy of Pediatrics 1983):

'To prevent vitamin K-dependent hemorrhagic disease and coagulation disorders, every neonate should receive a single parenteral dose of 0.5–1.0 mg of natural vitamin K1 oxide (phytonadione) within 1 hour of birth . . .'

Breastfed infants are recognized to be at greater than average risk of developing haemorrhagic disease of the newborn (Keenan *et al.* 1971). Failure to administer vitamin K to breastfed infants may predispose them to serious bleeding for example, intracranial haemorrhage (McNinch *et al.* 1983; Chaou *et al.* 1984). There is, however, a continuing debate about whether or not it is necessary to administer vitamin K to healthy formula-fed infants (Editorial Lancet, 1978; Van Doorm *et al.* 1977). The concentration of vitamin K in cow's milk or infant formula appears to be considerably greater than in human milk, and prothrombin levels in infants given parenteral vitamin K at birth are similar to those in comparable infants given only 24 hours of cow's milk feedings (Keenan *et al.* 1971).

The usually quoted incidence rates of haemorrhagic disease of the newborn in the absence of vitamin K administration range from 0.25 per cent to 0.50 per cent in most series (Oski 1972), but these rates are derived from studies done many years ago, at a time when traumatic deliveries were more common, and when first feedings were often delayed. Thus, the risk that healthy formula-fed infants cared for in present-day nurseries will develop haemorrhagic disease is likely to be considerably smaller. These considerations have led some paediatricians to abandon routine prophylaxis in normal infants.

The early studies of vitamin K prophylaxis were often poorly designed and used coagulation studies of uncertain validity and vitamin preparations and dosages which differ considerably from those used today. The clinical trials conducted during the last 35 years (Myer and Angus 1956; O'Connor and Addiego 1986; Shoskes *et al.* 1961; Sutherland *et al.* 1967; Vietti *et al.* 1960) have included virtually no infants with frank haemorrhagic disease of the newborn. Moreover, they have provided insufficient information about feeding and other factors to address the issue of whether vitamin K administration is warranted for infants who are free of known risk factors for haemorrhagic disease, such as illness, immaturity, circumcision, or maternal coumarin therapy (Aballi *et al.* 1959; Keenan *et al.* 1971; Vietti *et al.* 1960).

A very large study would be required to address these uncertainties. If the incidence of haemorrhagic disease of the newborn in healthy, formula-fed infants given no supplemental vitamin K were as great as 1 in 2000 infants, a sample size of approximately 50 000 infants would be required (accepting a one-sided alpha error of 0.05 and a beta error of 0.05 and assuming no diagnoses of haemorrhagic disease of the newborn in those assigned to vitamin K prophylaxis). It is unlikely that such a trial could ever be carried out in a setting where vitamin K is routinely used, but scope may exist for mounting a controlled trial to estimate its benefits, if any, in areas in which vitamin K is not yet in routine use.

Where a policy of routine vitamin K use is already in place, we consider that the weight of evidence justifies continuing that policy. Based on studies examining its effects on coagulation factors, oral administration of vitamin K1 has also been proposed as an effective alternative to parenteral administration (O'Connor and Addiego 1986), but until more information becomes available, we believe that intramuscular administration is preferable to oral administration.

2.5 Prophylactic measures to prevent eye infections

The Credé procedure of silver nitrate conjunctival prophylaxis, introduced in 1881, was credited with the control of gonococcal ophthalmia of the newborn in the past century. Many countries have a legal requirement that one of a list of approved chemical agents be routinely instilled into the eyes of all newborn infants, with the laudable aim of preventing infectious conjunctivitis. No controlled trials have been carried out to ascertain whether or not this is a more effective means of preventing blindness than clinical observation of the newborn, and adequate treatment of any conjunctivitis that should appear.

When routine chemical prophylaxis is advised or required, the next question is the choice of the most effective, and least harmful agent. The routine use of silver nitrate has been recently questioned, because it results in a higher frequency of conjunctivitis than do other agents (Christian 1960; Mathieu 1958; Wahlberg *et al.* 1982a; Yasunuga and Kean 1977), and because of its uncertain efficacy against the gonococcus, and its ineffectiveness against *chlamydia* (which in many areas is the most common cause of neonatal ophthalmia). None the less, 1 per cent silver nitrate solution in single-use ampoules continues to be included in a list of 'acceptable' agents (erythromycin 0.5 per cent ophthalmic ointment or drops in single-use tubes or ampoules and tetracycline 1 per cent ophthalmic ointment or drops in single-use tubes or ampoules complete the list) in semi-official guidelines—with the caveat that 'silver nitrate does not prevent chlamydial infections' (American Academy of Pediatrics 1983).

In addition to the 'official' three agents listed above, penicillin, sulfonamides, and bacitracin have at times been proposed. Recently, single-dose ceftriaxone has been suggested for African populations with a high incidence of penicillin-resistant gonococcal infections (Laga *et al.* 1986).

A rational choice of agents is difficult. There have been no recently completed trials involving an adequate number of infants with bacterial or chlamydial eye infections (Oriel 1984). Virtually no infants with gonococcal infections have been included with these trials, although a trial of silver nitrate and tetracycline ointment in the prevention of gonococcal and chlamydial ophthalmia is now being conducted in Africa by Laga and co-workers (personal communication). Maternal administration of sulfonamide as a strategy to prevent perinatal transmission of chlamydial infections (Schachter *et al.* 1986) deserves further investigation.

Concern has been voiced that immediate application of topical agents to the newborn's eyes would disrupt the visual interaction between mother and baby during the first hour of life, during much of which time the baby is in the 'quiet alert' state. While there is no evidence that this would have any long term detrimental effects on maternal–infant relationships (Butterfield *et al.* 1981; Wahlberg *et al.* 1982b,c,d), there is equally no evidence to suggest that topical agents must be given within the first minutes after birth.

3 Prophylactic measures in newborns considered to be at risk

3.1 Suctioning of infants who have passed meconium *in utero*

The obstetrician may be able to reduce the likelihood of postnatal aspiration of meconium by suctioning the nares and oropharynx of infants before the chest has been delivered and the umbilical circulation interrupted (Carson *et al.* 1976). Whether this strategy has

any important effect on the incidence of severe meconium aspiration syndrome is unknown, but it would seem to have somewhat less potential for doing harm than tracheal intubation of all infants born after meconium passage.

The recommended indications for tracheal suctioning for infants born after meconium has been observed in the amniotic fluid vary according to the Apgar score, the duration and thickness of the meconium, whether the infant's skin is stained, and whether meconium is present in the pharynx or at the vocal cords. In the absence of proper clinical trials, these recommendations are based on the findings of retrospective reviews or cohort analytic studies (Gregory *et al.* 1974; Ting and Brady 1975).

Those who advocate ready resort to endotracheal suctioning base that advice on the assumption that the low rate of morbidity following intubation reported by very experienced resuscitators can be reproduced by others with a lesser level of skill. The hazards of routine intubation in these circumstances may be greater than is often appreciated.

Meconium passage *in utero* occurs in a substantial proportion of infants born with pulmonary artery hypertension (Murphy *et al.* 1984) and even relatively mild stimuli may produce intense pulmonary vasospasm in these infants. Infection may also be a risk. Transmission of herpes simplex virus to a newborn infant during endotracheal suctioning has been documented by molecular analyses (Van Dyke and Spector 1984), and there is some evidence to suggest that the risk of cross-contamination of bacteria between newborns and physicians during airway suctioning may be high (Ballard *et al.* 1986). Hypoxia, bradycardia, and increased intracranial pressure are not unusual during intubation (Raju *et al.* 1980).

In the absence of demonstrated benefits, and because of the above-mentioned risks, we do not recommend that tracheal intubation be performed for non-depressed infants, simply because the baby has been born following meconium passage *in utero* (Linder *et al.* 1988). Tracheal suction is recommended for a depressed infant (heart rate less than 80–100 beats per minute at birth) born with meconium in the pharynx. The intubation should, of course, be performed as skilfully, atraumatically, and aseptically as possible, keeping in mind the potential hazards.

3.2 Elective tracheal intubation for very low birthweight infants

Some authors have recommended immediate intubation of all very low birthweight infants. A policy of elective tracheal intubation at birth has been compared with selective intubation in only one clinical trial, and this involved infants weighing 1500 g or less at birth, regardless of whether they showed signs of asphyxia or respiratory disease (Drew 1982). The policy of elective intubation was reported to have improved a variety of outcomes, including the incidence of pneumothorax and the overall mortality rate. However, the interpretation of this potentially very important study is difficult for several reasons. The physicians responsible for selective intubation were unspecified but were apparently often paediatric house staff; infants in the electively intubated group on the other hand were invariably intubated by a neonatologist. Indeed, infants assigned to the elective intubation group were excluded from the analysis if the neonatologist and resuscitation team were not present at birth. The better outcome of the electively intubated group may thus have resulted either from a 'skilled intubator' effect or from selection bias resulting from exclusion of infants who delivered precipitously or during times of the day or night when the resuscitation team was least available.

Because of the potential hazards of intubation, routine delivery room intubation of all infants below 1500 g is unjustified on the basis of current evidence.

3.3 Prophylactic administration of plasminogen to low birthweight infants

In 1977, Ambrus and his colleagues reported a large double-blind placebo-controlled trial of intravenous plasminogen administered in the immediate postnatal period to low birthweight infants to dissolve fibrin in the terminal airways, in an attempt to prevent surfactant inactivation. Although the overall incidence of respiratory distress was not diminished, severe respiratory distress syndrome and overall mortality was statistically significantly lower in the plasminogen-treated group.

Although the study has limitations, it remains one of the few reasonably well controlled attempts to evaluate a prophylactic manoeuvre given to infants soon after delivery. Its positive results should have provoked clinical interest and replication of the study, but the research appears to have been ignored by neonatologists. With the current interest in, and promise of, surfactant replacement it seems unlikely that methods by which surfactant inactivitation may be prevented will soon receive the attention that they have deserved ever since the results of the plasminogen trial were published more than a decade ago. This approach may, however, be explored further in infants who develop respiratory distress syndrome despite surfactant administration.

3.4 Prophylactic administration of surfactant to immature infants

A number of controlled trials of bovine, human, or artificial surfactant provide encouraging evidence that immediate postnatal administration of surfactant will prove to be an important intervention to reduce the mortality and morbidity of infants born before pulmonary maturation has occurred (Milner *et al.* 1984a; Halliday *et al.* 1984; Kwong *et al.* 1985; Wilkinson *et al.* 1985; Shapiro *et al.* 1985; Enhorning *et al.* 1985; Merritt *et al.* 1986; Ten Centre Study Group 1987). Another, non-randomized study by Morley *et al.* (1981) also provides support for the use of surfactant. The trials by Enhorning *et al.* (1985), Merritt *et al.* (1986), Kwong *et al.* (1985), and the Ten Centre Study Group (1987) were among the highest quality trials for any method of delivery room care.

The effects of prophylactic administration of calf surfactant at birth are shown in Table 75.1. Babies who received surfactant were less likely to develop moderate or severe respiratory distress and pneumothorax. They were also less likely to develop periventricular haemorrhage, but there were no clear effects on the rate of the most serious grades of haemorrhage. The numbers of cases were also insufficient to detect any effect which may exist on the risk of necrotising enterocolitis and patent ductus arteriosus. Most importantly, however, administration of calf lung surfactant was associated with an increased chance of survival without bronchopulmonary dysplasia.

With the exception of a trial in which an artificial surfactant consisting of a mixture of dipalmitoyl phosphatidylcholine and high-density lipoprotein was evaluated (Halliday *et al.* 1984), trials of prophylactic administration of other forms of exogenous surfactant have yielded similar results as those evaluating the effects of calf lung surfactant. In the trial of human lung surfactant (Table 75.2), the effects of the diagnosis of respiratory distress was not described; however, the requirements for respiratory support were significantly less among babies who had received surfactant. Further testing and use of human surfactant are likely to depend on whether practical methods to obtain and prepare it are developed, and whether it has important advantages over synthetic or animal surfactant administration. The results of all three trials in which prophylactic administration of some form of 'natural' surfactant has been evaluated are summarised in Table 75.3.

Prophylactic administration of 'artificial lung expanding compound' surfactant has been evaluated in two small and one very large trial and the results are presented in Table 75.4. These provide strong evidence that this preparation reduces the risk of severe respiratory distress and death. Unfortunately, no data about the proportions of infants who developed bronchopulmonary dysplasia are available.

The quality of the evidence which supports the adminstration of surfactant to high risk newborns is higher than for any other immediate prophylactic treatment method for newborn infants, or indeed for any other method of delivery room care. More research is required to compare the various kinds of surfactant, to

Table 75.1 Effect of prophylactic calf lung surfactant (vs. saline or air) in preterm infants on death before nursery discharge

Study	EXPT n	EXPT (%)	CTRL n	CTRL (%)	Odds ratio (95% CI)	Graph of odds ratios and confidence intervals
						0.01 0.1 0.5 1 2 10 100
Kwong *et al.* (1985)	1/14	(7.14)	2/13	(15.38)	0.45 (0.04–4.73)	
Enhorning *et al.* (1985)	2/39	(5.13)	7/33	(21.21)	0.23 (0.06–0.94)	
Typical odds ratio (95% confidence interval)					0.28 (0.08–0.92)	

Effect of prophylactic calf lung surfactant (vs. saline or air) in preterm infants on RDS (moderate to severe)

Study	EXPT n	EXPT (%)	CTRL n	CTRL (%)	Odds ratio (95% CI)	
Kwong *et al.* (1985)	1/14	(7.14)	5/13	(38.46)	0.17 (0.03–1.04)	
Shapiro *et al.* (1985)	5/16	(31.25)	7/16	(43.75)	0.60 (0.15–2.44)	
Enhorning *et al.* (1985)	8/39	(20.51)	16/33	(48.48)	0.29 (0.11–0.77)	
Typical odds ratio (95% confidence interval)					0.32 (0.16–0.67)	

Effect of prophylactic calf lung surfactant (vs. saline or air) in preterm infants on death or bronchopulmonary dysplasia

Study	EXPT n	EXPT (%)	CTRL n	CTRL (%)	Odds ratio (95% CI)	
Kwong *et al.* (1985)	7/14	(50.00)	11/13	(84.62)	0.22 (0.05–1.07)	
Enhorning *et al.* (1985)	22/39	(56.41)	28/33	(84.85)	0.27 (0.10–0.72)	
Typical odds ratio (95% confidence interval)					0.25 (0.11–0.59)	

Effect of prophylactic calf lung surfactant (vs. saline or air) in preterm infants on pneumothorax

Study	EXPT n	EXPT (%)	CTRL n	CTRL (%)	Odds ratio (95% CI)	
Kwong *et al.* (1985)	6/14	(42.86)	7/13	(53.85)	0.65 (0.15–2.88)	
Enhorning *et al.* (1985)	6/39	(15.38)	11/33	(33.33)	0.37 (0.13–1.11)	
Typical odds ratio (95% confidence interval)					0.46 (0.19–1.09)	

Effect of prophylactic calf lung surfactant (vs. saline or air) in preterm infants on periventricular haemorrhage (any grade)

Study	EXPT n	EXPT (%)	CTRL n	CTRL (%)	Odds ratio (95% CI)	
Enhorning *et al.* (1985)	11/39	(28.21)	20/33	(60.61)	0.27 (0.11–0.69)	
Typical odds ratio (95% confidence interval)					0.27 (0.11–0.69)	

Effect of prophylactic calf lung surfactant (vs. saline or air) in preterm infants on intraventricular haemorrhage (grade 3/4)

Study	EXPT n	EXPT (%)	CTRL n	CTRL (%)	Odds ratio (95% CI)	
Kwong *et al.* (1985)	5/14	(35.71)	4/11	(36.36)	0.97 (0.19–4.88)	
Enhorning *et al.* (1985)	4/39	(10.26)	3/33	(9.09)	1.14 (0.24–5.39)	
Typical odds ratio (95% confidence interval)					1.06 (0.35–3.23)	

Effect of prophylactic calf lung surfactant (vs. saline or air) in preterm infants on necrotizing enterocolitis

Study	EXPT		CTRL		Odds ratio	Graph of odds ratios and confidence intervals						
	n	(%)	*n*	(%)	(95% CI)	0.01	0.1	0.5	1	2	10	100
Kwong *et al.* (1985)	1/13	(7.69)	1/11	(9.09)	0.84 (0.05–14.42)							
Typical odds ratio (95% confidence interval)					0.84 (0.05–14.42)							

Effect of prophylactic calf lung surfactant (vs. saline or air) in preterm infants on PDA requiring treatment

Kwong *et al.* (1985)	3/13	(23.08)	1/11	(9.09)	2.62 (0.32–21.63)							
Typical odds ratio (95% confidence interval)					2.62 (0.32–21.63)							

Table 75.2 Effect of prophylactic human surfactant (vs. saline or air) in preterm infants on death before nursery discharge

Study	EXPT		CTRL		Odds ratio	Graph of odds ratios and confidence intervals						
	n	(%)	*n*	(%)	(95% CI)	0.01	0.1	0.5	1	2	10	100
Merritt *et al.* (1986)	7/31	(22.58)	17/29	58.62)	0.23 (0.08–0.64)							
Typical odds ratio (95% confidence interval)					0.23 (0.08–0.64)							

Effect of prophylactic human surfactant (vs. saline or air) in preterm infants on death or bronchopulmonary dysplasia

Merritt *et al.* (1986)	10/31	(32.26)	24/29	(82.76)	0.13 (0.05–0.36)							
Typical odds ratio (95% confidence interval)					0.13 (0.05–0.36)							

Effect of prophylactic human surfactant (vs. saline or air) in preterm infants on pneumothorax

Merritt *et al.* (1986)	2/31	(6.45)	7/29	(24.14)	0.26 (0.06–1.04)							
Typical odds ratio (95% confidence interval)					0.26 (0.06–1.04)							

Effect of prophylactic human surfactant (vs. saline or air) in preterm infants on periventricular haemorrhage (any grade)

Merritt *et al.* (1986)	19/31	(61.29)	21/29	(72.41)	0.61 (0.21–1.77)							
Typical odds ratio (95% confidence interval)					0.61 (0.21–1.77)							

Effect of prophylactic human surfactant (vs. saline or air) in preterm infants on intraventricular haemorrhage (grade 3/4)

Merritt *et al.* (1986)	8/31	(25.81)	10/29	(34.48)	0.67 (0.22–1.99)							
Typical odds ratio (95% confidence interval)					0.67 (0.22–1.99)							

Effect of prophylactic human surfactant (vs. saline or air) in preterm infants on necrotizing enterocolitis

Study	EXPT		CTRL		Odds ratio	Graph of odds ratios and confidence intervals						
	n	(%)	n	(%)	(95% CI)	0.01	0.1	0.5	1	2	10	100
Merritt et al. (1986)	2/31	(6.45)	4/29	(13.79)	0.45 (0.08–2.39)							
Typical odds ratio (95% confidence interval)					0.45 (0.08–2.39)							

Effect of prophylactic human surfactant (vs. saline or air) in preterm infants on PDA requiring treatment

Study	EXPT		CTRL		Odds ratio	
Merritt et al. (1986)	19/31	(61.29)	20/29	(68.97)	0.72 (0.25–2.06)	
Typical odds ratio (95% confidence interval)					0.72 (0.25–2.06)	

Table 75.3 Effect of prophylactic calf lung or human surfactant (vs. saline or air) in preterm infants on death before nursery discharge

Study	EXPT		CTRL		Odds ratio	Graph of odds ratios and confidence intervals						
	n	(%)	n	(%)	(95% CI)	0.01	0.1	0.5	1	2	10	100
Kwong et al. (1985)	1/14	(7.14)	2/13	(15.38)	0.45 (0.04–4.73)							
Merritt et al. (1986)	7/31	(22.58)	17/29	(58.62)	0.23 (0.08–0.64)							
Enhorning et al. (1985)	2/39	(5.13)	7/33	(21.21)	0.23 (0.06–0.94)							
Typical odds ratio (95% confidence interval)					0.25 (0.11–0.54)							

Effect of prophylactic calf lung or human surfactant (vs. saline or air) in preterm infants on RDS (moderate to severe)

Study	EXPT		CTRL		Odds ratio	
Kwong et al. (1985)	1/14	(7.14)	5/13	(38.46)	0.17 (0.03–1.04)	
Shapiro et al. (1985)	5/16	(31.25)	7/16	(43.75)	0.60 (0.15–2.44)	
Enhorning et al. (1985)	8/39	(20.51)	16/33	(48.48)	0.29 (0.11–0.77)	
Typical odds ratio (95% confidence interval)					0.32 (0.16–0.67)	

Effect of prophylactic calf lung or human surfactant (vs. saline or air) in preterm infants on death or bronchopulmonary dysplasia

Study	EXPT		CTRL		Odds ratio	
Kwong et al. (1985)	7/14	(50.00)	11/13	(84.62)	0.22 (0.05–1.07)	
Merritt et al. (1986)	10/31	(32.26)	24/29	(82.76)	0.13 (0.05–0.36)	
Enhorning et al. (1985)	22/39	(56.41)	28/33	(84.85)	0.27 (0.10–0.72)	
Typical odds ratio (95% confidence interval)					0.19 (0.10–0.37)	

Effect of prophylactic calf lung or human surfactant (vs. saline or air) in preterm infants on pneumothorax

Study	EXPT n	(%)	CTRL n	(%)	Odds ratio (95% CI)	Graph of odds ratios and confidence intervals
						0.01 0.1 0.5 1 2 10 100
Kwong et al. (1985)	6/14	(42.86)	7/13	(53.85)	0.65 (0.15–2.88)	
Merritt et al. (1986)	2/31	(6.45)	7/29	(24.14)	0.26 (0.06–1.04)	
Enhorning et al. (1985)	6/39	(15.38)	11/33	(33.33)	0.37 (0.13–1.11)	
Typical odds ratio (95% confidence interval)					0.39 (0.18–0.81)	

Effect of prophylactic calf lung or human surfactant (vs. saline or air) in preterm infants on periventricular haemorrhage (any grade)

Study	EXPT n	(%)	CTRL n	(%)	Odds ratio (95% CI)
Merritt et al. (1986)	19/31	(61.29)	21/29	(72.41)	0.61 (0.21–1.77)
Enhorning et al. (1985)	11/39	(28.21)	20/33	(60.61)	0.27 (0.11–0.69)
Typical odds ratio (95% confidence interval)					0.39 (0.19–0.78)

Effect of prophylactic calf lung or human surfactant (vs. saline or air) in preterm infants on intraventricular haemorrhage (grade 3/4)

Study	EXPT n	(%)	CTRL n	(%)	Odds ratio (95% CI)
Kwong et al. (1985)	5/14	(35.71)	4/11	(36.36)	0.97 (0.19–4.88)
Merritt et al. (1986)	8/31	(25.81)	10/29	(34.48)	0.67 (0.22–1.99)
Enhorning et al. (1985)	4/39	(10.26)	3/33	(9.09)	1.14 (0.24–5.39)
Typical odds ratio (95% confidence interval)					0.83 (0.38–1.83)

Effect of prophylactic calf lung or human surfactant (vs. saline or air) in preterm infants on necrotizing enterocolitis

Study	EXPT n	(%)	CTRL n	(%)	Odds ratio (95% CI)
Kwong et al. (1985)	1/13	(7.69)	1/11	(9.09)	0.84 (0.05–14.42)
Merritt et al. (1986)	2/31	(6.45)	4/29	(13.79)	0.45 (0.08–2.39)
Typical odds ratio (95% confidence interval)					0.53 (0.12–2.23)

Effect of prophylactic calf lung or human surfactant (vs. saline or air) in preterm infants on PDA requiring treatment

Study	EXPT n	(%)	CTRL n	(%)	Odds ratio (95% CI)
Kwong et al. (1985)	3/13	(23.08)	1/11	(9.09)	2.62 (0.32–21.63)
Merritt et al. (1986)	19/31	(61.29)	20/29	(68.97)	0.72 (0.25–2.06)
Typical odds ratio (95% confidence interval)					0.93 (0.36–2.38)

Table 75.4 Effect of prophylactic 'artificial lung expanding compound' surfactant (vs. saline or air) in preterm infants on death before nursery discharge

Study	EXPT n	(%)	CTRL n	(%)	Odds ratio (95% CI)	Graph of odds ratios and confidence intervals
Ten Centre study Group (1987)	30/159	(18.87)	44/149	(29.53)	0.56 (0.33–0.94)	
Wilkinson *et al.* (1985)	0/16	(0.00)	2/16	(12.50)	0.13 (0.01–2.12)	
Milner *et al.* (1984)	4/15	(26.67)	2/7	(28.57)	0.91 (0.13–6.53)	
Typical odds ratio (95% confidence interval)					0.55 (0.33–0.90)	

Graph axis: 0.01 0.1 0.5 1 2 10 100

Effect of prophylactic 'artificial lung expanding compound' surfactant (vs. saline or air) in preterm infants on RDS (moderate to severe)

Study	EXPT n	(%)	CTRL n	(%)	Odds ratio (95% CI)	
Ten Centre study Group (1987)	52/159	(32.70)	67/149	(44.97)	0.60 (0.38–0.94)	
Milner *et al.* (1984)	7/15	(46.67)	4/7	(57.14)	0.67 (0.12–3.87)	
Typical odds ratio (95% confidence interval)					0.60 (0.39–0.94)	

Effect of prophylactic 'artificial lung expanding compound' surfactant (vs. saline or air) in preterm infants on pneumothorax

Study	EXPT n	(%)	CTRL n	(%)	Odds ratio (95% CI)	
Ten Centre study Group (1987)	42/159	(26.42)	44/149	(29.53)	0.86 (0.52–1.41)	
Typical odds ratio (95% confidence interval)					0:86 (0.52–1.41)	

Effect of prophylactic 'artificial lung expanding compound' surfactant (vs. saline or air) in preterm infants on periventricular haemorrhage (any grade)

Study	EXPT n	(%)	CTRL n	(%)	Odds ratio (95% CI)	
Ten Centre study Group (1987)	54/154	(35.06)	61/143	(42.66)	0.73 (0.46–1.16)	
Typical odds ratio (95% confidence interval)					0.73 (0.46–1.16)	

Effect of prophylactic 'artificial lung expanding compound' surfactant (vs. saline or air) in preterm infants on intraventricular haemorrhage (grade 4)

Study	EXPT n	(%)	CTRL n	(%)	Odds ratio (95% CI)	
Ten Centre study Group (1987)	25/154	(16.23)	34/143	(23.78)	0.62 (0.35–1.10)	
Typical odds ratio (95% confidence interval)					0.62 (0.35–1.10)	

Effect of prophylactic 'artificial lung expanding compound' surfactant (vs. saline or air) in preterm infants on necrotizing enterocolitis

Study	EXPT n	(%)	CTRL n	(%)	Odds ratio (95% CI)	
Ten Centre study Group (1987)	14/152	(9.21)	17/139	(12.23)	0.73 (0.35–1.53)	
Typical odds ratio (95% confidence interval)					0.73 (0.35–1.53)	

Effect of prophylactic 'artificial lung expanding compound' surfactant (vs. saline or air) in preterm infants on PDA requiring treatment

Study	EXPT n	(%)	CTRL n	(%)	Odds ratio (95% CI)	
Ten Centre study Group (1987)	42/159	(26.42)	34/149	(29.53)	0.86 (0.52–1.41)	
Typical odds ratio (95% confidence interval)					0.86 (0.52–1.41)	

evaluate different dosage schedules, and to determine the relative value of administering surfactant prophylactically in the delivery room to all infants considered to be at high risk of developing respiratory distress syndrome compared to a policy of giving it only to those infants who develop respiratory distress syndrome. Many of these issues may be resolved by studies currently in progress. In addition it will be important to assess longer term morbidity (Halliday *et al.* 1986) in cohorts of high risk neonates with differential survival patterns.

4 Immediate resuscitation of ill newborn infants

The availability of professionals skilled in neonatal resuscitation has increased with the growth of neonatology as a specialty. This change has meant that the birth of an immature, asphyxiated, or otherwise high risk neonate is more likely to be attended by someone who is experienced in giving care to such infants. A proportion of ill and high risk infants will continue to present as unpredicted emergencies, however, and, as a recent national survey of neonatal resuscitation in Canadian hospitals has shown (Chance and Hanvey 1987), it will often fall to a midwife, nurse, general practitioner, or trainee specialist to initiate and continue neonatal resuscitation. In reviewing the immediate measures used to care for ill newborn infants we have taken account of the reality that people with varying levels of skill in resuscitation will continue to be called upon to provide short term emergency care.

4.1 Preparation for resuscitation

Whenever possible, a person skilled in resuscitation who can devote all his or her attention to the infant should be in attendance at high-risk deliveries, such as preterm deliveries, or when meconium-stained amniotic fluid or fetal heart rate abnormalities are detected.

Basic resuscitation equipment (e.g. a radiant warmer, resuscitation bags and masks, endotracheal tubes, laryngoscope, stethoscope, oxygen source, and tubing) should be readily available for every delivery room. Because the need for resuscitation is not recognized prior to the delivery of approximately half of all resuscitated infants (Chance and Hanvey 1987), the presence and proper working order of this equipment should be verified before each delivery.

Unfortunately, the medical literature provides little information useful in selecting the most effective of the equipment manufactured for the resuscitation of newborns. Some effort has been made to evaluate endotracheal tubes (Thibeault and Nelson 1979) and to compare commercially available face masks (Palme *et al.* 1985). We found only one clinical trial of reasonable

quality which evaluated resuscitation equipment. In this trial, use of the Laerdal resuscitation bag resulted in a more rapid improvement in blood pH than did use of the Sampson bag (Davies *et al.* 1985). Finer and colleagues (1986) have shown substantial variation among the widely used self-inflating resuscitation bags with respect to both oxygen concentration and maximum pressure delivered before a 'pop-off' valve automatically opens. Self-inflating bags, in contrast with anaesthesia bags, often do not allow delivery of a high concentration of oxygen.

While anaesthesia bags are likely to be required for the optimal resuscitation of severely asphyxiated infants, their hazards if used improperly (e.g. the application of dangerously high airway pressures) make them unsuitable for routine use by inexperienced personnel. Likewise, the hazards of umbilical artery catheters and trochars for endotracheal tubes (Thibeault and Nelson 1979; Tyson *et al.* 1976) should preclude their use in delivery rooms except by highly experienced resuscitators.

4.2 Resuscitation

In our textbook survey, the recommended indications for initiating resuscitation were frequently based upon low Apgar scores. However, Apgar scores appear to be a poor measure of the presence and degree of birth asphyxia, especially in preterm infants (Tooley *et al.* 1977; Catlin *et al.* 1986). Moreover, the resuscitation of some infants should not be delayed until the first Apgar score is obtained one minute after birth. In the absence of better measures of the need for resuscitation than Apgar scores, we recommend that artificial ventilation be promptly initiated for infants with a heart rate less than 100 beats per minute at or following birth, and that oxygen be administered to any infant with generalized cyanosis. Regardless of heart rate or colour, artificial ventilation is also recommended for infants with inadequate chest excursion and poor breath sounds, especially small preterm infants likely to have surfactant deficiency.

Proper ventilation of the infant is widely accepted as the most important aspect of neonatal resuscitation. Controversy remains as to when ventilation should be performed using an endotracheal intubation, rather than a face mask. In our textbook survey, a poor response to bag and mask ventilation was the most commonly noted indication for intubation. The response of the heart rate is the most useful and easily measured criterion for the success of resuscitation.

Before intubation is performed in an infant whose heart rate does not rise promptly with bag and mask ventilation, attention should be given to the following points: proper positioning of the head ('sniffing position'); ensuring that the upper airway is clear; using sufficient pressure to produce adequate chest excursions; and administering an adequate inspired oxygen concentration. Whether a proper head position and clear airway allow delivery of gas to the level of the glottis can be easily assessed by observing for distention of the neck as the resuscitation bag is squeezed. As noted earlier, the careful use of an anaesthesia bag may be required to deliver more pressure or a greater oxygen concentration than can be delivered by self-inflating bags. Persistent bradycardia may be caused by excessive pressure to the infant's head through the face mask.

Endotracheal intubation has been assessed in only two clinical trials (Hutchison *et al.* 1966; Wilson and Roscoe 1958), both of which have limited quality and relevance to modern delivery room care. Hutchison *et al.* compared hyperbaric oxygen therapy with resuscitation using endotracheal intubation; Wilson and Roscoe compared bag and mask ventilation using a Goddard–Bennet–Lovelace resuscitator with mouth-to-endotracheal tube ventilation and other resuscitation measures. There is evidence that ventilation by endotracheal tube is more efficient than ventilation by face mask (Milner *et al.* 1984b); however, given the known hazards of intubation and the absence of any clinical trials comparing intubation with use of a face mask, we recommend that except when quite skilled personnel are in attendance, resuscitation be initiated using a face mask rather than an endotracheal tube.

4.3 Ventilation regimens

The methods recommended and used for neonatal resuscitation vary and are not described in great detail. The American Academy recommends a rate of 40–60 breaths per minute with an initial pressure as high as 30–40 cm to produce adequate lung expansion during the first few breaths of some infants.

The ventilation regimens commonly used in delivery room are associated with a good outcome for the great majority of resuscitated newborns. Despite the fact that a number of studies have been mounted in an attempt to develop an improved basis for prescribing ventilatory regimens (Boon *et al.* 1972, 1979; Vyas *et al.* 1981), the adequacy of ventilation must still be assessed primarily by observing chest excursions and auscultating breath sounds and, for infants who respond poorly to resuscitation, by assessing blood gas status.

4.4 Oxygen

Supplemental oxygen (100 per cent concentration of the warm and humidified gas) is recommended for artificial ventilation of neonates who have not established effective spontaneous respiration by one minute of age. However, no comparative studies of the benefits and risks of various oxygen concentrations for the management of such infants have been reported. The rationale for the use of high oxygen concentrations is based on classic physiological studies in newborn mon-

keys, which demonstrated that decreased pulmonary blood flow during asphyxia (as the result of markedly elevated pulmonary vascular resistance) was a limiting factor in the animal's oxygen uptake (Dawes *et al.* 1968). Gaseous ventilation of the monkey, especially with high concentrations of oxygen, quickly reduced pulmonary vascular resistance; alveolar oxygen tension rose, alveolar and pulmonary arterial carbon dioxide tensions fell, and the acid–base balance, following the acidaemic consequences of asphyxia, was slowly restored. Direct measurements obtained during positive pressure resuscitation of asphyxiated human infants with oxygen confirmed rapid oxygen uptake (Hull and Segall 1966).

Some concern has been expressed that blowing oxygen across the face of a newborn infant would result in bradycardia (Brown *et al.* 1976). However, most concern has been focused on whether the risk of cicatricial retinopathy would be appreciably increased in immature infants who experience short periods of hyperoxaemia. This question is frequently raised and hotly debated, but there is no satisfactory evidence that the risk after short periods of hyperoxaemia ($PaO_2 > 100$ Torr) is any greater than that associated with the relative hyperoxaemia that occurs at birth in all babies (usual PaO_2 values of 20–25 Torr *in utero* and 45–110 Torr with the onset of air breathing). On the other hand, it must be recognized that the issue has not been explored systematically, and that there seems to be no good reason for attempting to produce hyperoxaemia.

At present, little attempt is made to measure either the inspired concentration of oxygen or the PaO_2 in most delivery rooms, largely because of the limited support required for most infants, the difficulty of performing an arterial puncture in the delivery room, and the potential hazards of inserting an umbilical artery catheter. The use of monitors to measure haemoglobin saturation (Durand and Ramanathan 1986) should be explored as a quick and non-invasive method for assessing oxygenation during resuscitation. The information derived in this way may permit more rational decisions concerning the provision of supplemental oxygen in the immediate postnatal period.

4.5 Cardiac massage

Cardiac massage, used for the infant born with an absent heart beat, can at times be a life-saving measure. The use of cardiac massage through the intact chest wall of the neonate was originally recommended by investigators who studied a small number of term infants, and noted that the procedure increased blood pressure without any evidence of trauma to the skeleton or viscera (Moya *et al.* 1962; Matthews *et al.* 1963). With more widespread use it became clear that the method occasionally causes rib fractures and trauma to the liver or lung. Since the original recommendation, cardiac massage of the neonate has received little systematic study (Todres and Rogers 1975), and there is little information of the kind needed to determine precise indications and methods.

4.6 Naloxone

Naloxone hydrochloride is considered to be a pure narcotic antagonist as a result of its marked opiate receptor affinity; the compound is believed to have no intrinsic agonist action and to be virtually free of side-effects. The formulation of the drug, which has been approved by the Food and Drug Administration for use in newborn infants, is 0.02 mg/ml. When given intravenously to a neonate in a dose of 0.01 mg/kg (the recommended route and dose), peak plasma concentrations can be expected within 40 minutes; the elimination half-life is approximately $2\frac{1}{2}$ hours.

The guidelines of the American Academy of Pediatrics (1980) suggest that naloxone may be administered as an adjunctive measure *after* assisted ventilation has been established if depression is thought to be the result of a narcotic drug given to the mother before delivery. A review committee has also advised against use of naloxone to infants of narcotic-dependent mothers for fear of precipitating withdrawal illness in the neonate (American Academy of Pediatrics 1980).

The recommended dosage of naloxone (0.01 mg/kg) is that reported to produce increased ventilatory drive during the first postnatal hour in narcotic-exposed infants (Gerhardt *et al.* 1977). Greater doses may be required to prevent the subtle neurobehavioural deficits that are sometimes observed for several days after birth in babies who have been exposed, as fetuses, to narcotics. Although some researchers (Bonta *et al.* 1979) have noted favourable neurobehavioural effects at a dose of 0.02 mg/kg, others (Welles *et al.* 1984) have failed to detect any benefits at an average dose of 0.03 mg/kg. The favourable effects reported by Wiener *et al.* (1977) were observed at an average intramuscular dose of nearly 0.06 mg/kg. Uncertainty about the proper naloxone dose is compounded by the fact that in these and in other studies (Evans *et al.* 1976; Dick *et al.* 1978) naloxone has been carefully evaluated only in term infants with high Apgar scores.

Concern has been raised about the potential importance of endogenous opioid substances in newborns (American Academy of Pediatrics 1983). Given this concern and the observations in one study (Welles *et al.* 1984) of less optimal maternal ratings of infant behaviour among naloxone-treated infants than among controls, we suggest that administration of naloxone should be restricted to infants who have not only been exposed to narcotics *in utero*, but who also require active resuscitation in the immediate neonatal period. While there has been some interest in other narcotic antagonists (Gupta and Moore 1973), only naloxone

has been studied sufficiently to make treatment recommendations.

4.7 Sodium bicarbonate

Despite the fact that almost all of the textbooks reviewed recommend the intravenous injection of sodium bicarbonate during resuscitation of asphyxiated neonates, randomized trials (Bland *et al.* 1976; Corbet *et al.* 1977) have failed to detect any benefit from either rapid or slow administration of sodium bicarbonate to neonates. The potential benefits of sodium bicarbonate therapy include improved myocardial performance and reduced asphyxial damage to the central nervous system. The potential hazards (evaluated principally in animal studies) include: a transient increase in $PaCO_2$ and fall in PaO_2; a sudden expansion of blood volume; an increase in venous pressure and reduction in cerebrospinal fluid pressure; a reduction in cerebral blood flow; and an increased incidence of intracranial haemorrhage (Kravath *et al.* 1970; Lou *et al.* 1978; Finberg 1977; Turbeville *et al.* 1976; Steichen and Kleinman 1977). These effects are increased by increasing the dosage and rate of administration, as well as by increasing the osmolality of the solution administered.

Recommendations that sodium bicarbonate be administered to asphyxiated neonates appear to be based largely on studies either of animals which are not susceptible to intraventricular haemorrhage (Dawes *et al.* 1964) or by reference to treatment regimens of uncertain efficacy used in resuscitating adults and older children. The investigators in a recent study conducted in adults with cardiopulmonary arrest concluded that arterial pH measurements may be misleading and that sodium bicarbonate administration 'may be counterproductive' (Weil *et al.* 1986). Rapid infusion of sodium bicarbonate in the first 20 minutes following birth was reported to be beneficial in one neonatal trial (Hobel *et al.* 1972). However, the comparison group consisted of infants who received delayed sodium bicarbonate therapy. No untreated control group was studied.

Both the frequency with which sodium bicarbonate is administered to neonates in the immediate postnatal period, and the dose and rate of administration appear to have diminished substantially following reports of an association between this intervention and periventricular haemorrhage in preterm infants (Simmons *et al.* 1974). Hypertonic sodium bicarbonate was previously used liberally and given in doses of up to 6 mEq/kg administered 'IV push'. The American Academy of Pediatrics now notes that sodium bicarbonate *may* be given to well-ventilated infants with persistent bradycardia and poor perfusion and that if used, the initial dose should be 2 mEq/kg given at a rate no greater than 1–2 mEq/kg/min of a solution. This treatment regimen is undoubtedly safer than those previously used. Nevertheless, in the absence of any demonstrated benefits of giving this drug in the immediate postnatal period, we cannot recommend that it be used.

4.8 Blood volume expanders

The only clear-cut indication for the use of volume expanders in the early neonatal period is the combination of unmistakable signs of shock with evidence of acute blood loss, including feto–maternal haemorrhage. In this circumstance, shock may be treated with repeated infusions of volume expanders (usually 5–10 ml) and the infant's response assessed after each infusion. The volume expander may be 5 per cent albumin, Ringer's lactate, saline, or heparinized placental blood (obtained aseptically from the umbilical cord, drawn into a 20-ml syringe containing no more than 50 units of heparin, and administered through a filter from a blood set).

The presence of hypotension unaccompanied by other signs of shock or blood loss has also been used as an indication for volume expanders. This practice is of far more dubious validity and can be challenged on several grounds: uncertainty about normal values for blood pressure shortly after birth, the likelihood that blood pressure is only a rough measure of blood volume, and the potential hazards of administering volume expanders, especially when hypotension might be due to asphyxial damage to the heart.

Blood pressure during the first postnatal hour is likely to be influenced by many factors, and blood pressure values during this time are thus especially difficult to interpret. The use of blood pressure standards derived from infants with delayed clamping of the umbilical cord (Kitterman *et al.* 1969) may explain why previously accepted values are now considered to exceed normal blood pressure in neonates (Versmold *et al.* 1981). There is both animal (Arant 1981) and human (Furzan *et al.* 1985) evidence suggesting that the use of volume expanders in neonates predisposes to patent ductus arteriosus. The possibility that volume expanders might increase the risk of intracranial haemorrhage has also been suggested by the results of both clinical and animal studies (Goldberg *et al.* 1980; Goodard-Finegold *et al.* 1982). The only clinical trial of volume expanders in neonates (Hambleton and Appleyard 1973) involved the administration of fresh frozen plasma to asphyxiated low-birth weight infants. This trial was conducted prior to the availability of sonographic measures to identify intracranial haemorrhage. Too few patients were studied to discriminate an important difference between groups in autopsy-proven intraventricular haemorrhage although the direction of the difference favoured the control group (intraventricular haemorrhage at autopsy was identified in 0 of 7 control infants and 3 of 7 infants treated with fresh frozen plasma).

Advances in echocardiography provide a means to evaluate cardiac function and output in response to the administration of volume expanders in infants with signs of hypovolaemia. However, changes in total cardiac output following volume expansion may not be a reliable indicator of blood flow to vital organs. In a recent study of dogs given volume expanders during resuscitation (Ditchey and Lindenfield 1984), volume expanders resulted in a decrease in cerebral and coronary flow despite an increase in total cardiac output. Other investigators (Laptook *et al.* 1982) have noted an increase in brain blood flow with volume expansion but important differences in flow to different regions of the brain.

Uncertainty about the proper clinical use of volume expanders is not likely to be resolved in the near future, in part because of the number of infants needed to distinguish the effects of volume expanders from the effects of a multitude of confounding factors which influence the mortality and morbidity of high risk infants. A more fundamental problem is that considerably more background information about the relation of the blood volume in neonates (which is not easily or routinely measured) to clinical problems may be required before appropriate clinical trials can be designed.

4.9 Adrenaline (epinephrine)

The proper use of adrenaline (epinephrine) during cardiopulmonary resuscitation of the asphyxiated neonate (for cardiac stimulation and to counteract electromechanical dissociation) remains controversial. The 'official' guideline advises the administration of 0.1 ml/kg of a 1:10 000 solution of adrenaline (following the use of sodium bicarbonate) for treatment of bradycardia that persists after adequate ventilation and cardiac massage (American Academy of Pediatrics 1983). The intracardiac route of adrenaline administration has been condemned unambiguously (Welch and Phillips 1984) because of the risk of pneumothorax, coronary laceration, cardiac tamponade and embolism. Administration of adrenaline by either intravenous infusion or endotracheal instillation has been proposed (Lindeman 1984) but these have not been evaluated in comparative trials.

4.10 Calcium gluconate and atropine sulphate

In the management of persistent bradycardia that does not respond to either sodium bicarbonate or to adrenaline, the 'official' guideline advises administration of a 10 per cent solution of calcium gluconate at a dose of 1 ml/kg, followed, if necessary, by atropine sulphate in a dose of 0.03 mg/kg to block parasympathetic inhibitory effects on intrinsic cardiac conduction and to increase the heart rate. There are no controlled studies supporting these measures for the treatment of neonatal asphyxia, nor for the use of isoproterenol (Isuprel) for cardiogenic shock (Lees 1980). Studies of bolus calcium administration in neonates have focused on infants with hypocalcaemia and have come to conflicting conclusions (Salsburey and Brown 1982; Scott *et al.* 1984; Venkataraman *et al.* 1985). While calcium therapy may have beneficial cardiac effects (Mirro and Brown 1984), the potential hazards include bradycardia, tissue necrosis following intravenous infiltration, intestinal necrosis following arterial injection (Book *et al.* 1978), and deposition of calcium in the central nervous system (Changaris *et al.* 1984).

4.11 Dopamine

The cardiovascular effects of dopamine (given at 2.5 micrograms/kg/minute) was investigated in a randomized, placebo controlled, double-blind comparative trial involving 14 severely asphyxiated infants (DiSessa *et al.* 1981). The findings suggest that low doses of dopamine raise systemic arterial pressure and improve cardiac performance. This treatment thus shows promise, although the trial should be replicated on a larger number of infants before valid recommendations can be made.

4.12 Indications for withholding or discontinuing resuscitation

The issue of when to withhold or discontinue resuscitation, despite its neglect in textbooks, concerns the most difficult treatment decision of all made in the delivery room. Outside the textbooks, however, the indications for withholding care from extremely high risk infants have been the subject of intense controversy (Stinson and Stinson 1983; Silverman 1981), especially in the United States where under the 'Baby Doe' regulations, withholding of care for severely impaired infants was regarded as a violation of the civil rights statutes (Angell 1986).

Few, if any, people would argue that aggressive methods of resuscitation should be applied to all infants born with a heart beat, for example, anencephalic infants or infants born at 22 weeks gestation. The factors most often considered in attempts to define when aggressive care is unwarranted (Britton *et al.* 1981; Campbell 1982; Milligan *et al.* 1984; Koops 1984; Whitelaw 1986) have included the likelihood of death, the likelihood of survival with what is considered an unacceptable quality of life, and the suffering and cost involved if intensive care is instituted.

The problems in defining appropriate indications for using intensive care are compounded by deficiencies in the information needed to apply such criteria: the effect of intensive care on mortality and the quality of life of survivors, and the cost of care for severely impaired or malformed infants. Furthermore, controversy continues about the process and persons involved in reaching such decisions. Some commentators recommend a decision-making process which only rarely involves people other than the parents and the physicians responsible for the care of their child. Others advocate active involvement of highly organized committees of lay, medical, and legal personnel.

Arguments about the criteria and methods which are appropriate in decisions to withhold intensive neonatal care have focused primarily on moral and ethical principles, with scant attention paid to the real world problems which have to be faced by parents, physicians, nurses, and others confronting these dilemmas at a more immediate level. We believe that the ultimate quality of these decisions may be improved by research efforts. Many follow-up studies fail to meet the majority of the standards and recommendations published by Kiely and Paneth (1981) (Tyson and Swanson 1987). These will need to include well-designed descriptive studies to document prognosis in various subgroups of infants, as well as experiments to assess how prognosis is affected by particular treatment modalities. Because it is unlikely that intensive care as a whole will be assessed in the context of randomized experiments, carefully controlled cohort studies are necessary. Such cohorts might be defined by the era in which the children were born relative to the introduction of intensive care (Horwood *et al.* 1982; Mutch *et al.* 1986), or perhaps on the basis of differences in the degree of aggressiveness of intensive care which reflected parental preferences—an approach which has already been used in the cancer field (Angell 1984).

Ultimately, decisions to withhold or withdraw aggressive care involve value judgements about what is considered an acceptable outcome and an acceptable cost (Boyle *et al.* 1983). Although much has been written to express the views of health care professionals, lawyers, and ethicists concerning aggressive care of extremely high risk infants, little has been done to explore the views of the parents who, apart from the child, have most at stake in such decisions. The values and attitudes of the general public require more study to allow more careful definition of society's priorities for health care expenditure and to avoid irrational use of resources; for example, by failing to provide adequate funds for programmes to reduce the disabilities caused by serious impairments in childhood while mandating programmes of neonatal intensive care to increase the survival of such children.

Given the limited amount of useful information which is available for reaching decisions about instituting or withholding aggressive neonatal care, a liberal policy of resuscitation must be recommended whenever doubt exists. This allows the physician time to gather important information about the infant. It also allows some time for distressed parents to participate more effectively in any joint decisions about subsequent therapy. Committees should not be routinely involved in this process unless the results of well-designed investigations suggest that they are more likely than the parents and the physicians responsible for sick infants to reach appropriate decisions.

4.13 Organization of efficient resuscitation

The previous discussion has emphasized the limited information that is available to guide decisions about both the place of active neonatal resuscitation and the methods which should be used to achieve it. In practice, however, the effectiveness of neonatal resuscitation may be compromised more by the failure to use basic principles of resuscitation properly than by limitations in our understanding about how to resuscitate severely immature or asphyxiated infants. We suspect that the most common serious error in resuscitation is a failure to ventilate the infant appropriately, resulting in hypoventilation, or less commonly, hyperventilation. Hypoventilation commonly results from failure to check that the upper airways are free, failure to evaluate breath sounds and chest excursions properly, the use of either an inappropriate airway pressure, or a malpositioned endotracheal tube, or inappropriate flexion of the infant's neck during resuscitation with a bag and mask.

More attention should be paid to ensuring that hospitals and their staff have effective training procedures in these basic elements of neonatal resuscitation. The limited attention given in most hospitals to the organization, training of personnel, and evaluation of neonatal resuscitation is apparent in the survey of Canadian Hospitals conducted by Chance and Hanvey (1987). Their findings supported the following recommendations:

1 'Written protocols should be developed and made available in the delivery room of all hospitals for neonatal resuscitation, use of drugs for emergencies, selection and maintenance of equipment and training of personnel for neonatal resuscitation.'

2 'Hospital staff should agree on and display lists of maternal and fetal conditions that indicate the need for additional personnel to be summoned to attend the birth of an infant likely to require resuscitation.'

3 'The training of family physicians . . . should include the use of suitable practice models to acquire expertise in neonatal resuscitation.'

4 'Regular practice of neonatal intubation by selected staff should be encouraged in all obstetric units . . .'

5 'The role and responsibilities of senior clinical nurses in neonatal resuscitation, including intubation, should be explored . . .'

These recommendations seem to be well-justified. Based on our experience in trying to ensure effective resuscitation procedures, we believe the following

measures also merit consideration and further evaluation: staff training, using cats anaesthetized with ketamine to teach intubation (Jennings *et al.* 1974); careful definition of the roles of each staff member when more than one person is involved in resuscitation; the use of periodic resuscitation drills using resuscitation dolls; the use of intercommunicating speakers to allow direct communication between each delivery room and the neonatal unit; the use of a resuscitation form which serves as both an order sheet and a coherent record of pertinent physical findings, resuscitation measures, and any laboratory results (blood glucose, haematocrit, and blood gas values) obtained; and, perhaps most important of all, a formal periodic review of the intrapartum and delivery room records of infants who required resuscitation.

5 Conclusions

Much of the above discussion about resuscitation procedures emphasizes the very limited information that is available about many of the treatment methods which are recommended and widely used. Indeed, it may not be possible to design appropriate management trials of neonatal resuscitation measures without a better understanding of the pathophysiology of asphyxia, hypovolaemia, meconium aspiration, pulmonary artery hypertension, pulmonary immaturity, and other neonatal problems presenting in the delivery room. Given the infrequency with which resuscitation is required and the problems of attempting controlled studies in the immediate neonatal period, animal studies will undoubtedly play a major role in improving the understanding of these problems.

Despite the very limited information from clinical trials of resuscitation, the great majority of ill or depressed infants can be successfully managed simply by appropriate ventilation, without the need to consider the use of drugs, volume expanders, or other adjuncts. We suspect that the most common serious error in neonatal resuscitation is the failure to recognize and correct hypoventilation, a problem which is preventable with sufficient staff training and experience. It is important that each hospital establish appropriate methods to facilitate the most effective care for asphyxiated or depressed neonates.

Careful consideration must be given to infants who are considered to have special risks of difficulties. Nasal and pharyngeal suction should be carried out on babies who have passed meconium *in utero*. Endotracheal suction should *not* be carried out on these babies unless they show clinical signs of depression (heart rate less than 100 beats per minute). There is no justification for routine intubation of all very low birthweight infants.

For the vast majority of infants, however, the only needs are vigilance, a clear airway, and a warm welcome.

References

Aballi AJ, Banus V, de Lamerens S, Rosengvaig S (1959). Coagulation studies in the newborn infant. III. Hemorrhagic disease of the newborn. Am J Dis Child, 97: 524–554.

Ambrus CM, Choi TS, Cunnanan E, Eisenberg B, Staub HP, Weintraub DH, Courey NG, Patterson RJ, Jockin H, Pickren JW, Bross ID, Jung OS, Ambrus J (1977). Prevention of hyaline membrane disease with plasminogen. A cooperative study. JAMA, 237: 1837–1841.

American Academy of Pediatrics Committee on Drugs (1980). Naloxone use in newborns. Pediatrics, 65: 667–669.

American Academy of Pediatrics and American College of Obstetrics and Gynecology (1983). Guidelines for Perinatal Care. Illinois: Evanston, pp 47–96.

Angell M (1984). Patient preferences in randomized clinical trials. New Engl J Med, 310: 1385–1387.

Angell M (1986). The Baby Doe rules. New Engl J Med, 314: 642–644.

Arant B (1981). Nonrenal factors influencing renal function during the perinatal period. Clin Perinatol, 8: 225–240.

Ballard J, Musial MJ, Myers M (1986). Hazards of delivery room resuscitation using oral methods of endotracheal suctioning. Pediatr Infect Dis, 5: 198–200.

Baum J, Scopes J (1968). The silver swaddler. Lancet 1: 672–673.

Besch NJ, Perlstein PH, Edwards NK, Keenan WJ, Sutherland JM (1971). The transparent baby bag—a shield against heat loss. New Engl J Med, 284: 121–124.

Bland R, Clarke T, Harden L (1976). Rapid infusion of sodium bicarbonate and albumin into high-risk premature infants soon after birth: A controlled, prospective trial. Am J Obstet Gynecol, 124: 263–267.

Bonta B, Gagliardi J, Williams V, Warshaw, J (1979). Naloxone reversal of mild neuro-behavioral depression in normal newborn infants after routine obstetric analgesia. J Pediatr, 94: 102–105.

Book L, Herbst J, Stewart D (1978). Hazards of calcium gluconate in newborn infant: Intraarterial injection producing intestinal necrosis in rabbit ileium. J Pediatr, 92: 793–797.

Boon A, Milner A, Hopkin I (1972). Physiologic responses of the newborn infant to resuscitation. Arch Dis Child, 54: 492–498.

Boon A, Milner A, Hopkin I (1979). Lung expansion, tidal exchange, and formation of the functional residual capacity during resuscitation of asphyxiated neonates. J Pediatr, 95: 1031–1036.

Boyle M, Torrance G, Sinclair J, Harwood S (1983). Economic evaluation of neonatal intensive care of very-low-birth-weight infants. New Engl J Med, 308: 1330–1337.

Britton S, Fitzhardinge P, Ashby S (1981). Is intensive care justified for infants weighing less than 801 gm at birth. J Pediatr, 99: 937–943.

Brown W, Ostheimer G, Bell G, Datta S (1976). Newborn response to oxygen blown over the face. Anesthesiology, 44: 535–536.

Butterfield P, Ende R, Platt BB (1978). Effect of silver nitrate on initial visual behavior. Am J Dis Child, 132: 426.

Butterfield PM, Ende RN, Svejda NJ (1981). Does the early application of silver nitrate impair maternal attachment? Pediatrics, 67: 737–738.

Campbell A (1982). Which infants should not receive intensive care? Arch Dis Child, 57: 569–571.

Carson B, Losey R, Bowes W, Simmons M (1976). Combined obstetric and pediatric approach to prevent meconium aspiration syndrome. Am J Obstet Gynecol, 126: 712–715.

Catlin E, Carpenter M, Brann B, Mayfield S, Shaul P, Goldstein M, Oh W (1986). The Apgar revisited: Influence of gestational age. J Pediatr, 109: 865–868.

Chance G, Hanvey L (1987). Neonatal resuscitation in Canadian Hospitals. Can Med Assoc J, 136: 601–606.

Changaris D, Purohit D, Balentine J, Levkoff A, Holden A, Dean D, Biggs P (1984). Brain calcification in severely stressed neonates receiving parenteral calcium. J Pediatr, 104: 941–945.

Chaou W, Chou M, Eitzman D (1984). Intracranial hemorrhage and vitamin K deficiency in early infancy. J Pediatr, 105: 880–884.

Christian JR (1960). Comparison of ocular reactions with the use of silver nitrate and erythromycin ointment in ophthalmia neonatorum prophylaxis. J Pediatr, 57: 55–60.

Corbet A, Adams J, Kenny J, Kennedy K, Rudolph A (1977). Controlled trial of bicarbonate therapy in high-risk premature newborn infants. J Pediatr, 91: 771–776.

Cordero L, Hon E (1971). Neonatal bradycardia following nasopharyngeal stimulation. J Pediatr, 78: 441–447.

Dahm L, James LS (1972). Newborn temperature and calculated heat loss in the delivery room. Pediatrics, 49: 504–513.

Davies VA, Rothberg AD, Argent AC, Cooper PA (1985). A comparison of two resuscitators in the management of birth asphyxia. S Afr Med J, 68: 19–22.

Dawes G (1968). Fetal and Neonatal Physiology. Chicago: Year Book.

Dawes G, Hibbard E, Windle W (1964). The effect of alkali and glucose infusion on permanent brain damage in rhesus monkeys asphyxiated at birth. J Pediatr, 65: 801–818.

Dick W, Knoche E, Traub E (1978). Clinical investigations of the influence of various naloxone doses on the newborn. J Perinat Med, 6: 95–101.

DiSessa T, Leitner M, Ching CT, Gluck L, Coen R, Friedman W (1981). The cardiovascular effects of dopamine in the severely asphyxiated neonate. J Pediatr, 99: 772–776.

Ditchey R, Lindenfield JA (1984). Potential adverse effects of volume loading on perfusion of vital organs during closed-chest resuscitation. Circulation, 69: 181–189.

Drew H (1982). Immediate intubation at birth of the very-low-birth-weight infant. Am J Dis Child, 136: 207–210.

Durand M, Ramanathan R (1986). Pulse oximetry for continuous oxygen monitoring in sick newborn infants. J Pediatr, 109: 1052–1056.

Editorial (1978). Vitamin K and the newborn. Lancet, 1: 755.

Enhorning G, Shennan A, Possmayer F, Dunn M, Chen C, Milligan J (1985). Prevention of neonatal respiratory distress syndrome by tracheal instillation of surfactant: a randomized clinical trial. Pediatrics, 76: 145–153.

Evans JN, Wiener PC, Hogg MIJ, Rosen M (1976). The use of naloxone in the neonate. Anaesthesia, 31: 145.

Fardig J (1980). A comparison of skin-to-skin contact and radiant heaters in promoting neonatal thermoregulation. J Nurs Midwifery, 25: 19–28.

Finberg L (1977). The relationship of intravenous infusions and intracranial hemorrhage a commentary. J Pediatr, 91: 777–778.

Finer N, Barrington K, Al-Fadley F, Peters K (1986). Limitations of self inflating resuscitators. Pediatrics, 77: 417–420.

Furzan J, Reisch J, Tyson J, Laird P, Rosenfeld C (1985). Risk factors for development of hemodynamically significant patent ductus arteriosus amongst in-born low-birth-weight-infants. Early Hum Dev, 12: 39–48.

Gandy G, Adamsons K, Cunningham N, Silverman W, James L (1964). Thermal environment and acid-base homeostasis in human infants during the first few hours of life. J Clin Invest, 43: 751–758.

Gardner S (1979). The mother as incubator—after delivery. J Obstet Gynecol Neonatal Nurs, May/June: 174–176.

Gellis S, White P, Pfeffer W (1949). A proposed additional technic for the prevention of asphyxia in infants delivered by cesarian section. New Engl J Med, 240: 533–536.

Gerhardt T, Bancalari E, Cohen H, Rocha L (1977). Use of naloxone to reverse narcotic respiratory depression in the newborn infant. J Pediatr, 90: 1009–1012.

Goldberg R, Chung D, Goldman S, Bancalari E (1980). The association of rapid volume expansion and intraventricular hemorrhage in the preterm infant. J Pediatr, 96: 1060–1063.

Goodard-Finegold J, Armstrong D, Zeller R (1982). Intraventricular hemorrhage following volume expansion after hypovolemic hypotension in the newborn beagle. J Pediatr, 100: 796–799.

Gregory G, Gooding C, Phibbs R, Tooley W (1974). Meconium aspiration in infants—a prospective study. J. Pediatr.

Gregory G (1977). Resuscitation of the newborn. In: Pediatrics. Rudolph A, Hoffman J (eds). Norwalk, Connecticut: Appleton-Century-Crofts, pp 148–152.

Gupta PK, Moore J (1973). The use of doxapram in the newborn. J Obstet Gynaecol Br Commnwlth, 80: 1002–1006.

Halliday HL, Reid MM, Meban C, McClure G, Lappin TRJ, Thomas PS (1984). Controlled trial of artificial surfactant to prevent respiratory distress syndrome. Lancet, 1: 476–478.

Halliday HL, McClure G, Reid MMcC (1986). Growth and development two years after artificial surfactant replacement at birth. Early Hum Dev, 13: 323–327.

Hambleton G, Appleyard WJ (1973). Controlled trial of fresh frozen plasma in asphyxiated low birthweight infants. Arch Dis Child, 48: 31–35.

Hobel C, Oh W, Hyvarinen M, Emmanouilides G, Erenberg A (1972). Early versus late treatment of neonatal acidosis in low birth weight infants. Relation to respiratory distress syndrome. J Pediatr, 81: 1178–1187.

Holzman I (1985). A method to maintain infant temperature. Am J Dis Child, 139: 390–392.

Horwood S, Boyle M, Torrance G, Sinclair J (1982). Mortality and morbidity of 500 to 1499 gram birthweight infants live-born to residents of a defined geographic region before and after neonatal intensive care. Pediatrics, 69: 613–620.

Hull D, Segall M (1966). Oxygen uptake during and after positive pressure ventilation for the resuscitation of asphyxiated newborn infants. Lancet, 2: 1096–1099.

Hutchison JH, Kerr MM, Inall JA, Shanks RA (1966). Controlled trials of hyperbaric oxygen and tracheal intubation in asphyxia neonatorum. Lancet, 1: 935–939.

Jennings P, Alden E, Brenz R (1974). A teaching model for pediatric intubation using ketamine-sedated kittens. Pediatrics 53: 283–284.

Keenan WJ, Jewett T, Glueck HI (1971). Role of feeding and vitamin K in hypoprothrombinemia of the newborn. Am J Dis Child, 121: 271–277.

Kitterman J, Phibbs R, Tooley W (1969). Aortic blood pressure in normal newborn infants during the first 12 hours of life. Pediatrics, 44: 959–968.

Kiely J, Paneth N (1981). Follow-up studies of low-birth-weight infants: suggestions for design, analysis, and reporting. Dev Med Child Neurol, 23: 96–99.

Kliot D, Silverstein L (1984). Changing maternal and newborn care. A study of the Leboyer approach to childbirth management. NY State J Med, 84: 169–174.

Koops B (1984). Extreme immaturity: A frontier in neonatology. Am J Dis Child, 138: 713–714.

Kravath R, Aharon A, Abal G, Finberg L (1970). Clinically significant physiologic changes from rapidly administered hypertomic solutions: Acute osmol poisoning. Pediatrics, 46: 267–275.

Kwong M, Egan E, Notter R, Shapiro D (1985). Double-blind clinical trial of calf lung surfactant extract for the prevention of hyaline membrane disease in extremely premature infants. Pediatrics, 76: 585–592.

Laga M, Namaara W, Brunham RC, Maitha G, D'Costa LJD, Mati JK, Ceang M, Plummer FA, Ndinya-Achola JO, Ronald AR, Bhullar VB, Fransen L, Piot P (1986). Single dose therapy of gonococcal ophthalmia neonatorum with ceftriaxone. New Engl J Med, 315: 1382–1385.

Laptook A, Stonestreet B, Oh W (1982). The effects of different rates of plasmanate infusions upon brain blood flow after asphyxia and hypotension in newborn piglets. J Pediatr, 100: 791–796.

Leboyer F (1975). Birth without Violence. New York: Alfred A Knopf.

Lees M (1980). Perinatal asphyxia and the myocardium. J Pediatr, 96: 675–677.

Linder N, Aranda JV, Tsur M, Matoth I, Yatsiv I, Mandelberg H, Rottem M, Feigenbaum D, Ezra Y, Tamir I (1988). Need for endotracheal intubation and suction in meconium-stained neonates. J Pediatr, 112: 613–615.

Lindeman R (1984). Resuscitation of the Newborn. Endotracheal administration of epinepherine. Acta Paediatr Scand, 73: 210–212.

Lou H, Lassen N, Friis-Hansen B (1978). Decreased cerebral blood flow after administration of sodium bicarbonate in the distressed newborn infant. Acta Neurol Scand, 57: 239–247.

Marks K, Naris E, Momin M (1986). Energy metabolism and substrate utilization in low birth weight neonates under radiant warmers. Pediatrics, 78: 465–472.

Mathews D, Avery M, Jude J (1963). Closed-chest cardiac massage in the newborn infant. JAMA, 183: 964–966.

Mathieu PL (1958). Silver nitrate and oxytetracycline in newborn eyes: conjunctivitis following instillation of silver nitrate or oxytetracycline into the eyes of newborn infants. Am J Dis Child, 95: 609–611.

McNinch A, Orme R, Tripp J (1983). Haemorrhagic disease of the newborn returns. Lancet, 1: 1089–1090.

Merritt T, Hallman M, Bloom B, Berry C, Bernischke K, Sahn D, Key T, Edwards D, Jarvenpaa A, Pohjavuori M,

Kankaanpaa K, Kunnas M, Paatero Rapola J, Jaaskelainen J (1986). Prophylactic treatment of very premature infants with human surfactant. New Engl J Med, 315: 785–790.

Meyer TC, Angus J (1956). The effect of large doses of 'Synkavit' in the newborn. Arch Dis Child, 31: 212–215.

Miller DL, Oliver TK (1966). Body temperature in the immediate neonatal period: the effect of reducing thermal losses. Am J Obstet Gynecol, 94: 964–969.

Milligan J, Shennan A, Hoskins E (1984). Perinatal intensive care: where and how to draw the line. Am J Obstet Gynecol 148: 499–503.

Milner AD, Vyas J, Hopkin I (1984a). Effect of exogenous surfactant on total respiratory system compliance. Arch Dis Child, 59: 369–371.

Milner A, Vyas H, Hopkin I (1984b). Efficacy of face mask resuscitation at birth. Br Med J, 289: 1563–1565.

Mirro R, Brown D (1984). Parenteral calcium treatment shortens the left ventricular systolic time intervals of hypocalcemic neonates. Pediatr Res, 18: 71–73.

Morley C, Bangham A, Miller N, Davis J (1981). Dry artificial surfactant and its effect on very premature babies. Lancet 1: 64–68.

Moya F, James LS, Burnard E, Hanks E (1962). Cardiac massage in the newborn infant through the intact chest. Am J Obstet Gynecol, 84: 798–803.

Murphy J, Vawter G, Reid L (1984). Pulmonary vascular disease in fetal meconium aspiration. J Pediatr, 104: 758–762.

Mutch L, Newdick M, Lodwick A, Chalmers I (1986). Secular changes in rehospitalization of very low birth weight infants. Pediatrics, 78: 164–171.

Nelson N, Enkin M, Saigal S, Bennett K, Milner R, Sackett D (1980). A randomized clinical trial of the Leboyer approach to childbirth. New Engl J Med, 302: 655–660.

O'Connor ME, Addiego JE (1986). Use of oral vitamin K1 to prevent hemorrhagic disease of the newborn infant. J Pediatr, 108: 616–619.

Oriel J (1984). Ophthalmia neonatorum: relative efficacy of current prophylactic practices and treatment. J Antimicrob Chemother, 14: 209–220.

Oski F (1972). Blood coagulation and its disorders in the newborn. In: Hematologic Disorders of the Newborn. Philadelphia: WB Saunders.

Palme C, Nystrom B, Tunell R (1985). An evaluation of the efficiency of face masks in the resuscitation of newborn infants. Lancet, 1: 207–10.

Perlstein P, Hersh C, Glueck C, Sutherland J (1974). Adaptation to cold in the first three days of life. Pediatrics, 54: 411–416.

Raju T, Vidyasagar D, Torres C, Grundy D, Bennett E (1980). Intracranial pressure during intubation and anesthesia in infants. J Pediatr, 96: 860–862.

Rappoport D (1976). Pour une naissance sans violence: resultants d'une premiere enquete. Bull Psychol, 29: 552–560.

de Saintonge DMC, Cross KW, Hathorn MKS, Lewis SR, Sothers JK (1979). Hats for the newborn infants. Br Med J, 2: 570–571.

Salsburey D, Brown D (1982). Effect of parenteral calcium treatment on blood pressure and heart rate in neonatal hypocalcemia. Pediatrics, 69: 605–609.

Schachter J, Sweet R, Grossman M, Landers D, Robbie M,

Bishop E (1986). Experience with the routine use of erythromycin for chlamydial infections in pregnancy. New Engl J Med, 314: 276–279.

Scott S, Ladenson J, Aquanna J, Walgate J, Hillman L (1984). Effect of calcium therapy in the sick premature infant with early neonatal hypocalcemia. J Pediatr, 104: 747–751.

Shapiro D, Notter R, Morin F, Deluga K, Golub L, Sinkin R, Weiss K, Cox C (1985). Double-blind randomized trial of calf lung surfactant extract administered at birth to very premature infants for prevention of respiratory distress syndrome. Pediatrics, 76: 593–599.

Shoskes M, Willner M, Pontoriero G, Chiong R (1961). 'Solubilized' vitamin K1 (phytonadione) in neonatal hypoprothrombinemia. J Pediatr, 58: 27–31.

Silverman WA (1981). Mismatched attitudes about neonatal death. Hastings Center Report. December, pp 12–16.

Simmons M, Adcock E, Bard H, Battaglia F (1974). Hypernatremia and intracranial hemorrhage in neonates. New Engl J Med, 291: 6–10.

Sinclair JC (1978). Temperature Regulation and Energy Metabolism in the Newborn. New York: Grune & Stratton.

Sorrells-Jones J (1983). A comparison of the effects of Leboyer delivery and modern 'routine' childbirth in a randomized sample. Presented at the 7th International Congress of Psychosomatic Obstetrics and Gynaecology, Dublin, Ireland, 1983.

Steichen J, Kleinman L (1977). Studies in acid-base balance. I. Effect of alkali therapy in newborn dogs with mechanically fixed ventilation. J Pediatr, 91: 287–291.

Stephenson JM, Du JN, Oliver TK (1970). The effect of cooling on blood gas tensions in newborn infants. J Pediatr, 76: 848–852.

Stinson R, Stinson P (1983). The Long Dying of Baby Andrew. Boston: Atlantic-Little Brown.

Sutherland J, Glueck J, Gleser G (1967). Hemorrhagic disease of the newborn. Breastfeeding as a necessary factor in the pathogenesis. Am J Dis Child, 113: 524–533.

Ten Centre Study Group (1987). Ten centre trial of artificial surfactant (artificial lung expanding compound) in very premature babies. Br Med J, 294: 991–996.

Thibeault D, Nelson P (1979). Pulmonary care of infants with endotracheal tubes. In: Neonatal Pulmonary Care. Thibeault D, Nelson P (eds). Menlo Park, California: Addison-Wesley.

Ting P, Brady J (1975). Tracheal suction in meconium aspiration. Am J Obstet Gynecol, 122: 767–771.

Todres ID, Rogers M (1975). Methods of external cardiac massage in the newborn infant. J Pediatr, 86: 781–782.

Tooley W, Phibbs R, Schlueter M (1977). Delivery room diagnosis and immediate management of asphyxia. In: Intrauterine Asphyxia and the Developing Fetal Brain. Gluck L (ed). London: Year Book, Medical Publisher.

Turbeville D, Bowen F, Killam A (1976). Intracranial hemorrhages in kittens: Hypernatremia versus hypoxia. J Pediatr, 89: 294–297.

Tyson J, De Sa D, Moore S (1976). Thromboatheromatous complications of umbilical arterial catheterization in the newborn period. Arch Dis Child, 51: 744–754.

Tyson J, Furzan J, Reisch J, Mize S (1983). An evaluation of the quality of therapeutic studies in perinatal medicine. J Pediatr, 102: 10–13.

Tyson J, Swanson M (1987). Problems of neonatal follow-up programs in the United States. Proceedings of the Seventh Annual Canadian Ross Conference in Paediatrics, Val David, Quebec, March.

Van Doorm J, Muller A, Hemker H (1977). Heparin-like inhibitor, not vitamin K deficiency in the newborn. Lancet, 1: 852–853.

Van Dyke R, Spector S (1984). Transmission of herpes simplex virus type 1 to a newborn infant during endotracheal suctioning for meconium aspiration. Pediatr Infect Dis, 3: 153–155.

Venkataraman P, Wilson D, Sheldon R, Rao R, Parker M (1985). Effect of hypocalcemia on cardiac function in very low birth weight preterm neonates: studies of blood ionized calcium, echocardiography, and cardiac effect of intravenous calcium therapy. Pediatrics, 76: 543–550.

Versmold H, Kitterman J, Phibbs R, Gregory G, Tooley W (1981). Aortic blood pressure during the first 12 hours of life in infants with birth weights 610–4220 grams. Pediatrics, 67: 607–613.

Vietti TJ, Murphy TP, James JA, Pritchard JA (1960). Observations on the prophylactic use of vitamin K in the newborn infant. J Pediatr, 56: 343–346.

Vyas H, Milner A, Hopkin I, Boon A (1981). Physiologic responses to prolonged and slow-rise inflation in the resuscitation of the asphyxiated infant. J Pediatr, 99: 635–639.

Wahlberg V, Kallings IM, Winberg J (1982a). Reconsideration of Crede prophylaxis I. Epidemiologic aspects of gonorrhoeal and chlamydial infection. Local effects of silver nitrate and hexarginum. Acta Pediatr Scand, 295 (Suppl): 27–57.

Wahlberg V, Lundh W, Winberg J (1982b). Reconsideration of Crede prophylaxis III. Effects of silver nitrate prophylaxis on visual alertness in neonates. Acta Pediatr Scand, 295 (Suppl): 43–48.

Wahlberg V, Lundh W, Winberg J (1982c). Reconsideration of Crede prophylaxis IV. Effects of silver nitrate prophylaxis on mother-infant relationship. Acta Pediatr Scand, 295 (Suppl): 49–57.

Wahlberg V (1982d). Reconsideration of crede prophylaxis. V. Long-term influences on conjunctival secreation, infant behavior, breast-feeding and maternal feelings. A descriptive study. Acta Paediatr Scand, Suppl. 59–67.

Weil M, Rackow E, Trevino R, Grundler W, Falk, J, Griffel M (1986). Difference in acid–base status between venous and arterial blood during cardiopulmonary resuscitation. New Engl J Med, 315: 153–156.

Welch K, Phillips J (1984). Management of the depressed newborn. Clin Obstet Gynecol, 27: 125–133.

Welles B, Belfrage P, de Chateau P (1984). Effects of naloxone on newborn infant behavior after maternal analgesia with pethidine during labor. Acta Obstet Gynecol Scand, 63: 617–619.

Whitelaw A (1986). Death as an option in neonatal intensive care. Lancet, 2: 328–331.

Widstrom A-M, Ransjo-Arvidson AB, Christensson K, Matthiesen A-S, Winberg J, Uvnas-Moberg K (1987). Gastric suction in healthy newborn infants: effects on circulation and developing feeding behaviour. Acta Paediatr Scand, 76: 566–572.

Wiener P, Hogg M, Rosen M (1977). Effects of naloxone on pethidine-induced neonatal depression. Br Med J, 2: 228–231.

Wilkinson A, Jenkins P, Jeffrey J (1985). Two controlled trials of dry artificial surfactant: early effects and later outcome in babies with surfactant deficiency. Lancet, 2: 287–291.

Wilson MG, Roscoe SN (1958). Resuscitation of newborn premature infants. A clinical study of the use of positive pressure respiration. California Medicine, 88: 312–315.

Yasunuga S, Kean EH (1977). Effect of three ophthalmic solutions on chemical conjunctivitis in the neonate. Am J Dis Child, 131: 159–161.

76 The effects of intrapartum care on the risk of impairments in childhood

Robert Bryce, Fiona Stanley, and Eve Blair

'Since the abnormal process of birth frequently produces no effect, one cannot exclude the possibility that, despite Little's anamnesis, diplegia might be of congenital origin. Difficult birth in itself in certain cases is merely a symptom of deeper effects that influenced the development of the fetus'.

Freud 1897

1 Introduction

In 1862, William Little published 'On the Influence of Abnormal Parturition, Difficult Labours, Premature Births and Asphyxia Neonatorum on the Mental and Physical Condition of the Child, Especially In Relation to Deformities'. He theorized that birth complications were the cause of spasticity. For reasons which are not clear, Freud's alternative hypothesis—that adverse events earlier in fetal development may cause *both* birth complications and impairments in childhood—failed to attract the attention of the medical profession. Little's theory has influenced both the aims and the methods of evaluation of perinatal care in this century.

When an impaired child is seen it is often assumed that this distressing situation has resulted from birth trauma or asphyxia after poor intrapartum care. Paneth and Fox (1983) confirmed that these assumptions were widely held when they found that health professionals overestimated by more than ten times the risk of cerebral palsy that accompanies a very low 5-minute Apgar score (Fig. 76.1). Their mean response was 58 per cent, while the correct figure is about 4 per cent. Many parents (and lawyers) also apparently believe that

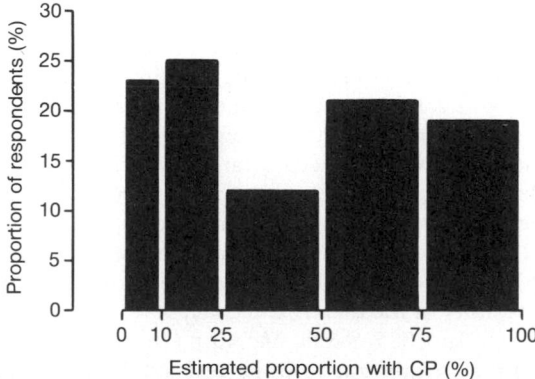

Fig. 76.1 Health professionals' estimates of proportion of infants with cerebral palsy after 5-minute Apgar score of 0–3 (Paneth and Fox 1983).

perinatal problems and obstetric mismanagement *often* result in major neurological impairments.

This overestimation of the risk of impairment may have led to the inappropriate use of some obstetrical interventions. For example, proponents of continuous electronic fetal heart rate monitoring have stated that 'early recognition and elimination of fetal distress should reduce by one-half the incidence of handicapping conditions or mental retardation' (Quilligan and Paul 1976). Leveno *et al.* (1985) concluded from observational data that a high caesarean section rate reduced the risk of neonatal seizures. Even courts of law have supported Little's theory when they have ruled obstetricians guilty of malpractice for not intervening during labour in cases where the resultant child was impaired.

Whether due to the increasing threat of legal action, to concern about maternal risks from over-intervention, or to a desire to ascertain the real causes of impairment, there is now a renewed interest among obstetricians, paediatricians and epidemiologists in Freud's alternative hypothesis (Niswander 1979; Illingworth 1979, 1985; Holm 1982; Nelson and Ellenberg 1984, 1986; Stanley 1984; Paneth 1986).

In order for interventions in labour to be capable of reducing childhood impairment significantly, two assumptions must both be correct. One is that a large proportion of impairments is due to adverse perinatal events. The other is that obstetric interventions can prevent, or significantly alter the effect of, adverse perinatal events. The evidence reviewed in this chapter challenges both these assumptions, with particular reference to non-progressive motor impairment (the cerebral palsies).

2 Historical background

The earliest descriptions and classifications of the cerebral palsies can be found in works by Little (1862), Osler (1889), and Freud (1897). All three avoided describing cerebral palsies as a disease entity, but rather considered them as a collection of motor disorders. All three authors believed that the 'lesions of the brain' resulting in cerebral palsies had occurred from the time of 'birth or early childhood' (Ingram 1984).

These authors were well aware of the *associations* of cerebral palsies with abnormal pregnancy, labour and delivery, and with anoxia in the newborn period. Little (1862) described the dangers of 'premature birth, unnatural labours, unnatural presentations, tedious labours from rigidity of the maternal passages and instrumental delivery'. In 1885 Sarah McNutt (1885a,b) ascribed congenital hemiplegia to unilateral subdural haemorrhage, and bilateral cerebral palsy to bilateral subdural haemorrhage. She attributed these subdural haemorrhages to difficult labour, especially breech delivery, and to the 'errors of obstetricians'. Ingram (1984) describes how 'this audacious lady toured widely lecturing obstetricians on their faults. When she reached Edinburgh it is reported that Sir James Young Simpson was not amused!'

Many early workers like Sachs and Peterson (1890), attempted to classify the cerebral palsies by the timing and nature of the brain injury. Freud (1897) objected to this classification on three grounds: first, it was often impossible to identify the timing or nature of the injury (many children with cerebral palsy syndromes had no relevant antenatal or birth histories); second, multiple causative factors might have operated; and third, such a classification was clinically useless. Apart from choreoathetosis, Freud's criticisms apply today, and classification based simply on a description of the motor and other impairments seems most appropriate until more is known about aetiology.

The idea that 'perinatal asphyxia', 'anoxia', or 'trauma' causes brain damage and subsequent cerebral palsy has been mentioned in almost every aetiological paper on the cerebral palsies published since 1900 (Stanley 1984). The observed association of cerebral palsies with perinatal problems in humans has been assumed to be causal, and rarely investigated further. For example, except for a study by Eastman and DeLeon in 1955, no comparison of cerebral palsied children with controls matched for the confounding effects of either preterm birth or low birthweight was published until the 1970s. Not surprisingly, therefore, 'asphyxia' was more common in the perinatal histories of cases than in those of controls. As these observations confirmed the dominant hypothesis at that time, no alternative explanations were sought.

Many clinicians, particularly those providing obstetric and neonatal care, still appear to believe that 'perinatal asphyxia' is, by itself, the sole cause of cerebral palsies, and that a normal and robust fetal brain can be irreversibly damaged by even a small degree of 'asphyxia'.

3 The epidemiology of impairments

An impairment is defined by the World Health Organization (1980) as a loss or abnormality of psychological, physiological, or anatomical structure or function. The major neuropaediatric impairments are intellectual, seizures (epilepsy), bilateral sensorineural defects (e.g. blindness or deafness), and the cerebral palsies.

At least 30 per cent of children with moderate to severe intellectual impairment (Intellectual Quotient < 50) have chromosomal anomalies (particularly Down's syndrome); a further 20 per cent have congenital malformations such as neural tube defects. Fewer than 10 per cent of cases are thought to be due to adverse perinatal events (Baird and Sadovnik 1985; Susser *et al.* 1985; Wellesley *et al.*, unpublished data).

Epilepsy, described as a non-febrile seizure disorder, occurs in up to 1 per cent of the population by the age of 20. Epilepsy in the absence of cerebral palsy does not appear to be associated with adverse perinatal events, but is associated with some genetically determined syndromes (Nelson and Ellenberg 1982, 1984; Susser *et al.* 1985).

The causes (probably various) of most intellectual impairment and epilepsy syndromes are currently unknown. The discovery of the X-linked fragile X mental retardation syndrome (Turner and Jacobs 1983) and the possible teratogenic effects of alcohol (Clarren and Smith 1978) has generated intense interest in the genetic and teratogenic causes of intellectual impairment and epilepsy. Current research is focused on factors disrupting developmental mechanisms including viral teratogenesis (e.g. rubella, cytomegalovirus) and specific severe nutritional deficiencies (e.g. iodine).

Some forms of sensorineural deafness and blindness do seem to be causally related to perinatal insults; for example, retinopathy of prematurity, and deafness after administration of some antibiotics to neonates (Silverman 1980). However, these conditions are still very rare and it is the cerebral palsies that are the impairments most commonly found to be associated statistically with perinatal events. The cerebral palsies are a diverse group of conditions defined as non-progressive disorders of movement and posture due to a defect or lesion of the immature brain (Bax 1964). The prevalence of cerebral palsy at the age of 5 years in children born in Western Australia is between 2 and 2.5 per 1000 (Stanley and Watson 1988). Similar rates have been found in the few developed countries in which population-based cerebral palsy data has been analysed (Paneth and Kiely 1984).

The birth cohort prevalence rate of cerebral palsies does not appear to have changed markedly with time in any country despite a marked fall in perinatal mortality

rates (Hagberg *et al.* 1984; Jarvis *et al.* 1985; Stanley and Watson 1988) (Fig. 76.2). This finding is in conflict with the popular theory of the 'continuum of reproductive casualty', i.e. that impairment and perinatal mortality are caused by similar perinatal insults, which are simply more severe in the case of mortality (Lilienfeld and Pasamanick 1955). In addition, the perinatal insults associated with cerebral palsy and perinatal mortality do not often overlap. Antepartum haemorrhage, for example, is associated with perinatal death but not with cerebral palsy.

4 Intrapartum events associated with impairments

Two intrapartum events have traditionally been believed to damage the brain—birth asphyxia and birth trauma.

4.1 Birth asphyxia

One of the major problems in studying the effects of 'intrapartum asphyxia' is the variety of ways in which it has been defined. The National Collaborative Perinatal Project in the United States, which involved 50 000 births between 1959 and 1966 in 12 hospitals, found a strong association between asphyxia (when defined as a low Apgar score at 1 or 5 minutes) and both cerebral palsy (Nelson and Ellenberg 1981) and lowered mean intelligence quotient at age 7 (Broman 1979). However, only 5 per cent of all infants with a 5-minute Apgar score of 0–3 had cerebral palsies at age 7 and only 15 per cent of all children with cerebral palsies had 5-minute Apgar scores of 0–3 (Nelson and Ellenberg 1981) (Table 76.1).

In Western Australia, the incidence of very low Apgar scores has fallen dramatically over the last 10 years (Fig. 76.3), yet no similar fall has been observed in the cerebral palsies (Fig. 76.2). Other measures of asphyxia such as abnormal intrapartum fetal heart rate patterns, acidotic fetal scalp blood gases, and delayed time to spontaneous respiration, are associated with low Apgar scores, but their relationship to impairment has not been adequately investigated (Bryce *et al.* 1985).

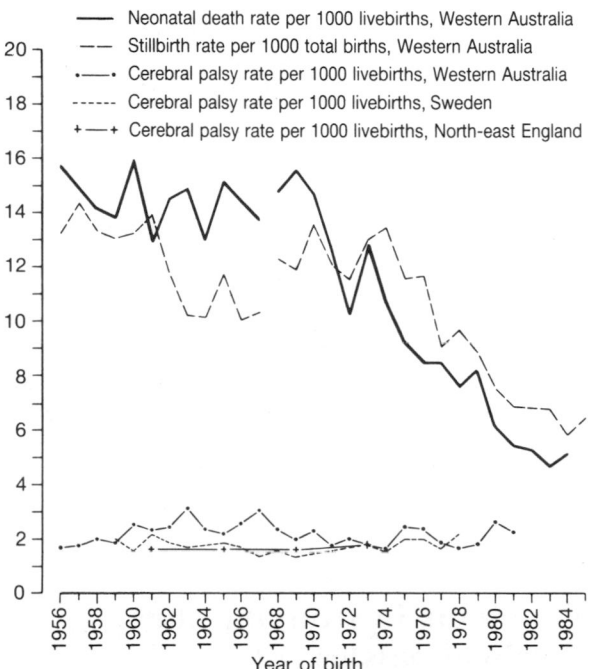

Fig. 76.2 Trends in perinatal mortality and cerebral palsy, 1956–85 (Stanley and Watson 1988; Hagberg *et al.* 1984; Jarvis *et al.* 1985). Gap in neonatal death and stillbirth rates between 1967–68 due to redefinition of 'birth' in Western Australia from one of >28 weeks gestation to one of >20 weeks in 1968. Cerebral palsy data for 1982–85 not yet available due to lag time to accurate diagnosis.

Table 76.1 Associations between Apgar scores and cerebral palsies (CP) in infants over 2500 g

Apgar score 5 min	Incidence of low Apgar %	Incidence of low Apgar in children with CP %	Incidence of CP in low Apgar children %	Relative risk of CP
0–6	3	23	2	9
0–3	1	14	4	22

(Nelson and Ellenberg 1981)

The legend within the figure reads:

— Neonatal death rate per 1000 livebirths, Western Australia
— — Stillbirth rate per 1000 total births, Western Australia
·—· Cerebral palsy rate per 1000 livebirths, Western Australia
----- Cerebral palsy rate per 1000 livebirths, Sweden
+—+ Cerebral palsy rate per 1000 livebirths, North-east England

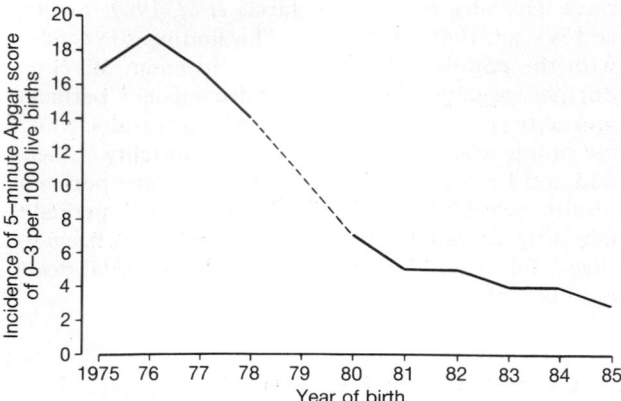

Fig. 76.3 Trends in 'asphyxia' in Western Australia, 1975–85. Data for 1979 are unreliable.

As Apgar scores reflect factors other than asphyxia, such as the effects of drugs administered to the mother, acidotic umbilical cord blood gases may better reflect the effects of oxygen deprivation. Sykes *et al.* (1982) demonstrated in a cohort of 1000 consecutive births in Oxford that acidotic cord gases frequently lead to a diagnosis of 'asphyxia' in different individuals from those diagnosed by low Apgar scores. Follow-up of this cohort to age 4 has not demonstrated an association between disturbed acid–base status at birth and developmental and behavioural dysfunction (Dennis *et al.*, in press).

In the Groningen Perinatal Project in The Netherlands, 3000 children born consecutively have been studied with respect to numerous perinatal features (including cord gases and Apgar scores) and by neurological examination during the neonatal period and subsequently. The conclusion from this project was that the difference in pH between maternal arterial blood and neonatal (up to 2 minutes of age) umbilical arterial blood is 'only slightly related' to neonatal neurological morbidity. The predictive ability of cord acidosis for neonatal neurological morbidity was slightly better in higher risk cases such as preterm births and light-for-gestational age infants (Dijxhoorn *et al.* 1985). These workers combined Apgar scores and pH for prediction of neurological abnormality in term infants, and found the highest frequency of neurologically abnormal neonates in the group with a normal pH, but a low Apgar score! (Dijxhoorn *et al.* 1986.)

Low *et al.* (1983) have conducted controlled follow-up to age 6 of a cohort of children born with high umbilical artery buffer bases, but they were unable to detect any increased risk of impairment compared with infants born with normal cord blood gases. It needs to be kept in mind, however, that all the follow-up cohorts mentioned had small numbers of acidotic infants and consequently only had the statistical power to demonstrate large differences in impairments between the groups.

Early neonatal seizures have been suggested as a marker of intrapartum asphyxia with a better prognostic value for impairments than previous markers (Dennis and Chalmers (1982). However, although seizures are associated statistically with other signs of birth 'asphyxia' such as fetal heart rate changes (Keegan *et al.* 1985) and low Apgar scores, seizures may occur in the absence of asphyxia, and many asphyxiated babies do not suffer seizures (Minchom *et al.*, in press). The presence of neonatal seizures does appear to be of better predictive value for impairments than other signs of 'asphyxia' (Minchom *et al.*, in press). New techniques of neonatal brain imaging such as ultrasound appear to be of even better predictive value for impairment for the small number of very low birthweight babies subjected to this method of screening (Stewart *et al.* 1987).

4.2 Birth trauma

Several authors have described follow-up studies of cohorts of infants born after mechanical birth trauma with or without birth asphyxia (Lilienfeld and Parkhurst 1951; Amiel-Tison 1969; Berendes 1975). The trauma occurred during prolonged, difficult births, breech deliveries or difficult forceps. Cerebral palsies or intellectual impairment were rarely seen after mechanical trauma except when the trauma was combined with birth asphyxia.

Mechanical trauma with a potential for brain damage is also rare in modern obstetrics. The National Collaborative Perinatal Project found only 12 children with skull fractures among 40 000 births, all of whom were neurologically normal at 1 year of age (Berendes 1975). Cephalohaematoma was seen in 1 per cent of births, and while these infants had a higher rate of mortality, none of the survivors had neurological abnormalities. We conclude that although mechanical birth trauma may have been a problem in the past, and may still be a problem in developing countries, its contribution to impairment in developed communities must now be very small.

5 Problems in studying the cerebral palsies

The major methodological problems in studying the causes of cerebral palsies include inadequate or inappropriate population samples, inadequate ascertainment of exposure (asphyxia or trauma) and inaccurate definition of outcome (cerebral palsy). In addition, many studies of the cerebral palsies have failed to recognize possible confounding factors or other expla-

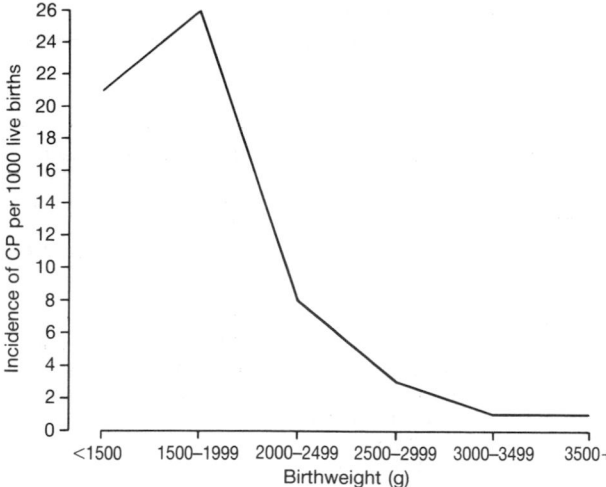

Fig. 76.4 Incidence of cerebral palsy by birthweight, 1968–81.

6 Asphyxia as a possible cause of the cerebral palsies

Paneth and Stark (1983) reviewed 6 prospective studies reported before 1980, of the association between 'perinatal asphyxia' and cerebral palsies. 'Asphyxia' was mainly defined as a low Apgar score, but poor clinical condition at birth was also used. They concluded that perinatal asphyxia was not a major cause of cerebral palsies. The majority of asphyxiated infants (75–98 per cent depending on the criteria used to define asphyxia) recovered without impairment. While very few asphyxiated infants developed cerebral palsies, those who did were severely affected and had other impairments. The asphyxia in these cases had usually been severe and followed by neonatal signs such as changes in conscious state, difficulties with respiratory control or seizures.

A review of the 9 controlled studies of the association between 'perinatal asphyxia' and cerebral palsies that have been reported since 1980 is presented in Table 76.2. Definitions of asphyxia varied and included abnormal fetal heart rate, and poor physical condition or abnormal biochemical parameters at birth. While two of the three studies in which the controls were matched for birthweight or gestation found no associations with indicators of perinatal asphyxia, all the unmatched studies did find associations.

Of the studies with matched controls, Low *et al.* (1983) had insufficient power to exclude an association between perinatal asphyxia and cerebral palsies; Shennan *et al.* (1985) found no associations; and Blair and Stanley (1988) found a positive association between perinatal asphyxia and cerebral palsies. A study in which multivariate analysis was attempted, (Taylor *et al.* 1985) did not have the statistical power to assess the effect of the antenatal factors it considered with respect to cerebral palsies, but Nelson and Ellenberg (1986) found that indicators of perinatal asphyxia were poor predictors of cerebral palsies when antenatal factors were also considered. Blair and Stanley (1988) came to similar conclusions. Assessing each of the 183 cases with cerebral palsies and 549 controls without cerebral palsies for any possible indication of asphyxia in labour or in the neonatal period, they concluded that cerebral palsies were possibly attributable to perinatal asphyxia in only 8 per cent of cases.

The recent literature therefore confirms the conclusions of Paneth and Stark (1983) that although the cerebral palsies are associated statistically with indicators of perinatal asphyxia, this association is confounded by gestational age and birthweight and is only rarely likely to be causal. A normally grown, term fetus is unlikely to be neurologically damaged by an episode of intrapartum asphyxia unless that episode is both prolonged and severe. Preterm or otherwise compromised infants may be affected by less severe

nations for associations observed. In choosing the sample of the population to be studied, bias can result if cases are selected which have a different distribution of confounding factors from that of controls.

Since low birthweight and preterm birth are associated with cerebral palsies (see Fig. 76.4) and, since both are also associated with measures of asphyxia, these constitute the two most important confounders. This selection bias may invalidate comparisons with inadequately matched controls. In addition as cerebral palsies are rare outcomes, imprecision often results when the sample size is not sufficiently large to have the power to demonstrate statistically any clinically significant differences in exposure (case-control studies) or outcome (cohort studies).

When ascertaining exposure retrospectively in case-control studies, recall bias is common where an abnormal outcome has sharpened the memory of an affected parent compared with that of the parent of a normal child. Misclassification of either exposure or outcome (cerebral palsy) can cause bias or imprecision, and the criteria used for exposures such as 'asphyxia' for example, are variable and often poorly defined.

The cerebral palsies are a diverse group of conditions, the expression of which varies with the stage of motor development. Thus length of follow-up is critical. This is often, however, less than the 5 years recommended for complete ascertainment of handicapping conditions (Stanley 1982), which may lead to misclassification. Furthermore, bias can result from selective loss to follow-up of children with or without impairment. In the light of these problems, it is not surprising that the literature attempting to describe the associations between cerebral palsies and antecedent factors is so confusing! (Stanley 1984).

Table 76.2 Controlled studies of perinatal asphyxia (PA) and cerebral palsies (CP) (1980–86)

Author and date	Sources of cases	Sample size	Study design	Controls	PA	Results
Nelson and Ellenberg (1981)	NCPP survivors* excluding post-neonatal causes of CP	45,559 (120 CP)	cohort	all non-CP	5-minute Apgar scores	CP strongly associated with PA Apgar 0–3, odds ratio (OR) = 17, population attributable risk (PAR) = 14%, Apgar 0–6, OR = 5, PAR = 15%
Nelson and Ellenberg (1984)	NCPP survivors* excluding all LBW (< 250 l/g) births	45,559 (125 CP)	cohort	all non-CP	Apgar < 6 and delivery complications (nuchal cord, fetal heart rate (FHR) < 100, breech, polyhydramnious)	CP strongly associated with PA (OR = 10), but only in the presence of delivery complications.
Nelson and Ellenberg (1986)	NCPP survivors* All CP	45,559 (189 CP) survivors	cohort	all non-CP	FHR ≦60 or 5 min Apgar <4 or TSR ≧5	CP associated with PA. 34% of CP predicted by non-PA factors, 37% predicted when PA added.
Dale and Stanley (1980)	All spastic CP b. 1966–75 from WA CP register†	208 CP 207 controls	case-control	matched by DOB and hospital	'fetal distress'	CP associated with PA
Stanley and English (1986)	All CP diagnosed by age 5 in 2.5 yr birth cohort, 1974–76 with birthweights 500–2000 g	21 CP in 512 LBW survivors	cohort	all non-CP	prolonged TSR	PA associated with CP. TSR 2–10, OR = 6, PAR = 70%, TSR > 10, OR = 13, PAR = 25%
Blair and Stanley (1988)	All spastic CP b. 1975–80 excluding post-neonatal causes from WA CP Register†	183 CP 549 controls	case control	matched by sex, race and birthweight	fetal distress or low Apgar or prolonged TSR	CP associated with PA. TSR > 3, OR = 7, PAR = 18%, 8% of cases attributable to PA
Low *et al.* (1983)	Asphyxiated, AGA,‡ term survivors of NICU. Follow-up to age 6	37 cases (1 CP) 57 controls	cohort	Term AGA; non-asphyxiated	Cord arterial buffer at birth of > 34 mEq/l	No associations
Shennan *et al.* (1985)	Survivors 26–30 wk gestation in NICU b. 1979–82. Follow-up to age 1	344 (34 handicapped including 27 CP)	cohort	matched by gestational age and DOB	1 and 5 min Apgar scores umbilical cord venous pH, or cord base deficit	No associations
Taylor *et al.* (1985)	All survivors b. Dundee 1974–75 Follow-up to 3 yr	4852 (12 CP)	case control	The two normally developed children born before and after each case	Meconium liquor, fetal bradycardia, fetal tachycardia	CP only associated with fetal tachycardia

* NCPP = National Collaborative Perinatal Project, USA. 56,000 pregnancies in 12 hospitals 1954–66 and followed to age 7.
† Western Australian Cerebral Palsy Register; population-based, multiple sources of ascertainment; follow-up to age 5 years.
‡ AGA = appropriate for gestational age.

asphyxic episodes, but they may also develop abnormally in the absence of asphyxia.

7 The effect of obstetric interventions on the cerebral palsies

As discussed earlier the justification for intervention in labour has often been the belief that death and impairment are both sequelae of the same insult—generally thought to be asphyxia. The evidence reviewed above suggests cerebral palsy is rarely caused by asphyxia. It is not surprising therefore, that evidence of a beneficial effect of obstetric intervention on the prevalence of cerebral palsies cannot be found. This calls into question the use of cerebral palsy rates to evaluate perinatal care (Stanley and English 1986).

Cohorts of patients who received or did not receive particular care have been compared retrospectively. For example, Pharaoh (1976) compared the incidence of cerebral palsies in low birthweight children born in 1966 in two hospitals, one of which pursued a more 'active' intervention policy with respect to perinatal care. The incidence of cerebral palsies was 4 per cent among low birthweight infants from the 'active' hospital and only 1 per cent in those from the hospital with a more conservative policy. This difference, however, was not statistically significant. Yu *et al.* (1984) compared disability rates in very low birthweight infants born by caesarean section or by vaginal delivery. They found a significantly lower incidence of disability at 2 years in very low birthweight children born by caesarean section (12 per cent) than in similar children who had been born vaginally (23 per cent). However, Kitchen *et al.* (1985) found no statistically significant difference in the incidence of cerebral palsies at age 2 in extremely preterm children born by caesarean section (13 per cent) and in those born vaginally (11 per cent). Such retrospective studies, however, are liable to be biased. For example, when the choice of route of delivery is made by the clinician (rather than in the context of a randomized trial), it must be based on assessments of fetal condition and chances of good outcome. Caesarean section may not, therefore, have been contemplated for the more severely compromised fetus.

One case-control study has examined the relationship between obstetric care and the cerebral palsies. Niswander et al. (1984) assessed the quality of obstetric care in cerebral palsy cases and controls without cerebral palsies, while blind to knowledge of their outcome.

Sub-optimal care was found in 3 per cent of cases of cerebral palsy and 4 per cent of controls. This study only had the power to demonstrate strong associations between sub-optimal care and the cerebral palsies. Such associations were detected, however, with respect to the death of normally formed fetuses and early neonatal seizures in infants born at term, in spite of the fact that, as for cerebral palsy, only relatively small samples of these outcomes were available.

A large (13 000 women) randomized controlled trial demonstrated a statistically significant decrease in neonatal seizures (12 compared with 27) in infants who were monitored by continuous fetal heart rate monitoring, with an option to assess acid–base status in labour, compared with those who were monitored by auscultation used intermittently. Follow-up at one year of age, however, revealed 3 children in each group who were diagnosed as having cerebral palsies (MacDonald *et al.* 1985).

Obstetric interventions have thus been shown to reduce the incidence of neonatal seizures, which are associated with asphyxia, but not the incidence of cerebral palsies. This may be either because asphyxia of this nature does not frequently cause cerebral palsies, or because the studies of these interventions lacked the power to demonstrate any important differences.

8 Conclusions

Those currently researching the causes of cerebral palsies believe that the majority of cerebral palsy syndromes are like congenital malformations and intellectual impairment. The majority of the causes of cerebral palsies are as yet unknown, but genetic, teratogenic, and early pregnancy influences are thought to be the main avenues worth pursuing. Brain damage from asphyxia appears to be very rare.

The evidence for this conclusion is mainly negative. There are, however, a few studies which suggest a relationship between cerebral palsies and congenital malformations and other markers of prenatal damage (Stanley 1984; Nelson and Ellenberg 1986). The main thrust of our own cerebral palsy research is towards elucidating *non-perinatal* risk factors for spastic cerebral palsy syndromes. These include genetic and familial factors, undiagnosed central nervous system malformations, inborn errors of metabolism and cytogenetic anomalies (like the X-linked fragile X mental retardation syndrome) as well as maternal illnesses and pregnancy complications. This is a challenging prospect. It is worth remembering that Freud gave up research into cerebral palsies because it was so difficult, and went into psychoanalysis!

References

Amiel-Tison C (1969). Cerebral damage in fullterm newborn. Aetiological factors, neonatal status and longterm follow up. Biologia Neonatorum, 14: 234–250.

Baird PA, Sadovnik AD (1985). Mental retardation in over half-a-million consecutive livebirths: an epidemiological study. J Ment Defic Res, 89: 323–330.

Bax M (1964). Terminology and classification of cerebral palsy. Dev Med Child Neurol, 6: 295–297.

Berendes HW (1975). The epidemiology of Perinatal Injury. In: Preventability of perinatal injury. Adamsons K, Fox HA (eds). New York; Liss, pp 1–33.

Blair, EM, Stanley FJ (1988). Intrapartum asphyxia: a rare case of cerebral palsy. Pediatrics 112: 515–519.

Broman SH (1979). Perinatal anoxia and cognitive development in early childhood. In: Infants born at risk: behaviour and development. Field TM (ed). New York: SP Medical and Scientific Books, pp 29–52.

Bryce RL, Halperin ME, Sinclair JC (1985). Association between indicators of perinatal asphyxia and adverse outcome in the term infant: a methodological review. Neuroepidemiology, 4: 24–38.

Clarren SK, Smith DW (1978). The fetal alcohol syndrome. New Engl J Med, 298: 1063–1067.

Dale A, Stanley FJ (1980). An epidemiological study of cerebral palsy in Western Australia 1956–75. II: Spastic cerebral palsy and perinatal factors. Dev Med Child Neurol, 22: 13–25.

Dennis J, Chalmers I (1982). Very early neonatal seizure rate: a possible epidemiological indicator of the quality of perinatal care. Br J Obstet Gynaecol, 89: 418–426.

Dennis J, Johnson MA, Mutch LMM, Yudkin PL, Johnson P (in press). Acid base status at birth in term infants and outcome at $4\frac{1}{2}$ years of age. Proceedings of 59th Annual Meeting of the British Paediatric Society, April 1987.

Dijxhoorn MJ, Visser GHA, Fidler VJ, Touwen BCL, Huisjes HJ (1986). Apgar score, meconium and acidaemia at birth in relation to neonatal neurological morbidity in term infants. Br J Obstet Gynaecol, 93: 217–222.

Dijxhoorn MJ, Visser GHA, Huisjes HJ, Fidler V, Touwen BCL (1985). The relation between umbilical pH values and neonatal neurological morbidity in full-term appropriate-for-dates infants. Early Hum Dev, 11: 33–42.

Eastman NJ, DeLeon M (1955). The etiology of cerebral palsy. Am J Obstet Gynecol, 69: 950–961.

Freud S (1897). Infantile cerebral paralysis. (Translation by Russin LA (1968) of 'Die Infantile Cerebrallähmung Wien: A Holder'). Florida: University of Miami Press.

Hagberg B, Hagberg G, Olow I (1984). The changing panorama of cerebral palsy in Sweden. Acta Paediatr Scand, 73: 433–440.

Holm VA (1982). The causes of cerebral palsy. JAMA, 247: 1473–1477.

Illingworth RS (1979). Why blame the obstetrician? A review. Br Med J, 1: 797–801.

Illingworth RS (1985). A paediatrician asks—why is it called birth injury? Br J Obstet Gynaecol, 92: 122–130.

Ingram TTS (1984). A historical review of the definition and classification of the cerebral palsies. In: The Epidemiology of the Cerebral Palsies. Stanley F, Alberman E (eds). Oxford: Blackwell, pp 1–11.

Jarvis SN, Holloway JS, Hey EN (1985). Increase in cerebral palsy in normal birthweight babies. Arch Dis Child, 60: 113–121.

Keegan KA, Waffarn F, Quilligan DJ (1985). Obstetric characteristics and fetal rate patterns of infants who convulse during the newborn period. Am J Obstet Gynecol, 153: 732–737.

Kitchen W, Ford GW, Doyle LW, Rickards AL, Lissenden JV, Pepperell RJ, Duke JE (1985). Cesarean section or vaginal delivery at 24–28 weeks' gestation: comparison of survival and neonatal and two-year morbidity. Obstet Gynecol, 66: 149–157.

Leveno KJ, Cunningham FG, Pritchard JA (1985). Cesarean section: an answer to the House of Horne. Am J Obstet Gynecol, 153: 838–844.

Lilienfeld AM, Pasamanick B (1955). The association of maternal and fetal factors with the development of cerebral palsy and epilepsy. Am J Obstet Gynecol, 70: 93–101.

Lilienfeld AM, Parkhurst E (1951). A study of the association of factors of pregnancy and parturition with the development of cerebral palsy. Am J Hygiene, 53: 262–282.

Little WJ (1862). On the influence of abnormal parturition, difficult labours, premature births and asphyxia neonatorum on the mental and physical condition of the child, especially in relation to deformities. Trans Obstet Soc Lond, 3: 293–344. (Reprinted in Cerebral Palsy Bulletin 1958, 1: 5–34).

Low JA, Galbraith RS, Killen H, Pater EA, Karchmar EJ (1983). Intrapartum fetal hypoxia: a study of long-term morbidity. Am J Obstet Gynecol, 145: 129–134.

MacDonald D, Grant A, Sheridan-Pereira M, Boylan P, Chalmers I (1985). The Dublin randomized controlled trial of intrapartum fetal heart rate monitoring. Am J Obstet Gynecol, 152: 524–539.

McNutt S (1885a). Double infantile spastic hemiplegia with the report of a case. Am J Med Sci, 89: 58.

McNutt S (1885b). Apoplexia neonatorum. Am J Obstet Gynecol, 1: 73.

Minchom P, Niswander K, Chalmers I, Dauncey M, Newcombe R, Elbourne D, Mutch L, Andrews J, Williams G (1987). Antecedents and outcome of very early neonatal seizures in infants born at or after term. Br J Obstet Gynaecol (in press).

Nelson KB, Ellenberg JH (1981). Apgar scores as predictors of chronic neurologic disability. Pediatrics, 68: 36–44.

Nelson KB, Ellenberg JH (1982). Maternal seizure disorder, outcome of pregnancy, and neurologic abnormalities in the children. Neurology, 32: 1255–1259.

Nelson KB, Ellenberg JH (1984). Obstetric complications as risk factors for cerebral palsy or seizure disorders. JAMA, 251: 1843–1848.

Nelson KB, Ellenberg JH (1986). Antecedents of cerebral palsy. Multivariate analysis of risk. New Engl J Med, 315: 81–86.

Niswander KR (1979). The obstetrician, fetal asphyxia, and cerebral palsy. Am J Obstet Gynecol, 133: 358–361.

Niswander K, Henson G, Elbourne D, Chalmers I, Redman C, Macfarlane A, Tizard JPM (1984). Adverse outcome of pregnancy and the quality of obstetric care. Lancet, ii: 827–831.

Osler W (1889). The Cerebral Palsies of Children. London: HK Lewis.

Paneth N, Fox HE (1983). The relationship of Apgar score to neurological handicap: a survey of clinicians. Obstet Gynecol, 61: 547–550.

Paneth N (1986). Etiologic factors in cerebral palsy. Pediatr Ann, 15: 191–201.

Paneth N, Kiely J (1984). The frequency of cerebral palsy: a review of population studies in industrialised nations since 1950. In: The Epidemiology of the Cerebral Palsies. Stanley F, Alberman E (eds). Oxford: Blackwell, pp 46–56.

Paneth N, Stark RI (1983). Cerebral palsy and mental retardation in relation to indicators of perinatal asphyxia. An epidemiologic overview. Am J Obstet Gynecol, 147: 960–966.

Pharaoh POD (1976). Obstetric and neonatal care related to outcome. Br J Prev Soc Med, 30: 257–261.

Quilligan E, Paul RH (1976). Fetal monitoring: is it worth it? Obstet Gynecol, 45: 96–100.

Sachs B, Peterson F (1890). A study of cerebral palsies of early life. J Nerv Ment Dis, 17: 295–332.

Shennan AT, Milligan JE, Hoskins EM (1985). Perinatal factors associated with death or handicap in very preterm infants. Am J Obstet Gynecol, 151: 231–238.

Silverman WA (1980). Retrolental Fibroplasia: A Modern Parable. New York: Grune & Stratton.

Stanley FJ (1984). Perinatal risk factors in the cerebral palsies. In: The Epidemiology of the Cerebral Palsies. Stanley F, Alberman E (eds). Oxford: Blackwell, pp 98–115.

Stanley FJ (1982). Using cerebral palsy data in the evaluation of neonatal intensive care: a warning. Dev Med Child Neurol, 24: 93–94.

Stanley FJ, English DR (1986). Prevalence of and risk factors for cerebral palsy in a total population cohort of low-birthweight (< 2000 g) infants. Dev Med Child Neurol, 28: 559–568.

Stanley FJ, Watson L (1988). The cerebral palsies in Western Australia: Trends, 1968–1981. Am J Obstet Gynecol 158: 89–93.

Stewart AL, Reynolds EOR, Hope PL, Hamilton PA, Baudin J, Costello AM de L, Bradford BC, Wyatt JS (1987). Probability of neurodevelopmental disorders estimated from ultrasound appearance of brains of very preterm infants. Dev Med Child Neurol, 29: 3–11.

Susser M, Hauser WA, Kiely JL, Paneth N, Stein Z (1985). Quantitative estimates of prenatal and perinatal risk factors for perinatal mortality, cerebral palsy, mental retardation and epilepsy. In: Prenatal and Perinatal Factors Associated with Brain Disorders. Freeman JM (ed). US Dept of Health and Human Services, Bethesda, pp 359–439.

Sykes GS, Molloy PM, Johnson P, Gu W, Ashworth F, Stirrat GM, Turnbull AC (1982). Do Apgar scores indicate asphyxia? Lancet, i: 494–496.

Taylor DJ, Howie PW, Davidson J, Davidson D, Drillien CM (1985). Do pregnancy complications contribute to neurodevelopmental disability? Lancet, i: 714–716.

Turner G, Jacobs P (1983). X-linked mental retardation. In: Advances in Human Genetics, Vol 13. Harris H, Hirchorn K (eds). New York: Plenum Press, pp 83–111.

Wellesley D, Hockey A, Stanley F (unpublished data).

World Health Organization (1980). International Classification of Impairments, Disabilities, and Handicaps. Geneva: World Health Organization, p 47.

Yu VYH, Bajuk B, Cutting D, Orgill AA, Astbury J (1984). Effect of mode of delivery on outcome of very-low-birthweight infants. Br J Obstet Gynaecol, 91: 633–639.

77 Restriction of mother–infant contact in the immediate postnatal period

Molly Thomson and Ruta Westreich

1 Introduction

Immediate postnatal social interaction between newly delivered mothers and their babies seems likely to be the rule for most births throughout the world (see Chapter 6). The situation in contemporary industrialized society is the outstanding exception to this rule. In association with the move of births to hospitals, Western society embarked on a large-scale experiment (with vast numbers of experimental subjects and very few controls) in which early separation of mother and baby became the rule.

Although it is obviously possible that a larger proportion of new mothers in more traditional societies might prefer to delay contact with their newborn infant if they had the opportunity to do so, it hardly seems likely that a majority would deliberately choose separation. The interactive behaviour that occurs between mothers and their newborn infants appears to have deep biological and social roots (see Chapters 6 and 48).

The progressive shift from domiciliary to institutional birth has influenced this pattern in two ways. First, women giving birth in unfamiliar surroundings and attended by caregivers with whom they are not familiar may feel inhibited. They may thus not behave towards their newborn child in the way that they would have done had they been at home among familiar faces. Second, however, institutions often have rules and policies that obstruct or actually prohibit immediate postnatal social interaction between newly delivered mothers and their babies. In 11 of 24 countries surveyed within the European Region of the World Health Organization, for example, separation of babies from their mothers in the immediate postnatal period was found to be the rule rather than the exception (World Health Organization 1985).

In this, as in many other fields of care during pregnancy and childbirth, individual women and their babies will vary in their needs and wishes. Early social interaction with their babies will be impossible for some women because they are too exhausted, in too much pain, or actually unconscious in the immediate postnatal period. Other mothers may not wish to have their babies with them at this time for less obvious reasons that are nevertheless important to them. Our purpose in this chapter is to assess the possible effects of the still widespread practice of routinely separating most babies from their mothers in the immediate postnatal period.

2 Possible advantages of restricting early mother-infant contact

In the past the usual rationale for routine early separation of mothers and their newborn infants seems to have been couched in terms of preventing infection in the baby. Ironically, the small amount of evidence available (see Chapter 78) suggests that the policy of separation may actually have led to an increase in the risks of cross-infection, possibly because of reduced colonization of the infant with maternal commensals which may confer a degree of protection against infection with pathogenic organisms.

Policies of routine separation of mothers and babies may have advantages for either the institutions concerned or the staff working in them. The physical arrangement of the institutional accommodation may impose constraints, as may the division of labour between various categories of staff. Like others (Brimblecombe *et al.* 1978), however, we have been unable to identify any research providing empirical justification for routine restriction of mother–infant contact for reasons such as these.

Any advantages that routine separation of mothers and babies may offer could only be justified if the routines either conferred positive advantages on mothers, their babies or both, or, at the very least, had no deleterious effects. We have already referred to the evidence suggesting that routine separation may actually increase the risks of neonatal infection. There is persuasive evidence that this policy also has other adverse consequences.

3 The effects of restricted contact on maternal affectionate behaviour

Evidence concerning the possible adverse consequences of routine separation of mothers and their newborn infants in the early postnatal period has been accumulating throughout the period of thirty years or more during which this practice has become widespread. Although this research has been inspired mainly by the work of Klaus and Kennell (Klaus *et al.* 1972), relevant data is available from controlled trials published as long ago as 1952 (Illingworth *et al.* 1952). In general, the pertinent controlled trials have compared the effects of the restricted early contact that is standard in most forms of institutional care with those of more liberal early contact between mothers and their newborn infants. The relative effect on maternal affectionate behaviour has been the focus of much of this research.

3.1 Restricted contact within two hours of birth

Table 77.1 gives details of the controlled trials in which standard institutional policies resulting in restricted interaction between mothers and their newborn babies within two hours of delivery were compared with the encouragement of such interaction at that time. Among

these trials, subsequent maternal affectionate behaviour was assessed at different periods of time after delivery using a total of 55 different indicators.

For 23 of these 55 indicators of maternal behaviour, statistically significantly less affectionate behaviour was observed in the group receiving standard institutional care. In no trial was any statistically significant increase in affectionate behaviour associated with the policy that involved greater separation. Chance alone might account for 3 statistically significant differences among 55 measures (in 55 two-tailed *t*-tests at $p = 0.05$), but it is extremely unlikely to account for 23 such differences. Furthermore, the high proportion of trials in which statistically significant differences were reported is remarkable because the samples studied were all small (the median number of participants in the 14 trials was only 52 (range 20–202)). It is possible that these observations may reflect a tendency among investigators to report selectively those outcomes for which statistically significant differences were observed, but we have no way of investigating this possibility.

Among the nine trials that we judged to be methodologically particularly sound (see Chapter 2), six (Klaus *et al.* 1972; de Chateau and Wiberg 1977a,b; Hales *et al.* 1977; Grossmann *et al.* 1981; Anisfield and Lipper 1983; Gomes-Pedro *et al.* 1984) reported that maternal affectionate behaviour was significantly less common among mothers who had received routine care involving restricted early contact between mother and baby. The fact that no statistically significant differences were observed in the remaining three studies (Svejda *et al.* 1980; Curry 1982; Craig *et al.* 1982) may reflect either lack of statistical power because of small numbers, or that there were actually no differences. It is worth noting, however, that the three studies in which statistically significant differences were not observed differed from the others in two respects that may be important. First, the contrasts in the types of care compared tended to be less marked in these studies. Second, the women involved in these trials were of higher socioeconomic status and more likely to have other children than the women in the six trials that yielded statistically significant differences.

It seems plausible that a woman's circumstances may influence whether or not early separation from her baby has any detectable effects on her subsequent behaviour. This possibility is supported by the observations of Anisfield and Lipper (1983) that primiparae and women lacking social support show the greatest increases in affectionate behaviour, while multiparae and women whose social support networks appeared to be adequate show little increase in such behaviour.

3.2 Restricted contact more than two hours after birth

Table 77.2 outlines seven controlled trials in which

Table 77.1 Trials in which the effect of restricting mother–infant contact within two hours of birth on subsequent affectionate maternal behaviour has been assessed.

Report	Participants	Restricted contact group	Enhanced contact group	Outcome measures	Effect in restricted contact group
Klaus et al. (1972)	28 primiparae, low income, USA	No contact until 6 hr postpartum, then feedings every 4 hr	1 hr in recovery room then 5 hr contact daily	(at 4 weeks) Watching–soothing at physical exam Fondling–'enface'	Decreased ($p = 0.02$) Decreased ($p < 0.05$)
Kennell et al. (1974)	Same trial as above			(at 1 year) Soothing at physical exam Behaviours at developmental exam Interview Picture-taking Free play	Decreased ($p < 0.05$) Similar Similar Similar Similar
Ringler et al. (1975)*	Same trial as above			(at 1 year) Maternal speech patterns with child	More statements but other speech elements similar
Ringler et al. (1976)	Same trial as above			(at 2 years) Maternal speech patterns with child	Fewer adjectives and questions with more commands
de Chateau and Wiberg (1977a)	42 primiparae, middle income, Sweden	No contact until 4 hr postpartum, then feedings every 4 hr	15 min in delivery room, then routine contact	(at 36 hr) Holding Encompassing Loving touch Close contact Looks 'Enface' Kisses	Decreased ($p < 0.01$) Incr. trend ($p < 0.1$) Similar Similar Similar Similar Similar
de Chateau and Wiberg (1977b)	Same trial as above			(at 3 months) Holding Encompassing Loving touch Close contact Looks 'Enface' Kisses	Similar Similar Similar Similar Similar Decreased ($p < 0.01$) Decreased ($p < 0.01$)
de Chateau and Wiberg (1984)	Same trial as above			(at 1 year) Holding positively Loving touch	Decreased ($p < 0.01$) Decreased ($p < 0.01$)
Hales et al. (1977)†	60 primiparae, low income, Guatemala	No contact until 12 hr postpartum, then modified rooming-in	45 min in delivery room, then routine contact	(at 36 hr) Affectionate behaviour score	Decreased ($p < 0.01$)
Carlsson et al. (1978)‡	62 primiparae, middle income, Sweden	5 min in delivery room then no contact until 4 hr postpartum, modified rooming-in	1 hr in delivery room then routine contact	(at 2 days) Contact behaviour score (at 4 days) Contact behaviour score	Decreased ($p < 0.05$) Decreased ($p < 0.01$)

Study	Population	Restricted contact	Extended contact	Contact behaviour score	
Hwang, C.-P. (1981)	reworked data from above trial				
Kontos (1978)*	48 primiparae, middle income, Canada	7 min in delivery room then no contact until 6 hr postpartum, feedings every 4 hr or rooming-in	1 hr in delivery room then routine contact	(1 and 3 months) Summed attachment score	Decreased ($p<0.01$)
McClellan and Cabianca (1980)	40 multiparae having repeat caesarean sections, middle income, USA	No contact until 12 hr postpartum, then rooming-in	1 hr in recovery room then routine contact	(at 36 hr) Holding–touching–looking score	(Decreased ($p=0.001$))
				(at 1 month) Holding–touching–looking score	Decreased ($p=0.002$)
Siegel et al. (1980)	202 mixed parity, low income, USA	Routine contact at feedings	45 min during first 3 hr postpartum, then 5 hr daily	(at 4 months) Factor analysis of home observations Acceptance	Decreased ($p=0.04$)
Svejda et al. (1980)	29 primiparae, middle income, USA	Up to 5 min during transfer from delivery room then feedings every 4 hr	15 min in delivery room, then 45 min in own room, then routine care	(at 36 hr) Affectionate behaviour score in interaction	Similar
				Affectionate behaviour score at feeding	Similar
Ali and Lowry (1981)	100 of mixed parity, low income, Jamaica	No contact until 9 hr postpartum	45 min in delivery room, then routine contact	(at 6 weeks) Proximity at physical exam	Similar
				Gazing	Similar
Grossmann et al. (1981)⊙	54 of mixed parity, middle income, West Germany	Feedings every 4 hr in one group; 5 hr extra contact daily in other group	30 min in delivery room, then routine contact	(at 2, 5, and 8 days) Summer scores for tender touches: Duration	Decreased ($p=0.06$)
				Frequency	Decreased ($p=0.06$)
Craig et al. (1982)	60 primiparae, low income, USA	Up to 10 min in delivery room	Over 1 hr in delivery room	(at 1 month) Neonatal perception	Similar
Curry (1982)	20 primiparae, middle income, USA	15 min in delivery room, wrapped infants	15 min in delivery room, skin-to-skin	(at 36 hr) Attachment behaviour	Similar
Anisfield and Lipper (1983)	49 of mixed parity, low–middle income, USA	No contact until 3 hr postpartum, then at feedings every 4 hr	45 min in delivery room, then routine contact	(at 2 days) Affectionate contact score	Decreased ($p<0.005$)
Gomes-Pedro et al. (1984)	60 primiparae, low–middle income, Portugal	No contact until 6 hr postpartum, then rooming-in	30 min in delivery room, then routine contact	(at 3 days) Affectionate behaviour score	Similar
Taylor et al. (1985a)	78 primiparae, middle income, USA	In delivery room majority touched or held infant; in transfer to recovery room all held infant about 5 min	Average of 46 min in delivery room, then routine contact	(at 2 days) Mother–infant feeding profile	Similar
				(at 1 month) Mother–infant feeding profile	Similar

* A further publication (Ringler et al. 1976), measured the child's speech patterns at 5 years of age.
† A third group was given extra contact at 12 hours postpartum, as listed in Table 77.2.
‡ One group was given supportive nursing care, with little measurable effect as compared to the group given routine nursing care.
* The 'routine (restricted) contact group' comprised a rooming-in group and a scheduled feeding group which are compared in Table 77.2.
⊙ The 'routine (restricted) contact group' comprised a group given extra 5 hours' contact daily and a group given scheduled feedings which are compared in Table 77.2.

Table 77.2 Trials in which effect of restricting mother–infant contact two or more hours after birth on affectionate maternal behaviour has been assessed

Report	Participants	Restricted contact group	Enhanced contact group	Outcome measures	Effect in restricted contact group
Leifer et al. (1972)	44 primiparae with premature infants, middle class, USA	No proximal contact until 3–12 weeks postpartum	Caretaking in intensive care nursery after 2–7 days postpartum	(at hospital discharge, 1 week after, and 1 month after discharge) Observed behaviours	Similar
Leiderman and Seashore (1975)	Same trial as above			(at 1 week, 1 month, 6 months, 1 year) Observed behaviours Infant performance	Similar Similar
Greenberg et al. (1973)	100 women of mixed parity, Sweden	Scheduled feedings	Rooming-in 8 hr per day after 12–36 hr	(at 6 days) Feelings of competence Feelings of self-confidence	Decreased ($p < 0.01$) Decreased ($p < 0.01$)
Hales et al. (1977)	60 primiparae, low income, Guatemala	Modified rooming-in after 12 hr postpartum	1 hr contact at 12 hr postpartum, then routine contact	(at 36 hr) Affectionate behaviour score	Similar
Kontos (1978)	48 primiparae, middle income, Canada	7 min contact in delivery room then scheduled feedings after 6 hr postpartum	7 min contact in delivery room then rooming-in after 6 hr postpartum	(at 1 and 3 months) Summed attachment score	Decreased ($p < 0.05$)
Jones et al. (1980)	40 primiparae, low income, USA	No instructions, scheduled feedings	Subjects instructed to hold and stroke infants for 15 min after each feeding, scheduled feedings	(at hospital discharge) Maternal behaviour	Similar
Grossmann et al. (1981)	54 of mixed parity, middle income, West Germany	Scheduled feedings	5 hr extra contact daily after 24 hr postpartum	(at 2, 5, and 8 days) Summed scores for tender touches: Duration Frequency	Similar Similar
O'Connor et al. (1980b, 1981)	152 of mixed parity, low income, USA	Not described	About 9 hr extra contact during first 48 hr postpartum	(at 1, 3, 6, 12, and 18 months) Many measures of mother–infant interaction	Inconsistent

standard hospital practices were compared with attempts to encourage mother–infant interaction after the immediate postnatal period (more than two hours after delivery). The additional interaction in these trials ranged from, in one trial, a small amount of caretaking in the intensive care nursery by mothers of premature infants, to full rooming-in for mothers of normal infants. Not only do these studies differ in the nature of the policies compared; in addition, the effects of the policies were evaluated using a variety of different outcomes. As a consequence of this heterogeneity, is less possible to assess the effects of reduced interaction between mothers and their children than with the more coherent body of research relating to immediate postnatal separation.

Having said this, no study generated findings which suggested that policies which restricted mother–child interaction have any advantages. On the contrary, the few statistically significant differences that were observed suggested that restrictive policies were associated with less affectionate maternal behaviour (Kontos 1978) and maternal feelings of incompetence and lack of confidence (Greenberg *et al.* 1973).

Perhaps most important of all, the results of one well-conducted study suggested that, compared with a policy of rooming-in, the routine hospital policy of separating mothers from their babies led to an increase in the subsequent risk of child abuse and neglect among socially deprived, first time mothers (O'Connor *et al.* 1980a,b; 1981).

Table 77.3 Trials in which effect of restricting mother–infant contact on subsequent breastfeeding has been assessed

Report	Participants	Restricted contact group	Enhanced contact group	Months postpartum at time infant feeding method ascertained
Illingworth *et al.* (1952)	227 women of mixed parity, UK	Rigid feeding schedule from 6 to 12 hr postpartum	Demand feeding after 48 hr postpartum	1
Sousa *et al.* (1974)	200 women of mixed parity, Brazil	No feeding until 12–24 hr postpartum then 3 hr schedule	Breastfeeding immediately after birth, then rooming-in	2
Johnson (1976)	12 primiparae, USA	No feeding until 16 hr postpartum	Breastfeeding within 1 hr of delivery	2
Sosa *et al.* (1976)*	40 primiparae, Social Security Hospital, Guatemala	No feeding until 24 hr postpartum, then schedule	Breastfeeding in delivery room	3
Sosa *et al.* (1976)†	60 primiparae, Roosevelt Hospital, Guatemala	No feeding until 24 hr postpartum, then schedule	Breastfeeding in delivery room	2 or 3
Sosa *et al.* (1976)*	64 primiparae, Roosevelt Hospital, Guatemala	No feeding until 12 hr postpartum, then schedule	Breastfeeding in delivery room	3
de Chateau and Wiberg (1977b)	40 primiparae, Sweden	No feeding until 4 hr postpartum, then 4 hr schedule	Breastfeeding in delivery room	3
Salariya *et al.* (1978)‡	108 primiparae, UK	No feeding until 4 hr postpartum, then 2 hr or 4 hr schedule	Breastfeeding in delivery room	3
Thomson *et al.* (1979)	30 primiparae, Canada	No feeding until 12 hr postpartum, then 4 hr schedule	Breastfeeding in delivery room	2
Taylor *et al.* (1985b)*	53 primiparae, USA	Majority touched or held infant in delivery room, then held infant in transfer to recovery room	Breastfeeding in recovery room	2

* Data extrapolated from Fig. 2, Sosa *et al.* (1976).
  † Data extrapolated from Klaus and Kennell (1982), p. 49.
  ‡ The 4-hour schedule group was compared with the 2-hour schedule group: 51 per cent in the 4-hour schedule group were breastfeeding at 3 months compared to 60 per cent in the 2-hour schedule group.
  * Data are given here only for women who initiated breastfeeding. Fewer women initiated breastfeeding in the group randomized to restricted contact (29/39) than in the group randomized to enhanced contact (31/39).

4 The effects of restricted contact on subsequent breastfeeding

The effect of policies tending to restrict early or frequent mother–infant interaction on subsequent breastfeeding has been examined in ten trials (Table 77.3). The women participating in these trials all wished to breastfeed their babies and, in all but two of the trials, they were having their first child. The restrictive policies were characterized by delays in permitting mother–infant interaction for anything between 4 and 48 hours after delivery. These delays were then followed (in most studies) by scheduled breastfeeding.

In the comparison groups in nine of these ten trials, mother–infant interaction was encouraged within the first hour after delivery and this interaction probably included suckling; in the remaining trial the extra contact consisted of demand feeding beginning 48 hours postpartum (Illingworth *et al.* 1952).

Although these ten trials involved women from a range of socioeconomic backgrounds and a variety of countries, the results were remarkably consistent: the proportion of women who had discontinued breastfeeding 1 to 3 months after delivery was substantially higher in the women who had been subject to the more restrictive policies (Table 77.4).

5 Conclusions

We have been unable to find any evidence suggesting that the restriction of early postnatal mother–infant interaction which has been such a common feature of the care of women giving birth in hospitals has any beneficial effects. On the contrary, the available evidence suggests that any effects that these restrictive policies have are undesirable. The data suggest the plausible hypothesis that women of low socioeconomic status may be particularly vulnerable to the adverse effects of restricting contact.

It may be thought surprising that disruption of maternal–infant interaction in the immediate postnatal period may set some women on the road to breastfeeding failure and altered subsequent behaviour towards their children. Paediatricians, psychologists, and others have indeed debated this issue (Lozoff *et al.* 1977; Rutter 1979; Chess and Thomas 1982; Klaus and Kennell 1982; Lamb 1982; Siegel 1982; Anisfield *et al.* 1983; Elliott 1983; Goldberg 1983; Thomson and Kramer 1984; Richards 1985). This scepticism does not, however, constitute grounds for acquiescing in hospital routines which lead to unwanted separation of mothers from their babies. In the light of the evidence that such policies may actually do harm, they should be changed forthwith.

Table 77.4 Effect of restricted mother–infant contact after delivery on discontinuation of breastfeeding at 1–3 months

Study	Retricted contact		Enhanced contact		Odds ratio	Graph of odds ratios and confidence intervals						
	n	(%)	*n*	(%)	(95% CI)	0.01	0.1	0.5	1	2	10	100
Thomson *et al.* (1979)	12/15	(80.00)	6/15	(40.00)	5.01 (1.19–21.06)							
De Chateau *et al.* (1977b)	15/20	(75.00)	8/20	(40.00)	4.04 (1.17–13.94)							
Salariya *et al.* (1978)	26/53	(49.06)	22/55	(40.00)	1.44 (0.68–3.06)							
Sosa *et al.* (1976)	12/20	(60.00)	5/20	(25.00)	4.04 (1.17–13.94)							
Sosa *et al.* (1976)	3/30	(10.00)	8/30	(26.67)	0.33 (0.09–1.22)							
Sosa *et al.* (1976)	17/32	(53.13)	13/32	(40.63)	1.64 (0.62–4.34)							
Taylor *et al.* (1985b)	9/22	(40.91)	9/31	(29.03)	1.68 (0.54–5.27)							
Illingworth *et al.* (1952)	34/96	(35.42)	33/131	(25.19)	1.63 (0.92–2.90)							
Sousa *et al.* (1974)	73/100	(73.00)	23/100	(23.00)	7.34 (4.22–12.76)							
Johnson (1976)	5/6	(83.33)	1/6	(16.67)	11.52 (1.32–99.99)							
Typical odds ratio (95% confidence interval)					2.62 (1.98–3.48)							

The importance of maternal caretaking behaviour is so essential to the newborn baby that a variety of biological and social mechanisms must have evolved to promote it. The mutually reinforcing affectionate behaviour which appears to occur during early postnatal mother–infant contact is only one such mechanism.

Because it is not the only mechanism, it is important to recognize that many mothers who are constrained from early contact with their babies, whether through illness, misguided hospital policies, or personal preference, are likely to overcome any effects of this separation.

References

Ali Z, Lowry M (1981). Early maternal–child contact: Effects on later behaviour. Dev Med Child Neurol, 23: 337–345.

Anisfield E, Lipper E (1983). Early contact, social support and mother–infant bonding. Pediatrics, 72: 79–83.

Anisfield E, Curry MA, Hales DJ, Kennell JH, Klaus MH, Lipper E, O'Connor S, Siegel E, Sosa R (1983). Maternal–infant bonding: A joint rebuttal. Pediatrics, 72: 569–572.

Brimblecombe FSW, Richards MPM, Roberton NRC (1978). Separation and Special Care Baby Units, Clinics in Developmental Medicine No. 68. London: Spastics International Medical Publications.

Carlsson SG, Hagerberg H, Horneman G, Hwang C-P, Larsson K, Rodholm M, Schaller J, Danielsson B, Gundewall C (1978). Effects of amount of contact between mother and child on the mother's nursing behavior. Dev Psychobiol, 11: 143–150.

Carlsson SG, Larsson K, Schaller J (1980). Early mother–child contact and nursing. Reprod Nutr Dev, 20: 881–889.

Chess S, Thomas A (1982). Infant bonding: mystique and reality. Am J Orthopsychiat, 52: 213–223.

Craig S, Tyson JE, Samson J, Lasky RE (1982). The effect of early contact on maternal perception of infant behavior. Early Hum Dev, 6: 197–204.

Curry MA (1982). Maternal attachment behavior and the mother's self-concept: the effect of early skin-to-skin contact. Nursing Res, 31: 73–78.

de Chateau P, Wiberg B (1977a,b). Long term effect on mother infant behaviour of extra contact during the first hour postpartum. I. First observation at 36 hours. II. A follow-up at 3 months. Acta Paediatr Scand, 66: 137–143, 145–151.

de Chateau P, Wiberg B (1984). Long-term effect on mother–infant behaviour of extra contact during the first hour post partum. III. Follow-up at one year. Scand J Soc Med, 12: 91–103.

Elliott MR (1983). Maternal infant bonding: taking stock. Can Nurse, 79: 28–31.

Goldberg S (1983). Parent–infant bonding: another look. Child Dev, 54: 1355–1382.

Gomes-Pedro J, Bento de Almeida J, Silveira da Costa C, Barbarosa A (1984). Influence of early mother-infant contact on dyadic behaviour during the first month of life. Dev Med Child Neurol, 26: 657–664.

Greenberg M, Rosenberg I, Lind J (1973). First mothers rooming-in with their newborns: its impact upon the mother. Am J Orthopsychiat, 43: 783–788.

Grossmann K, Thane K, Grossman KE (1981). Maternal tactual contact of the newborn after various postpartum conditions of mother–infant contact. Dev Psych, 17: 158–169.

Hales DJ, Lozoff B, Sosa R, Kennell JH. (1977) Defining the limits of the maternal sensitive period. Dev Med Child Neurol, 19: 454–461.

Hwang C-P (1981). Aspects of the mother-infant relationship during nursing, 1 and 6 weeks after early extended postpartum contact. Early Hum Dev, 5: 279–287.

Illingworth RS, Stone DGH, Jowett GH, Scott JF (1952). Self-demand feeding in a maternity unit. Lancet, 1: 683–687.

Johnson NW (1976). Breast-feeding at one hour of age. Am J Matern Child Nurs, 1: 12–16.

Jones FA, Green V, Krauss DR (1980). Maternal responsiveness of primiparous mothers during the postpartum period: age differences. Pediatrics, 65: 579–584.

Kennell JH, Jerauld R, Wolfe H, Chesler D, Kreger NC, McAlpine W, Steffa M, Klaus MH (1974). Maternal behavior one year after early and extended post-partum contact. Dev Med Child Neurol, 16: 172–179.

Klaus MH, Jerauld R, Kreger NC, McAlpine W, Steffa M, Kennell JH (1972). Maternal attachment: importance of first post-partum days. New Engl J Med, 286: 460.

Klaus MH, Kennell JH (1982). Labor, birth and bonding. In: Parent-Infant Bonding (2nd edn). Klaus MH, Kennell JH (eds). St Louis: Mosby, pp 22–109.

Kontos D (1978). A study of the effects of extended mother–infant contact on maternal behavior at one and three months. Birth Family J, 5: 133–140.

Lamb ME (1982). Early contact and maternal–infant bonding: one decade later. Pediatrics, 70: 763–768.

Leiderman PH, Seashore MJ (1975). Mother–infant neonatal separation: some delayed consequences. In: Parent–Infant Interaction, Ciba Foundation Symposium 33. Amsterdam: Associated Scientific Publishers, pp 213–239.

Leifer AD, Leiderman PH, Barnett CR, Williams JA (1972). Effects of mother–infant separation on maternal attachment behavior. Child Dev, 43: 1203–1218.

Lozoff B, Brittenham GM, Trause MA, Kennell JH, Klaus MH (1977). The mother–newborn relationship: limits of adaptability. J Pediatrics, 91: 1–12.

McClellan MS, Cabianca WA. (1980). Effects of early mother–infant contact following caesarean birth. Obstet Gynecol, 56: 52–55.

O'Connor S, Vietze PM, Sherrod KB, Sandler HM, Altemeier WA (1980a). Reduced incidence of parenting inadequacy following rooming-in. Pediatrics, 66: 176–182.

O'Connor S, Vietze PM, Sandler HM, Sherrod KB, Altemeier WA (1980b). Quality of parenting and the mother–infant relationship following rooming-in. In: Parent–Infant Relationships. Taylor PM (ed). New York: Grune & Stratton, pp 349–369.

O'Connor S, Altemeier WA, Vietze PM, Gerrity PS, Sandler HM, Sherrod KA (1981). Responsivity of mother-infant interaction after extended postpartum contact. Pediatr Res Abstr, 15: 484.

Richards MPM (1985). Bonding babies. Arch Dis Childhood, 60: 293–294.

Ringler NM, Kennell JH, Jarvella R, Navojosky BJ, Klaus MH (1975). Mother to child speech at 2 years—effects of early postnatal contact. J Pediat, 86: 141–144.

Ringler NM, Trause MA, Klaus MH (1976). Mother's speech to her two-year old, its effect on speech and language comprehension at 5 years. Pediatr Res, 10: 307.

Rutter M (1979). Separation experiences: a new look at an old topic. J Pediatr, 95: 147–154.

Salariya EM, Easton PM, Cater JI (1978). Duration of breast-feeding after early initiation and frequent feeding. Lancet 2: 1141–1143.

Siegel E (1982). Early and extended maternal–infant contact. Am J Dis Child, 136: 251–257.

Siegel E, Bauman KE, Schaefer ES, Saunders MM, Ingram DD (1980). Hospital and home support during infancy: impact on maternal attachment, child abuse and neglect, and health care utilization. Pediatrics, 66: 183–190.

Sosa R, Kennell JH, Klaus M, Urrutia JJ (1976). The effect of early mother–infant contact on breast-feeding, infection and growth. In: Breast-feeding and the Mother. Ciba Foundation Symposium 45. Amsterdam: Associated Scientific Publishers, pp 179–187.

Sousa PLR, Barros FC, Gazalle RV, Begeres RM, Pinheiro GN, Menezes ST, Arruda LA (1974). Attachment and lactation. Pediatria XIV. Vol 3. XIV Int Congr Pediat, Buenos Aires: Editorial Medica Panamericana SA, pp 136–138.

Svejda MJ, Campos JJ, Emde RN (1980). Mother-infant 'bonding': failure to generalize. Child Dev, 51: 775–779.

Taylor PM, Taylor FH, Campbell SB, Maloni JA, Cannon M (1985a). Effects of extra-early mother–infant contact. I. Extra early physical contact and aspects of the early mother-infant relationship. Acta Pediatr Scand (Suppl), 316: 3–14

Taylor PM, Maloni JA, Taylor FH, Campbell SB (1985b). Effects of extra-early mother–infant contact. II. Extra early mother–infant contact and duration of breast-feeding. Acta Pediatr Scand (Suppl), 316: 15–22.

Thomson ME, Kramer MS (1984). Methodologic standards for controlled clinical trials of early contact and maternal-infant behavior. Pediatrics, 73: 294–300.

Thomson ME, Hartsock TG, Larson C (1979). The importance of immediate postnatal contact: its effect on breast-feeding. Can Family Physician, 25: 1374–1378.

World Health Organization (1985). Having a Baby in Europe. Public Health in Europe 26. Copenhagen: WHO Regional Office for Europe. pp 26–27.

Part IX

Care of the mother and newborn infant

78 Care of the new mother and baby

Janet Rush, Iain Chalmers, and Murray Enkin

1 Introduction

In almost all societies, women rely on other people for some sort of practical and emotional support after childbirth. In some societies birth is followed by a set period of prescribed rest, during which the new mother is helped in a number of practical ways to recover physically from childbirth and to adapt to the presence of a new child (see Chapters 6 and 86). In North American and European cultures, the stress and new duties associated with becoming a mother are officially acknowledged by the state in a variety of dispensations connected with a woman's usual responsibilities at work (see Chapter 14). These arrangements vary widely from country to country, as does the amount of practical help made available to women.

In The Netherlands, for example, whether a mother delivers in hospital or at home (as over a third of them do), care from either a midwife or a doctor is provided for another 5 days. In addition, unless mothers stay in hospital, maternity aides are available to help them in caring for older children and in coping with household duties for a week after delivery.

In the United Kingdom, mothers who have had an uncomplicated childbirth are discharged from hospital after periods ranging from 5 or 6 hours to over a week. Regardless of how long a mother spends in hospital after giving birth, however, she must be visited at least once daily by a midwife for a minimum of ten days after delivery. On the tenth day, the midwife usually hands over professional responsibility for continuing care to the health visitor (whose main responsibilities relate to care of the child). But the midwife may go on visiting the new mother for as long as four weeks after delivery if she judges this to be necessary. Although paid home help in coping with domestic tasks is available on a limited scale in Britain, it is very unusual for this kind of practical help to be made available in the way that it is for Dutch women.

In Canada and the United States the specific provisions of health insurance policies and the high direct costs associated with hospital care may often result in less flexibility than exists in the United Kingdom concerning the duration of postnatal hospital stay. Although home care programmes have been organized in some places in North America (see below), there is relatively little organized care for mothers after they have been discharged from hospital.

This variety of arrangements not only serves to emphasize the uncertainty about what is 'right', and the diversity of expectations which exists across Europe and North America; it also inevitably constrains any generalizable discussion of what constitutes effective care for mothers and their new babies in the early postpartum period. One feature of early postpartum care that is shared by most women in Europe and North America, however, is that this care is provided primarily in hospitals. Sufficient evidence exists both about women's views of this care (see Chapter 8), and about its nature and content, to allow some generalizable conclusions to be made.

2 Regulating 'lying-in'

It is really not surprising that, as an increasing proportion of women came to give birth in hospitals, and as anaesthesia and operative delivery became more common, women who had recently given birth came to be treated as sick patients. Routines of postpartum care developed that were similar to those in surgical wards. Justifiable fear of maternal and newborn infection led to a zealous approach to strict environmental control (Wertz and Wertz 1977).

This type of postpartum care was firmly in place by the 1950s. Typical practices at that time included separation of the baby and mother immediately after birth, separate wards for the mother and baby (Mac-Echern 1962), and strictly scheduled infant feedings (Davis and Shekler 1951). Nurseries were out of bounds to visitors, including the baby's own mother (Williams and Oliver 1969). For the mother, 'standing orders' were in place for a variety of medications and treatments, including analgesics, laxatives, lactation suppressants, sitz baths, heat lamps, foments, enemas, perineal irrigations and sprays—whether or not the woman had any need for them. Abdominal binders, breast binders, and T-binders were the usual undergarments (Van Blarcom 1930). Regular physical assessments of fundal height, lochia, stitches, and vital signs were a constant reminder to the new mother that she was a patient in a hospital. Contacts with the outside world were minimized and visiting hours were rigidly restricted (Davis and Shekler 1951; Eastman 1950; Myles 1958).

Needless to say, the infant also did not escape this regimentation. Breastfeeding, if it was attempted at all, was regulated by the clock rather than the baby's needs. Supplementary infant feeding with formula or glucose water was the standard practice. Routines for feeding, bathing, changing, recording vital signs, and treating eyes and umbilical cords were implemented with military precision in the nurseries.

These rigid regimens of postpartum care, inherent in the institutional approach to birth, gained further acceptance during the post-war baby boom when large numbers of births put pressure on the available facilities. Deliveries and postpartum care had to be efficiently 'processed'.

Two facts about this period are particularly worth noting. First, these practices developed and were widely implemented without any evidence that they contributed to the well-being of either mothers or babies. Second, rigorous and regimented as these practices were, there were few if any complaints voiced about them from women at the time (see Chapter 7).

A number of trends during the 1950s and 1960s contributed to a growing dissatisfaction with the rigid hospital approach to postpartum care. Society's values during the 1960s included increased self-reliance, defiance of authority, and a return to more 'natural' ways (see Chapters 7 and 9). Population growth and urbanization resulted in the dispersal of the extended family and loss of the support which the new mother might have received at home when she left hospital. The public became more skilled at asking questions. The civil rights movement served as an example to those who felt victimized, and women began to assert their rights in childbirth as well as in the wider sphere (Haire 1963; Elkins 1976; Arms 1977).

Although much of the emphasis and pressure for change was at first directed toward intrapartum procedures, the postpartum period did not escape the general demand for change in childbirth practices. The 'old' care was satisfactory to some women, but it did not meet the needs of many. Women began to complain that they felt as if they were taking a stranger home rather than their own baby. They were no longer satisfied with unclear and inconsistent answers to their questions. 'That's the way we've always done it' or 'Doctors's orders' were no longer acceptable responses to requests for something different. A number of alternatives to traditional hospital postpartum care practices were suggested (Haire and Haire 1968; Jordan 1973; Paukert 1979; Young 1982; McKay 1982).

Mainstream medical, midwifery, and nursing views (and the institutional policies which they controlled and implemented) were somewhat slower to change. Although pressure for 'humanizing' postpartum care was recognized, it was not taken too seriously. A number of studies on mother–newborn interaction, however, beginning with Bowlby's (1951) work on attachment, began to attract professional attention. The concept of 'bonding' between mother and newborn (Klaus and Kennell 1976) seemed to provide professionals with a medical reason to support change (see Chapters 9 and 77).

This combination of consumer pressure and professional acceptance stimulated a number of changes in postpartum routines aimed at facilitating the mother–baby relationship. 'Family-centred maternity care' became the watchword. Many professional groups in North America, such as the American Medical Association (1977), and a task force including representatives of the American College of Obstetricians and Gynecologists, the American Hospital Association, and the American Academy of Pediatrics (Interprofessional Task Force on the Care of Women and Children 1978), issued position statements endorsing the concept of maternity care that was more orientated to the needs of the new mother and her family. Their recommendations included rooming-in, more judicious use of drugs, support for breastfeeding, and involvement of husbands, partners and other family members. 'Family-centered' maternity care included education and responsiveness to the individual needs of families, while at the same time providing safe care.

3 Current patterns of care

The pattern of postpartum care varies widely, not only from country to country, but also within each country. A survey of Canadian hospitals conducted in 1980 (Post 1981) demonstrated wide variations in postpartum programmes. Written information about labour and delivery and postpartum practices was available and distributed to new parents in just over a third of the settings. Although rooming-in was permitted in all but 1 per cent of the hospitals, less than half of them allocated more than 50 per cent of their maternity beds for use in this way. Just under half of the hospitals stated that they had an 'open visiting policy', but many had separate rules for grandparents and other close relatives and friends. Sibling visiting was not allowed in some hospitals, and was by appointment or only on special days in others. In over half of the hospitals that did allow the mother's other children to visit her, the new baby was removed to the nursery for the duration of the visit. Length of hospital stay ranged from 3 to 7 days with an average of 4 to 5 days. Formal early discharge programmes were developed in only a fifth of the hospitals surveyed (Post 1981).

The survey was repeated 5 years later (Post and Hanvey 1986). The results showed definite, but very variable progress towards more flexible options. Written information to parents about hospital practices was now given out in more than half of the hospitals. Eighty-five per cent of the responding hospitals in the second survey reported that more than half of their beds were available for rooming-in: just over half the surveyed hospitals reported that 24 hour rooming-in was permitted. Open visiting for fathers was allowed in 58 per cent of hospitals and 27 per cent reported that siblings were welcome at any time. The average length of postnatal hospital stay remained unchanged, and formal early discharge programmes were reported in a somewhat lower proportion of hospitals (16 per cent) than 5 years previously. While these findings represented some major changes in hospital practices and regulations, the authors of the report noted that in 7 per cent of hospitals siblings were allowed to visit by appointment only, and a few hospitals never allowed siblings to visit their mothers. Many present-day postpartum settings exhibit a discordant melange of new liberal and residual old inflexible practices.

Postnatal care in Canada is not particularly inflexible when compared with many other countries. Postpartum care in many hospitals in Europe (Phaff 1986) and North America still continues to follow a pattern of care that is more suitable for sick people than for new mothers. Hospital practices appropriate for sick patients, such as regularly measuring and recording vital signs, and routinely analysing specimens of blood and urine, continue almost unabated. Non-prescription medications, which women could take as desired outside the hospital, can only be administered by professionals within the hospital walls.

If we are to have any credible basis for retaining restrictive practices in the postpartum period, the onus of proof is on us, as professionals, to show that our continuing restriction of women's autonomy, freedom of choice, and access to their babies is likely to do more good than harm.

4 Control of infection

Many of the regulations and routines in postpartum care in hospital have been instituted in attempts to prevent or contain cross-infection. Until the decline in virulence of the streptococcus, and the arrival of effective antimicrobial therapy in the late 1940s, the major risk associated with institutional delivery was maternal death from infections contracted during childbirth in hospitals (Loudon 1987; Campbell and Macfarlane 1987). As hospital nurseries began to fill up with members of the baby boom that followed World War II, staphylococcal skin disease among neonates, particularly after the emergence of penicillin-resistant organisms in the mid-1960s, became the major infectious problem. A variety of measures, including isolation, segregation, rules of dress and entry to the nursery, medicated bathing, special treatment of the umbilical cord, and even routine vaccination against staphylococcal disease (Burkinshaw 1964) were taken in attempts to deal with this problem.

4.1 Segregation and isolation

The inflexible use of central nurseries, with little or no provision for babies to 'room-in' with their mothers, has jeopardized breastfeeding (see Chapters 80 and 81), eroded maternal self-confidence and happiness, and compromised the development of an attachment between mothers and their newborn babies (see Chapters 77 and 81). It has also had a significant effect on the spread of infection. Indeed, the extent of the problem presented by infection among babies who were apparently healthy at the time of birth has almost certainly been greater than it should have been, precisely because of the measures taken to avoid it.

Housing babies in central nurseries, in which a number of babies are kept in close proximity, may have actually increased the very risk which its adoption as a policy was intended to decrease. In a comparison of babies who spent between 8 and 12 hours a day with their mothers (on a public ward) with babies who were kept in the nursery and were rarely in contact with their mothers (who were in a private ward), Montgomery *et al.* (1959) found lower rates of colonization and infection in the rooming-in group.

It is sad that the results of this controlled study conducted in the late 1950s appeared to have had so little impact on the almost universal policy of routinely separating mothers and babies in this way.

Probably because the results of the controlled comparison conducted by Montgomery and colleagues posed such a fundamental challenge to the way in which postnatal care was organized, it provoked neither change in practice nor any attempts to replicate the study using randomization, either of mother–infant pairs, or wards. Instead, the problem of cross-infection and nursery epidemics of staphylococcal infection was addressed using a variety of more technological approaches. The use of gowns, hats, and masks in normal newborn and intensive care nurseries became routine in spite of the lack of any evidence from controlled trials, conducted either at that time (Forfar and MacCabe 1958) or subsequently (Silverman and Sinclair 1967; Renaud 1983; Rush *et al.*, unpublished data), that these practices had any beneficial effect on infant colonization and infection rates. Routine medication (Harris 1960) and isolation of babies (Kozinn *et al.* 1959) were used in (unsuccessful) attempts to control the spread of candidiasis, another infectious problem in the newborn. The mainstay of infection prophylaxis, however, involved the use of medicated bathing and treatment of the umbilical cord.

4.2 Bathing and cord care

In the first controlled trial mounted to assess any of these new regimens, Jellard (1957), in Cardiff, Wales, showed that staphylococcal colonization of the skin could be reduced by daily applications of triple dye (brilliant green, proflavine hemisulphate, and crystal violet in aqueous solution) to the umbilical cord stump, and this effect was confirmed in a number of studies conducted over the subsequent two decades (Table 78.1).

On the other side of the Atlantic a rather more radical and complex approach to the problem was being recommended (Simon *et al.* 1961): full strength, 3 per cent hexachlorophene in detergent was used to wash babies immediately after birth, and then daily until (and sometimes after) discharge from hospital. Bathing carried a risk of inducing hypothermia (Henningson *et al.* 1981) (this may have been the explanation for the exclusion of 20 per cent of the bathed group in the first published report of a controlled trial of this regimen (Gluck and Wood 1963)). Compared with dry care or care with medicated soap, 3 per cent hexachlorophene bathing was subsequently shown to reduce staphylococcal skin colonization (Table 78.2) and, more importantly, pyoderma (Table 78.3).

Again, however, an opportunity was missed to evaluate these emerging policies more thoroughly. No direct comparisons were made at that time between the simpler (and probably less expensive) regimen of painting the umbilical cord with triple dye, and the more elaborate policy of daily bathing with hexachlorophene (with its known attendant risk of hypothermia) for controlling staphylococcal disease in neonates. Evidence derived more than a decade later (Table 78.4) suggests that the two regimens have similar effects on staphylococcal skin colonization rates, but this was not until after 1971, when the Food and Drug Administration issued a warning that hexachlorophene could be neurotoxic in the newborn, and advised that it should no longer be used for routine bathing in hospital nurseries (Food and Drug Administration 1971).

Table 78.1 Effect of prophylactic triple dye on the umbilical cord on staphylococcal skin colonization

Study	EXPT		CTRL		Odds ratio	Graph of odds ratios and confidence intervals						
	n	(%)	*n*	(%)	(95% CI)	0.01	0.1	0.5	1	2	10	100
Barrett *et al.* (1979)	15/100	(15.00)	72/100	(72.00)	0.10 (0.06–0.17)							
Jellard (1957)	10/50	(20.00)	26/49	(53.06)	0.24 (0.11–0.55)							
Pildes *et al.* (1973)	56/531	(10.55)	148/207	(71.50)	0.05 (0.03–0.07)							
Speck *et al.* (1977)	17/62	(27.42)	25/63	(39.68)	0.58 (0.28–1.21)							
Coyer (1975)	110/270	(40.74)	36/52	(69.23)	0.32 (0.18–0.58)							
Typical odds ratio (95% confidence interval)					0.11 (0.09–0.14)							

Table 78.2 Effect of prophylactic neonatal bathing with 3% hexachlorophene on staphylococcal skin colonization

Study	EXPT n	(%)	CTRL n	(%)	Odds ratio (95% CI)	Graph of odds ratios and confidence intervals
						0.01 0.1 0.5 1 2 10 100
Gezon *et al.* (1964)	108/450	(24.00)	241/463	(52.05)	0.31 (0.23–0.40)	
Hnatko (1977)	1/25	(4.00)	6/50	(12.00)	0.39 (0.08–2.03)	
Kwong *et al.* (1973)	9/166	(5.42)	21/166	(12.65)	0.42 (0.20–0.88)	
Gluck and Wood (1963)	9/114	(7.89)	97/284	(34.15)	0.26 (0.16–0.43)	
Pildes *et al.* (1973)	156/379	(41.16)	148/207	(71.50)	0.30 (0.21–0.42)	
Coyer (1975)	114/283	(40.28)	36/49	(73.47)	0.26 (0.14–0.48)	
Typical odds ratio (95% confidence interval)					0.30 (0.25–0.36)	

Table 78.3 Effect of prophylactic neonatal bathing with 3% hexachlorophene on pyoderma

Study	EXPT n	(%)	CTRL n	(%)	Odds ratio (95% CI)	Graph of odds ratios and confidence intervals
						0.01 0.1 0.5 1 2 10 100
Gezon *et al.* (1964)	26/363	(7.16)	51/363	(14.05)	0.48 (0.30–0.78)	
Kwong *et al.* (1973)	2/166	(1.20)	9/166	(5.42)	0.27 (0.08–0.89)	
Typical odds ratio (95% confidence interval)					0.45 (0.29–0.69)	

Table 78.4 Effect of triple dye on umbilical cord vs. 3% hexachlorophene bathing on staphylococcal skin colonization

Study	EXPT n	(%)	CTRL n	(%)	Odds ratio (95% CI)	Graph of odds ratios and confidence intervals
						0.01 0.1 0.5 1 2 10 100
Pildes *et al.* (1973)	56/531	(10.55)	156/379	(41.16)	0.18 (0.13–0.25)	
Coyer (1975)	110/270	(40.74)	114/283	(40.28)	1.02 (0.73–1.43)	
Typical odds ratio (95% confidence interval)					0.40 (0.32–0.50)	

In spite of evidence that staphylococcal colonization of the newborn skin is controlled equally effectively using a lactoserum-lactic acid compound to change the pH of the skin surface (McHattie *et al.* 1974), hexachlorophene remains in use in some neonatal nurseries. This is because of a view that its advantages in controlling staphylococcal colonization outweigh its likely disadvantages in the concentrations at which it is currently in contact with neonatal skin (Alder *et al.* 1980). However, as Hnatko has observed (1977), neither current concentrations of hexachlorophene, nor the various bath additives which were introduced after hexachlorophene came under suspicion, are known to be free of unwanted effects. As with the assumptions underlying the separation of babies from their mothers and families in an attempt to prevent infection, however, a more fundamental question is raised by these observations: is routine medicated bathing of neonates justified at all in the light of the available evidence? A controlled trial (Bhakoo *et al.* 1969) showed that infants bathed routincly in a bath with 'Savlon' (which contains cetrimide and chlorhexidine) were statistically significantly more likely than controls to develop an infection subsequently, an effect of 'Savlon' which is consistent with observations made in other studies (Hnatko 1977).

Taking into account the evidence derived from the controlled trials cited above and others (Henningson *et al.* 1981; Cowan and Frost 1986; Rush 1986), and the fact that triple dye applied to the umbilical cord appears to be more effective than medicated bathing in reducing staphyloccal skin colonization (Table 78.4), our conclusion is that routine medicated bathing of newborn infants is not justified.

The controlled trials which have assessed routine treatment of the umbilical cord with triple dye do not provide adequate information on which to assess the effect of this policy on the frequency of frank infection, but they do demonstrate a significant reduction in staphylococcal skin colonization associated with this policy (Table 78.1). This effect was first demonstrated more than thirty years ago (Jellard 1957) and has been confirmed in 4 subsequent controlled trials, the most recent of which was reported in 1978.

Of the variety of methods used to treat the umbilical cord, only neomycin has been shown to reduced colonization rates more effectively than triple dye (Table 78.5). Convincing evidence exists that silver sulphadiazine offers no advantage over triple dye with respect to colonization rates (Table 78.6); the available evidence on their relative effects on infection rates is consistent with the conclusion that there is little if any difference between them (Table 78.7). Other preparations currently in use for treating the umbilical cord have simply not been adequately compared with the triple dye 'standard' and their introduction into clinical practice probably reflects commercial interests rather than scientific evidence.

The irrationality of current practice can be illustrated by the results of a survey of policies for umbilical cord care in English Health Districts (Table 78.8). A variety

Table 78.5 Effect of prophylactic neomycin vs. triple dye on the umbilical cord on staphylococcal skin colonization

Study	EXPT		CTRL		Odds ratio	Graph of odds ratios and confidence intervals						
	n	(%)	*n*	(%)	(95% CI)	0.01	0.1	0.5	1	2	10	100
Coyer (1975)	74/271	(27.31)	110/270	(40.74)	0.55 (0.39–0.79)			⊢—⊣				
Typical odds ratio (95% confidence interval)					0.55 (0.39–0.79)			⊢—⊣				

Table 78.6 Effect of prophylactic silver sulphadiazine vs. triple dye on the umbilical cord on umbilical colonization at 48 hours

Study	EXPT		CTRL		Odds ratio	Graph of odds ratios and confidence intervals						
	n	(%)	*n*	(%)	(95% CI)	0.01	0.1	0.5	1	2	10	100
Barrett *et al.* (1979)	81/100	(81.00)	55/100	(55.00)	3.28 (1.82–5.94)					⊢—⊣		
Speck *et al.* (1980)	38/82	(46.34)	12/80	(15.00)	4.30 (2.21–8.37)					⊢—⊣		
Speck *et al.* (1977)	31/89	(34.83)	25/89	(28.09)	1.36 (0.73–2.56)				⊢—⊣			
Typical odds ratio (95% confidence interval)					2.66 (1.85–3.83)					⊢—⊣		

Table 78.7 Effect of prophylactic silver sulphadiazine vs. triple dye on the umbilical cord on bacterial infections

Study	EXPT		CTRL		Odds ratio	Graph of odds ratios and confidence intervals						
	n	(%)	*n*	(%)	(95% CI)	0.01	0.1	0.5	1	2	10	100
Speck *et al.* (1977)	4/89	(4.49)	3/89	(3.37)	1.34 (0.30–6.07)							
Typical odds ratio (95% confidence interval)					1.34 (0.30–6.07)							

Table 78.8 Policies for umbilical care in English Health Districts (Mugford *et al.* 1986)

	Number (%)
Powder (*N* = 104)	
Routine 'Sterzac'*	76 (73.0)
Routine chlorhexidine	4 (3.8)
Routine other powder	6 (5.7)
Only if necessary	14 (13.5)
Other treatment	4 (3.8)
Cleansing method (*N* = 103)	
Spirit	79 (76.7)
Water	11 (10.7)
Nothing	6 (5.8)
Other	7 (6.8)
Frequency (*N* = 100)	
Every napkin change	14 (14.0)
Daily or more often	58 (58.0)
As necessary	24 (24.0)
Once only	3 (3.0)
Not at all	1 (1.0)

*hexachlorophene 0.0033, zinc oxide 0.03, starch 0.08, talc 0.8867.

of practices was reported, but in three out of four health districts a powder containing hexachlorophene ('Sterzac') was used to dust the cord after spirit (usually isopropyl alcohol) had been used as a cleansing agent (Mugford *et al.* 1986). Neither the adoption of this new formulation of hexachlorophene, nor the use of alcohol in this way is based on good evidence that these policies are likely to do more good than harm. In fact, the available evidence suggests that both the hexachlorophene powder and alcohol predispose to delayed healing of the umbilical cord (Mugford *et al.* 1986).

4.3 Conclusions

The various restrictive and interventionist policies that have been introduced in the care of hospitalized mothers and babies in an attempt to control nosocomial infection were conceptualized through induction based on theoretical considerations, rather than through deduction from empirical evidence derived from controlled trials—that is, they were based on what *should* work rather than what *does* work. Gradually the various elements of this wholesale and poorly controlled experiment on women and their babies have been challenged with evidence from randomized controlled trials, and studies using other designs. Williams and Oliver (1969), for example, described how in one nursery some of the long standing procedures were removed sequentially while monitoring colonization rates in newborn infants. The removal, one after the other, of rules for wearing caps, masks, and hairnets; for delivery room baby bathing; for restricting access of mothers and students to the nursery; and for initial scrub brushing of hands and gowning while doing incubator care, was not associated with any significant rise in colonization rates.

Yet, many restrictive and costly practices remain in force today. For example, recent survey data from 712 American doctors and institutions revealed that the gowning rule persists in 73 per cent of newborn nursery settings, despite the lack of evidence that this ritual has any beneficial effect (Cloney and Donowitz 1986). As mentioned earlier, many hospitals invoke concern about infection as a reason for restricting or forbidding siblings to visit, although studies using concurrent and historical control groups have been unable to detect any adverse effect of sibling visiting on infant colonization rates (Umphenour 1980; Wranesh 1982; Maloney *et al.* 1983; Kowba and Schwirian 1985). This segregation is particularly ironic in the light of the evidence already presented suggesting that earlier and longer contact between babies and their mothers after birth may well have contributed to the welcome decline in staphylococcal infection in newborn infants. Observational data continue to give support to the notion that early and increased contact between mothers and their newborn infants reduces the risk of bacterial colonization. In a recent study (Rush *et al.* 1987), colonization rates were more than twice as high among babies who had spent less than 50 per cent of their hospital stay with their mothers than among those who spent more than 50 per cent of the time rooming-in.

Because the available evidence suggests that most of the restrictive practices still perpetuated in some hospitals are ineffective if not harmful, the ball is in their court to provide good evidence to justify their continuation. Unless or until they do so, mothers should have unrestricted access to their babies; caps and masks should be abolished, and aprons and gowns used only by those who wish to protect their own clothing from the various kinds of messes which babies make. Bathing the baby should be seen, not as a measure for preventing infection, but as an opportunity for a mother to interact with and gain confidence in handling her child.

There is no solid scientific basis upon which to select from the variety of measures used to treat the umbilical cord, because the available trials have not been large enough to distinguish differences in infection rates (as opposed to colonization rates). Based on the available evidence concerning colonization rates, triple dye is an inexpensive and effective prophylactic for routine use. Neomycin powder is a somewhat more expensive and effective alternative. There is currently no evidence to justify the use of alcohol, powders containing hexachlorophene, or other medications, outside the context of randomized controlled trials to assess whether they offer any advantages over triple dye or neomycin powder.

Choice of cord treatment (Arad *et al*. 1981; Mugford *et al* 1986) affects the rate at which the cord stump heals. Because dusting powders formulated with talc, starch or alum, and zinc oxide have been shown to promote relatively rapid healing of the umbilical stump compared with powders containing hexachlorophene (Mugford *et al*. 1986), and because they are inexpensive and less messy than triple dye, there is scope for a large trial comparing the effects of these two approaches on colonization and infection rates.

We do not wish do give the impression that a cavalier attitude to the undoubted reality of nosocomial infections among normal newborn infants is justified, but we do wish to emphasize that the introduction of inadequately validated policies in this area of practice in the past has sometimes had effects which were quite the opposite of those intended. The emergence of threats posed by organisms other than the staphylococcus, including the streptococcus and upper respiratory tract viruses and enteroviruses, implies that the means for preventing or containing nosocomial infection must be kept under constant review.

The policy variations in this field may reflect, in part, variations in bacteriological and other circumstances, but these policy differences certainly also reflect differences in unsubstantiated opinions (Gillam 1978; Wang *et al*. 1987). Until those who wish to translate their opinions into clinical routines can show that their introduction is likely to reduce the incidence of important infections, policy should be guided by simplicity. This approach, in addition to being less likely to do more harm than good, is likely to conserve valuable resources. Mugford and her colleagues (1986), for example, have estimated that, because the effect of current cord treatment policies is to delay the healing of the umbilical stump, the annual extra cost to the British National Health Service is at least 45,000 midwife hours.

5 Routine observations

Making and recording regular measurements of temperature, pulse, blood pressure, fundal height, and observations of lochia and the various wounds that a woman may sustain during delivery is still common practice in the days following childbirth. The intensity of this screening activity varies arbitrarily and depends more on the hospital in which a mother happens to give birth, and on the length of time she happens to spend in it, than on her individual need. It would certainly seem prudent to screen women in this way if they are known to be at increased risk of either infection (see Chapter 73) or haemorrhage (see Chapter 67). It is more difficult to see how this deployment of resources could be justified as a routine for all women.

In addition to the variation from hospital to hospital in the extent to which mothers are examined routinely following childbirth, there is a marked variation in the extent to which doctors, rather than midwives or nurses, are involved. A survey of English obstetric specialist units conducted in 1984 (Garcia *et al*. 1986) showed that in 17 per cent of units a doctor became involved only after referral by a midwife. In most of the remaining units, women were examined routinely by a doctor on one or two occasions. In 1 in 5 units a doctor was expected to examine every woman daily until discharge from hospital. Judged by almost any criterion, this would seem to be an inappropriate use of scarce resources for a screening process that lacks any support from good evidence.

Unfortunately, no research has been conducted to evaluate screening and diagnostic activities (see Chapter 3) during the days following childbirth. Particularly because of the differences in resource implications of different postnatal maternal screening policies, there is an urgent need for systematic evaluation of the various options currently in place.

6 Drugs for relief of symptoms

The postpartum period is often accompanied by a number of discomforts. Pain in the perineum and breasts is common and women not infrequently count these symptoms among the most unpleasant memories they have of childbirth. Other chapters in this book (Chapters 79–82) discuss in some detail the relief of perineal and breast discomfort respectively. But it is worth considering the general issue of access to drugs for relief of unpleasant symptoms.

In most hospitals medication of women after childbirth tends to be under the direct control and supervision of hospital personnel. This policy is obviously valid in the case of dangerous drugs, drugs that might interact with other medications, or those that would normally be available only on a doctor's prescription. It is hardly rational in the case of drugs which, outside hospital, are readily available to the woman without a prescription. Because these medications are usually for the relief of symptoms, it would seem more sensible for women to use them when they feel the need.

In many hospitals, however, non-prescription drugs intended for the relief of symptoms are still administered routinely and at set times. Professional belief in the value of early and regular bowel evacuation, for example, has led to some rather obsessional concerns on this matter. Laxatives, stool softeners, enemas, and anal ointments remain routine components of postpartum care in some hospitals. Controlled trials have confirmed that, in the puerperium, as at other times, routinely prescribed laxatives (Zuspan 1960; Diamond *et al.* 1968; Shelton 1979) and medicated enemas (Rosenfield *et al.* 1958) do result in earlier bowel movements, and that bulk-forming laxatives are less likely to cause unpleasant cramps and diarrhoea than are irritant laxatives (Greenhalf and Leonard 1973; Raatikainen and Silvennoinen 1974). None of the reported results in this small body of research, however, could be regarded as justification for administering any of these preparations routinely.

In an attempt to provide a more rational basis for care (including self-care), a number of hospitals have developed programmes to provide mothers with information about the drugs they may use, and have given them access to their own supply of medications (Herman 1974; Taylor 1976; Mynick 1981). These descriptive studies all suggest that women are usually pleased with these arrangements, and that staff time was used more efficiently after their introduction.

7 General support and education

Fragmentation of care is almost inevitable when the care of mothers is the responsibility of midwives or postpartum nurses and obstetricians, while that of the babies is the responsibility of nursery nurses and paediatricians. Consistent advice and as much continuity of care as possible are prerequisites for giving effective support to mothers and their newborn babies. Common sense would suggest that the desired consistency of care would be easier to achieve if mother and baby were accommodated together (Vestal 1982; Fraleigh 1984; Watters 1985), or if at the least, mother and baby were looked after by the same personnel. The implementation of such programmes at the present time, however, is far from easy.

A number of observational studies have described attempts to implement changes in the direction of greater coherence and continuity of care, as well as pointing out some of the difficulties and pitfalls encountered (Vestal 1982; Barickman and Kraning 1983; Man-

sell 1984; Watters 1986). The only controlled study (Fraleigh 1984) described the difficulties involved in instituting a major change in nursing assignment. Nursing staff had concerns about their workload, their knowledge, and their competence to carry out the procedures that would be necessary to provide more comprehensive care to both mothers and babies postpartum. The enthusiasm for change in this direction among the head nurses and consultant was not shared by the core nursing staff. After implementation of the programme, women in the experimental ward required less formal instruction in feeding and cleansing their babies than women in a control ward, but no differences were detected between the two groups of women in terms of enjoying their time with their babies, obtaining rest, or their feelings of readiness for discharge home.

The postpartum stay in hospital presents obvious opportunities for imparting information that may be of help to the new mother. Although there is little agreement on what should be the content of formal postpartum educational programmes, a number of studies, several of them controlled trials, have addressed methods of postpartum education (Sayegh and Mosley 1976; Hall 1980; Adam *et al.* 1985; Petrowski 1981; Riesch and Munns 1984; Field *et al.* 1980; Holtzman *et al.* 1983; Lakhani *et al.* 1984; Christophersen and Sullivan 1982; Herrera *et al.* 1983; Maisels *et al.* 1983; Krozy and McColgan 1985; Buffett 1986; Shapiro and Katcher 1987). These studies concern educational programmes relating to subjects ranging from contraception, through feeding and immunization advice, to information about child safety. Although the demonstrable effects of teaching were rarely as dramatic as the investigators had hoped, this body of research shows that postpartum educational programmes can and do affect parental behaviour and health outcomes.

8 Length of hospital stay

How long should a healthy woman and baby remain in hospital after childbirth? The generally accepted 'correct' length of postnatal stay has varied greatly from time to time, and at present it varies equally widely from place to place: it appears to be determined more by fashion and the availability of beds than by any systematic assessment of the needs of recently delivered women and their new babies.

As noted at the beginning of this chapter, most societies have quite precise prescriptions and proscriptions for women following childbirth. The period of 'lying in' in Western societies had its institutional foundations with the establishment of charitable lying-in hospitals in the mid-eighteenth century. In these first maternity hospitals, women were, quite literally, confined to bed for a period of 28 days following delivery (Versluysen 1981). By the 1950s the usual hospital lying-in period was 12–14 days, but since then it appears to have been falling in a number of countries. The average length of postnatal stay in Canada fell from 10 days in the 1940s to the present 4–5 days in the 1980s (McIntosh 1984). Swedish statistics show a similar trend, from an average of 8.4 days in 1950 to 6.5 days in 1975 (Jonsson and Lindgren 1980). In the United States there was a fall from an average stay of 4.1 days in 1968 to 3.3 days in 1978 (Office of Technology Assessment 1983). The average length of postnatal stay in the United Kingdom dropped slightly from 6.3 days in 1970 to 5.5 days in 1978 (Macfarlane and Mugford 1984). These widely reported trends in the average length of postnatal hospital stay have occurred in spite of the fact that women having their first babies (who tend to stay in hospital rather longer than multiparae) have come to constitute an increasing proportion of all women giving birth.

The recent fall in the average time that a woman stays in hospital after giving birth may reflect a decrease in the proportion of women who spend a relatively long time in hospital, rather than an increase in the proportion discharged very soon after childbirth. In England, for example, the decline in the average length of stay was largely attributable to a decrease in the proportion of women staying for nine days or more, from over 25 per cent to less than 15 per cent (Macfarlane and Mugford 1984). Nevertheless, several formal early discharge programmes, often with strict inclusion criteria, have been instituted as a deliberate change from standard hospital policies. The most common impetus for initiating such programmes seems to have been the needs of the institution, either because of a shortage of beds (Theobald 1959; Hellman *et al.* 1962; Power *et al.* 1980; McIntosh and Ure 1984) or because of a shortage of personnel (Thurston and Dundas 1985). Other programmes appear to have been inspired by the preferences of women using the maternity services (Yanover *et al.* 1976; Scupholme 1981; Avery *et al.* 1982; Burnell *et al.* 1982).

A number of observational studies (Theobald 1959; Power *et al.* 1980; Scupholme 1981; Avery *et al.* 1982; Regan 1984; McIntosh 1984; Jansson 1985; Thurston and Dundas 1985; James *et al.* 1987) have shown that few women or babies are readmitted to hospital after early discharge (Table 78.9). These low readmission rates demonstrate that early discharge from hospital is feasible, and that healthy mothers and babies who have help at home, and follow-up care and guidance available may safely go home within 6 to 48 hours of birth.

These findings are supported by the results of two randomized controlled trials of early discharge programmes. In the first of these, following an administrative mandate to decrease length of stay, Hellman *et al.* (1962) randomly allocated one in ten newly delivered

Table 78.9 Hospital readmission rates associated with early postpartum discharge programmes

Study	Mother n/N (%)	Baby n/N (%)
Theobald *et al.* (1959)	2/741(0.3)	4/741(0.6)
Power *et al.* (1980)	2/323(0.6)	
Scupholme *et al.* (1981)		1/35(2.9)
Avery *et al.* (1982)	3/154(1.9)	8/154(5.2)
McIntosh and Ure (1984)		1/109(0.9)
Thurston and Dundas (1985)	2/267(0.7)	2/267(0.7)

women to remain in hospital for the previously standard period of five days, discharging the remainder within 48 hours as required by the hospital administration. A nurse visited the parents in the early discharge group once while they were still in hospital, twice during the first week at home, and again 3 weeks postpartum. Mothers in the delayed discharge group had the same number of nurse visits as the mothers in the early discharge group, the first two while still in the hospital. Reports of complications, advice required, and readmission to hospital showed no statistically significant differences.

In another controlled trial involving women and babies selected because of their low predicted risk of problems (Yanover *et al.* 1976), the intervention involved more than just early discharge, as it included extra antenatal visits, hospital and home visits, earlier mother–baby contact and rooming-in, as well as discharge home at an average of 26 hours after delivery. The control group received 'traditional care', including central nursery care for the baby for 24 hours before rooming-in was permitted, and discharge after an average of 3 days. There were no statistically significant differences in the rates of problems experienced by either the mothers or the infants in the two groups over the subsequent six weeks, suggesting that early discharge is unlikely to predispose to harmful effects in these terms. Indeed, the results of a more recently reported randomized trial suggest that early discharge from hospital may lead to more successful breastfeeding (Waldenstrom *et al.* 1987).

Although there have been no demonstrable adverse consequences of early postnatal discharge from hospital in terms of maternal and child health, it is important to note that there is also no evidence that such programmes, on balance, save money or scarce resources if care continues in a domiciliary setting. Indeed, Yanover *et al.* (1976) estimated that the costs of the home support given to women discharged early were about the same as the savings in hospital costs that resulted from earlier discharge.

Craig and Muirhead (1967) also pointed out that when healthy women go home earlier, those remaining in hospital are, on average, more sick, require more intensive care, and involve additional work and strain for the staff. Moreover, as the greatest portion of the cost of hospitalization for childbirth occurs at the beginning of the hospital stay, over the period when decisions about early discharge are being made, the average cost per day is falling. Early hospital discharge programmes inevitably put an additional load on the primary care sector and on the family or friends of the woman (Jonsson and Lindgren 1980). The additional resources required to cope with this load must obviously be assessed in any credible attempt to assess the costs of early discharge from hospital (see Chapter 5).

Demands for increased early discharge programmes have been made by a variety of commentators who believe themselves to be speaking on behalf of child-bearing women (Regan 1984; Elkins 1985; Mehl *et al.* 1976; McCarty 1980), but when such programmes have been instituted they have not always been popular with women. In Canada, this may have been one of the reasons why the availability of early discharge pro-grammes declined somewhat between 1980 and 1985 (Post and Hanvey 1986). For example, an early dis-charge programme was instituted in the Hamilton–Wentworth region (Ontario, Canada) in 1982. A woman who meets the criteria and is registered with the programme will have two visits from a public health nurse within 24 hours of returning home with her baby, and a daily visit for four days, or for longer if necessary. If she needs extra help, a home helper can also be provided to help care for other children, make meals and do light housekeeping. There is no means test, and the cost of the programme is covered by the Ministry of Health. Despite wide and positive publicity in the media and in antenatal classes, and the apparent sup-port of local physicians, hospitals, public health and home care authorities, less than 100 women of the more than 6000 women giving birth annually in the region take advantage of the programme.

Similarly, although early discharge is a widely avail-able option for women in England, between 1975 and 1985 the proportion of women leaving hospital within two days of delivery remained low (between 11 and 17 per cent, although it has tended to be at the upper end of this range in more recent years) (Department of Health and Social Security 1986).

The apparently limited popularity of early discharge programmes may be partly a reflection of a lack of awareness among women that flexibility in the length of postnatal hospital stay is possible (Williams 1985). It may also reflect attempts to force a decision about these matters during pregnancy when it is still difficult for women (and professionals) to take all the relevant factors into account. An abortive attempt to conduct a third randomized trial to compare earlier with later

discharge emphasises this: women who, during preg-nancy, stated that they had no preferences about their length of postnatal stay were randomly assigned to a hospital stay of either 6–14 days, or to a stay of less than 5 days. So many women were unwilling or unable to abide by their allocated length of hospital stay that no analysis by randomized allocation was carried out (Bur-nell *et al.* 1982). Other studies (Williams 1985) have confirmed that a substantial minority of women may have to, or may decide to change the plans for postnatal hospital stay which they had made tentatively during pregnancy.

But even allowing for the particular difficulties of making postnatal plans antenatally, the extent to which women who have recently given birth in hospital want early discharge may have been overestimated. Women participating in the trial conducted by Hellman and his colleagues (1962), for example, were less satisfied if they had been discharged early, both with the length of their hospital stay and with their hospital care in general. In the other randomized trial (Yanover *et al.* 1976), women in the early and later discharge groups were equally likely to feel that their length of stay was appropriate, and 60 per cent of the women allocated to the longer hospital stay reported that they would not participate in an early discharge programme in a subse-quent pregnancy if given the choice.

Women's physical, social and psychological circum-stances after delivery vary greatly (see Chapter 86). It would seem sensible for professionals to be as flexible as possible in trying to respond to this variation. The exercise of choice may well be the crucial issue. The greater dissatisfaction expressed by women discharged early in the trial conducted by Hellman and his col-leagues may well have reflected the fact that they had no choice about the length of their postnatal stay. Williams (1985), in another comparative, but non-randomized study, interviewed women who had given birth in two hospitals which did and did not give women an option concerning the length of postnatal stay. She found a somewhat higher proportion of women satisfied with the length of their postnatal stay among those who had given birth at the hospital with a more liberal approach. Even so, a substantial proportion of women in both hospitals felt that the length of their hospital stay had been 'wrong', usually because it had been too long, but also because, for some women, it had been too short. Some of the latter felt that a more extended escape from duties at home would have helped them to recover from childbirth more effectively (Williams 1985).

The available evidence suggests that although early discharge from hospital is obviously feasible and appar-ently safe, it is neither clearly beneficial (in health or economic terms), nor wanted by the majority of women. Firm decisions about when a particular woman should go home after childbirth should be delayed until after she has delivered and, as far as possible, be based on her particular needs and preferences rather than by any predetermined formula. Even with such a policy, it seems likely that a not inconsiderable proportion of women will feel, in retrospect, that they should have stayed in hospital for either a longer or a shorter time.

9 Conclusions

For some women, the postpartum period in hospital can serve a valuable function. The physical, emotional, and educational needs of the new mother can be met. Incipient problems, whether physical, psychological, or social, can be recognized, identified, resolved, or referred appropriately. The role of the caregiver can change from that of performer of tasks to that of teacher

and counsellor. This can only be accomplished, however, by a flexible approach to care, recognizing the special needs of each individual woman. To accomplish this, many long-standing routines and attitudes must be challenged.

The standard hospital setting, with its orientation towards sickbed protocols and procedures, and its division of care along the lines of the separate medical disciplines of obstetrics and paediatrics, is not conducive either to helping the new mother develop the skills and self-confidence she needs to care for herself and her new baby, or to enhancing her sense of personal worth and self-esteem. It is unlikely that any single scheme of care will prove to be right for all women. Treating the new mother as a responsible adult, giving her accurate and consistent information, letting her make her own decisions and supporting her in those decisions is the essence of effective postpartum care.

References

Adam H, Stern EK, Stein REK (1985). Anticipatory guidance: a modest intervention in the nursery. Pediatrics, 76: 781–786.

Alder VG, Burman D, Simpson RA, Fysh J, Gillespie WA (1980). Comparison of hexachlorophene and chlorhoxidane powders in prevention of neonatal infection. Arch Dis Child, 55: 277–280.

American Medical Association (1977). Statement on Parent and Newborn Interaction. Chicago.

Arad I, Eyal F, Fainmeiser P (1981). Umbilical care and cord separation. Arch Dis Child, 56: 887–888.

Arms S (1977). Immaculate Deception (Bantam Edition). Boston, Massachusetts: Houghton Mifflin.

Avery MD, Fournier LC, Jones PL, Sipovic CP (1982). An early postpartum hospital discharge program. J Obstet Gynecol Neonatal Nurs, 11: 233–235.

Barickman C, Kraning MJ (1983). Combined mother-baby nursing care: Guidelines for a successful transition. Cybele Report, 4, Suppl 4: 3–6.

Barrett FF, Mason EO, Fleming D (1979). The effect of three cord care regimens on the bacterial colonization of normal newborn infants. J Pediatr, 94: 796–800.

Bhakoo ON, Lall JC, Agarwall KC (1959). Prevention of hospital infection in neonates: an evaluation of no bath regime. Indian Pediatr, 6, suppl 11: 597–700.

Bowlby J (1951). Maternal care and mental health. Geneva: World Health Organization.

Buffett C (1986). Restrain infants, secure kids: a community program to teach parents to buckle up their children. Can Family Physician 32: 379–381.

Burkinshaw J (1964). Subsequent infection of infants born in a maternity hospital. Arch Dis Child, 39, 485–491.

Burnell I, McCarthy M, Chamberlain GVP, Hawkins DF, Elbourne D (1982). Patient preference and postnatal hospital stay. J Obstet Gynaecol, 3: 43–47.

Campbell R, Macfarlane A (1987) Where to be born: the debate and the evidence. Oxford: National Perinatal Epidemiology Unit.

Christophersen ER, Sullivan MA (1982). Increasing the protection of newborn infants in cars. Pediatrics, 70 Suppl 1: 21–25.

Cloney DL, Donowitz LG (1986). Overgown use for infection control in nurseries and neonatal intensive care units. Am J Dis Child, 140: 680–683.

Cowan ME, Frost MR (1986). A comparison between a detergent baby back additive and baby soap on the skin flora of neonates. J Hosp Infect, 7: 91–95.

Coyer WF (1975). Neonatal skin care and the prevention of staphylococcus aureus colonization. Pediatr Res, 9: 339.

Craig GA, Muirhead JMB (1967). Obstetric aspects of the early discharge of maternity patients. Br Med J, 3: 520–522.

Davis ME, Shekler CE (1951). DeLee's Obstetrics (15th edn). Philadelphia: WB Saunders.

Department of Health and Social Security (1986). Nursing Services 1975–1985. Summary information from form LHS 27/3: 1985. London: DHSS.

Diamond RA, Hall SA, Spellacy WA (1968). Bisoxatin acetate as a postpartum oral laxative: a random double blind controlled experiment in 106 subjects. Lancet, 88: 16–17.

Eastman JN (1950). William's Obstetrics (10th edn). New York: Appleton-Century-Crofts.

Elkins VH (1976). The Rights of the Pregnant Parent. New York: Waxwing Productions.

Elkins VH (1985). The Rights of the Pregnant Parent. New York: Schocken Books.

Field TM, Wedmayer SM, Stringer S, Dgnatoff E (1980). Teenage, lower-class black mothers and their preterm infants: an intervention and developmental follow-up. Child Dev, 51: 426–436.

Food and Drug Administration (1971). Hexachlorophene and Newborns. Food and Drug Administration Bulletin. US Dept. of Health, Education and Welfare, Public Health Service, Rockville, Md.

Forfar JO, MacCabe, AF (1958). Masking and gowning in nurseries for the newborn infant. Br Med J, 1: 76–79.

Fraleigh D (1984). Combined mother–baby care: an experiment in patient assignment. Canadian Nurse 80: 25–28.

Garcia J, Garforth S, Ayers A (1986). Midwives confined? Labour ward policies and routines. Proceedings of the 1985

Conference on Research and the Midwife, University of Manchester, pp 2–30.

Gezon HM (1969). Should nursery environmental control measures be re-examined? Pediatrics, 44 Suppl 5: 636–638.

Gezon HM, Thompson DJ, Rogers KD, Hatch TF, Taylor PM (1964). Hexachlorophene bathing in early infancy. Effect on stapylococcal disease and infection. New Engl J Med 270: 379–386.

Gillam GL (1978). Infections and diseases of the newborn. Austral Family Physician, 7: 1363–1369.

Gluck L, Wood HF (1963). Staphyloccal colonization in newborn infants with and without antiseptic skin care. Pediatrics, 268: 1265–1268.

Greenhalf JO, Leonard HSD (1973). Laxatives in the treatment of constipation in pregnant and breast-feeding mothers. Practitioner, 210: 259–263.

Haire D (1963). The Pregnant Patient's Bill of Rights. International Childbirth Education Association, Minneapolis.

Haire D, Haire J (1968). Implementing Family-centered Maternity Care with a Central Nursery. International Childbirth Education Association, New Jersey.

Hall LA (1980). Effect of teaching on primiparas' perceptions of their newborn. Nurs Res, 29 Suppl 5: 317–321.

Harris LJ (1960). Further observations on a simple procedure to eliminate thrush from hospital nurseries. Am J Obstet Gynecol, 80 Suppl 1: 30–31.

Hellman LM, Kohl SG, Palmer J (1962). Early hospital discharge in obstetrics. 1: 223–232.

Henningson A, Nystrom B, Tunnell R (1981). Bathing or washing babies after birth? Lancet, 2: 1401–1403.

Herman K (1974). Self-administration of medication. J Obstet Gynecol Nurs, 3: 27–30.

Herrera AJ, Cochran B, Herrera A, Wallace B (1983). Parental information and circumcision in highly motivated couples with higher education. Pediatr, 71 Suppl 2: 233–234.

Hnatko SI (1977). Alternatives to hexachlorophene bathing of newborn infants. Can Med Assoc J, 117: 223–226.

Holtzman NA, Faden R, Chwalow AJ, Horn SD (1983). Effect of informed parental consent on mothers knowledge of newborn screening. Pediatr, 72 Suppl 6: 807–812.

Interprofessional Task Force on Health Care of Women and Children: Joint Position Statement on the Development of Family-Centered Maternal/Newborn Care in Hospitals. (1978). Chicago. American College of Obstetricians and Gynecologists

James ML, Hudson CN, Gebski VJ, Browne LH, Andrews GR, Crisp SE, Palmer D, Beresford JL (1987). An evaluation of planned early postnatal transfer home with nursing support. Med J Austral, 147: 434–438.

Jansson P (1985). Early postpartum discharge. Am J Nurs 85: 547–550.

Jellard J (1957). Umbilical cord as a reservoir of infection in a maternity hospital. Br Med J, 20: 925–928.

Jonsson B, Lindgren B (1980). Five common fallacies in estimating the economic gains in early discharge. Soc Sci Med, 14: 27–33.

Jordan AD (1973). Evaluation of a family-centered maternity care hospital program. J Obstet Neonatal Nurs, 2: 13–34.

Klaus MH, Kennell JH (1976). Maternal-infant bonding. St. Louis: Mosby.

Kowba MD, Schwirian PM (1985). Direct sibling contact and bacterial colonization in newborns. J Obstet Gynecol Neonatal Nurs, 14: 412–417.

Kozinn PJ, Wiener H, Taschdjian CL (1959). Isolation of infants with thrush necessary. JAMA, 170 Suppl 10: 1172–1174.

Krozy RE, McColgan JJ (1985). Auto safety. Pregnancy and the newborn. J Obstet Neonatal Nurs, 14: 11–15.

Kwong MS, Loew AD, Anthony FA, Oh W (1973). The effect of hexachlorophene on staphylococcal colonization rates in the newborn infant: a controlled study using a single bath method. J Pediatr, 82: 982–986.

Lakhani AD, Avery A, Gordon A, Tait N (1984). Evaluation of a home based health record booklet. Arch Dis Child, 59: 1076–1081.

Loudon I (1987). Puerperal fever, the streptococcus, and the sulphonamides, 1911–1945. Br Med J 295: 485–490.

MacEchern T (1962). Hospital Organization and Management (3rd edn). Berwyn, Illinois: Physician's Record Co.

Macfarlane A, Mugford M (1984). Birth Counts. Statistics of Pregnancy and Childbirth. London: Her Majesty's Stationery Office.

Maisels MJ, Hayes B, Conrad S, Chez RA (1983). Circumcision: the effect of information on parental decision making. Pediatrics, 71 Suppl 3: 453–455.

Maloney MJ, Ballard JL, Hollister L, Shank M (1983). A prospective, controlled study of scheduled sibling visits to a newborn intensive care unit. J Am Acad Child Psychiatry, 22 Suppl 6: 565–570.

Mansell KA (1984). Mother–baby units: a concept that works. Matern Child Nurs J 9: 132–133.

McCarty E (1980). Early postpartum nursing care of mother and infant in the home care setting. Nurs Clin North Am, 15 Suppl 2: 361–372.

McHattie JC, Crossan M, Talukdor C, Elder R, Murdock AI (1974). A comparison of hexachlorophene and lactacyd on growth of skin flora in healthy term newborn infants. Can Med Assoc J 110: 1248–1250.

McIntosh ID (1984). Hospital effects of maternity early discharge. Medical Care, 22: 611–619.

McIntosh ID, Ure D (1984). Maternity early discharge in a local health authority. Can J Publ Health, 75: 445–449.

McKay S (1982). Humanizing Maternity Services Through Family-centred Care. International Childbirth Education Association, Minneapolis.

Mehl LE, Peterson GH, Sokolosky W, White MC (1976). Outcomes of early discharge after normal birth. Birth, 2 Suppl 3: 101–107.

Montgomery TL, Wise RI, Lang WR, Mandle RJ, Fritz MA (1959). A study of staphylococcal colonization of postpartum mothers and newborn infants. Comparison of central care and rooming-in. Am J Obstet Gynecol, 78: 1227–1233.

Mugford M, Somchiwong M, Waterhouse IL (1986). Treatment of umbilical cords: a randomized trial to assess the effect of treatment methods on the work of midwives. Midwifery, 2: 177–186.

Myles MF (1958). A Textbook for Midwives. Edinburgh: Churchill Livingstone.

Mynick A (1981). Instituting a postpartum self-medication program. Matern Child Nurs J. 6: 422–424.

Office of Technology Assessment (1983). Variations in hospital length of stay: their relationship to health outcomes. Health Technology Case Study 24. Washington DC: US Congress, Office of Technology Assessment, OTA-HCS-23.

Paukert SE (1979). One hospital's experience with implementing family-centered maternity care. J Obstet Gynecol Neonatal Nurs, 8: 351–358.

Petrowski DD (1981). Effectiveness of prenatal and postnatal instruction in postpartum care. J Obstet Gynecol Neonatal Nurs, 10: 386–389.

Phaff JML (1986). Perinatal Health Services in Europe. London: Croom Helm.

Pildes RS, Ramamurthy RS, Vidyasagar D (1973). Effect of tripled dye on staphylococcal colonization in newborn infant. J Pediatr, 82: 987–990.

Post S (1981). Family-centred maternity care: the Canadian picture. Dimens Health Serv, June 58: 26–31.

Post SE, Hanvey L (1986). Family-centered maternity care—what has happened in five years? Dimens Health Serv, 63: 14–16.

Power DJ, Wolf E, Van Coeverden de Groot HA (1980). Early discharge from maternity units in cape town. S Afr Med J, 58: 1156–1162.

Raatikainen OR, Silvennoinen R (1974). Constipation after delivery: comparative study of two laxative preparations. Katilolenti, 79: 421–422.

Regan K (1984). Obstetrical Discharge: a program that works. Canadian Nurse, 80: 32–35.

Renaud MT (1983). Effects of discontinuing cover gowns on a postpartal ward upon cord colonization of the newborn. J Obstet Gynecol Neonatal Nurs, 12: 399–401.

Riesch SK, Munns SK (1984). Promoting awareness: the mother and her baby. Nurs Res, 33: 271–276.

Rosenfield HH, Burke L, Rubin H (1958). Disposable enema unit in obstetrics. Obstet Gynecol, 11: 222–225.

Rush J (1986). Routine newborn bathing as a means of reducing staphylococcus aureus colonization rates: a randomized trial. Birth, 13: 18–22.

Rush JP, Hempal V, Dotzert L (1987). Rooming in and visiting on the maternity ward: effects on newborn colonization rates. Infect Control, 2 Suppl 3: 10–15.

Rush JP, Fiorino-Chioviti R, Kaufman K, Mitchell A (In press). The effects of discontinuing individual cover gowns in a family centered maternity setting. Birth.

Sayegh J, Mosley WH (1976). The effectiveness of family planning education on acceptance of contraception by postpartum mothers. Johns Hopkins Med J, 139 (Suppl): 31–37.

Scupholme A (1981). Postpartum early discharge—an inner city experience. J Nurs Midwifery, 26: 19–22.

Shapiro MM, Katcher ML (1987). Injury-prevention education during postpartum hospitalization. Am J Dis Child, 141: 382.

Shelton MG (1979). Standardized senna in the management of constipation in the puerperium. A clinical trial. S Afr Med J, 57: 78–80.

Silverman WA, Sinclair JC (1967). Evaluation of precautions before entering a neonatal unit. Pediatrics, 40: 900–901.

Simon HJ, Yaffe SJ, Gluck L (1961). Effective control of staphylococci in a nursery. New Engl J Med, 265: 1171–1176.

Speck WT, Driscoll JM, Polin RA, O'Neill J, Rosenkranz HS (1977). Staphylococcal and streptococcal colonization of the newborn infant. Am J Dis Child, 131: 1005–1008.

Speck WT, Driscoll JM, O'Neill J, Rosenkranz HS (1980). Effect of antiseptic cord care on bacterial colonization in the newborn infant. Chemotherapy, 26: 372–376.

Taylor HP (1976). Conservation of postpartum nurses' time—bedside self-medication and patient control of visiting. Am J Obstet Gynecol, 76: 215–217.

Theobald G (1959). Home on the second day: The Bradford experiment. Br Med J, 2: 1364–1367.

Thurston NE, Dundas JB (1985). Evaluation of an early post partum discharge program. Can J Publ Health, 76: 384–387.

Umphenour JH (1980). Bacterial colonization in neonates with sibling visitation. J Obstet Gynecol Neonatal Nurs, 9: 73–75.

Van Blarcom CC (1930). Obstetrical Nursing (2nd edn). New York: Macmillan.

Versluysen MC (1981). Midwives, medical men and poor women labouring of child: lying in hospital in eighteenth century London. In: Women, Health and Reproduction. Roberts H (ed). London: Routledge and Kegan Paul. Cited in Williams, Lorraine, 'The Policy and Practice of Midwifery'; Parents views of maternity discharge policies, BASS (Sociology) Dissertation.

Vestal K (1982). A proposal: primary nursing for the mother–baby dyad. Nurs Clin North Am, 17: 3–9

Waldenstrom U, Sundelin C, Lindmark G (1987). Early and late discharge after hospital birth: breastfeeding. Acta Paediatr Scand, 76: 727–732.

Wang EL, Elder D, Mishkel N (1987). Staphylococcal and colonization and infection after discharge from a term newborn nursery. Infect Control, 8 Suppl 1: 30–33.

Watters NE (1985). Combined mother–infant nursing care. J Obstet Neonatal Nurs, 14: 478–483.

Watters N (1986). Combined nursing care caters to parents needs. Dimens Health Serv, 63: 17–18.

Wertz RW, Wertz DC (1977). Lying-In: A History of Childbirth in America. London: Collier Macmillan.

Williams L (1985). Parents' views of maternity discharge policies. Dissertation prepared for the Degree of Bachelor of Arts, Middlesex Polytechnic, London.

Williams CPS, Oliver KK (1969). Nursery routines and staphyloccal colonization of the newborn. Pediatrics, 44: 640–646.

Wranesh EBl (1982). The effect of sibling visitation on bacterial colonization rate in neonates. J Obstet Gynecol Neonatal Nurs, 11: 211–213.

Yanover MJ, Jones D, Miller MD (1976). Perinatal care of low risk mothers and infants—early discharge with home care. New Engl J Med, 294: 702–705.

Young D (1982). Changing Childbirth. New York: Childbirth Graphics.

Zuspan FP (1960). A double blind laxative study on postpartum patients. Am J Obstet Gynecol, 80: 548–550.

79 Relief of perineal pain and discomfort after childbirth

Adrian Grant and Jennifer Sleep

1 Introduction

Prevention and treatment of perineal pain following childbirth was the subject of what may have been the first controlled trial of British obstetric practice. In 1923 it was common practice at the Royal Maternity Hospital, Glasgow to manage perineal trauma by tying the woman's knees together. This was done in the belief that it enhanced healing and reduced pain. Because of the obvious disadvantages of the method, Dugald Baird, then a young house-officer, conducted an evaluation in which alternate mothers did not have their knees tied together following delivery. Subsequent comparison of these women with those who had had their knees tied together as usual did not suggest that the accepted practice conferred any advantage in terms of less pain or more successful perineal healing. This led to discontinuation of the practice in the hospital (Baird, personal communication).

Perineal pain remains a major problem for mothers in the early days following vaginal delivery, especially if they have sustained perineal trauma. In addition to the pain in the immediate postpartum period, as many as a quarter report discomfort 10 days postpartum, and this persists until at least 3 months later for 8 per cent of all women (Sleep *et al.* 1984). Furthermore, dyspareunia as long as 3 years after delivery may have its origin in suboptimal postpartum care (see Chapter 68).

Avoidance of trauma when possible (see Chapter 66), and proper repair when trauma occurs (see Chapter 68) are the obvious primary approaches to avoiding or reducing these problems. In addition, a wide range of postpartum measures and active treatments are advocated for secondary prevention, or relief. In this chapter we review the evidence from controlled studies of the effectiveness of these measures and assess whether current practice is consistent with this evidence.

2 Local applications

2.1 Non-pharmacological applications

Sprays, gels, creams, solutions, ice packs, baths, and douches are all commonly recommended for the relief of perineal discomfort following vaginal delivery, but they have had little, if any formal evaluation. The few studies that have been reported evaluate the use of these agents as vehicles for pharmacologically more active substances such as anaesthetics, antiseptics, and anti-inflammatory agents. In 'blinded', placebo-controlled studies it is only possible to assess the usefulness of the additional agent and this begs the question of whether the vehicle alone has any effect. In open 'unblinded' studies it is also impossible to separate the effect of either the vehicle or the 'active ingredient' from placebo effect or observer bias.

Although there has been little formal evaluation, there is anecdotal evidence to suggest that some of these inert treatments may relieve some perineal discomfort. Cooling with ice or sprays, for example, is often used in postnatal care in the belief that pain and oedema are reduced. In 1987 we conducted a telephone survey of 50 randomly selected English maternity units and enquired about the management of postpartum perineal discomfort. Icepacks were used in 42 of the units and were the most common locally applied therapy. Icepacks in the puerperium do give immediate symptomatic relief by numbing the perineum, but this is usually short-lived and there is no evidence of any longer-term benefit. Furthermore, there are worries about causing perineal 'ice-burns', particularly if solid rather than crushed ice is used in direct contact with tissues (which may be some distance from the perineal birth trauma). For these reasons crushed ice applied between the layers of a pad should be preferred. Sprays have also been reported to relieve perineal discomfort, probably by a cooling effect, although they occasionally cause a stinging discomfort (Harrison *et al.* 1982, 1987c).

Bathing in cold sitz baths has also been prescribed for this reason. There is evidence from a randomized trial that cold sitz baths are more effective than warm sitz baths in relieving perineal discomfort, but the differential effect is limited to the first half-hour after bathing (Ramler and Roberts 1986). The cold baths were not popular with women; of the 159 approached to enter the trial 119 refused to participate, and for 112 of these the reason was that they did not feel like having a cold bath!

The warmth of a hot bath may give some comfort in the immediate puerperium. In a recent survey (Sleep and Grant 1988), 93 per cent of women when questioned on the tenth day following vaginal delivery reported that bathing had relieved perineal discomfort; but this observation was uncontrolled and there is no knowing whether a similar proportion of women would have gained relief if they had not bathed at all or had used showers rather than baths. With the current trend towards showers and bidets rather than baths in modern maternity hospitals the question of the difference in comfort resulting from these different approaches is important.

Our survey revealed that 12 per cent of English maternity units used local heat therapy. We know of no controlled evaluation of this therapy other than as a component of therapeutic ultrasound (see below).

After the puerperium, simple gel is commonly prescribed for symptomatic relief of persistent dyspareunia. Twenty-three per cent of women report pain during intercourse 3 months after delivery (Sleep *et al.* 1984). We have attempted to assess the value of simple gel for this problem in a randomized controlled trial, but its very small size (13 allocated to gel and 16 allocated to no gel), together with the fact that a number of women allocated 'no gel' actually used it, severely limit the trial's usefulness. The severity of dyspareunia was very similar in the two groups one week after recruitment. A month after recruitment, 4 women in each group reported that they no longer had dyspareunia.

The growing popularity of herbal substances for relief of perineal pain (Bunce 1987; Ehudin-Pagano *et al.* 1987) probably reflects both a belief that 'time honoured natural medicines must be safe', and their easy availability from many retail outlets (Drugs and Therapeutics Bulletin 1986). Solutions and creams have been used as vehicles for herbal substances for both prevention and treatment of perineal symptoms.

Witch hazel soaked into gauze swabs or other pads and applied directly to the perineal tissues is commonly recommended for the relief of pain. Two randomized trials have assessed this practice. Spellacy (1965) conducted a randomized comparison of pads soaked in a witch hazel and glycerin solution with pads soaked in tap water. The majority of women in both groups reported some relief of their symptoms (the author wondered whether this was a cooling effect) but there was no evidence that witch hazel and glycerin was any more effective in this respect than tap water. The second trial was conducted in Bristol during 1986 and has yet to be fully reported. 300 women who had been delivered with forceps were randomly allocated to one of three treatment groups: witch hazel, icepacks, and pramoxine and hydrocortisone spray ('Epifoam') (see below). There was some evidence that the most satisfactory analgesic on the first day was witch hazel and on the third day was icepacks; there were no clear differences thereafter up to the final assessments, 6 weeks postpartum (W Moore, personal communication).

Swabbing of the perineum with tincture of calendula (Marigold) has also been recommended because it is thought to have antiseptic properties, hence its advocated use also on the cord stump of the neonate. Rare cases of hypersensitivity have been reported (Drugs and Therapeutics Bulletin 1986). Bruising may be treated by the local application of a poultice steeped in comfrey. However, to the best of our knowledge, there has been no formal evaluation of these practices.

Another suggestion is that the addition of a herbal infusions of Shepherd's Purse, garlic, comfrey, and sea salt to bath water may help to soothe pain, promote healing, and reduce the risk of infection (Bunce 1987; Ehudin-Pagano *et al.* 1987). Again, these claims have not been formally assessed.

Salt on its own added to bath water is, in fact, one of the oldest claimed 'remedies' for perineal and other trauma. It is still very popular: in a recent survey (Sleep *et al.* 1984) as many as 33 per cent of women were adding salt to their bath water 10 days after normal vaginal delivery. The salt is believed to soothe discomfort and to promote healing, although a precise mode of action is unclear. Claims that it has antiseptic or antibacterial properties have not been confirmed (Ayliffe *et al.* 1975). There is no consensus as to the type of salt preparation or quantity which should be used, recommendations about the quantity ranging from a heaped tablespoon in a small bath (Marks and Ribeiro 1983) to 3 lb in 30 gallons of water (Houghton 1940). In a randomized controlled trial (Sleep and Grant 1988), 600 women were asked to add a standard measure of salt equivalent to 42 g to their bathwater for 10 days (89 per cent actually complied) and 600 women were asked not to add anything to their baths (only 7 per cent actually added salt). As mentioned earlier, the majority of women felt that bathing had given them some relief of discomfort (Table 79.1), but there was no detectable difference between the two groups in terms of perineal pain or symptomatic relief afforded at either 10 days or 3 months postpartum (Table 79.1). The patterns of wound healing were also similar when assessed on the 10th day after delivery. This trial therefore provided no support for this common practice.

2.2 Local antiseptics

The addition of antiseptic solution, particularly 'Savlon' concentrate (chlorhexidine gluconate 1.5 per cent w/v and cetrimide 15 per cent w/v in aqueous solution) to the bath water is also a common practice during the postnatal period. 'Savlon' has now become available on the retail market and so is more accessible to women at home. The value of 'Savlon' bath concentrate in the 10 days following delivery was also evaluated in the study

mentioned above in which salt was evaluated (Sleep and Grant 1988). In addition to the groups of women asked to add salt or asked not to add anything, a further 600 women were given ten 25 ml sachets of 'Savlon' concentrate and asked to add the contents of one sachet to a daily bath for the first 10 days after delivery. There was no evidence that the addition of 'Savlon' improved symptomatic relief from bathing or reduced perineal discomfort at either 10 days or 3 months postpartum (Table 79.2). On the debit side, 4 per cent of women complained that the 'Savlon' made the bath slippery; furthermore, a 10 day course of 'Savlon' has a cost (£3.20, 1986 prices). A study comparing local swabbing using antiseptic solution for the women in one-half of a ward with 'jug douching' using tap water for those in the other half of the ward reached similar conclusions in respect of symptoms and signs (Martin *et al.* 1957). The rates of bacterial colonization of perineal skin, genital

Table 79.1 Effect of adding salt to bath water for perineal trauma on perineal pain on 10th day

Study	EXPT		CTRL		Odds ratio	Graph of odds ratios and confidence intervals
	n	(%)	*n*	(%)	(95% CI)	
Sleep and Grant (1988)	238/565	(42.12)	256/565	(45.31)	0.88 (0.69–1.11)	
Typical odds ratio (95% confidence interval)					0.88 (0.69–1.11)	

Effect of adding salt to bath water for perineal trauma on oral analgesia use on 10th day

Study	EXPT		CTRL		Odds ratio	
Sleep and Grant (1988)	44/558	(7.89)	32/561	(5.70)	1.41 (0.89–2.25)	
Typical odds ratio (95% confidence interval)					1.41 (0.89–2.25)	

Effect of adding salt to bath water for perineal trauma on 'bathing did not help'

Study	EXPT		CTRL		Odds ratio	
Sleep and Grant (1988)	24/391	(6.14)	26/376	(6.91)	0.88 (0.50–1.56)	
Typical odds ratio (95% confidence interval)					0.88 (0.50–1.56)	

Effect of adding salt to bath water for perineal trauma on perineal pain at 3 months

Study	EXPT		CTRL		Odds ratio	
Sleep and Grant (1988)	61/531	(11.49)	65/536	(12.13)	0.94 (0.65–1.36)	
Typical odds ratio (95% confidence interval)					0.94 (0.65–1.36)	

Effect of adding salt to bath water for perineal trauma on not resumed pain-free intercourse at 3 months

Study	EXPT		CTRL		Odds ratio	
Sleep and Grant (1988)	379/518	(73.17)	386/527	(73.24)	1.00 (0.76–1.31)	
Typical odds ratio (95% confidence interval)					1.00 (0.76–1.31)	

Table 79.2 Effect of adding 'Savlon' concentrate to bath water for perineal trauma on perineal pain on 10th day

Study	EXPT		CTRL		Odds ratio	Graph of odds ratios and confidence intervals						
	n	(%)	n	(%)	(95% CI)	0.01	0.1	0.5	1	2	10	100
Sleep and Grant (1988)	264/563	(46.89)	256/565	(45.31)	1.07 (0.84–1.35)							
Typical odds ratio (95% confidence interval)					1.07 (0.84–1.35)							

Effect of adding 'Savlon' concentrate to bath water for perineal trauma on oral analgesia use on 10th day

Sleep and Grant (1988)	44/558	(7.89)	32/561	(5.70)	1.41 (0.89–2.25)							
Typical odds ratio (95% confidence interval)					1.41 (0.89–2.25)							

Effect of adding 'Savlon' concentrate to bath water for perineal trauma on 'bathing did not help'

Sleep and Grant (1988)	26/425	(6.12)	26/376	(6.91)	0.88 (0.50–1.54)							
Typical odds ratio (95% confidence interval)					0.88 (0.50–1.54)							

Effect of adding 'Savlon' concentrate to bath water for perineal trauma on perineal pain at 3 months

Sleep and Grant (1988)	51/528	(9.66)	65/536	(12.13)	0.78 (0.53–1.14)							
Typical odds ratio (95% confidence interval)					0.78 (0.53–1.14)							

Effect of adding 'Savlon' concentrate to bath water for perineal trauma on not resumed pain-free intercourse at 3 months

Sleep and Grant (1988)	370/519	(71.29)	386/527	(73.24)	0.91 (0.69–1.19)							
Typical odds ratio (95% confidence interval)					0.91 (0.69–1.19)							

tract infection, puerperal pyrexia, delayed healing, and the need for resuturing were almost identical for the two policies.

In the early 1950s vaginal creams containing sulphonamides were recommended for routine use in the postpartum period (Palm 1951). Two controlled studies have assessed claims that this practice reduced puerperal morbidity and wound breakdown, as well as the claim that it 'almost eliminates endocervicitis' (Palm 1951). In the first study, Bischoff and colleagues (1956) studied 300 multigravid women whose deliveries had been managed with episiotomies. By alternate allocation, these women either were given sulphisoxazole cream or acted as controls. In the intervention group cream was applied with a vaginal applicator each night from the 7th day postpartum for two to three weeks. Outcome was assessed 6 weeks after delivery. Equal proportions of women in each group (25 per cent) had resumed sexual intercourse, but twice as many of the controls had used douches. It is not clear whether the assessment of outcome was made without knowledge of the group to which the women had been allocated. Although abnormalities were reported for 39 per cent in the control group compared with 20 per cent of the group managed with sulphisoxazole cream, most of the difference was in asymptomatic abnormalities of the cervix such as erosion, ectropion, and cervicitis, which are of uncertain clinical significance.

In the second trial, Rubin (1961) prescribed triple sulphonamide cream to women who delivered on certain days of the week; women delivering on alternate days acting as controls and were prescribed no vaginal cream. Rates of cervical erosion, vaginal discharge and vaginal discomfort were similar in the two groups. There was a suggestion of less puerperal pyrexia in the sulphonamide group but the differences were not statistically significant.

2.3 Local anaesthetics

Local anaesthetics are commonly applied as sprays, gels, creams, or foams. In 1982, Harrison and his colleagues reported an evaluation of the anaesthetic fomocaine applied as an aerosol spray. Following delivery, 70 women were randomly allocated ('double-blind') either canisters of active spray or canisters of inactive spray; that is, propellant and perfume only. Nine women in the active group and 13 in the control group did not complete the pre-specified 4-day course and were subsequently removed from the analysis; it is not stated why they failed to comply, or what their outcome was. Although women allocated to use the 'active' spray seemed to be somewhat less likely to use it than those allocated to the placebo spray, the actively treated women used consistently less oral analgesia in the first 4 days postpartum. More recently, Harrison and Brennan have reported a series of three randomized trials assessing which is the best vehicle for lignocaine when this local anaesthetic is used in a spray. In the first of these studies (Harrison and Brennan 1987a), 5 per cent lignocaine was compared with 2 per cent cinchocaine (both as alcoholic preparations) and with a spray of distilled water, all as single administrations. Both local anaesthetics were clearly better than the water spray. Of the two anaesthetics, lignocaine performed marginally better. In the second trial (Harrison and Brennan 1987b), an aqueous formulation of 5 per cent lignocaine appeared to have some advantage over the alcoholic preparations of lignocaine and cinchocaine. The results of the third study, an apparently well-conducted double-blind trial (Harrison and Brennan 1987c), are consistent with this. Again, the aqueous preparations appeared to be the best of these three spray formulations. Aqueous 5 per cent lignocaine had an analgesic effect which was comparable to a single oral administration of 500 mg of mefenamic acid; although the effect was seen somewhat more quickly it was however, less well sustained. Both were clearly better than placebo. The only side-effect reported was transitory stinging after spraying. This was more commonly associated with the alcoholic formulations and the rate for the aqueous spray was only slightly higher than that for the placebo spray. These trials were, however, single application studies and stinging from sprays may deter women from repeated applications. Serum concentrations of all the local anaesthetics were negligible.

Hutchins and his colleagues (1985) compared lignocaine in a gel with aqueous cream (BNF). Women in the lignocaine group had less pain and better pain relief on the first two days after delivery. There was a suggestion that this difference persisted and was reflected in less use of oral analgesia but these differences were not statistically significant.

Although we have heard claims that repeated application of local anaesthetics in close proximity to mucous membranes can produce local sensitization and irritation, which in turn may increase local discomfort, we can find no evidence to substantiate these suggestions. On the evidence of the studies discussed above there is reason to believe that local anaesthetics alone are useful for relief of perineal pain in the immediate postpartum period. Aqueous 5 per cent lignocaine spray or lignocaine gel would appear to be the most rational first choice of agent and formulation.

2.4 Combinations of local anaesthetics and topical steroids

Based on the assumption that much of the pain from perineal trauma arises from local oedema and inflammation, a local anaesthetic has recently been combined with a steroid as a single topical agent. Pramoxine hydrochloride 1 per cent and hydrocortisone acetate 1 per cent in a water miscible muco-adhesive foambase has been used for the local treatment of proctitis for a number of years (marketed in Britain as 'Proctofoam'). Recently, it has been remarketed under a new name (Epifoam, Stafford-Miller Ltd) for use following perineal trauma. Early uncontrolled (Nenno and Loehfelm 1973; Bouis *et al.* 1981) and unsatisfactorily controlled (Goldstein *et al.* 1977) studies produced very encouraging results. Two well-controlled studies have recently been published which give conflicting results (Greer and Cameron 1984; Hutchins *et al.* 1985). The study by Hutchins and his colleagues was mentioned above and included a third group randomly allocated to pramoxine/hydrocortisone foam. The Greer and Cameron study is somewhat the more satisfactory of the two: it is truly double-blind, the control group using a simple aqueous foam identical to the vehicle for the pramoxine/hydrocortisone foam, and there were fewer post-randomization exclusions. In both studies, outcome was assessed by an observer who did not know the trial allocation. Whereas Hutchins *et al.* reported less pain, better pain relief and less use of oral analgesia in their pramoxine/hydrocortisone group, Greer and Cameron reported more oedema and a greater use of oral analgesia, particularly after the 3rd day. Wound breakdown was also more common in the actively treated group in this study. Steroids are known to impair wound healing (Walter and Israel 1979) so this latter finding is biologically plausible. Pramoxine/hydrocortisone (Epifoam, Stafford-Miller Ltd) is costly: £4.20 per canister (1987 price), and Hutchins and his colleagues did not feel that the advantages suggested by their study were sufficient to warrant this expense. In the light of the Greer and Cameron study it is very questionable whether it does have the advantages claimed for it and we suggest that it should not be used in clinical practice unless in the context of further properly-controlled trials.

2.5 Local infiltration

There are historical reports of local anaesthetic infiltration around perineal trauma at the time of repair. The enzyme, hyaluronidase, also used in this way, was assessed in a trial conducted during the early 1950s (Weber *et al.* 1952). The hope was that dispersion of oedema would be encouraged by fibrin degradation. The trial has major methodological limitations. Taken at face value, oedema and pain were lower in the hyaluronidase group. The authors, however, expressed some concern about a possible adverse effect of hyaluronidase in wound healing (which is unclear from the data provided) and did not recommend its use in these circumstances.

3 Local physiotherapies

3.1 Relief of pressure on the perineum

A variety of simple aids may be used during sitting or lying as a means of relieving pressure on the sore perineum. When a mother is resting in bed, a wedge or pillow may be used to support her on her side. These should be covered in a waterproof fabric so they may easily be cleaned. Rubber or foam rubber rings have been widely advocated in the past, especially for mothers needing to sit comfortably to feed their babies. Foam rubber is less satisfactory in practice because it is absorbent and therefore difficult to keep clean. Rubber rings have anyway now largely been withdrawn from use in the National Health Service as they are believed to compress venous return, so increasing the risk of thrombosis in women already at higher risk postpartum. The fact that they are no longer supplied in hospitals does not prevent many women from buying their own or substituting children's swimming rings. The popularity of this simple aid suggests that it does give relief to many women.

3.2 Ultrasound and pulsed electromagnetic energy

Recent developments in the physical treatments of soft tissue injuries have lead to the increased use of electrical therapies for the traumatized perineum. Two such treatments are currently in common usage—ultrasound, and pulsed electromagnetic energy. Evidence about the effectiveness of therapeutic ultrasound for other soft-tissue injuries is not totally consistent. In apparently well-conducted randomized trials, ultrasound treatment appeared to hasten recovery from tennis elbow (Binder *et al.* 1985) but not from frozen shoulder (Downing and Weinstein 1986). Randomized trials of ultrasound following oral surgery (El Hag *et al.* 1985) and for the treatment of venous leg ulcers (Dyson *et al.* 1976; Roche and West 1984), however, have all

suggested a beneficial effect. The precise mode of action is not properly understood but postulated mechanisms include improved healing as a result of increased fibroblast activity and protein synthesis (Harvey *et al.* 1975), reduction in oedema due to increased cell wall permeability (Lehmann *et al.* 1958), enhanced vascularity (Hogan *et al.* 1982), and reduction in scar tissue formation due to interference with collagen deposition (Dyson *et al.* 1968). Application of ultrasound in 'pulses' rather than as a continuous wave minimizes the risks of heating and cavitation in the tissues. Nevertheless, ultrasound therapy does require constant operator attendance during treatment and hence is costly in physiotherapists' time. The transducer is applied directly to the skin and must be moved during transmission as a safeguard against tissue damage; conduction is aided by a couplant jelly or cream. This gentle movement of the transducer head over the injured tissues may alone provide some therapeutic or psychological benefit; this possible placebo effect must be taken into account in the design of evaluative studies.

Similar benefits to those seen following ultrasound therapy have been claimed on the basis of observational studies, for pulsed electromagnetic energy in the treatment of inversion injury of the ankle (Wilson 1972), as well as the traumatized perineum and haemorrhoids (Frank 1985). The interrupted transmission of the energy enables waves of high intensity to be used while minimizing local heating. Pulsed electromagnetic energy is believed to have a therapeutic effect by restoring the electrical balance in damaged cells (Bentall 1976).

The advantage of pulsed electromagnetic energy in the context of perineal injury is its ease of application. It may be transmitted through a sanitary towel, so obviating the need for constant operator attendance. As far as we are aware, the effects of this therapy on perineal healing have been assessed in only two controlled trials. A preliminary report of the first has recently been reported (Bird, personal communication; Bewley 1986). Following vaginal delivery, 100 mothers were randomly allocated to receive a treatment from one of two machines: one active and the other inactive. Maternal reporting of perineal pain before and after treatment failed to reveal any benefit from the active therapy in this respect. The physiotherapists who operated the machines, however, observed a reduction in the extent of perineal bruising which they ascribed to pulsed electromagnetic energy. One of the difficulties in assessing these results is that the author acknowledges that by the third day of the trial it was 'obvious' by results which machine was active. This may have influenced the mothers' expectations of the therapy and the subsequent assessments of outcome is also likely to be subject to observer bias.

Because of this dearth of evidence we and others have

recently mounted a randomized controlled trial to compare ultrasound, pulsed electromagnetic energy and placebo therapy given in the immediate postpartum period for the treatment of the 'severely traumatized' perineum. Women were eligible for entry to the trial if they required operative vaginal delivery; or sustained severe perineal trauma involving extensive damage to the anal sphincter or to the rectal or anal mucosa; or developed severe perineal oedema, bruising, or haematoma within 24 hours of delivery; a total of 414 women eventually participated. 'Operator', 'subject', and 'assessor' biases were minimized by comparing each mode of treatment 'double-blind' with 'placebo' treatment. This was achieved by using 12-point dials on each machine: 8 settings were active, 4 were mock-insonated. The codes for the switches were changed at 2 monthly intervals to minimize the risk of participants breaking the operating code and thereby introducing bias. The ultrasound was transmitted at an operating frequency of 3 MHz, an intensity of 0.5 watts/cm and a pulse interval of 1:4. Treatment was given for 2 minutes to each area of trauma equal to the size of the transmitting head. The output of the pulsed electromagnetic energy machine was set at an operating frequency of 27 MHz, a pulse repeat rate of 100 pulses/sec, and pulse width 65 seconds. The duration of each treatment was set at 10 minutes.

Trial 'therapy' was initiated 12 hours following delivery, a maximum of three treatments being given during a 36-hour period. Pre- and post-treatment assessments were carried out by both the mother (in terms of perineal pain), and a midwife co-ordinator who documented the presence of oedema, bruising, haemorrhoids, and the amount of analgesia taken during the course of the three therapies. Both the mother and the midwife observer were unaware of the trial allocations. Maternal morbidity was assessed at 10 days and at 3 months postpartum.

Preliminary analyses have recently been performed. The two placebo groups were amalgamated to give a single control group of the same size as the two actively treated groups. The three groups were generally similar at the time of entry and there was very good compliance with the trial allocation. No clear differences were seen between the groups in respect of the major measures of outcome either immediately following treatment, or at 10 days or at 3 months postpartum. About 90 per cent of women in each group, including the placebo group, felt that the treatment had made the pain better, underlining the necessity for well-designed comparative studies, the natural history of the condition and the possibility of a placebo effect. These preliminary analyses provide no basis for the widespread use of these two expensive physiotherapies in the treatment of perineal problems. Further randomized trials would be needed to justify any continued use of these technologies in the postnatal ward and would provide an opportunity to assess the size of the placebo effect.

3.3 Pelvic floor exercises

The usual rationale for advising postnatal exercises of the pelvic floor muscles is the belief that they will reduce the risk of urinary stress incontinence and genital prolapse. In the only large controlled trial in which the effects of postnatal exercises on incontinence rates has been assessed (Sleep and Grant 1987), the rate of incontinence (3 months after delivery) experienced by women who had received intensive instruction and reinforcement for pelvic floor exercises was similar to that among other women who had received the usual level of information and no special reinforcement. Although no prophylactic effects of postnatal exercises on subsequent incontinence rates were detected, however, some other outcomes did appear to be affected. Women who received the intensive postnatal exercise programme and reinforcement were significantly less likely to have perineal pain. They were also less likely to be depressed. This latter difference may have been mediated either by the greater attention paid to their progress postpartum (see Chapter 86), or simply because they were in less pain.

4 Treatments taken by mouth

4.1 Herbal preparations

A range of herbal preparations, aimed at relieving perineal symptoms, is available. For example, arnica (Leopard's Bane) supplied as tablets and also comfrey as a tablet or a tea are claimed to reduce bruising (Ehudin-Pagano *et al.* 1987). As far as we know, these have never been formally evaluated.

4.2 Proteolytic enzymes

Some of the pharmacologically more active proteolytic enzymes also occur naturally; ananase, for example, is an extract of Hawaiian pineapple plants. Three such enzyme preparations (bromolain, chymotrypsin alone, and chymotrypsin plus trypsin) have been evaluated in 10 controlled trials, of varying quality (Zatuchni and Colombi 1967; Roberts and McKay Hart 1983; Howat and Lewis 1973; Huntsinger and Lebherz 1966; Bumgardner and Zatuchni 1965; Schmitz and Pavlic 1961; Soule *et al.* 1966; Sherman and Ellison 1961; Bare and Fine 1963; Harvo-Noponen and Seppala 1968). Generally speaking, the enzymes are taken orally in tablet form 6-hourly, over 3 to 5 days. One mechanism by which these preparations might relieve perineal discomfort is by reducing oedema. Relevant data are available from 8 of the trials. There is wide variation in the point estimates of the odds ratios in these trials: the results of four studies suggest a beneficial effect, whereas in four others there were no clear differences

(Table 79.3). The typical odds ratio in the overview (0.71) reflects this distribution and has an upper 95 per cent confidence interval of 0.87. Generally speaking, there is close correspondence within the individual trials between the differences in oedema and differences in pain when sitting (Table 79.4) and walking (Table 79.5). There were no clear differences detected between the four enzyme preparations compared. The findings in this overview suggest that oral proteolytic agents may have an important effect on perineal discomfort. Nevertheless, the trials are of such heterogeneity in terms of quality, prevalence of outcomes and estimates of treatment effect that this conclusion can be only tentative. Further, better controlled studies should be mounted.

Table 79.3 Effect of oral proteolytic enzymes for perineal trauma on oedema on the 3rd day

Study	EXPT n	(%)	CTRL n	(%)	Odds ratio (95% CI)	Graph of odds ratios and confidence intervals
Zatuchni and Colombi (1967)	4/80	(5.00)	23/80	(28.75)	0.19 (0.08–0.42)	
Howat and Lewis (1972)	53/80	(66.25)	44/70	(62.86)	1.16 (0.59–2.26)	
Huntsinger and Lebherz (1966)	63/496	(12.70)	48/476	(10.08)	1.29 (0.87–1.92)	
Roberts and McKay Hart (1983)	30/84	(35.71)	35/88	(39.77)	0.84 (0.46–1.56)	
Bumgardner and Zatuchni (1965)	13/156	(8.33)	36/155	(23.23)	0.33 (0.18–0.60)	
Schmitz and Pavlic (1961)	64/250	(25.60)	93/250	(37.20)	0.58 (0.40–0.85)	
Bare and Fine (1963)	8/38	(21.05)	21/34	(61.76)	0.19 (0.07–0.48)	
Harvo-Noponen and Seppala (1968)	35/76	(46.05)	15/47	(31.91)	1.79 (0.86–3.74)	
Typical odds ratio (95% confidence interval)					0.71 (0.59–0.87)	

Table 79.4 Effect of oral proteolytic enzymes for perineal trauma on pain when sitting—3rd day

Study	EXPT n	(%)	CTRL n	(%)	Odds ratio (95% CI)	Graph of odds ratios and confidence intervals
Zatuchni and Colombi (1967)	6/80	(7.50)	43/80	(53.75)	0.11 (0.06–0.22)	
Huntsinger and Lebherz (1966)	57/496	(11.49)	62/476	(13.03)	0.87 (0.59–1.27)	
Roberts and McKay Hart (1983)	24/84	(28.57)	28/88	(31.82)	0.86 (0.45–1.64)	
Bumgardner and Zatuchni (1965)	51/156	(32.69)	91/155	(58.71)	0.35 (0.23–0.55)	
Schmitz and Pavlic (1961)	141/250	(56.40)	126/250	(50.40)	1.27 (0.90–1.81)	
Bare and Fine (1963)	5/38	(13.16)	24/34	(70.59)	0.09 (0.04–0.24)	
Harvo-Noponen and Seppala (1968)	70/76	(92.11)	42/47	(89.36)	1.40 (0.39–4.97)	
Typical odds ratio (95% confidence interval)					0.64 (0.52–0.77)	

Table 79.5 Effect of oral proteolytic enzymes for perineal trauma on pain when walking—3rd day

Study	EXPT		CTRL		Odds ratio	Graph of odds ratios and confidence intervals						
	n	(%)	*n*	(%)	(95% CI)	0.01	0.1	0.5	1	2	10	100
Zatuchni and Colombi (1967)	4/80	(5.00)	21/80	(26.25)	0.20 (0.09–0.47)							
Huntsinger and Lebherz (1966)	164/496	(33.06)	119/476	(25.00)	1.48 (1.12–1.95)							
Roberts and McKay Hart (1983)	64/84	(76.19)	74/88	(84.09)	0.61 (0.29–1.29)							
Bumgardner and Zatuchni (1965)	37/156	(23.72)	90/155	(58.06)	0.24 (0.15–0.38)							
Schmitz and Pavlic (1961)	57/250	(22.80)	112/250	(44.80)	0.37 (0.26–0.54)							
Bare and Fine (1963)	4/38	(10.53)	18/34	(52.94)	0.14 (0.05–0.38)							
Typical odds ratio (95% confidence interval)					0.62 (0.52–0.75)							

4.3 Oral analgesics

There is a bewildering choice of pharmacologically active preparations which can be taken by mouth to relieve perineal pain. Given the large number of randomized trials in which these agents have been evaluated (National Perinatal Epidemiology Unit 1985), it is surprising that the experimental evidence is relatively unhelpful. There are two main reasons for this. First, most trials show that the active preparations are superior to placebo but fail to distinguish clinically important differences between alternative analgesics. Second, many of the drugs included in the trials are no longer commercially available.

One factor which needs to be taken into account when making a choice is the severity of the pain being treated. It is useful to categorize pain as mild, moderate or severe (Wallenstein and Hood 1975) and limit the choice to preparations with sufficient analgesic potency for each type of pain. Postpartum perineal pain is usually mild or moderate when classified on this scale. Another factor which should be considered is whether the formulation is likely to cause constipation, something which is particularly important to avoid when treating perineal pain.

A further consideration is whether the drug or drugs are carried in breast-milk and if so, whether this has any potential danger for the baby. Also, some oral preparations can cause gastric upset and this should obviously be avoided if possible. In addition, some drugs have more serious, albeit rare, adverse effects. Finally, the relative costs of the alternative preparations should be taken into account.

On the basis of these criteria, paracetamol (acetominophen) is probably the drug of choice for mild perineal pain; it has a useful analgesic effect and is largely free of unwanted side-effects. Effervescent paracetamol (sulpadene) has a quicker action but is more expensive. Aspirin is less satisfactory because it can cause gastric irritation and prolong bleeding time, and poses a potential risk to the baby because of its carriage in breast-milk. The mild opioid dextropropoxyphene (especially in combination with paracetamol) is much less popular than it used to be. Dependence is common and it carries risks when taken in an overdose, particularly in combination with alcohol.

Of the other non-steroidal anti-inflammatory drugs which also have a potent analgesic effect, ibuprofen would seem to be the most appropriate alternative to paracetamol for treating perineal pain. Unlike some of the other non-steroidal anti-inflammatory drugs it appears to be largely free of unwanted side-effects and very little is excreted in breast-milk.

The choice of analgesics is less satisfactory when perineal pain is insufficiently relieved by paracetamol or ibuprofen. One option is to give paracetamol in combination with lower doses of codeine or dihydrocodeine than would be the case if the latter were being used on their own. Although it seems reasonable to combine the two types of analgesia it is uncertain whether the analgesic effect is greater than paracetamol on its own. The addition of codeine or dihydrocodeine can, however, cause nausea and vomiting and may lead to constipation.

The actual choices of oral analgesics in clinical practice reflect these theoretical considerations. The telephone survey of 50 English maternity units which we conducted in 1987 revealed that paracetamol was the oral analgesic used for mild perineal pain in almost every hospital. Use of aspirin on its own was not reported, although its use in combination with codeine was reported. There was no consensus concerning the management of pain that was not adequately controlled by paracetamol. Of the 32 maternity units which specified an oral analgesic for more severe pain, 9 combined paracetamol with codeine or dihydrocodeine, 6 gave a combination of aspirin with codeine, 9 prescribed Distalgesic (paracetamol and dextropropoxyphene) and 2 used dihydrocodeine on its own. Of the remaining 6 of these 32 units, 3 reported that they used a non-steroidal anti-inflammatory agent (ibuprofen or mefenamic acid), 1 used the opioid, butrenorphine, and 2 used the combination of papaveretum and aspirin.

If perineal pain does not respond adequately to paracetamol it seems sensible to consider the additional use of local therapies such as heat and local anaesthetics. The pain is likely to be associated with local inflammation and a non-steroidal anti-inflammatory agent such as aspirin or ibuprofen may be helpful. If stronger analgesia is still required there is no obvious first choice. It should be recognized that there are differences in individual susceptibility to different analgesia formulations. Codeine derivatives are less suitable for perineal pain than for other types of pain because they predispose to constipation. For this reason the combinations of paracetamol (acetominophen) with a stronger opioid analgesic may have a special place for the relief of perineal pain.

5 Conclusions

5.1 Implications for current practice

Local cooling with crushed ice, witch hazel, or tap water gives short term symptomatic relief from perineal pain and discomfort. Locally applied anaesthetics such as aqueous 5 per cent lignocaine spray or lignocaine gel are also effective and may last longer. There is no good reason, however, for adding a steroid to such local anaesthetics; indeed, this may do more harm than good in the longer term. The addition of salt or antiseptic solution to bathwater appears to have no effect on perineal pain and healing.

The quality of personal care during the puerperium is likely to be a major determinant of postpartum perineal discomfort. On the basis of currently available evidence sympathetic support may be the mechanism by which personalized physiotherapies, such as therapeutic ultrasound, pulsed electromagnetic energy, and the teaching of postnatal exercises, have a therapeutic effect, rather than via the treatment modalities themselves.

Paracetamol (acetominophen) is the oral analgesic of choice for mild perineal pain. If paracetamol in conjunction with the local therapies mentioned above, fails

to control the pain, a non-steroidal anti-inflammatory agent, such as aspirin or ibuprofen, is a useful alternative. The oral proteolytic enzymes may also be considered for relatively intractable perineal pain, although their effectiveness is still not clearly established. There is no obvious oral analgesic for more severe pain which is inadequately controlled by paracetamol. The tendency for codeine derivatives to cause constipation makes these drugs less suitable for perineal pain than for pain in other sites. For this reason, the addition of an oral opioid (such as papaveretum) may have a special place in the management of postpartum pain.

5.2 Implications for future research

Until recently, the prevention and treatment of perineal pain following childbirth using approaches other than systemic analgesia have been the subject of little formal evaluative research. Unlike many of the problems discussed in this book, postpartum perineal pain is so common that alternative strategies can be compared in statistically powerful, single-centre, randomized controlled trials. For this reason there are many opportunities to mount useful evaluative research.

There are three areas that need urgent attention. First, there is a need for well-conducted randomized trials to evaluate further the combination of a local anaesthetic and a topical steroid (as in 'Epifoam'). In our survey of English maternity units, over half reported that they used this preparation. The short term pain relief observed in some studies of 'Epifoam' may solely reflect the local anaesthetic pramoxine hydrochloride (other trials have shown that local anaesthetics have this effect). But other evidence suggests that the hydrocortisone component of 'Epifoam' may cause wound breakdown in the longer term.

Second, a series of randomized trials is required to clarify the place (if any) and optimal lengths and intensity of treatment of therapeutic ultrasound and pulsed electromagnetic energy. Judged by our survey results, these locally applied physiotherapies, particularly ultrasound, are in use in nearly 50 per cent of English maternity units, despite the lack of any evidence that they have anything other than a possible placebo effect in preventing or alleviating perineal pain.

Third, the review of the controlled trials of oral proteolytic enzyme therapy suggests that these preparations may have a useful place in the management of perineal trauma. Further trials are needed before their use in everyday practice can be recommended.

In respect of oral analgesia the main challenge is to find an agent for the more severe pain which is not adequately controlled by paracetamol. There are special considerations when choosing an oral analgesic for perineal pain, but as for moderate pain in other sites the ideal agent has not yet been identified.

References

Ayliffe GAB, Babb JR, Collins RJ, Davies J, Deverill C, Varney J (1975). Disinfection of baths and bathwater. Nurs Times Suppl, 22–23.

Bare WW, Fine ES (1963). Prophylaxis of episiotomy pain: a controlled study of oral trypsins on the post partum course. Am J Obstet Gynecol, 87: 268–271.

Bentall R (1976). Healing by electromagnetism—fact or fiction? New Scientist, 22 April: 166–167.

Bewley EL (1986). The Megapulse trial at Bristol. Association of Chartered Physiotherapists in Obstetrics and Gynaecology Journal, 58: 16.

Binder A, Hodge G, Greenwood AM, Hazleman BL, Page Thomas DP (1985). Is therapeutic ultrasound effective in treating soft tissue lesions? Br Med J, 290: 512–514.

Bischoff PA, Upchurch KP, Carter JJ (1956). The use of sulfisoxazole cream in the post partum patient. Am J Obstet Gynecol, 71: 113–115.

Bouis PJJ, Martinez LA, Hambrick TL (1981). Epifoam (Hydrocortisone acetate) in the treatment of post episiotomy patients. Curr Ther Res, 30: 912–916.

Bumgardner HD, Zatuchni GI (1965). Prevention of episiotomy pain with oral chymotrypsin. Am J Obstet Gynecol, 92: 514–517.

Bunce KL (1987). The use of herbs in midwifery. J Nurs Midwifery, 32: 255–259.

Downing DS, Weinstein A (1986). Ultrasound therapy for subacromial bursitis. Physical Therapy, 66: 194–199.

Drugs and Therapeutics Bulletin (1986). Herbal medicines—safe and effective? 24: 97–100.

Dyson M, Pond JB, Joseph J, Warwick R (1968). The stimulation of tissue regeneration by means of ultrasound. Clin Sci, 35: 273–285.

Dyson M, Franks C, Suckling J (1976). Stimulation of healing of varicose ulcers by ultrasound. Ultrasonics, 14: 232–236.

Ehudin-Pagano E, Paluzzi PA, Ivory LC, McCartney M (1987). The use of herbs in nurse–midwifery practice. J Nurs Midwifery, 32: 260–262.

El Hag M, Coghlan K, Christmas P, Harvey W, Harris M (1985). The anti-inflammatory effects of dexamethazone and therapeutic ultrasound in oral surgery. Br J Oral Maxillofacial Surg, 23: 17–23.

Frank R (1985). Treatment of the perineum by pulsed electro magnetic therapy. Midwives' Chron & Nursing Notes, November: 297–298.

Goldstein PJ, Lipmann M, Luebehusen J (1977). A controlled trial of two local agents in postepisiotomy pain and discomfort. South Med J, 70: 806–808.

Greer IA, Cameron AD (1984). Topical pramoxine and hydrocortisone foam versus placebo in relief of post partum episiotomy symptoms and wound healing. Scot Med J, 29: 104–106.

Harrison RF, Brennan M (1987a). Evaluation of two local anaesthetic sprays for the relief of post-episiotomy pain. Curr Med Res Opin, 10: 364–369.

Harrison RF, Brennan M (1987b). A comparison of alcoholic and aqueous formulations of local anaesthetic as a spray for the relief of post-episiotomy pain. Curr Med Res Opin, 10: 370–374.

Harrison RF, Brennan M (1987c). Comparison of two formulations of lignocaine spray with mefanamic acid in the relief of post-episiotomy pain: a placebo-controlled study. Curr Med Res Opin, 10: 375–379.

Harrison RF, Tayob Y, Brennan M (1982). The use of a local anaesthetic aerosol spray for the relief of pain after episiotomy. Irish Med J, 75: 190-191.

Harvey W, Dyson M, Pond JB, Grahame R (1975). The stimulation of protein synthesis in human fibroblasts by therapeutic ultrasound. Rheumatology and Rehabilitation, 14: 237.

Harvo-Noponen M, Seppala M (1968). Double blind study of oral chymotrypsin in patients with episiotomy. Ann Chir Gynaecol Fenn, 57: 444–446.

Hogan RD, Burke KM, Franklin TD (1982). The effect of ultrasound on microvascular haemodynamics in skeletal muscle: effects during ischaemia. Microvascular Res, 23: 370–379.

Houghton M (1940). Aids to Practical Nursing. Eastbourne: Ballière, Tindall & Cox.

Howat RCL, Lewis GD (1972). The effect of bromelain therapy on episiotomy wounds—a double blind controlled clinical trial. J Obstet Gynaecol Br Commnwlth, 79: 951–953.

Huntsinger LA, Lebherz TB (1966). Double-blind study of the use of oral chymotrypsin in episiotomy. Obstet Gynecol, 27: 268–270.

Hutchins CJ, Ferreira CJ, Norman-Taylor JQ (1985). A comparison of local agents in the relief of discomfort after episiotomy. J Obstet Gynaecol, 6: 45–56.

Lehmann JF, Erickson DJ, Martin GM, Krusen FH (1958). Comparison of ultrasonic and microwave diathermy in the physical treatment of periarthritis of the shoulder. Arch Phys Med, 35: 627–638.

Marks J, Ribeiro D (1983). Silicone foam dressings. Nursing Times, 79: 58–59.

Martin RT, Reiss HE, Milne SE (1957). Vulval and perineal toilet in the puerperium. Br Med J, 3: 670–673.

National Perinatal Epidemiology Unit (1985). A Classified Bibliography of Controlled Trials in Perinatal Medicine 1940–1984. Oxford: Oxford University Press.

Nenno DJ, Loehfelm G (1973). Clinical trial of a topical foam for episiotomies. Medical Times, 101: 123–125.

Palm JM (1951). The use of a multiple sulphonamide vaginal cream in postpartum care. Am J Obstet Gynecol, 61: 680–682.

Ramler D, Roberts J (1986). A comparison of cold and warm sitz baths for relief of postpartum perineal pain. J Obstet Gynecol Neonatal Nurs, 15: 471–474.

Roberts ADG, McKay Hart D (1983). Polyglycolic acid and catgut sutures, with and without oral proteolytic enzymes, in the healing of episiotomies. Br J Obstet Gynaecol, 90: 650–653.

Roche C, West J (1984). A controlled trial investigating the effect of ultrasound on venous ulcers referred from general practitioners. Physiotherapy, 70: 475–477.

Rubin A (1961). Use of a sulfonamide vaginal cream post partum. A controlled 'blind' study of 700 patients. Am J Obstet Gynecol, 82: 860–862.

Schmitz HE, Pavlic RS (1961). Control of oedema and pain in episiotomy. Use of oral proteolytic enzymes. Obstet Gynecol, 17: 260–262.

Sherman E, Ellison RS (1961). Subjective evaluation of an

enzyme preparation in episiotomy pain. Am J Obstet Gynecol, 82: 863–864.

Sleep JM, Grant A (1987). Pelvic floor exercises in post-natal care—the report of a randomised controlled trial to compare an intensive exercise regime with the programme in current use. Midwifery, 3: 158–164.

Sleep JM, Grant A (1988). Routine addition of salt or Savlon bath concentrate during bathing in the immediate post-partum period. A randomised controlled trial. Nursing Times, 84: 55–57.

Sleep J, Grant A, Garcia J, Elbourne D, Spencer JAD, Chalmers I (1984). West Berkshire perineal management trial. Br Med J, 289: 587–590.

Soule SD, Wasserman HC, Burstein R (1966). Oral proteolytic enzyme therapy (chymoral) in episiotomy patients. Am J Obstet Gynecol, 95: 820-823.

Spellacy W (1965). A double blind control study of a medicated pad for relief of episiotomy pain. Am J Obstet Gynecol, 92: 272.

Wallenstein SL, Hood RW (1975). The clinical evaluation of analgesic effectiveness. In: Narcotic Research. Ehrenpreis S, Neidl A (eds). New York: Marcel Dekker, pp 127–145.

Walter JB, Israel M (1979). General Pathology (5th edn). Edinburgh, Churchill Livingstone, p 104.

Weber JE, Fletchko AM, Carroll JH (1952). The use of hyaluronidase in episiotomies. Am J Obstet Gynecol, 64: 194–196.

Wilson DH (1972). Treatment of soft tissue injuries by pulsed electrical energy. Br Med J, 2: 269–270.

Zatuchni GI, Colombi DJ (1967). Bromelains therapy for the prevention of episiotomy pain. Obstet Gynecol, 29: 275–278.

80 Establishing and maintaining breastfeeding

Sally Inch and Sally Garforth

1 Introduction

Any consideration of how best to help recently delivered mothers to establish and maintain breastfeeding must begin with a recognition that a wide variety of the elements of care during pregnancy and childbirth can foster or jeopardize the successful accomplishment of these objectives. For example, among the various dividends resulting from efforts made to provide social and psychological support to mothers during pregnancy is an increased likelihood that mothers so supported will breastfeed their babies successfully (see Chapter 15). In contrast, sedative and analgesic drugs given during labour, by altering the behaviour of the newborn infant, can compromise the crucial role of the baby in the initiation of lactation (Kron et al. 1966; see Chapter 57). Similarly, although there is no evidence that a single dose of an ergot alkaloid given during the third stage of labour has adverse effects on the establishment of lactation (see Chapter 67), these drugs are known to suppress the release of prolactin (Varga et al. 1972;

Shane and Naftolin 1974; Weiss et al. 1975; Symes 1984) and reduce the likelihood of successful breastfeeding if they are continued beyond the third stage of labour (Table 80.1).

Drugs administered to the mother are not the only way in which the establishment of lactation may be jeopardized at the time of delivery. Controlled trials have shown, for example, that routine gastric suctioning (Widstrom et al. 1987) and administration of silver nitrate eye drops (Wahlberg et al. 1982) in the immediate postnatal period alter infant behaviour in a way which prejudices the infant's role in establishing lactation (see Chapter 75). Similarly, separating babies from their mothers, either for no good reason at all other than entrenched hospital routines (see Chapter 77), or during treatment of the baby (Elander and Lindberg 1986), reduces the likelihood that breastfeeding will be established successfully.

This chapter examines the important factors in establishing and maintaining breastfeeding after birth. These include the time of the first feed, positioning,

Table 80.1 Effect of oral ergometrine for four weeks postpartum on primary lactation failure

Study	EXPT		CTRL		Odds ratio	Graph of odds ratios and confidence intervals						
	n	(%)	n	(%)	(95% CI)	0.01	0.1	0.5	1	2	10	100
Arabin et al. (1986)	57/444	(12.84)	38/436	(8.72)	1.53 (1.00–2.35)							
Typical odds ratio (95% confidence interval)					1.53 (1.00–2.35)							

feeding frequency and duration, supplements for babies and mothers, and support for breastfeeding mothers.

2 Early versus later suckling

It is remarkable that the spontaneous feeding behaviour of a new mother and her newborn infant has only recently been considered a matter worthy of formal observation and description by researchers. Anne-Marie Widstrom and her colleagues (1987) recently reported their observations of 10 infants placed in a prone position between the mother's breasts after delivery (none of the mothers received drugs for pain relief or sedation during labour). After 15 minutes of comparative inactivity, spontaneous sucking and rooting movements occurred. These reached maximal intensity at 45 minutes after delivery. The first hand-to-mouth movement was observed at an average age of 34 minutes. By an average age of 55 minutes, the infants had spontaneously found the nipple and started to suckle.

The issue of early versus late suckling has been confounded by the issues surrounding separation of mother and baby at delivery. If mother and baby are separated, they clearly cannot breastfeed spontaneously. Neither can they engage in the variety of behaviours, such as touching and gazing, that are important to the whole mother-baby relationship of which breastfeeding is one part.

A number of studies have demonstrated that early contact has beneficial effects on breastfeeding among other important outcomes (Table 80.2). For obvious reasons it is virtually impossible to examine the effects of early or late breastfeeding in mothers and babies who are together at birth. Many studies (for example, Sousa et al. 1974; Sosa et al. 1976; Woolridge et al. 1985; de Chateau et al. 1977; and Thomson et al. 1979) have examined the combined effects of early contact and early suckling. All these studies demonstrate beneficial effect on breastfeeding.

The one study in which contact between mothers and babies appeared to be similar in both experimental and control groups, was carried out in Scotland by Salariya et al. (1978). One hundred and sixty primiparous women who had chosen to breastfeed were randomized into 4 comparable groups by the use of envelopes coded for age and social class variables. The 4 groups were given different feeding instructions as follows: Group 2E gave their babies an early breastfeed within 10 minutes of delivery and subsequently fed every 2 hours; those in Group 4E gave the same early feed and then followed a 4-hourly schedule; Group 2L followed the routine practice for the first feed (approximately 4–6 hours postpartum) and then 2-hourly thereafter; while Group 4L had the routine first feed and then adopted the 4-hourly pattern. Feeding in all 4 groups was supervised by a midwife and individual feeds were not kept to a strict time limit.

Table 80.2 Effect of restricted mother–infant contact after delivery on discontinuation of breastfeeding at 1–3 months

Study	EXPT n	EXPT (%)	CTRL n	CTRL (%)	Odds ratio (95% CI)	Graph of odds ratios and confidence intervals
Thomson et al. (1979)	12/15	(80.00)	6/15	(40.00)	5.01 (1.19–21.06)	
De Chateau et al. (1977)	15/20	(75.00)	8/20	(40.00)	4.04 (1.17–13.94)	
Salariya et al. (1978)	26/53	(49.06)	22/55	(40.00)	1.44 (0.68–3.06)	
Sosa et al. (1976)	12/20	(60.00)	5/20	(25.00)	4.04 (1.17–13.94)	
Sosa et al. (1976)	3/30	(10.00)	8/30	(26.67)	0.33 (0.09–1.22)	
Sosa et al. (1976)	17/32	(53.13)	13/32	(40.63)	1.64 (0.62–4.34)	
Taylor et al. (1985)	9/22	(40.91)	9/31	(29.03)	1.68 (0.54–5.27)	
Illingworth and Stone (1952)	34/96	(35.42)	33/131	(25.19)	1.63 (0.92–2.90)	
Sousa et al. (1974)	73/100	(73.00)	23/100	(23.00)	7.34 (4.22–12.76)	
Johnson (1976)	5/6	(83.33)	1/6	(16.67)	11.52 (1.32–99.99)	
Typical odds ratio (95% confidence interval)					2.62 (1.98–3.48)	

The graph scale (odds ratios and confidence intervals): 0.01 0.1 0.5 1 2 10 100

The results showed 'immediate postpartum suckling resulted in mothers feeding for longer periods than mothers whose infants were not put to the breast until a few hours after delivery'. The authors report that the 4-hourly early initiation groups weaned their babies at a later time than the 2-hourly later initiation group, suggesting that the early suckling had a stronger influence in extending the nursing period than did the increased frequency of feeds. Further follow-up carried out at 18 months substantiated these findings.

No research has demonstrated a 'critical period' for the first feed in terms of breastfeeding success. In other words, there is no evidence to suggest that if a mother does not feed her baby immediately after birth, then her subsequent breastfeeding will suffer. Indeed, in some societies breastfeeding is not practised at all for the first few days as colostrum is considered poisonous (Jelliffe and Jelliffe 1978) yet lactation proceeds well. There are therefore no research-based grounds for replacing traditional dogma ('no baby should breastfeed until 4 hours after delivery') with new dogma ('all babies should feed immediately after delivery'). The findings of the only study to date of spontaneous feeding behaviour after delivery (Widstrom *et al.* 1987) show that babies have a wide range of behaviour following spontaneous delivery and are ready to feed from 15 to 55 minutes after delivery. More work is required to describe further the support that mothers and babies need at this point. In the meantime, interventions aimed either at delaying or speeding up the time of the first feed should be avoided (Woolridge *et al.* 1985).

These findings would suggest that a skilled professional helping session given at the first *feed* after delivery (as opposed to the immediate post-delivery nuzzle at the breast) would be useful. This should be done at a time when the baby is receptive, in privacy, and after the newly delivered mother and baby have been attended to and made comfortable (Houston 1985). If possible, it should be done while the father or someone else whom the mother has found supportive, is still present. The baby's behaviour and needs can be explained to new parents, who will usually be very receptive at this time. A brief explanation of the importance of correct positioning and the concept of supply and demand can be given before the mother (with help if necessary) positions the baby accurately at the breast (see Section 3, below). This can be followed by a little more information, including the importance of unrestricted feeding (see Section 4, below), potential problems, and how (and why) to summon prompt help (M J Houston 1985, quoted in Minchin 1985).

3 The importance of correct positioning

Most of the mothers who abandon their attempts to breastfeed within a few weeks of starting do so because of sore nipples or insufficient milk (Martin and Monk 1982). The diagnosis and treatment of these problems will be discussed in detail in the next chapter (see Chapter 81). A variety of different approaches have been used in attempts to prevent sore and cracked nipples. For example, various vitamins and hormones have been administered prophylactically. No beneficial effects of either systemic supplements of ascorbic acid (Gunther 1945) or local application of vitamin A and D ointment (Newton 1952) were detected in the controlled trials in which they were evaluated. Furthermore, vitamin A and D concentrate (Newton 1952) and stilboestrol ointment (Gans 1958), far from reducing the incidence of cracked nipples, resulted in significantly more pain and nipple damage than occurred among untreated controls. The fact that sore nipples affect so many women (Martin and Monk 1982), coupled with the observation that in the majority of cases the condition resolves spontaneously (Gans 1958; Rotch 1985), tends to suggest that the underlying cause may be something that women and babies get wrong to start with, and then get right with practice. Some mothers and babies, on the other hand, take longer to get it right, and go on to develop cracked nipples in the process. Still others never get it right and either abandon their attempts to breastfeed, or struggle on with problems and lose the potential enjoyment of breastfeeding both for themselves and their families.

A factor which appears to play a crucial role both in the prevention of sore nipples and in the successful establishment of breastfeeding is the positioning of the baby on the breast.

As Woolridge (1986a) has suggested, the ability of a woman to position her baby correctly on her breast seems likely to be a learned, and predominantly manual skill, which the mother must acquire from observation and practice. Industrialized societies, on the whole, do not provide women with the opportunity to make any useful observations of other breastfeeding women before they come to attempt breastfeeding themselves. This deficiency is compounded by the frequent lack of experienced breastfeeding mothers in the woman's immediate social sphere.

Similarly, before professionals can be of real value to the mother, they have to understand the underlying mechanisms of suckling, and acquire the skill and experience to help a mother to position her baby correctly. The fragmentation or, in some countries, total lack of postnatal care, means that many professionals are unable to acquire these skills: hospital midwives never see the results of their attempts to help mothers, while community midwives and health visitors are unable to influence the initiation of breastfeeding.

A better understanding of the importance of correct

positioning and the dynamic process of suckling has come from careful observations, including cineradiographic (Adran *et al.* 1958) and ultrasound (Weber *et al.* 1986) visualization of events inside the infant's mouth (Woolridge 1986a). When the baby is properly attached to the breast (see Fig. 80.1), the nipple, together with some of the surrounding breast tissue, is drawn out into a teat by the suction created within the baby's mouth. Breaking this suction causes the nipple to recoil abruptly. The teat thus created extends as far back as the junction of the baby's hard and soft palate, with the nipple itself forming only about one-third of the teat. At its base, the teat is held between the upper gum and the tongue, which covers the lower gum. It lies in a central trough formed by the raised edges of the tongue, which directs the expressed milk backwards into the pharynx, using a roller-like, peristaltic movement of the tongue. The peristaltic action begins as the front edge of the tongue curves upwards, closely followed by the raising of the lower jaw, which follows the tongue's movement with pressure from the lower gum. This wave of compression moves progressively backwards

beyond the tip of the nipple, thus directing the milk into the pharynx and on into the oesophagus. Meanwhile, a fresh cycle of compression by the tongue has been initiated from its tip.

It is thus the breast tissue opposed to the baby's lower jaw and tongue which is the critical region in the transfer of milk: the tongue applies peristaltic force to the underside of the teat. The hard palate simply provides the necessary resistance to the tongue's action (Woolridge 1986a). Once sufficient breast tissue has been formed into the 'teat', there should be virtually no movement of this teat in and out of the baby's mouth. Similarly, friction from the tongue and gums against the skin of the breast and nipple should be minimal; only the milk within the sinuses of the breast should move across the border of the baby's mouth, not the breast tissue itself. If, on the other hand, the baby is incorrectly positioned at the breast and is unable to form a teat out of the breast tissues as well as the nipple, then the nipple is likely to incur frictional damage as the teat is repeatedly drawn in and out of the mouth between the tongue and gums by the cyclical application of suction.

It has been postulated that the two most likely functions of the suction exerted by the baby while feeding are to maintain the shape and position of the nipple in the mouth, and to aid refilling of the nipple by milk from the ducts and sinuses that enter it. When the baby first goes to the breast, short fast bursts of sucking can be observed. During this period no milk is flowing and unrelieved suction is applied to the surface of the nipple. Once the milk begins to flow it fills the oral cavity and relieves the negative pressure. As soon as this happens the sucking pattern changes, and long, slow, continuous, sucking supervenes. Very little milk transfer is necessary to cause the shift away from short, fast, continuous sucking. If the baby has an inadequate mouthful of breast tissue (Fisher 1981), however, or milk flow is impaired (often for the same reason), the nipple will be subjected to unrelieved negative pressure. In addition, Gunther (1945) has demonstrated that an inadequate mouthful of breast tissue, because of the breast's elasticity, has a tendency to slip out of the baby's mouth. The baby may counter this tendency by sustaining negative pressure during periods of rest. It has been suggested that the effects of sustained negative pressure due to incorrect positioning may also contribute to nipple damage (Woolridge 1986b).

The mother needs to be taught how to elicit and use the two components of the baby's rooting reflex, namely the moving of the head towards the source of stimulation when the skin around the mouth is touched, and the accompanying gaping of the mouth, preparatory to receiving the breast. At the moment that the baby's mouth gapes widely, the mother must then be shown how to move the baby towards the breast and

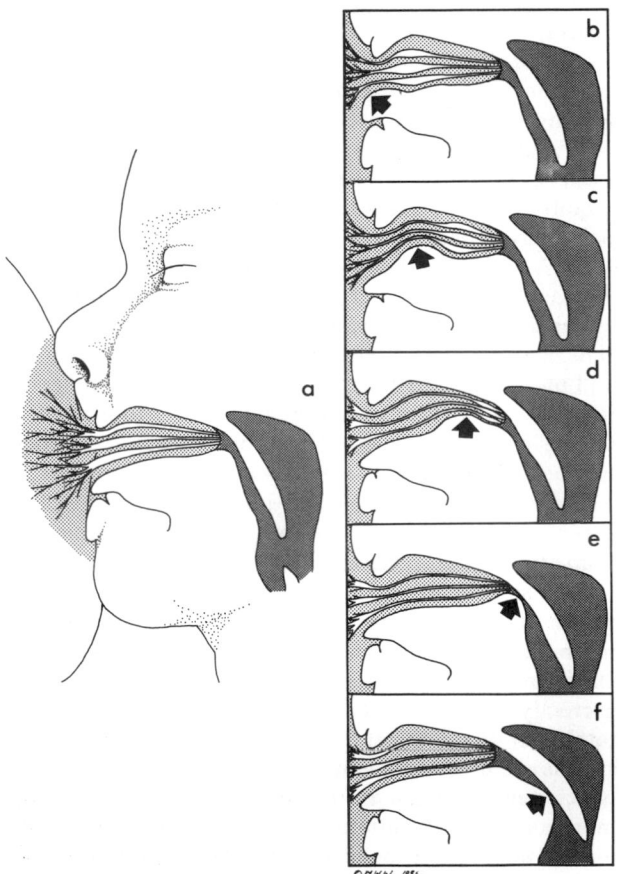

Fig. 80.1 (a–f): Diagrams of accurate positioning of the baby on the breast (from Woolridge 1986a).

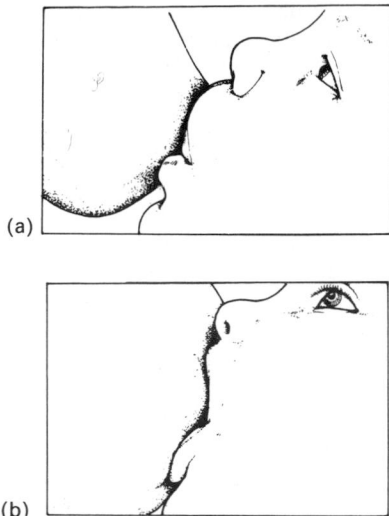

Fig. 80.2 (from Fisher 1981):
  (a) Baby incorrectly positioned at breast.
  (b) Baby correctly positioned at breast.

'plant' the lower rim of the baby's mouth well below the nipple, and follow this by moving the baby close to the breast as it takes a good mouthful of breast tissue. The mother cannot rely, as her helper does, on seeing where the baby's lower lip and jaw are in relation to her nipple, for the critical area of attachment (the underside of the breast) is one of which the mother herself has the poorest view. Observation of the baby's sucking pattern, as well as the sensations that the mother herself experiences (she should feel no pain), will serve to confirm that the baby is correctly positioned (see Fig. 80.2).

More widespread acquisition and use of the skills needed to achieve correct positioning of the baby on the breast would probably do more than anything else to reduce the frequency of the problems currently experienced by so many breastfeeding mothers.

4 The importance of flexibility in breastfeeding practices

4.1 Historical background to current practices

Until the beginning of this century almost all medical writing on the subject of breastfeeding was descriptive rather than prescriptive. One of the responses to the increasing public concern about the high infant mortality rates in the late nineteenth and early twentieth centuries, however, was to try and make infant feeding 'scientific' and therefore safe (Fisher 1987). This meant paying close attention to the composition and preparation of bottle feeds. A relatively small number of doctors began to emerge as 'experts' on infant feeding

and they then wrote about this subject prolifically. Unfortunately, their books also contained much advice about breastfeeding, a subject on which it was expected that they would be equally knowledgeable.

In 1904, one of the most influential authorities on infant feeding, Eric Pritchard, expressed his regret that human milk could not have its chemical composition altered to make it 'scientific and exact'; ominously, he noted that 'we can on the other hand control the quantity'. In the same year, Ralph Vincent (1904) opined that '... too frequent nursing and too prolonged intervals so disturb the quality of human milk as to transform a perfectly good milk into one entirely unfitted for the infant's power of digestion'. Two years later Chavasse (1906) 'explained' why this was so: 'If too frequent applications are made to the breast, the milk is too rich; if the interval prolonged, the milk is too thin and weak'. Helen Serjeant (1905), on the other hand, felt it had more to do with the necessity of providing 'resting time to the infant's stomach'. Her view was endorsed by Pritchard (1907) who suggested that 'It is essential not only that the food should be given at regular intervals, but that these intervals should be sufficiently spaced out to give the stomach time to become empty and to recover from fatigue'.

During the first 25 years of this century, the interpretation of 'sufficiently spaced out' intervals at which babies should be offered the breast changed dramatically from $1\frac{1}{2}$ or 2 hours (Serjeant 1905; Vincent 1913), to at least 3 or 4 hours (Langmead 1916; King 1924).

Over the same period, many of these 'experts' encouraged mothers to establish, from the outset, a feeding schedule with no night feeds (Pritchard 1907; King 1913). As prescribed feeding intervals became longer and longer, more and more mothers despaired of persuading a breastfed baby to last for the duration of the prescribed interval. Not surprisingly, many abandoned their attempts and began feeding formula to their babies (Hardyment 1983).

The manuals on infant feeding that contained all this unsubstantiated advice may not have been widely read by mothers, at least among working-class women (Lewis 1980). But they do appear to have been taken seriously by many health professionals. As an increasing proportion of women gave birth in hospital, so more and more babies were subjected to the recommended routines. Four-hourly feeding became widely endorsed (Langton 1929) and continued to be advocated for over a generation by professionals who had accepted these unsubstantiated 'expert opinions' at face value. The consequence of restricting the frequency of feeds to 4-hourly intervals was that babies who required feeding more frequently were underfed. Liddiard (1924), who was an advocate of 4-hourly feeding, noted that many breastfed babies took 6 months to double their birthweight. Mothers were given to understand that if their babies required feeding more often than 4-hourly it must be because they were producing insufficient milk. This was a self-fulfilling prophecy, of course, because lactation was eventually inhibited by the artificial suppression of demand that resulted from the policies that had been adopted (Kochenour 1980; Carvalho *et al.* 1983).

At the same time that restrictions on the interval between feeds were being imposed, the 'experts' on infant feeding were also recommending that the duration of feeds should be limited. In 1904, Vincent advocated only 2–3 minutes at the breast, for he considered it a 'serious mistake to allow the baby to take freely of the colostrum. In anything but a small amount, colostrum seriously disturbs the infant—a fact that is not at all surprising when its chemical constitution is considered'. The reason for Pierre Budin's (1907) and Truby King's (1918) promotion of restricted feeding times was their belief that 'overfeeding' led to diarrhoea, vomiting, and failure to thrive. Even more widespread, however, was the belief that it was necessary to limit sucking time in order to prevent sore nipples (King 1913; Naish 1913; Liddiard 1924).

4.2 Frequency and duration of feeds

Until relatively recently, professional opposition to policies which limit feeding frequency and duration has been rare. There has been sporadic dissent since the beginning of the century (Cran 1913). In 1939, for example, Aldrich noted that the 'thoughtful observer' must come to recognize that a baby needs 'to eat, sleep and eliminate according to his own individual rhythms rather than by those imposed by arbitrary regimes'. The results of studies in which these 'individual rhythms' have been observed are summarized in Table 80.3. It can be seen from these data that feeds are usually infrequent in the first day or so, but the frequency rapidly increases between the 3rd and 7th day, and then decreases more slowly. Although some babies with feeding frequencies at the lower end of the range would be content to feed as infrequently as 4-hourly, the data show that the vast majority communicate a desire to be fed more frequently than this. Further-

more, these studies demonstrate that the interval between feeds, for the first few weeks of life at least, is very variable, ranging from 1 to 8 hours.

Babies who are permitted to regulate the frequency of their feeds themselves gain weight more quickly (Illingworth and Stone 1952; Salber 1956; Carvalho *et al.* 1983), and remain breastfed for longer than those who have external limitations imposed on them (Illingworth and Stone 1952; Martin and Monk 1982) (Table 80.4). There are no data providing any justification for the imposition of breastfeeding schedules.

Similar comments apply in respect of the duration of feeds. The fact that limitation of sucking time is still being advocated in books addressed both to mothers (Close 1976; Stoppard 1982; Rice 1987) and to professionals (Ajayi 1980; Arneil and Stroud 1984) reflects the deeply ingrained belief that the nipples need to be 'toughened' to permit pain-free feeding. Mothers and professionals are thus instructed that the baby should be permitted to feed for only 2 minutes at each breast for the first day, increasing the time by 2–3 minutes daily, so that at the end of the first week the baby has reached a maximum of 10 minutes on each side. These admonitions are based on the belief that this practice will 'break the nipples in gradually', prevent their exposure to prolonged sucking, and thus prevent nipple soreness and cracks.

Slaven and Harvey (1981) tested this theory in their hospital, where the policy at the time for each of the four postnatal wards was to allow 'demand feeding' but to restrict the duration of the feed in the manner just outlined. Subsequently, two postnatal wards continued with the timed regimen; the other two allowed the mothers to feed for as long as they wished. There were no significant differences between the two groups in the proportion of women who developed sore or cracked nipples, but significantly more mothers in the regulated group had given up breastfeeding altogether by 6 weeks. These conclusions were supported by the findings of a study conducted by Carvalho *et al.* (1984).

Similar conclusions were reached over 30 years ago by Illingworth and Stone (1952). They had divided all the babies on the two postnatal floors of their hospital

Table 80.3 Number of feeds per day taken by unsupplemented infants with unrestricted access to the breast during the first week of life

Study (*n*)	Day 1	Day 2	Day 3	Day 4	Day 5	Day 6	Day 7
Simsarian and McLendon (1942) (*n* = 1)	3	6	7	9	11	9	9
Simsarian and McLendon (1945) (*n* = 1)	0	5	8	11	11	11	10
Olmsted and Jackson (1950) (*n* = 100)	2–12	2–12	3–15	4–17	4–17	5–12	4–14
Inch (1980) (*n* = 1)	NA	8	10	9	10	10	9
Hawken (1982) (*n* = 1)	3	15	9	12	10	7	6
Carvahlo *et al.* (1982) (*n* = 46)	4–10	6–12	6–12	6–13	6–12	7–14	6–12

Table 80.4 Effect of restricted breastfeeding on not regaining birthweight 1 week postpartum

Study	EXPT		CTRL		Odds ratio	Graph of odds ratios and confidence intervals
	n	(%)	*n*	(%)	(95% CI)	0.01　0.1　0.5　1　2　10　100
Illingworth and Stone (1952)	79/98	(80.61)	84/116	(72.41)	1.57 (0.84–2.94)	
Typical odds ratio (95% confidence interval)					1.57 (0.84–2.94)	

Effect of restricted breastfeeding on stopping breastfeeding 4–6 weeks postpartum

Study	EXPT		CTRL		Odds ratio	Graph
Salariya *et al.* (1978)	19/53	(35.85)	17/56	(30.36)	1.28 (0.58–2.83)	
Illingworth and Stone (1952)	34/96	(35.42)	24/122	(19.67)	2.23 (1.22–4.08)	
Typical odds ratio (95% confidence interval)					1.82 (1.13–2.94)	

Effect of restricted breastfeeding on not fully breastfed on discharge

Study	EXPT		CTRL		Odds ratio	Graph
Illingworth and Stone (1952)	12/101	(11.88)	7/124	(5.65)	2.23 (0.87–5.73)	
Typical odds ratio (95% confidence interval)					2.23 (0.87–5.73)	

Effect of restricted breastfeeding on stopping breastfeeding 12 weeks postpartum

Study	EXPT		CTRL		Odds ratio	Graph
Salariya *et al.* (1978)	26/53	(49.06)	22/55	(40.00)	1.44 (0.68–3.06)	
Typical odds ratio (95% confidence interval)					1.44 (0.68–3.06)	

Effect of restricted breastfeeding on babies not having complementary formula

Study	EXPT		CTRL		Odds ratio	Graph
Salariya *et al.* (1978)	16/57	(28.07)	5/56	(8.93)	3.50 (1.36–9.00)	
Typical odds ratio (95% confidence interval)					3.50 (1.36–9.00)	

into two groups. After the 3rd postnatal day, all the babies on one floor were fed on a 4-hourly regimen, and no limitation on duration was placed on those on the other floor. Daily assessments, until the 9th postnatal day, were carried out by the staff on each floor, both floors being under the same paediatric supervision. Mothers who had been encouraged to feed their babies flexibly were less likely to experience breast engorgement and sore nipples, and their babies were more likely to have regained their birthweight by the time of discharge home and to be fully breastfed one month after delivery. Given the importance of these findings it is surprising that harmful policies have persisted for so many years after they were reported.

Unfortunately, the still commonly given advice to limit sucking time to 10 minutes on each breast has repercussions beyond its failure to prevent nipple damage. When a baby is nursed at the breast, the composition and the rate of flow of milk changes over time. The fat content increases and the flow rate decreases as the feed progresses (Hytten 1954). The result of this is that, at the start of a feed, the baby takes a large volume of low calorie foremilk; this changes to a smaller volume of high calorie hindmilk at the end of the feed (Hall 1975). Babies feed for vastly differing lengths of time at the breast if left undisturbed (Woolridge *et al.* 1982; Howie *et al.* 1981). The length of the feed is probably determined by the effectiveness and rate of milk transfer between mother and baby. While it may be true that there are many babies who will terminate a feed spontaneously in under 10 minutes, those who have a slow rate of intake may well take longer than this;

and even though the volume of milk that they consume after 10 minutes have elapsed may not be very great, it may be sufficiently high in calories to make a significant contribution in energy value (Lucas 1979). The external imposition of a time limit for feeding will thus result in some babies having their calorie intake significantly curtailed. There are a number of ramifications of this as the infant responds to, and/or seeks to compensate for, a low calorie feed.

It was demonstrated by Fomon *et al.* (1972) that babies were driven to feed by the need to obtain calories, and would take much larger volumes of low calorie milk than they would of high calorie milk, in an attempt to gain the required number of calories. It is possible, therefore, that a baby who is taken from the first breast before it spontaneously terminates the feed, will take a much larger volume of milk from the second breast than it might otherwise have done, in order to try to 'make up' its calories. For the same reason the baby might also require feeding much more frequently, in order to gain the required calories, than it would if it were allowed to finish feeding spontaneously. It is not difficult to envisage a situation in which a baby was taking large volumes of milk at very frequent intervals in order to compensate for imposed feeding restrictions.

In addition, interference with spontaneous feeding patterns may result in the baby being deprived of essential vitamins. Recent evidence shows that vitamin K, for example, is especially concentrated in colostrum and hindmilk (von Kries *et al.* 1987), and this may explain the increased incidence of haemorrhagic disease of the newborn in breastfed babies (Sutherland 1967).

4.3 Promoting flexible breastfeeding practices

Hospital policies do now appear to be changing in the light of a wider appreciation of just how profoundly professionals have jeopardized successful lactation by imposing misconceived and unvalidated regulations. In a national survey of English mothers in 1975, 23 per cent of mothers said they had been 'allowed' to feed their babies flexibly; a repeat survey in 1980 showed that this proportion had risen to 66 per cent (Martin and Monk 1982). Correspondingly, the proportion of mothers who said that they had been required to breastfeed 'at set times' fell by half, from 64 per cent in 1975 to 32 per cent in 1980. This change was felt by the authors of the survey to have contributed significantly to the fall in the number of women who had stopped breastfeeding within two weeks of giving birth. The results of a national survey of policy and practice in midwifery in England in 1984 (Garcia *et al.* 1987), suggested that the policy in nearly all specialist obstetric units (97 per cent) was to encourage 'demand feeding' (Inch 1987; Garforth and Garcia, in press).

Although policies have moved in the right direction, however, their implementation still leaves considerable scope for improvement. Women are still being encouraged to believe that regular, 4-hourly feeding is the 'norm' for breastfed babies (see, for example, Culley *et al.* 1979). Similarly, copies of the breastfeeding policies enclosed with the completed questionnaires in the national survey conducted by Garcia *et al.* (1987) revealed many interpretations of the term 'demand feeding'. These ranged from instructions that babies should be fed whenever they wished for as long as they wished; to the imposition of restrictions concerning both the frequency and duration of feeds, and feeding at night. Discrepancies were found not only between policies and practise, but in practises in different parts of a single institution.

It would appear, therefore, that even if policy makers are convinced by the evidence that individual babies know better than anyone else when they need to be fed, there is still a need, in some institutions, for more intensive policy discussions and in-service training to ensure that a policy that supports and encourages flexible breastfeeding is translated effectively into practice.

5 'Supplementing' the baby

The practice of giving normal breastfeeding babies supplementary feeds of water, glucose, or formula is widespread (Martin and Monk 1982; Nicoll *et al.* 1982; Winikoff 1986; Garforth and Garcia, in press). In a survey of babies under the care of 20 paediatricians selected at random, Nicoll *et al.* (1982) found that 79 per cent of breastfed babies aged between 2 and 6 days had received some kind of supplementary feed. The survey conducted by Garcia and her colleagues (1987) revealed that it was the policy to give normal breastfed infants additional fluids of some sort in 70 per cent of the specialist obstetric units in England (Garforth and Garcia, in press).

The professionals surveyed in these two studies gave a variety of reasons for their prescription of additional fluid or formula. These included thirst (and hot weather); jaundice; and hunger—either because lactation had not yet been established, or because it had been deemed to have 'failed'.

There is no evidence to support the use of supplements of fluids or formula routinely for any of these reasons. A healthy baby has no need for large volumes of fluid any earlier than these become available physiologically from the breast (Houston *et al.* 1983; Saint *et al.* 1984; Casey *et al.* 1986). The idea that breastfed babies require extra fluid in hot weather is contradicted by the results of research showing that healthy babies who are entirely breastfed are able to regulate their own fluid intake and urine osmolarity successfully under extreme climatic conditions (Amroth 1978; Goldberg and Adams 1983; Brown *et al.* 1986). Neither is there any evidence to support the widespread belief that giving additional fluids to breastfed babies prevents or helps to resolve physiological jaundice. In the only randomized controlled trial to have examined the question (Nicoll *et al.* 1982), there was no statistically significant reduction in mean plasma bilirubin levels associated with giving water supplements, nor any evidence that babies receiving extra fluids were any less likely to develop 'breast-milk jaundice' or require

phototherapy. Non-randomized cohort studies have come to similar conclusions (Carvalho *et al.* 1981; Herrera 1984).

The practice of giving breastfed babies formula while lactation is becoming established is also misconceived and unsupported by evidence. De Chateau and his colleagues (1977) reported a randomized evaluation of 'routine care', which involved test weighing followed by supplementation with breast milk substitute or pasteurized breast-milk to a predetermined amount; the care received by the comparison group consisted of

Table 80.5 Effect of provision of formula supplements to breastfed newborns on stopping breastfeeding before 9 weeks postpartum

Study	EXPT n	(%)	CTRL n	(%)	Odds ratio (95% CI)	Graph of odds ratios and confidence intervals
Gray-Donald *et al.* (1985)	121/393	(30.79)	151/388	(38.92)	0.70 (0.52–0.94)	
Typical odds ratio (95% confidence interval)					0.70 (0.52–0.94)	

Effect of provision of formula supplements to breastfed newborns on not fully breastfeeding 9 weeks postpartum

Study	EXPT n	(%)	CTRL n	(%)	Odds ratio (95% CI)	
Gray-Donald *et al.* (1985)	255/393	(64.89)	248/388	(63.92)	1.04 (0.78–1.40)	
Typical odds ratio (95% confidence interval)					1.04 (0.78–1.40)	

Table 80.6 Effect of giving free formula samples to breastfeeding mothers on stopping breastfeeding 4–6 weeks postpartum

Study	EXPT n	(%)	CTRL n	(%)	Odds ratio (95% CI)	
Bergevin *et al.* (1983)	47/212	(22.17)	31/194	(15.98)	1.49 (0.91–2.44)	
Frank *et al.* (1987)	57/167	(34.13)	42/157	(26.75)	1.41 (0.88–2.27)	
Evans *et al.* (1986)	19/55	(34.55)	10/40	(25.00)	1.56 (0.65–3.76)	
Feinstein *et al.* (1986)	12/76	(15.79)	11/90	(12.22)	1.35 (0.56–3.25)	
Typical odds ratio (95% confidence interval)					1.45 (1.07–1.96)	

Effect of giving free formula samples to breastfeeding mothers on stopping breastfeeding 10–14 weeks postpartum

Study	EXPT n	(%)	CTRL n	(%)	Odds ratio (95% CI)	
Bergevin *et al.* (1983)	85/212	(40.09)	74/194	(38.14)	1.09 (0.73–1.62)	
Frank *et al.* (1987)	155/167	(92.81)	122/157	(77.71)	3.37 (1.82–6.25)	
Feinstein *et al.* (1986)	21/76	(27.63)	25/90	(27.78)	0.99 (0.50–1.96)	
Typical odds ratio (95% confidence interval)					1.39 (1.03–1.88)	

encouraging mothers to feel that their own milk and colostrum were quite adequate and to withhold supplements from their babies. Women receiving the 'routine' care were five times more likely to give up breastfeeding in the first week, and twice as likely to abandon it during the second week (Table 80.5). It is interesting to note that mothers in the 'no supplement' group were ready to accept that breastfeeding alone was adequate, even though the midwifery staff were very uncertain about this when the practice was first introduced. The results of this randomized trial have been supported by similar observations made in non-randomized studies (Herrera 1984; Gray-Donald *et al.* 1985).

The psychological effect upon the mother of any practice which suggests that her milk may not be sufficient will undermine her confidence, a factor which is undoubtedly crucial to breastfeeding success but difficult to quantify. The use of supplements sets a precedent for acceptable feeding patterns which a vulnerable new mother is likely to continue at home (Neifert and Seacat 1985).

Finally, giving breast-milk substitutes derived from cows' milk may interfere with the operation and development of normal immunological mechanisms (McClelland *et al.* 1978; Chandra 1985).

The fact that the practice of giving formula feeds to breastfed babies is more likely to do harm than good means that resources used in this way are wasted. Nicoll *et al.* (1982) have estimated that, at 1980 prices, a hospital which delivered 5000 babies per year, of which 70 per cent were initially breastfed, paid £7000 per year for prepacked supplementary feeds in disposable bottles.

Those hospitals which allow breastfeeding mothers to be given free samples of formula also prejudice the chances of successful establishment and maintainance of breastfeeding. The four randomized evaluations of this policy show that it increases the chances that breastfeeding will have been abandoned within a few weeks of delivery (Table 80.6).

6 'Supplementing' the mother

Advice given to breastfeeding women concerning their own fluid intake has been inconsistent and has led to confusion and misinformation. As early as 1940, Olsen began to question the widespread advice given to breastfeeding women to drink more than their thirst dictated. He observed that if ingesting additional fluid is a logical way of making mammary glands produce more milk, then it should similarly be expected to make the lachrimal glands produce floods of tears. He added that in his home country of Denmark, where great efforts were being made to maximize dairy milk production, it had never been suggested that milk yield could be increased by forcing cows to consume more

water than their thirst led them to drink spontaneously.

Olsen (1940) went on to conduct the earliest of a number of controlled studies, none of which has produced any support for the idea that increased fluid intake by breastfeeding mothers results in improved lactation (Illingworth and Kilpatrick 1953; Dearlove and Dearlove 1981; Dusdieker *et al.* 1985). Some women find drinking when they are not thirsty positively unpleasant (Dusdieker *et al.* 1985); indeed, Olsen (1940) reported that women felt 'turgid' and 'unwell' during fluid loading. Furthermore, Dearlove and Dearlove (1981) note that women with perineal and labial trauma may have their discomfort increased by the increased diuresis associated with greater fluid intake.

7 The effects of combined oestrogen/progestogen contraceptives

The effects of combined oestrogen/progestogen contraceptives on lactation and breastfeeding have been studied in 7 controlled trials (Semm 1966; Kaern 1967; Abdel Kader *et al.* 1969; Miller and Hughes 1970; Kamal *et al.* 1970; Borglin and Sandholm 1971; Koetsawang *et al.* 1972). Combined oestrogen/progestogen contraceptives may affect the composition of breastmilk: in the trial reported by Abdel Kader *et al.* (1969), contraceptive use was associated with statistically significant reductions in the protein, fat, sodium, potassium, magnesium, phosphorus, and calcium content of milk.

The results of trials in which attempts were made to estimate milk volume in women using combined oestrogen/progestogen contraceptives and controls are confusing, probably because of the limitations inherent in the methods used to estimate milk volume (see Chapter 81). The available data from the trials that have assessed the effects of combined oestrogen/progestogen contraceptives on breastfeeding success are consistent, however. These drugs increase the incidence of both breastfeeding failure and supplementation with breastmilk substitutes (Table 80.7). Although the report of the trial conducted by Miller and Hughes (1970) provided no details of the number of women in the comparison groups who gave supplements, they reported that, 4–5 weeks postpartum, the mean calorie intake provided in supplements was at least twice as great in babies whose mothers were taking combined oestrogen/progestogen contraceptives as it was among controls.

All the evidence from the 7 available controlled trials suggests that combined oestrogen/progestogen contraceptives are unsuitable for women who wish to breastfeed their babies. This finding is obviously of particular importance in parts of the world in which use of breastmilk substitutes poses a threat to infant life and health. It is also important to remember that lactation itself,

Table 80.7 Effect of combined oestrogen/progestogen contraceptive in breastfeeding on stopping breastfeeding within 3–4 months

Study	EXPT		CTRL		Odds ratio	Graph of odds ratios and confidence intervals						
	n	(%)	n	(%)	(95% CI)	0.01	0.1	0.5	1	2	10	100
Koetsawang *et al.* (1972)	4/40	(10.00)	0/20	(0.00)	4.86 (0.57–41.03)							
Miller and Hughes (1970)	19/24	(79.17)	13/48	(27.08)	8.01 (3.01–21.31)							
Typical odds ratio (95% confidence interval)					7.34 (3.01–17.87)							

Effect of combined oestrogen/progestogen contraceptive in breastfeeding mothers on introduction of breast-milk substitutes

Study	EXPT		CTRL		Odds ratio							
Kaern (1967)	26/212	(12.26)	7/206	(3.40)	3.37 (1.66– 6.87)							
Koetsawang *et al.* (1972)	6/40	(15.00)	0/20	(0.00)	5.15 (0.87–30.36)							
Typical odds ratio (95% confidence interval)					3.58 (1.85–6.92)							

particularly if breastfeeeding is unrestricted, has a contraceptive effect (Potter *et al* 1965; Berman *et al* 1972; Howie *et al*. 1982a,b; Howie and McNeilly 1982; Glasier *et al*. 1984). Indeed, Rosa (1975) has estimated that, in developing countries, breastfeeding prevents more pregnancies than all other methods of contraception combined. If women wishing to breastfeed also wish to enhance the contraceptive effect of lactation itself, they should do so without recourse to hormonal preparations containing both oestrogens and progestogens.

8 Supporting breastfeeding mothers and babies

Since only a very small minority of women and babies are physiologically incapable of breastfeeding successfully (Neifert 1983; Chetley 1986), it might be presumed that the initial decision to breastfeed was the most crucial determinant of whether or not full breastfeeding continues for the widely recommended period of 4–5 months. Yet it is clear that a large proportion of women who wish to breastfeed begin to do so, but discontinue long before their babies are 4 months old (Sjolin *et al.* 1979; Martin and Monk 1982; Kaplowitz and Olson 1983; Ross *et al.* 1983). Perhaps the most important factor in the efforts to achieve successful breastfeeding is that those who attempt it should succeed. The evolutionary advantages of such positive feedback are seen in other areas of social behaviour (Dawkins 1986). As shown above, many of the problems that confront women who are trying to breastfeed are avoidable. The evidence suggests that fewer women would experience these problems if all breastfeeding women had access to accurate information, and appro-

priate and practical help and support when required. More pregnant women would then know of others who had breastfed and succeeded, and might be more confident that they themselves would succeed.

Although some of the knowledge required to breastfeed successfully is instinctive, much of it is socially acquired by observation and experience; in other words it is a learned activity. Success will therefore depend to a large extent both on what women learn, and on the support and skilled teaching that they receive while they are learning (Morgan 1985; Jones *et al.* 1986a). Both the baby and the baby's father can be important sources of encouragement to the mother in her breastfeeding attempts (Beske and Garvis 1982; Wiles 1984; Jones *et al.* 1986b). Similarly, the mother's own mother has been identified as an important source of encouragement if she herself has breastfed (and conversely, an important source of discouragement if she has not) (Jones *et al.* 1986b; Beske and Garvis 1982).

There have been few formal attempts to evaluate the effectiveness of alternative methods of conveying information about breastfeeding. The results of one randomized trial (Johnson *et al.* 1984) are uninterpretable because of differential and substantial losses to follow-up from the three randomized cohorts. In another controlled trial, mothers who attended a 20–30 minute group meeting (supported by an information sheet then and at the first postnatal visit) were less likely than controls to have introduced solids to their babies' diets within 4 months of birth (Adam *et al.* 1985).

A number of controlled trials have assessed the effects of various forms of support for breastfeeding mothers (Sjolin *et al.* 1979; Bloom 1982; Jones and West 1985, 1986; Lynch *et al.* 1986; Grossman *et al.* 1987; Frank *et al.* 1987; Moore *et al.* 1987). Two of

Table 80.8 Effect of postnatal support for breastfeeding mothers on stopping breastfeeding before 8–12 weeks

Study	EXPT		CTRL		Odds ratio	Graph of odds ratios and confidence intervals
	n	(%)	n	(%)	(95% CI)	0.01 0.1 0.5 1 2 10 100
Lynch *et al.* (1986)	47/135	(34.81)	47/135	(34.81)	1.00 (0.61–1.65)	
Frank *et al.* (1987)	105/163	(64.42)	122/161	(75.78)	0.58 (0.36–0.94)	
Grossman *et al.* (1987)	28/38	(73.68)	25/38	(65.79)	1.45 (0.55–3.82)	
Sjolin *et al.* (1979)	16/75	(21.33)	24/71	(33.80)	0.54 (0.26–1.11)	
Jones and West (1985)	87/228	(38.16)	180/355	(50.70)	0.60 (0.43–0.84)	
Moore *et al.* (1985)	192/250	(76.80)	210/275	(76.36)	1.02 (0.68–1.53)	
Typical odds ratio (95% confidence interval)					0.75 (0.62–0.91)	

these trials (Grossman *et al.* 1987; Moore *et al.* 1987) failed to detect any short term beneficial effect of the supportive interventions on breastfeeding success or duration; indeed, in the trial involving women of low socioeconomic status reported by Grossman *et al.* (1987), the intervention group were less likely than controls to be breastfeeding 3 months after delivery. The results of the remaining 5 trials, however, suggest that the duration of breastfeeding can be increased by regular and frequent contact with mother by the same caretaker, either in person or by visits followed by telephoning. In the light of these findings (Table 80.8) it seems reasonable to conclude that advice and support for mothers who wish to breastfeed can be important in helping them to achieve their objectives, but that this this may not necessarily always be the case. Obviously, if the advice given is flawed (in the ways described earlier in this chapter) it is unlikely to be helpful. Furthermore, helping women of low socioeconomic status to establish and maintain breastfeeding may present a particular challenge (Beske and Garvis 1982).

9 Conclusions

9.1 Implications for current practice

Those who care for women during pregnancy and childbirth have a crucial role to play in enabling a woman to breastfeed successfully. Now that sound, research-based information is readily available to them, the professional ignorance which may have been acceptable in the past is no longer tolerable (Minchin 1985). If the potential for helping women to breastfeed their babies is to be realized, professionals must reject much of the received wisdom in this field and pass on to women only those practices which have been demonstrated to be effective.

Those who are most likely to be closely involved with mothers at the time that breastfeeding is becoming established should have a clear understanding of how a baby breastfeeds. They should recognize that although separation of babies from their mothers after delivery jeopardizes the successful establishment of lactation, there is no evidence to suggest that the timing of the first feed, in itself, is crucial to success.

Professionals should know how a mother can be helped to position her baby correctly on the breast. They should impose no restrictions on the duration or the frequency of feeds, and neither offer nor recommend additional fluids or formula for healthy breastfed babies, particularly by giving free samples of formula to women in hospital.

Normal lactating women with access to adequate fluid can depend on their thirst to regulate fluid intake effectively. Urging women to drink more than their thirst dictates has no justification.

Use of combined oestrogen/progestogen contraceptives compromises lactation. If women wishing to breastfeed also wish to enhance the contraceptive effect of lactation itself, they should do so without recourse to hormonal preparations containing both oestrogens and progestogens.

Women can be helped to establish and maintain breastfeeding in a number of ways, but the experimentally-derived evidence suggests that continuity of personal support from an individual who is knowledgeable about breastfeeding is most effective.

9.2 Implications for future research

This review has demonstrated that little is known about the spontaneous breastfeeding behaviour of mothers and babies. Women have been subjected to a series of practices many of which have been shown to be ineffective. Future research should therefore concentrate on two areas of investigation. First, there is a need to expand the existing observations on the normal spontaneous breastfeeding behaviour of mothers and babies. This would result in a growth of knowledge about the range of normal feeding behaviour which would be important, both in helping normal mothers and babies, and in identifying and treating mothers and babies with genuine problems.

Second, there is need to ascertain why professional behaviour has remained so deeply affected by unfounded assumptions, in spite of the obvious detrimental effect these assumptions have had on breastfeeding. This would provide a basis for studies examining how best to change clinical behaviour so that it takes account of knowledge and understanding rather than received 'wisdom'.

When both these areas have been thoroughly investigated, it will become possible, for the first time this century, to measure the incidence of problems with breastfeeding that are not attributable to the misguided practices that are still so widespread. Treatments for these problems could then be tested.

References

Abdel Kader MM, Abdel Hay A, El-Safouri S, Abdel Aziz MT, Saad El-din J, Kamal I, Hefnawi F, Ghoneim M, Talaat M, Younis N, Tagui A, Abdalla M (1969). Biochemical and experimental studies on lactation. III. Clinical changes induced in human milk be gestagens. Am J Obstet Gynaecol, 105: 978–985.

Adam HM, Stern EK, Stein REK, (1985). Anticipatory guidance: A modest intervention in the nursery. Pediatrics, 76: 781–786.

Adran GM, Kemp FH, Lind J (1958). A cineradiographic study of breast feeding. Br J Radiol, 31: 156–162.

Ajayi V (1980). The normal infant. In: Textbook of Midwifery. London: Macmillan International College Edns., p 145.

Aldrich CA (1939). Role of gratification in early development. J Pediatr, 15: 578–582.

Amroth SG (1978). Water requirements of breast-fed infants in a hot climate. Am J Clin Nutr, 31: 1154–1157.

Arabin B, Ruttgers H, Kubli F (1986). Effects of routine administration of methylergometrin during the puerperium on involution, maternal morbidity and lactation. Geburtsh Frauenheilkd, 46: 215–220.

Arneil G, Stroud C (1984). Infant feeding. In: Textbook of Paediatrics (3rd edn) Vol. I. Forfar JO, Arneil G (eds). Edinburgh: Churchill Livingstone, pp 259–277.

Bergevin Y, Dougherty C, Kramer MS (1983). Do infant formula samples shorten the duration of breast feeding? Lancet, 1: 1148–1151.

Berman ML, Hanson K, Hellman IL (1972). Effect of breastfeeding on postpartum menstruation, ovulation and pregnancy in Alaskan Eskimos. Am J Obstet Gynecol, 114: 524–534.

Beske EJ, Garvis MS (1982). Important factors in breastfeeding success. Matern Child Nurs J, 7: 174–179.

Bloom K, Goldbloom RB, Robinson SC, Stevens SE (1982). Factors affecting the continuance of breastfeeding. Acta Paediatr Scand (Suppl), 300: 9–14.

Borglin NE, Sandholm LE (1971). Effect of oral contraceptives on lactation. Fertil Steril, 22: 39–41.

Brown KH, Creed de Kanashiro H, Aguila R, Lopez de Romana G, Black R (1986). Milk consumption and hydration status of exclusively breastfed infants in a warm climate. Pediatrics, 108: 677–680.

Budin PC (1907). The Nursling. London: Caxton.

Carvalho M, Hall M, Harvey D (1981). Effects of water supplementation on physiological jaundice in breast-fed babies. Arch Dis Child, 56: 568–569.

Carvalho M, Robertson S, Merkatz R, Klaus M (1982). Milk intake and frequency of feeding in breastfed infants. Early Hum Dev, 7: 155–163.

Carvalho M, Robertson S, Friedman A, Klaus M (1983). Effect of frequent breastfeeding on early milk production and infant weight gain. Pediatrics, 72: 307–311.

Carvalho M, Robertson S, Klaus M (1984). Does the duration and frequency of early breastfeeding affect nipple pain? Birth, 11: 81–84.

Casey CE, Neifert MR, Seacat JM, Neville MC (1986). Nutrient intake by breastfed infants during the first five days after birth. Am J Dis Child, 140: 933–936.

Chandra RK, Puri S, Cheema PS (1985). Predictive value of cord blood IgE in the development of aptoic disease and role of breastfeeding in its promotion. Clin Allergy, 15: 517–522.

Chavasse J (1906). Chavasse's Advice to Mothers (16th edn). London: Churchill.

Chetley A (1986). The Politics of Babyfood—Successful Challenges to International Marketing Strategy. London: Francis Pinter.

Close S (1976). The Know-How of Breastfeeding. Bristol: John Wright, p 17.

Cran DHD (1913). Breastfeeding: Dr. Variot's teaching. Lancet, 14 June: 1659.

Culley P, Milan P, Roginski C, Waterhouse J, Wood B (1979). Are breastfed babies still getting a raw deal in hospital? Br Med J, 2: 891–893.

Dawkins R (1986). The Blind Watchmaker. Essex: Longman, pp 196–199.

de Chateau P, Holmberg H, Jakobsson K, Winberg J (1977). A study of factors promoting and inhibiting lactation. Dev Med Child Neurol, 19: 575–584. (See also Winberg and de Chateau 1979.)

Dearlove JC, Dearlove BM (1981). Prolactin, fluid balance and lactation. Br J Obstet Gynaecol, 88: 652–654.

Dusdieker LB, Booth BM, Stumbo PJ, Eichenberger JM (1985). Effect of supplemental fluids on human milk production. J Paediatr, 106: 207–211.

Elander G, Lindberg T (1986). Hospital routines in infants with hyperbilirubinemia influence the duration of breastfeeding. Acta Paediatr Scand, 75: 708–712.

Evans CJ, Lyons NB, Killien MG (1986). The effect of infant

formula samples on breastfeeding practices. J Obstet Gynecol Neonatal Nurs, 15: 401–405.

Feinstein JM, Berkelhamer JE, Gruszka ME, Wong CA, Carey AE (1986). Factors related to early termination of breastfeeding in an urban population. Pediatrics, 78: 210–215.

Fisher C (1981). Breastfeeding. Midwife's view. J Matern Child Health, Feb: 52–56.

Fisher C (1987). Difficulties with breastfeeding—midwives in disarray? J R Soc Med, 80: 53–58. (Cited in Inch 1987.)

Fomon SJ, Filer LJ, Thomas LN, Anderson TA, Nelson SE (1972). Influence of formula concentration on caloric intake and growth of normal infants. Acta Paediatr Scand, 64: 172–181.

Frank DA, Wintz SJ, Sorenson JR, Heeren T (1987). Commercial discharge packs and breast-feeding counselling: Effects on infant-feeding practices in a randomized trial. Pediatrics, 80: 845–854.

Gans B (1958). Breast and nipple pain in early stages of lactation. Br Med J, 4: 830–834.

Garcia J, Garforth S, Ayers S (1987). The policy and practice of midwifery study: Introduction and methods. Midwifery, 3: 2–9.

Garforth S, Garcia J (1989). Breastfeeding policies in practice: no wonder they get confused. Midwifery, 5: 75–83.

Glasier AS, McNeilly AS, Howie PW (1984). The prolactin response to suckling. Clin Endocrinol, 21: 109–116.

Goldberg NM, Adams E (1983). Supplementary water for breast-fed babies in a hot and dry climate—not really a necessity. Arch Dis Child, 58: 73–74.

Gray-Donald K, Kramer MS, Munday S, Leduc DG (1985). Effect of formula supplementation in the hospital on the duration of breast-feeding: A controlled clinical trial. Paediatrics, 75: 514–518.

Grossman LK, Harter C, Kay A (1987). Postpartum lactation counseling for low-income women. Am J Dis Child, 141: 375.

Gunther M (1945). Sore nipples: Causes and prevention. Lancet, 2: 590–593.

Hall B (1975). Changing composition of milk and early development of an appetite control. Lancet, 1: 779–781.

Hardyment C (1983). Dream Babies. London: Cape, p 125.

Hawken J (1982). Unpublished observations.

Herrera AJ (1984). Supplemented versus unsupplemented breastfeeding. Perinatology-Neonatology, 8: 70–71.

Houston MJ, Howie PW, McNeilly AS (1983). Factors affecting the duration of breastfeeding; I. Measurement of breast milk intake in the first week of life. Early Hum Dev, 8: 49–54.

Howie PW, McNeilly AS (1982). Effect of breastfeeding patterns on human birth intervals. J Reprod Fertil, 65: 545–557.

Howie PW, Houston MJ, Cook A, Smart L, McArdle T, McNeilly AS (1981). How long should a breastfeed last? Early Hum Dev, 5: 71–77.

Howie PW, McNeilly AS, Houston MJ, Cook A, Boyle H (1982a). Fertility after childbirth: Infant feeding patterns, basal prolactin levels and postpartum ovulation. Clin Endocrinol, 17: 315–322.

Howie PW, McNeilly AS, Houston MJ, Cook A, Boyle H (1982b). Fertility after childbirth: Postpartum ovulation and menstruation in bottle and breastfeeding mothers. Clin Endocrinol, 17: 323–332.

Hytten F (1954). Clinical studies in lactation; II: Variation in the major constituents during a feeding. Br Med J, 1: 176–179.

Illingworth RS, Stone DG (1952). Self-demand feeding in a maternity unit. Lancet, 1: 683–687.

Illingworth RS, Kilpatrick B (1953). Lactation and fluid intake. Lancet, 2: 1175–1177.

Inch S (1980). Unpublished observations

Inch S (1987). Difficulties with breastfeeding—midwives in disarray? J R Soc Med, 80: 53–58.

Jelliffe DB, Jelliffe EFP (1978). Human Milk in the Modern World. Oxford: Oxford University Press, p 6.

Johnson CA, Garza C, Nichols B (1984). A teaching intervention to improve breastfeeding success. J Nutr Educ, 16: 19–22.

Johnson NW (1976). Breast feeding at one hour of age. Am J Matern Child Nurs, 1: 12–16.

Jones DA, West RR (1985). Lactation nurse increases duration of breastfeeding. Arch Dis Child, 60: 772–774.

Jones DA, West RR (1986). Effect of a lactation nurse on the success of breast-feeding: A randomized controlled trial. J Epidemiol Community Health, 40: 45–49.

Jones DA, West RR, Newcombe RG (1986). Maternal characteristics associated with the duration of breastfeeding. Midwifery, 2: 141–146.

Kaern T (1967). Effect of an oral contraceptive immediately post-partum on initiation of lactation. Br Med J, 3: 644–645.

Kamal I, Hefnawi F, Ghoneim M, Abdallah MS, Abdel Razek S (1970). Biochemical and experimental studies on lactation. IV. Clinical effect of steroids on the initiation of lactation. Am J Obstet Gynecol, 108: 655–658.

Kaplowitz DD, Olson CM (1983). The effect of an education program on the decision to breastfeed. J Nutr Educ, 15: 61–65.

Koetsawang S, Bhiraleus P, Chiemprajert T (1972). Effects of oral contraceptives on lactation. Fertil Steril, 23: 24–28.

King FT (1913). Feeding and Care of the Baby. London: Macmillan.

King FT (1918). The Natural Feeding of Infants. London: Whitcombe & Tombs.

King FT (1924). The Expectant Mother and Baby's First Month. London: Macmillan.

Kochenour NK (1980). Lactation suppression. Clin Obstet Gynaecol, 23: 1045–1059.

Kron RE, Stein M, Goddard KE (1966). Newborn sucking behaviour affected by obstetric sedation. Pediatrics, 37: 1012–1015.

Langmead F (1916). Mothercraft. Chapter 5: Breastfeeding. The National League for Physical Education and Improvement.

Langton JH (1929). Our Baby for Mothers and Nurses. Bristol: John Wright.

Lewis J (1980). The Politics of Motherhood. London: Croom Helm, pp 71–73.

Liddiard M (1924). The Mothercraft Manual. London: Churchill.

Lucas A, Lucas PJ, Baum JD (1979). Patterns of milk flow in breastfed babies. Lancet, 2: 57–59.

Lynch SA, Koch AM, Hislop TG, Goldman AJ (1986). Evaluating the effect of a breastfeeding consultant on the duration of breastfeeding. Can J Public Health, 77: 190–195.

Martin J, Monk J (1982). Infant Feeding 1980. Office of Population Censuses and Surveys, Social Survey Division, pp 40–44.

McClelland DBL, McGrath J, Samson RR (1978). Antimicrobial factors in human milk. Acta Paediatr Scand (Suppl): 271.

Miller GH, Hughes LR (1970). Lactation and genital involution effects of a new low-dose oral contraceptive on breastfeeding mothers and their infants. Obstet Gynecol, 35: 44–50.

Minchin M (1985). Breastfeeding Matters. Victoria, Australia: Alma Publications and Australia: Allen & Unwin.

Morgan E (1985). The Descent of Woman. London: Souvenir Press.

Moore WJ, Midwinter RE, Morris AF, Colley JRT, Soothill JF (1985). Infant feeding and subsequent risk of atopic eczema. Arch Dis Child, 60: 722–726.

Naish L (1913). Breastfeeding—its management and mismanagement. Lancet, 1: 1657–1659.

Niefert MR (1983). Infant problems in breastfeeding. In: Lactation. Neville MC, Niefert MR (eds). New York: Plenum Press.

Neifert MR, Seacat JM (1985). Contemporary breastfeeding management. Clin Perinatol, 12: 319–342.

Newton N (1952). Nipple pain and nipple damage. J Paediatr, 41: 411–423.

Nicoll A, Ginsburg R, Tripp JH (1982). Supplementary feeding and jaundice in newborns. Acta Paediatr Scand, 72: 759–761.

Olmsted RW, Jackson EB (1950). Self demand feeding in the first week of life. Pediatrics, 6: 396–401.

Olsen A (1940) Nursing under conditions of thirst or excessive ingestion of fluids. Acta Obstet Gynaecol Scand, 20: 313–343.

Potter RG, New ML, Wyon JB, Gordon JE (1965). Appreciations of field studies to research in physiology of human reproduction. J Chronic Dis, 18: 1125–1140.

Pritchard EL (1904). The Physiological Feeding of Infants. London: Henry Kempton.

Pritchard EL (1907). Infant Education. London: Marylebone Health Society.

Rice I (1987). Breastfeeding: A Heartstart. New York: Dell Books.

Rosa FW (1975). The role of breastfeeding in family planning. Protein Advisory Group, Bulletin 5, Part 3: 5–10.

Ross SM, Loening WEK, van Middlekoop A (1983). Breastfeeding—evaluation of a health education programme. SA Medlese Tydskrif Deel, 64: 361–362.

Rotch TM (1895). Paediatrics—the hygienic and medical treatment of children. Philadelphia: Lippincott, p 162.

Saint L, Smith M, Hartman PE (1984). The yield and nutrient content of colostrum and milk of women giving birth to one month postpartum. Br J Nutr, 52: 87–95.

Salariya EM, Easton PM, Cater JI (1978). Duration of breastfeeding after early initiation and frequent feeding. Lancet, 2: 1141–1143.

Salber EJ (1956). The effect of different feeding schedules on the growth of Bantu babies in the first week of life. J Trop Pediatr, Sept: 97–102.

Semm K (1966). Contraception and lactation. In: Social and Medical Aspects of Lactation. Round Table Conference held in Scheveningen, The Netherlands, May 1966. Amsterdam: Excerpta Medica Foundation, pp 98–101.

Serjeant H (1905). Hints For Infant Feeding. London: Elliot Stock, p 4.

Shane JM, Naftolin F (1974). Effect of ergonovine maleate on puerperal prolactin. Am J Obstet Gynecol, 120: 129–131.

Simsarian FP, McLendon PA (1942). Feeding behaviour of an infant during the first twelve weeks of life on a self-demand schedule. J Pediatr, 20: 93–103.

Simsarian FP, McLendon PA (1945). Further records of the self-demand schedule in infant feeding. J Pediatr, 27: 109–114.

Sjolin S, Hofvander Y, Hilleervik C (1979). A prospective study of individual courses of breastfeeding. Acta Paediatr Scand, 68: 521–529.

Slaven S, Harvey D (1981). Unlimited sucking time improves breastfeeding. Lancet, 1: 392–393.

Sosa R, Kennell JH, Klaus MH, Urrutia JJ (1976). The effect of early mother infant contact on breast feeding, infection and growth. In: Breastfeeding and The Mother. Ciba Foundation Symposium 45, Amsterdam, pp 179–187.

Sousa PLR, Barros FC, Gazelle RV, Begeres RM, Pinheiro GN, Menezes ST, Arruda LA (1974). Attachment and Lactation. Proceedings of the 14th International Congress of Pediatricians, Buenos Aires, South America, pp 136–138.

Stoppard M (1982). Your Baby. London: Octopus Books, pp 75–76.

Sutherland JM, Glueck HI, Gleser G (1967). Hemorrhagic disease of the newborn: Breast feeding as a necessary factor in the pathogenesis. Am J Dis Child, 113: 524–433.

Symes JB (1984). A study on the effect of ergometrine on serum prolactin levels following delivery. J Obstet Gynaecol, 5: 36–38.

Taylor PM, Taylor FH, Campbell SB, Maloni JA, Cannon M (1985). 1. Extra early physical contact and aspects of the early mother-infant relationship. Acta Paediatr Scand, 1416: 3–14.

Thomson ME, Hartsock TG, Larson C (1979). The importance of immediate postnatal contact: Its effect on breastfeeding. Can Family Physician, 25: 1374–1378.

Varga L, Lutterbeck PM, Pryor JS, Wenner R, Erb H (1972). Suppression of puerperal lactation with an ergot alkaloid: A double-blind study. Br Med J, 2: 743–744.

Vincent R (1904). The Nutrition of the Infant (3rd edn). London: Baillière Tindall.

Vincent R (1913). The Nutrition of the Infant (4th edn). London: Baillière Tindall.

Von Kries R, Shearer M, McCarthy PT, Haug M, Harzer G, Gobel U (1987). Vitamin K1 content of maternal milk: Influence of the stage of lactation, lipid composition, and vitamin K1 supplements given to the mother. Paediatr Res, 22: 513–517.

Wahlberg V, Lundh W, Winberg J (1982). Reconsideration of Crede's prophylaxis: IV. Effects of silver nitrate on mother-infant relationship. Acta Paediatr Scand, (Suppl) 295: 49–57.

Weber F, Woolridge MW, Baum JD (1986). An ultrasographic analysis of sucking and swallowing in newborn infants. Dev Med Child Neurol, 28: 19–24.

Weiss G, Facog SK, Shenkman L, Kataoka K, Hollander CS (1975). Effect of methylergonovine on puerperal prolactin secretion. Obstet Gynaecol, 46: 209–210.

Widstrom A-M, Ransjo-Arvidson AB, Christensson K, Mattiesen A-S, Winberg J, Uvnas-Moberg K (1987). Gastric suction in healthy newborn infants: Effects on circulation and developing feeding behaviour. Acta Paediatr Scand, 76: 566–572.

Wiles LS (1984). The effect of prenatal breastfeeding education on breastfeeding success and maternal perception of the infant. J Obstet Gynecol Neonatal Nurs, 13: 253–257.

Winberg J, de Chateau P (1979). Attempts to increase breastfeeding. In: Psychosomatic Medicine in Obstetrics and Gynaecology, 5th International Congress: Rome. Zichella (ed). pp 851–854.

Winikoff B, Laukaran VH, Meyers D, Start R (1986). Dynamics of infant feeding, mothers, professionals and the institutional context in a large urban hospital. Pediatrics, 77: 357–365.

Woolridge MW, Baum JD, Drewett RF (1982). Individual patterns of milk intake during breastfeeding. Early Hum Dev, 7: 265–272.

Woolridge MW, Greasley V, Silpiornkosol S (1985). The initiation of lactation: The effect of early versus delayed contact for suckling on milk intake in the first week postpartum. A study in Chiang Mai, Northern Thailand. Early Hum Dev, 12: 269–278.

Woolridge MW (1986a). The anatomy of infant suckling. Midwifery, 2: 164–171.

Woolridge MW (1986b). Aetiology of sore nipples. Midwifery, 2: 172–176.

World Health Organization (1980). Provisional Summary Record of the 8th Meeting of Committee A, at the 33rd World Health Assembly, Geneva 1980. Geneva: World Health Organization, Document No. A33/A/SR/8, p 11 (cited in Chetley 1986).

81 Common breastfeeding problems

Sally Inch and Mary J. Renfrew

1 Introduction

Over the past two decades the incidence of initiation of breastfeeding has increased in many countries (World Health Organization 1982; Martin and Monk 1982; Fieldhouse 1984), but there is now evidence that it may be declining for the first time in twenty years (Martin and White 1988). This decline has been predicted by a number of authors (see, for example, Minchin 1985); if women try to breastfeed, and experience difficulty and pain, then it is likely that they will not choose to breastfeed again. In addition, their friends, family, and neighbours may be influenced by watching them struggling. Prevention and rapid, effective treatment of breastfeeding problems is thus of great importance.

The chapter on establishing and maintaining breastfeeding described how many of the common problems with breastfeeding are preventable because they are often caused by unnecessary interventions and inappropriate treatment (see Chapter 80). This chapter addresses the common problems of nipple trauma, engorgement, mastitis, and insufficient milk.

2 Nipple trauma

The most widely held explanation for the prevalence of nipple pain in industrialized cultures is the supposed thinness or sensitivity of the nipple epithelium. This probably explains the widespread belief that women with fair skin or red hair are more likely to experience problems, and there is some evidence to suggest that these beliefs may influence women's decisions about breastfeeding (Brockway 1986). Two of the four studies that have examined the association between hair and skin colour and nipple trauma reported that no relationship had been found, but no actual data were presented (Gans 1958; Brown and Hurlock 1975). One survey found no difference in the distribution of hair colour between mothers who had nipple problems and those who did not (Brockway 1986). The association reported in a small study reported by Atkinson (1978) was not statistically significant. There is no evidence to support the commonly held belief that fair-skinned and red-haired women are more vulnerable to nipple trauma than dark-haired or dark-skinned women. All women, regardless of the colour of their skin or hair, should receive skilled help with learning to breastfeed so that problems can be prevented.

As shown in the previous chapter, careful observations have demonstrated that sore nipples are a direct result of poor positioning of the baby at the breast (Ardran *et al.* 1958; Weber *et al.* 1986; Woolridge 1986a, 1986b; also Chapter 21). If the baby is not well-positioned, friction is applied to the nipple, and pain and trauma result. If the baby is well-positioned, breastfeeding should not hurt at all. The skill of positioning is not one that has been taught in midwifery, nursing, or medical training until very recently. It is unlikely that a new mother will be able to acquire this skill for herself as it is rare in industrialized cultures to see women breastfeeding. A further complicating factor is that virtually all diagrams of babies at the breast in books for midwives, doctors, and mothers are inaccurate (see, for example, Lawrence 1985; Riordan 1983; Messenger 1982). It is therefore not surprising that skill in positioning is now rare, as neither professionals nor mothers can learn from teaching, from example, or from reading.

There is no indication from any studies of the proportion of sore and damaged nipples that may be caused by positioning problems. Clinical experience in this field would suggest that this problem is the major cause of nipple damage (Fisher 1981). If this is the case then it follows that most nipple damage could be prevented by skilled and available care from the very first feed. The results of a recently completed controlled trial (Righard, personal communication) confirm the strong clinical impression that the treatment of sore and damaged nipples which result from positioning problems is simple: correct the positioning and the nipple trauma resolves rapidly.

If professionals have neither the time nor the experience necessary to pass on good breastfeeding techniques and prevent most nipple trauma, it is not surprising that, in their desire to do something, they turn to methods of treating the condition when it has occurred. These 'treatments' often take the form of mechanical aids, ointment, or sprays. Neither the methods of antenatal preparation, nor the postnatal use of ointments, tinctures, or sprays that have been evaluated have been shown to be of benefit in preventing nipple problems. Indeed, some may actually increase the possibility of damage (see Chapter 80). Some women and some professionals feel that they need to care for damaged nipples in some active way in addition to learning and implementing good positioning. In these circumstances putting colostrum or breastmilk on the damaged nipple is unlikely to do harm and may be of psychological benefit.

In a controlled trial comparing different approaches to the management of nipples that had become sore and damaged, Nicholson (1985) randomly allocated 90 women who were experiencing such problems to one of three treatment groups: discontinuation of breastfeeding with expression of milk from the affected breast until the nipple healed; the use of a nipple shield on the affected breast until the nipple healed; or continuation of breastfeeding on the affected breast with supervision and information on positioning the infant at the breast. No statistically significant differences in nipple healing were detected, but the nipple shield was less acceptable to women than the other two methods. As well as being unacceptable to the majority of women, the thick rubber nipple shields that are in common use have also been shown to reduce the amount of milk available to the baby. A randomized controlled trial which compared the effects of the traditional nipple shield with that of a thinner, latex one, and with no shield at all (Woolridge *et al.* 1980) found that milk transfer was reduced by 56 per cent in the case of the traditional shield (a statistically significant reduction) and 22 per cent in the case of the latex shield. Thus the use of a nipple shield for any length of time, even by those who find its use acceptable, may ultimately add to a mother's problems by gradually suppressing her milk production.

The only factor that has been shown to both prevent and treat nipple trauma is good positioning of the baby at the breast. Breastfeeding is a learned skill, and in common with other learned skills, it is unlikely that there will be any short cuts to its acquisition, and mothers, midwives, and other professionals should therefore devote their energies to ensuring they acquire the skill of good positioning as quickly as possible.

3 Problems with milk flow

A number of problems result from interference with milk flow from the breasts and the stasis of milk, blood, and lymph that results. The most common of these problems are engorgement and mastitis.

3.1 Engorgement

As with nipple soreness, the problems associated with breast engorgement have been documented for considerable time. Fildes (1979) notes that engorgement was recognized at least 200 years ago. At that time it was considered to be responsible for milk fever, abscesses, and even maternal death. Furthermore, then (Nelson 1753, cited in Fildes 1979) as now (Applebaum 1977), it was seen as being almost always iatrogenic—due to the hospital staff's management of mother and baby—as it was and is common only when mothers are restricted in responding to the spontaneous feeding behaviour of their babies (Minchin 1985).

If the milk is not removed as it is formed (as regulated by the baby's need to go to the breast) it is quite likely that, as milk production rapidly increases, the volume of milk in the breast will exceed the capacity of the alveoli to store it comfortably. Over-distension of the alveoli with milk 'engorgement' causes the individual milk-secreting cells to become flattened, drawn out, and even to rupture (Hammond 1936; Dawson 1935). In addition, the distension also partly or completely occludes the capillary circulation surrounding the alveolar cells, further reducing cellular activity (Dawson 1935). It might also, if severe, cause a secondary vascular engorgement, giving rise to what Waller described as 'engorgement with obstruction' (Waller 1946). Once the alveoli become distended, further milk production begins to be suppressed. As Minchin (1985) remarks 'failure to remove milk has only one significance in nature: the baby has died and the milk is therefore not required. It may take days of frequent suckling to reverse that message and build up an adequate supply'.

The evidence reviewed in the chapter on establishing and maintaining breastfeeding (see Chapter 80) demonstrates that engorgement results from limitations on feeding frequency and duration, and from problems with positioning the baby at the breast. Both Illingworth and Stone (1952) and L'Esperance (1980) found a positive association between sore nipples and engorgement. It might therefore be the case that either nipples become sore because the baby is not able to take an adequate mouthful of an engorged breast, or that the baby who is incorrectly positioned at the breast will not only make the nipples sore, but will cause the breast to become engorged due to inefficient drainage of milk and stimulation of the milk ejection reflex. Babies who are not properly positioned at the breast will not 'switch' quickly from the short bursts of sucking evident when they first go to the breast to the longer, slow sucking which begins when the milk ejection reflex is stimulated (see Chapter 80). The results of the controlled study by Illingworth and Stone (1952) suggest that in the absence of any restrictions on feeding frequency, the latter mechanism is more likely to operate. The most appropriate form of treatment for engorgement (as well as prevention) is thus to ensure that the baby is correctly positioned at the breast when feeding.

A number of different treatments for engorgement have been advocated. In addition to allowing the baby unrestricted access to the breast, these include: moist heat and icepacks (neither of which have been rigorously tested); oxytocin; manual expression of milk; proteolytic enzymes; stilboestrol; and binding of the breasts. The only published controlled evaluation of the effects of oxytocin on engorgement (Ingelman-Sundberg 1953) failed to find any beneficial effect of oxytocin in relieving engorgement, and another, unreported trial arrived at similar conclusions (D Hawkins, personal communication). The studies reported by Waller (1946) and Blaikeley *et al.* (1953) seem to indicate that manual expression, started antenatally and continued postnatally, will help to relieve engorgement and increase the duration of breastfeeding (see Chapter 80). However, both of these studies were carried out under conditions where feeding was restricted and engorgement was, as a result, very common.

Two interesting studies suggest that oral proteolytic enzymes may provide effective relief for women with engorged breasts. Murata *et al.* (1965) and Koshiishi (1971), who subscribed to the view that early postnatal engorgement was largely venous and lymphatic in origin, treated the women in their double-blind trials with oral doses of two proteolytic enzymes in a single tablet, and compared the outcomes with that experienced by women who were given a placebo of enteric-coated lactose. Although the therapeutic effectiveness of the enzymes in question (Bromelain 20 000 units, Trypsin 2500 units) is in doubt (British National Formulary 1981a), these enzymes are claimed to relieve soft-tissue inflammation caused by bruising, swelling, or trauma, by removing exudate as well as coagulated blood and

necrotic tissue. In both trials, women who had evident breast pain, swelling, and tenderness between days 2 and 4 (Koshiishi *et al.* 1971) or 3 and 5 (Murata *et al.* 1985), were randomly allocated to receive three daily doses of active or placebo tablets. Both trials found a statistically significant improvement in the groups receiving the proteolytic enzymes.

Allowing the baby unrestricted access to the breast appears to be the most effective method of preventing and treating engorgement (Illingworth and Stone 1952; see Chapter 80). If the baby is given unrestricted access to the mother's breast from birth, prolactin levels are increased (Tyson *et al.* 1977) and small quantities of milk are removed through milk ejection as soon as they are formed. Just as importantly, mother and infant have an opportunity to learn to breastfeed effectively while the breasts are still soft, the baby still has nutritional reserves, and the elevated prolactin levels are not yet wholly dependent on efficient suckling.

Treatment of severe engorgement has included both administration of stilboestrol and binding of the breasts. In the 1940s and 1950s, if expression did not prevent or cure engorgement, stilboestrol, up to 20 to 25 mg every 4 hours was the treatment of choice (Blaikeley *et al.* 1953; Waller 1946; Gunther 1958). The mechanism of action of oestrogens in lactation is not clearly established (Kochenour 1980), but they appear to suppress lactation by acting locally on breast tissue (Bruce and Ramirez 1970). This is discussed further in Chapter 82. No randomized controlled trials have evaluated the efficacy of oestrogens in the treatment of breast engorgement in breastfeeding women, and there is no mention of the potential complications of thromboembolism in any of the studies that advocate their use.

Another treatment of severe engorgement that was recommended by Waller (1946) was to 'raise and firmly support the breasts and allow no attempt at feeding'. Unfortunately this is the treatment that is noted by Kochenour (1980) to successfully suppress lactation in 60 to 70 per cent of women. Brooten (1983) considers that binding the breasts mimics total distension and causes lactation to subside quickly; useful when this is desired, but counterproductive when it is not.

3.2 Mastitis

The other common difficulty caused by milk flow problems is mastitis. Milk flow can be limited by restriction of feeding or by a badly positioned baby, or when some obstacle is placed in the way of milk draining from one section of the breast. This obstacle (either internal or external) can result from such factors as blocked ducts, compression from fingers holding the breast, bruising from trauma, or rough handling, or because a brassiere is too small or too tight. In consequence, the milk collects in the alveoli and the pressure rises. The distension of the alveoli can often be felt as a lump in the breast tissue, which is tender when palpated. If this distension is unrelieved the pressure in the glandular system may be high enough to force substances from the milk through the cell walls and into the capillaries or connective tissue. The woman then begins to exhibit symptoms of an immune response to a foreign substance, similar in some ways to those observed in patients having an incompatible blood transfusion (Gunther 1973). The mother has a swollen, red, and painful area on her breast, her pulse and temperature rise, and she has an aching, flu-like feeling, often accompanied by shivering attacks and rigors. At this stage blood cultures are consistently negative (Gunther 1958, 1973), and it is still possible to resolve the problem by relieving the obstruction and draining the breast (Thomsen *et al.* 1984). If this is not speedily accomplished, however, bacterial infection may supervene and may ultimately give rise to a breast abscess (Devereux 1970).

It is clear, however, that a substantial proportion of women with mastitis do not have 'infective' mastitis: in 50 per cent or more of women with inflamed breasts no pathogenic organisms can be isolated from milk cultures (Marshall *et al.* 1975; Neibyl *et al.* 1978). Furthermore, positive cultures are quite common in women with no symptoms (Marshall *et al.* 1975) indicating that contamination of samples with skin commensals is a frequent occurrence. Perhaps understandably, the immediate response of the professional confronted with the symptoms of localized breast tenderness, redness, and fever in breastfeeding women is often the prescription of antibiotics. What begins as a non-infective, inflammatory process may, if inappropriately treated, rapidly progress to an infective process (Gunther 1958; Thomsen *et al.* 1984) and delay in treating an infective process will adversely affect the outcome (Devereux 1970; Thomsen *et al.* 1984).

Thomsen *et al.* (1984) present the best evidence supporting the need to differentiate between the infective and non-infective stages of mastitis. They compared the effectiveness of different forms of treatment for women presenting with similar symptoms of 'mastitis'. Their condition was classified, not on the basis of milk cultures, but by using leucocyte and bacterial counts. Women whose milk contained $< 10^6$ leucocytes and $< 10^3$ bacteria per millilitre of milk were deemed to be suffering from milk stasis (engorgement); those with $> 10^6$ leucocytes but $< 10^3$ bacteria per millilitre from non-infectious inflammation (obstructive mastitis); and those with $> 10^6$ leucocytes and $> 10^3$ bacteria per ml from infective mastitis. Out of 213 women and 339 inflamed breasts (each breast being considered as a separate case), 126 (37 per cent) of the cases were of milk stasis, 48 (14 per cent) were of non-infectious

inflammation, and 165 (49 per cent) were of infective mastitis. The cases in the first two categories were randomly allocated to two treatment regimens: either simply continuing to breastfeed; or breastfeeding supplemented by manual or mechanical expression of milk after feeds. The outcome was judged to be good if the symptoms disappeared and were followed by normal lactation for two weeks after the attack.

In the milk stasis group, breast expression additional to breastfeeding conferred no extra benefit, and the outcome was equally good for almost all cases. In the non-infectious inflammation group, those who had expressed as well as continuing to breastfeed fared statistically significantly better in terms of both the duration of the symptoms and the outcome ($p < 0.001$). The most frequent complication in the breastfeeding only group was a progression to infective mastitis.

In the third group, all of whom had been diagnosed as having infective mastitis, the outcome was very poor for those who just continued to breastfeed. Eighty-five per cent of these women had either poor lactation, recurrence or persistence of symptoms, and 6 of the 55 in this subgroup developed breast abscesses, from which *Staphylococcus aureus* was isolated in each instance. Those with infective mastitis who expressed as well as continuing to breastfeed fared better; 51 per cent had a good outcome and none developed abscesses. Those who received antibiotics in addition to breast expression did best, 96 per cent having a good outcome.

4 Problems with milk supply

Mothers and health professionals are likely to become concerned about breastfeeding on the basis of a number of signs, including failure of the baby to gain weight adequately, changes in behaviour (such as crying), and changes in the colour and consistency of the baby's stools. Common explanations for these symptoms are that the mother does not have enough milk, or that her milk is too 'thin', or 'weak', to sustain her baby.

Unfortunately, there is currently no basis for making accurate diagnoses in this field. Not only is it not possible to differentiate between problems that are solely subjective and those that can be confirmed objectively (Behar 1986): there is not even any way of being certain that the abnormal signs mentioned above relate to breastfeeding. There are good theoretical reasons to think that there are at least two distinct kinds of problem: one relating to the volume of the milk, the other to the ratio of foremilk to hindmilk in the feed (Williams *et al.* 1985; Woolridge and Fisher 1988). Unfortunately, because there are as yet no readily available ways of distinguishing between these two potential sources of difficulty in practice (although it is possible for research purposes (Jackson *et al.* 1987)), those who try to help women and babies who experience these problems must therefore recognize that the symptoms and signs referred to above may have a variety of origins.

4.1 Insufficient milk

The most common reason given for discontinuing breastfeeding is insufficient milk (World Health Organization 1979; Starling *et al.* 1979; West 1980; Martin and Monk 1982; Martin and White 1988). There is no information, however, about the extent to which this insufficiency is inevitable, as opposed to iatrogenic and thus preventable. Objective evidence of insufficient milk is hard to obtain, but it is likely that the high reported incidence (68 per cent of mothers who stopped breastfeeding between 2 and 8 weeks after birth in the national survey conducted by Martin and Monk (1982) gave insufficient milk as the reason) reflects over-diagnosis of the problem. Neifert (1983), on the basis of physiological evidence, suggests a figure of 1 to 5 per cent of women would be incapable of producing an adequate milk supply. Observations in traditional societies suggest an even lower figure (Behar 1986). One small study (Houston *et al.* 1981) found that in a group of women who received regular and consistent support, no mothers stopped breastfeeding as a result of insufficient milk, as compared to 19 per cent of women in a contemporary control group.

Adequate milk production is dependent on three main factors: prolactin release from the anterior pituitary, which then binds to the prolactin receptors in the milk glands and stimulates milk manufacture; oxytocin release from the posterior pituitary, which enables the manufactured and stored milk to be released; and efficient removal of milk from the breast. The effective functioning of all three aspects of milk production is accomplished in the majority of women by means of unrestricted and efficient suckling of the baby. Prolactin release, unlike oxytocin release, is in normal circumstances entirely dependent on suckling. Although the breast is 'primed' for milk production during pregnancy by the progressive rise from 30 ± 20 ng prolactin per millilitre in the first trimester to a mean of 200 ng per millilitre at term, so that it is effective as soon as the placental hormone levels fall, prolactin levels will only remain high after the first week if the baby is put to the breast (Hwang *et al.* 1971). Each suckling episode results in a release of prolactin, which reaches a peak between 15 and 60 minutes later and falls away again equally rapidly to reach basal levels within about 2 hours of a feed (suggesting that the half-life of prolactin in serum is less than 30 minutes) (Hwang *et al.* 1971; Glasier *et al.* 1984). This response to suckling can be demonstrated as late as 55 weeks postpartum (Madden *et al.* 1978; Gross *et al.* 1979) despite the fact that basal prolactin levels (Howie 1985) and the amplitude of the prolactin response also decrease over time (Glasier *et al.*

1984). Even so, significant amounts of milk are still produced, sufficient to sustain good growth in infants up to 8 months of age (Ahn and McLean 1980).

It would seem that once lactation is well-established milk yield is not dependent on high levels of prolactin. Possibly the prolactin receptors become increasingly sensitive to prolactin over time, so that ever-increasing levels of serum prolactin are not necessary. Both Carvahlo and colleagues (1983, 1985) and Martin (1983) suggest that in the first two weeks after parturition the frequency and duration of breastfeeds significantly affect milk production (prolactin) mechanisms, but that later (35–40 days postpartum) this is no longer the case. Others have postulated that a high milk yield in the first week has some predictive value for the long term success of lactation (Hytten 1954; Houston *et al.* 1983). There is some support from animal studies (Lincoln and Renfree 1981; Sernia and Tyndale-Biscoe 1979; Hinds and Tyndale-Biscoe 1982) for the suggestion that there may be a critical period during which the ability of the breast to produce the quantities of milk that will be required in later weeks or months is established in response to suckling frequency. If this is the case, then it becomes even more important that no artificial restrictions are placed on feeding intervals, and that good feeding technique is established in the first two weeks (the time that in Britain mothers and babies receive statutory care from midwives).

Although not yet fully understood, the mechanisms involved in milk production seem to be potentially effective in the vast majority of women (World Health Organization 1980, cited in Chetley 1986). As with all physiological functions, however, there are variations in efficiency between individuals. It is conceivable that milk production may be truly inadequate (as opposed to 'badly managed') in a few women (Neifert 1983).

It would seem to be fundamentally important to be able to diagnose the occurrence and aetiology of insufficient milk accurately. However, at present, the techniques available are limited. Three techniques for estimating breast-milk intake have been described in the literature: test weighing; the use of deuterium oxide (Coward *et al.* 1982); and measurement by Doppler ultrasound (How *et al.* 1979). The latter two require access to expensive and sophisticated equipment and have been used for research purposes only.

Test weighing of the baby before and after feeds, then calculating the breast-milk intake by the difference in weights, has been a common practice for many years. It has been used to estimate the baby's intake in case of anxiety about milk supply, and as a routine practice in some hospitals. The rationale for routine test weighing is to determine whether babies are taking 'too much' or 'too little'. On the basis of the test weigh results babies may either be given complements of cows' milk, formula, glucose, or donated breast-milk if it is deemed that they have taken too little, or have the length of subsequent breastfeeds limited in duration if they are deemed to have taken too much (Myles 1981). This response to a test weigh presupposes that the weighing is accurate, that it is representative of the 24-hour volume, and that professionals 'know' how much milk a particular baby should consume. It also raises the question of whether the action taken as a result of test weighing will do more good than harm. (The hazards associated with giving cows' milk to breastfed infants, and limiting the duration of feeds are discussed in Chapter 80.)

The results may still be of little value unless the weighing itself is accurate. This will depend on several factors, including whether the same person does the weighing on each occasion, their accuracy, the accuracy of the scales, and the degree to which the baby moves about while being weighed (see Chapter 3).

Researchers collecting normative data, (Lucas *et al.* 1979; Houston *et al.* 1983; Saint *et al.* 1984; Butte *et al.* 1984) have used an integrated electronic balance, which takes the mean value of a number of weighings over 2–4 second periods, and provides readings which are reproducible to within 2 g, even if the baby moves vigorously. A digital readout further facilitates accurate recording of the weight. Such sophisticated (and expensive) equipment is not commonly found on postnatal wards for routine clinical use. Most ward scales cannot generally be read to an accuracy of more than 10 g, and this accuracy is further reduced if the baby is agitated.

An investigation conducted to determine the accuracy of test weighing in a clinical context, using standard (Salter Trent) scales, was undertaken by Stevens and Whitfield (Stevens and Whitfield 1980; Whitfield *et al.* 1981). They compared the test weight of 96 bottle-fed babies with a known feed weight. The feed weights varied from 25 to 100ml. If test weighing were a reliable procedure, there should have been a 1:1 relationship between the test weight and the feed weight. The 'test weight error' (the difference between the result of the test weighing and the weight of formula actually consumed by the baby) exceeded 10 per cent in nearly three-quarters of the measurements; 20 per cent in nearly half, and exceeded 30 per cent in a quarter of them. They found a large variation in test feed values in infants who appeared, from test weighing, to have consumed the same amount of milk; for example, babies with a test weight of 40 g had consumed between 32.5 and 88.4 g of formula. Conversely, infants who had in fact taken the same amount of feed had widely varying test weight values; when the amount of formula actually consumed was 60 g, test weight results varied from 21 to 90 g. This poor correlation was also found by Culley *et al.* (1979) in their preliminary validation of test weighing, though their results were somewhat

improved by having the same observer for all 115 weighings, a situation which is not likely to apply in the usual clinical setting.

The degree of error was most marked when the volume of feed was less than 60 ml. In some instances the test weight error was greater than the test weight itself! At test weight values over 80 ml there was a tendency to overestimate the feed weight, but the percentage error in these cases did not exceed 20 per cent. To a lesser degree the infant's body weight appeared to affect the accuracy of the test weight, which increased as body weight decreased. Below 2.5 kg the error was in the order of 30 per cent.

A procedural error of 20–30 per cent strongly suggests that test weighing using standard baby scales in a routine clinical context is a poor indication of feed intake, especially of small volumes in small babies. This conclusion is further supported by Winberg and Wesser (1971), who showed that in a hospital where babies were routinely test weighed and were expected to take 10 ml and 20 ml respectively per feed in the first two days, 98.5 per cent of them were deemed not to have taken the required amount and were thus given supplements.

This concern over accuracy is compounded by whether or not one or two test weighed feeds are representative of the 24-hour intake. The evidence on this point is that feed volumes vary widely from feed to feed (Forsyth 1913; Carvalho *et al.* 1982; Dewey and Lönnerdal 1983). One study (Houston *et al.* 1983), using accurate electronic scales and measuring breast-milk intake for research purposes, found a strong association in the first three days between the estimates of the volumes of single feeds and 24-hour volumes. However, the association was even stronger between the estimates of the volumes of two feeds and the 24-hour volumes. The authors noted that care should be taken when using a single feed to assess milk intake, that it should never be done on normal scales, and that early feed volumes may be more consistent than feed volumes after the first week.

In 1977 de Chateau *et al.* examined the effect of routine test weighing and supplementary feeding during the first week of life on the total duration of breastfeeding. One hundred and nineteen infants born during February and March were subjected to routine test weighing, and the 203 infants born during April and June of the same year were neither weighed or supplemented. They found the total duration of breastfeeding was almost the same in both groups, (42 vs. 47 days), but that the mothers in the test weigh group were five times more likely to stop breastfeeding in the first week, and twice as likely to stop in the second week as those in the group whose babies were not test weighed. On the basis of these results routine test weighing was abandoned in that hospital. A year later, when the researchers wished to repeat the experiment and compare a third group of 68 babies born during May with a (fourth) control group who would be test weighed in the previously traditional manner, the staff raised objections with which the researchers could only agree. They therefore compared the total duration of breastfeeding in their new group with the historical control group, and found that the total duration of breastfeeding was now 95 days, compared with the previous 42 days. Mothers who had previous experience of the test weighing regimen said spontaneously that they felt themselves to be under less pressure this time. Others have noted that mothers may find the test weighing procedure to be threatening, especially if it is being used to assess their performance—which it so often is (Kitzinger 1979).

The decision to give a healthy term breastfed baby supplementary feeds as a result of information gained by assessing milk intake is based on an assumption that it is possible to know how much breast-milk an individual baby needs. An infant's total energy requirements will depend on its basal metabolic rate, body configuration, rate of growth, sex, age, and the degree to which thermogenesis is diet-dependent (Butte *et al.* 1984). Thus, although it may be acceptable to use the best available estimate of the average energy requirements for infants as a *group*, the actual energy requirements of a specific individual (of any age) are very difficult to assess, and may differ quite considerably from the average. Furthermore, the recommended averages themselves are currently the focus of some discussion, as recent investigations suggest that they may have been considerably overestimated (Whitehead and Paul 1981; Butte *et al.* 1984; Wood *et al.* 1988). The situation is further complicated by the fact that the calorific value of milk in a breast, unlike milk in a bottle, is not constant, because the fat content rises throughout the feed (Hall 1975; Baum 1980), and it cannot therefore be calculated easily (Woolridge *et al.* 1983; Saint *et al.* 1984).

Pyke (1975) refers to Widdowson's study in which she calculated the exact energy value of the dietary intake of 20 18-year-old males, all with similar lifestyles and doing similar work; it ranged from 9773 kJ (2335 kcals) per day to 25 113 kJ (6002 kcals) per day. He concluded that 'the most direct way of finding out whether an individual energy intake is nutritionally adequate is to ask him whether he has had enough to eat. If he says "Yes" and his body weight is satisfactory, his energy intake is satisfactory too'.

Similarly, it may be more relevant to monitor the general condition of a baby (health, contentment/behaviour, colour and consistency of stools, colour of urine, etc.) and, having allowed for some adjustment to the infant's genetic growth potential after the prenatal effects on birthweight have subsided (Butte *et al.* 1984),

note his or her progress (change in body weight) in relation to the appropriate centile growth curve.

4.2 Treatment of insufficient milk

4.3.1 Primary measures

In the light of the evidence presented and discussed in Chapter 80, it is clear that the best means of preventing the occurrence of insufficient milk is unrestricted feeding by a well-positioned infant while giving good practical and emotional support to the breastfeeding mother. This is also the basis for the treatment of insufficient milk and is likely to solve the problem in a high proportion of mothers. Mothers and babies need reassurance and careful attention at this time, and professionals should be alive to the possibility that milk insufficiency may persist. It is not unknown for babies to have become seriously undernourished because of a dogged, but mistaken belief that the problem will always be resolved by these means (Roddey *et al.* 1981; Neifert and Seacat 1987). When mothers and babies do not respond to the fundamental elements of good breastfeeding practice other treatments should be seriously considered.

4.3.2 Drug treatment

In the past, when a baby's life depended on breast-milk, many remedies were sought for those who seemed unable to produce enough milk. These galactogogues included: blow-fly larvae, dried goat's udder, and cuttle-fish soup (Platt and Gin 1938). Herbal infusions, such as the seeds of fennel (*Foeniculom vulgare*) and the flowers of goat's rue (*Galega officinalis*) were, and still are, recommended to increase milk production (Culpeper 1983). We have been unable to identify any controlled evaluation of the effects of these preparations. Four main types of drugs have, however, been evaluated in attempted treatment of insufficient milk: dopamine antagonists, iodine, thyrotropin-releasing hormone, and oxytocin.

4.3.2.1 Dopamine antagonists Since dopamine has been shown to have a critical role in the mechanisms which control prolactin production (Duech *et al.* 1976; McLeod and Robyn 1977), several researchers have experimented with drugs that block dopamine receptors, including metoclopramide (Maxalon), sulpiride (Dolmatil), and domperidone (Motilium).

Metoclopramide and sulpiride are both antipsychotic drugs belonging to the orthopramide class. As well as producing hyperprolactinaemia, they may also give rise to side-effects such as dystonia (which may appear after only a few doses), sedation, elevations in blood pressure, as well as akathisia and a parkinson-like syndrome following prolonged use. All these symptoms usually remit if the drug is withdrawn (Martindale 1982).

Extrapyramidal dystonia has also been observed in infants (Casteels-van Daele *et al.* 1970; Silb and Glass 1978). Tardive dyskinesia (an involuntary movement disorder with an estimated prevalence rate of 10-15 per cent in those making prolonged use of antipsychotic drugs, and usually affecting those over 50 years of age) does occasionally occur after short term use with low dosage (British National Formulary 1981b). The cause is unknown and no satisfactory treatment is currently available (Tarsy and Baldessarini 1984). Domperidone, although a dopamine antagonist, acts peripherally rather than centrally. It does not cross the blood–brain barrier, and does not provoke extrapyramidal side effects (Reyntjens *et al.* 1978).

Four studies have examined the administration of sulpiride to enhance lactation (Aono *et al.* 1979; Ylikorkala *et al.* 1982, 1984; Aono *et al.* 1982). In all of these studies, sulpiride, in doses of either 100 or 150 mg daily

was given to women with inadequate lactation. The two studies by Ylikorkala *et al.*, although ostensibly placebo-controlled and double-blind, excluded some women from the control group because of 'lack of effect of the treatment'. These studies have therefore not been included in the summary tables or the overview.

The results presented in Tables 81.1, 81.2 and 81.3, indicate that, in women with 'inadequate lactation', sulpiride given in early lactation increases both basal serum prolactin and daily milk yield, but only by small amounts which are unlikely to be of practical importance. Aono *et al.* (1979) did show an increase in mean daily milk yield of 112 ml by the 5th day postpartum. However, their 1982 study failed to show any effect on the rate of discontinuation of breastfeeding by 4 weeks postpartum. So far therefore, there is no basis for using this drug in practice.

Table 81.1 Mean basal serum prolactin in breastfeeding women treated with oral sulpiride

Authors and year	Dose	Group	Time of measurement	Mean basal serum prolactin (ng/ml)* Experimental	Controls	Difference
Aono *et al.* (1982)	50 mg × 2 daily from 3rd day postpartum for 4 days	Women with 50 ml total milk secretion in 1st 3 days. Controls $n = 10$; Exp. $n = 10$	3rd day postpartum	162.5 ± 13.5	105 ± 5	+57
			6th day postpartum	133.2 ± 12.1	102 ± 8	+31.2
Aono *et al.* (1979)	50 mg × 2 daily 1st 7 days postpartum	'tended to complain of lactational insufficiency'. Controls $n = 10$; Exp. $n = 10$	4th day post-partum	157 ± 10	105 ± 3	+52
			6th day post-partum	140 ± 10	92 ± 5	+48

* Derived from figure

Table 81.2 Estimated daily milk yield in breastfeeding women treated with oral sulpiride

Authors and year	Dose	Group	Time of measurement	Estimated daily milk yield (ml) Experimental	Controls	Difference
Aono *et al.* (1982)	50 mg × 2 daily from 3rd day postpartum for 4 days	Women with 50 ml total milk secretion in 1st 3 days Controls $n = 10$; Exp. $n = 10$	3rd day postpartum	111.4 ± 17	86.6 ± 14.7	+24.8
			4th day postpartum	224.5 ± 21	143.5 ± 19.6	+81
			5th day postpartum	325.8 ± 31.7	211.1 ± 72.9	+114.7
Aono *et al.* (1979)	50 mg × 2 daily 1st 7 days postpartum	'tended to complain of lactational insufficiency'. Controls $n = 10$; Exp. $n = 10$	1st day postpartum	26.7 ± 7.9	$12.5 + 4.6$	+14.2
			3rd day postpartum	247.1 ± 15.4	188.1 ± 18.2	+59
			5th day postpartum	483.1 ± 24	370.9 ± 24.5	+112.2

Table 81.3 Effect of giving oral sulpiride 50 mg twice daily to women with poor milk secretion on primiparae stopping breastfeeding 4 weeks postpartum

Study	EXPT n	(%)	CTRL n	(%)	Odds ratio (95% CI)	Graph of odds ratios and confidence intervals
Aono *et al.* (1982)	4/20	(20.00)	4/20	(20.00)	1.00 (0.22–4.62)	
Typical odds ratio (95% confidence interval)					1.00 (0.22–4.62)	

Effect of giving oral sulpiride 50 mg twice daily to women with poor milk secretion on multiparae stopping breastfeeding 4 weeks postpartum

Study	EXPT n	(%)	CTRL n	(%)	Odds ratio (95% CI)	Graph of odds ratios and confidence intervals
Aono *et al.* (1982)	3/20	(15.00)	4/20	(20.00)	0.71 (0.14–3.57)	
Typical odds ratio (95% confidence interval)					0.71 (0.14–3.57)	

(Graph axis values: 0.01 0.1 0.5 1 2 10 100)

The studies on the effects of domperidone on prolactin levels and daily milk yield are summarized in Tables 81.4 and 81.5. These studies (Petralgia *et al.* 1985; Hofmeyr *et al.* 1985) indicate that domperidone given at a dose of 20–30 mg daily raises basal serum prolactin levels marginally in women with 'inadequate lactation'. In healthy women whose infants were temporarily unable to take breast-milk, Hofmeyr *et al.* (1985) showed an increase of 105 ng/ml in mean basal serum prolactin after only one dose of 20 mg. Only Petralgia *et al.* (1985) estimated milk yield. They found an increase of 275 ml on the 10th treatment day in women with inadequate lactation. This observation is encouraging, but, taken alone, it does not provide an adequate basis for recommending use of the drug without further evaluation.

Three controlled trials have examined the effects of oral metoclopramide on prolactin and milk yield in breastfeeding women (Guzman *et al.* 1979; De Gezelle *et al.* 1983; Kauppila *et al.* 1985). The study by Guzman *et al.* (1979) had a crossover design with results which are difficult to interpret, and it has therefore not

Table 81.4 Mean basal serum prolactin in breastfeeding women treated with oral domperidone

Authors and year	Dose	Group	Time of measurement	Mean basal serum prolactin (ng/ml)* Experimental	Controls	Difference
Petralgia *et al.* (1985)	10 mg×3 daily 2nd–5th postpartum day: Group A	Group A Multiparae with history of failure of lactogenesis in previous puerperium	Group A Day 3 postpartum	155	98	+57
	10 postpartum days: Group B	Controls n=7; Exp. n=8	Day 5 postpartum	150	70	+80
		Group B Primiparae affected by inadequate lactation 2 weeks after delivery. Controls n=8; Exp. n=9	Group B 2nd day of treatment	169±27	84+17	+85
Hofmeyr *et al.* (1985)	20 mg, 1 dose only	Women whose infants were temporarily unable to take breast-milk. Controls n=5; Exp. n=5	2 hours after treatment	255	150	+105

* Derived from figure.

Table 81.5 Estimated daily milk yield in breastfeeding women treated with oral domperidone

Authors and year	Dose	Group	Time of measurement	Estimated daily milk yield (ml)		Difference
				Experimental	Controls	
Petralgia *et al.*(1985)	10 mg × 3 daily for 10 days	Primiparae affected by inadequate lactation 2 weeks after delivery. Controls *n* = 8 Exp. *n* = 9	2nd treatment day	347 ± 36	335 ± 30	+ 12
			6th treatment day	636 ± 59	440 ± 27	+ 196
			10th treatment day	672 ± 44	398 ± 45	+ 275

been included in the summary Tables 81.6 and 81.7. Of the other two trials, that by De Gezelle and his colleagues referred to normal mothers and babies. Although 30 mg of metoclopramide daily was associated with small increases in mean basal serum prolactin levels and estimated daily milk yield, these were trivial. The trial by Kauppila *et al.* (1985) has greater potential relevance in that they studied women who wished to improve their milk production. In this trial the increases in mean basal serum prolactin levels were more substantial, and after two weeks during which there was no detectable increase in estimated milk production, an estimated increase of 100 ml was detected.

These results indicate little benefit, in terms of milk yield or breastfeeding continuation, of any of the dopamine antagonists in the types of women studied. Further work, however, is required to clarify the possible role of these drugs in women with insufficient milk. There is some evidence that these drugs may be of use for women who are temporarily unable to feed their sick or premature babies. Further research is required to clarify this.

4.3.2.2 Iodine, thyrotropin-releasing hormone, and oxytocin Nearly a century has passed since iodine containing substances were recommended for milk insufficiency (Hertoghe 1896) and, more recently, they have been evaluated in controlled trials. Dried thyroid was given with apparent success by Robertson (1947a), who later reported that iodine gave equally good results (Robertson 1947b). Following an unsuccessful attempt by Nicholson (1948) to confirm these findings, a small trial was conducted in Wuppertal in Germany by Dean (1950). He was unable to show that the iodine treatment conferred any benefit on lactation for any of the outcomes measured, and reluctantly concluded that the improvements in lactation reported by Robertson were not due to the administration of iodine.

In 1974, Zarate and colleagues noted that the administration of synthetic thyrotropin releasing hormone induced a significant release of prolactin. They carried out a placebo-controlled evaluation of the effects of 60 mg of thyrotropin-releasing hormone (Table 81.8). The drug or the placebo was given from 2 days postpartum until the 4th postpartum week to 16 healthy women who had previously breastfed successfully.

Table 81.6 Mean basal serum prolactin in breastfeeding women treated with oral metoclopramide

Authors and year	Dose	Group	Time of measurement	Mean basal serum prolactin		Difference
				Experimental	Controls	
Kauppila *et al.* (1985)	10 mg × 3 daily starting at 4–20 weeks postpartum for 3 weeks	Women who wanted to improve milk production. Controls *n* = 14; Exp. *n* = 11	1 week after therapy started	315 ± 300*	89.6 ± 60.1*	+ 225.4*
			3 weeks after therapy started	210.7 ± 131.4*	68.5 ± 58.3*	+ 142.2*
De Gezelle *et al.* (1983)	10 mg × 3 daily from 1st–8th day postpartum	Normal mothers and babies. Controls *n* = 6; Exp. *n* = 7	Day 3	240.9 ± 89.3†	225 ± 148.1†	+ 15.9†
			Day 7	132 ± 130.9†	120.4 ± 97.2†	+ 12†
			Day 21	57.6 ± 67.5†	47.8 ± 48.6†	+ 9.8†
			Day 28	64.1 ± 84.9†	70.5 ± 81†	− 6.4†

* Units are μl; † units are ng/ml.

Table 81.7 Estimated daily milk yield of breastfeeding women treated with oral metoclopramide

Authors and year	Dose	Group	Time of measurement	Estimated daily milk yield (ml)		Difference
				Experimental	Controls	
Kauppila *et al.* (1985)	10 mg × 3 daily starting at 4–20 weeks postpartum for 3 weeks	Women who wanted to improve milk production. Controls $n = 14$; Exp. $n = 11$	1 week after therapy started	480*	480	0
			2 weeks after therapy started	500	500	0
			3 weeks after therapy started	520	420	+100
De Gezelle *et al.* (1983)	10 mg × 3 daily from 1st–8th day postpartum	Normal mothers and babies. Controls $n = 6$; Exp. $n = 7$	Day 3	50.7 ± 14.6	41.7 ± 24	+9
			Day 5	82.9 ± 11.1	52.5 ± 10.8	+30.4
			Day 7	81.4 ± 17.7	59.2 ± 18.6	+22.2
			Mean	75.4 ± 13.2	51.1 ± 10.9	+24.3

* Derived from figure

Table 81.8 Mean basal serum prolactin in breastfeeding women treated with thyrotropin-releasing hormone (TRH)

Authors and year	Dose	Group	Time of measurement	Mean basal serum prolactin (ng/ml)*		Difference
				Experimental	Controls	
Zarate *et al.* (1976)	20 mg × 3 daily from 2 days postpartum until 4th postpartum week, 30 min before breastfeeding	Healthy puerperal women, with adequate lactation in previous puerperium. Controls $n = 8$; Exp. $n = 8$	Day 7 postpartum	550	155	+395
			Day 14 postpartum	540	120	+420
			Day 21 postpartum	230	100	+130
			Day 28 postpartum	170	80	+90

* Derived from figure

They measured basal serum prolactin and milk protein, fat, and lactose, but not milk volume. The mean basal serum prolactin was increased by 420 ng/ml by day 14 in the women receiving thyrotropin-releasing hormone: by day 28 the difference was only 90 ng/ml. No differences were found in milk composition.

A further study was carried out by these investigators, (Zarate *et al.* 1976) in which thyrotropin-releasing hormone or placebo was given to 8 women with 'inadequate lactation'. In these women thyrotropin releasing hormone did not elicit an increase in basal serum prolactin, and no increase was seen in milk supply. These results suggest that although thyrotropin-releasing hormone may increase prolactin levels in early lactation in healthy, normally breastfeeding women, it is unlikely to increase milk supply and no therapeutic effect has been demonstrated for women with milk insufficiency.

As previously described (see Chapter 80) the letdown reflex, which is primed by oxytocin release from the posterior pituitary, is essential for successful breastfeeding. Some investigators have therefore reasoned that to give oxytocin may improve problems with milk supply.

Reports of six double-blind randomized controlled evaluations of the effects of oxytocin on breastfeeding are available. A variety of outcomes have been studied, but the most crucial information concerns weight changes in the baby. This information is available for the five published comparisons presented in the papers by Friedman and Sachtleben (1961), Huntingford (1961) and Luhman (1963). Data are presented in

Table 81.9 The effects on infant weight-loss of giving oxytocin to breastfeeding women

Authors and year	Dose (IU) (route)	Weight loss (g) Oxytocin	Control	Difference	p
Friedman and	10 × 5 (buccal)	67.7	89.2	−21.5	NS
Sachtleben	100	89.1	122.7	−33.6	NS
(1961)	100	112.7	90.0	+22.7	NS
Huntingford (1961)	40 (nasal)	142	207	−65	<0.02
Luhman (1963)	40 (nasal)	208	207	+1	NS

NS = not significant

Table 81.9. In only one of the trials was weight-loss greater in the babies whose mothers had used oxytocin than in controls. In one trial there was no difference. In the remaining three trials the weight-loss was less after maternal use of oxytocin, and this difference was statistically significant in one of these (Huntingford 1961). We are aware of one unpublished trial in which no differences were noted (D Hawkins, personal communication). In summary, there is no strong evidence that oxytocin administration has a beneficial effect on milk supply, but a real effect may await discovery.

5 Conclusions

5.1 Implications for current practice

The main reasons women give for discontinuing breast-feeding are nipple trauma, breast engorgement, mastitis, and insufficient milk. Evidence reviewed in this and the previous chapter (Chapter 80) suggests that the majority of these problems can be prevented by unrestricted breastfeeding by a baby who has been well-positioned from the first feed on, and by giving mothers excellent practical and emotional support (Fig. 81.1).

If a woman does sustain nipple trauma, she should continue to breastfeed, express milk if necessary, and receive help with positioning. Discontinuing breast-feeding, and the application of any of a variety of preparations to the nipple, does not help. Indeed, some of these interventions have been shown to be prejudice to the success of breastfeeding.

Problems with milk flow can result in engorgement and possibly in mastitis. The best means of preventing both of these problems is ensuring unrestricted feeds with the baby well-positioned at the breast. These measures are also the basis for treating these problems when they do occur, with the possibility that breast expression may also help. Oral proteolytic enzymes may help in the treatment of engorgement. If mastitis does not resolve rapidly with good feeding and expression, then antibiotic treatment should be instituted. Although routine antibiotic administration for mastitis is not justified, a simple method of differentiating

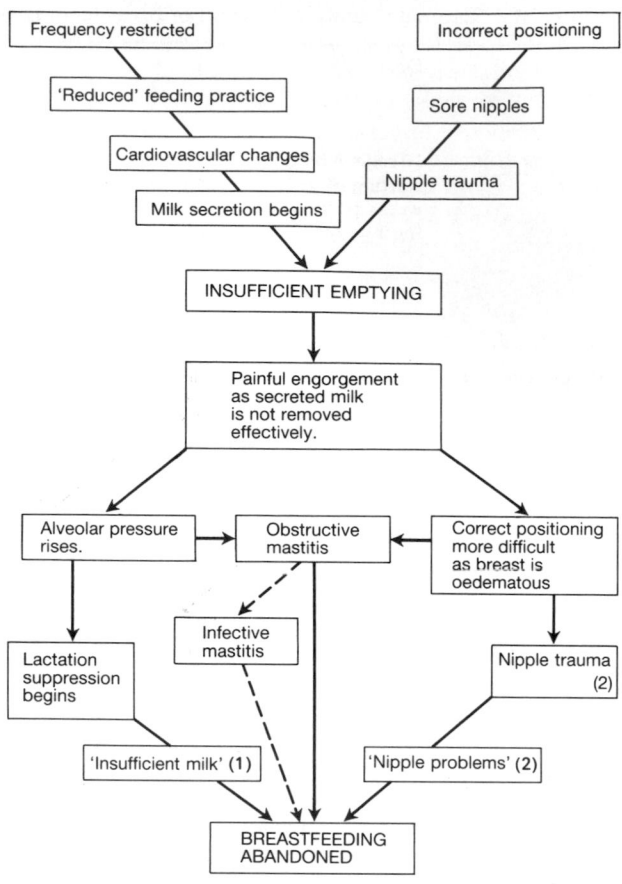

Fig. 81.1 Possible consequences of a restrictive feeding schedule and insufficient early attention to the way in which the baby is positioned at the breast.

(1) and (2): the most common reasons given for giving up breastfeeding. (Whichelow 1982; Sloper *et al.* 1977; Martin and Monk 1982; Martin and White 1988.)

between infective and non-infective mastitis could help to make management more rational. In all cases of engorgement and mastitis, however, the key to successful treatment is good drainage of the breast. This is best achieved by unlimited feeds by a well-positioned baby.

Mothers and health professionals who suspect insufficient milk as a result of signs and symptoms in the baby or the mother face a challenging problem because identifying the problem and its cause is always difficult and often impossible. Until diagnostic precision improves, the basis of the treatment offered when insufficient milk is suspected remains unrestricted breast-feeding by a well-positioned baby, together with practical and emotional support for the mother. If the problem does not resolve, ill health of either the mother or the baby should be suspected. So far there is no good evidence that administration of dopamine antagonists, or other drugs, improves milk production in women with problems of milk supply.

5.2 Implications for future research

In spite of the large volume of research in this field, there is currently a dearth of sound evidence on such basic matters as the incidence of the problems faced by breastfeeding mothers and their babies. This area will only be enlightened, however, by studying populations of women who have had access to consistently good care, and avoided preventable problems. Thus research is required to enable a differentiation to be made between milk insufficiency that is inevitable, and that which is iatrogenic and thus preventable. Identifying women who experience problems in spite of having received and implemented sound advice about positioning and unrestricted feeding patterns is of particular importance because it is among these that it will be necessary to identify the aetiologies of less tractable problems. Randomized trials will be required to evaluate the effectiveness and safety of the solutions proposed for their problems.

References

Ahn CH, McLean WC (1980). Growth of the exclusively breast fed infant. Am J Clin Nutr, 33: 183–192.

Aono T, Shiojo T, Aki T, Hirota K, Nomura A, Kurachi K (1979). Augmentation of puerperal lactation by oral administration of sulpiride. J Clin Endocrinol Metab, 48: 478–482.

Aono T, Aki T, Kolke K, Kurachi K (1982). Effect of sulpiride on poor puerpural lactation. Am J Obstet Gynecol, 143: 927.

Applebaum RM (1977). The modern management of successful breastfeeding. Pediatr Clin North Am, 24: 37–47.

Ardran GM, Kemp FH, Lind J (1958). A cineradiographic study of breastfeeding. Br J Radiol, 31, 156–162.

Atkinson LD (1978). Prenatal nipple conditioning for breastfeeding. Nursing Res, 28: 267–271.

Baum JD (1980). Flow and composition of suckled breast milk. In: Human Milk, Its Biological and Social Value. Proceedings of the International Symposium on Breastfeeding, Tel Aviv, Israel. Freier S, Edelman AI (eds). Amsterdam: Excerpta Medica.

Behar M (1986). Factors influencing breastfeeding in relation to infant and maternal health. Geneva: World Health Organization, Document No. WHO/MCH/NUT/85.1 Rev.1 February.

Blaikeley J, Clarke S, MacKeith R, Ogden KM (1953). Breastfeeding: factors affecting success. J Obstet Gynaecol Br Empire, 60: 657–669.

British National Formulary Number 2 (1981a). Drugs for the relief of soft tissue inflammation. 10.3.1: Enzymes. London: British Medical Association/The Pharmaceutical Society of Great Britain, p 265.

British National Formulary Number 2 (1981b). London: British Medical Association/The Pharmaceutical Society of Great Britain, p 107.

Brockway L (1986). Hair colour and problems in breastfeeding. Midwives' Chron & Nursing Notes, March: 66–67.

Brooten DA (1983). A comparison of 4 treatments to prevent and control pain and engorgement in non-nursing mothers. Nursing Res, 32: 225–229.

Brown MS, Hurlock JT (1975). Preparation of the breast for breastfeeding. Nursing Res, 24: 448–451.

Bruce JO, Ramirez VD (1970). Site of action of the inhibitory effect of oestrogen upon lactation. Neuroendocrinology, 6: 19.

Butte NF, Garza C, O'Brian Smith E, Nichols BL (1984). Human milk intake and growth in exclusively breast-fed infants. J Pediatr, 104: 187–195.

Carvalho M, Anderson DM, Giangreco A, Pittard WB (1985). Frequency of milk expression and milk production by mothers of non-nursing premature neonates. Am J Dis Child, 139: 483–485.

Carvalho M, Robertson S, Merkatz R, Klaus M (1982). Milk intake and frequency of feeding in breastfed infants. Early Hum Dev, 7: 155–163.

Carvalho M, Robertson S, Friedman A, Klaus M (1983). Effect of frequent breastfeeding on early milk production and infant weight gain. Pediatrics, 72: 307–311.

Casteels-van Daele M, Jacken J, Van Der Schueren P, Zimmerman A, Van Den Bon P (1970). Dystonic reaction in children caused by metaclopramide. Arch Dis Child, 45: 130.

Chetley A (1986). The politics of baby food: successful challenges to an international marketing strategy. London: Francis Pinter.

Coward WA, Cole TJ, Sawyer MB, Prentice AM, Orr-Ewing AK (1982). Breastmilk intake and measurement in mixed fed infants by administration of deuterium oxide to their mothers. Hum Nutr, 36: 141–148.

Culley P, Milan P, Roginski C, Waterhouse J, Wood B (1979). Are breastfed babies still getting a raw deal in hospital? Br Med J, 2: 891–893.

Culpeper (1983). Colour Herbal. London: W Foulsham, pp 71, 76.

Dawson EK (1935). Histological study of normal mamma in relation to tumour growth; mature gland in lactation and pregnancy. Edinburgh Med J, 42: 569.

de Chateau P, Holmberg H, Jakobsson K, Winberg J (1977). A study of factors promoting and inhibiting lactation. Dev Med Child Neurol, 19: 575–584.

De Gezelle H, Ooghe W, Ghiery M, Dhont M (1983). Metoclopramide and breast milk. Eur J Obstet Gynecol Reprod Biol, 15: 31–36.

Dean RFA (1950). Iodine as an aid to lactation. Lancet, 1: 762–763.

Devereux DP (1970). Acute puerperal mastitis. Am J Obstet Gynecol, 108: 78.

Dewey KG, Lönnerdal B (1983). Breastmilk intake: variations in breastfeeding practices. Am J Clin Nutr, 38: 152–153.

Duech AJ, Simon P, Boissier JR (1976). Antogenism by sulpiride of three apomophin-reduced effects in rodents. Eur J Pharmacol 36: 139.

Fieldhouse P (1984). A revival in breastfeeding. Can J Publ Health 75: 128–132.

Fildes V (1979). Putting mum in the picture. Nursing Mirror, 149: 22–24.

Fisher C (1981). Breastfeeding—a midwife's view. Matern Child Health, February: 52–55.

Forsyth D (1913). Breastfeeding: the consumption of breast milk. Lancet, June 14: 1656–1657.

Friedman EA, Sachtleben MR (1961). Oxytocin in lactation. Am J Obstet Gynecol, 82: 846–855.

Gans B (1958). Breast and nipple pain in the early stages of lactation. Br Med J, 4: 830–834.

Glasier A, McNeilly AS, Howie PW (1984). The prolactin response to suckling. Clin Endocrinol, 21: 109–116.

Gross BA, Eastman CJ, Bowen KM, McElduff AP (1979). Integrated concentrations of prolactin in breastfeeding mothers. Austral NZ J Obstet Gynaecol, 19: 150–153.

Gunther M (1958). Discussion of the breast in pregnancy and lactation. Proc R Soc Med, 51: 306–309.

Gunther M (1973). Infant Feeding. Harmondsworth: Penguin Books, p 107.

Guzman V, Toscano G, Canales ES, Zarate A (1979). Improvement of defective lactation by using metoclopramide. Acta Obstet Gynecol Scand, 50: 53–55.

Hall B (1975). Changing composition of milk and early development of an appetite control. Lancet, 1: 779–781.

Hammond J (1936). Vet J, 16: 519. Cited in Waller H (1946).

Hertoghe E (1896). 'De l'influence des produits thyroidiens sur les organes genitaux pelviens et thoraciques chez femme; applications a la theraputique gynecologique'. Bull Acad R Med Belg: Brux, 4.5 x: 380–391. Cited in Dean RFA (1950).

Hinds LA, Tyndale-Biscoe CH (1982). Prolactin in the marsupial Macropus eugenii, during the oestrus cycle, pregnancy and lactation. Biol Reprod, April 26: 391–398.

Hofmeyr GJ, Van Iddekinge B, Blott JA (1985). Domperidone: secretion in breastmilk and effect on puerperal prolactin levels. Br J Obstet Gynaecol, 92: 141–144.

Houston MJ, Howie PW, Smart L, McArdle T, McNeilly AS (1983). Factors affecting the duration of breastfeeding. Early Hum Dev, 8: 55–63.

Houston MJ, Howie PW, Cook A, McNeilly AS (1981). Do breastfeeding mothers get the home support they need? Health Bull, 39: 166–172.

How TV, Ashmore MP, Rolfe P, Lucas A, Baum JD (1979). A Doppler ultrasound technique for measuring human milk flow. J Med Eng Technol, 3: 66–71.

Howie PW (1985). Breastfeeding: a new understanding. Midwives' Chron & Nursing Notes, July: 184–192.

Huntingford PJ (1961). Intranasal use of synthetic oxytocin in management of breastfeeding. Br Med J, 2: 709–711.

Hwang P, Guyda H, Friesen H (1971). A radio immunoassay for human prolactin. Proc Natl Acad Sci USA, 60: 1902–1906.

Hytten FE (1954). Clinical and chemical studies in lactation. Br Med J, 1: 1410.

Illingworth RS, Stone DGH (1952). Self-demand feeding in a maternity unit. Lancet, 1: 683–687.

Ingelman-Sundberg A (1953). Early puerperal breast engorgement. Acta Paediatr Scand, 32: 399–402.

Jackson DA, Woolridge MW, Imong SM *et al.* (1987). The automatic sampling shield: a device for sampling suckled breastmilk. Early Hum Dev, 15: 295–306.

Kauppila A, Anunti P, Kivinen S, Koivisto M, Ruokonen A (1985). Metoclopramide and breastfeeding: efficacy and anterior pituitary responses of the mother and the child. Eur J Obstet Gynecol Reprod Biol, 19: 19–22.

Kitzinger S (1979). The Experience of Breastfeeding. Harmondsworth: Penguin Books, p 22.

Kochenour NK (1980). Lactation suppression. Clin Obstet Gynecol, 23: 1052–1059.

Koshiishi T, Furusawa Y, Iseki H, Iwasaki Y (1971). A double blind study of the effects of Kimotab on engorgement of the breast. Acta Obstet Gynecol Japan, 18: 222–228.

L'Esperance CM (1980). Pain or pleasure: The dilemma of early breast feeding. Birth Family J, 7: 21–26.

Lawrence R (1985). Breastfeeding: a guide for the medical profession (2nd edn). St. Louis: Mosby.

Lincoln DW, Renfree MB (1981). Mammary gland growth and milk ejection in the agile wallaby, macropus agilis, displaying concurrent assynchronous lactation. J Reprod Fertil, 63: 193–196.

Lucas A, Lucas PJ, Baum JD (1979). Patterns of milk flow in breastfed babies. Lancet, 2: 57–59.

Luhman LA (1963). The effect of intranasal oxytocin on lactation. Obstet Gynecol, 21: 713–717.

Madden JD, Boyar RM, MacDonald PC, Porter JC (1978). Analysis of secretory patterns of prolactin and gonadotrophins during 24 hours in a lactating woman before and after resumption of menses. Am J Obstet Gynecol, 132: 430–441.

Marshall BR, Hepper JK, Zirbel CC (1975). Sporadic puerperal mastitis: an infection that need not interrupt lactation. JAMA, 233: 1377–1379.

Martin RH (1983). The place of prolactin in human lactation. Clin Endocrinol, 18: 295–299.

Martin J, White A (1988). Infant Feeding 1985. London: Her Majesty's Stationery Office.

Martin J, Monk J (1982). Infant Feeding 1980. London: Her Majesty's Stationery Office.

Martindale (1982). The Extra Pharmacopia (28th edn). London: London Pharmaceutical Press, p 1557.

McLeod RM, Robyn C (1977). Mechanism of increased prolactin secretion by sulpiride. J Endocrinol, 72: 273.

Messenger M (1982). The Breastfeeding Book. London: Century Publishing Co.

Minchin M (1985). Breastfeeding Matters. Sydney: George Allen & Unwin.

Murata T, Hanzawa M, Nomura Y (1965). The clinical effects of 'protease complex' on post-partum breast engorgement (based on the double blind method). J Japan Obstet Gynecol Soc, 17: 10–15.

Myles M (1981). Textbook for Midwives. Edinburgh: Churchill Livingstone, pp 507–508.

Neibyl JR, Spence MR, Parmley TH (1978). Sporadic (non-epidemic) puerperal mastitis. J Reprod Med, 20: 97–100.

Neifert MR, Seacat JM (1987). Lactation insufficiency: a rational approach. Birth, 14: 182–188.

Neifert MR (1983). Infant problems in breastfeeding. In: Lactation. Neville MC, Neifert MR (eds). New York: Plenum Press.

Nicholson W (1985). Cracked nipples in breastfeeding mothers: a randomized trial of three methods of management. Nursing Mothers of Australia Newsletter, 21: 7–10.

Nicholson DP (1948). Lugol's solution in failing lactation. Br Med J, i: 1029–1030.

Petraglia F, DeLeo V, Sardelli S, Pieroni ML, D'Antona N, Genazzani AR (1985). Domperidone in defective and insufficient lactation. Eur J Obstet Gynecol Reprod Biol, 19: 281–287.

Platt BS, Gin SY (1938). Chinese methods of infant feeding and nursing. Arch Dis Child, 13: 343–354.

Pyke M (1975). Success in Nutrition. London: John Murray.

Reyntjens AJ, Niemegeers CJE, Van Neuten JM, Laduron P (1978). Domperidone: a novel and safe gastrokinetic antinauseant for the treatment of dyspepsia and vomiting. Arzneimittelforschung, 28: 1194–1196.

Riordan J (1983). A Practical Guide to Breastfeeding. St. Louis: Mosby.

Robinson M (1947a). Hormones and lactation (dried thyroid gland). Lancet, 2: 385.

Robinson M (1947b). Iodine and failing lactation. Br Med J, 2: 126.

Roddey OF, Martin ES, Swetenberg RL (1981). Critical weight loss and malnutrition in breastfed infants. Am J Dis Child, 135: 597–599.

Saint L, Smith M, Hartmann PE (1984). The yield and nutrient content of colostrum and milk of women giving birth to one month postpartum. Br J Nutr, 52: 87–95.

Sernia C, Tyndale-Biscoe CH (1979). Prolactin receptors in the mammary gland corpus leteum and other tissues of the tammar Wallarby, Macropus eugenii. J Endocrinol, 83: 79–89.

Silb JA, Glass EJ (1978). Metoclopramide in young children. Br Med J, 2: 431.

Sloper K, Elsden E, Baum JD (1977). Increasing breastfeeding in a community. Arch Dis Child, 52: 700–702.

Starling J, Ferguson DM, Horwood LJ, Taylor B (1979). Breastfeeding success and failure. Austral Paediatr J, 15: 271–274.

Stevens S, Whitfield MF (1980). How accurate is clinical test weighing of the newborn? Midwives' Chron & Nursing Notes, May: 148–149.

Tarsy D, Baldessarini RJ (1984). Tardive dyskinesia. Annual Rev Med, 35: 605–623.

Thomsen AC, Espersen T, Maigaard S (1984). Course and treatment of milk stasis, non-infectious inflammation of the breast and infectious mastitis in nursing women. Am J Obstet Gynecol, 149: 492–495.

Tyson JE, Wang PH, Guyda H, Friesen HG (1977). Studies of prolactin secretion in human pregnancy. Am J Obstet Gynecol, 129: 454.

Waller H (1946). The early failure of breastfeeding. Arch Dis Child, 21: 1–12.

Weber F, Woolridge MW, Baum JH (1986). An ultrasonographic analysis of sucking and swallowing in newborn infants. Dev Med Child Neurol, 28: 19–24.

West CP (1980). Factors influencing the duration of breastfeeding. J Biosoc Sci, 12: 325–331.

Whichelow MJ (1982). Factors associated with the duration of breastfeeding in a privileged society. Early Hum Dev, 7: 273–280.

Whitehead RG, Paul AA (1981). Infant growth and human milk requirements. Lancet, ii: 161–163.

Whitfield MF, Kay R, Stevens S (1981). Validity of routine clinical test weighing as a measure of the intake of breastfed babies. Arch Dis Child, 56: 919–921.

Williams AF, Akinkugbe FM, Baum JD (1985). A comparison of two methods of milk sampling for calculating the fat intake of breastfed babies. Hum Nutr: Clin Nutr 1985 39C 193–202.

Winberg J, Wesser G (1971). Does breastmilk protect against septicaemia in the newborn? Lancet, i: 1091–1094.

Wood CS, Isaacs PC, Jensen M, Hilton HG (1988). Exclusively breastfed infants: growth and caloric intake. Pediatr Nurs, 14: 117–125.

Woolridge MW, Fisher C (1988). Colic 'overfeeding' and symptoms of lactose malabsorption in the breastfed baby: A possible artifact of feeding management? Lancet, 13 Aug: 382–384.

Woolridge MW, Baum JD, Drewett RF (1980). Effect of a traditional and of a new nipple shield on sucking patterns and milk flow. Early Hum Dev, 4: 357–364.

Woolridge MW (1986a). The anatomy of infant sucking. Midwifery, 2: 164–171.

Woolridge MW (1986b). Aetiology of sore nipples. Midwifery, 2: 172–176.

World Health Organization (1979). Collaborative Study on Breastfeeding. Geneva: World Health Organization.

World Health Organization (1980). Provisional Summary Record of the 8th Meeting of Committee A, at the 33rd World Health Assembly, Geneva 1980. Geneva: World Health Organization, Document No. A33/A/SR/8, p 11 (cited in Chetley 1986).

World Health Organization (1982). The prevalence and duration of breastfeeding: a critical review of available information. World Health Stat Qtly, 2: 91–117.

Ylikorkala O, Kauppila A, Kivinen S, Viinikka L (1984). Treatment of inadequate lactation with oral sulpiride and buccal oxytocin. Obstet Gynecol, 63: 57–60.

Ylikorkala O, Kauppila A, Kivinen S, Viinikka L (1982). Sulpiride improves inadequate lactation. Br Med J, 285: 249–251.

Zarate A, Schally AV, Soria J, Jacobs LS, Canales ES (1974). Effect of thyrotrophin releasing hormone (TRH) on the menstrual cycle in women. Obstet Gynecol, 43: 487–489.

Zarate A, Villalobos H, Canales E, Soria J, Arcovedo F, MacGregor C (1976). The effect of oral administration of thyrotropin-releasing hormone on lactation. J Clin Endocrinol Metab, 43: 301–305.

82 Relief of breast symptoms in women who are not breastfeeding

Fabio Parazzini, Flavia Zanaboni, Alessandro Liberati, and Gianni Tognoni

1 Introduction

Women do not breastfeed their babies after childbirth for a variety of reasons which range from stillbirth to personal wishes. The decision not to breastfeed may lead to considerable breast pain and engorgement during the days following childbirth until the time that lactation eventually becomes suppressed naturally. A number of approaches (apart from analgesics) have been adopted in attempts to hasten the suppression of lactation and reduce the symptoms that are associated with this process.

2 Non-pharmacological approaches

Until 40 years ago, only non-pharmacological methods were used in these circumstances. Tight binding of the breasts and fluid restriction were probably the most common of these approaches then, and they probably remain among the most frequently adopted of the non-pharmacological methods. The relative merits of these non-pharmacological methods have been the subject of almost no formal investigation. Indeed, as far as we know, it was not until 1983 that binding, fluid restriction, and simply wearing a brassiere were compared in a small randomized trial (Brooten *et al.* 1983). Most of the differences observed in the trial can easily be ascribed to chance because of the small sample size, but women who restricted their fluid intake were statistically significantly less likely than those wearing brassieres to have experienced breast pain.

Non-pharmacological methods of inhibiting lactation have probably been implicitly compared with pharmacological methods in many of the trials reviewed below. Yet the comparison has only rarely been conceptualized and reported in these terms. In two studies (De Gezelle *et al.* 1979; Shapiro and Thomas 1984) in which breast binders were explicitly compared with a drug (bromocriptine), the drug was shown to be more effective in controlling symptoms during the first week postpartum (Table 82.1). Only one of these two trials provides data on longer term follow-up. By the second week the two groups were equally likely to be experiencing symptoms, and three weeks postpartum nearly all the women who experienced problems were in the group that had received the drug (Table 82.2). It seems probable, therefore, that there may be short term costs, but longer term benefits of at least some of the non-pharmacological approaches to suppressing lactation.

3 Pharmacological approaches

A number of pharmacological agents have been used in attempts to inhibit lactation and reduce the pain that is often associated with it. We reviewed a total of 72

Table 82.1 Effect of bromocriptine vs. breast binders for lactation suppression on continuing lactation 1 week postpartum

Study	EXPT		CTRL		Odds ratio	Graph of odds ratios and confidence intervals						
	n	(%)	*n*	(%)	(95% CI)	0.01	0.1	0.5	1	2	10	100
Shapiro and Thomas (1984)	2/25	(8.00)	18/25	(72.00)	0.07 (0.02–0.22)							
De Gezelle *et al.* (1979)	2/18	(11.11)	17/18	(94.44)	0.04 (0.01–0.14)							
Typical odds ratio (95% confidence interval)					0.06 (0.02–0.13)							

Effect of bromocriptine vs. breast binders for lactation suppression on breast pain 1 week postpartum

| Shapiro and Thomas (1984) | 1/25 | (4.00) | 16/25 | (64.00) | 0.07 (0.02–0.23) | | | | | | | |
| Typical odds ratio (95% confidence interval) | | | | | 0.07 (0.02–0.23) | | | | | | | |

Effect of bromocriptine vs. breast binders for lactation suppression on breast engorgement 1 week postpartum

Shapiro and Thomas (1984)	1/25	(4.00)	10/25	(40.00)	0.13 (0.03–0.48)							
De Gezelle *et al.* (1979)	5/18	(27.78)	18/18	(100.0)	0.05 (0.01–0.18)							
Typical odds ratio (95% confidence interval)					0.08 (0.03–0.20)							

Table 82.2 Effect of bromocriptine vs. breast binders for lactation suppression on continuing lactation 2 weeks postpartum

Study	EXPT		CTRL		Odds ratio	Graph of odds ratios and confidence intervals						
	n	(%)	*n*	(%)	(95% CI)	0.01	0.1	0.5	1	2	10	100
Shapiro and Thomas (1984)	4/25	(16.00)	3/25	(12.00)	1.38 (0.28–6.73)							
Typical odds ratio (95% confidence interval)					1.38 (0.28–6.73)							

Effect of bromocriptine vs. breast binders for lactation suppression on breast pain 2 weeks postpartum

| Shapiro and Thomas (1984) | 3/25 | (12.00) | 2/25 | (8.00) | 1.55 (0.25–9.63) | | | | | | | |
| Typical odds ratio (95% confidence interval) | | | | | 1.55 (0.25–9.63) | | | | | | | |

Effect of bromocriptine vs. breast binders for lactation suppression on breast engorgement 2 weeks postpartum

| Shapiro and Thomas (1984) | 2/25 | (8.00) | 2/25 | (8.00) | 1.00 (0.13–7.56) | | | | | | | |
| Typical odds ratio (95% confidence interval) | | | | | 1.00 (0.13–7.56) | | | | | | | |

Effect of bromocriptine vs. breast binders for lactation suppression on continuing lactation 3 weeks postpartum

Study	EXPT		CTRL		Odds ratio	Graph of odds ratios and confidence intervals						
	n	(%)	*n*	(%)	(95% CI)	0.01	0.1	0.5	1	2	10	100
Shapiro and Thomas (1984)	6/25	(24.00)	1/25	(4.00)	5.09 (1.05–24.77)							
Typical odds ratio (95% confidence interval)					5.09 (1.05–24.77)							

Effect of bromocriptine vs. breast binders for lactation suppression on breast pain 3 weeks postpartum

Study	EXPT		CTRL		Odds ratio	
Shapiro and Thomas (1984)	3/25	(12.00)	0/25	(0.00)	8.05 (0.80–81.12)	
Typical odds ratio (95% confidence interval)					8.05 (0.80–81.12)	

Effect of bromocriptine vs. breast binders for lactation suppression on breast engorgement 3 weeks postpartum

Study	EXPT		CTRL		Odds ratio	
Shapiro and Thomas (1984)	2/25	(8.00)	0/25	(0.00)	7.70 (0.47–99.99)	
Typical odds ratio (95% confidence interval)					7.70 (0.47–99.99)	

potentially relevant reports of controlled trials published in English. We excluded two studies because only biochemical endpoints had been considered (David *et al.* 1977; Osbourne *et al.* 1978). We also excluded 21 reports of studies involving comparisons for which there were only one or two trials in total. These included evaluations of the effects of oral contraceptives, tamoxifen, bromelain/trypsin combinations, non-hormonal tranquillizers, and clomiphene, as well as comparisons of different dosage schedules of bromocriptine and oestrogen/androgen preparations (Garry 1956; Stenchever 1962; Semm 1966; Booker *et al.* 1970; Lee 1971; Koshiishi *et al.* 1971; Ng and Lee 1972; Zuckerman and Carmel 1973; Utian *et al.* 1975; Kalir *et al.* 1975; Shaaban 1975; Canales *et al.* 1977; MacLeod *et al.* 1977; Yuen *et al.* 1977; Masala *et al.* 1978; De Cecco *et al.* 1979; Boes 1980; Venturini *et al.* 1981; Thorbert and Akerlund 1983; Caballero *et al.* 1987; Defoort *et al.* 1987). Of the 49 studies that remained, five did not present data in a usable form (Binns 1967; Grant *et al.* 1978; Hutchinson and Sill 1981; Kulski *et al.* 1978; Walker *et al.* 1975). The remaining 42 reports form the basis of the analyses that follow. Efficacy in terms of lactation suppression was generally measured as the effect of treatment by the end of the first postpartum week, because this was the most commonly adopted period of follow-up. We comment on the disadvantages of using this short period of follow-up later in the chapter.

3.1 Sex hormones

Stilboestrol has been compared with placebo in 14 studies (Primrose and Tremblay 1957; Weinstein *et al.* 1976; De Gezelle *et al.* 1979; Hodge and Carlisle 1969; Fleming 1977; Llwewllyn-Jones 1963; Markin and Wolst 1960; Stirrat *et al.* 1968; Kirkland *et al.* 1960; Foukas 1973; MacDonald *et al.* 1965; Winter and Robinson 1964; Steele 1968; Varga *et al.* 1972). Table 82.3 shows that the drug reduces the incidence of continuing lactation, breast pain and engorgement during the first week postpartum. Quinoestrol, a long-acting oestrogen, has similar, but apparently less marked effects (Table 82.4). As indicated above, however, there appear to be longer term costs of this short term efficacy. In one large study, for example, 37 per cent of women given stilboestrol compared with only 21 per cent of women given placebo required additional treatment after discharge from hospital, and 30 per cent of the stilboestrol group but only 7 per cent of the placebo group reported abnormal bleeding after the end of treatment (Winter and Robinson 1964). Indeed, the authors of this report concluded that these unwanted effects of the drug outweighed its short term benefits.

The suggestion from the indirect comparisons of stilboestrol and quinoestrol shown in Tables 82.3 and 82.4, that the former suppresses lactation and pain more effectively than the latter, is supported by the results of the five trials in which the two drugs have been compared directly (Gillibrand and Huntingford 1968; Kuku 1968; Watson 1969; Bergsjø and Brodtkorb 1974; and Mann 1971, not included in the tables because it reports only on breast engorgement) (Table 82.5).

Chlorotrianisene, another stilboestrol analogue, has

Table 82.3 Effect of stilboestrol for suppression of lactation on continuing lactation 1 week postpartum

Study	EXPT		CTRL		Odds ratio	Graph of odds ratios and confidence intervals						
	n	(%)	*n*	(%)	(95% CI)	0.01	0.1	0.5	1	2	10	100
Primrose and Tremblay (1957)	8/48	(16.67)	37/45	(82.22)	0.07 (0.03–0.17)							
Weinstein *et al.* (1976)	11/15	(73.33)	8/15	(53.33)	2.30 (0.53–9.90)							
De Gezelle *et al.* (1979)	3/18	(16.67)	17/18	(94.44)	0.05 (0.01–0.17)							
Hodge and Carlisle (1969)	14/178	(7.87)	131/365	(35.89)	0.24 (0.16–0.36)							
Fleming (1977)	14/165	(8.48)	129/162	(79.63)	0.06 (0.04–0.09)							
Llewellyn-Jones (1963)	15/36	(41.67)	25/37	(67.57)	0.36 (0.14–0.89)							
Markin and Wolst (1960)	16/52	(30.77)	153/218	(70.18)	0.19 (0.10–0.35)							
Stirrat *et al.* (1968)	8/50	(16.00)	42/50	(84.00)	0.07 (0.03–0.15)							
Kirkland *et al.* (1960)	16/39	(41.03)	11/12	(91.67)	0.14 (0.04–0.49)							
Foukas (1973)	12/68	(17.65)	71/86	(82.56)	0.07 (0.04–0.14)							
Typical odds ratio (95% confidence interval)					0.12 (0.10–0.15)							

Effect of stilboestrol for suppression of lactation on breast pain 1 week postpartum

Study	EXPT		CTRL		Odds ratio							
MacDonald and O'Driscoll (1965)	13/250	(5.20)	27/250	(10.80)	0.47 (0.25–0.89)							
Primrose and Tremblay (1957)	6/48	(12.50)	37/45	(82.22)	0.06 (0.03–0.14)							
Weinstein *et al.* (1976)	11/15	(73.33)	8/15	(53.33)	2.30 (0.53–9.90)							
Winter and Robinson (1964)	20/400	(5.00)	160/400	(40.00)	0.13 (0.10–0.19)							
Markin and Wolst (1960)	4/52	(7.69)	118/218	(54.13)	0.15 (0.08–0.28)							
Stirrat *et al.* (1968)	0/50	(0.00)	28/50	(56.00)	0.06 (0.03–0.15)							
Kirkland *et al.* (1960)	2/39	(5.13)	4/12	(33.33)	0.07 (0.01–0.51)							
Steele (1968)	7/47	(14.89)	19/44	(43.18)	0.25 (0.10–0.63)							
Typical odds ratio (95% confidence interval)					0.16 (0.13–0.20)							

Effect of stilboestrol for suppression of lactation on breast engorgement 1 week postpartum

Study	EXPT		CTRL		Odds ratio							
Varga *et al.* (1972)	1/20	(5.00)	18/20	(90.00)	0.04 (0.01–0.12)							
Primrose and Tremblay (1957)	12/45	(26.67)	46/48	(95.83)	0.05 (0.02–0.12)							
Winter and Robinson (1964)	60/400	(15.00)	190/400	(47.50)	0.22 (0.16–0.30)							
Markin and Wolst (1960)	44/218	(20.18)	39/52	(75.00)	0.08 (0.04–0.15)							
Typical odds ratio (95% confidence interval)					0.15 (0.12–0.20)							

Table 82.4 Effect of quinoestrol for suppression of lactation on continuing lactation 1 week postpartum

Study	EXPT		CTRL		Odds ratio	Graph of odds ratios and confidence intervals						
	n	(%)	n	(%)	(95% CI)	0.01	0.1	0.5	1	2	10	100
Morris (1967)	14/23	(60.87)	11/20	(55.00)	1.27 (0.38–4.20)							
Cruttenden (1971)	3/33	(9.09)	12/30	(40.00)	0.19 (0.06–0.59)							
McGlone (1969)	14/22	(63.64)	22/22	(100.0)	0.09 (0.02–0.42)							
Typical odds ratio (95% confidence interval)					0.32 (0.15–0.66)							

Effect of quinoestrol for suppresion of lactation on 'failure' (to suppress lactation/engorgement/pain) 1 week postpartum

Vischi *et al.* (1975)	23/132	(17.42)	55/66	(83.33)	0.06 (0.04–0.12)							
Firth (1969)	33/50	(66.00)	50/50	(100.0)	0.09 (0.03–0.26)							
Cruttenden (1971)	8/33	(24.24)	17/30	(56.67)	0.26 (0.10–0.72)							
Typical odds ratio (95% confidence interval)					0.09 (0.06–0.15)							

Table 82.5 Effect of stilboestrol vs. quinoestrol for suppression of lactation on continuing lactation 1 week postpartum

Study	EXPT		CTRL		Odds ratio	Graph of odds ratios and confidence intervals						
	n	(%)	n	(%)	(95% CI)	0.01	0.1	0.5	1	2	10	100
Watson (1969)	10/49	(20.41)	29/50	(58.00)	0.21 (0.09–0.47)							
Bergsjø and Brodtkorb (1974)	11/18	(61.11)	13/23	(56.52)	1.20 (0.35–4.14)							
Typical odds ratio (95% confidence interval)					0.35 (0.18–0.69)							

Effect of stilboestrol vs. quinoestrol for suppresion of lactation on 'failure' (to suppress lactation/engorgement/pain) 1 week postpartum

Gillibrand and Huntingford (1968)	2/21	(9.52)	18/27	(66.67)	0.10 (0.03–0.31)							
Kuku (1968)*	19/52	(36.54)	17/52	(32.69)	1.18 (0.53–2.64)							
Typical odds ratio (95% confidence interval)					0.52 (0.27–1.01)							

*quinoestrol vs. ethinyloestradrol

Table 82.6 Effect of chlorotrianisene for suppression of lactation on continuing lactation 1 week postpartum

Study	EXPT		CTRL		Odds ratio	Graph of odds ratios and confidence intervals
	n	(%)	n	(%)	(95% CI)	0.01 0.1 0.5 1 2 10 100
Morris *et al.* (1970)	89/220	(40.45)	47/72	(65.28)	0.37 (0.22–0.63)	
Primrose and Tremblay (1957)	35/68	(51.47)	37/45	(82.22)	0.27 (0.12–0.58)	
Tyson (1966)	5/27	(18.52)	7/20	(35.00)	0.43 (0.12–1.59)	
Phillips (1975)	18/98	(18.37)	23/98	(23.47)	0.74 (0.37–1.46)	
Typical odds ratio (95% confidence interval)					0.42 (0.29–0.60)	

Effect of chlorotrianisene for suppression of lactation on breast pain 1 week postpartum

Study	EXPT		CTRL		Odds ratio	
Morris *et al.* (1970)	91/220	(41.36)	60/72	(83.33)	0.19 (0.11–0.32)	
Primrose and Tremblay (1957)	25/68	(36.76)	37/45	(82.22)	0.16 (0.08–0.34)	
Tyson (1966)	2/27	(7.41)	5/20	(25.00)	0.26 (0.05–1.28)	
Phillips (1975)	18/98	(18.37)	23/98	(23.47)	0.74 (0.37–1.46)	
Typical odds ratio (95% confidence interval)					0.27 (0.19–0.38)	

Effect of chlorotrianisene for suppression of lactation on breast engorgement 1 week postpartum

Study	EXPT		CTRL		Odds ratio	
Morris *et al.* (1970)	112/220	(50.91)	55/72	(76.39)	0.35 (0.21–0.61)	
Niebyl *et al.* (1979)	4/25	(16.00)	1/21	(4.76)	3.11 (0.49–19.66)	
Primrose and Tremblay (1957)	16/68	(23.53)	33/45	(73.33)	0.13 (0.06–0.29)	
Tyson (1966)	9/27	(33.33)	8/20	(40.00)	0.75 (0.23–2.48)	
Phillips (1975)	18/90	(20.00)	23/98	(23.47)	0.82 (0.41–1.63)	
Typical odds ratio (95% confidence interval)					0.41 (0.29–0.58)	

also been shown to reduce lactation, breast pain, and engorgement in the short term in placebo-controlled trials (Morris *et al.* 1970; Primrose and Tremblay 1957; Tyson 1966; Phillips 1975; Niebyl *et al.* 1979; and King 1958, not included in the table since it presents data as an overall index of efficacy) (Table 82.6).

Various combinations of an oestrogen and testosterone have been assessed and these have been shown to have dramatic short term effects on lactation, breast pain, and breast engorgement (Primrose and Tremblay 1957; Kirkland *et al.* 1960; Markin and Wolst 1960; Roser 1966; Morris *et al.* 1970; and Barns 1961, not included in the table since it reports data only on an overall index of efficacy) (Table 82.7). The only trial in which longer term effects have been reported, however, shows a reversal of the short term effects by the end of the second postpartum week (Table 82.8).

Among the more than 2000 women treated with oestrogens in the context of trials, there have been 3 reported cases of superficial thrombophlebitis compared with 1 reported case among the 1500 or so 'controls'. This is consistent with the increased risk of thromboembolic complications associated with oestrogen use that was first reported by Daniel *et al.* (1967), but suggests that the risk may be quite low. Withdrawal bleeding after hormonal treatment is reported by about

Table 82.7 Effect of oestrogen/testosterone combination for suppression of lactation on continuing lactation 1 week postpartum

Study	EXPT		CTRL		Odds ratio	Graph of odds ratios and confidence intervals						
	n	(%)	n	(%)	(95% CI)	0.01	0.1	0.5	1	2	10	100
Roser (1966)	4/86	(4.65)	55/89	(61.80)	0.08 (0.04–0.15)							
Morris *et al.* (1970)	19/96	(19.79)	63/96	(65.63)	0.16 (0.09–0.27)							
Primrose and Tremblay (1957)	33/54	(61.11)	37/45	(82.22)	0.36 (0.15–0.87)							
Markin and Wolst (1960)	51/268	(19.03)	153/218	(70.18)	0.12 (0.09–0.18)							
Kirkland *et al.* (1960)	23/41	(56.10)	11/12	(91.67)	0.22 (0.06–0.83)							
Typical odds ratio (95% confidence interval)					0.13 (0.10–0.17)							

Effect of oestrogen/testosterone combination for suppression of lactation on breast pain 1 week postpartum

Study	EXPT		CTRL		Odds ratio	
Iliya *et al.* (1966)	1/102	(0.98)	65/90	(72.22)	0.04 (0.02–0.08)	
Morris *et al.* (1970)	22/96	(22.92)	84/96	(87.50)	0.07 (0.04–0.13)	
Louviere and Upton (1975)	92/235	(39.15)	177/215	(82.33)	0.17 (0.11–0.24)	
Primrose and Tremblay (1957)	27/54	(50.00)	37/45	(82.22)	0.25 (0.11–0.56)	
Markin and Wolst (1960)	36/268	(13.43)	118/218	(54.13)	0.15 (0.10–0.22)	
Kirkland *et al.* (1960)	7/41	(17.07)	4/12	(33.33)	0.38 (0.08–1.82)	
Typical odds ratio (95% confidence interval)					0.13 (0.10–0.16)	

Effect of oestrogen/testosterone combination for suppression of lactation on breast engorgement 1 week postpartum

Study	EXPT		CTRL		Odds ratio	
Iliya *et al.* (1966)	6/102	(5.88)	79/90	(87.78)	0.04 (0.02–0.07)	
Roser (1966)	8/86	(9.30)	83/89	(93.26)	0.04 (0.02–0.06)	
Morris *et al.* (1970)	22/96	(22.92)	83/96	(86.46)	0.08 (0.04–0.14)	
Louviere and Upton (1975)	105/235	(44.68)	193/215	(89.77)	0.13 (0.09–0.20)	
Primrose and Tremblay (1957)	24/54	(44.44)	33/45	(73.33)	0.31 (0.14–0.69)	
Markin and Wolst (1960)	52/268	(19.40)	174/218	(79.82)	0.09 (0.06–0.13)	
Typical odds ratio (95% confidence interval)					0.08 (0.07–0.10)	

Table 82.8 Effect of oestrogen/testosterone combination for suppression of lactation on continuing lactation 2 weeks postpartum

Study	EXPT		CTRL		Odds ratio	Graph of odds ratios and confidence intervals						
	n	(%)	*n*	(%)	(95% CI)	0.01	0.1	0.5	1	2	10	100
Markin and Wolst (1960)	84/268	(31.34)	0/218	(0.00)	8.92 (5.56–14.30)						—·—	
Typical odds ratio (95% confidence interval)					8.92 (5.56–14.30)						—·—	

Effect of oestrogen/testosterone combination for suppression of lactation on breast pain 2 weeks postpartum

| Markin and Wolst (1960) | 82/268 | (30.60) | 0/218 | (0.00) | 8.82 (5.47–14.21) | | | | | | —·— | |
| Typical odds ratio (95% confidence interval) | | | | | 8.82 (5.47–14.21) | | | | | | —·— | |

Effect of oestrogen/testosterone combination for suppression of lactation on breast engorgement 2 weeks postpartum

| Markin and Wolst (1960) | 76/268 | (28.36) | 0/218 | (0.00) | 8.54 (5.23–13.97) | | | | | | —·— | |
| Typical odds ratio (95% confidence interval) | | | | | 8.54 (5.23–13.97) | | | | | | —·— | |

Table 82.9 Effect of bromocriptine for suppression of lactation on continuing lactation 1 week postpartum

Study	EXPT		CTRL		Odds ratio	Graph of odds ratios and confidence intervals						
	n	(%)	*n*	(%)	(95% CI)	0.01	0.1	0.5	1	2	10	100
Dewhurst *et al.* (1977)	8/20	(40.00)	16/17	(94.12)	0.10 (0.03–0.38)		—·—					
Weinstein *et al.* (1976)	4/15	(26.67)	8/15	(53.33)	0.34 (0.08–1.44)			—·——				
De Gezelle *et al.* (1979)	2/18	(11.11)	17/18	(94.44)	0.04 (0.01–0.14)		—·—					
Shapiro and Thomas (1984)	2/25	(8.00)	18/25	(72.00)	0.07 (0.02–0.22)		—·—					
Willmott *et al.* (1977)	4/16	(25.00)	13/14	(92.86)	0.07 (0.02–0.29)		—·—					
Typical odds ratio (95% confidence interval)					0.09 (0.05–0.16)		—·—					

Effect of bromocriptine for suppression of lactation on breast pain 1 week postpartum

Dewhurst *et al.* (1977)	1/20	(5.00)	13/17	(76.47)	0.05 (0.01–0.19)		—·—					
Weinstein *et al.* (1976)	0/15	(0.00)	8/15	(53.33)	0.07 (0.01–0.35)		—·—					
Shapiro and Thomas (1984)	1/25	(4.00)	16/25	(64.00)	0.07 (0.02–0.23)		—·—					
Willmott *et al.* (1977)	3/16	(18.75)	11/14	(78.57)	0.10 (0.02–0.40)		—·—					
Typical odds ratio (95% confidence interval)					0.07 (0.04–0.14)		—·—					

Table 82.9—*continued* Effect of bromocriptine for suppression of lactation on breast engorgement 1 week postpartum

Study	EXPT		CTRL		Odds ratio	Graph of odds ratios and confidence intervals
	n	(%)	n	(%)	(95% CI)	0.01 0.1 0.5 1 2 10 100
Dewhurst *et al.* (1977)	6/20	(30.00)	15/17	(88.24)	0.10 (0.03–0.36)	
Rolland and Schellekens (1973)	2/30	(6.67)	9/10	(90.00)	0.02 (0.00–0.08)	
Varga *et al.* (1972)	1/20	(5.00)	18/20	(90.00)	0.04 (0.01–0.12)	
Weinstein *et al.* (1976)	0/15	(0.00)	8/15	(53.33)	0.07 (0.01–0.35)	
Shapiro and Thomas (1984)	1/25	(4.00)	10/25	(40.00)	0.13 (0.03–0.48)	
De Gezelle *et al.* (1979)	5/18	(27.78)	18/18	(100.0)	0.05 (0.01–0.18)	
Willmott *et al.* (1977)	3/16	(18.75)	13/14	(92.86)	0.06 (0.01–0.23)	
Bhardwaj (1979)	2/21	(9.52)	15/24	(62.50)	0.11 (0.03–0.36)	
Typical odds ratio (95% confidence interval)					0.06 (0.04–0.10)	

Table 82.10 Effect of bromocriptine for suppression of lactation on continuing lactation 2 weeks postpartum

Study	EXPT		CTRL		Odds ratio	Graph of odds ratios and confidence intervals
	n	(%)	n	(%)	(95% CI)	0.01 0.1 0.5 1 2 10 100
Dewhurst *et al.* (1977)	6/20	(30.00)	13/16	(81.25)	0.14 (0.04–0.50)	
Shapiro and Thomas (1984)	4/25	(16.00)	3/25	(12.00)	1.38 (0.28–6.73)	
Willmott *et al.* (1977)	4/16	(25.00)	12/14	(85.71)	0.09 (0.02–0.39)	
Typical odds ratio (95% confidence interval)					0.22 (0.10–0.51)	

Effect of bromocriptine for suppression of lactation on breast pain 2 weeks postpartum

Study	EXPT		CTRL		Odds ratio	
Dewhurst *et al.* (1977)	3/20	(15.00)	3/16	(18.75)	0.77 (0.14–4.38)	
Shapiro and Thomas (1984)	3/25	(12.00)	2/25	(8.00)	1.55 (0.25–9.63)	
Willmott *et al.* (1977)	2/16	(12.50)	3/14	(21.43)	0.54 (0.08–3.56)	
Typical odds ratio (95% confidence interval)					0.87 (0.30–2.47)	

Effect of bromocriptine for suppression of lactation on breast engorgement 2 weeks postpartum

Study	EXPT		CTRL		Odds ratio	
Dewhurst *et al.* (1977)	3/20	(15.00)	3/16	(18.75)	0.77 (0.14–4.38)	
Shapiro and Thomas (1984)	2/25	(8.00)	2/25	(8.00)	1.00 (0.13–7.56)	
Willmott *et al.* (1977)	2/16	(12.50)	13/14	(92.86)	0.04 (0.01–0.18)	
Typical odds ratio (95% confidence interval)					0.22 (0.08–0.57)	

15 per cent of women without any apparent differences in frequency for different drugs.

3.2 Bromocriptine

Eight studies compared bromoergocriptine with placebo (Dewhurst *et al.* 1977; Weinstein *et al.* 1976; De Gezelle *et al.* 1979; Shapiro *et al.* 1984; Willmott *et al.* 1977; Rolland *et al.* 1973; Varga *et al.* 1972; Bhardwaj 1979), and the drug schedules evaluated in these trials were generally comparable. Taken individually and together, the results suggest that bromoergocriptine greatly decreased (about 90 per cent) lactation, breast

pain, and engorgement in the first postpartum week (Table 82.9). When the analysis was performed on data referring to the 14th postpartum day, the differences were less dramatic (Table 82.10).

No major adverse effect has been reported in women treated with bromoergocriptine for suppression of lactation. The reported frequency of nausea is less than 5 per cent.

Although indirect comparisons of bromoergocriptine and stilboestrol suggest that the former may suppress lactation and breast engorgement more effectively than the latter, the available data from controlled trials in

Table 82.11 Effect of bromocriptine vs. stilboestrol for suppression of lactation on continuing lactation 1 week postpartum

Study	EXPT		CTRL		Odds ratio	Graph of odds ratios and confidence intervals
	n	(%)	*n*	(%)	(95% CI)	0.01 0.1 0.5 1 2 10 100
Steenstrup and Steenstrup (1977)	2/20	(10.00)	8/21	(38.10)	0.23 (0.06–0.93)	
Seppala *et al.* (1975)	2/20	(10.00)	1/19	(5.26)	1.92 (0.19–19.61)	
Nilsen *et al.* (1976)	3/20	(15.00)	0/18	(0.00)	7.45 (0.72–76.61)	
Weinstein *et al.* (1976)	4/15	(26.67)	11/15	(73.33)	0.16 (0.04–0.67)	
De Gezelle *et al.* (1979)	2/18	(11.11)	3/18	(16.67)	0.64 (0.10–4.10)	
Typical odds ratio (95% confidence interval)					0.46 (0.21–0.99)	

Effect of bromocriptine vs. stilboestrol for suppression of lactation on breast engorgement 1 week postpartum

Study	EXPT		CTRL		Odds ratio	Graph
Steenstrup and Steenstrup (1977)	1/20	(5.00)	3/21	(14.29)	0.36 (0.05–2.74)	
Seppala *et al.* (1975)	4/20	(20.00)	3/19	(15.79)	1.32 (0.26–6.64)	
Nilsen *et al.* (1976)	1/20	(5.00)	1/18	(5.56)	0.90 (0.05–14.96)	
Varga *et al.* (1972)	1/20	(5.00)	1/20	(5.00)	1.00 (0.06–16.58)	
Weinstein *et al.* (1976)	0/15	(0.00)	11/15	(73.33)	0.05 (0.01–0.20)	
De Gezelle *et al.* (1979)	5/18	(27.78)	3/18	(16.67)	1.87 (0.40–8.80)	
Typical odds ratio (95% confidence interval)					0.47 (0.22–1.00)	

Table 82.12 Effect of pyridoxine for suppression of lactation on continuing lactation 1 week postpartum

Study	EXPT		CTRL		Odds ratio	Graph of odds ratios and confidence intervals
	n	(%)	*n*	(%)	(95% CI)	0.01 0.1 0.5 1 2 10 100
Fleming (1977)	110/155	(70.97)	129/162	(79.63)	0.63 (0.38–1.05)	
Foukas (1973)	5/75	(6.67)	71/86	(82.56)	0.05 (0.03–0.09)	
Typical odds ratio (95% confidence interval)					0.22 (0.15–0.33)	

which direct comparisons between the two drugs have been made do not provide strong evidence for a large differential effect of the two drugs (Table 82.11).

3.3 Pyridoxine

Pyridoxine has been compared with placebo in three studies (Foukas 1953; Fleming 1977; and MacDonald *et al.* 1976, not included in the table because data not presented in a suitable form), the few data available show a limited effect on lactation (Table 82.12).

3.4 Oxytocin

In the early 1960s the effects of spraying of synthetic oxytocin intranasally on lactation and breast symptoms was studied in at least three trials, one of them unpublished (Ryan and Brown 1962; Winter and Robinson 1964; D Hawkins, personal communication). None of these studies provided any evidence that the treatment was effective.

4 Discussion

Although a total of more than 3000 women are represented in published reports of controlled trials of lactation suppression published over the last 30 years, the quality of the available evidence is very unsatisfactory. Not only have many of the trials been poorly executed and reported, but most have been unimaginatively designed. First of all, very few formal comparisons between non-pharmacological and pharmacological approaches to suppression of lactation and control of breast pain have been conducted. Second, the periods of follow-up have, in general, been very short, so that the relative efficacy beyond the first week postpartum, both of non-pharmacological and pharmacological methods, and of different pharmacological methods, is not clear.

Furthermore, it is difficult to estimate the real frequency of adverse reactions to these various drugs because although quantitative estimates of side-effects were reported in about the 40 per cent of the studies reviewed, many studies had a large proportion of dropouts, perhaps because of unrecorded side-effects. Rebound lactation and prolonged leakage after pharmacological attempts to suppress lactation appear to affect between a quarter and a third of women given hormones, and a somewhat lower proportion of women given bromocriptine, yet, as we have already noted, the available information is inadequate to quantify these problems with any confidence.

Another note of caution is appropriate about the research done in this field. A large proportion of it is supported by the drug industry (such support was acknowledged explicitly in 58 per cent of the reports reviewed here). This is known to decrease the chances of 'negative studies' in this field being reported in print (D Hawkins, personal communication), and may also result in the selective presentation of results relative to one end point, but not to another, simply to increase the 'impact' of a study.

5 Conclusions

5.1 Recommendations for current practice

The available evidence suggests that fluid restriction may reduce symptoms compared with a less active intervention among women who do not wish to breastfeed. Non-pharmacological methods of lactation suppression, like breast binding, are associated with more pain in the first week after delivery than pharmacological methods, but they may be more effective in the longer term. Women should be made aware of these relative advantages and disadvantages when a method to suppress lactation is chosen.

If it is decided to use one of the pharmacological approaches, a variety of drugs that reduce lactation, breast pain, and breast engorgement during the first week postpartum are available. Relatively few studies have compared these different preparations directly, so no firm answers can be given to questions about their relative merits for suppressing lactation and controlling breast pain. The available evidence suggests that, in the short term, stilboestrol may be superior to quinoestrol, and bromoergocriptine superior to stilboestrol in suppressing lactation and reducing breast pain in women who do not wish to breastfeed. The thrombogenic potential of oestrogens, although small, is another reason for selecting bromoergocriptine from among the various pharmacological options available.

5.2 Recommendations for future research

Bromoergocriptine, and newer drugs like di-hydroergocriptine, should be compared formally with nonpharmacological methods of suppressing lactation in well-designed trials that have adequate sample sizes and duration of follow-up. Women's views of the relative merits and disadvantages of the alternative methods should constitute an essential element in the evaluation, and more serious attention should be given to documenting the frequency of short and long term adverse reactions.

References

Barns DH (1961). Suppression of postpartum lactation and prevention of breast engorgement in non-nursing mothers. Am J Obstet Gynecol, 81: 339–343.

Bergsjo P, Brodtkorb C (1974). Comparison between quinestrol and diethylstilbestrol for the inhibition of lactation. Acta Obstet Gynecol Scand, 53: 77–80.

Bhardwaj N (1979). Inhibition of puerperal lactation: evaluation of bromocriptine and placebo. Austral NZ J Obstet Gynaecol, 19: 154–157.

Binns DT (1967). A double-blind trial of chlorotrianisene in the suppression of lactation. Practitioner, 199: 685–688.

Boes EGM (1980). Inhibition of puerperal lactation: a comparative study of bromocryptine and pyridoxine. S Afr Med J, 57: 900–903.

Booker DE, Pahl IR, Forbes DA (1970). Control of postpartum breast engorgement with oral contraceptives: II. Am J Obstet Gynecol, 108: 240–242.

Brooten DA, Brown LP, Hollingsworth AO, Tanis JL, Donlen J (1983). A comparison of four treatments to prevent and control breast pain and engorgement in nonnursing mothers. Nursing Res, 32: 225–229.

Caballero A, Mena P, Caballero-Diaz JL, Caballero-Asensi A (1987). Metergoline as an inhibitor of prolactin release. J Reprod Med, 32: 115–119.

Canales ES, Lasso P, Soria J, Zarate A (1977). Effect of clomiphene on prolactin secretion and lactation in puerperal women. Br J Obstet Gynaecol, 84: 758–759.

Cruttenden LA (1971). Inhibition of lactation. Practitioner, 206: 248.

Daniel DG, Campbell H, Turnbull AC (1967). Puerperal thrombo-embolism and suppression of lactation. Lancet, 2: 287–289.

David A, Romen I, Lunenfeld B, Kaufman M, Serr DM (1977). Stilbestrol administration in the puerperium and its effect on the prolactin excretion of non-lactating patients. Acta Obstet Gynecol Scand, 56: 211–215.

De Cecco L, Venturini PL, Ragni N, Rossato P, Maganza C, Gaggero G, Horowski R (1979). Effect of lisuride on inhibition of lactation and serum prolactin. Br J Obstet Gynaecol, 86: 905–908.

Defoort P, Thiery M, Baele G, Clement D, Dhont M (1987). Bromocriptine in an injectable retard form for puerperal lactation suppression: comparison with estradon prolongatum. Obstet Gynecol, 70: 866–869.

De Gezelle H, Dhont M, Thiery M, Parewyck W (1979). Puerperal lactation suppression and prolactin. Acta Obstet Gynecol Scand, 58: 469–472.

Dewhurst CJ, Harrison RF, Biswas S (1977). Inhibition of puerperal lactation: a double blind study of a bromocriptine and placebo. Acta Obstet Gynecol Scand, 56: 327–331.

Firth PS (1969). Inhibition of lactation. Br Med J, 1: 254–255.

Fleming JS (1977). Inhibition of puerperal lactation: pyridoxine of no benefit. Austral NZ J Obstet Gynaecol, 17: 131–132.

Foukas M (1973). An antilactogenic effect of pyridoxine. J Obstet Gynecol Br Commnwlth, 80: 718–720.

Garry J (1956). Estrogen–androgen preparation for prevention of postpartum breast engorgement and lactation. Obstet Gynecol, 7: 422–432.

Gillibrand PN, Huntingford PJ (1968). Inhibition of lactation with combined oestrogen and progestogen. Br Med J, 4: 769.

Grant K, Rabello Y, Freeman AG, Freeman RK, Baumgardner AS (1978). Comparison of quinestrol and TACE for relief of postpartum breast discomfort. Obstet Gynecol, 51: 636–639.

Hodge C, Carlisle JS (1969). Relief of pain during suppression of lactation. J Obstet Gynaecol Br Commnwlth, 76: 66–68.

Hutchinson P, Sill H (1981). Lactation suppression with bromocriptine. NZ Med J, 94: 309–310.

Iliya FA, Safon L, O'Leary JA (1966). Testosterone enanthate (180mg) and estradiol valerate (8mg) for suppression of lactation: a double-blind evaluation. Obstet Gynecol, 27: 643–645.

Kalir R, David MP, Kraicer PF (1975). Clomiphene citrate in suppression of puerperal lactation. Am J Obstet Gynecol, 22: 570–572.

King AG (1958). Prevention of puerperal breast engorgement with large doses of long-acting estrogen. Am J Obstet Gynecol, 78: 80–85.

Kirkland JA, Greenberg BG, Flowers CE (1960). Suppression of lactation: a double-blind hormone study. Obstet Gynecol, 15: 292–298.

Koshiishi T, Furasawa Y, Iseki H, Iwasaki Y (1971). A double blind study of the effects of Kimotab on engorgement in the breast. Acta Obstet Gynecol Japan, 18: 222–228.

Kuku SB (1968). Inhibition of lactation with quinestrol. J Obstet Gynaecol Br Commnwlth, 75: 103–104.

Kulski JK, Hartmann PE, Martin JD, Smith M (1978). Effects of bromocriptine on blood coagulation, serum prolactin and serum FSH levels in puerperal women. Br J Obstet Gynaecol, 85: 687–691.

Lee KH (1971). A trial of chlormezanone, a non-hormonal tranquillizer for inhibition of postpartum lactation. Austral NZ J Obstet Gynaecol, 11: 99–102.

Llewellyn-Jones D (1963). Inhibition of lactation using hormones. Med J Malaysia, 18: 13–15.

Louviere RL, Upton RT (1975). Evaluation of Deladumone OB in the suppression of postpartum lactation. Am J Obstet Gynecol, 121: 641–642.

MacDonald D, O'Driscoll K (1965). Suppression of lactation. A double-blind trial. Lancet, 2: 623–625.

MacDonald HN, Collins YD, Tobin MJW, Wijayratne DN (1976). The failure of pyridoxine in the suppression of puerperal lactation. Br J Obstet Gynaecol, 83: 54–55.

MacLeod SC, Scott J, Lord L, Brodie G, Perlin I, Simpson AA (1977). Prevention and suppression of post-partum lactation with 2-bromo-alpha-ergocryptine (CB-154). Clin Endocrinol, 6: 65s–70s.

Mann CW (1971). Lactation inhibition in the Outer Hebrides. Practitioner, 206: 246–247.

Markin KE, Wolst MD (1960). A comparative controlled study of hormones used in the prevention of postpartum breast engorgement and lactation. Am J Obstet Gynecol, 80: 128–137.

Masala A, Delitala G, Lo Dico G, Stoppelli I, Alagna S, Devilla L (1978). Inhibition of lactation and inhibition of prolactin release after mechanical breast stimulation in puerperal women given tamoxifen or placebo. Br J Obstet Gynaecol, 85: 134–137.

McGlone J (1969). An assessment of quinestrol in the inhibition of lactation. Practitioner, 203: 187–188.

Morris JA (1967). Lactation inhibition with quinestrol. Int J Fertil, 12: 261–265.

Morris JA, Creasy RK, Hohe PT (1970). Inhibition of puerperal lactation. Double-blind comparison of chlorothianesene, testosterone enanthate with estradiol valerate and placebo. Obstet Gynecol, 36: 107–114.

Ng KH, Lee KH (1972). Inhibition of postpartum lactation with single-dose drugs. Austral NZ J Obstet Gynaecol, 12: 59–61.

Niebyl JR, Bell WR, Schaaf ME, Blake DA, Dubin NH, King TM (1979). The effect of chlorotrianisene as postpartum lactation suppression on blood coagulation factors. Am J Obstet Gynecol, 134: 518–522.

Nilsen PA, Meling AB, Abildgaard U (1976). Study of the suppression of lactation and the influence on blood clotting with bromocriptine (CB 154) (Parlodel): a double-blind comparison with diethylstilboestrol. Acta Obstet Gynecol Scand, 55: 39–44.

Osbourne GK, Whigham KAE, Howie PW, England P, Kelly A, Prentice CRM (1978). The effects of quinestrol and bromocriptine on blood coagulation, serum prolactin and serum FSH levels in puerperal women. Br J Obstet Gynaecol, 85: 687–691.

Phillips WP (1975). Prevention of postpartum breast engorgement: double-blind comparison of chlorotrianisene 72mg and placebo. J Arkansas Med Soc, 72: 163–167.

Primrose T, Tremblay P (1957). Studies on the suppression of lactation by hormones. Am J Obstet Gynecol, 73: 1218–1224.

Rolland R, Schellekens LA (1973). A new approach to the inhibition of puerperal lactation. J Obstet Gynaecol Br Commnwlth, 80: 945–951.

Roser DM (1966). Breast engorgement and postpartum fever. Obstet Gynecol, 27: 73–77.

Ryan GM Jr, Brown DAJ (1962). Intranasal syntocinon and postpartum breast engorgement. Obstet Gynecol, 20: 582–584.

Semm K (1966). Contraception and lactation. In: Social and medical aspects of oral contraception. Amsterdam: Excerpta Medica Foundation, pp 98–101.

Seppala M, Ylinen O, Sternthal V, Soiva K, Vara P (1975). Suppression of established puerperal lactation with 2-Br-alpha-ergocryptine methane sulphonate (CB 154). Int J Gynaecol Obstet, 13: 1–5.

Shaaban MM (1975). Suppression of lactation by an antiestrogen, tamoxifen. Eur J Obstet Gynecol Reprod Biol, 4: 167–169.

Shapiro AG, Thomas L (1984). Efficacy of bromocriptine versus breast binders as inhibitors of postpartum lactation. South Med J, 77: 719–721.

Steele SJ (1968). Inhibition of lactation by oestrogens. Br Med J, 4: 578.

Steenstrup EK, Steenstrup OR (1977). Prevention of puerperal lactation with bromocriptin (CB 154): a double-blind comparison with diethylstilbestrol. Curr Ther Res, 21: 327–332.

Stenchever MA (1962). Evaluation of chlorprophenpyridamine for prevention of postpartum breast engorgement. Am J Obstet Gynecol, 840: 969–971.

Stirrat GM, Anderson GE, Grant O (1968). The effectiveness of stilboestrol in the suppression of postpartum lactation. J Obstet Gynaecol Br Commnwlth, 75: 313–315.

Thorbert G, Akerlund M (1983). Inhibition of lactation of lactation by cyclofenil and bromocriptine. Br J Obstet Gynaecol, 90: 739–742.

Tyson JEA (1966). A high-dosage estrogen for lactation suppression. Obstet Gynecol, 27: 729–732.

Utian WH, Begg G, Vinik AI, Paul M, Schuman L (1975). Effect of bromocriptine and chlorotrianisene on inhibition of lactation and serum prolactin. A comparative double-blind study. Br J Obstet Gynaecol, 82: 755–759.

Varga L, Lutterbeck PM, Pryor JS, Wenner R, Erb H (1972). Suppression of puerperal lactation with an ergot alkaloid: a double-blind study. Br Med J, 2: 743–744.

Venturini PL, Horowski R, Maganza C, Morano S, Pedretti E, Ragni N, Semino F, De Cecco L (1981). Effects of lisuride and bromocriptine on inhibition of lactation and on serum prolactin levels: comparative double-blind study. Eur J Obstet Gynecol Reprod Biol, 11: 395–400.

Vishi F, Mandruzzato GP, Dell'acqua S, Bruni G (1975). Further evaluation of quinestrol in the inhibition of lactation: a double-blind comparison of two dose levels against placebo. Arch Int Pharmacodyn Ther, 214: 62–67.

Yuen BH, Pendleton HJ, Blair S (1977). Efficacy of bromocriptine and chlorotrianisene in preventing postpartum lactation. Can Med Assoc J, 117: 919–921.

Walker S, Hibbard BM, Groom G, Griffiths K, Davis RH (1975). Controlled trial of bromocriptine, quinestrol and placebo in suppression of puerperal lactation. Lancet, 2: 842–845.

Watson PS (1969). Instant inhibition of lactation. Practitioner, 203: 184–186.

Weinstein D, Ben-David M, Polishuk WZ (1976). Serum prolactin and the suppression of lactation. Br J Obstet Gynaecol, 83: 679–682.

Willmott MP, Colhoun EM, Bolton AE (1977). The suppression of puerperal lactation with bromocryptine. Acta Obstet Gynecol Scand, 56: 145–149.

Winter RW, Robinson SC (1964). Prevention of lactation. Obstet Gynecol, 23: 906–909.

Zuckerman H, Carmel S (1973). The inhibition of lactation by clomiphene. J Obstet Gynaecol Br Commnwlth, 80: 822–823.

83 Clinical examination of the newborn infant

Howard Berger

1 Introduction

The large majority of babies are perfectly healthy at birth. All they require is warmth and tender loving care followed by feeding at appropriate times. For the minority who present with problems either at birth or in the immediate postnatal period, quick and reliable recognition of the problem may be essential to prevent delay in correcting the problem and thereby forestall further impairment. This chapter attempts to give a systematic approach to the clinical examination of the newborn, illustrating its special features but keeping, as much as possible, to a scheme used in adult examinations. With some common problems, such as cyanosis, the aetiology and clinical clues to their diagnosis are briefly discussed and references for further reading given.

Warm hands and the use of a pacifier help to keep the baby calm. Particular attention must be paid to room temperature, e.g. doors closed; an overhead radiant heater is useful to prevent heat loss. The parents may appreciate a running commentary on the examination, and when the baby is ill it is particularly important also to mention the normal findings.

A thorough examination can, with practice, be carried out rapidly but the extent of the examination of each system should be altered according to the postnatal age and clinical condition of the baby. Thus immediately after birth, if there are no worrying features in the maternal and fetal history, the bonding of baby and parents should be a priority. In term babies the Apgar score can be performed (and subsequently major congenital malformations excluded) without separating the baby from the mother. Detailed examination should be carried out within the next 24 hours. A repeat examination prior to discharge in the term baby who is feeding and growing well should in particular assess the level of jaundice, and check for the presence of cardiac murmurs which may not initially be present (see cardiovascular examination).

2 Sequence of examination

Many excellent schemes for the examination of the newborn have been published (Gandy 1986; Lawrence 1984) and several variations of such schemes are practised in various neonatal units. Most of these are adequate when continuously practised by the expert. Retaining the order of examination practised in older children and adults has a major advantage, however. Although it is clear that opportunities to assess clinical signs, such as the urine stream or the cry, must be taken as they arise, the examination is more likely to be complete when it is conducted in a sequence that is familiar to the examiner. For most caregivers, the order of examination learnt in adult medicine or in general paediatrics, will be familiar and there is little reason to change that sequence in the examination of the newborn. Even if the order of the examination is changed, it is worth documenting the findings in a uniform way to facilitate exchange of information with co-workers.

The plan of examination followed in this chapter is: first the general examination, followed by examination of neck, thorax, abdomen, and then head and limbs including the neurological signs. A similar sequence of examination (craniocaudal, anteroposterior, or mediolateral) is followed for each system. The sequence of inspection, palpation, percussion, and auscultation is followed for every part of the examination, including the head and neck. As exclusion of congenital abnormalities is a major aim of the examination of a newborn, attention should be given to minor external malformations that may provide clues to the presence of major internal abnormalities (Smith 1977).

3 General examination

The most essential part of the general examination is to establish that the baby does not require emergency treatment and can safely undergo a detailed examination. The five measurements (respiration, colour, pulse, responses, and tone) that make up the Apgar score (Catlin *et al.* 1986) should be assessed at the start of every examination, instead of being performed only at birth. These tests, if normal, suggest that adequate transport of oxygen to the vital centres is occurring and that no resuscitation is needed and the rest of the examination may be performed.

3.1 Respiration

The main question at this stage is whether the baby is breathing adequately. A quick assessment of frequency and depth of respiration as a clinical measure of minute ventilation is sufficient.

3.2 Colour

The colour helps to indicate whether there is adequate oxygen uptake and transport by the red cells. It gives an indication of the haemoglobin level (anaemia or polycythaemia) and its degree of oxygenation (cyanosis or hyperoxygenation). Although pallor and cyanosis usually receive more attention than plethora due to polycythaemia and hyperoxygenation, these 'opposite' signs must be included in the examination scheme. They are not rare findings, and may signal potential problems. Polycythaemia, commonly seen in babies who are light for their gestational age, in babies of diabetic mothers, and in twin-to-twin transfusion, can cause cyanosis, hypoglycaemia, and jaundice (Black 1987). The excessively pink baby is commonly seen in the aftermath of a successful resuscitation, and reduction of the ambient oxygen concentration may be required.

In a pale baby, the palms of the hands and soles of the feet should be examined, and then the tongue to estab-

lish whether the pallor is peripheral or central. Peripheral pallor is caused by vasoconstriction of skin arterioles, and usually occurs because the baby has been exposed to a cold environment. It may, however, be the first indication of a poor cardiac function due to asphyxia, myocarditis, or a hypoplastic left ventricle, or may be a sign of blood loss or sepsis. Central pallor, although also seen in severe circulatory failure, mainly suggests anaemia. In the newborn this is rarely due to inadequate red cell production and the cause is either haemorrhage or haemolysis (Letsky 1986). The haemorrhage may be obvious, such as bleeding from the umbilicus, or 'hidden' (e.g. feto-maternal or internal bleeding) in which case the problem may be misdiagnosed as asphyxia neonatorum. A useful clue that haemorrhage is the cause of the 'white asphyxia' is that the baby remains pale despite adequate ventilation, and has a tachycardia rather than the bradycardia associated with anoxia. The presence or rapid development of jaundice in the first hours after birth supports a diagnosis of haemolytic anaemia.

Mild cyanosis can be difficult to detect, as its intensity is markedly influenced by the lighting conditions of the room (Lees and Sunderland 1983). The light from an overhead examination lamp may turn a blue baby pink. If the baby is severely anaemic, cyanosis will not be detected, even if there is hypoxaemia. Inspection of the palms, soles, and tongue helps to determine whether cyanosis is peripheral or central. Peripheral cyanosis develops when haemoglobin oxygen desaturation occurs in the skin because of a reduced blood flow rate. This can occur in cardiac shock (e.g. the 'grey' baby with hypoplasia of the left ventricle), or peripheral vasoconstriction (e.g. blood loss or hypothermia), or with increased viscosity of the blood (e.g. polycythaemia in twin-to-twin transfusion). There are many causes of central cyanosis (Lees and Sunderland 1983) but a clinically useful approach for the generalist is to search for clinical clues suggesting poor pulmonary ventilation or poor pulmonary perfusion (Table 83.1). Methaemoglobinaemia also presents with cyanosis and no marked respiratory distress, but the chocolate-brown colour of a heelprick blood sample which does not turn pink when exposed to oxygen is a useful differentiating clue (Lees and Sunderland 1983).

Jaundice, although usually less of an acute problem than pallor and cyanosis, is nevertheless, for convenience, assessed at the same time. Jaundice usually shows first in the face. Facial jaundice becomes clinically detectable when the bilirubin level is 5 mg per cent, while jaundice of the hands and feet occurs last and is seen when the bilirubin is above 14 mg per cent (Kramer 1969). These are, of course, crude estimates that are easily influenced by the room lighting and other skin coloration caused by cyanosis, pallor, or racial colour. The level of jaundice must be assessed under standard conditions: by the window, using natural

Table 83.1 Causes of central cyanosis

(a) *Inadequate ventilation*
(1) poor respiratory effort
    respiratory centre: e.g. pethidine, hypoglycaemia, cerebral
    haemorrhage
    spinal cord injury
    peripheral nerve: Werdnig Hoffman disease
    myoneural junction: maternal myasthenia gravis
    muscle: myotonia, congenital dystrophica, myopathies

(2) obstructed airway
    choanal atresia
    retrognathia: Pierre Robin syndrome
    large tongue: glycogen storage disease, haemangioma
    upper airway: aberrant large vessels
    lower airway: meconium aspiration

(3) alveolar problem
    hypoplasia: compression in utero (oligohydramnios,
    ascites, diaphragmatic hernia)
    atelectasis: hyaline membrane disease, compression due to
    pneumothorax, pleural fluid, or diaphragmatic hernia
    fluid: wet lung, meconium or milk aspiration, pneumonia,
    cardiac failure, total anomalous pulmonary venous
    drainage

(b) *Inadequate pulmonary perfusion*
    atrium: tricuspid atresia
    ventricle: Fallot's Tetralogy
    artery: pulmonary atresia
    arteriole: persistent fetal circulation
    capillary: excess CPAP, polycythaemia

(c) *Inadequate O_2 uptake by red cells*
    e.g. methaemoglobinaemia

(d) *Mixing pulmonary and systemic blood*
    e.g. transposition of the great vessels, truncus arteriosus

light, and after gentle pressure on the nose. The icter-ometer, a plastic strip with a graded yellow colour scale, helps the reliable estimation of jaundice even in artificial light (Schumacher *et al.* 1985). The use of skin colour to assess jaundice is invalid when the baby is receiving phototherapy.

Clinical jaundice is so common (up to 50 per cent of term babies and an even higher proportion of preterm babies) that the diagnosis of pathological causes can be delayed. Criteria on clinical examination suggesting non-physiological causes are development of jaundice in the first 24 hours (usually haemolytic), very rapid increase in intensity, and persistence for more than 7 days and 14 days in the term and preterm baby respectively (Maisels 1981).

3.3 Pulse and circulation

The circulation is assessed by measuring the blood pressure, palpating the pulses, and checking the capillary flow.

The recently developed oscillometric method for the measurement of blood pressure is much more convenient than the older flush and palpation methods (Dar-

nall 1985). The blood pressure increases with gestational and postnatal age (Wilkinson and Cooke 1986) and an average systolic/diastolic pressure in a 1500 g and a 3000 g baby is 40/25 and 70/40 respectively. It is important to use the appropriate cuff size, i.e. the cuff bladder should completely encircle the limb and its width should be equal to two-thirds of the length of the upper arm (or thigh if comparing the upper and lower limb pressures in suspected coarctation). Hypertension, defined as a systolic pressure greater than 100 mm Hg in a resting baby (Wilkinson and Cooke 1986) is rare in the newborn but must always be checked for in a baby with suspected coarctation or renal disease. Hypotension is more commonly encountered, and asphyxia, blood loss, sepsis, and hypoplastic left ventricle are important causes.

The normal pulse rate of a newborn is 120 to 160 beats per minute, although rates as low as 100 beats per minute in the term baby and as high as 180 beats per minute in the preterm baby are common. Sinus tachycardia, most commonly due to crying and also found with fever, shock, or hyperthyroidism, does not usually rise above 200 beats per minute, and a higher rate may indicate a supranodal tachycardia (Lees and Sunderland 1983). Occasional extrasystoles are common in the first week of life, and are usually benign, but require careful clinical assessment as they may be a sign of congenital heart disease (Wilkinson and Cooke 1986). The pulses in the arm (radial and or brachial) must always be compared with the pulses in the leg (dorsalis pedis and/or femoral artery), to exclude a coarctation of the aorta. These pulses may initially be equal because of an open ductus arteriosus, which allows the right ventricle to pump blood to the legs. Poorly palpable pulses are an important sign of shock, and easily palpable collapsing pulses are found in left to right shunting due to an open ductus arteriosus and arteriovenous fistulas.

Refilling of the capillaries after compression of the skin of the palm or sole normally occurs within 3 seconds, and when this occurs it is a useful sign of adequate tissue perfusion. However, delayed refilling is more difficult to assess as the skin is then often cold, and it may be difficult to decide whether this is the cause or the result of the perfusion problem.

3.4 Response to stimuli; muscle tone

If ventilation and circulation are normal the brain should receive an adequate oxygen supply, and the baby will respond to stimuli and have normal muscle tone. These last two signs are rapidly assessed at this stage, just as in the Apgar score, and it is important to take gestational age into account (Catlin *et al.* 1986) in deciding if the findings are abnormal (see neurological examination).

Disturbances in response and tone despite adequate ventilation and circulation should alert one to problems such as infection, sedation, or hypoglycaemia.

3.5 Temperature

Changes in temperature rapidly influence the baby's energy balance, and it is thus appropriate to check this next. Whether hyperthermia is due to overheating or infection is a common diagnostic problem. Neonatal infections may also result in hypothermia, and these should be considered along with other possible causes of decreased heat production or excess heat loss. In a baby who is undergoing prolonged resuscitation it is wise to assess frequently the temperature of the abdominal skin (central) and sole of the foot (peripheral) with the back of the hand.

3.6 Hydration

Disturbances in fluid balance are not uncommon problems in newborn babies (Table 83.2). Change in weight is a sensitive index of the state of hydration, but it can be difficult to repeatedly weigh the ill baby, and the results are easily influenced by a feed, passage of urine and faeces, or by using different scales. Dehydration is therefore also checked by the fontanelle pressure, overlapping of the skull sutures, skin turgor, and the colour and volume of the urine. It is useful to acquire the habit of using a single site, such as the pectoralis area, for examining skin turgor, because the elasticity varies at different sites and is influenced by the amount of subcutaneous fat.

Oedema is often detectable around the eyes in the baby, but dependent sites such as the sacrum and ankle must be palpated. Local oedema of the scalp or limbs after difficult deliveries should be differentiated from more generalized oedema. Turner's syndrome frequently presents with marked puffiness of the dorsum of the feet. Generalized pitting oedema is most commonly seen in preterm babies. There are many other causes (Etches 1986) and careful examination (e.g. presence of anaemia, other signs of cardiac failure, and proteinuria) must be performed. Non-pitting oedema

Table 83.2 Causes of dehydration can be approached by following a simple input/output model

---

(a) *Decreased input*:
(1) inadequate breast-milk
(2) miscalculated daily increments if not demand feeding
(3) vomiting

(b) *Increased output*:
(1) skin: preterm
hyperthermia: fever
         phototherapy
         incubator
(2) renal: renal or endocrine disease
        osmotic diuresis (glycosuria)
        diuretic drugs
(3) intestinal: diarrhoea
(4) respiratory: hyperventilation

---

in the newborn is usually sclerema occurring because of severe illness, but a thick rubbery skin associated with coarse facial features can occur in the inborn errors of connective tissue metabolism (Burton 1987).

3.7 Odour

The breath of the adult patient is routinely checked for the smell of ketones and alcohol. In the newborn, the equivalent is to sniff the skin (the 'sweaty feet' odour of isovaleric acidaemia) and the urine (the smell of burnt sugar in maple syrup urine disease). If this is done routinely these rare conditions may be diagnosed earlier (Burton 1987).

4 Specific examination

4.1 Skin

The red, thin skin of the preterm baby becomes thicker and paler, and the vernix and lanugo disappear as gestation progresses. Desquamation is seen in the postmature and malnourished baby. The skin over the entire body must be inspected thoroughly for any lesions. It is therefore convenient to include the skin with the examination of each system. A useful review of neonatal skin lesions for the general clinician is given by Esterley and Solomon (1983).

Forceps marks indicate the need to check for underlying nerve involvement or tissue damage. Lacerations due to blood gas measurements or invasive skin electrodes are usually minor, but must always be checked for signs of secondary infection. Petechiae are common, on the face and neck in vertex deliveries and on the legs and buttocks in breech deliveries. Bruising of the sacrococcygeal area is usually easily distinguished from the pigmentation of a mongolian spot, which is so common in dark-skinned races. If there is concern about the distribution and extent of the bleeding, consider the possibility of an underlying coagulation defect and observe carefully for the development of jaundice.

The commonest congenital lesions are the benign telangiectasia of the nape of the neck and upper eyelids ('stork bites'). These are easily distinguished from the flat 'port wine' capillary haemangiomas or the raised 'strawberry' cavernous haemangiomas.

Macules, papules, vesicles, and pustules often worry both the mother and doctor. Infection should always be considered, although the majority are benign. The commonest rash is erythema toxicum, which develops 24 hours after birth in 20 per cent of term babies but rarely in preterm babies. Typically, the lesions are 1–3 mm papules on an erythematous base, and are easy to diagnose. If they are atypical, present at birth, and are vesiculopustular, other causes such as herpes simplex or bacterial and fungal infections should be considered. Finding eosinophils and no bacteria or candida in a stained preparation of the fluid helps confirm the diagnosis. The presence of associated mucosal lesions can be important clues in the diagnosis of herpetic and monilial infections.

Milia is a fine white papular rash seen on the nose, and miliaria a fragile vesicular 'sweat' rash on the forehead and in skin folds of the neck and axilla. Common rashes such as these require only reassurance of the parents.

4.2 Neck

Systematic inspection of the neck should begin in the midline, looking for enlargement of the thyroid and thyroglossal cysts. Laterally, one looks anterior to the sternomastoid muscle for branchial cysts and clefts, and posterior to the muscle for the larger cystic hygromas. The cysts transilluminate brightly unless secondary haemorrhage or infection has occurred. Posteriorly, redundant skin may be noted in trisomy 21, or because of an excessively short neck due to defective vertebral growth (Klippel–Feil syndrome). The latter syndrome may also cause a torticollis at birth. When torticollis is due to a sternomastoid haemorrhage it usually takes 2–3 weeks to become obvious. Webbing of the neck is typical of Turner's syndrome, but is also seen in Down's syndrome and trisomy 17–18 (for details of clinical features see Smith 1977). Finally, the clavicles should be inspected, and gently palpated to reveal fractures, especially in large babies, and after breech deliveries or shoulder dystocia. There is usually little displacement and swelling may only become apparent when callus develops, but it is tender, crepitus is often palpable, and pseudoparalysis of the arm may be present.

4.3 Pulmonary system

The sounds of breathing and the cry should always be noted, since they help to localize the anatomical site of a pulmonary problem. Inspiratory stridor (as in croup in older children) occurs when some obstruction is present in the larynx or trachea, e.g. post-intubation oedema or compression due to aberrant large vessels. A hoarse cry further helps to localize the lesion to the vocal cords. Expiratory wheeze (as in bronchiolitis and asthma in older children) occurs with bronchial or bronchiolar obstruction (e.g. meconium aspiration). Grunting is typically described in idiopathic respiratory distress syndrome, but also occurs with other alveolar diseases, and with cerebral causes of respiratory distress. Crying is used to assess the 'vital capacity'; a loud cry is a rough, but good, index of the pulmonary reserve in an ill child.

The size of the breast buds increases with gestational age; obvious swelling and discharge of 'witches milk' is common in the term baby. Abnormally wide placement of the nipple can be seen in Turner's syndrome, and a

flattened chest wall due to a missing pectoralis major muscle occurs in Poland's syndrome. The thorax is often hyperinflated at birth and the visible respiratory excursions are mainly abdominal. Normally the respiratory rate is 40–60 times per minute, and the rhythm irregular, i.e. 'periodic': apnoea for 5–10 seconds alternating with breathing. Periodic breathing is a benign disorder, because the pause between respirations is short, and is very common in the preterm baby. If a pause between breaths is greater than 10 seconds in a term baby or 20 seconds in a preterm baby, and/or results in bradycardia and/or cyanosis, it is considered pathological, and requires monitoring and further investigation to exclude causes such as hypoglycaemia and infection (Rigatto 1986). The most important sign of respiratory distress is an increased respiratory rate. Other signs include flaring alae nasi, and retraction of suprasternal, supraclavicular, and intercostal spaces, and also the ribs and sternum in the preterm baby. Retraction, however, is not uncommon in normal babies on crying.

The thin chest wall of the newborn baby allows the use of transillumination with bright light (fibre optic) and this is a rapid and sensitive clinical test (Donn and Faix 1985) for the diagnosis of a pneumothorax. It is an essential part of the examination of a baby with respiratory distress or at risk of developing a pneumothorax (Table 83.3). The test is also positive (over the sternum) if the baby has a pneumomediastinum or pneumopericardium. The test must be performed in a dark room. Oedema of the skin can produce a false positive result, and excess subcutaneous fat, as seen in the baby of a diabetic mother, a false negative result.

The maximal cardiac impulse is in the 4th intercostal space in the midclavicular line. It is essential to localize

Table 83.3 Factors predisposing to development of a pneumothorax

---

(a) Lung too weak

    Prematurity

(b) Pressure too great

    1. Air volume too large because:

        (a) excess air inspired: spontaneous or during resuscitation

        (b) decreased air expired: air trapping due to meconium aspiration

    2. Lung volume too small because of poor growth *in utero*:
        (a) external compression: oligohydramnios

        (b) internal compression: diaphragmatic hernia, ascites or intra-abdominal blood transfusion.

Table 83.4 Shift of the apex beat: causes and diagnosis

Reason for shift	Aetiology	Useful clinical clues
(a) *Pushed due to increased pressure*		
excess air	pneumothorax lobar emphysema	transillumination
excess tissue	diaphrag. hernia	scaphoid abdomen, audible peristalsis over chest
excess fluid	chylothorax hydrops	dull to percussion oedema generalized
(b) *Pulled due to decreased pressure*		
	agenesis atelectasis	deformed chest meconium aspiration

the apex beat, especially in babies with respiratory distress. A shift to the left is difficult to detect, but a shift to the right is an important diagnostic clue and the pulmonary causes are shown in Table 83.4. This finding may allow appropriate therapy to be undertaken in a pneumothorax or diaphragmatic hernia long before a roentgen diagnosis is possible. In a pneumothorax, important additional clues are provided by the history and by transillumination. The development of respiratory distress in a term baby with no predisposing factors makes it essential to exclude a diaphragmatic hernia. A scaphoid abdomen, though not always obvious, is a further clue. With pleural effusions the chest will be dull to percussion. Of course, a heart on the right may also be due to cardiac malformation, and this may be isolated or associated with complete situs inversus (the liver position should be checked by palpation and percussion).

It is necessary to use a neonatal-sized stethoscope to obtain adequate contact with the chest wall. The patency of the choanae (choanal atresia or post-intubation trauma) can easily be checked without disturbing the baby with a tube insertion by listening to the air expired from each nostril with the bell of the stethoscope. The air entry into the chest is then controlled, comparing the right and left side. Air entry may be decreased on one side (pneumothorax, atelectasis, diaphragmatic hernia, pleural effusion) or on both sides (decreased compliance of the lung in idiopathic respiratory distress syndrome, lung hypoplasia, abdominal distension). Bronchial breathing is rarely heard in the newborn, but crepitations (cardiac failure, aspiration, and pneumonia) and rhonchi (meconium or bronchial secretion) must be checked for. The moist sounds due to excess secretions in the nose and throat are easily transmitted to the lungs and may be confused with rhonchi.

For a detailed description of the the clinical diagnosis of pulmonary problems see the review by Guthrie and Hodson (1986).

4.4 Cardiovascular system

The amount of blood shunting between the pulmonary and systemic circulations (right to left or left to right) determine the clinical signs of many of the congenital heart lesions. Because of the rapid postnatal changes in the circulation (rise in systemic and fall in pulmonary pressures, and closure of the ductus arteriosus) the signs can vary, and they require frequent and careful assessment if abnormalities are suspected. Despite these difficulties, clinical examination is essential for prompt and appropriate referral for specialist attention.

In the first hours after birth a left parasternal heave is often visible. Although it is an indication for serial observations, if it is an isolated finding it is usually not associated with cardiac disease and usually soon disappears.

After checking the position of the apex, the force of the impulse and the presence of thrills (rare) must be assessed. The precordium is often not abnormal in severe heart defects at birth, as the potential haemodynamic consequences have been limited *in utero* because of the high pulmonary pressure in the fetus. In the normal baby the visible left parasternal heave is easily palpable after birth and then subsides. The hyperactivity may persist or increase in certain pathological conditions of the heart.

Soft heart sounds can occur in cardiac shock or because of overlying air due to a pneumopericardium or pneumomediastinum. Abnormalities in rhythm already detected on palpation of the pulse can be rechecked. The second heart sound is single in the first week of life because of the raised pulmonary pressure. Even after this time the split is still difficult to hear because of the fast heart rate in the newborn, and is therefore less useful in the differential diagnosis of congenital heart disease than in older children. The presence of extra heart sounds is usually only detected if a gallop rhythm is present.

Murmurs are harder to interpret in the newborn than at any other time (Wilkinson and Cooke 1986). Because of the rapid changes in the pressure gradient between the pulmonary and systemic circulation, and the patency of the ductus arteriosus, murmurs may be transiently heard in normal babies and be absent in babies with serious heart defects. Attempting to diagnose the cause of the murmur by assessing its site of maximal intensity and radiation is not easy, but some simple clinical rules of thumb may be found helpful. A very loud murmur in early neonatal life suggests a stenotic lesion of the pulmonary artery or aortic valve, as cardiac shunts are not yet large (Wilkinson and Cooke 1986). A continuous murmur is typical of a patent ductus arteriosus. One should always check if a murmur is not originating from the head, as the rare cerebral arteriovenous fistulas are even more rarely diagnosed without a lot of time being wasted. It is essential to search for other clues of cardiac disease (cyanosis, a poor peripheral circulation, respiratory distress and other signs of cardiac failure), and for other congenital anomalies or dysmorphic features.

4.5 Abdomen

Any opportunity to examine gastrointestinal fluids and urine must be taken. Excessive and frothy saliva is seen in oesophageal atresia, and bile-stained vomit must be considered as due to intestinal obstruction below the duodenum until proved otherwise. The black-green colour of meconium is usually easily distinguished from melaena. Breastfed babies have more frequent and looser stools than formula-fed babies.

In a male the dribbling of urine, or more rarely an extremely long stream, may indicate a urethral stenosis. The colour of the urine may also provide clues to dehydration, direct hyperbilirubinaemia, or haematuria. When indicated, the simple tests for urine (specific gravity, microscopy, and testing for reducing sugars, pH, direct bilirubin, haemoglobin, and protein) should be regarded as part of the clinical examination and rapidly performed 'at the bedside'.

Slight distension is normal in the newborn, but pathological causes are not infrequently encountered at or soon after birth. Distension due to intestinal gas is the most frequently encountered cause and can occur because of excess input, i.e. air swallowed due to crying, mask ventilation, or a tracheo-oesophageal fistula, or decreased outflow, i.e intestinal obstruction in, for example, meconium ileus or Hirschsprung's disease. The degree of distension is a clue to how distal the obstruction is.

Other causes of distension in the newborn are less common. Ascites is usually encountered as part of hydrops fetalis and the most common cause of isolated ascites is hydronephrosis. Large tumours and intraperitoneal haemorrhage due to birth trauma are uncommon causes of distension.

Transillumination is of value in abdominal problems (Donn and Faix 1985), and in distension the presence of a perforation is suggested by the loss of the dark liver shadow. Ventilation may be impaired by distension and may be relieved by gastric suction, or in an emergency by a peritoneal tap. Redness and isolated oedema of the abdominal wall can be presenting signs of peritonitis, as in necrotizing enterocolitis.

Peristalsis is frequently visible in the preterm baby because of the thin abdominal wall, but may be a sign of intestinal obstruction.

The umbilical cord must be checked for meconium-staining, infection, and other abnormalities. If a single artery is present the possibility of other congenital abnormalities, especially of the genitourinary tract, must be considered. A cord thick with jelly is typical in the baby of a diabetic mother. Leakage of urine through a patent urachus, or meconium through a Meckel's fistula, are rare findings. An umbilical hernia is common and needs no treatment but an omphalocoele is a surgical emergency (a check should always be made immediately for associated hypoglycaemia—Beckwith's syndrome) using a capillary blood test stick).

The external genitalia are then checked. In the male the size of the penis, the position of the meatus, and the position of the testes must be noted. The testes descend into the scrotum at 36 weeks' gestation. The prepuce is not retractile in infancy and a pearl white (sebaceous) cyst at its tip is a normal finding. A hypospadias, especially if situated in the shaft, may be associated with other urinary abnormalities, and if associated with undescended testes (it is necessary to check that the testes are not just retracted) may indicate an abnormality in sexual differentiation. Swelling of the scrotum may be cystic, due to a hydrocoele or an inguinal hernia (note that the thin-walled intestine may also transilluminate), or solid (due to torsion, a tumour, or in breech deliveries, a haematoma) and requires careful assessment as urgent surgery may be needed.

In the female the size of the clitoris and labia, the degree of labial fusion, and the hymen are checked. The labia majora cover the labia minora at 36 weeks' gestation. A white mucous discharge is common and is sometimes bloodstained. An imperforate hymen may obstruct the flow of these secretions and present as an obvious bulge through the labia. Hernias are very uncommon in the female and may indicate other abnormalities such as testicular feminizing syndrome.

The patency of the anus and its tone (gentle stimulation) are then assessed. Anal fissures can occur and may present with streaking of the faeces with blood. Even in the term baby, gentle examination using the little finger may produce an anal skin tear, and this rarely needed examination should be left to the consultant.

For convenience, the palpation of the groin is performed during inspection of the area. Diastasis of the rectus abdominis muscles is common. Guarding and tenderness are often subtle signs and, in the newborn, best checked by gently palpating with just the index finger over the whole abdomen if local early peritonitis is not to be missed. Rigidity is a late sign of peritonitis.

The organs are systematically felt for, starting with the liver, then the spleen, kidneys, bladder, and then other masses. In the normal baby, the liver edge can be palpated up to 2 cm below the right costal margin, and the liver is firm and smooth. The spleen tip may also be palpable normally, but not more than just the tip. If the edge of the liver or tip of the spleen are lower it may be due to downward displacement by hyperinflation of the lungs or a pneumothorax. The more common causes of hepatomegaly are congestion (cardiac failure), swelling of the cells due either to chronic infection (cytomegalovirus and syphilis) or acute infection (herpes virus or bacterial sepsis), or hyperplasia of the reticuloendothelial cells as in extramedullary haemopoiesis in haemolytic disease (Walker and Mathis 1975). The accumulation of glycogen in babies of diabetic mothers is the commonest metabolic cause, as inborn errors of carbohydrate, fat, or mucopolysaccharides metabolism are very rare (Burton 1987 and see Chapter 84). In the baby who develops hepatomegaly in the neonatal period (after receiving milk) it is surprising how often the diagnosis of galactosaemia is delayed because the urine is not immediately checked at the 'bedside'. A positive Clinitest tablet reaction, i.e. Benedict's reagent for a reducing sugar which is not glucose (negative Clinistix, i.e. glucose oxidase test) is good reason to immediately stop milk feeds until the diagnosis is confirmed (Burton 1987). Very rare, but needing consideration especially if the liver enlargement is irregular, are liver tumours and traumatic haemorrhage. Splenomegaly is also found in many of the above conditions (Walker and Mathis 1975).

Normal-sized kidneys can be difficult to palpate even if the technique of bimanual palpation is correctly used. Enlarged kidneys are more easily detected. Bilateral enlargement is usually due to distension with urine in polycystic renal disease or hydronephrosis. In unilateral enlargement a tumour or a renal vein thrombosis must also be considered. The bladder must be palpated for. A distended bladder will help localize the site of a urinary obstruction (bladder paralysis or meatal stenosis), and if it can be emptied with steady pressure a flaccid paralysis (spina bifida) is most probably present. The clinical examination of the abdomen and diagnostic features of abdominal masses in the neonate is dealt with in detail by Henderson and Torch (1977).

Percussion is at times useful, in distinguishing between distension of the abdomen due to excess gas or fluid, localization of the liver in a suspected situs inversus, and in delineating the upper border of the bladder. Bowel sounds may be scanty in the well baby, especially if preterm. Decreased sounds can occur in the baby ill from any cause, but the possibility of necrotizing enterocolitis must always be considered. Increased bowel sounds are typical of intestinal obstruction, although in meconium ileus the sounds are often absent because the meconium is so sticky.

4.6 Nervous system

It is essential to remember that not only disease or medication, such as pethidine or phenobarbitone, but also the gestational and postnatal age, the sleep state of the baby, and time of the last feed may influence the neurological findings. There are now excellent schemes for detailed neurological examination of the newborn (Dubowitz and Dubowitz 1981), but the examination sequence often differs from the sequence for the examination of adults and children, and the non-specialist is constantly having to look up what comes next. Volpe (1987) has emphasized that an 'adult' scheme can largely be followed in the newborn. This makes the important aspects of the neonatal examination easier for the general practitioner and obstetrician. The following scheme combines the anatomical and the functional features into one examination; for example, examination of the eye combines looking at the shape of eye and colour of the sclera with testing of cranial nerves 2, 3, 4, and 6. The basic order of the examination is: first, central: head, cerebral function including autonomic system, 'speech', cranial nerves; and second, peripheral: spine, motor, sensory, and autonomic systems.

4.6.1 Central nervous system

This examination should include measurement of the head circumference (see section on anthropometry). A guide to the causes of a large or small head circumference is given in Table 83.5. Transillumintion may help differentiate between hydrocephaly and a sudural haemorrhage (Donn and Faix 1985). The head shape can vary because of compression before or during birth, or because of craniostenosis of various sutures. The hair pattern, birth marks, and evidence of trauma must be noted.

Caput succedaneum (oedema of the scalp) is the commonest scalp lesion. A cephalhaematoma (subperiosteal bleeding), because of its clear delineation by the sutures, is easily diagnosed, but the less commonly

Table 83.5 Small and large heads

SMALL HEAD
(1) limited skull expansion: craniostenosis
(2) limited brain growth: chromosomal abnormalities
                                   congenital infections
                                   maternal alcoholism
                                   phenylketonuria

LARGE HEAD
(1) pseudo-enlargement: scaphocephaly in preterm
(2) extracranial: subaponeurotic haemorrhage
(3) subdural: haemorrhage or effusion
(4) cerebral: tumours or storage diseases
(5) ventricles: hydrocephalus, e.g. post-haemorrhagic, infection, congenital

Large fontanelles or wide sutures occur due to excess expansion of the intracranial content (see large head) or limited bone growth.

Limited bone growth
- preterm and small for gestational age babies
- hypothyroidism
- maternal rickets
- craniocleidodysostosis, osteogenesis imperfecta
- syndromes: e.g. trisomy 17–18, nephrotic syndrome

occurring subaponeurotic (subgaleal) haematoma is easily misdiagnosed. Bleeding under this fascia, which extends from its attachment to the facial muscle anteriorly to the occipital bone posteriorly, can lead to haemorrhagic shock. It should always be considered in the differential diagnosis of large scalp swelling after a vacuum extraction (Kappy 1981). It presents with non-pitting diffuse thickening of the scalp, impalpable sutures, and puffiness (and later bruising) of the eyes and occipital region in an often pale child.

Palpation should begin with the metopic suture and should be followed posteriorly to the diamond-shaped anterior fontanelle and the parietal sutures, then continued posteriorly along the sagittal suture to the triangular posterior fontanelle, and the occipital sutures. The tension, size, and shape of the fontanelles, and the width of the sutures must be noted. Kaiser and Whitelaw (1987) have recently shown that estimation of elevated intracranial pressure by palpation of the fontanelle can be inaccurate. A large fontanelle or wide sutures may be due to increased cerebral pressure (see Table 83.5: large heads) or limited skull bone growth (Table 83.5). It is convenient to test for neck stiffness at the end of 'palpation', but this sign is only positive in a very late stage of meningitis in the newborn.

Percussion of the skull for hyperresonance due to separation of the sutures is not of value in the newborn, since the sutures are normally not fused. On auscultation bruits can be heard in normal babies but may occur with compression of vessels in cerebral oedema. The most important reason for listening is to exclude an arteriovenous fistula.

Assessment of the mental state is based on observing spontaneous eye opening, gross movements, and crying, and their occurrence after gentle stimulation (Dubowitz and Dubowitz 1981; Volpe 1987). The state of wakefulness is difficult to assess prior to 28 weeks' gestation unless active stimulation is used. By 32 weeks, however, the typical alternation between sleep and waking states becomes clearer (Table 83.6) (Prechtl 1977; Dubowitz and Dubowitz 1981). The diagnosis of lethargy or hyper-irritability must be related to the gestational age, time of the last feed and sleep state. The ability to console a crying child by cuddling or use of a soother or a feed is a reassuring sign when trying to determine what the problem is in an irritable baby. There are many causes of lethargy (Volpe 1987) (Table 83.7), and it should always be carefully assessed when reported by the mother or nursing staff. The rare inborn errors of metabolism must always be considered (Burton 1987) (see Chapter 84) as they so closely imitate infections. These inborn errors are unfortunately often misdiagnosed until they present again in a following pregnancy.

The strength of the cry ('speech') and the amount of crying is also an important clue to the mental state. The

Table 83.6 Grading the state of wakefulness

1. Deep sleep:	Eyes closed, regular respiration and no movements
2. Active sleep:	Eyes closed, irregular respiration and no gross movements
3. Quiet wakefulness:	Eyes open, no gross movements
4. Active wakefulness:	Eyes open, gross movements, no crying
5. Crying:	Eyes open or closed

Table 83.7 Lethargy: causes, and guide to the diagnosis

Immaturity

Overfeeding

Infection: sepsis, meningitis (bacterial and viral) urinary infection, enterocolitis

Metabolic: (1) anoxia: asphyxia, respiratory distress, shock
(2) hypoglycaemia
(3) hyperaminoacidaemia, hyperammonaemia, acidaemia
(4) hypothyroidism and kernicterus

Haemorrhage: trauma (subdural)
post-anoxia and prematurity (intraventricular)
bleeding diathesis

Drugs: maternal drugs via placenta and breast-milk

pitch may also indicate cerebral damage, e.g. the high-pitched cry of meningeal irritation, and the mewing cry of babies with the *Cri-du-Chat* syndrome.

It is useful to note the general appearance of the face before details of the features are assessed with the related cranial nerves. An unusual facies may be related to the race and personal appearance of the parents, the position of the fetus *in utero* (Clarren and Smith 1977), and the mode of delivery as well as various syndromes (Smith 1977).

The eyes are often difficult to assess in the first days because of the puffiness of the eyelids. The eyebrows and eyelashes are poorly developed in the newborn, and thick eyebrows meeting in the midline are found in the Cornelia de Lange syndrome. The size and slant of the eyes and the presence of epicanthic folds or ptosis are noted (Smith 1977). Then the conjunctiva are checked, and also, with the help of a torch and fundoscope, the cornea, the iris, and finally the lens and the fundus, by looking for the presence of a red retinal reflex. This is normally sufficient for general screening to exclude a 'white eye' due to a cataract or retinal pathology. An excellent problem-orientated approach to the examination and diagnosis of eye lesions is given by Read and Goldberg (1983).

Movement of the eyelids and eyes must be carefully examined, since normal movements may be difficult to distinguish from those seen in subtle seizures. In a lower motor lesion of the facial nerve, usually caused by forceps trauma, the branch to the upper face is involved and the eyelid cannot close. Repetitive spontaneous blinking or fluttering of the eyelids is abnormal. The pupillary reflex is only consistently present by 32 weeks' gestation, but blinking in response to the bright light begins at 28 weeks. Bilateral fixed dilated pupils are seen after asphyxia and also with intoxication from maternal epidural anaesthesia, while unilateral dilatation can occur in a subdural haemorrhage (Volpe 1987). Extraocular movements normally occur spontaneously or in response to rotating the head from side to side ('doll's eye' movement) from about the 30th week. Fixed deviation of the eyes occurs in paralysis of nerves 3, 4, or 6. Tonic deviation, horizontal or vertical, is a subtle sign of convulsions, but unsustained horizontal nystagmus is normal.

The normal ear has the helix top in line (horizontal) with the outer canthus of the eye. Abnormal position, size, and form can be seen with renal agenesis and chromosomal abnormalities (Smith 1977). Malformations such as skin tags (often familial), or sinuses, must be looked for. The eardrum is difficult to examine because of the narrowness of the external canal in the neonate and is not routinely checked, but in a baby with possible infection otitis media should be excluded (Gravel *et al.* 1988). The auditory function is tested simply by observation of blinking or a Moro response after a loud noise.

The mouth and chin are assessed, and then the gums (retention cysts, erupted teeth), inside of the cheeks (thrush, herpes ulcers), hard and soft palate (cleft, high arch, and the normal presence of small white inclusion cysts, Ebstein's pearls), and the tongue.

By 32–34 weeks' gestation the normal infant is able to co-ordinate the action needed for feeding. Continuous sucking, smacking of the lips, tongue thrusting, and drooling may be signs of 'subtle seizures'. Finally, atrophy or persistent fasciculation of the tongue (bag of worms), seen in degeneration of the anterior motor neurone, may be present in Werdnig–Hoffman disease.

4.6.2 Peripheral nervous system

The spine is usually checked during the examination of the neck, chest, and abdomen. After the curvature is noted, the skin from the base of the skull to the coccyx is checked for dimples (sacrococcygeal pits are common and harmless); sinuses (which may communicate with the spinal cord); and any naevi, abnormal hair growth, or swellings (which are commonly associated with underlying spinal malformations).

Examination of the sensory system is generally limited to evaluating the response to touch by assessing and comparing the withdrawal of the arms and legs on gentle stimulation with a blunt stick. If there is any doubt about the response, then pain reaction is assessed by pinprick. This may be necessary in the case of severe cerebral depression, or to locate the affected dermatomes in peripheral nerve lesions such as Erb's palsy and spina bifida. In a baby who is hypotonic due to a pure motor pathway lesion (anterior motor neurone, myoneural junction, or muscle disease) the pain response is still present, although it may only show by facial grimacing.

4.6.3 Locomotor system

The examination of the locomotor system for malformations or deformations is made in combination with the neurological examination (movements, tone, and reflexes). The examination of the hips for dislocation which often causes crying, however, should be left to the very end of the whole examination.

It is important to note the symmetry of the response of the right and left side for movement, tone, and reflexes, and therefore the baby must be tested with the head in the midline position to obviate the effects of the tonic neck reflexes (using rolled-up nappies (diapers) to support the head if necessary). It must be remembered that the sleep state influences the tone and movement.

The length of the limbs in proportion to the body should be judged and a comparison made of the size of the right and left side. A wide carrying angle of the elbow is seen in Turner's syndrome. The hands, fingers, and nails should be examined. Polydactyly and syndactyly are often innocent findings, but may be associated with major abnormalities such as Holt–Oram syndrome and trisomy 13–14, and Apert's syndrome respectively (Smith 1977).

The lower limbs must similarly be examined. Talipes equinovarus is often an isolated finding, but the possibility of neuromuscular disease or intrauterine compression should be considered, especially if it is associated with limited movement of hip and elbow joints (Clarren and Smith 1977). Calcaneovalgus is usually due to compression *in utero*, and will be spontaneously corrected in a few days without manipulation. Rocker bottom feet are a typical finding in trisomy 17–18, and puffiness of the feet with hypoplastic nails is a useful clue in Turner's syndrome. Overriding of the toes is usually self-correcting.

Wasting of the muscles due to neuromuscular disease may not be detected in babies because of their thick subcutaneous fat layer. Because of this fat layer in babies also, fasciculation of muscle is best checked for in the tongue when lower motor neurone disease must be excluded.

Many movements (stretches, twitches, clonus, and startles) are seen in the normal newborn baby (Prechtl *et al.* 1979). These are more frequent in the preterm baby, and the assessment that they are excessive must be related to the gestational age of the baby, associated findings, and sleep state. Rowing movements of the arms and pedalling movements of the legs occur in subtle seizures. More easily diagnosed as convulsions are the generalized tonic (usually extension of all limbs) and/or clonic fits. The clonic movements are distinguished from tremor in that they have a fast and slow component, are induced by stimuli and stop on flexing the limb, and are not associated with abnormal gaze or eye movements (Volpe 1987). The causes of convulsions are similar to those for lethargy (Table 83.7). Pseudoparalysis is the common presenting sign of fractures of the clavicle and humerus and sometimes of periostitis, e.g. syphilis.

As well as measuring tone of the muscle groups by assessing their resistance to passive movement it is useful to use special tests developed for babies. These tests, which are already commonly used to assess gestational age (Dubowitz *et al.* 1970; Ballard *et al.* 1979), have now also been included in the neurological examination of the newborn (Dubowitz and Dubowitz 1981). With the help of diagrams the tone of various muscle groups is scored, allowing more accurate serial observations and decreasing inter-observer variations (see Chapter 3). The typical outstretched posture of the hypotonic preterm baby under 28 weeks' gestation gradually changes to the flexed position of the arms and legs of the term baby. The position of the head at rest is checked for extensor hypertonia (remember that opisthotonus is not only seen with neurological damage but also in upper airway obstruction or because of an abnormal fetal position (Clarren and Smith 1977)). Hypotonia of the neck (head lag) is tested by gently pulling the child into the sitting position, when in the term baby the head keeps in line with the body. The tone in the shoulder is tested by the 'scarf sign' and in the elbow and in the hip by traction and recoil on release. The tonus of the knee is tested by gently extending the knee, and of the ankle by testing for sustained clonus.

Hypertonia, normally seen in the crying baby, is a rarer sign of neonatal neurological disease than hypotonia (Volpe 1987), but is seen in hypoxic-ischaemic damage, kernicterus, tetany and tetanus, and is a feature of trisomy 17–18. The central causes of hypotonia are similar to those listed for lethargy (Table 83.7), and the peripheral causes similar to those for hypoventilation because of inadequate respiratory effort (Table 83.1a). The central causes, characteristically, have less effect on the movement and reflexes than the more peripheral lesions.

The primitive neonatal reflexes are examined together with the tendon reflexes, again following a cranio-caudal sequence. Only a limited number of primitive reflexes are described (rooting, sucking, Moro, and grasp), because performing all of them does not provide extra information (Dubowitz and Dubowitz 1981). The primitive reflexes described all begin to appear around the 26–28th week, and gradually increase in strength as the baby matures. The triceps and ankle tendon reflexes are often difficult to elicit because of the baby's increased flexor tone.

Rooting: With the head in the midline, the corners of the mouth are stroked, observing at the same time whether the mouth opens and the head turns. The reflex is often absent in lethargic infants.

Sucking: The finger (in a stall) or a rubber teat are used, and the strength and rhythmicity of the sucking documented. If the response is inappropriate, useful information on sucking during feeds can be obtained from the mother and nursing staff. The influence of sleep state and gestational age, the time since the last feeding, and the mother's use of sedatives (including postnatally if breastfeeding) should not be overlooked. Weak sucking is seen in central and peripheral nervous system problems; however, strong sucking may occur despite gross brain damage, and may be a manifestation of 'subtle' convulsions.

Moro reflex: As the reflex matures, the arm extension is followed by adduction. The most common cause of an absent or depressed Moro reflex is a generalized central nervous system disturbance. If asymmetrical, the commonest neurological cause is an Erb's palsy, but again the possibility of a 'pseudoparalysis' should not be forgotten. Focal cerebral damage does not affect the Moro reflex (Volpe 1987).

Palmar grasp: This shows similar responses to the Moro reflex in central and peripheral lesions.

Tendon reflexes: The biceps and triceps jerk are often difficult to elicit in the baby even with the use of an appropriately sized reflex hammer, but the knee and ankle jerk are easier to test. Only the knee jerk can be consistently elicited in the normal baby. Attention must be paid to the degree and symmetry of the response.

5 Special examinations

5.1 Gestational age

Formal assessment of gestational age is unnecessary if the maternal dates are reliable. However, if there is any uncertainty, it is important to assess the gestational age in the possibly preterm or undersized baby in order to anticipate possible problems (see Chapter 74). There is often large variation between the maturity score of individual signs and therefore they are best used by combining them into a total score. The various scoring systems (reviewed by Robertson 1979 and Gandy 1986) use the assessment of anatomical and or neurological features. They are still only accurate to plus or minus 2 weeks (Gandy 1986). The 'Dubowitz score' is widely used (Dubowitz *et al.* 1970). It is, however, very detailed and all its tests should not be carried out on an ill baby. A simpler scheme (Ballard *et al.* 1979) using fewer items is not less accurate but should also be performed within 40 hours of birth. Any scheme using tone of the baby can be unreliable when the baby is ill. Note that the minimal age scored in these schemes is 26 weeks' gestation, and the only physical assessment for more immature babies is that the eyelids are fused until 25–26 weeks.

5.2 Anthropometry

The measurements of weight, length, and head circumference must be performed routinely, and the percentile for gestational age can be plotted on appropriate charts (Gairdner and Pearson 1971). The percentiles for the three measurements must always be compared. For example, a head circumference on the 75th percentile may indicate a large head due to hydrocephaly if the other measurements are on the 10th percentile. The underweight baby may be proportionately smaller in length and head circumference after longstanding intrauterine problems such as chromosomal abnormalities or congenital infections, but may be disproportionately larger in length and head circumference after short term intrauterine malnutrition (see Chapter 26).

Large for gestational age babies must be carefully assessed. Well-known causes are large parents, miscalculated maternal dates, and maternal diabetes. The role of oedema (and dehydration) on the weight must be taken into account, especially since it may result in excess drug dosages being administered as the water balance changes. Whenever possible one scale should be used for repeating the measurements. The contributions of movements by the baby, scale inaccuracy, and observer error can be minimized by using an electronic balance, which averages a series of measurements (Whitfield 1982). The accuracy and reproducibility of measurement of length has been improved with the development of 'neonatometers' (Davies and Holding 1972). Inaccuracies due to difficulty in 'straightening' the baby must be accepted, as there is concern that excessive extension during length measurement may damage the hip joint (Standard Medical Advisory Committee 1986). The head circumference is an accurate and reproducible measurement once the initial oedema of the scalp and moulding of the skull has subsided.

5.3 Hips

The hips must always be checked for instability or subluxation, and a detailed description of a method adapted from the Ortulani (1937) and the Barlow (1962) methods has been published (Standard Medical Advisory Committee 1986). Congenital dislocation of the hip is present when the head of the femur is, or can be, partially or completely displaced from the acetabulum.

Predisposing factors are a positive family history, breech presentation, oligohydramnios (often associated with other postural deformities, see Clarren and Smith 1977), and neuromuscular disorders such as spina bifida. The condition is commoner in females, and more frequently affects the left hip. The baby must be in the supine position and relaxed (a pacifier helps). Using warm hands, the examiner first checks for the classical signs of dislocation: initially, with the baby supine the position of the legs is inspected for differences in the angle of abduction. Then, with the hips and knees flexed the hip–knee length is compared, the symmetry of the buttock creases checked, and the limitation of abduction is tested; the thighs can normally be abducted to 75° in the term baby.

The second stage of the examination tests each hip separately. As shown (Fig. 83.1), while the one hand steadies the pelvis, the upper thigh of the flexed hip is grasped with the middle digit over the trochanter, and the thumb on the inner side of the thigh. The hip is first tested for an already present posterior dislocation by pressing on the greater trochanter and by feeling the movement of the head of the femur (sometimes with a palpable 'clunk') anteriorly into the acetabulum. If this part of the test is normal, the hip is finally tested for dislocatibility. Backward and lateral pressure is applied by the thumb and the head of the femur moves (+/-0.5 cm) over the rim of the acetabulum into the posterior part of the joint capsule, and back into the acetabulum when the pressure is released (again a clunk may be felt). Note that a ligamentous 'click' is commonly felt during the above procedure: it is not associated with movement of the femoral head, and although not of

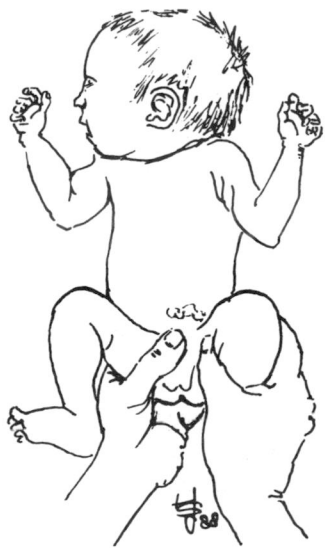

Fig. 83.1 Examination for congenital dislocation of the hip. The position of the hands for testing the left hip are shown.

clinical significance, it accounts for many referrals to orthopaedic surgeons.

The most favourable time for performing the test is in the first 24 hours, as some affected hips 'temporarily lose the sign of instability after birth' (Standard Medical Advisory Committee 1986). The examination should therefore be carried out by the immediate care staff. The examination is best learnt by a clinical demonstration, and should not be done by inexperienced staff without supervision, as the examination may damage the hip. The babies often cry during the examination, making the procedure more difficult, and a training aid ('baby hippy', Medical Plastics Laboratory Inc., Export Department, Medica International, 205 West Wacker Drive, Chicago, Illinois 60606, USA) is now available.

6 Conclusions

The above examination scheme attempts to combine the general approach designed for older patients with the specific examination requirements of the newborn. It, like all schemes, has disadvantages, and should be modified as deemed necessary. More important than any specific order is the constant repetition of a chosen order by the examiner and her or his colleagues. In this way the accuracy and reproducibility of clinical signs can be checked, and the quality of the examinations monitored and improved.

In adult medicine there has been a very welcome resurgence in interest in the value of clinical signs in differential diagnosis, and their accuracy and reproducibility is being assessed (Craige 1988, Spiteri *et al.* 1988). Similar studies are more difficult in the neonate because of ethical considerations hindering repeated examinations by different observers in the ill baby, but the example set by Kaiser and Whitelaw (1987) should be followed. Siegel and Parrino (1988) stress that the rapid development and use of computerized medical diagnosis is another reason making it imperative to assess the accuracy and reproducibility of bedside skills.

References

Ballard JL, Novak KK, Driver M (1979). A simplified score for assessment of fetal maturation of newly born infants. J Pediatr, 95: 769–774.

Barlow TG (1962). Early diagnosis and treatment of congenital dislocation of the hip. J Bone Joint Surg, 448: 292–301.

Black VD (1987). Neonatal hyperviscosity syndromes. Curr Probl Pediatr, 17: 73–130.

Burton BK (1987). Inborn errors of metabolism: The clinical diagnosis in early infancy. Pediatrics, 79: 359–369.

Catlin EA, Carpenter MW, Brann BS, Mayfield SR, Shaul PW, Goldstein M, Oh W (1986). The Apgar sore revisited: Influence of gestational age. J Pediatr, 109: 865–868.

Clarren SK, Smith DW (1977). Congenital deformities. Pediatr Clin North Am, 24: 665–677.

Craige E (1988). Should auscultation be rehabilitated? N Engl J Med, 318: 1611–1613.

Darnall RA (1985). Noninvasive blood pressure measurement in the neonate. Clin Perinatol, 12: 31–49.

Davies DP, Holding RE (1972). Neonatometer: A new infant length measure. Arch Dis Child, 938–940.

Donn SM, Faix RG (1985). Transillumination in neonatal diagnosis. Clin Perinatol, 12: 3–20.

Dubowitz LMS, Dubowitz V, Goldberg C (1970). Clinical assessment of gestational age in the newborn infant. J Pediatr, 77: 1–10.

Dubowitz L, Dubowitz V (1981). The Neurological Assessment of the Preterm and Fullterm Infant. Clinics in Developmental Medicine No. 79. London: Heinemann.

Etches PC (1986). Hydrops foetalis. In: Textbook of Neonatology. Roberton NRC (ed). Edinburgh: Churchill Livingstone, pp 484–494.

Esterley NB, Solomon LM (1983). The skin. In: Neonatal-Perinatal Medicine. Fanaroff AA, Martin RJ (eds). St. Louis: Mosby, pp 939–966.

Gairdner D, Pearson J (1971). A growth chart for premature and other infants. Arch Dis Child, 46: 783–787.

Gandy GM (1986). Examination of the newborn including gestational age assessment. In: Textbook of Neonatology. Roberton NRC (ed). Edinburgh: Churchill Livingstone, pp 131–147.

Gravel JS, McCarton CM, Ruben RJ (1988). Otitis media in neonatal intensive care graduates: A 1 year prospective study. Pediatrics, 82: 44–49.

Guthrie RD, Hodson WA (1986). Clinical diagnosis of pulmonary insufficiency: History and physical. In: Neonatal Pulmonary Care. Thibeault DW, Gregory GA (eds). Norwalk, Connecticut: Appleton-Century-Crofts, pp 175–193.

Henderson KG, Torch EM (1977). Differential diagnosis of abdominal masses in the neonate. Pediatr Clin North Am, 24: 557–578.

Kappy KA (1981). Vacuum extractor. Clin Perinatol, 8: 79–86.

Kaiser AM, Whitelaw AGL (1987). Intracranial pressure estimation by palpation of the anterior fontanelle. Arch Dis Child, 62: 516–517.

Kramer KI (1969). Advancement of dermal icterus in the jaundiced newborn. Am J Dis Child, 118: 454–459.

Lawrence RA (1984). Physical examination. In: Assessment of the Newborn. A Guide for the Practitioner. Ziai M, Clarke TA, Merrit TA (eds). Boston: Little Brown, pp 86–111.

Lees MH, Sunderland CO (1983). The cardiovascular system. In: Neonatal-Perinatal Medicine. Fanaroff AA, Martin RJ (eds). St Louis: Mosby, pp 536–631.

Letsky EA (1986). Anaemia in the newborn. In: Textbook of Neonatology. Roberton NRC (ed). Edinburgh: Churchill Livingstone, pp 449–464.

Maisels MJ (1981). Neonatal jaundice. In: Neonatology: Pathophysiology and Management of the Newborn. Ziai M, Clarke TA, Merrit TA (eds). Philadelphia: Lippincott, pp 473–543.

Ortulani M (1937). Un segno poco noto e sua importanza per la diagnosi precoce de prelussazione congenita dell'anca. Pediatrica (Napoli), 45: 129–136.

Prechtl HFR (1977). The Neurological Examination of the Fullterm Newborn Infant. Clinics in Developmental Medicine No. 63. London: Heinemann.

Prechtl HFR, Fargel JW, Weinmann HM, Bakker HH (1979). Postures, motility and respiration of low risk preterm infants. Dev Med Child Neurol, 21: 3–27.

Read JE, Goldberg MF (1983). The eye. In: Neonatal-Perinatal Medicine. Fanaroff AA, Martin RJ (eds). St Louis: Mosby, pp 967–1003.

Rigatto H (1986). Apnoea. In: Neonatal Pulmonary Care. Thibeault DW, Gregory GA (eds). Norwalk, Connecticut: Appleton-Century-Crofts, pp 641–655.

Robertson A (1979). Gestational age. J Pediatr, 95: 732–734.

Schumacher RE, Thornberry JM, Gutcher GR (1985). Transcutaneous bilirubinometry: A comparison of old and new methods. Pediatrics, 76: 10–14.

Siegel JD, Parrino TA (1988). Computerized diagnosis: Implications for clinical education. Med Educ, 22: 47–54.

Smith DW (1977). Recognisable Patterns of Human Malformations. Philadelphia: WB Saunders.

Spiteri MA, Cook DG, Clarke SW (1988). Reliabilty of eliciting clinical signs in examination of the chest. Lancet, 1: 873–875.

Standard Medical Advisory Committee and the Standard Nursing and Midwifery Advisory Committee for the Secretaries of State for Social Services and Wales (1986). Screening for the Detection of Congenital Dislocation of the Hip. London: Department of Health and Social Security.

Volpe JJ (1987). Neurology of the Newborn (2nd edn). Philadelphia: WB Saunders.

Walker WA, Mathis RK (1975). Hepatomegaly, an approach to differential diagnosis. Pediatr Clin North Am, 22: 929–942.

Whitfield MF (1982). Accuracy of routine clinical test weighing. Arch Dis Child, 57: 810.

Wilkinson JL, Cooke RWI (1986). Cardiovascular disorders. In: Textbook of Neonatology. Roberton NRC (ed). Edinburgh: Churchill Livingstone, pp 340–382.

84 Biochemical screening for disease in the newborn infant

Michael Daker and Martin Bobrow

1 Introduction

Neonatal screening serves two main purposes. First, the care of some conditions, such as phenylketonuria or congenital hypothyroidism, can be greatly improved by early diagnosis and prompt institution of effective treatment. Second, certain forms of genetic disease may not become clinically manifest for a considerable time. In such cases, even when no treatment is available, early detection makes it possible to warn patients of the risks to subsequent pregnancies and possibly avoid having a second affected child.

In a previous chapter (Chapter 23) we outlined a general background to genetic screening, covering in particular, screening of adults and screening during pregnancy. Neonatal screening forms a third, natural group for consideration. The basic principles discussed in the earlier chapter apply equally here. In addition, the reader is referred back to the section outlining the use of recombinant DNA technology, which is also of relevance to certain aspects of neonatal screening.

Many of the metabolic disorders are difficult to detect in the neonatal period. Exceptions to this are phenylketonuria and congenital hypothyroidism, but for others the onset of diagnostic symptoms may not occur until later in infancy. Diagnosis is made more difficult by the fact that the majority of inborn errors have a low birth incidence (of the order of 0.1 to 0.01 per 1000), and it is only the specialist who can hope to become familiar with the manifestations and range of these rare disorders. Again, because of their rarity, general population screening for the majority of metabolic disorders is not possible, the test being limited to individual families for which there is an established risk, usually by virtue of the previous birth of an affected child.

Most inborn errors of metabolism are characterized by an enzyme deficiency which may be detected by a specific biochemical assay. Nowadays, many of these diagnostic tests may be carried out prenatally for those pregnancies known to have a high risk of producing an affected child. There are, however, certain areas where neonatal population screening has been established as routine practice. These include the disorders of amino acid metabolism, congenital hypothyroidism, and cystic fibrosis, each of which is covered in this chapter. The final section consists of a brief discussion of neonatal screening for Duchenne muscular dystrophy. (See also Chapter 23, where Duchenne muscular dystrophy is discussed in relation to heterozygote testing.)

2 Disorders of amino acid metabolism

The classical example of screening for this type of disorder is phenylketonuria, and this is discussed at some length, together with brief accounts of other disorders of amino acid metabolism, including maple syrup urine disease, histidinaemia, homocystinuria, and tyrosinaemia (see Table 84.1).

2.1 Phenylketonuria

Phenylketonuria (PKU) is a disorder largely restricted to Caucasian populations. The overall incidence is

Table 84.1 Biochemical screening in the newborn

Disorder	Incidence/1000 births	Test	Comments
1. Disorders of amino acid metabolism			
(a) Phenylketonuria	0.016 to 0.25	Assay of blood levels of phenylalamine	In general use for neonatal screening
(b) Maple syrup urine disease	0.005		
(c) Histidinaemia	0.05 to 0.125	Standard assays using thin layer chromatography	Screening policies vary—very rare disorders
(d) Homocystinuria	0.005		
(e) Tyrosinaemia	0.008 to 1.46		
2. Congenital hypothyroidsim	0.24	T4 or TSH tests or combination	All neonates
3. Cystic fibrosis	0.5	Immunoreactive trypsin levels: DNA probes for family studies	Mass screening not widely practised
4. Duchenne muscular dystrophy	0.3 (male births)	Serum creatine phosphokinase levels: DNA probes	Mass screening not widely practised

about 0.09 per 1000 live births, but reported figures show a range of variation from 0.25 per 1000 in Northern Ireland to 0.016 in Denmark (Veale 1980). The disorder is due to a lack of the enzyme phenylalanine hydroxylase, required to convert phenylalanine into tyrosine. The resulting accumulation of phenylalanine and phenolic derivatives, including the ketoacid phenylpyruvate, from which the disorder gets its name, are manifested by a general failure to thrive, developmental delay, and increasing mental retardation.

Newborn screening programmes for the detection of phenylketonuria are accepted as a normal component of neonatal care throughout a large part of the world. Early detection followed by the appropriate dietary control, allows the affected child to develop normally. Cost–benefit analyses (detailed by Komrower 1984) show substantial savings to the community as a whole by undertaking neonatal screening for phenylketonuria.

Early recognition of the condition is important because treatment is effective in preventing the sequelae. It revolves around dietary control of the intake of phenylalanine, and the provision of adequate amounts of tyrosine. The survival rate is quite good: Komrower *et al.* (1979a) reported an average of 39.5 years, with a range of 19–64 years in the Manchester population.

The microbiological assay for blood phenylalanine (Guthrie test), described by Guthrie and Susi (1963), has been adapted very successfully for mass screening. The test is normally carried out on the 5th or 6th day after delivery, thus allowing time for levels of phenylalanine to build up in affected individuals. A spot of blood from a heelprick is taken up on to filter paper, which is dried and sent to the laboratory. Here a disc of the filter paper is punched out from the area of the bloodspot, and, together with control discs, it is placed on an agar containing beta-2-thienylalanine and spores of the bacterium *Bacillus subtilis*. Growth of the bac-

terium is inhibited by the beta-2-thienylalanine, except around those discs that contain phenylalanine. This is a very sensitive test, and can detect 0.15 mmol/l of phenylalanine. One-dimensional chromatography using paper or thin-layer techniques are slightly more expensive, but equally good, and have the advantage that levels of other amino acids may be checked at the same time. Fluorometric methods may also be used, but are more costly still.

Komrower (1984) gives data from the Manchester survey showing very good discrimination between affected and unaffected infants for serum phenylalanine levels, with no overlap. The cut-off point is taken at 0.24 mmol/l. Repeat tests will be required in about 0.22 cases/1000, of which most will be found to be normal on re-testing. Confirmation of phenylketonuria is usually made by demonstrating low serum tyrosine, and the presence of phenylpyruvic acid and other phenyl compounds in the urine.

Where both parents are known to be heterozygous for the mutant allele, prenatal testing of the fetus is theoretically feasible, by doing a fetal liver biopsy to assess phenylalanine hydroxylase activity. Recently, Lidsky *et al.* (1985a,b) have reported the prenatal diagnosis of phenylketonuria by DNA analysis, and this would seem the method of choice for the future.

Lenke and Levy (1980) present data showing that the stillbirth rate for mothers who have the disorder themselves (with blood phenylalanine levels equal to or greater than 20 mg/dl) is approximately 25 per cent. Of the surviving infants, approximately 70 per cent are microcephalic, and 12 per cent have congenital heart disease, while 90 per cent have an intelligence quotient below 75. Phenylketonuric mothers with lower levels of blood phenylalanine are less at risk of having affected offspring. Lipson *et al.* (1984) showed that maternal hyperphenylalaninaemia appears to be teratogenic in its effect on the fetus. Smith *et al.* (1979) have shown that fetal damage occurs despite a low phenylalanine diet after conception, in a phenylketonuric woman, and Komrower *et al.* (1979b) suggest that dietary control must be exercised before conception, as well as through pregnancy, if the fetus is to have a reasonable chance of being normal. Data on this aspect of dietary control is very sparse, but a report by Lenke and Levy (1982) cites two cases where treatment was initiated prior to conception which both resulted in an apparently normal child at birth.

The technique used for phenylketonuria screening may also be adapted for the other disorders of amino acid metabolism mentioned above (maple syrup urine disease, histidinaemia, homocystinuria, and tyrosinaemia). The feasibility of screening for each of these disorders has been shown by various programmes over the years, but probably the most effective approach is to use thin-layer chromatographic techniques (Bittles *et al.* 1983), which enable a wide range of errors of amino acid metabolism to be tested on a single specimen.

2.2 Maple syrup urine disease

Maple syrup urine disease is due to a deficiency of branched-chain ketoacid decarboxylase. Urine of affected infants has a distinctive smell of maple syrup, which gives the disorder its name. Screening of over 12 million newborn infants has revealed an incidence of approximately 0.005 per 1000 births (Naylor 1980). Affected infants show a very rapid deterioration soon after birth, and if the appropriate dietary treatment (limitation of the intake of the three branched-chain amino acids and the administration of vitamins and minerals) is to be successful, it should be initiated as soon as possible. Prenatal diagnosis can be offered if required.

2.3 Histidinaemia

Histidinaemia is not the rare disorder it was once thought to be. Screening programmes for the newborn have shown it to occur with an incidence in the range of 0.125 per 1000 in Japan (Tada *et al.* 1982) to 0.05 per 1000 in the United States (Levy *et al.* 1974). The disorder is due to a deficiency of the enzyme histidase. The clinical features usually involve only relatively mild brain damage, if, indeed, any at all, and the treatment, which consists of a reduced histidine intake, is not always carried out. Contrary to the situation found in phenylketonuria, histidinaemic mothers do not seem to require dietary control during pregnancy.

2.4 Homocystinuria

Homocystinuria is usually caused by deficiency of the enzyme cystathionine beta-synthase. There is considerable clinical heterogeneity. Ninety per cent of patients develop dislocation of the optic lens, while other symptoms include varying degrees of skeletal changes, and mental retardation. The most serious complications result from arterial or venous thromboses. Treatment of the disorder involves the administration of pyridoxine, coupled with dietary restriction of methionine.

Mass screening of about 2.6 million infants indicates a frequency of about 0.005 per 1000 (Benson and Polani 1978). Heterozygote detection is not reliable, but prenatal diagnosis may be carried out by assaying cystathionine beta-synthase activity in cultured amniotic fluid cells. Similarly, first trimester diagnosis of the disorder may be made using chorionic villi, but only after culture; uncultured villi show very little or no enzyme activity (Benson *et al.* 1983).

2.5 Tyrosinaemia

Tyrosinaemia varies widely in its incidence, from 0.008 per 1000 in Sweden (Alm and Larsson 1979), to 1.46 per 1000 in Quebec (Bergeron *et al.* 1974). The most serious clinical feature is liver damage. Probably the best method of population screening is to use a thin-layer chromatographic technique to assay the tyrosine levels in the blood, at the age of about four weeks. Prenatal diagnosis is possible, either by demonstrating an increase in succinylacetone in amniotic fluid or by estimating the level of the enzyme fumaryl acetoacetate hydrolase in amniotic fluid cells.

3 Congenital hypothyroidism

A congenital deficiency of unbound circulating thyroid hormone results in impaired intellectual and motor function, which, if untreated, will lead to the classical picture of cretinism. Deficiency of the thyroid hormone, which is essential for brain development, may be compensated for by the administration of thyroxine. The normality of final intelligence depends on the age at which treatment begins, but although treatment ensures that the children are not at risk for mental retardation, a prospective investigation (Rovet 1986) of children with congenital hypothyroidism showed that affected children have a slightly lower intelligence quotient than their unaffected siblings. Rovet's study also confirmed the observation of previous workers, that these children have problems with language ability, neuromotor skills, and perceptual performance, presumably the result of hypothyroidism despite early treatment. This emphasizes the great importance of having an efficient neonatal screening programme, so that affected infants can be identified early, and treatment initiated without delay.

The true incidence of congenital hypothyroidism is uncertain. Data from Holland (de Jonge 1976) and Sweden (Alm *et al.* 1978), on unscreened populations, indicated a frequency of approximately 0.15 per 1000 live births, whereas the mean frequency determined from screening programmes is 0.24 per 1000 (Layde 1984). The differences between these two figures may reflect either under-detection in the case of the non-screened population, in spite of a 2-year follow-up period, or it may be that a proportion of those cases detected by screening would never develop symptomatic disease. Early mortality without diagnosis could also be a factor.

There are two tests that are used to screen for congenital hypothyroidism: the measurement of thyroid-stimulating hormone, (TSH), and of the total level of both bound and unbound thyroxine (T$_4$). When thyroxine screening is carried out, equivocal results are normally checked using the thyroid-stimulating hormone assay.

The time of testing is important. Immediately after birth there is normally a surge in the level of thyroid-stimulating hormone, which stimulates the production of thyroxine. For thyroid-stimulating hormone testing, therefore, it is necessary to wait until the infant is at least 4 days old before obtaining a blood sample. Alternatively, cord blood could be used. For thyroxine testing, it is, again, probably wise to wait until about day 5, since the thyroid-stimulating hormone surge may elevate the thyroxine levels to within the normal range in hypothyroid infants with some residual thyroid function.

The thyroids-stimulating hormone test is more sensitive than that for thyroxine, and gives fewer false positive screening results (Layde 1984). On the other hand, thyroxine screening is cheaper and technically less difficult, which are important considerations in implementing screening programmes. It has the additional advantage that secondary and tertiary hypothyroidism resulting from an abnormality of the pituitary or a deficiency of thyroid-stimulating hormone releasing factor from the hypothalamus can also be detected. Thyroxine testing also results in the detection of the benign condition of thyroxine-binding globulin deficiency (Lee *et al.* 1978). Both tests may now be carried out using radioimmunoassay techniques on small quantities of capillary blood, dried on to filter papers, (Dussault *et al.* 1975; Larsen and Broksin 1975; Dussault *et al.* 1976; Foley *et al.* 1977). This means that screening for hypothyroidism may be carried out on the same sample that is taken for phenylketonuria screening, thus minimizing costs. Many screening programmes for congenital hypothyroidism use thyroxine screening as the main test, supplemented by thyroid-stimulating hormone testing where the thyroxine values are considered borderline. There is, however, considerable variation from centre to centre in the thyroxine levels below which thyroid-stimulating hormone testing is carried out, thus making it difficult to arrive at a consistent figure for the false positive rate. Layde (1984) summarized data from five centres showing that

out of 1 046 362 infants screened, 249 cases of congenital hypothyroidism were detected and 8 were missed. The majority of infants with low levels of thyroxine are, in fact, normal on re-testing, including infants who appeared to be severely hypothyroid on neonatal screening: so-called transient hypothyroidism, which seems to be associated with factors such as prematurity, caesarian section and respiratory distress (Layde 1984).

4 Cystic fibrosis

Cystic fibrosis (CF) is the commonest of the clinically important single gene disorders. It is inherited as an autosomal recessive condition, occurring with a frequency of about 0.5 per 1000 live births in Caucasian populations. It is less common in other ethnic groups. The underlying molecular basis of cystic fibrosis is not yet understood, but clinically the disorder, which is essentially one of widespread dysfunction of exocrine glands, is characterized by chronic progressive pulmonary disease which eventually results in respiratory insufficiency and death by about the age of 30. Pancreatic insufficiency is also typical of most affected individuals, and children in particular often show symptoms of malabsorption. Males affected by the condition are normally sterile due to obliteration of the vas deferens. An important finding in affected individuals are the abnormally elevated levels of sweat electrolytes which provide the basis for a diagnostic test.

This test (quantitative pilocarmine iontophoresis) (Gibson *et al.* 1975), measures the concentration of sodium and/or chloride ions in the sweat. The test is really only satisfactory in prepubertal children, where there are usually clear separations between the values for healthy children and affected individuals (20 mEq/l in normal; 100 to 110 mEq/l in affected, Lobeck 1972). After puberty the clear distinction between affected and unaffected is lost. In newborn infants it is difficult to carry out the sweat test, and the most widely used procedure has been to measure the albumin content of meconium. The BM-meconium (using a dip-stick marketed by Boehringer-Mannheim) is a very simple test where the meconium is applied directly to an indicator paper, which shows a colour change when the concentration of albumin exceeds 20 mg/g. A multicentre study, combining data from 15 groups in Europe and America, reported on a total of 296 484 tests, of which 109 were positive (confirmed with the sweat test). A false positive rate of 0.6 per cent was recorded (Stephan 1980). The main disadvantage of this test is that only 85 per cent of newborn babies with cystic fibrosis appear to have a pancreatic insufficiency and hence, an increased concentration of albumin in their meconium.

Following a report that serum immunoreactive trypsin levels are almost always elevated in infants with cystic fibrosis (Crossley *et al.* 1979), it is now possible to carry out neonatal screening using blood clots dried on to filter paper. Dodge (1984) presents collective data for seven prospective studies of immunoreactive trypsin screening on a total of 263 000 individuals, that indicate it to be a highly specific test with a final low false positive rate of less than 0.005 per cent. The false negatives that occur seem to be associated with those infants with meconium ileus. The reasons for this are not known, but the occurrence of such false negatives is of little consequence since meconium ileus in itself is an indication of cystic fibrosis.

The measurement of amniotic fluid microvillar enzymes (alpha-glutamyl transpeptidase; aminopeptidase; alkaline phosphatase) (Carbarns *et al.* 1983; Brock *et al.* 1984a) gives important, though far from perfect information for prenatal diagnosis of cystic fibrosis, with approximately 5 per cent of pregnancies escaping detection. More recently, Brock *et al.* (1984b), has attempted to measure immunoreactive trypsin in amniotic fluid. At the present time, however, interest is focused on DNA studies and the use of genetic markers.

Although the molecular mechanism of cystic fibrosis is not known, and no gene products have been convincingly identified, the location of the gene has been narrowed down to a short region in the middle of the long arm of chromosome 7. It is, therefore, now possible to identify variations in DNA sequences (restriction fragment length polymorphisms (RFLPs) generated by the action of restriction enzymes) that are closely linked to the gene locus. Already, three groups have isolated RFLPs that are within about 1 000 000 base pairs of the cystic fibrosis gene (White *et al.* 1985; Wainwright *et al.* 1985; Knowlton *et al.* 1985). The methods as they stand are not suitable for population screening because the technique does not identify the defective gene directly, but merely closely linked markers. Family studies are, therefore, necessary to identify which specific markers are associated with the cystic fibrosis carrying chromosome in each individual.

This information can then be used for carrier detection and prenatal diagnosis, in most families. The existing probes are sufficiently informative to allow full diagnosis in about two-thirds of couples presenting with at least one affected child (Farrall *et al.* 1986).

5 Duchenne muscular dystrophy

Neonatal screening for affected males (based on levels of creatine phosphokinase—CPK) is feasible (Skinner *et al.* 1982), but the wide-scale detection of heterozygous females in the population is not. The question of neonatal screening is open to debate on ethical grounds. To some, it is unacceptable to screen for a disorder that is untreatable. On the other hand, delay in diagnosis until the disease becomes manifest may result in further affected children being conceived before the parents are aware of the risks. Up to 15 per cent of affected children may be born in this way (Gardner-Medwin 1979). An assessment of the views of parents of children with Duchenne muscular dystrophy with regard to newborn screening are given by Firth and Wilkinson (1983), who found that in 75 per cent of families (90 per cent of those who expressed an opinion) the parents were in favour of neonatal screening. At the present time, however, neonatal screening is not widely practised, and testing at the family level will normally be set in motion as a result of the birth of an affected child.

6 Conclusions

The value of total population neonatal screening for some conditions, and screening of selected individuals for others has been well established. New technologies are likely to produce more sensitive and specific tests, leading to an expansion of the range of disorders for which neonatal screening is feasible. The application of screening programmes depends on a careful balance of ethical, practical, and cost–benefit arguments.

References

Alm J, Larsson A (1979). A follow-up of a nationwide neonatal metabolic screening programme in Sweden. Pediatr Res, 13: 79.

Alm J, Larsson A, Zetterström R (1978). Congenital hypothyroidism in Sweden. Acta Paediatr Scand, 67: 1–3.

Benson PF, Fensom AH, Crees MJ, Lam STS, Coleman D, Heaton D, Rodeck C (1983). Recent advances in prenatal diagnosis for inborn errors of metabolism. In: Progress in Perinatal Medicine. Albertini A, Crosignani PG (eds). Amsterdam: Excerpta Medica.

Benson PF, Polani PE (1978). Appendix A: an estimate of the number of amniocentesis for metabolic disorders required per year. In: The Provision of Services for the Prenatal Diagnosis of Fetal Abnormality in the United Kingdom. Report of the Clinical Genetics Society Working Party on prenatal diagnosis in relation to genetic counselling. Bull Eugenics Soc Suppl., 3: 30.

Bergeron P, Laberge C, Grenier A (1974). Hereditary tyrosinemia in the province of Quebec. Prevalence at birth and geographic distribution. Clin Genet, 5: 157–162.

Bittles AH, Radha Rama Devi A, Vankat Rao S, Appaji Rao N (1983). A newborn screening programme for the detection of amino acid disorders in South India. Biochem Rev, 52: 20–24.

Brock DJH, Bedgood D, Hayward C (1984a). Prenatal diagnosis of cystic fibrosis by assay of amniotic fluid microvillar enzymes. Hum Genet, 65: 248–251.

Brock DJH, Hayward C, Gosden C, Rodeck C (1984b). Immune reactive trypsin and the prenatal diagnosis of cystic fibrosis. Br J Obstet Gynaecol, 91: 449–452.

Carbarns NJB, Gosden C, Brock DJH (1983). Microvillar

peptidase activity in amniotic fluid: possible use in the prenatal diagnosis of cystic fibrosis. Lancet, 1: 329–331.

Crossley JR, Elliott RB, Smith PA (1979). Dried blood spot screening for cystic fibrosis in the newborn. Lancet, 1: 472–474.

de Jonge GA (1976). Congenital hypothyroidism in the Netherlands. Lancet, 2: 143.

Dodge JA (1984). Screening for cystic fibrosis. In: Screening and Management of Potentially Treatable Genetic Metabolic disorders. Benson PF (ed). MTP Press, Lancaster, pp 9–16.

Dussault JH, Parlow A, Letarte J, Guyda H, Laberge C (1976). TSH measurement from blood spots on filter paper: a confirmatory screening test for neonatal hypothyroidism. J Pediatr, 89: 550–552.

Dussault JH, Coulombe P, Laberge C, Letarte J, Guyda H, Khoury K (1975). Preliminary report on a mass screening program for neonatal hypothyroidism. J Pediatr, 86: 670–674.

Farrall M, Law HY, Rodeck CH, Warren R, Stanier P, Super M, Lissens W, Scrambler P, Watson E, Wainwright B, Williamson R (1986). First trimester prenatal diagnosis of cystic fibrosis with linked DNA probes. Lancet, 1: 1042–1045.

Firth MA, Wilkinson EJ (1983). Screening the newborn for Duchenne muscular dystrophy: parents' views. Br Med J, 286: 1933–1934.

Foley TP Jr, Klein AH, Agustin AV (1977). Adaptation of TSH filter paper method for regionalized screening for congenital hypothyroidism. J Lab Clin Med, 90: 11–17.

Gardner-Medwin D (1979). Controversies about Duchenne muscular dystrophy. 1: Neonatal screening. Dev Med Child Neurol, 21: 390–393.

Gibson LE, Di Sante' Agnese PA, Schwacmann H (1975). Procedure for the Quantitative Iontophoretic Sweat Test for Cystic Fibrosis. Atlanta: Cystic Fibrosis Foundation.

Guthrie R, Susi A (1963). A simple phenylalanine method for detecting phenylketonuria in large populations of newborn infants. Pediatrics, 32: 338–343.

Knowlton RG, Cohen-Haguenauer O, Vancong N, Frezal J, Brown VA, Barker D, Draman JC, Schumm JW, Tsui LC, Buchwald M, Donis-Kelleb H (1985). A polymorphic DNA marker linked to cystic fibrosis is located on chromosome 7. Nature, 318: 380–382.

Komrower GM (1984). Phenylketonuria and other inherited metabolic defects. In: Antenatal and neonatal screening. Wald NJ (ed). Oxford: Oxford University Press, pp 221–238.

Komrower GM, Sardharwalla IB, Fowler B, Bridge C (1979a). The Manchester regional screening programme: a 10 year exercise in patient and family care. Br Med J, 2: 635–638.

Komrower GM, Sardharwalla IB, Coutts JMJ, Ingham D (1979b). Management of maternal phenylketonuria: an emerging clinical problem. Br Med J, 1: 1383–1387.

Larsen PR, Broksin K (1975). Thyronine immunoassay using filter paper blood samples for screening of neonates with hypothyroidism. Pediatr Res, 9: 604–608.

Layde PM (1984). Congenital hypothyroidism. In: Antenatal and neonatal screening. Wald NJ (ed). Oxford: Oxford University Press, pp 239–257.

Lee T, McNaughton WM, Wellby ML (1978). Thyroxine binding globulin deficiency which mimics neonatal hypothyroidism. Med J Austral, 2: 161.

Lenke RR, Levy HL (1980). Maternal phenylketonuria and hyperphenylalaninaemia. New Engl J Med, 303: 1202–1208.

Lenke RR, Levy HL (1982). Maternal phenylketonuria: results of dieting therapy. Am J Obstet Gynecol, 142: 548–553.

Levy HL, Shih VE, Madigan PM (1974). Routine newborn screening for histidinaemia: clinical and biochemical results. New Engl J Med, 291: 1214–1219.

Lidsky AS, Ledley FD, Di Lella AG, Kwok SCM, Daiger SP, Robson KJH, Woo SLC (1985b). Extensive restriction site polymorphism at the human phenylalanine hydroxylase locus and application in prenatal diagnosis of phenylketonuria. Am J Hum Genet, 37: 619–634.

Lidsky AS, Guttler F, Woo SLC (1985a). Prenatal diagnosis of classic phenylketonuria by DNA analysis. Lancet, 1, 549–551.

Lipson A, Beuhler B, Bartley J, Walsh D, Yu J, O'Halloran M, Webster W (1984). Maternal hyperphenylalaninaemia: fetal effects. J Pediatr, 104: 216–220.

Lobeck CC (1972). Cystic fibrosis. In: The Metabolic Basis of Inherited Disease (3rd edn). Stanbury JB, Wyngaarden JS, Frederickson DS (eds). New York: McGraw-Hill, pp 1605–1606.

Naylor EW (1980). Newborn screening for Maple syrup urine disease. In: Neonatal Screening for Inborn Errors of Metabolism. Bickel H, Guthrie R, Hammersen G (eds). Berlin: Springer-Verlag, pp 19–28.

Rovet JF (1986). A prospective investigation of children with congenital hypothyroidism identified by neonatal thyroid screening in Ontario. Can J Publ Health, 77 (Suppl 1): 164–173.

Skinner R, Emery AEH, Schuerbrandt G, Syme J (1982). Feasibility of neonatal screening for Duchenne muscular dystrophy. J Med Genet, 19: 1–3.

Smith I, Erdohazi M, MacArtney FJ, Pincott JR, Wolff OH, Brenton DP, Biddle SA, Fairweather DVI, Dobbing J (1979). Fetal damage despite low phenylalanine diet after conception in a phenylketonuric woman. Lancet, 1: 17–19.

Stephan U (1980). Neonatal screening for cystic fibrosis. In: Neonatal Screening for Inborn Errors of Metabolism. Bickel H, Guthrie R, Hammersen G (eds). Berlin: Springer-Verlag, pp 81–87.

Tada K, Tateda H, Arashima S, Sakai K, Kitagawa T, Aoki K, Suwa S, Kawamura M, Oura T, Takesada M, Kuroda Y, Yamashita F, Matsuda I, Maruse H (1982). Intellectual development in patients with untreated histidinaemia: a collaborative study group of neonatal screening for inborn errors of metabolism in Japan. J Pediatr, 101: 562–563.

Veale AMO (1980). Screening for phenylketonuria. In: Neonatal Screening for Inborn Errors of Metabolism. Bickel H, Guthrie R, Hammersen G (eds). Berlin: Springer-Verlag, pp 7–18.

Wainwright BJ, Scambler PJ, Schmidtke J, Watson EA, Law HY, Farrall M, Cooke HJ, Eiberg H, Williamson R (1985). Localization of cystic fibrosis locus to human chromosome 7cen-q22. Nature, 318: 384–385.

White R, Woodward S, Leppert M, O'Connell P, Hoff M, Herbst J, Jalovel JM, Dean M, Van de Woude G (1985). A closely linked genetic marker for cystic fibrosis. Nature, 318: 382–384.

85 Care of the bereaved after perinatal death

Gillian Forrest

1 Introduction

This chapter is concerned with one of the most challenging aspects of care in pregnancy and childbirth— the care of families whose baby is born dead, malformed, or gravely ill. There have been great changes in attitude towards perinatal death and childhood illness and impairment over the past few decades. Improvements in perinatal and infant mortality rates have been accompanied by ever-increasing expectations by parents that their children will be born safely and survive. Nowadays, most couples choose to have only two or three children, making each pregnancy and delivery a very significant experience. When things do go wrong therefore, it comes as a great shock, and many parents suffer not only a sense of the loss of the healthy baby they had anticipated, but also the loss of their faith in modern medicine and doctors. It is often similarly shattering for members of the maternity unit staff to witness the apparent failure of their technical skills. To compound the difficulties further, in industrialized Western societies today, we have lost our day-to day familiarity with death and bereavement, along with the mourning rituals that used to play an important part in meeting the psychological needs of the bereaved. Thus we have become poorly equipped to cope with a situation which will continue to occur even in the best maternity units.

Our knowledge of bereavement is based partly on descriptive accounts of bereaved patients in psychiatric treatment, and partly on objective studies of bereaved people. The following account of the psychology of bereavement is based on the work of many authors, but principally Freud (1917), Lindemann (1944), Parkes (1972), and Raphael (1984).

The two components of normal grief are the 'pangs of grief, (episodes of restlessness, angry pining, and anxiety), set against a chronic background disturbance (Worden 1982). This background disturbance consists of chronic low mood, loss of purpose in life, social withdrawal, impaired memory and concentration, and disturbances of appetite, weight, and sleep. These symptoms occur as bereaved people go through the process of coming to terms with the reality of their loss, and of withdrawing psychologically from their relationships with those who have died in order to continue with their own lives in a positive manner. This process may take months or years to complete, and a successful outcome depends on the personalities and life experiences of the people concerned; the circumstances of the death; the relationship with the dead person; and on the effectiveness of the supportive network surrounding bereaved people (Raphael 1977). The style of an individual's grief reaction will be determined by personality traits; for example, whether emotions are expressed openly, or grief is expressed only in private.

As far as abnormal grief reactions are concerned, a longitudinal study (Parkes and Weiss 1983) has distinguished three common types. These are: the unexpected grief syndrome, when the death was sudden and numbness or shock with much anxiety is seen; the ambivalent grief syndrome, where the relationship with the deceased was stormy, and the grief reaction is delayed and characterized by much guilt; and chronic grief, which is seen after the loss of a dependent relationship.

A number of generalizations have been made about the needs of people coping with loss (Marris 1974):

- They are in a state of intense emotional turmoil, which temporarily overthrows their normal coping strategies, particularly if they have no previous experience.

- Having an object to mourn (a body), facilitates grief work as the bereaved are thereby confronted with the painful reality of their loss.

- Escaping confrontation with the painfulness of the loss (not attending the funeral, never speaking of the dead person, or never revisiting the place of death) hinders rather than helps mourning.

- In trying to cope, the bereaved seek facts as anchor points of reality, although any information offered to them while they are shocked and numb, will need to be repeated later.

- Recovery from bereavement is marked by a gradual return to a normal pattern of life, free of depression or anxiety and with a regained capacity for enjoyment.

2 Perinatal bereavement

2.1 Perinatal death

It will come as no surprise to read that losing a baby late in pregnancy or soon after delivery is, today, accompanied by the same sort of grief reactions as those described in the Introduction. However, this may not always have been the case. As recently as 1970 there was a widely held belief that perinatal death was a relatively minor trauma, recovery taking only a few weeks. Kennell *et al.* (1970) and Giles (1970) published two of the first studies of grief reactions following perinatal death, dispelling this idea. Since then there has been a great deal of descriptive literature, with some objective studies on care and outcome, and it is clear that grief after perinatal death is no different qualitatively from that following the death of any loved person. There are some special features however.

Anxiety and anger is frequently described, with blame being directed at the staff, other members of the family, or at the self, as guilt. This may be due in part to the suddenness of the death, and is probably compounded when no 'scientific' explanation is available to help the parents understand exactly what has gone wrong (Newton *et al.* 1986). Desperately seeking for a cause of the baby's death is also commonly described. It is clearly easier for those parents who have an explanation, such as malformations or extreme immaturity. 'Empty arms' is another common and distressing symptom after the phase of numbness has passed, and mothers are frequently tormented by hearing their dead baby crying. Some bereaved parents experience very

negative feelings towards other babies and are fearful of losing control, while others long to hold a baby—any baby—however painful this might be. Many mothers do not expect to lactate once the baby has died and find the fact that they do very upsetting. Most authors emphasize the great sense of loss of self-esteem experienced by the mothers; their sense of being failures both as women and as wives.

Most young parents will not have been bereaved before, and difficulties in coping with the complicated registration and funeral procedures are often reported. Many are unprepared for the emotional turmoil of their grief reaction, and often feel they should be 'over it' after a few weeks. This view may be reinforced by well-meaning friends and relatives, and even some medical practitioners, who may advise the couple to go ahead with another pregnancy long before they have recovered sufficiently from their loss. There is evidence that the fathers recover from their grief more quickly than the mothers (Helmrath and Steinitz 1978; Clyman *et al.* 1980; Rowe *et al.* 1978; Forrest *et al.* 1982) and this in itself may lead to problems with their relationship, particularly if the couple are not used to sharing their feelings, or if one of them is blaming the other for the baby's death. Meyer and Lewis (1979) report that sexual and marital difficulties are common sequelae, although it is hard to separate any specific effect of perinatal bereavement from the loss of libido that accompanies many forms of bereavement.

Another difficult area is the reaction of other young children in the family to the loss of the baby. They may be very confused about what has happened to the baby, and even feel responsible for the disappearance (Bowlby 1979). Behavioural changes are common, and may take the form of over-activity, naughtiness, regression and school problems, as well as emotional problems, (Van Eerdewegh *et al.* 1985). These reactions are usually fairly short-lived (a few weeks or months is the time noted by most authors) unless the emotional state of the parents is such that there is an absence of normal warmth in family relationships for an extended period of many months (Black and Urbanowicz 1985) or if serious difficulties develop in the relationships between the mother and her living children (Halpern 1972; Lewis 1983).

There are some particular problems associated with miscarriages and stillborn babies, in which iatrogenic factors undoubtedly play a part. Miscarriages are frequently regarded by professionals, and others, as minor setbacks in successful childbearing. For some women, however, they represent a loss as painful as the loss of a full term baby (Oakley *et al.* 1984). This is particularly so if there have been difficulties in conceiving, previous miscarriages, or if the pregnancy was terminated because of fetal abnormalities (Lloyd and Laurence 1985). In these circumstances there is often a sense of double loss of the baby and of the perceived chance of childbearing. A previous termination of pregnancy has been reported by many clinicians as a complicating factor for normal grieving, because of the associated guilt and sense of retribution that is experienced by the mothers.

Much has been written, notably by Lewis (1976, 1983), about unresolved grief after a baby has been stillborn. Lewis attributes this to the 'painful emptiness' of the experience. There is no real object to mourn as the baby has never lived outside the womb and because there are no memories to help. It is similar to the situation in which someone is 'missing, believed dead'. The problems are accentuated if the stillborn baby is rapidly removed from the delivery room before the parents have a chance to see or hold him or her, and if the hospital, for whatever reason, takes over the funeral arrangements without involving the parents (as has been common practice in the UK since 1975). Until recently in the UK it was not even possible to register a first name for a stillborn baby, and they are still often buried in unmarked graves. The attitudes of friends and relations may also contribute to the difficulties with comments such as, 'You can't have postnatal depression, you haven't got a baby!'. For these reasons, successful mourning after stillbirth may be harder to achieve without the guidance of well-informed staff to compensate for the lack of understanding on the part of society in general.

2.2 Long term effects of perinatal death

There have been few studies on the long term effects of perinatal death. Cullberg (1971) interviewed 56 women 1 to 2 years after a perinatal death. Nineteen were found to be suffering from serious maladaptive psychological symptoms. Wolff *et al.* (1970) followed up 40 women for 3 years after a stillbirth. Although all of them experienced a typical grief reaction, 8 were resolved never to have another pregnancy, and, of these, 4 had been sterilized. Nicol *et al.* (1986) followed up 110 women for 6 to 36 months after a perinatal death. She found 21 per cent suffering from a pathological grief reaction with continuing severe psychological symptoms (depression, anxiety, tiredness, etc.), social adjustment problems and marital difficulties; and a resolve to have no further children. Nicol also found that a poor psychological outcome was associated with a crisis in the pregnancy, an unsupportive family network, and only seeing but not holding the baby. We followed up 35 women for 14 months after a perinatal death (Forrest *et al.* 1982), and they have now been interviewed again 3 to 5 years later. At this most recent interview, 5 of these mothers were still showing pathological grief reactions characterized by high scores for depression and anxiety on standardized rating scales, psychosomatic symptoms, and problems with relation-

ships within the family. We found that poor outcome was associated with an unsupportive marriage and social isolation. Of the remaining 30 women in our sample who were free of psychiatric symptoms and functioning well, return to good health had taken on average 24 months, and was marked by a successful pregnancy. Most of these mothers reported high anxiety levels during this pregnancy and were over-protective towards the new baby in the first few months. These findings were also reported by Phipps (1985).

There have been reports of problems with parental relationships with babies conceived too quickly after a loss (Cain and Cain 1964; Poznanski 1972; Lewis and Page 1978; Bourne and Lewis 1984). It seems that if the dead child has been incompletely mourned before the start of a new pregnancy, mourning may be postponed until after the delivery of the baby, when it can reappear as 'postnatal depression' (Lewis 1979). The new baby's identity can become confused with that of the idealized baby, causing great emotional problems. The new child may never be able to live up to the parents' expectations, and may become the focus of any unresolved anger that the parents have as a result of their loss. The survivor of a twin pregnancy may be involved in very similar problems, if the dead twin is not properly mourned at the time.

It seems, therefore, that about one in five bereaved families are likely to suffer adverse long term effects after losing a baby. Although at this stage, we are not able to identify with great confidence those most at risk of developing problems subsequently, the most frequently reported markers are not seeing or holding the baby, having an unsupportive partner or social network, and embarking immediately on another pregnancy.

2.3 Illness and impairment

The reaction of parents to a newborn baby who is gravely ill or impaired is a form of grief reaction to the loss of the healthy child that the parents had expected. Bicknell (1983), writing about the diagnosis of impairment in a child, calls this the 'bereavement response'. She describes its component parts as shock; panic ('I can't look after a handicapped child'); denial ('He's not my baby'); grief, guilt, and anger. This is followed by a phase of bargaining ('I will look after him if he can be taught to be clean and dry'); and finally acceptance, when parents cope with the reality of the situation. Klaus and Kennell (1976) base their observations on studies of different types of impairment and report very similar stages in the grief reactions (shock, denial, sadness, anger, equilibrium, and reorganization). They point out that some parents fail to adapt and remain in a state of chronic sorrow. They also stress the importance of staff forming an effective alliance with the parents, on which plans for care can be based. In addition to a grief reaction, most parents of ill or impaired babies suffer high levels of anxiety, which appear to be increased by contact with the baby. This does not mean that separation of mother and baby is to be recommended (see Chapter 77; Davis *et al.* 1983). Apart from the emotional stress of the situation, parents have the physical and financial stress of visiting their baby in hospital, particularly if the baby has recurrent medical crises, and needs care over a long period of time. Some parents withdraw emotionally and physically from their baby before the medical staff have given up hope of the baby's survival. This is termed 'anticipatory mourning' and can be precipitated by giving an unrelievably gloomy prognosis, or even by a casual remark indicating a possible bad prognosis (Klaus and Kennell 1976). It carries with it a risk of rejection if the baby does eventually survive.

3 Care by the hospital

In many countries now recommendations for the care of bereaved parents emphasize the important role to be played by maternity unit staff (National Stillbirth Study Group 1979; Royal College of Obstetricians and Gynaecologists 1985; Fetus and Newborn Committee, Canadian Paediatric Society 1983; Giles 1970; Klaus and Kennell 1976; Kowalski 1980; Rousseau and Moreau 1984).

A planned programme of care based on the recommendations of the National Stillbirth Study Group has been evaluated in a randomized study (Forrest *et al.* 1982). The recommendations include encouraging the parents to see, hold, and name their baby and hold a funeral; arranging for them to see senior obstetric and paediatric staff to discuss what went wrong; obtaining genetic and obstetric counselling; and ensuring that the parents receive the autopsy results. In addition, a short series of counselling sessions with a child psychiatrist was included in the care offered to the index group. Parents were seen on an average of three occasions. At follow-up at 6 months, only 2 out of the 16 index mothers had high scores on measures of depression and anxiety, compared with 10 of the 19 comparison group of mothers ($p = 0.01$). By 14 months, this statistically significant difference between the groups had disappeared. We concluded that the provision of informed, compassionate care significantly facilitated the recovery process after a perinatal death.

As the majority of the group had had a normal grief reaction, it was not felt that bereavement counselling services had been required routinely. Thus, effective care for most families can, and should, be provided by the maternity unit staff. Indeed, it can be argued that these professionals are in the ideal position to help bereaved families by facilitating the establishment of normal grieving from the start, thus preventing abnormal reactions.

3.1 Immediate and early care

In order that mourning can begin parents must be enabled to overcome their fear of death and dying so that they can experience the painful reality of their loss. This involves encouraging them to have as much contact as possible with their baby, both before and after death, and there is widespread agreement that it is particularly important for parents of a stillborn baby to see, hold, and name their baby.

When an intrauterine death is suspected, the fears for the baby's condition should not be denied, but shared with the parents, together if at all possible. If the mother is at the clinic, efforts should be made to contact her partner or a friend, so that she is not left to travel home alone and unsupported. The technicians in the ultrasound scanning room have an important role to play when the confirmatory scan is done. They need to be sympathetic to the situation, relaxing any rules to allow the mother to be accompanied by anyone she chooses. Most women are very frightened at the prospect of delivering a dead baby, as well as shocked by their loss. It helps if staff take time to explain carefully what will happen, that adequate pain relief will be available, and what the baby will look like at delivery. This is usually very successful in overcoming any reluctance that the parents may have about seeing or holding their baby. It may help to show a very malformed or macerated baby to the parents wrapped up at first. A few parents will not be able to cope with seeing and holding the baby at the time of delivery. A photograph should be taken and kept in the medical notes for possible use later, and further opportunities for seeing the baby should be offered to parents over the next few days, as they often change their minds. Photographs and other mementos of the baby are very important, as they provide tangible evidence of the reality of the baby's existence and loss. They should be available for parents as keepsakes, if they wish.

When the baby lives long enough to be transferred to an intensive care unit, it is, again, very important for staff to make time to keep parents as fully informed as possible about the baby's condition, and encourage them to share in any way possible in the care. Photographs of the baby are very helpful, particularly for fathers to keep at home, or if the mother is too unwell herself to visit the unit. In a randomized trial of the use of routine polaroid photographs of sick neonates in the first week of life (Pareira *et al.* 1980), there was a significant increase in visiting by the parents of the photographed babies, compared with the non-photographed group. When the baby's condition is known to be terminal, it is important to try to involve the parents in the decision to cease life support, and then to let them take their dying baby in their arms, free, if at all possible, of all equipment that has been necessary until then. In describing this, authors quote parents saying such things as, 'It was all I could do for her to hold her in my arms as she died'. Feelings of guilt about removing the baby from the life support system have not been reported.

Many parents like to help with the laying out of the baby's body, and this should be encouraged. Often they have selected special clothes or toys to be placed in the coffin with the baby. Facilitating the parents' contact with the reality of the death of their baby in these ways will facilitate their grief reaction, too. They will need privacy to express their grief, though, and this should be provided, however busy the unit happens to be.

The choice of site of the aftercare of the mother is important, as mothers differ in their requirements at this time. Some want to be on their own, far away from the sound of babies crying; others long to return to familiar faces on the ward. It is helpful if as much flexibility as possible is offered to them and if, at least for the first night, partners are allowed to remain with them. Ideally, the hospital should provide a couch in the mother's room so that their grief can be shared together. Lactation and help with its suppression (see Chapter 82) has already been mentioned as an important issue for the mother whose baby has died. If the mother is physically fit to return home immediately, and wishes to do so, it is essential to ensure, as far as possible, that she has a supportive network of family, friends and professionals before discharging her.

3.2 Autopsy

Consent for an autopsy and chromosome studies should always be requested after a perinatal death, as they may well provide invaluable information about the cause of death, helping parents not only with their grief, but also assisting the planning of future pregnancies. Most parents do agree, although it is often a painful decision for them. One mother expressed her feelings about the autopsy like this: 'She's been through enough, must she be cut up now as well?'. There are, however, a small number of parents whose religious practices forbid this, and the dilemma with which these parents are confronted needs to be acknowledged, to avoid intolerable pressure being placed upon them in order to obtain their consent. Having consented, parents cherish great hopes that the results will provide the answers to their questions about why the baby died, and so it is very important that they not only receive the results, but do so in a form which makes sense to them. The best person to do this would seem to be a senior member of staff who can interpret the pathologist's findings, and this can be done as part of the follow-up interview, along with advice about future pregnancies.

3.3 Death registration and funeral arrangements

Fundamental to good care is not only a knowledge of the bereavement process but also of the legal procedures required when a baby dies or is stillborn. It is also necessary to be familiar with the registration and funeral arrangements operating in one's own unit or locality as these are often complicated and baffling for parents still suffering from the shock of their baby's death (Forrest *et al.* 1981). Religious practices vary greatly, too, and an awareness of these and sensitivity to the wishes of individual parents is crucial. The funeral may involve considerable expense, and assisting parents in making difficult choices and helping those in financial straits, besides encouraging them to attend, are therapeutic aspects of care. The maternity unit should ensure that someone is available for this task.

Many units have prepared leaflets outlining their own procedures and giving helpful advice on various aspects of losing a baby and these can be helpful for parents.

3.4 Communication

Good care hinges around good communication, and parents frequently comment on communication failures when describing their experiences. Staff need to be able to give bereaved parents opportunities for talking together about the loss of their baby and need to listen sympathetically to their expressions of grief. (It is much harder to listen than talk oneself.) In addition to this, staff need to try and help parents with their search for a cause of death, and the senior obstetric or paediatric staff will need to create opportunities for discussing this with the parents. Seeing both parents together not only helps to strengthen their relationship as they share the experience of their baby's loss, but also helps to prevent misunderstandings and inconsistencies in explanation. Arranging for the same members of staff to attend regularly to the parents also helps this. Any information given in the first few days of the loss will probably have to be repeated later, as the initial shock of the bereavement passes. (A follow-up interview a few weeks later seems to be the best way of overcoming this difficulty; see below.) Good communication between staff about the loss of the baby is also vital, to prevent painful situations such as a member of staff being unaware that the baby had died, and breezily asking the mother when she was to be delivered. Communication between the hospital and the primary health care team also needs to be good. The primary care team should be informed about the baby's loss immediately, so that they can make contact with the family as soon as, or even before, the mother is discharged. Parents may want the support of their own religious adviser, and the hospital will need to check on this and contact him or her if required.

3.5 Follow-up

Most mothers will be discharged home within a few days of their baby's death, still too shocked by it to properly grasp what has happened and why. Careful and supportive follow-up is extremely important. Parents should be able to contact the staff who cared for them by telephone after they leave the hospital. Some units are able to offer home visits by their social worker. An appointment should be made for both parents to see a senior member of staff 2 to 6 weeks later, as soon as the chromosomes and autopsy results are available, and some form of perinatal mortality conference has taken place. The follow-up visit should aim to give the parents the opportunity of going over the events around the loss of their baby and of releasing their emotions about these; to allow clarification, if at all possible, of why the baby died, giving the autopsy results to parents in an appropriate form; to give further counselling and in particular to advise about the timing of future pregnancies (see below); and to make arrangements for genetic counselling, if necessary.

Returning to visit the maternity unit for these appointments is usually a harrowing prospect for parents, but they almost always find it helpful to have kept them. Perhaps this is because they move a step further in their grief work by facing the painful memories once again.

As has already been discussed, the timing of the next pregnancy is important, to allow for the dead baby to be mourned first. The Stillbirth and Neonatal Death Society from their members' experience, recommend waiting 6 to 8 months. It has been found that an early pregnancy (less than 6 months after the loss) was strongly associated with high depression and anxiety scores at an assessment made 14 months after the baby's death (Forrest *et al.* 1982). However, the enormous individual variation of bereavement response means that it is inappropriate to recommend a fixed time interval. The best advice appears to be to wait 'a while' until the parents have had a chance to say goodbye to the dead baby, and until the mother feels emotionally as well as physically strong enough to cope with another pregnancy. The next pregnancy will inevitably be an extremely anxious time, and she will need extra support during pregnancy and in the first few months after delivery.

3.6 Check-lists

Some units have found it useful to develop check-lists to ensure that all the practical aspects of care have been covered (e.g. White *et al.* 1984). The example reproduced here (Appendix 85.1) is in use at Queen Charlotte's Maternity Hospital, London. Although these can be very helpful as *aides-mémoire*, it is important that check-lists do not come to replace personal, compassionate contact with bereaved parents.

4 Care in the community

4.1 Health professionals

The general practitioner, health visitor, and the other primary health care workers form the professional supportive network around the family once the mother has been discharged home. These professionals can be very helpful by continuing to facilitate the expression of emotion, informing parents about the symptoms of bereavement, and putting them in touch with any local support groups for parents who have lost a child (see Appendix 85.2).

The general practitioner can watch for signs of pathological grief reactions, and refer the parents for specialist help if necessary. These are most likely to take the form of an inhibited reaction, with no sign of any sense of loss; or a prolonged reaction, with unremitting symptoms of depression, severe anxiety, or the appearance of psychosomatic illness. There may also be drug or alcohol abuse. Unremitting anger is another feature of a pathological reaction, and the general practitioner may need to deal with anger focused on the maternity unit. To do so, he or she will need to have good relationships with the obstetric and paediatric staff, and be fully informed about the course of events which led to the baby's loss. The parents may blame the general practitioner, too, of course. When this happens, it is essential that he or she meets with the family as soon as possible so that they can ventilate their feelings, and, hopefully, re-establish their relationship. Many parents remain angry simply because they were denied any compassionate response to their situation: no one on the staff said 'I'm so sorry your baby died'.

The general practitioner or health visitor will probably be the person to whom the family will turn to for help with the reactions of their other children to the baby's death (and again, it is vitally important for them to be informed by the maternity unit as soon as the baby has died). Black and Urbanowicz (1985) described the reactions of 80 bereaved children in a study of family intervention after the death of a parent, and found an association between crying and talking about the dead parent with good outcome after a year. They concluded that the expression of mourning by children was helpful. Parents may need help to allow their children to ventilate their feelings about so painful a subject, however, and it must be remembered that young children will use play as a vehicle for doing so. Explaining death to the under-5-year-olds is difficult, because they are not yet able to grasp the concept (Lansdown and Benjamin 1985). Even very simple statements like 'The baby's gone' will be interpreted literally and lead to questions about where the baby has gone, and when a visit can be made. The parents will need to add more information as the child's capacity for understanding develops.

4.2 Self-help groups

Self-help can be very effective in providing the right kind of support for parents facing many different kinds of problems, and perinatal bereavement is no exception. It is important though, that the people running the group have recovered sufficiently from their own loss to be able to help others (2 years is the usual time required) and that they have access to professionals for help and advice as and when necessary. There are several national organizations in the United Kingdom; for example, the Stillbirth and Neonatal Death Society (SANDS), and the Compassionate Friends, and there are often locally based groups as well. Parents can benefit from sharing their experiences together, from discovering that they are not alone in their suffering, and from learning that time does help to heal the wounds. However, not everyone can cope with group support, and it is unwise to rely on a local self-help group to meet the needs of all bereaved families. So while it is invaluable to give parents the telephone number or address of a local contact, this should not replace follow-up by the hospital and general practitioner.

5 The role of specialist counsellors

So far, this chapter has concentrated on the management of normal grief reactions, and the prevention of abnormal (pathological) ones through the care of the normal staff of the maternity unit and primary health care team. However, about one in five families will show pathological reactions. All of these reactions are likely to be accompanied by problems in family relationships. The help of specialist counsellors trained in grief work will be needed in these situations, either to advise other colleagues giving care, or by taking over responsibility for care themselves. The treatment required is often protracted, and antidepressant drugs and psychiatric surveillance may be necessary for severe depressive symptoms. Child and family psychiatrists may be particularly helpful in dealing with the relationship problems within families. Specialist counsellors can also try and promote normal grieving in parents most at risk of pathological reactions. Risk markers that have been identified so far are: a crisis in the pregnancy; an unsupportive partner or spouse; and lack of a supportive social network.

Specialist counsellors can also be useful in supporting the staff of the unit (through regular staff meetings, case discussions, or training sessions) and can offer help and advice to self-help groups (Lake *et al.* 1983; Kellner *et al.* 1981). The training of staff in the care of families who lose their baby, or who are faced with a baby with a severe impairment, deserves as much emphasis as the development of their technical expertise. Because we have lost our familiarity with death and bereavement at a personal level, staff will need to be given information about the process of mourning as well as training in basic interviewing and counselling skills. They will also need to explore their own feelings about death if they are to understand and help others. A good training programme should therefore combine formal teaching with informal methods, such as group discussion and role play. In addition, junior staff can learn a great deal from watching and listening while more experienced members of staff handle difficult and painful situations.

6 Conclusions

Good care does not end with a baby's stillbirth or death. Much can be done to help the family cope with their loss and to facilitate their recovery from their bereavement. In this chapter, an attempt has been made to set out some guidelines for care, but the successful implementation of these will depend on the attitudes of individual staff members and the importance that is attached to training in this area.

Effective care also has implications for both maternity unit staff and professionals working in the community. Time will need to be spent with parents whose baby dies or is impaired, listening to them as well as talking; attention needs to be given to the details of follow-up in individual cases; the unit may well have to review its procedures for postnatal care in order to offer appropriate flexibility; the senior members of staff need to play a central role in caring for the parents, sharing their experience and expertise with the junior staff; the unit must pay attention to the practical aspects of the registration and funeral arrangements for babies; and the primary health care team will need to accept the role of monitoring and supporting the bereavement process. The results of such changes in care will almost certainly lead to greatly improved rapport with grieving families; to staff who cope much better with the painfulness of perinatal death because they feel able to help; and last and most important of all, to families who will, on the whole, emerge from their grief able to continue functioning well, with positive attitudes towards the professionals who shared the loss of their baby.

To improve care further, we need research to clarify the effects of recommending that all parents see and hold their babies; which individuals and families are most at risk of pathological grief reactions; and how best to treat them. We also need to study the mother–child relationship problems associated with 'replacement babies', and develop ways of preventing and treating these.

References

Bicknell J (1983). The psychopathology of handicap. Br J Med Psychol, 56: 167–178.

Black D, Urbanowicz A (1985). Bereaved children—family intervention. In: Recent Research in Developmental Psychopathology. Stevenson JE (ed). Oxford: Pergamon Press.

Bourne S, Lewis E (1984). Pregnancy after stillbirth or neonatal death. Lancet, 2: 31–33.

Bowlby H (1979). Attachment and Loss. Vol. 3: Loss. London: Hogarth Press.

Cain AC, Cain BS (1964). On replacing a child. J Am Acad Child Psychiatry, 3: 443–445.

Clyman R, Green C, Rowe J, Mikkelsen C, Ataide L (1980). Issues concerning parents after the death of their newborn. Crit Care Med, 4: 215–218.

Cullberg J (1971). Mental reactions of women to perinatal death. In: Psychosomatic medicine in obstetrics and gynaecology. 3rd Int Congress of Psychosomatic Obstetrics and Gynaecology. London/Basel, Karger, pp 326–329.

Davis JA, Richards MPM, Robertson NCR (1983). Parent–baby attachment in premature infants. London: Croom Helm.

Fetus and Newborn Committee, Canadian Paediatric Society (1983). Support for parents experiencing perinatal loss. Can Med Assoc J, 129: 335–339.

Forrest GC, Claridge RS, Baum JD (1981). The practical management of perinatal death. Br Med J, 282: 31–33.

Forrest GC, Standish E, Baum JD (1982). Support after perinatal death: a study of support and counselling after perinatal bereavement. Br Med J, 285: 1475–1479.

Freud S (1917). Mourning and melancholia. In: Sigmund Freud Collected Papers, Vol. 4. New York: Basic Books.

Giles P (1970). Reactions of women to perinatal death. Austral NZ J Obstet Gynaecol, 10: 207–210.

Halpern W (1972). Some psychiatric sequence in crib death. Am J Psychiatry, 129: 398–402.

Helmrath TA, Steinitz EM (1978). Parental grieving and the failure of social support. J Family Practice, 6: 785–790.

Kellner KR, Kirkley-Best E, Chessborough S, Donnelly W (1981). Perinatal mortality counselling program for families experiencing stillbirth. Death Education, 5: 29–40.

Klaus MH, Kennell JH (1976). Maternal infant bonding. St. Louis: Mosby.

Kennell JH, Slyter J, Klaus MH (1970). The mourning responses of parents to the death of a newborn infant. New Engl J Med, 283: 344–349.

Kowalski K (1980). Managing perinatal loss. Clin Obstet Gynaecol, 23: 1113–1123.

Lake M, Knuppel RA, Murphy J, Johnson T (1983). The role of a grief support team following stillbirth. Am J Obstet Gynecol, 146: 877–881.

Lansdown R, Benjamin G (1985). The development of the concept of death in children aged 5–9 years. Child Care Health Dev, 11: 13–20.

Lewis E (1976). Management of stillbirth coping with an unreality. Lancet, 2: 619–620.

Lewis E (1979). Inhibition of mourning by pregnancy: psychopathology and management. Br Med J, 11: 27–28.

Lewis E (1983). Stillbirth: psychological consequences and strategies of management. In: Advances in Perinatal Medicine, Vol. 3. Milunsky A, (ed). New York: Plenum Press.

Lewis E, Page A (1978). Failure to mourn a stillbirth: an overlooked catastrophe. Br J Med Psychol, 51: 237–241.

Lindemann E (1944). Symptomatology and management of acute grief. Am J Psychiatry, 101: 141–148.

Lloyd J, Laurence KM (1985). Sequelae and support after termination of pregnancy for fetal malformation. Br Med J, 290: 907–909.

Marris P (1974). Loss and Change. London: Routledge & Kegan Paul.

Meyer R, Lewis E (1979). Impact of stillbirth on a marriage. J Fam Ter, 1: 361.

National Stillbirth Study Group (1979). The Loss of Your Baby. London: Health Education Council/MIND.

Newton RW, Bergin R, Knowles D (1986). Parents interviewed after their child's death. Arch Dis Child, 61: 711–715.

Nicol MT, Tompkins JR, Campbell NA, Syme GJ (1986). Maternal grieving response after perinatal death. Med J Austral, 144: 287–289.

Oakley M, McPherson A, Roberts H (1984). Miscarriage. London: Fontana.

Pareira GR, Talbot YR, Boatwell WR, Parina PA, Musholt KS (1980). Photographs of sick neonates prior to transport: the effect on parental visiting pattern. Pediatr Res 14: 2662–2673.

Parkes CM (1972). Bereavement: Studies of Grief in Adult Life. London: Tavistock Publications.

Parkes CM, Weiss RS (1983). Recovery from Bereavement. New York: Basic Books.

Phipps S (1985). The subsequent pregnancy after stillbirth: anticipatory parenthood in the face of uncertainty. Int J Psychiatry Med, 15: 243–263.

Poznanski EO (1972). The 'replacement child': a saga of unresolved parental grief. Behav Pediatr, 81: 1190–1193.

Raphael B (1977). Preventive intervention with the recently bereaved. Arch Gen Psychiatry, 34: 1450–1454.

Raphael B (1984). The Anatomy of Bereavement. London: Hutchinson.

Rousseau P, Moreau K (1984). Le devil perinatal. Extrait de la Revue l'Enfant de l'ONE no. 5.

Rowe J, Clyman R, Green C, Mikkelsen C, Haight J, Ataide L (1978). Follow up of families who experience a perinatal death. Pediatrics, 62: 166–170.

Royal College of Obstetricians and Gynaecologists (1985). Report of the Royal College of Obstetricians and Gynaecologists Working Party on the Management of Perinatal Deaths. London: Royal College of Obstetricians and Gynaecologists.

Van Eerdewegh MM, Clayton P, Ban Eerdewegh P (1985). The bereaved child: variables influencing early psychopathology. Br J Psychiatry, 147: 188–194.

Wolff JR, Nielson PE, Schiller P (1970). The emotional reaction to a stillbirth. Am J Obstet Gynecol, 108: 73–77.

White MP, Reynolds B, Evans TJ (1984). Handling of death in special care nurseries and perinatal grief. Br Med J, 289: 167–169.

Worden W (1982). Grief counselling and grief therapy. London: Tavistock Publications.

Appendix 85.1 Check-list for staff following a stillbirth or neonatal death

Here is a suggested procedure to be followed, following a stillbirth or neonatal death before the mother leaves hospital. All concerned are responsible for ensuring that all the items are attended to. It is not necessary to keep to the order listed. This sheet may be stapled to the front of the notes.

Hospital contact person for parents:

Name	Please tick, sign and date
Mother informed of death by	
Father informed of death by	
Parents given opportunity to handle baby	
Consultant Obstetrician informed	
Consultant Paediatrician informed	
Consent for Post-mortem requested given/refused (please delete)	
Post-mortem form completed	
Date and time of Post-mortem	
Preliminary PM results explained to mother and father	
General practitioner informed of stillbirth	
Death or stillbirth certificate completed and given to parents	
Information re funeral arrangements	
Parents offered booklet "Loss of Your Baby"	
Mother seen by consultant obstetrician / Father seen by consultant obstetrician	
Mother seen by consultant paediatrician / Father seen by consultant paediatrician	
Mother seen by cons. paediatrician / Father seen by consultant paed.	
Religious adviser notified (if desired by patient)	
Chapel service requested/not requested (please delete)	
Community midwives notified and/or health visitor	
Post-natal visit date. Clinic Sister notified (re link with Consultant)	
Informed of Book of Remembrance	
Follow-up visit or 'phone call	
Photograph taken yes/no / Photograph given to parents or kept in case notes	
Case sheet specially marked	

We are grateful to the North Middlesex Hospital and Queen Charlotte's Maternity Hospital for permission to reproduce this check list.

Appendix 85.2 Addresses of self-help bereavement groups in the United Kingdom

Compassionate Friends,
6 Denmark Street,
Bristol BS1 5DQ

Stillbirth and Neonatal Death Society,
28 Portland Place,
London W1 3DE

86 Unhappiness after childbirth

Patrizia Romito

1 Introduction

'The medicalization of unhappiness as depression is one of the great disasters of the twentieth century'.

Oakley 1986.

The unhappiness that so many mothers experience after childbirth has traditionally been considered a medical subject; it is defined as an illness and given the label 'postpartum depression' (Day 1982). Some features of the medical model are retained even when the subject is studied by sociologists and psychologists. This illness-dominated way of defining reality interferes with a valid understanding of maternal unhappiness after childbirth.

There is widespread agreement among mental health professionals that women are at increased risk of mental disturbances in the reproductive period. Three different entities are recognized on empirical grounds: postpartum blues, postpartum depression and postpartum psychosis.

The frequently seen transient experience of weepiness, mood instability, anxiety and irritability is called 'postpartum blues' (or 'baby-blues'). Most mothers (up to 80 per cent in some studies) experience some or all of these feelings in the first few days after childbirth. 'Postpartum blues' is widely recognized because, in addition to being so common, it happens during the stay in hospital, and thus under the professional eye (Oakley 1980; McIntosh 1986).

At the opposite end of the spectrum, 'postpartum psychosis' describes a severe illness characterized by thought disorders and/or severe depression, affecting one to two in every thousand new mothers (Kendell 1985). Psychosis appearing postpartum is easily recog-

nized; it is impossible to ignore the acute distress of women suffering from it, their often strange behaviour, and their need for help. These women are frequently admitted to psychiatric hospitals. There is no agreement, however, about when a psychosis should be classified as a 'postpartum psychosis'. After reviewing the literature on the subject and searching for an acceptable definition Thomas and Gordon (1959) could only conclude that: 'Those psychoses which have an onset prior to emptying of the uterus would definitely be excluded'.

Postpartum depression is even more difficult to delineate and define. It emerges as 'a catch-all diagnosis, defined differently by different authors' (Affonso and Domino 1984). In the words of Pitt (1968), it is 'what lies between the extreme of severe puerperal depression, with the risk of suicide and infanticide, and the trivial weepiness of "the Blues"; something occurring frequently, much less dramatic than the former, yet decidedly more disabling than the latter'.

The fundamental question is whether or not an entity that we label postpartum depression actually exists. The research in this field seems to assume that postpartum depression is something that pre-exists the research process (Day 1982), and that all the researchers have to do is discover and describe it. Their results inevitably 'confirm' this assumption.

The variety of conceptual descriptions and definitions of postpartum depression suggest that the phenomenon labelled 'postpartum depression', rather than being an actual entity, is not only defined by, but actually constructed by the instruments used to measure it.

1.1 Frequency and duration

In view of the vague and varying definitions used, it is

not surprising that the reported incidence of postpartum depression varies so widely, depending on the measuring instruments used, the people who use them, the criteria for diagnosis, the time after birth at which depression is assessed, and the characteristics of the women studied (Watson *et al.* 1984; Arizmendi and Affonso 1984). Estimates of its frequency range from 7 per cent to 30 per cent, depending on whether the criterion for diagnosis is women seeking psychiatric help (Dalton 1971), scores achieved using psychological depression scales (Raskin *et al.* 1970; Paykel *et al.* 1980), or 'emotional problems' as assessed by obstetricians (Gordon *et al.* 1965).

Little is known about the duration of postpartum depression, because there have been relatively few longitudinal studies. Most articles leave the reader with the impression that the duration of postpartum depression has been measured effectively.

For example, Hopkins *et al.* (1984) quote a personal communication of O'Hara, asserting that the average duration of postpartum depression may be between 6 and 8 weeks and suggest that, 'confirmation of this finding would indicate that the average duration of postpartum depression is shorter than that of non postpartum depression'. A closer look at O'Hara's work (1982) reveals that he interviewed women by telephone, over a period of time ranging from 5 to 20 weeks after childbirth. The conclusion that postpartum depression lasts 6–8 weeks is possibly the result of his simply calculating the mean time after birth at which the interviews took place, rather than the actual duration of depression.

Looking at the few longitudinal studies that have been reported, it would seem that researchers find a more or less conspicuous minority of depressed women for as long as they are willing to continue the follow-up.

Six weeks after birth, Pitt (1968) found that 11 per cent of mothers were depressed; half of these were still depressed 1 year later.

In a recent prospective study of emotional disorders in childbearing women (Kumar and Mordecai Robson 1984; Cogill *et al.* 1986), 16 per cent of mothers were assessed as depressed three months after childbirth; the percentage rose to 22 per cent when any period of depression within the first year postpartum was taken into account. Eight per cent were still depressed four years after childbirth.

Wolkind and Zajicek (1981), who studied 247 primiparous women from a working-class area, found that most of the women in the small subgroup who had been depressed before their pregnancies remained so throughout the first years of motherhood. They were joined by a group of women who had their first experience of depression after the birth of their child. In all, 1 in every 10 new mothers was depressed throughout the first 3½ years of her child's life.

Cutrona (1983) followed 85 primiparae from the third trimester of pregnancy through the second month postpartum. She assessed 'major depression' with the Hamilton Rating Scale of Depression (Hamilton 1960) at three separate time points: once before and twice after the birth. Of these 85 women, 3.5 per cent were depressed during the third trimester of pregnancy; 4.7 per cent were depressed 2 weeks postpartum; and 3.5 per cent were depressed 8 weeks postpartum. Only one woman (1.2 per cent) was diagnosed as depressed on more than one of the three occasions. Overall, 7 of the 85 women (8.2 per cent) were assessed as having a 'major depression' at some time in the two months following the birth of their child; milder symptoms of depression were much more common.

A similar result was found by Romito (1988) who interviewed a sample of 44 French primiparae once during their pregnancy, twice postpartum (at 1 and 4 months) and by postal questionnaire when their children were around 9 months old. While the prevalence of depression, assessed with Pitt's depression questionnaire (Pitt 1968), was fairly stable in the three time points after the birth (around 12 per cent), there was only a partial overlap between women depressed at these three times: only one woman remained depressed from the birth until 9 months later. Overall, however, 11 women, a quarter of the sample, were depressed at some time or other during the 9 months following the birth of their first child.

The results of longitudinal studies, and especially those of the last two cited, clearly point out that depression after childbirth is not a condition that the researcher may or may not find by interviewing mothers at some arbitrarily chosen time during the months following birth, but rather a process, in which women will be more or less involved. Most studies limit themselves to the first 6–8 weeks postpartum (Watson *et al.* 1984). Yet it is clear that mothers are depressed at different times and/or for periods of longer duration than this.

Research focusing on depression in mothers of young children (apparently a different academic field, for few cross-references are made) has yielded similar findings. A high proportion of the mothers studied are depressed, whether or not they have recently given birth. Richman (1974), for example, studied a sample of 75 mothers with at least two young children: she found that 41 per cent had depressive symptoms of a moderate to severe degree, and that 17 per cent were judged to be suffering from quite severe psychiatric illness. In another study, Richman compared 100 mothers of 3-year-old children with problem behaviour with a further 100 mothers whose 3-year-old children had no such problems: 39 per cent of the former mothers and 26 per cent of the latter showed symptoms of 'depressive psychiatric illness' (Richman 1977, quoted by

Table 86.1 Factors associated with postpartum depression

Factor	Evidence of association	No evidence of association
Postnatal blues	Pitt (1968) Kendell et al. (1981) Oakley (1980) (only with depressed mood, not with ppd) Buesching et al. (1986) Romito (1988)	
Past history of psychiatric disorder	Gordon and Gordon (1960) Todd (1964) Wolkind and Zajicek (1981) Ballinger et al. (1979) Paykel et al. (1980) Watson et al. (1984) O'Hara (1980)	Pitt (1968) Dalton (1971) Kumar and Robson (1984)
Obstetric difficulties and complications	Oakley (1980) Romito (1988) (only between unexpected complications and baby-blues)	Pitt (1968) Paykel et al. (1980)[1] Elliott et al. (1984)
Complications of pregnancy		Paykel et al. (1980) Pitt (1968)[1] Dalton (1971)[1]
Age	Hayworth et al. (1980)[2] Paykel et al. (1980)[2] Gordon and Gordon (1960)[3]	Pitt (1968)
Anxiety during pregnancy	Todd (1964) Dalton (1971) Meares et al. (1976) Hayworth et al. (1980) Watson et al. (1984)	Pitt (1968) Kumar and Robson (1984)
Parity	Pitt (1968)[4] Gordon et al. (1965)[4] Todd (1964)[5] Kaij et al. (1967)[5]	Paykel et al. (1980) Hayworth (1980) Cox et al. (1983) Watson et al. (1984)
Marital conflict	Todd (1964) Ballinger et al. (1979) Paykel et al. (1980) Oakley (1980) Kumar and Robson (1984) Watson et al. (1984) Field et al. (1985) Romito (1988a) O'Hara et al. (1983) Braverman and Roux (1978) Bookman-Livingood et al. (1983)	
Poor relationship with own mother	Kumar and Robson (1984)	Paykel et al. (1980)
Unplanned pregnancy		Paykel et al. (1980) Breen (1975)[6] Dalton (1971)
Considered termination of pregnancy	Kumar and Robson (1984) Field et al. (1985)	Pitt (1968) Watson et al. (1984)
History of previous termination		Paykel et al. (1980) Kumar and Robson (1984)
Social class		Paykel et al. (1980) Hayworth et al. (1980) Watson et al. (1984) Romito (1988a)
Housing problems	Oakley (1980) Paykel et al. (1980)	
'Undesirable Life Events' in previous year; social or psychological stress	Paykel et al. (1980) Watson et al. (1984) Gordon and Gordon (1960) Grossman et al. (1980)[7]	Pitt (1968)
Being unmarried	O'Hara (1980)[8]	Pitt (1968) Hayworth et al. (1980) Paykel et al. (1980)

[1]They actually reported a significantly decreased risk
[2]More depression among younger mothers
[3]More depression among older mothers
[4]More depression among primiparae
[5]More depression among multiparae
[6]Actually, an inverse relationship was found
[7]Relationship holds only for experienced mothers
[8]More divorced among depressed

Moss and Plewis 1977).

Brown and Harris (1978) looked at psychiatric disturbances in a random sample of 220 London women and found that 27 per cent of mothers with children under 6 were judged to have suffered from a 'definite psychiatric disorder' at some time in the 3 months prior to the interview. Similarly, Moss and Plewis (1977) assessed mental 'distress' in a sample of 180 mothers with preschool children in Inner London and found that 52 per cent had suffered moderate or severe distress in the 12 months prior to interview.

These studies make it clear that a high proportion of mothers of young children are distressed and unhappy and that their suffering sometimes approaches what professionals define as 'psychiatric illness'. There does not seem to be any theoretical or practical reason for trying to separate (or to construct) different categories of suffering, labelling what happens in the first year after birth as 'postpartum depression' and what happens later as 'mental distress in mothers of preschool children'. Indeed, the studies cited cast grave doubts on the utility of 'postpartum depression' as a concept, irrespective of how it is defined. Mothers of young children do suffer. It is important to know more about the conditions in which this suffering occurs in order to be able to help them.

1.2 Associated factors

As different authors study different samples of women, with different instruments and criteria for depression, and at different times after birth, it is hardly surprising that many factors have been proposed as associated with postpartum depression (Table 86.1). For example, some research (Oakley 1980; Garel *et al.* 1987a,b) has suggested that the use of technology in the care of women during childbirth predisposes to postpartum depression; other research has have found no such correlation (Elliott *et al.* 1984); while still other research actually showed an inverse relationship between obstetric complications and depression, with depressed women having fewer complications (Paykel *et al.* 1980). The association between postpartum depression and the method of infant feeding is also far from clear: two investigators (Kumar and Robson 1978; Paykel *et al.* 1980) found no relationship, while others (Dalton 1971; Alder and Cox 1983; Alder and Bancroft 1988; Romito 1988b) reported that breastfeeding mothers were more likely to be depressed.

Such conflicting findings stress the difficulties that exist in trying to unravel the tangled web of causal relationships in this field. Nevertheless, one finding deserves particular attention because of its consistency. At least eleven research reports (see Table 86.2) have documented a significant link between postpartum depression and 'marital difficulties' or a 'poor relationship

Table 86.2 Assessment of 'marital difficulties' and 'poor relationship with husband' in studies in which a relationship with postpartum depression is found

Watson *et al.* (1984)
Information about the marital relationship was obtained with a joint interview with the couple, early in pregnancy.

Kumar and Robson (1984)
Marital conflict is assessed antenatally, via a semi-structured clinical interview.

Bookman-Livingood *et al.* (1983)
'Marital adjustment' was measured by the Marital Adjustment Scale (Locke and Wallace 1959), self-administered in the first days postpartum.

Field *et al.* (1985)
'Marital difficulties' were assessed in the third trimester of pregnancy with the Braverman and Roux (1978) questionnaire.

Paykel *et al.* (1980)
The variable was assessed 6 weeks postpartum, by means of a semi-structured interview, tapping different aspects of 'marital adjustment' such as adequacy of communication between spouses, feelings of affection, degree of help provided by husband with household chores, shopping, and older children.

O'Hara *et al.* (1983)
'Marital happiness' was assessed prenatally and postnatally with a 7-point rating scale; relationship with postpartum depression was found with postnatal assessment.

Oakley (1980)
'Segregated marital role relationship' was assessed by means of a semi-structured interview.

Romito (1988a)
The variables were assessed 5 weeks postpartum via a semi-structured questionnaire in which several aspects were tapped, such as husbands' participation in baby-care, women's disappointment about this issue, women's evaluation of marital relationship as compared to the period before the birth of the child.

with the husband': no one who has looked for such a link has failed to find it.

Different authors have adopted different theoretical frameworks and methodologies to assess 'marital difficulties': in some cases, the variable is assessed during pregnancy as well as after birth; in others it is assessed only after the birth. Sometimes it refers to the practical help (or the lack of such help) offered by husbands; at other times it is concerned only with the psychological aspects of the relationship (communication, confidence, and affection, for example).

Even though different authors use the term 'marital difficulties' to describe somewhat different phenomena, the consistency with which the role of the husband is associated with postpartum depression is striking. While these correlations do not, in themselves, establish that an unhappy marital relationship causes postpartum depression, it is surprising that some authors completely dismiss this possibility. Others note it but suggest that it is the woman's mental state which is responsible for the marital problems. Leigh *et al.*

(1977), for example, in their *Concise Encyclopaedia of Psychiatry*, state that: 'Puerperal neurosis may *cause* family and marital discord'.

It must be stressed that even statistically significant associations between 'risk factors' and depression are not very helpful in understanding what really happens to mothers who become depressed. Interestingly, the few studies describing the experience of new mothers, and sometimes of depressed mothers (Oakley 1980; Welburn 1980), are seldom quoted in the research on postpartum depression. It is as if the description of the experience and the search for its 'associated factors' were two completely different fields of study.

2 Limitations of traditional explanations

2.1 The medical model

Some doctors state quite unambiguously that postpartum depression is a disease ('postpartum mental illness, in its inception, is an acute disease' Hamilton 1962) or an illness ('depressed mothers were not always identified ... as having an illness' Cox 1986). Many medical writers have postulated a biological basis for postpartum depressive disorders based on the important hormonal and endocrinological changes that occur after parturition (Hamilton 1962, 1982; Coppen 1969; Treadway *et al.* 1969; Dalton 1971, 1980; Handley *et al.* 1977). This has led to attempts to demonstrate hormonal or other biochemical differences between a history of women who do and women who do not become depressed, or whose mood is unstable in the first few days after the birth. Some investigators have sought associations between menstrual difficulties and postpartum mood alterations (Pitt 1968 and 1973; Yalom *et al.* 1968; Dalton 1971; Davidson 1972; O'Hara *et al.* 1982). Others, seeking more direct evidence for the involvement of hormones in postpartum depression have studied the role of oestrogens and progesterone (Nott *et al.* 1976), norepinephrine (Treadway *et al.* 1969), tryptophan (Handley *et al.* 1977; Stein *et al.* 1976), plasma cortisol (Handley *et al.* 1980), and cyclic AMP (Ballinger *et al.* 1979). Because some antidepressant drugs have appeared to alleviate 'symptoms', this fact has stimulated investigations into the possible association of monoamines and depression (Sandler 1978). (For a more thorough review of this literature, see Gelder 1978; Hopkins *et al.* 1984; Kendell 1985.)

To date no evidence of any direct or indirect link between hormones and postpartum depression has been found (Weissman and Klerman 1977; Gelder 1978; Brockington and Kumar 1982; Hopkins *et al.* 1984; Kendell 1985.)

The only consistent association found is that between changes in tryptophan metabolism and postpartum blues (Stein *et al.* 1976; Handley *et al.* 1977), but as these biochemical studies have limited their research to the first days after the birth it is very difficult to make generalizations on the basis of the results.

In addition to the doubts engendered by the lack of correlation between postpartum mood and the results of hormone assays, further doubts about the supposed role of hormones in the aetiology of postpartum depression are raised by the findings from other fields of research. For example, the fact that new fathers can also become depressed (Atkinson and Rickel 1984) and emotionally upset (Quadagno *et al.* 1986) suggests that the social and psychological fact of having to care for a child can, in at least some cases, be more important in the genesis of depression than the biological aspects of reproduction. The results of cross-cultural anthropological research also suggest that postpartum depression is not an inevitable concomitant of childbirth and the hormonal changes which follow it in all human populations. Stern and Kruckman (1983), for example, examined many elements of what they call 'the social structuring of the postpartum period' both in their own observations and by reviewing the relevant cross-cultural literature. They describe the habit of 'secluding' the new mother with her baby, which is common in many non-industrialized societies. The seclusion is usually related to notions of vulnerability and pollution: it can last from a few days (as in the Punjab) to 2 to 3 months (as in Nigeria). It is worth noting that during this period the new mother is absolved of her normal duties, which are taken over by female relatives, ensuring that she rests. On the basis of their research, Stern and Kruckman (1983) suggest that Western researchers have until now never considered the simple fact that a mandatory rest period might possibly be a major contributor to postpartum well-being.

Notwithstanding the absence of any well-founded empirical basis, the hormonal explanation still holds an important place in the medical construct of postpartum depression. A look through the proceedings of the 'Conference on Motherhood and Mental Illness' held in London, 21–23 July 1982, reveals that 45 per cent of the papers presented took the hormonal theory for granted.

One of the dangers inherent in this approach is its reductionism. Many authors restrict their analysis to endocrinological changes, and ignore other aspects pertaining to the biological domain, such as the very real physical consequences that pregnancy, childbirth, lactation, and obstetrical interventions have on the physical and psychological well-being of new mothers. These possible consequences are all too well-known: painful stitches, incontinence, piles, breast engorgement, cracked nipples and breast abscesses, painful intercourse, backache, tiredness, lack of sleep, and so on (see, for instance, Robert 1971). By taking such a narrow approach, some authors end up explaining not only mood instability in the puerperium but much more complex phenomena. Kaij and Nilsson (1972) state for instance that,

> 'in the second half of the first postpartum month ... many women become more easily fatigued, need much more sleep than usual, feel tired, irritable and complain of a number of psychosomatic symptoms. These complaints are often explained as a consequence of caring for the child. The fact that some overburdened women do not complain ... suggests that exogenous factors are relatively unimportant. We feel that the main cause of this postpartum 'hang-over' is to be found in physiological factors, perhaps in the hormonal readjustment.' (pp 371–372.)

Dalton (1980) goes even further when she affirms:

> 'Irritability is of chemical origins. The irritability is reflected on the husband ... He finds she has changed from the elated, vivacious, person she was during pregnancy into the ever moaning bitch of today. Can you blame him if he stops for a quick pick-me-up on his journey home?' (p 34.)

These examples, while they may seem extreme, simply state explicitly what is often assumed implicitly in the medical model of postpartum depression. For Kaij and Nilsson (1972) and for Dalton (1980), tiredness, need of sleep, and irritability are wholly attributable to some (still undemonstrated) abnormality in the biochemical balance.

In the same vein they, like other authors, define the women's 'inability to cope' with her motherly duties as a 'symptoms' of her 'illness':

> 'the *symptoms* reported by the depressed women also included tearfulness, despondency, labile mood and feelings of inadequacy and inability to cope, particularly with the baby.' (Hopkins *et al.* 1984, p 502.)

> 'Only careful enquiry about the presence or absence of certain depressive *symptoms* will enable this disorder to be recognized. The symptoms of postnatal depression ... include somatic symptoms such as headache or palpitations, excessive anxiety about the baby, sadness and difficulty to cope with household tasks.' (Cox 1986, p 14.)

> 'The inability to cope is part of the *illness*. (p 16) ... it may result from the body's supply of potassium being too low ... or from thyroid deficiency.' (Dalton 1980, p 18) (emphasis added.)

If the inability to cope with housework is defined as a symptom, or an illness (depression), little room is left for other, concurrent, explanations of new mothers' capabilities and incapabilities. Some 'researchers' seem not to recognize that a woman's organism may not yet have recovered from the hard work of parturition and lactation, and that having a baby to care for at the same time as looking after older children and her husband and performing household chores, is simply too much.

As Graham (1982) argues convincingly, what society expects from mothers is that they will be able to cope, however difficult the conditions are in which they have to perform this task. The endocrinological model of postpartum depression plays its part in supporting this point of view, claiming that incapacity to cope is a symptom of an illness, which requires pharmacological cures. Fromhagen (1963) employed benzodiazepine for his 'emotionally unstable postpartum patients'; more recently, the use of tricyclic antidepressants and monoamine oxidase inhibitors have been advocated to 'cure' postpartum depression (Dominion 1976; Cox 1986). It has to be remembered that all these drugs have adverse side-effects (see Cooperstock and Hill 1982; Goodman and Gillman 1985).

The foregoing account does not suggest that biochemical mechanisms may not have some part to play in mothers' mood postpartum and the possibility that endocrinological factors may play a role in the genesis or course of depression should certainly continue to be studied. But the interacting effects of physical, social, and psychological factors in women's lives must be taken into account as well. The danger is that the reductionism inherent in the biochemical model of postpartum depression is used to legitimize unrealistic social expectations about mothers' duties.

2.2 The psychoanalytic perspective

When considering psychoanalytic formulations about postpartum depression, earlier reviewers have pointed out that, apart from anecdotal clinical evidence, the model suffers from a lack of empirical support and is impossible to test (Oakley 1980; Hopkins *et al.* 1984). For this reason, other authors have not even considered it (Arizmendi and Affonso 1984; Kendell 1985). Moreover, psychoanalytic doctrine in general, and not only its accounts of mothers' depression, has been convincingly criticized. Its lack of empirical support has been stressed, and alternative, empirically grounded, explanations have been proposed for the phenomena observed (Timpanaro 1974; Van Rillaer 1980; Eysenck 1985).

There are two reasons for considering the psychoanalytic point of view on postpartum depression. First, although the psychoanalytic model has been criticized and is now disregarded in most academic and research circles, many health care professionals still regard it as important. Psychoanalytic concepts have become part of 'common knowledge' about pregnancy and motherhood, scattered through magazines and books for expectant and new mothers (see, for instance, the review by Jaubert (1979) of French literature for expectant mothers). Thus, although it is impossible to regard psychoanalytic studies as scientific investigations, they should be considered because of their strong social influence.

Secondly, the psychoanalytic model of postpartum depression might be taken as a kind of magnifying glass, or caricature of the medical interpretation of mothers' depression. Some of the more extreme versions of this interpretation make it easier to perceive more subtly expressed social beliefs about motherhood.

Briefly, the psychoanalytic account of postpartum depression is as follows: regression occurs in all women during pregnancy and in the first months of motherhood. This regression may re-evoke earlier conflicts (such as the alleged Oedipus complex), particularly when there are inadequate maternal role models, or when the maternal role models are rejected. Depression then results from unresolved conflicts (such as an unconscious incestuous desire for one's own father), or from an unsuccessful adaptation of the woman to motherhood (Deutsch 1945; Bibring *et al.* 1961; Racamier 1961, 1978; Chertok 1969; Blum 1978; Pazzagli *et al.* 1981).

First consider the key concept: that women regress when they are pregnant. According to the *Penguin Dictionary of Psychology*, 'regression' means:

'the opposite of progression. Thus 1. A reverting to an earlier, more primitive or more childlike behaviour ... a) in psychoanalytic theories, it has a negative implication, i.e. the notion that a stress or anxiety is causing the individual to flee from anxiety into a more infantile state.' (Reber 1985.)

The technical formulation of an unproven concept is easily translated into popular knowledge. According to some successful French books for mothers-to-be:

'Few pregnant women know it, but during their pregnancy they re-live the story of their own early childhood ... they are in a state of regression. Confronted by this extraordinary event which throws their organism and their daily routine into confusion, they look for security by simply becoming little girls again ... the father-to-be should not be irritated by the infantile attitude of his young wife, nor should be jealous if she draws nearer to her family, particularly to her mother.' (Dana and Marion 1975 translated by J. Moss.)

'Before she actually becomes a mother, a woman feels as though she has become a child again, a child who has everything still to learn. Moreover, she is often unconsciously happy in this role, which allows her to let herself be pampered.' (Pernaud 1979, quoted by Jaubert 1979, translation by J. Moss.)

Thus, according to psychoanalytic theory, women revert to more primitive or childlike behaviour when expecting a child; their psychological organization undergoes significant disintegration and closely resembles the structure of psychotics. Furthermore, these changes, which would be considered pathological at other times, are seen as normal during pregnancy. One is logically led to the conclusion, both that expectant mothers are mentally disturbed, and that it is normal that they should be so.

Is the condition of being childless then the 'normal one'? Indeed not, because psychoanalysts have labelled women who prefer not to have children as infantile, immature, selfish, narcissistic, and neurotic (Deutsch 1945; Bettelheim 1965; Chertok 1969). The only conclusion we can draw is that, in the psychoanalytic model, one cannot even be a woman without being mentally disturbed!

Let us now briefly consider the psychoanalytic interpretation of postpartum depression as the result of unresolved conflicts or of the mother's failure to 'adapt'. One psychoanalyst's description of the successful adaptation of a previously depressed new mother under his care speaks volumes:

'She had six months of regular psychotherapeutic sessions twice a week and then attended twice more during the next month. By this time she knew what hard work was involved in running a home and caring for a child, but she had come to find it satisfying.' (Douglas 1963.)

Oddly enough, in both psychoanalytic and biochemical studies, the social circumstances to which women are expected to adapt (being a full-time mother and a housewife with housework to do) are exactly the same.

As with the biochemical model, the most flagrant internal inconsistency in the psychoanalytic model is the persistent confusion between what is considered as 'natural' and therefore unchangeable, and what is social. Both models assume that the cause of postpartum depression lies in the hypothetical failure of some inner mechanism (biochemical or intrapsychic), when in fact the true failure is women's incapacity or unwillingness to adapt to the social institution of motherhood. This failure, and its consequences, are defined by these models as an illness, namely depression.

In conclusion, although neither the medical/biochemical nor the psychoanalytic explanations of postpartum depression are useful for understanding mothers' unhappiness after childbirth, they help to highlight some of the ideological assumptions inherent in these widely espoused conceptualizations of the problem of unhappiness after childbirth.

3 The social context of maternal unhappiness

The first person to investigate the role of social factors in postpartum depression systematically was a medical doctor, Richard Gordon, working in collaboration with his wife (Gordon 1958; Gordon and Gordon 1960; Gordon *et al.* 1959, 1965). Their results indicate that postpartum depression was positively associated with the amount of 'social strains' reported by women, such as the presence of cultural differences between husband and wife, physical complications in pregnancy, the mother's lack of experience with babies, and no help being available to her (Gordon *et al.* 1959). On the basis of these findings, the authors organized 'experimental' antenatal classes, in which expectant mothers were informed about the social and psychological aspects of having a new baby. Different topics were covered in these talks. Some were quite general: 'The responsibilities of being a mother, and not a martyr, are learned; hence get help and advice'. Others were more practical: 'Make friends of other couples who are experienced with young children'; 'get plenty of rest and sleep'; 'arrange for a baby-sitter in advance'; and 'learn to drive a car' (Gordon and Gordon 1960). Their preventive programme proved to be successful, since the women in the experimental group reported significantly more changes in the suggested direction than women attending ordinary parenting classes. They also underwent significantly less subsequent emotional upset; 15 per cent of experimental mothers were depressed postpartum, compared with 37 per cent in the control group. Moreover, classes with husbands attending appeared to be more effective than those in which husbands did not attend. These findings are consistent with the previous conclusion of the same authors (Gordon *et al.* 1959) who, evaluating the results of psychotherapy for depressed new mothers, suggested that an intervention that focussed on the analysis and resolution of social and practical problems was far more effective than one that employed classic psychodynamic therapy.

The Gordons' work suffers from several methodological problems (failure to create control groups by random allocation, non-standardized assessment measures, vague definitions, unblinded rating of emotional disorders, and so on); moreover, some of the solutions proposed to new mothers are very much in conformity with traditional expectations. Nevertheless, the Gordons were the first researchers to provide challenging evidence of a relationship between postpartum emotional problems and the lack of practical as well as emotional support after childbirth. Even more important, the new mothers who are described in the reports of this research stand out as human beings, faced with natural, understandable difficulties (such as being isolated in a new house with a crying baby, with no friends nearby, and being unable to drive a car), rather than being mere containers in which the battle of intrapsychic conflicts or hormonal adjustments is taking place.

Notwithstanding the quality and importance of the research, the Gordons' social approach to postpartum depression was largely neglected until the 1980s, when Paykel *et al.* (1980), albeit in a somewhat different context, studied the effects of life events and social support on puerperal depression. The theoretical context of Paykel's work is the previously mentioned model of depression developed by Brown and Harris (1978) in which clinical depression is considered to be an understandable response to adversities. The presence of 'vulnerability factors' (such as lack of a supportive relationship with the husband, lack of paid employment, having other children at home, and loss of the woman's mother in early childhood) appear to make things worse by lowering woman's self-esteem; thus, faced with the occurrence of a negative 'life event' (such as the loss of a loved one, or of employment), women tend to generalize their feelings of hopelessness and then to become depressed. Brown and Harris' (1978) results show that negative life events, vulnerability factors and depression were more frequent in the lives of working class women than in those of middle-class women (23 per cent of the former were depressed compared with only 6 per cent of the latter). When the stage of the family life cycle was controlled in the analysis, however, class differences were restricted to difference between women with children. The work of Brown and Harris clearly shows the widespread scale of working class mothers' emotional impairment. However, it must be pointed out that some 'vulnerability factors' merely correspond to the main requirements of womanhood and motherhood in our culture (Oakley 1980). Thus, these results actually show that women are made unhappy mostly by their ordinary conditions of life, which are then technically defined as 'vulnerability factors'.

The work of Paykel and his colleagues (1980) is very much in the same vein. They studied the effects of recent stressful life events retrospectively in a sample of 120 recently delivered women. Their results showed statistically significant relationships between postpartum depression and recent stressful life events, previous psychiatric history, poor marital support and housing problems. Poor marital support acted as a 'vulnerability factor', maintaining its link with depression only in presence of stressful life events.

Even if the sociological work on depression in women is somewhat overshadowed by the technical terminology of 'life event' and of 'vulnerability factors', it does indicate that 'mild and severe forms of mental suffering are related to the lived experience, the actual practice of being a woman and a mother in contemporary society' (Day 1985).

4 The realities of early motherhood

Although the experience of early motherhood is certainly influenced by many factors, the help that a woman receives following childbirth seems likely to be the most important of all. The work entailed in being a new parent is substantial. Newborn babies are helpless human beings and in order to survive they need to be cared for, completely and continuously, by one or more concerned adults. Five-week-old babies, for example, have anything between 4 and 10 feeds every 24 hours, each of which may last anything from 5 minutes to an hour and a half; in addition, every day they cried for an average of 90 minutes (range 30–300 minutes) (Romito 1988a). The 'average' baby thus needs around five hours a day of an adult's time just to be fed and comforted. In addition, they have to be bathed and kept clean. Oakley (1976) estimated that each child required about 4000 or 5000 nappy changes in total); their clothes have to be washed and sometimes ironed; unless they are breast fed, their food has to be bought and prepared; and these are only some of the more concrete and well-defined tasks.

The tasks associated with being a new parent must often be accomplished in addition to those expected of a housewife and mother of older children. Food has to be bought and prepared at least twice a day; dishes have to be washed; the house has to be cleaned; clothes have to be washed, ironed, and sometimes mended; and older children have to be cared for, both materially and psychologically.

These activities are often soulless and boring; but even if this is not always the case, they add up to a substantial amount of hard work. Bearing in mind that, in our society, this work usually has to be performed when the mother has not yet fully recovered from childbirth, it seems reasonable to ask what kind of help new mothers receive during this time, and from whom.

A number of studies conducted in North America and Europe have shown that, in the first few weeks after discharge from hospital, new mothers receive a certain amount of 'special' help, either from their husbands, or from another woman, often the maternal grandmother or aunt of the new baby (Oakley 1979; Moss *et al.* 1982; Entwistle and Doering 1981; Romito 1988a). Withdrawal of this special help sometimes seems to precipitate mild depression (Entwistle and Doering 1981).

The 'special' help that is sometimes provided by the husband during very early parenthood is not, in general, sustained for very long (Oakley 1979 1980; Entwistle and Doering 1981; Moss *et al.* 1982; Romito 1988). Husbands actually tend to do less housework after the birth of the baby than they did while their wives were pregnant (Meissner 1975; Cowan *et al.* 1978; Oakley 1980; Kellerhals *et al.* 1982; Moss *et al.* 1982; Romito 1988). Although some of them appear to be willing to play with the new baby, they tend to shun the more mundane tasks of child care, the most uncongenial one being changing a nappy, especially a dirty

one (Richards *et al.* 1977; Oakley 1979; Parke 1981; Moss *et al.* 1982; Romito 1988a). By five weeks after delivery, a majority of new mothers are receiving little or no extra help with child care (Oakley 1979, 1980; Entwistle and Doering 1981; Romito 1988a). Considering that women tend to overestimate the amount of practical help actually provided by their husbands (Kellerhals *et al.* 1982; Wilson 1986; Romito 1988a), we must conclude that mothers take on most of the baby care and housework very soon after childbirth.

Surprisingly, few studies have explored the effects of postnatal work on the physical and psychological wellbeing of new mothers. Nevertheless, both Paykel *et al.* (1980) and Romito (1988a) found that mothers were more likely to be depressed when husbands offered no help with the baby, older children, or housework, especially when this lack of help coincided with some negative life event.

Even when considering outcomes other than maternal depression, what men do (or do not do) in the house seems to be important. Oakley (1980) found that women were more likely to have positive feelings about their babies if their husbands helped with housework. She suggested that release from too much domestic work may well be a condition of nurturant maternal behaviour. In the same vein, Entwistle and Doering (1981) showed a positive relationship between mothers' enjoyment of baby care and motherhood and the amount of time fathers spent with the child in activities other than caretaking. These data are consistent with the results of studies in the field of child development which show that fathers' involvement with their children and the affectionate support they provided for their wives enhanced maternal competence and enjoyment in caring for the baby. A competent and happy mother goes on to have a positive influence on the social and cognitive development of her infant (Pedersen *et al.* 1978; Price 1977; Crnic *et al.* 1983; Easterbrooks and Goldberg 1984; Belsky 1981, 1984; Yogman 1984).

5 Minimizing maternal unhappiness

It may seem all too obvious that maternal happiness after delivery is so intimately related to a mother's social circumstances and family dynamics. Yet, as we have seen, it is remarkable how the persuasive data that exist have been ignored by so many people, particularly health professionals. That 'transition to parenthood' represents a 'crisis' is an idea which has been put forward repeatedly over the last three decades. The results of research conducted over this period consistently show that the birth of a child, no matter how welcome it may be, implies for many couples a deterioration in their relationship and a decrease in marital satisfaction (LeMasters 1957; Hobbs 1965, 1968; Feldman 1974; Oakley 1980; Moss *et al.* 1982; Belsky *et al.* 1983; Scott-Heyes 1983; Nordio *et al.* 1983). Moreover, it seems that the process of 'traditionalization of roles' that occurs at this time entails a shift of power within the couple from the relative equality of the childless couple to a more patriarchal family organization (Meyerowitz and Feldman 1966; Campbell 1967; Cowan 1978; Entwistle and Doering 1981). It is not surprising that women are consistently more negative than their husbands in their evaluations of these changes (Dyer 1963; Hobbs 1965, 1968; Ryder 1973; Russell 1974; Hobbs and Cole 1976; Hobbs and Wimbush 1977; Miller and Sollie 1980; Moss *et al.* 1982).

Identifying and implementing effective strategies to influence family dynamics in ways that are likely to minimize maternal unhappiness presents a challenge to society as a whole, rather than to individual caregivers working in the maternity services. Those providing care to women during pregnancy and childbirth, however, still have an important role to play. After all, they have often been responsible for the rosy expectations women have about some aspects of motherhood. Moreover, they often seem to ignore the wishes, experience, and day-to-day social circumstances of many mothers (see Chapters 8, 14 and 22). There is a gap to bridge between what professionals think mothers do, think, and want, and what mothers, in reality, do think and want. If they are prepared to do so, professionals can bridge this gap by acquiring a better knowledge of the findings of research on the subject and, even more importantly, by listening to what mothers say and by 'taking them seriously' (Oakley 1983). The important beneficial effects on postpartum unhappiness that can result from simply encouraging women to talk about their feelings to a non-judgemental person have recently been demonstrated clearly in a randomized trial (Holden *et al.* 1989).

Professionals should also take into account that some elements of their practice may influence the chances of a mother becoming unhappy. The fact that obstetric intervention is not consistently related to postpartum unhappiness (see Table 86.1) may not be as paradoxical as might first appear. For individual women, the interventions concerned may have entirely different meanings. The conflicting results of research in this field might be reconciled by taking into account the woman's personal feelings of control over the situation. For example, Garel *et al.* (1987a,b) found that women who had a planned caesarean section were less depressed than women who had an unexpected operation. Women who had epidural anaesthesia, and who therefore remained aware of what was going on, were also less likely to be depressed than mothers who had general anaesthesia. A suggestion by Day (1982) provides a reasonable explanation for these findings: women undergoing a planned caesarean section are more likely to have played a part in the decision to operate. An

unexpected intervention, sometimes made under general anaesthesia, after a normal pregnancy and early labour, can shatter a woman's expectations and put her into a situation over which she has no feeling of control.

The importance of this feeling of control has been suggested by the results of research in a variety of fields. More than three decades ago, Janis (1958) showed that pre-operative patients who had been prepared for the reality of surgery (and especially for its negative aspects, such as post-operative pain) reacted better and recovered faster than patients who had not been so realistically prepared. Subsequent research has supported the conclusions reached in this pioneering work. An impressive body of literature on psychological preparation for surgery, recently reviewed by Wallace (Wallace 1984, 1986) and discussed by King (1986), shows that when patients are told what to expect from their surgery and are given pre-operative counselling, they tend to show less anxiety both before and after operation, request fewer analgesics, stay in hospital for shorter periods, and report increased feelings of control and ability to cope. Studies of mothers' satisfaction with the experience of childbirth have come to similar conclusions: the most important factors enabling women to experience satisfaction appear to be awareness, and the possibility of being in control during birth (Doering and Entwistle 1975; Norr *et al.* 1977; Doering *et al.* 1980; Entwistle and Doering 1981).

The likely importance of predictability and a sense of control raises questions about the possible adverse effects of the 'rosy' picture of pregnancy, childbirth, and early parenthood which is painted in many antenatal classes and in most books and magazines for expectant mothers (Jaubert 1979; Romito and Chatelanat 1981). The available evidence suggests that efforts made (and time taken) by professionals to give women more accurate information throughout the course of their care during pregnancy and childbirth will help new mothers react more appropriately to the realities of early parenthood. This in turn should lead to a reduction in the unhappiness and emotional distress suffered by so many new mothers.

6 Conclusions

This review of the literature on postpartum depression allows some general conclusions. Postpartum depression is a not a special category of depression: mothers of young children are often depressed, and are no less likely to be so six months or a year after delivery than in the first few weeks or months following childbirth. There is no persuasive evidence to support traditional explanations of postpartum depression: no intrinsic, biochemical explanation of women's unhappiness after childbirth has been uncovered, and psychoanalytic explanations of postpartum depression cannot be validated empirically. Although unsupported with evidence, however, these traditional explanations have reinforced some conventional social beliefs about women. By contrast, sociological and psychological studies have provided strong empirical evidence of a relationship between some social conditions and postpartum depression: the social conditions linked with depression are only rarely 'out of the ordinary'; more often, they correspond to social expectations about what normal womanhood and normal motherhood must be.

The continuing belief in an entity named 'postpartum depression' still constitutes an obstacle standing in the way of a better understanding of unhappiness following childbirth. The results of psychosocial research using empirical data can be expected to continue to enlarge our understanding of women's lives and of their difficulties.

Because many of the social factors leading to postpartum unhappiness are rooted in society's expectations of new mothers, the solutions lie mainly in social change. Based on what is already known, however, there is considerable scope for professionals working in the maternity services to reduce the difficulties and unhappiness experienced by women after childbirth. In particular, they should be more ready to listen to women and learn about their social circumstances, and to provide them with information which will lead to more realistic predictions about the experience of pregnancy, childbirth, and early parenthood.

[The author is grateful to Judy Moss, who revised the English and translated the quotations from French.]

References

Alder E, Cox J (1983). Breast feeding and post-natal depression. J Psychosom Res, 27: 139–144.

Alder E, Bancroft J (1988). The relationship between breast feeding persistence, sexuality and mood in postpartum women. Psychol Med, 18: 389–396.

Affonso D, Domino G (1984). Postpartum depression: A review. Birth, 11: 231–235.

Arizmendi T, Affonso D (1984). Research on psychosocial factors and postpartum depression: A critique. Birth, 11: 237–240.

Atkinson A, Rickel A (1984). Postpartum depression in primiparous parents. J Abnorm Psychol, 93: 115–119.

Ballinger B, Buckley DE, Naylor GJ, Stansfield DA (1979). Emotional disturbance following childbirth. Psychol Med, 9: 293–300.

Belsky J (1981) Early human experience: A family perspective. Dev Psychol, 17: 3–23.

Belsky J (1984). The determinants of parenting: A process model. Child Dev, 55: 83–96.

Belsky J, Spanier GB, Rovine M (1983). Stability and change in marriage across the transition to parenthood. J Marriage and the Family, August: 567–577.

Bettelheim B (1965). Women in scientific professions. Proceedings of the Massachusetts Institute of Technology MIT Symposium on American Women in Science and Engineering. Cambridge.

Bibring BL, Thomas FD, Huntington D, Valenstein A (1961). A study of the psychological processes in pregnancy and the earliest mother-child relationship. Psychoanal Study Child, 16: 9–72.

Blum HP (1978). Reconstruction in a case of post-partum depression. Psychoanal Study Child, 33: 335–362.

Bookman-Livingood A, Daen P, Smith B (1983). The depressed mother as a source of stimulation for her infant. J Clin Psychol, 39: 369–375.

Braverman J, Roux J (1978). Screening for the patient at risk of postpartum depression. Obstet Gynecol, 52: 731–736.

Breen D (1975). The Birth of a First Child. London: Tavistock.

Brockington I and Kumar R (eds) (1982). Motherhood and Mental Illness. London: Academic Press.

Brown B, Harris T (1978). Social Origins of Depression. London: Tavistock.

Buesching D, Glasser M, Frate D (1986). Progression of depression in the perinatal and postpartum periods. Women and Health, 11: 61–78.

Campbell F (1967). Demographic Factors in Family Organizations. Unpublished Ph D thesis, University of Michigan.

Chertok L (1969). Motherhood and Personality. London: Tavistock.

Cogill SR, Caplan HL, Alexandra H, Mordecai Robson K, Kumar R (1986). Impact of maternal postnatal depression on cognitive development in young children. Br Med J, 292: 1165–1167.

Cooperstock R, Hill J (1982). Les effets de l'usage de tranquillisants. Ministère de la Santé et du Bien-être Social, Ottawa (Ontario) Canada.

Coppen AJ (1969). Biochemical aspects of depression. In: Aspects of Depression. International Psychiatry Clinics 6. Shneidman E, Ortega M (eds). Boston: Little Brown.

Cowan CP, Cole L, Cole JD (1978). Becoming a family: The impact of a first child's birth on the couple's relationship. In: The First Child and Family Formation. Miller WB, Newman LF (eds). Chapel Hills Carolina Population Center, University of North Carolina, pp 296–324.

Cox JL (1986). Postnatal Depression: A Guide for Health Professionals. Edinburgh: Churchill Livingstone.

Crnic K, Greenberg M T, Ragozin A, Robinson N, Bahsam R (1983). Effect of stress and social support on mothers and premature and full-term infants. Child Dev, 54: 209–217.

Cutrona C (1983). Causal attributions and perinatal depression. J Abnorm Psychol, 92: 161–172.

Dalton K (1971). Prospective study into puerperal depression. Br J Psychiatry, 118: 689–692.

Dalton K (1980). Depression after Childbirth. Oxford: Oxford University Press.

Dana J, Marion S (1975). Donner La Vie. 9 Mois de La Vie du Couple. Paris: Seuil.

Davidson JR (1972). Postpartum mood change in Jamaican women. A description and discussion of its significance. Br J Psychiatry, 121: 659–663.

Day S (1982). Is obstetric technology depressing? Radical Sci J, 12: 17–45.

Day S (1985). Puerperal Insanity: The Historical Sociology of a Disease. Ph D dissertation, Darwin College, Cambridge.

Deutsch H (1945). The Psychology of Women. Vol. II: Motherhood. New York: Grune & Stratton.

Doering S, Entwistle D (1975). Preparation during pregnancy and ability to cope with labor and delivery. Am J Orthopsychiatry, 45: 825–837.

Doering S, Entwistle D, Quinlan D (1980). Modelling the quality of women's birth experience. J Health Soc Behav, 21: 12–21.

Dominion J (1976). Depression. Glasgow: Fontana.

Douglas G (1963). Puerperal depression and excessive compliance with the mother. Br J Med Psychol, 36: 271–278.

Dyer ED (1963). Parenthood as a crisis: A re-study. Marriage and Family Living, 25: 196–201.

Easterbrooks M, Goldberg WA (1984). Toddler development in the family: Impact of father involvement and parenting characteristics. Child Dev, 55: 740–752.

Elliott S, Anderson M, Brough D, Watson G, Rugg A (1984). Relationship between obstetric outcome and psychological measures in pregnancy and the postnatal year. J Reprod Infant Psychol, 2: 18–32.

Entwistle D, Doering G (1981). The First Birth. Baltimore: Johns Hopkins University Press.

Eysenck H (1985). Decline and Fall of the Freudian Empire. New York: Viking.

Feldman H (1974). Change in marriage and parenthood: A methodological design. In: Pronatalism: The Myth of Mom and Apple Pie. Peck E, Senderowitz J (eds). New York: Thomas Crowell, pp 206–226.

Field T, Sandberg D, Garcia R, Vega-Lahr N, Goldstein S, Guy L (1985). Pregnancy problems, postpartum depression and early mother–infant interactions. Dev Psychol, 21: 1152–1156.

Fromhagen C (1963). Management of emotional disturbances in obstetrical and gynecological patients. Am J Obstet Gynecol, 15: 183–189.

Garel M, Lelong N, Kaminski M (1987a). Consequences de l'analgésie péridurale sur l'experience de la césarienne et les premières réactions mère-enfant. J Gynecol Obstet Biol Reprod, 16: 219–228.

Garel M, Lelong N, Kaminski M (1987b). Psychological consequences of caesarian childbirth in primipares. J Psychosom Obstet Gynaecol. 6: 197–209.

Gelder M (1978). Hormones and post-partum depression. In: Mental Illness in Pregnancy and the Puerperium. Sandler M (ed). Oxford: Oxford University Press.

Goodman A, Gillman L (1985). The Pharmacological Basis of Therapeutics (7th edn). New York: Macmillan.

Gordon RE (1958). Psychiatric problems of a rapidly growing suburb. AMA Archives Neurology Psychiatry, 79: 543–548.

Gordon RE, Gordon KK, Englewood N (1959). Social factors in the prediction and treatment of emotional disorders of pregnancy. Am J Obstet Gynecol, 77: 1074–1083.

Gordon RE, Gordon KK (1960). Social factors in prevention of postpartum emotional problems. Obstet Gynecol, 15: 433–437.

Gordon RE, Kapostius EE, Gordon KK (1965). Factors in postpartum emotional adjustment. Obstet Gynecol, 25: 158–166.

Graham H (1982). Coping: Or how mothers are seen and not heard. In: On the Problem of Men. Friedman S, Sarh E (eds). London: Women's Press.

Grossman F, Eichler L, Winickoff S (1980). Pregnancy, Birth and Parenthood. San Francisco: Jossey-Bass.

Hamilton J (1960). A rating scale of depression. J Neurol Neurosurg Psychiatry 23: 56–61.

Hamilton J (1962). Post-partum Psychiatric Problems. St Louis: Mosby.

Hamilton J (1982). The identity of post-partum psychosis. In: Motherhood and Mental Illness. Brockington I, Kumar R (eds). London: Academic Press.

Handley SL, Dunn TL, Baker JM, Cockshott C, Gould S (1977). Mood changes in puerperium and plasma tryptophan and cortisol concentrations. Br Med J, 2: 18–22.

Handley SL, Dunn TL, Waldron G, Baker J (1980). Tryptophan, cortisol and puerperal mood. Br J Psychiatry, 136: 490–506.

Hayworth J, Little B, Bonham Carter S, Raptopoulos P, Priest R, Sandler M (1980). A predictive study of postpartum depression. Br J Med Psychol, 53: 161–167.

Hobbs DF (1965). Parenthood as a crisis: A third study. J Marriage and the Family, 27: 367–372.

Hobbs DF (1968). Transition to parenthood: A replication and an extension. J Marriage and the Family, 30: 413–417.

Hobbs DF, Cole SP (1976). Transition to parenthood: A decade replication. J Marriage and the Family, 38, 723–731.

Hobbs DF, Wimbish JM (1977). Transition to parenthood by black couples. J Marriage and the Family, 39: 677–689.

Holden JM, Sagovsky R, Cox JL (1989). Counselling in a general practice setting: controlled study of health visitor intervention in treatment of postpartum depression. Br Med J, 298: 223–226.

Hopkins J, Marcus M, Campbell SB (1984). Postpartum depression: A critical review. Psychol Bull, 95: 498–515.

Janis I (1958). Psychological Stress. New York: John Wiley.

Jaubert MJ (1979). Les bateleurs du mal joli. Paris: Balland.

Kaij L, Jacobson L, Nilsson A (1967). Postpartum mental disorder in an unselected sample. The influence of parity. J Psychosom Res, 10: 317–325.

Kaij L, Nilsson A (1972). Emotional and psychotic illness following childbirth. In: Modern Perspectives in Psycho-Obstetrics. Howells J (ed). London: Oliver & Boyd.

Kellerhals J, Perrin JF, Steinauer-Cresson G, Vonèche L, Wirth G (1982). Mariages au quotidian. Lausanne: Favre.

Kendell RE, Rennie D, Clarke J, Dean C (1981). The social and obstetric correlates of psychiatric admission in the puerperium. Psychol Med, 11: 341–350.

Kendell RE (1985). Emotional and physical factors in the genesis of puerperal mental disorders. J Psychosom Res, 29: 3–11.

King J (1986). Informed consent. Bull Inst Med Ethics. Suppl No. 3. 1–19.

Kumar R, Robson KM (1978). Neurotic disorders during pregnancy and puerperium. In: Mental Illness in Pregnancy and the Puerperium. Sandler MJ (ed). Oxford: Oxford University Press.

Kumar R, Robson KM (1984). A prospective study of emotional disorders in childbearing women. Br J Psychiatry, 144: 35–47.

Leigh D, Pare C, Marks J (1977). A Concise Encyclopaedia of Psychiatry. Lancaster: MTP Press.

LeMasters EE (1957). Parenthood as a crisis. Marriage and Family Living, 19: 352–355.

Locke HJ, Wallace KM (1959). Short marital adjustment and prediction tests. Marriage and Family Living 21: 251–255.

McIntosh J (1986). Postnatal blues; A bio-social phenomenon? Midwifery, 2: 187–192.

Meares R, Grimwade J, Wood C (1976). A possible relationship between anxiety in pregnancy and puerperal depression. J Psychosom Res, 20: 605–610.

Meissner M (1975). Sur la division du travail et l'inégalité des sexes. Sociologie du Travail, 4: 329–350.

Miller BC, Sollie DL (1980). Normal stresses during the transition to parenthood. Family Relation, 29: 459–465.

Meyerowitz JH, Feldman H (1966). Transition to parenthood. Psychiatric Research Reports, 20: 78–84.

Moss P, Plewis I (1977). Mental distress in mothers of pre-school children in Inner London. Psychol Med, 7: 641–652.

Moss P, Bolland G, Foxman R (1982). Transition to Parenthood (Report). London: Department of Health and Social Security.

Nordio S, Piazza G, Stefanini P (1983). Diventar padri. Milano: Angeli.

Norr K, Block C, Charles A, Meyering S, Meyers E (1977). Explaining pain and enjoyment in childbirth. J Health Soc Behav, 18: 260–275.

Nott PN, Franklin M, Armitage C, Gelder MG (1976). Hormonal change and mood in the puerperium. Br J Psychiatry, 128: 279–283.

Oakley A (1976). Housewife. Middlesex, England: Pelican Books.

Oakley A (1979). Becoming a Mother. Oxford: Martin Robertson.

Oakley A (1980). Women Confined. Oxford: Martin Robertson.

Oakley A (1986). Beyond the yellow wallpaper, or taking women seriously. In: Telling the Truth about Jerusalem. Oakley A (ed.). Oxford: Blackwell Publications.

O'Hara MW (1980). A Prospective Study of Postpartum Depression. A test of cognitive and behavioural theories. Unpublished PhD dissertation, University of Pittsburgh.

O'Hara MW, Rehm LP, Campbell SB (1982). Predicting depressing symptomatology: Cognitive behavioural models and postpartum depression. J Abnorm Psychol, 91: 457–461.

O'Hara MW, Rehm LP, Campbell SB (1983). Postpartum depression. A role for social network and life stress variables. J Nerv Ment Dis, 171: 336–341.

Parke R (1981). Fathering. Glasgow: Fontana.

Paykel ES, Emms EM, Fletcher J, Rassaby ES (1980). Life events and social support in puerperal depression. Br J Psychol, 136: 339–346.

Pazzagli A, Benvenuti P, Rossi Monti M (1981). Maternità come crisi. Roma: Il Pensiero Scientifico Editore.

Pedersen F, Yarrow L, Anderson B, Cain R (1978). Conceptualisation of father influence in the infancy period. In: The Social Network of the Developing Infant. Lewis M, Rosenblum L (eds). New York: Plenum Press.

Pitt B (1968). 'Atypical' depression following childbirth. Br J Psychiatry, 114: 1325–1335.

Pitt B (1973). Maternity Blues. Br J Psychiatry, 122: 431–433.

Price G (1977). Factors influencing reciprocity in early mother–infant interaction. Paper presented to the Society for Research in Child Development, March 1977, New Orleans.

Quadagno D, Dixon L, Denney N, Buck H (1986). Postpartum moods in men and women. Am J Obstet Gynecol, 154: 1018–1023.

Racamier PC (1961). La mère et l'enfant dans la psychose du postpartum. Evolution Psychiatrique, 4: 525–570.

Racamier PC (1978). A propos des psychoses de la maternalité. In: Mère mortifère, mère meurtrière, mère mortifiée. Soulé M (ed.). Paris: Editions Sociales Françaises.

Raskin A, Schulterbrandt J, Reatig N, McKeon J (1970). Differential response to chlorpromazine, imipramine and placebo. Arch Gen Psychiatry, 23: 164–173.

Reber A (1985). Dictionary of Psychology. England: Penguin Books.

Richards M, Dunn J, Antonis B (1977). Caretaking in the first year of life: The role of fathers' and mothers' social isolation. Child Care Health Dev, 3: 23–36.

Richman N (1974). The effects of housing on pre-school children and their mothers. Dev Med Child Neurol, 16: 53–58.

Robert HS (1971). Le préjudice corporel de la maternité. Paris: Baillière.

Romito P (1988a). Etude de l'environnement psychologique et social de la maternité et de son influence sur la dépression post-partum. Unpublished PhD dissertation, University of Geneva.

Romito P (1988b) Mother's experience of breast feeding. J Reprod Infant Psychol, 6: 89–99.

Romito P, Chatelanat G (1981). Quelques propos sur l'information concernant grossesse et accouchement dans le magazine 'Parents'. Revue Médicale de la Suisse Romande, 101: 395–401.

Russell C (1974). Transition to parenthood: Problems and gratifications. J Marriage and the Family, 18: 29–46.

Ryder RG (1973). Longitudinal data relating marriage satisfaction and having a child. J Marriage and the Family, 35: 604–607.

Sandler M (1978). Some biological correlates of mental illness in relation to childbirth. In: Mental Illness in Pregnancy and in the Puerperium. Sandler M (ed). Oxford: Oxford University Press.

Scott-Heyes G (1983). Marital adaptation during pregnancy and after childbirth. J Reprod Infant Psychol, 1: 18–28.

Stein G, Milton F, Bebbington P, Wood K, Coppen A (1976). Relationship between mood and free and total plasma tryptophan in postpartum women. Br Med J, 2: 457.

Stern S, Kruckman L (1983). Multi-disciplinary perspective on post-partum depression: An anthropological critique. Soc Sci Med, 17: 1027–1041.

Timpanaro S (1974). Il lapsus freudiano. Firenze: LaNuova Italia. (English translation: The Freudian Slip: Psychoanalysis and Textual Criticism. London: New Left Books, 1976)

Thomas CL, Gordon JE (1959). Psychosis after childbirth:

Ecological aspects of a single impact stress. Am J Med Sci, 238: 363–388.

Todd E (1964). Puerperal depression. A prospective epidemiological study. Lancet, 2: 1264–1266.

Treadway CR, Kane F, Jarrahi-Zadeh A, Lipton M (1969). A psychoendocrine study of pregnancy and puerperium. Am J Psychiatry, 125: 1380–1386.

Van Rillaer J (1980). Les Illusions de la psychanalyse. Bruxelles: Mardaga.

Wallace L (1984). Psychological preparation as a method of reducing the stress of surgery. J Human Stress, Summer: 62–77.

Wallace L (1986). Informed consent to elective surgery: The 'therapeutic' value? Soc Sci Med, 22: 29–33.

Watson JP, Elliott SA, Rugg AJ, Brough DI (1984). Psychiatric disorder in pregnancy and in the first postnatal year. Br J Psychiatry, 14: 453–462.

Weissman M, Klerman G (1977). Sex differences and epidemiology of depression. Arch Gen Psychiatry, 34: 98–110.

Welburn V (1980). Postnatal Depression. Glasgow: Fontana.

Wilson G (1986). Background paper. International Conference 'Housework and Household Production', 4 March 1986, Centre Nationale de Reacherches Scientifiques, Paris.

Wolkind S, Zajicek E (1981). Pregnancy: A Psychological Study. London: Academic Press.

Yalom ID, Lunde D, Moos R, Hamburg D (1968). 'Postpartum blues' syndrome. Arch Gen Psychiatry, 18: 16–27.

Yogman M (1984). Competence and performance of fathers and infants. In: Progress in Child Health. MacFarlane JA (ed). London: Churchill Livingstone.

Part X

Promoting effective care during pregnancy and childbirth

87 National strategies for promoting effective care

David Banta

1 Introduction

For care to be effective, it must be not only efficacious, that is, of demonstrable benefit in an ideal situation; it must also be available, affordable, and acceptable to both providers and consumers of care. This book opened with a group of chapters that began by considering the kind of evidence that should lead to valid inferences about the effectiveness of care during pregnancy and childbirth. In subsequent chapters, most of the elements of care commonly given during pregnancy and childbirth have been considered in the light of the available evidence about their effects. The results of surveys of clinical practice have also been cited throughout the book. These have made it clear that current practice is often 'out-of-line' with the best available evidence about the effects of practice. Mothers and babies thus sometimes receive care which is of dubious benefit or actually harmful, while on other occasions they are not being provided with care from which they could benefit. This state of affairs is clearly unsatisfactory and must be addressed not only on behalf of those using the maternity services, but also in the pursuit of more cost-effective use of resources within the health services.

The promotion of effective and cost-effective health care is at or near the top of the list of policy issues for most industrialized countries. This is primarily because the cost of care at the national level has risen in virtually all of these countries, and it has often proved difficult to demonstrate clear-cut benefits from these increased expenditures. These rising costs have caused policy makers to focus on the various technologies which comprise health care. The word 'technology' is used here in a broad sense, implying 'the systematic applica-tion of scientific or other organized knowledge to practical tasks' (Galbraith 1977). Health care technology thus includes the drugs, devices, and medical and surgical procedures used in health care, as well as the organizational and supportive systems within which such care is provided (Office of Technology Assessment 1978).

2 Obtaining information about the effects of care

The first problem confronting anyone who wishes to promote effective care, whether at national or any other level, is that the relevant information is often not available (Institute of Medicine 1985). No country has a fully developed national effort in health care technology assessment which goes beyond the assessment of drugs. Faced with the problems outlined in the Introduction, however, several countries are moving to develop such a system. Perhaps the furthest ahead is Sweden. The Swedish Planning and Rationalization Institute (SPRI) in Stockholm has been carrying out health care technology assessments to assist national and regional policy-making for more than a decade and it has grown in recent years. With the demonstration of the usefulness of the information produced, the Swedish Medical Research Council declared in 1984 that technology assessment was a priority in its programmes. Simultaneously, the University of Linkoping, with the support of the county council of that area, decided to establish a centre for health care technology assessment headed by a professor of technology assessment. In 1985, the Swedish government appointed a committee to make recommendations on how to develop health care technology assessment activities. The committee recommended a national programme in health care technology assessment, and that recommendation was accepted by the government, which set aside US $1.5 million for the first year of the programme, to begin in June 1986 as a free-standing and independent function. The programme, since named the Swedish Council on Technology Assessment in Health Care, actually began functioning in 1987.

The situation in The Netherlands shares some similarities with that in Sweden. The government has been interested in health care technology assessment for some years, and the Health Council, an independent advisory structure, has issued reports on both specific technologies and on aspects of technology assessment as a field. In 1985, the Steering Committee on Future Health Scenarios appointed a special commission on future health care technology, one of whose tasks was to analyse policies toward health care technology in The Netherlands. The commission was itself a mechanism for identifying future technology, and carried out future-oriented assessments of several technological areas, including genetic screening. The commission was seen by the government as a step toward a national programme in health care technology assessment. At the same time, the government has established a policy that technology assessment will be an integral part of policy making in all areas of science and technology. A programme to implement this policy is being organized by the Ministry of Education and Science, which has cited the programme at the National Academy of Sciences with a first year budget of Dfl. 1.5 million. The programme will include consideration of health care technologies, focusing on those with potentially large social and ethical consequences. The Ministry of Welfare, Public Health and Cultural Affairs has also established a small co-ordinating office for technology assessment which could grow into a national effort.

In the United States, where technology assessment began, no truly national programme or institution has resulted from more than 10 years of effort, but some progress is being made. The Office of Technology Assessment has been working in the health area for more than 10 years, producing policy analyses for the United States Congress. In 1978, legislation established the National Centre for Health Care Technology in the Executive Branch, but it was abolished in 1981. A small part of the centre survived in the National Centre for Health Services Research. In 1985 the Congress passed legislation to change the name of that Centre to include 'Health Care Technology Assessment' and to set aside US $3 million a year for technology assessment. The legislation also established a Council on Health Care Technology at the Institute of Medicine of the National Academy of Sciences to serve as a clearing house for assessment information. In May 1988, the Council held a forum to discuss the assessment of neonatal intensive care.

Other countries, such as Finland, France, and Norway, are discussing the advisability of establishing national efforts, but there is little sign of serious interest in some others. In the United Kingdom, the country of origin of the kind of well-controlled trials upon which inferences about the effects of health care can be based most firmly, responsibility for technology assessment falls in the 'no man's land' between the Department of Health and Social Security (DHSS) and the Medical Research Council (MRC). The Department of Health and Social Security, which is nominally responsible for giving the lead in health services research, maintains that controlled trials are the responsibility of the Medical Research Council. The Medical Research Council, which is nominally responsible for giving the lead in biomedical research, regards controlled trials as health services research, and thus the responsibility of the Department of Health and Social Security.

In the United States, T Chalmers (1982) has been active in promoting the idea that those paying for health care should fund the controlled trials that are so necessary to provide a more rational basis for resource deployment. He points out that cost-containment strategies that refuse to pay for unproven care are already having a beneficial effect on the quality of health care. He proposes that insurance companies and other third party payers should fund controlled trials, since these may lead to monetary savings as ineffective care is discarded. He proposes that for the United States, at least, legislation is needed to assure that this happens.

There has been one move in the United States that is consistent with Chalmers' proposal. The legislation establishing the Diagnosis Related Groups (DRG) system also established the Prospective Payment Assessment Commission (ProPAC), an independent commission, established to advise and assist the government in maintaining and updating the payment system. One part of Prospective Payment Assessment Commission's responsibilities is to assess new health technologies. However, with a 1985 budget of only US $2.4 million, Prospective Payment Assessment Commission has, not surprisingly, been slow to take on this task.

In The Netherlands, the Sick Fund Council has begun technology assessment activities to assist it in making decisions as to whether a technology should be allowed in the benefit package. The Council has funded cost-effectiveness analyses of several organ transplant programmes, most recently for heart transplant. More recently, the Council funded a clinical trial and cost-effectiveness study of *in vitro* fertilization.

The genesis, synthesis, and dissemination of valid information about the effects of health care is obviously a crucial prerequisite if more rational deployment of health service resources is to be achieved and the need for this information will be a recurring theme throughout this chapter. The promotion of effective use of health technologies using the information that is available can be tackled at a number of different levels, and by using a variety of different strategies. The remaining sections of this chapter discuss some strategies that might be pursued by governments and others at national level in attempts to make care more effective and cost-effective (Banta *et al*. 1981).

3 National strategies for promoting effective care

3.1 Strengthening regulatory programmes

The most frequent approach governments have taken to controlling health care technologies is regulatory. When regulation is considered in the health care field, it is usually thought of as being aimed at correcting problems in the 'medical market'. Regulatory interventions involve prohibitions, and are usually directed at the supply side of technology, including industry, hospitals, and health care providers (Russell 1982).

Regulatory programmes have not, in general, been very successful. They are usually born out of substantial political compromise and tend to be weak from the outset. In addition, they must deal with health care technologies one by one, despite a general lack of expertise and access to specific and adequate information. An examination of the effects of health planning law on the adoption of electronic fetal monitoring in United States hospitals, for example, found that most planning agencies did not even deal with the technology (Banta and Thacker 1979a,b). A final problem is that laws and regulations inevitably contain loopholes and other opportunities for evasion (Banta and Russell 1982). One example of the weakness of such programmes is the health planning programme in the United States which functioned from 1974, in part to regulate large investments; another is the 'Article 18' programme in The Netherlands, which regulates the siting of certain large health care technologies, such as equipment for magnetic resonance imaging. Neither of these programmes has been very effective because the counter pressures to adopt and use new technology are very strong.

There is, however, one major exception to this generalization about the relative weakness of regulatory programmes, namely the regulation of drugs for efficacy and safety. All industrialized countries have national programmes for this purpose. Indeed, the case for such programmes has been strengthened by the disastrous consequences of using both diethylstilbestrol (DES) and thalidomide during pregnancy prior to careful assessment and regulation. Drug regulation programmes usually require industry to present data on the efficacy and safety of drugs before they can be marketed. Although these requirements sometimes lead to delays in marketing useful drugs, they are constructive overall (Temin 1980) and generally function well, with reasonably good co-operation from industry. Not only do they help to keep useless and harmful drugs off the market, but they lead to the production of much important information on the efficacy and safety of drugs.

The debates about drug regulation are not usually about whether or not it is desirable in general terms—most commentators seem to think that it is. Discussions tend instead to revolve around the role of drug regulation: should it merely assure that a drug is efficacious and safe (as in the United States), or should it also require that a drug also be an improvement over what is on the market, or even that it is cheaper?

This is not to say that drug regulatory programmes are perfect. They too are subject to political and other pressures. The greatest problem with such programmes, however, is that they may have little influence on actual use of licensed drugs. Once a drug is on the market, physicians tend to use it as they like. Furthermore, and of particular relevance to the promotion of effective care during pregnancy and childbirth, drugs are seldom tested in pregnant women. All drugs should be considered potentially hazardous for the fetus, yet drug prescribing during pregnancy, for example, of oral betamimetics (see Chapter 44), is apparently done without much consideration of such risks.

In most industrialized countries, medical equipment and devices are generally not regulated in the same way that drugs are. Only the United States has a premarketing programme that systematically assesses and regulates all devices for efficacy and safety. The medical devices programme in the United States is analogous to the programme for drugs: companies are required to present evidence of efficacy and safety before the equipment can be marketed. Countries such as The Netherlands are considering what to do about the problem of medical devices, but it is a difficult problem for a small country, which cannot undertake the assessment of thousands of devices on its own. Co-operative arrangements for the sharing of information are developing. Perhaps this is a step toward active regulation.

Some have proposed that other medical and surgical practices be regulated in the same way that drugs are (Chalmers I 1986). Of course, both professional providers and hospitals are regulated in all countries. The typical arrangements require physicians, nurses, and other professionals to be licensed to practice. Hospitals must often be licensed or accredited. These licensing arrangements assure a minimum standard of quality and their importance should not be underestimated. But some current proposals to regulate practice go far beyond present programmes. Under such proposals, a procedure could not be used until the national regulatory programme had examined the evidence for efficacy and safety, and drugs and devices could only be used for approved indications.

Such proposals seem likely to meet a number of difficulties. Although the public is likely to support regulation of products, it is far less likely to support such specific regulation of physicians. Physicians are certainly likely to resist such regulation by all means within their power. Finally, it is difficult to see how monitoring and enforcement could be carried out. Quite apart from these probable difficulties, however, it is probably not desirable to replace professional judgement so completely with bureaucratic judgement, with all that this is likely to imply in terms of conservatism and delays. Nevertheless, even if regulation on the scale proposed by some may be both unfeasible and undesirable, proposals for greater regulation can be linked constructively to payment strategies. This option will be examined in the next section.

3.2 Making use of the financing system

It is natural to consider the use of the financing system to control costs of health technologies. The amount spent on health care by a particular society is more a reflection of the level of its development and wealth than of its health needs. Every society has ways of deciding how much to spend on health care. In some countries, this decision is taken centrally and the total amount budgeted explicitly. This process is followed in the United Kingdom, which has had more success in controlling health care expenditure than most other countries.

Few industrialized countries have health care financing systems with inherent control over expenditures as is the case in the United Kingdom, however. Nevertheless, whatever financing system is in place, every system has inherent incentives. In general, the payment systems in industrialized countries encourage excessive reliance on technology by patients, physicians, and hospitals. In part, this reflects the more general priorities in these societies. Still, many health technologies are used when they have little or no useful effect, provide only duplicative information, or add unnecessary costs.

One example is that of electronic fetal monitoring. In the United States in 1978, a separate fee (usually US $25) for use of the monitor was common, and this encouraged its use in circumstances in which it was unlikely to be useful (Banta and Thacker 1979a,b). Caesarean section provides another example. In countries using fee-for-service payment to physicians, fees for caesarean section tend to be much higher than those paid for attendance at a normal delivery. Marieskind (1979) concluded that high fees for caesarean sections in the United States were one of the main factors generating the high operative delivery rates in that country.

Several papers from Brazil appear to demonstrate the importance of payment. In São Paulo, 75 per cent of private patients (where the physician collects a fee) are delivered by caesarean section, while less than 25 per cent of indigent patients are delivered using the operation (Janowitz et al. 1984). In Fortaleza (Janowitz et al. 1982), a study examined the care of about 6000 women. About half of the 600 private patients were delivered by caesarean section, whereas only 1 in 10 insured patients (for whom the physician received no additional fee for a caesarean delivery) were delivered in this way. Public patients, where the physicians were salaried, had a caesarean section rate of 8 per cent.

A more global approach to payment, such as prospective reimbursement, eliminates financial incentives for use of health technologies in this way. Under prospective reimbursement systems, the rates are set in advance of the time period in which they apply. This limits total revenue, forcing providers to choose among alternative services and among alternative methods of providing those services. A simple kind of prospective reimbursement scheme is a global budget. Romeo et al. (1984) examined the impact of three such schemes on the diffusion of five technologies, three judged to be cost-increasing and two judged to be cost-decreasing. One of the cost-increasing technologies was electronic fetal monitoring. The adoption of the cost-increasing technologies was generally found to be slowed by the budget system.

The philosophy of prospective payment was followed in the development of the Diagnostic Related Groups (DRG) System for hospital payment in the United States Medicare programme in 1983. United States policy makers hope that this system will control costs and affect the use of technology. Predicted effects of the programme on technological change are exceedingly complex (Office of Technology Assessment 1985). What does seem clear is that the incentives within the programme have been changed dramatically. For example, the incentive is now to shorten length of stay in the hospital; to reduce the use of diagnostic services; and to lower staffing levels. Some of the changes flowing from these incentives could benefit those using the health services; others might result in less effective and even harmful forms of care. The Diagnosis Related Groups programme, or one like it, could foster the development of services that are less labour intensive and this might reduce the quality of care in circumstances (intrapartum care, for example) in which machines are sometimes seen as acceptable alternatives to human beings.

A national budgetary system for hospitals has been developed in Canada and appears to have worked reasonably well in controlling costs without adverse effects on health. But some of the changes taking place and being contemplated may not be for the better.

A mechanism often proposed for inclusion in the financing system, with the goal of reducing technology use and expenditures, is cost-sharing. Perhaps the best examination of the effects of this policy was done in the Rand Health Insurance Experiment, in which 7700 persons were randomly assigned to one of several experimental health insurance plans (Lohr *et al.* 1986). Plans which included cost sharing led to decreased services across the entire spectrum of illness and problems, with no discernable encouragement to cost-effective care or selective discouragement to ineffective care. Cost-sharing reduced inappropriate hospital use, but also reduced appropriate use (Siu *et al.* 1986). However, the adverse effect on health was small, although greater among the poor, except for hypertension control, myopia, and for those with conditions requiring hospitalization (Brook *et al.* 1983). Perhaps adverse effects of cost-sharing were offset by benefits of the reduction of inappropriate procedures and hospitalization (Siu *et al.* 1986).

3.3 Modifying the structure of medical practice

Governments sometimes attempt to influence the structure and organization of medical practice. For example, the Health Maintenance Organization (HMO) strategy of the Nixon Administration in the late 1960s was aimed at promoting group practice and other collective arrangements between physicians in the United States. The organizational structure of medical practice has received little attention in the context of the adoption and use of effective health care.

Prepaid group practices in the United States are known to use some technologies, especially hospitalization and certain surgical procedures, at lower rates than fee-for-service practice (Luft 1981). However, it is not clear whether the care provided is more cost-effective as a result, since studies have generally not attempted to measure effectiveness of care (Banta *et al.* 1981). One exception is the Rand Health Insurance Experiment which randomly assigned participants to fee-for-service or Health Maintenance Organization practice in Seattle, Washington (Lohr *et al.* 1986). The study found that medical care costs were strikingly reduced for economically advantaged people and that their health ratings also improved. For low income people, however, although costs were reduced, health outcomes were worse in the Health Maintenance Organization (Ware *et al.* 1986). This implies that Health Maintenance Organizations have a tendency to under-provide services and that low income people may not be able to overcome obstacles to care. Further analysis, with additional health status measures, found consistent results, but with less evidence of a worsened health status for low income people (Sloss *et al.* 1987). This issue obviously needs further examination on other sites.

The research does give striking evidence of the effects of organization on technology and cost-effectiveness of care.

Because the general trend around the world is toward group practice, the implications for the promotion of effective care of encouraging this trend should be further evaluated. It may well be, for example, that some types of organizations, such as prepaid group practices, make more judicious decisions about the adoption and use of new health technologies. Large prepaid group practices such as the Kaiser-Permanente system in the United States certainly have the resources to develop research and evaluation programmes. However, these and other organized systems of care, although sometimes promoting activities such as peer review of practice and monitoring of hospital admissions, have invested little in attempts to generate or synthesize information on effectiveness or cost-effectiveness of care (Office of Technology Assessment 1980). A citizen's commission organized by the Harvard Community Health Plan, an Health Maintenance Organization in Boston, has strongly recommended that such activities be expanded in that Health Maintenance Organization (Loran Commission 1988).

In a broader sense, the organization of services must influence the effectiveness of health services. What are the implications of retaining a strong role for general practitioners, as has been done in Canada, the United Kingdom, and The Netherlands? What are the implications of solo versus group practice? What are the implications of allowing community practitioners direct access to diagnostic services versus requiring patient referral to a specialist? These questions and many others deserve research. A strategy based on evidence of the effects of organization on the quality of care could provide an alternative to an increase in direct regulatory activities. The central problem seems to be that policy makers continue to be interested primarily in controlling costs and pay little attention to issues of effectiveness, and thus the quality of health services.

3.4 Linking reimbursement to evidence of effectiveness

One proposal which combines some elements of all the strategies mentioned so far and which appears to be gaining ground is that payment for a health technology should be conditional on the existence of a satisfactory evaluation of efficacy and safety. If a particular form of care has been shown to be effective its cost should be reimbursed; if it has either been shown to be ineffective, or its value is unknown, the cost of using it should not be reimbursed (Brook *et al.* 1984). This proposal has been partly implemented in the United States Medicare programme. When the programme is not certain about the efficacy and safety of a technology, it turns for guidance to the Office of Health Technology

Assessment, which has prepared over 100 assessments for Medicare since 1981. Many of these assessments have advised against including the technology in the health care package which is covered by the scheme.

In The Netherlands and the United Kingdom, drugs are handled in an analogous way. The drugs may be licensed for sale, but the Sick Fund Council and Department of Health and Social Services respectively make an independent decision as to whether or not to list the drug. If the drug is not listed, it will not be paid for. Thus, although the drug can be purchased if prescribed, it must be purchased out of pocket. Not surprisingly, these drug lists are the most important instruments effecting drug use in The Netherlands and the United Kingdom. In the United Kingdom, for example, there were 13 million less prescriptions written for minor ailments in the 12 months following introduction of the selected drug list than in the year prior to its introduction (Cuthbert 1988). This global reduction was mainly accounted for by reduced prescribing of drugs of questionable efficacy (like cough and cold remedies and vitamins), drugs which are widely regarded as being over-prescribed (like bezodiazepine sedatives and tranquillizers), and analgesics for mild to moderate pain. Reduced prescribing in these categories resulted in an estimated £75 million for other uses within the National Health Service (Newton 1987).

This and similar restricted drug lists are seen not only as a way of reducing the expenditure on drugs, but as an aid to good prescribing and better patient care (Cuthbert 1988). But the major problem with any technology (drug or otherwise), even when its availability is restricted, is to know how to maximize the possibility that it will be used appropriately. In some instances (haematinics during pregnancy, for example), there seems to be over-use (see Chapter 19); in others (antenatal corticosteroids, for example), the problem appears to be under-use (see Chapter 45).

In addition to making *any* reimbursement of the cost of care dependent on evidence of cost-effectiveness, the *amount* of reimbursement can obviously be adjusted with the promotion of effectiveness in mind. For example, payment levels for new technologies are often well above their actual costs, thus providing incentives to provide the technologies in question. Because these payment levels are seldom reduced later, they might reasonably be held down while evidence is assembled concerning the effectiveness and safety of the technologies concerned. Another possibility is to provide larger fees for technologies known to be particularly beneficial, so that providers have an incentive to use them. General practitioners in the United Kingdom, for example, are paid separately for preventive procedures such as cervical smears, immunizations, and other services and this gives them an incentive to provide them.

Linking reimbursement for particular elements of health care to evidence that they can deliver the desired effects is a principle which has obvious appeal. Translating it into practice, however, will require not only endorsement of the principle, but also agreement on the goals of health care and the kind of evidence that should be considered in assessing whether they can be achieved (see Chapter 88).

3.5 Educational strategies

Educational strategies used alone in an attempt to promote effective use of health technologies tend to have a rather limited effect on clinical practice in the short term (Lomas and Haynes 1987; Mugford 1987). In the longer term, however, they may represent the soundest investment of the various attempts to promote more effective care. It would be highly desirable, for example, if physicians were trained to interpret evidence more effectively and to be more discerning in their choice of health care technologies (Jonas 1978). Despite the development of innovative medical schools such as McMaster University in Hamilton, Ontario, and Newcastle, New South Wales, however, medical education has been slow to change in this direction.

Better continuing education for physicians is also needed, especially with the pace of technological change, but good evidence that continuing education has been successful is hard to come by. One example of an exception may be the national programme in Sweden. Before a physician can move up in the administrative hierarchy, he or she must take courses in management organized by the county councils. During the past decade, these courses have increasingly emphasized health technology assessment as a necessary tool for effective management. While no systematic evaluation has been done, observers feel that it has had an impact on technology at the practice level. Another recent trend is to feed back information to physicians on their own practice patterns; perhaps such mechanisms facilitated by the computer age, will be more effective (Hershey *et al.* 1986; Wennberg 1984).

Dissemination of results of assessments of health care technologies is generally poor. Effective dissemination of results depends on knowing how physicians get information. Medical journals and textbooks, continuing medical education courses, and discussions with colleagues appear to be influential sources (Office of Technology Assessment 1982). Manufacturers take other steps toward disseminating information about their products, their two main methods of reaching practitioners being advertising and the use of representatives who visit physician offices. Such information, which is oriented to increasing use, needs to be counterbalanced with information oriented to promoting appropriate use and effectiveness. The Drugs and Therapeutics Bulletin published by the Consumers' Association in the United Kingdom is an example of an attempt to disseminate such counterbalancing information.

A national strategy that includes satisfactory attention to dissemination of valid information about the effects of health care has not been developed in any country. However, some interesting attempts have been made. The National Heart, Lung and Blood Institute of the United States National Institutes of Health pays special attention to the dissemination of the results of the clinical trials that it funds. The vehicles of community dissemination that it recommends are conferences, activities of professional societies, workshops, and articles in less specialized medical publications and the popular press. Professional societies often help disseminate information. The American College of Physicians (the professional society of those practicing internal medicine), for example, has a programme on clinical efficacy. It synthesizes information on efficacy and safety of selected technologies and actively disseminates the results to its membership.

An educational strategy which has been adopted more widely during recent years has been the consensus development process. This generally involves bringing together a group of experts to discuss the evidence concerning a particular technology or practice with the intention of developing recommendations for its appropriate use. This model was developed by the National Institutes of Health in the United States, which has relied primarily on scientific and medical experts for its panels and which has targeted its results primarily to the medical community. The National Institutes of Health programme has carried out consensus development exercises on such subjects as electronic fetal monitoring and caesarean section (National Institutes of Health 1980, 1981). Both of these exercises implied, although they did not state, that these technologies were over-used in the United States.

The effects of the consensus development programmes in different countries have not been evaluated. However, the National Institutes of Health has contracted with the Rand Corporation to carry out an evaluation of the impacts of its programme. The recommendations of the Canadian Consensus Conference Report (1986) on caesarean section are being disseminated and promoted in a number of ways, and their relative success in influencing obstetric practice are being formally evaluated (Lomas 1986).

In some countries, such as the United Kingdom and Denmark, the consensus development process has been conceived far more broadly than the model initiated by the National Institutes of Health. There has been more varied membership on consensus development panels and they have reached out to a broader audience. In the series of consensus conferences organized by the King's Fund Centre in Britain, half of the panel membership has been lay, and the professionals involved have not included any experts on the subject in question. Written and oral evidence is received from expert 'witnesses' as well as from any person who wishes to attend the open sessions. The panel is required to draft a consensus statement in the light of this input. The draft statement is considered again at a public session before being finalized and printed for wide distribution to the lay and professional press, and to lay and professional organizations and individuals likely to be interested in the issue examined.

The public has generally not been considered sufficiently in the educational strategies that have been used in attempts to promote more effective use of health technologies. The area of pregnancy and birth is something of an exception to this general rule. Lay voluntary associations and women's groups have helped to ensure that information on the efficacy and safety of technologies has been prominent in the debates which, in some countries at least, have raged about care during pregnancy and childbirth (see Chapter 7). For example, the book produced by the Boston Women's Health Collective, *Our Bodies, Ourselves* has apparently had a worldwide impact on women's approaches to choices in pregnancy and birth care.

Again, formal evidence that these educational strategies have been effective in promoting better care is not available. But one of the factors which anecdotal evidence suggests may have prompted some British maternity units to abandon some routine practices unsupported by any good evidence was an idea first proposed by the Editor of the *Journal of the Association for Improvements in Maternity Services* (Taylor 1977). The idea was implemented by a popular writer on childbirth, Sheila Kitzinger, who compiled a consumers' guide to British maternity hospitals from information provided both by mothers who had experienced care at each of the hospitals, and (when it was made available) by the hospitals themselves (Kitzinger 1979). The *Good Birth Guide*, as it was called, was an immediate bestseller and gave maternity hospitals a far more explicit public image than they had been used to. One newly appointed obstetrician at a hospital which attracted some rather unfavourable comment asked the editor of the guidebook to make it clear to her readers that, during the interval between her receipt of the comments and their publication, the hospital had 'come under new management'. As new editions of the guidebook are published, British maternity hospitals have opportunities to demonstrate that they have taken steps to attend to the causes of a previously poor public image earned by imposing forms of health care which have never been shown to be effective.

No government has taken an active role in developing such information for lay people, probably because of fears that the implicit encroachment on professional territory would result in a politically unacceptable backlash from the professions. This political timidity may change as it becomes clearer that containing the costs of health care is an issue that no government can escape, and that the resources available should be deployed on forms of health care that have been shown to be effective. The signs that the public may accept this rationale are encouraging. A group practice with consumer control, such as the Group Health Cooperative of Puget Sound in Seattle, Washington provides an interesting model of how health service users who are better informed about issues of effectiveness could have a positive impact on the content of health services. In the Puget Sound Cooperative, consumers interact continually with administrative and clinical staff in attempts to improve care. In 1970, dissatisfied with services for women's needs, a group of members in the plan forced a referendum on the question of expanding such services. After the members had decided to support the general idea, the prepaid package was changed to cover certain services, including contraception for both men and women (Putnam and Banta 1976). Subsequently, the plan responded to consumer concerns about preventive services by setting up a joint provider-consumer committee to examine evidence about the effectiveness of these services and to suggest additions to coverage.

4 Conclusions

Societies have a number of strategies to choose from in attempting to improve the use of health care technology and promote effective care. The need for change soon because of the inexorable rise in health care costs, together with disenchantment with the regulatory approach, has led to financing and technology assessment—and the links between them—receiving more and more attention.

The system of payment for health care in most countries has remained relatively untouched during the past decade. That situation is changing. The concern now is that cost containment strategies will be developed without adequate attention to effectiveness. It seems clear that the most effective strategy for the future must involve linking payment with more controlled assessment of the effects of health care.

Naturally, no strategy can apply to every country. Nevertheless, every country needs a national capability to support health technology assessments. Given the growth of national programmes, international communication in this field will be more and more useful to prevent duplication and to assure efficient use of available resources.

Educational strategies to effect change in the direction of more effective care have not, as yet, been demonstrated to be very effective in the short term. In the long run, however, such strategies offer great potential for having a profound and enduring effect, particularly if there is active involvement of health service users and other members of the public.

References

Banta HD, Kemp K (eds) (1982). The Management of Health Care Technology in Nine Countries. New York: Springer.

Banta HD, Russell LB (1982). Summary and analysis. In: The Management of Health Care Technology in Nine Countries. Banta D, Kemp K (eds). New York: Springer, pp 193–237.

Banta HD, Thacker SB (1979a). Assessing the costs and benefits of electronic fetal monitoring. Obstet Gynecol Surv, 34: 627–642.

Banta HD, Thacker SB (1979b). Policies toward medical technology: The case of electronic fetal monitoring. Am J Public Health, 69: 931–935.

Banta HD, Behney CJ, Willems JS (1981). Toward Rational Technology in Medicine. New York: Springer.

The Boston Women's Health Collective (1984). The New Our Bodies, Ourselves. New York: Simon & Schuster.

Brook RH, Ware JE, Rogers WH, Keeler EB, Davies AR, Donard CA, Goldberg GA, Lohr KN, Masthay PC, Newhouse JP (1983). Does free care improve adults' health? Results from a randomized controlled trial. New Engl J Med, 309: 1426–1434.

Brook RH, Lohr K, Chassin M, Kosecoff J, Fink A, Solomon D (1984). Geographic variations in the use of services: Do they have any clinical significance? Health Aff (Millwood), 3: 62–73.

Chalmers I (1986). Minimizing harm and maximizing benefit during innovation in health care: Controlled or uncontrolled experimentation. Birth, 13: 51–60.

Chalmers T (1982). Who will fund clinical trials? The Sciences, March: 6–8.

Consensus Conference Report (1986). Indications for cesarean section: Final statement of the panel of the National Consensus Conference on Aspects of Cesarean Birth. Can Med Assoc J, 134: 1348–1352.

Cuthbert MF (1988). Répertoire des produits sélectionnes du Royaume-Uni. Industrie Santé 129, February: 19–21.

Galbraith J (1977). The New Industrial State. New York: New American Library, p 31.

Hershey CO, Porter DK, Breslau D, Cohen DI (1986). Influence of simple computerized feedback on prescription charges in an ambulatory clinic. Medical Care, 24: 472–481.

Institute of Medicine (1985). Assessing medical technologies. Report of the Committee for Evaluating Medical Technologies in Clinical Use. Washington DC: National Academy Press.

Janowitz B, Nakamura M, Lins F, Brown M, Clapton D (1982). Cesarean section in Brazil. Soc Sci Med, 16: 19–25.

Janowitz B, Wallace S, Araujo G, Araujo L (1984). Method of payment and the cesarean birth rate in a hospital in Northeast Brazil. J Health Politics Policy and Law, 9: 515–526.

Jonas S (1978). Medical Mystery. New York: Norton.

Kitzinger S (1979). The Good Birth Guide. London: Fontana.

Lohr KN, Brook RH, Kamberg CJ, Goldberg GA, Leibowitz A, Keesey J, Reboussin D, Newhouse JP (1986). Use of medical care in the Rand Health Insurance Experiment, diagnosis and service specific analyses in a randomized controlled trial. Medical Care (Suppl), 24: S71–S87.

Lomas J (1986). The consensus process and evidence dissemination. Can Med Assoc J, 134: 1340–1341.

Lomas J, Haynes RB (1987). A typology and critical review of tested strategies for the application of clinical practice recommendations. Paper presented at the Conference on 'Preventive Services in Primary Care', Ville D'Esterel, Quebec, Canada, 4–7 October.

Loran Commission (1988). Report to the Harvard Community Health Plan. Boston, Massachusetts.

Luft HS (1981). Health Maintenance Organizations: Dimensions of Performance. New York: John Wiley.

Marieskind H (1979). An evaluation of caesarean section in the United States. Final Report submitted to the DHEW Office of the Assistant Secretary for Planning and Evaluation/Health, Washington DC, June.

Mugford M (1987). Effects of feedback of information on clinical practice. Paper presented at a meeting entitled Changing Clinical Practice, King's Fund, 17 June 1987.

National Institutes of Health (1980). National Institute of Child Health and Human Development: Task Force on Predictors of Fetal Distress. Consensus Development Conference on Antenatal Diagnosis. Bethesda, Maryland.

National Institutes of Health (1981). Consensus development conference on cesarean childbirth. Report of the Task Force on Cesarean Childbirth. Bethesda, Maryland.

Newton T (1987). Selected list. Hansard, 113: 75.

Office of Technology Assessment (1978). Assessing the Efficacy and Safety of Medical Technologies. Washington DC: US Government Printing Office.

Office of Technology Assessment (1980). The Implications of Cost-effectiveness Analysis of Medical Technology. Washington DC: US Government Printing Office.

Office of Technology Assessment (1982). Strategies for Medical Technology Assessment. Washington DC: US Government Printing Office.

Office of Technology Assessment (1985). Medicare's Prospective Payment System. Washington DC: US Government Printing Office.

Putnam SM, Banta HD (1976). The consumer and primary care. In: Primary Care and the Practice of Medicine. Noble J (ed). Boston: Little Brown, pp 141–157.

Romeo AA, Wagner JL, Lee RH (1984). Prospective reimbursement and the diffusion of new technologies in hospitals. J Health Economics, 3: 1–24.

Russell LB (1982). Planning and regulation in the allocation process. In: Resources for Health. David Banta (ed). New York: Praeger, pp 175–177.

Siu AL, Sonnenberg FA, Manning WG, Goldberg GA, Bloomfield ES, Newhouse JP, Brook RH (1986). Inappropriate use of hospitals in a randomized trial of health insurance plans. New Engl J Med, 315: 1259–1266.

Sloss EM, Keeler EB, Brook RH, Operskalski BH, Goldberg GA, Newhouse JP (1987). Effect of a health maintenance organization on physiologic health, results from a randomized trial. Ann Intern Med, 106: 130–138.

Taylor A (1977). Maternity matters. Mother and Baby, July: 34.

Temin P (1980). Taking Your Medicine, Drug Regulation in the United States. Cambridge, Mass: Harvard University Press.

Ware JE, Rogers WH, Davies AR, Goldberg GA, Brook RH, Keeler EB, Sherbourne CD, Camp P, Newhouse JP (1986). Comparison of health outcomes at a health maintenance organization with those of fee-for-service care. Lancet, 2: 1071–1022.

Wennberg JE (1984). Dealing with medical practice variations: A proposal for action. Health Aff (Millwood), 3: 6–32.

88 Prospects and problems in promoting effective care at the local level

Sally Macintyre and Maureen Porter

1 Introduction

In this chapter we wish to stress that many of the barriers to the promotion of effective maternity care lie in the social, rather than in the technical or financial, sphere. This is true at the national level, but is particularly so at the local level of maternity care provision. Managers, care providers, and lay persons seeking to promote effective care therefore need to be sensitive to the social factors and processes which are critical in shaping the provision of maternity care.

However appropriate the national standards devised for maternity care might be, it is what happens at a local level—whether that be in an antenatal or a postnatal ward, a labour suite, a nursery, a hospital, or a city— that is really important for the providers and recipients of care. National pronouncements about appropriate or effective care (for example, in Britain, Central Health Services Council 1961; Social Services Committee 1980; Royal College of Obstetricians and Gynaecologists 1982; Munro 1983) are useless unless translated into local, 'coal-face' action. It is sometimes assumed, however, that making national pronouncements is sufficient of itself, and that no monitoring or persuasion is required in order to have the recommendations implemented. In this regard the Social Services Committee of the House of Commons was unusual in following up its Report on Perinatal and Neonatal Mortality (1980) by asking government and other organisations what they had done to implement their recommendations, and then publishing a follow-up report (1984).

The book of which this chapter forms a part has been concerned mainly with reviewing evidence concerning the effectiveness of maternity care, rather than with its efficiency. This is relatively unusual for, historically, there has been more interest in the efficiency of maternity care than in its effectiveness. It has tended to be taken for granted that maternity care does good; the main issue has been how to make the best use of scarce resources. Major national policy decisions—for example, recommendations for increasing the proportion of hospital deliveries (Cranbrook 1959; Peel 1970)— have been made with little or no reference to evidence concerning the effectiveness of such a policy in reducing perinatal death or handicap (Campbell and Macfarlane 1987). Similarly, whether or not domiciliary deliveries have been legalized in various States in the USA seems to have varied according to the personal experiences and views of influential individuals such as Attorney-Generals rather than by reference to the results of evaluative studies (de Vries 1985; Reid M, personal communication). Local administrators have tended to be more concerned with the management of resources—whether to close down or amalgamate small maternity units, for example—than with assessing the effectiveness of such units in promoting certain desired perinatal outcomes. This tradition of taking effectiveness for granted is not peculiar to maternity care but is common to many areas of health care and medical practice (Cochrane 1972).

More recently, there appears to have been a major shift at national and academic level, towards questioning the effectiveness of many routine practices and procedures. The results of such questioning—findings from controlled clinical trials or the recommendations of expert bodies—may, however, fail to percolate through to the local level. It would be interesting to know, for example, how many local units have responded to the results of controlled trials evaluating the effects of enemas at the beginning of labour (see Chapter 51), liberal use of episiotomies (see Chapter 66), hospitalization for bed rest of women with twin pregnancies (see Chapter 39), or to the important recommendations contained in reports such as that on 'Human Relations in Obstetric Care' produced by the Ministry of Health (Central Health Services Council 1961) and that on 'Antenatal and Intrapartum Care' produced by the Royal College of Obstetricians and Gynaecologists (1982).

The more sceptical attitudes to some aspects of maternity care that have become more fashionable at a national and academic level may diffuse to the coal-face. Certainly there is evidence that some providers are becoming more interested in evaluating the effectiveness of various components of their work (Robinson *et al.* 1981; Enkin and Chalmers 1982; Hall *et al.* 1985). Possibly the single most important factor in promoting effective maternity care at a local level is the creation of sceptical and self-critical attitudes on the part of local maternity care managers and providers.

2 Goals

The effectiveness of components of local maternity care provision can only be judged in the light of the goals they are supposed to achieve. But goals for maternity care may be unclear or conflicting. The ultimate goal of maternity care—a happy, healthy baby in a happy, healthy family (Porter 1982)—is pitched at so general a level that everyone can assent to it (and indeed, it would be a brave person who would dissent from it). But how this worthy ultimate goal is operationalized in terms of more specific objectives may be the subject of considerable dissent.

For example, do we want to ensure that no labour lasts longer than 12 hours (O'Driscoll *et al.* 1973), or that obstetric intervention be kept to a minimum (Rakusen and Davidson 1982)? Is it our objective that women be scanned routinely in early pregnancy (see Chapter 27), or that unnecessary visits to hospital should be reduced (Hall *et al.* 1985)? Do we wish to ensure that doctors in training see enough interesting cases to learn from, or that women attending a specialist hospital should always see a fully trained specialist (Hall *et al.* 1985)? Is it more important that new mothers have every opportunity to rest, or that mother–baby and mother–family separation be kept to a minimum and all babies be breastfed (Central Health Services Council 1961)?

The list could go on. The main point is that there are many possible objectives that can be pursued by providers, managers, and users of care; these may differ within and between these three main groups, and may often be mutually incompatible. Promoting effective care at the local level involves clear specification of the goals to be achieved, and then securing agreement both on the goals themselves and on the means to achieve them. This may be difficult when one person's (or professional group's) desirable goal may be another person's (or professional group's) undesirable outcome.

It should also be noted that even if there is agreement on goals, different groups may have different views about the best means of achieving them. The public outcry in Britain about the Medical Research Council's randomized controlled trial of periconceptional multivitamin supplements for women at risk of having babies with neural tube defects arose partly from conflict over the appropriate means—swift implementation of new interventions versus their careful evaluation—of achieving the agreed goal of preventing neural tube defects. There are other instances in which an agreed goal—ensuring that new procedures are introduced only when they have been shown to be effective and safe, for example—is difficult to achieve because research workers, practitioners, and lay people may disagree about the ethics of the evaluative studies proposed.

Some of these conflicts of goals may be deeply embedded both in professional ethos and training, and in organizational exigencies. The legitimate requirements of managers for predictability, clear-cut rules, and order, for example, may conflict with the equally legitimate desires of some providers and users of services for flexibility and variation of treatment according to individual needs. Restricted visiting hours in maternity hospitals may assist ward routines and provide some in-patients with more opportunities for rest, but may be inconvenient and stressful for other mothers and their families. Ensuring that no doctor in an outpatient clinic is kept waiting between seeing successive women may mean that women are, on average, kept waiting longer. Having the woman's partner present throughout labour might be good for the couple's relationship but may make the relationship between the attending midwife and the woman more difficult. Increasing the role of midwives in antenatal care may decrease the role of general practitioners; and indeed both Hall *et al.* (1985) and Draper *et al.* (1984) have argued that there may be no arrangement of antenatal care as between general practitioners, midwives, and obstetricians that is satisfactory to all these professions.

These conflicts of interest arise not (merely) from the whims of individuals, but from structural differences in interests that have to be taken seriously and thought through. They constitute a major problem in any attempts to promote effective care, since care which is effective from one person's viewpoint may have knock-on effects and reduce the effectiveness of care from someone else's viewpoint.

3 Evaluation

Many practices and procedures in maternity care (as in other walks of life and other sectors of health care) can develop a taken-for-granted quality as 'the way things are done'. This has indeed been the response given to both of us in replies to our queries about the reasons for policies or practices as diverse as episiotomies, childbirth preparation classes, annual vaginal examinations for women seeking contraception, a limit of 30 minutes on second stage of labour, perineal shaving, fasting in labour, the administration of milk of magnesia in labour, or health visitors not telephoning clients to make appointments. Many of these procedures and practices were introduced without any evidence of either their effectiveness or their efficiency (McKinlay 1981).

It is interesting to note, however, that while such procedures and practices may not have been evaluated before being introduced, many of them are being evaluated now. This poses the question of why evaluation has recently become so much more popular. Is it because of political and economic trends such as the need for cost containment, the increasing power and influence of consumer pressure groups, the threat of litigation, or the desire of professionals to enhance their scientific credibility? Whatever the reasons, the trend towards more systematic evaluation is to be applauded.

Considerable resistance to systematic evaluation continues to exist, however. We all have a vested psychological interest in believing that what we are doing is valuable and that we are doing it in the best way possible. Doing something differently from one's colleagues may be taken as implying that what your colleagues are doing is wrong, and this can be very threatening for the colleagues and render the 'deviant' unpopular. The recent attempt to suspend a British woman obstetrician, Wendy Savage, is a case in point (Inch 1988). Even simple descriptive statistics, such as the duration of consultations, can be seen as threatening by those whose practices are being described (Macintyre 1984). Professionals or administrators may refuse to believe that complaints about maternity care could be applicable to their own practices or localities—atrocities are always assumed to have been perpetrated by someone else or on someone else's patch—and this refusal can be a tremendous barrier confronting those trying to improve care. Any form of audit or evaluation can potentially be seen as very threatening, and people may thus be reluctant to engage in, permit, or believe the results of any evaluations (Cochrane 1972; Stocking and Morrison 1978; Challah and Mays 1986).

Furthermore, innovators may be so convinced of the value of their innovations, and so impatient to see improvements in patient care, that they may be particularly dismissive of the need for thorough evaluation of their proposals. The reformer's temperament is often very different from that of the evaluator: the latter needs a degree of scepticism and caution that does not sit well with the desire to improve the world, and to do so quickly. The maternity services (and the health services in general) need both types of temperament if effective care is to be promoted.

Where the two types of temperament often clash is in the running of randomized controlled trials. Those who desire to do the best by their patients and to improve the world may be impatient with those who would urge the necessity of painstakingly designed randomized controlled trials to protect patients from unsuspected adverse effects of new treatments. They may urge the abandonment of such trials half-way through, when preliminary results point in a particular direction, even if this means the trial will be inconclusive.

Nevertheless, the involvement of staff in a research project to evaluate the effects of routine practices will sometimes bring about change. A British midwife had experienced difficulty in persuading her colleagues to support her proposal that they should evaluate the routine use of enemas in a randomized controlled trial: they told her that it would be unethical to deny women in the control group the assumed benefits of the policy. The trial was mounted after a grudging acknowledgement that there was no evidence to support their assumption. It was stopped earlier than anticipated because the midwives became convinced by their experience during the trial that it had become unethical to subject women in the experimental group to enemas routinely (Romney and Gordon 1981). This is not the only example of the fluid nature of many ethical judgements about treatment options in health care.

Given the current fashion for evaluation and audit, proposals for change in maternity care tend to gain in credibility and respectability if they are accompanied by plans to evaluate new procedures or practices. However, such evaluations can take on an entirely ritual quality, as if undertaking an evaluation in itself guarantees the success of the new procedure or practice, irrespective of the results of the evaluation. Procedures introduced on a 'trial' basis may thus gradually come to be seen as 'standard practice', with people believing that evaluation has shown them to be beneficial, without this actually being the case (McKinlay 1981).

The results of evaluation may be selectively interpreted by different individuals or interest groups as supporting their own position or preferences. Perceptions of the same study—for example, the Dublin trial of fetal heart monitoring (Macdonald *et al.* 1985) or the Aberdeen test of a new system of antenatal care (Hall *et al.* 1985)—may differ markedly as people take what they want out of the findings. If existing or new procedures and practices are to be evaluated in order to promote effective care, steps therefore have to be taken to surmount the many barriers to systematic evaluation, and to ensure that the evaluation is more than ritualistic.

4 Innovation

It is interesting to note that there are certain aspects of maternity care about which people complain for years but about which nothing whatsoever is done (for example, hospital food, waiting times, waiting lists, being woken at 6 am in hospital, poor communications between professionals and their clients, and so on). Whether or not something is eventually done about these complaints seems to depend less on the rationality or volume of the complaints, and more on social processes that are very complex (Fuller and Myers 1941; Becker 1966; Blumer 1971).

In general, there is a great deal of inertia associated with innovation in medical care (Stocking 1985). There are many good reasons for this. As Coleman, Katz and Menzel wrote in 1966: 'The medical practitioner ... has to be sceptical of the host of major and minor innovations that are urged on him each year. He builds up a certain amount of resistance to innovations, for their advantages are sometimes dubious, often minor by comparison to the cost in new uncertainties, in money, and in mental tooling up, and they occasionally prove to be accompanied by harmful effects. But even "good" changes—innovations that later prove to be of inestimable value in the prevention and treatment of disease—are often resisted. The annals of medical history provide numerous and dramatic examples... And, in almost every case, there was some highly respected scientific leader to head the opposition.' (p. 9, 1966).

Nevertheless, it is usually easier to innovate by adding things to medical practice than to innovate by taking them away, even if the former costs more money or involves more time and resources. This appears to stem from the desire to do something, and to be seen to be doing something, which characterizes the helping professions (Scheff 1963). This can be illustrated by the tendency for all Royal Commissions, Government committees, and similar bodies, to recommend that more things be done rather than that less things be done. It is much more difficult to subtract possibly ineffective practices than it is to add practices which may also be ineffective. 'I am not going to conduct routine vaginal examinations at every antenatal visits any more', or 'let us stop screening pregnant women for glycosuria', earns less 'brownie points' than, 'I have started pre-pregnancy counselling' or 'let us do routine ultrasound screening at *n* weeks' gestation'—even if the demonstrated effectiveness or efficiency of the latter are no greater than of the former. Once some policy or procedure becomes established people develop a vested

interest in it; if one wants to subtract it, one has to deal with their interests and recognize the threat that this subtraction poses to people's positions. If one wants to promote effective care, however, it is important to stop ineffective or inefficient things as well as to add effective things, despite the former often being harder to achieve than the latter.

Professionals and managers often have a low opinion of their patients or clients, and seem to expect the worst of them—for example, that they do not understand technical terminology (McKinlay 1975), will lose their case notes if allowed custody of them (Lovell and Elbourne 1987), will steal toys left in waiting areas (Reid 1983), or be incapable of correctly reporting their menstrual cycle (Porter 1986). This poor view of the moral and intellectual capabilities of their clientele may discourage professionals from introducing otherwise sensible reforms. Single instances of derelictions by their clients ('I had a patient once who ...') can be used for years to justify this resistance. It may thus be necessary to demonstrate, experimentally, that, for example, women are no more likely to lose their case notes than are hospital records departments (Draper *et al.* 1986; Baldry *et al.* 1986), before professionals or managers can be convinced of the reliability of their clientele. Even then however, the experiment may be inconclusive because it is subverted by some of the professionals not giving women the benefit of the doubt even during the experiment (Reid 1983). There is also the problem of getting professionals and managers to allow the experiment to take place in the first place.

People lower down in professional and other hierarchies are often more protective of the status quo and more threatened by change than people at the top. Although juniors may invoke rules imposed on them by their seniors as the reason for certain practices, the seniors may be unaware of these rules or perfectly willing to change them. This greater caution on the part of juniors is perfectly understandable in the light of their vulnerability to criticism and censure from above—particularly in relatively strict hierarchies such as those characteristic of medicine, midwifery, and nursing. The implication of this observation is that in order to institute change it may be necessary to go to the top of the relevant local hierarchies. Whether or not change is then instituted may depend on the personality, style, or politics of these senior people.

A midwife in London had been convinced by the available evidence (see Chapter 51) that the only effects of a policy of routinely shaving the perineum were unwanted effects. She spoke to each of the six senior obstetricians in the maternity unit in which she worked to secure their agreement to the policy being abandoned in respect of the women for whose care each of them was nominally responsible. Five of the six obstetricians, having considered the evidence presented to them by the midwife, concurred in her request that the policy of routine shaving be discontinued. The sixth obstetrician began by insisting that, regardless of the evidence, he wished women admitted under his name to continue to be shaved. His obstructionism collapsed when the midwife made it clear to him that, unless he could provide good evidence to justify routine perineal shaving, she and her colleagues would call him to do the shaving himself every time a woman for whose care he was responsible was admitted to the labour ward!

As Kitzinger (1983) has pointed out, attempts to initiate change may fall prey to 'the patchwork quilt syndrome'. That is, professionals or managers may misunderstand the essence of some complaint about care or proposal for change, and agree to certain peripheral or trivial changes that totally miss the point of the original complaint or proposal. When the misconceived change is criticized, the professionals or managers may then feel hurt or betrayed, feeling that their efforts at improvement are scorned, and in subsequent debates follow the line that 'we gave them what they asked for and they still complained'. Such misperceptions may cause severe problems for the promotion of effective care. Another problem is that administrators or providers may assume that users of maternity care are a homogeneous group with unanimous preferences; they may then be hurt because innovations intended to please clients are not greeted with universal approval (Riley 1977).

Many shifts in policy or practice in maternity care do not stem from gradual, incremental reform, or from collective decision-making. Rather, as with shifts in scientific paradigms (Kuhn 1970; Ravetz 1971), they seem more likely to be triggered by somewhat maverick figures and to occur in large rather than small steps (Mackinlay 1981). Perhaps unlike the situation in science, however, the 'paradigm shifters' in the health professions tend to be placed reasonably high up their professional hierarchies—or at least they have to be so placed if they are to be successful in their efforts to have paradigms shifted. Many of those in the UK who have initiated changes in, or radical shifts in thinking about maternity care are not only strong-minded and sometimes charismatic figures, but have also operated from reputable power bases such as professorships or consultantships. Some innovations have been introduced by firm, centralized, and sometimes autocratic leadership; for example, the Mastership system at the National Maternity Hospital in Dublin facilitated the introduction of a uniform policy for the active management of labour as well as the Dublin randomized trial of fetal monitoring (see Chapter 54). Other innovations have involved a well-placed individual quietly getting on with something; for example, Dr Elizabeth McGregor initiated and organized a model system for call and recall of women for cervical cytology in Aberdeen.

In sum, then, innovation in maternity care is frequently not a rational, incremental, process but may instead involve complex social processes such as the redefinition of a practice or procedure as being problematic; the existence of people high enough up a hierarchy assenting to the change; or the overcoming of professionals' low views of their clientele—all of which can be summarized in the perhaps depressing formula of having the right person in the right place at the right time. In trying to promote effective care, the trick is perhaps to identify that right person.

5 Resources

Lack of money for staffing, equipment, tests, and other facilities is often cited as the reason for less-than-optimally-effective care. This may stem from the assumption that effective care is necessarily expensive care, effectiveness often being equated with heavy use of costly, often centralized, facilities. Often, however, the refusal to contemplate certain changes on the grounds that they will be too expensive is not based on rational calculations about the actual costs. As noted in Chapter 5, very few 'evaluations' of maternity care have had any serious cost–benefit analyses incorporated in them. Having continuity of midwife care during the antenatal or intrapartum periods, for example, has often been dismissed as impracticable or expensive because of duty rotas, but has been shown to be more practicable and less costly than is often thought (O'Driscoll *et al.* 1973; see Chapter 10).

The appeal to lack of resources also derives from the tendency to assume that improvements always involve adding rather than subtracting something from a package of services. If some components of maternity care which are ritualistically adhered to, despite lack of evidence about effectiveness, were to be abolished, then more resources could perhaps be released for other forms of care. Earlier chapters in this book offer many examples of resource-consuming practices that could be safely abandoned on the basis of the available evidence. Similarly, managers and professionals may have to be convinced that not all innovations are more expensive than the forms of care, currently provided, that they are intended to replace.

Many aspects of effective maternity care may not, in any case, depend on the total volume of resources (staffing, hospital beds, etc.), but rather on how these resources are used. In spite of this, there is a tendency to see extra resources—rather than a more effective or efficient deployment of existing resources—as the only solution to perceived problems of local provision. Not unnaturally this may lead to pessimism about the possibility of any improvements. Although to be deplored on other grounds, cuts in health service spending may force a change of perspective and a realization that shifts in the allocation of resources may be possible and beneficial. Midwife care, for example, may be more appropriate and less expensive than obstetric medical care.

6 Collaboration

Collaboration between professionals, whether of the same or different professional affiliation, is extremely important if maternity care is to be effective. Problems in intra-professional collaboration can arise for mundane reasons such as 'busy-ness', tiredness, differences in personal style, communication failures, differences in training, and so on. Difficulties in inter-professional collaboration can also arise from deeper, structural reasons such as differing professional perspectives, orientations and goals; different positions in power hierarchies of status or gender; different information held by various professionals about the same client(s); and differential access to resources. All these, and other factors, may militate against fruitful co-operation (McIntosh and Dingwall 1978). In particular, when the number of births is decreasing, different professional groups may all be protecting their corner and fighting to maintain their share of resources and status.

The tradition of professional autonomy, particularly marked among the medical profession, may create problems for collaboration. Senior doctors may have evolved their own patterns of practice and clinical routines, or may simply continue the practices they were taught in medical school. They may only rarely encounter different ways of doing things because they do not observe their colleagues' practices, nor are they observed by their colleagues. This may lead to very varied practices even among members of the same department or partnership, and this may hinder collaboration, teamwork, and the development of uniform policy. Although there is usually more visibility and uniformity among nursing and midwifery staff in any one setting than there is among medical practitioners, there can be differences in policy and practice between different nursing or midwifery sectors. Midwives taking childbirth preparation classes, for example, may be out of touch with contemporary or local labour ward practice. Policies with regard to breastfeeding on post-natal wards may differ from those prevailing among community midwives who visit new mothers on their discharge from post-natal wards (Macintyre 1981).

Although it would be productive in the long run to foster sceptical attitudes about the efficacy of local practices, this may cause conflict in the short run unless sensitively handled. Scepticism about prevailing patterns may be perceived to be criticism directed towards colleagues in one's own or related professions, and this may be seen as highly threatening and engender defensive reactions. Criticism across professional boundaries may be particularly resented. Supportive mechanisms may thus have to be fostered in order to permit non-threatening self- and mutual criticisms.

Collaboration and co-operation within and between professional groups—and between these groups and users and managers of services—are extremely important. However, there are a number of barriers to, and processes militating against, successful teamwork. Collaboration is thus something that has to be worked at rather than just expected to happen.

7 Conclusions

'Effective care during pregnancy and childbirth' implies different things to different people. It is important to recognize that different people may have different goals, and that the means of achieving these differing goals may be mutually incompatible. Those who wish to promote effective care must thus clarify and agree the goals of care during pregnancy and childbirth having asked and answered the question 'Effective for whom?'

Scepticism about the effectiveness (however this may be defined) of all aspects of maternity care should be fostered, but efforts are required to ensure that this questioning attitude is not experienced as threatening to individual practitioners or particular professions. It should not be assumed that policies and practices automatically have the desired effect, nor that recommended changes necessarily occur in the manner or have the impact envisaged.

Effective maternity care takes place in a social context, and is not simply the delivery of well-validated forms of care with technical excellence. There is always a need to take into account social relationships, social and psychological processes, and concepts such as hierarchy, autonomy, status, power, vested interests, and charisma.

References

Baldry M, Cheal C, Fisher B, Gillett M, Huet V (1986). Giving patients their own records in general practice: experience of patients and staff. Br Med J, 292: 596–598.

Becker HS (ed) (1966). Social Problems: A Modern Approach. New York: John Wiley.

Blumer H (1971). Social Problems as Collective Behaviour. Social Problems, 18: 298–306.

Campbell R, Macfarlane AM (1986). Place of delivery: a review. Br J Obstet Gynaecol, 93: 675–683.

Central Health Services Council (1961). Standing Maternity and Midwifery Advisory Committee: Human Relations in Obstetrics. London: Her Majesty's Stationery Office.

Challah S, Mays NB (1986). The randomised controlled trial in the evaluation of new technology: a case study. Br Med J, 292: 877–879.

Cranbrook Committee (1959). Report of the Maternity Services Committee. London: Her Majesty's Stationery Office.

Cochrane A (1972). Effectiveness and Efficiency: Random Reflections on Health Services. Nuffield Provisional Hospitals Trust, London.

Coleman J, Katz E, Menzel H (1966). Medical Innovation: A Diffusion Study. Indianapolis: Bobbs-Merrill.

De Vries R (1985). Regulating Birth: Midwives, Medicine and the Law. Arizona: Temple University Press.

Draper J, Fields S, Thomas H (1986). The Early Parenthood Project: An Evaluation of a Community Antenatal Clinic. Hughes Hall, Cambridge University (mimeo).

Draper J, Fields S, Thomas H, Hare MJ (1986). Should women carry their antenatal records? Br Med J, 292: 603.

Enkin M, Chalmers I (eds) (1982). Effectiveness and Satisfaction in Antenatal Care. London: Spastics International Medical Publications, Heinemann Medical Books.

Fuller RC, Myers RR (1941). The Natural History of a Social Problem. Am Sociol Rev, June 321–28.

Hall M, Macintyre S, Porter M (1985). Antenatal Care Assessed. Aberdeen: Aberdeen University Press.

Inch S (1988). The Savage suspension: its significance and implications. J R Soc Med, 81: 178–182.

Kitzinger S (1983) The New Good Birth Guide. Harmondsworth: Penguin, p 104.

Kuhn T (1970). The Structure of Scientific Revolutions (2nd edn). Chicago: University of Chicago Press.

Lovell A, Elbourne D (1987) Holding the baby—and your notes. Health Services J, 19 March, 335.

MacDonald D, Grant A, Sheridan-Pereira M, Boylan P, Chalmers I (1985). The Dublin randomized controlled trial of intrapartum fetal heart rate monitoring. Am J Obstet Gynecol, 152: 524–539.

McIntosh J, Dingwall R (1978). Teamwork in Theory and Practice. In Dingwall R and McIntosh J (eds). Readings in the Sociology of Nursing. Edinburgh: Churchill Livingstone.

Macintyre S (1981). Expectations and Experiences of Pregnancy: Report of a Prospective Study of Married Primigravidae. Institute of Medical Sociology, Occasional Paper Number 5, University of Aberdeen.

Macintyre S (1984). Professionals' views of maternity care—a neglected topic? Paper presented to Forum on Maternity and Neonatal Care, Royal Society of Medicine. Reported in J R Soc Med.

McKinlay J (1975). Who is really ignorant—physician or patient? J Health Social Behav, 16: 3–11.

McKinlay J (1981). From 'Promising Report' to 'Standard Procedure'. Seven stages in the career of a Medical Innovation. Milbank Mem Fund Qtrly/Health and Society, 59: 374–411.

Munro Report (1983). First Report of the Maternity Services Advisory Committee, Maternity Care in Action Part I: Antenatal Care. London: Her Majesty's Stationery Office.

O'Driscoll K, Stronge JM, Minoghue M (1973). Active management of labour. Br Med J, 3: 135.

Peel Committee (1970). Standing Maternity and Midwifery Advisory Committee, Domiciliary Midwifery and Maternity Bed Needs. London: Her Majesty's Stationery Office.

Porter M (1982). Interim report in antenatal care in general practice: G.P.s and health visitors in Aberdeen City and Suburbs. University of Aberdeen (mimeo).

Porter M (1986). Professional–client relationships in reproductive health care consultations. Presented at B.S.A. Medical Sociology Group's Scottish Meeting at Pitlochry, March, mimeo, University of Aberdeen.

Rakusen J, Davidson N (1982). Out of Our Hands: What Technology Does to Pregnancy. London: Pan Books.

Ravetz JR (1971). Scientific Knowledge and its Social Problems. Oxford: Clarendon Press.

Reid M (1981). Helping those mothers: antenatal care in a Scottish peripheral housing estate. In Glasgow Women's Studies Group (eds). Uncharted Lives, pp. 163–180, Glasgow: Pressgang.

Riley EMD (1977). 'What do women want?' The question of choice in the conduct of labour. In T Chard and M Richards, Benefits and Hazards of the New Obstetrics. London: Heinemann.

Robinson S, Thomson A (1981). Research and the Midwife: Conference Proceedings 1979 and 1980, Chelsea College of Nursing Research (mimeo).

Romney M, Gordon H (1981). Is your enema really necessary? Br Med J, 282: 1269.

Ross A (1986). The case against showing patients their records. Br Med J, 292: 578.

Royal College of Obstetricians and Gynaecologists (1982) .Report of the RCOG Working Party on Antenatal and Intrapartum Care. London: RCOG.

Scheff T (1963). Decision rules and types of error and their consequences. Behav Sci, 8: 97–107.

Social Services Committee (1980). Perinatal and Neonatal Mortality, Vol. 1. London: Her Majesty's Stationery Office.

Social Services Committee (1984). Perinatal and Neonatal Mortality Report: Follow-Up. London: Her Majesty's Stationery Office.

Stocking B (1985). Initiative and Inertia: Case Studies in the NHS Nuffield Hospitals Provisional Trust. London.

Stocking B, Morrison SL (1978) The Image and the Reality. Oxford: Oxford University Press (for the Nuffield Provincial Hospitals Trust).

89 Effective care in pregnancy and childbirth: a synopsis for guiding practice and research

Iain Chalmers, Murray Enkin, and Marc J. N. C. Keirse

The underlying thesis of this book is that evidence from well-controlled comparisons provides the best basis for choosing among alternative forms of care for pregnancy and childbirth. This evidence should encourage the adoption of useful measures and the abandonment of those that are useless or harmful. It is probably worth noting that the systematic review of evidence on which the book has been based has, at times, shattered our own preconceptions about the effects of care.

In this final chapter we have tried to summarize the main conclusions reached in earlier chapters. This summary takes the form of four Appendices which list, respectively, forms of care that have been shown to reduce negative outcomes of pregnancy and childbirth; forms of care that appear promising, but require further evaluation; forms of care that have unknown effects; and finally, forms of care that we think should be abandoned in the light of the available evidence. The strength of the evidence on which these conclusions are based is discussed in earlier chapters (to which reference is made with each entry in the Appendices).

We hope that the explicit form in which these conclusions have been stated will be useful, and that the advantages of the Appendices will outweigh their drawbacks. A tabulated summary such as this is necessarily selective and, to some extent, subjective. Nuances discussed in earlier chapters cannot find expression in tables. A few of the apparently causal associations listed may have arisen by chance; others may appear to be implausible. Many of the conclusions will be controversial. Our conclusions must obviously be judged in the light of the methods used by our collaborators and ourselves to assemble and review the evidence on which they are based. These were described in the first two chapters of the book.

Before discussing the Appendices in more detail, we would like to reiterate some of the points made in the opening chapters of the book about ways in which the results of research may, and may not, be applicable in practice. First, because research based on the study of groups generates evidence about how people respond to particular forms of care on average, they may be relevant in guiding the development of broad policies for care during pregnancy and childbirth. For example, there is strong evidence that continuity of personal care, combined with efforts to provide social and psychological support during pregnancy and childbirth, is preferred by women, and that it has a number of other beneficial effects; furthermore, there is no evidence that it has any adverse effects. This evidence should be used to support efforts to ensure that continuity of care and the provision of social and psychological support is pursued as a matter of policy. Similarly, there is strong evidence that, compared with other suture materials, catgut used to repair perineal trauma leads to more short-term perineal discomfort, and that it has no compensating advantages. As a matter of policy, therefore, catgut should be abandoned for suturing perineal trauma.

Second, the results of research must be considered in relation to decisions about the care of individuals. Once again, evidence from controlled comparisons will usually identify the form of care that is best for most women and babies. Nevertheless, forms of care that appear to be desirable for the majority of women and babies may be wrong for some of them; conversely, forms of care that do not appear to be effective overall may be effective for some women or babies. Improvements in diagnostic accuracy should help caregivers to identify individual women and babies who are likely to respond in an atypical way to particular forms of care. Although advances in diagnostic accuracy will undoubtedly occur, however, tailoring care to meet the specific needs of individuals will continue to be more of an art than a science. This art can be improved by listening more carefully to what women have to say, and by involving them to a greater extent in decisions about their care.

Lastly, there is an important additional dimension to be considered in assessing the implications for care of the results of the reviews presented earlier. This is that different people will use the evidence presented in this book in different ways because of the different values they assign to particular forms of care and their effects. Their judgements will differ when it comes to assessing whether the benefits of a particular form of care are sufficient to outweigh its costs, whether the latter are assessed in terms of unwanted physical or psychological effects, inconvenience, or resource consequences. In other words, the differing circumstances and values of different individuals may provoke different reactions to the same quality of evidence—as common sense would suggest they should. Knowledge of the effects of care, however, is a necessary prerequisite if the choices made by individuals about care are to be properly informed. We hope that the four Appendices that follow, used in conjunction with the chapters on which they have been based, will assist this process of informed choice.

Appendix 1 lists forms of care that, in our opinion, have been shown to reduce negative outcomes of pregnancy and childbirth. We do not pretend that it is comprehensive because there are many aspects of care (transfusions for haemorrhagic shock, for example) that are so obviously worthwhile that their inclusion would have appeared trite. Our decision to include forms of care in Appendix 1 was usually made because the estimates of their beneficial effects derived from controlled trials were statistically significant. Other evidence was used when we considered it to be sufficiently strong.

The inclusion of a particular form of care in Appendix 1 does not necessarily imply that it should be adopted in practice. Whether the forms of care included in this Appendix are adopted will depend on assessments of the importance of the likely benefits weighed against the importance of the likely costs. For a variety of reasons, as noted above, perceptions of this relationship between benefits and costs will vary from individual to individual, and from situation to situation. Although the available evidence suggests that the forms of care included in Appendix 1 do indeed reduce the negative outcomes listed, these welcome effects are sometimes achieved at the cost of increasing unwanted effects. Thus, genetic amniocentesis, although it leads to improved detection of fetal chromosomal abnormalities, increases the risk of miscarriage and neonatal respiratory morbidity; epidural anaesthesia, while providing very effective relief of pain during labour, increases the chances that instrumental assistance will be used for delivery; and pharmacological suppression of lactation, although reducing unpleasant symptoms in the short term, may result in 'rebound' lactation and breast symptoms two or three weeks after delivery.

In addition, although a certain form of care may well be able to reduce the frequency of a particular negative outcome, the outcome may already be so rare (or be considered so trivial) that adoption of this form of care would seem unwarranted. These considerations might

apply to screening for gonorrhoea during pregnancy to reduce the incidence of gonococcal ophthalmia; or to the routine use of continuous electronic fetal heart rate monitoring with fetal scalp blood sampling during labour to reduce the incidence of early neonatal seizures; or to routine ultrasonography in early pregnancy to reduce the incidence of induction of labour for 'post-term' pregnancy.

Appendix 2 lists those forms of care that appear to be promising in the light of the available evidence, but which, in our opinion, require further evaluation before informed decisions can be made about whether or not they should be adopted in practice. Some of the forms of care in Appendix 2 were included because the estimates of their effects did not quite reach conventional levels of statistical significance; others were included because we felt that a statistically significant reduction in negative effects may have reflected bias because of the quality of the available evidence. Some of the possible effects of forms of care included in Appendix 2 could be of great relevance for improving the effectiveness of care, and it is important that they should receive some priority in future research.

Appendix 3 lists forms of care for which we feel there is simply too little good evidence to permit an informed judgement about their effects one way or the other. Some of the forms of care listed may reduce the likelihood of substantive negative outcomes of pregnancy and childbirth; others may have valuable placebo effects. Other forms of care included in Appendix 3 may have no important beneficial effects, or may, on balance, actually do more harm than good. Because of these uncertainties, those who use or advocate the forms of care listed in Appendix 3 should be aware of their inadequately evaluated status, and should collaborate in well-designed studies to assess their effects. This should apply especially to those forms of care that are costly in terms of resources. Those who do not use these forms of care should not introduce them, unless this is done within the context of properly controlled trials to assess whether they do more good than harm. Such assessment should be made in terms of substantive, not intermediate outcomes. A reasonable 'rule of thumb' for deciding whether a particular outcome should be regarded as substantive is to ask whether parents regard it as important.

Finally, Appendix 4 lists those forms of care which, in our view, should be abandoned. Inclusion of a form of care in this table does not imply that no woman or baby could ever derive benefit from it. Forms of care have been included in Appendix 4 either because we feel that the evidence suggests that their adverse effects are likely to outweigh any conceivable beneficial effects that they may have; or because alternative forms of care, which we judge to be preferable, are available. Many of the forms of care included in Appendix 4 are unjustified routines and policies, which, applied inflexibly, result in the differing needs of individual women being ignored.

As stated in our Preface, there is still scope for considerable disagreement about many of the conclusions that we and our collaborators have reached. While we have made great efforts to ensure that the data presented are comprehensive and accurate, it is likely that some important studies have been overlooked, and that errors and misinterpretations have crept in. We conclude by reiterating our invitation to readers to bring omissions and mistakes to our attention for inclusion and correction in later editions of this book. We shall ensure that those who help us in this way are appropriately acknowledged.

Appendix 1 Forms of care that reduce negative outcomes of pregnancy and childbirth

Intervention	Effects	Chapters
Enhanced social and psychological support from caregivers	Reduced: —poor communication with staff —dissatisfaction with care —not feeling 'in control' —worries and unhappiness —feeding problems with baby —feeling physically unwell 6 weeks postpartum	6–15
Various anti-smoking interventions, particularly behaviour modification techniques and psychological support	Reduced: —smoking during pregnancy —low average birthweight	16
Carbohydrate supplements for malnourished women	Reduced: —low average birthweight	17
Antenatal classes	Reduced: —use of pharmacological analgesia in labour	16, 20
Serum alpha-feto-protein estimation	Improved: —detection of neural tube malformations —detection of Down's syndrome	23
Genetic amniocentesis	Diagnosis of: —chromosomal disorders —neural tube malformations	23
Measurement of blood pressure during pregnancy	Improved: —detection of pre-eclampsia	24
Selective use of ultrasonography	Improved: —confirmation of fetal life —estimation of gestational duration —estimation of fetal size —estimation of amniotic fluid volume —detection of fetal malformation —location of placenta —investigation of pelvic masses —establishment of fetal presentation	27
High vs. low feedback to mother during ultrasonography	Reduced: —negative feelings about examination	27
Routine ultrasonography in early pregnancy	Reduced: —induction of labour for 'post-term' pregnancy	27
Antiemetics (antihistamines, Debendox/Bendectin) for nausea/vomiting	Reduced: —nausea and vomiting	32
Antacids for heartburn	Reduced: —heartburn	32
Increased dietary fibre intake	Reduced: —constipation	32
Bulking agents and stool softeners	Reduced: —constipation	32
Prophylactic diuretics for woman at increased risk of pre-eclampsia	Reduced: —hypertension	33
Methyldopa for hypertension	Reduced: —severe hypertension	33

Appendix 1 Forms of care that reduce negative outcomes of pregnancy and childbirth—*continued*

Intervention	*Effects*	*Chapters*
Beta blockers for hypertension	Reduced: —severe hypertension	33
Antihypertensive therapy for severe hypertension	Reduced: —hypertensive encephalopathy —cerebral haemorrhage	33
Screening and treatment for asymptomatic bacteriuria	Reduced: —persistent/recurrent bacteriuria —pyelonephritis	34
Screening and treatment for syphilis	Reduced: —congenital syphilis	34
Screening and treatment for gonorrhoea	Reduced: —gonococcal disease in mother and baby	34
Clotrimazole for candidiasis	Reduced: —persistent candidiasis —infant colonization	34
Imidazoles vs. nystatin for candidiasis	Reduced: —persistent candidiasis	34
Metronidazole (after organogenesis complete) for symptomatic trichomonal vaginitis	Reduced: —symptomatic vaginitis	34
Intrapartum antibiotics for group B strep. colonization	Reduced: —infant colonization —infant sepsis with group B strep.	34, 43
Rubella vaccination postpartum	Reduced: —rubella embryopathy in subsequent pregnancy	34
Anti-D postpartum for Rh negative women with Rh positive babies	Reduced: —isoimmunization after 6 months —isoimmunization in subsequent pregnancy	35
Screening for Rh status and anti-D Rh globulin for Rh negative women during pregnancy	Reduced: —positive Kleihauer test at 32–35 weeks —positive Kleihauer test at delivery —isoimmunization 6 months postpartum	35
Tight vs. moderate control of diabetes	Reduced: —urinary tract infection —caesarean section —preterm birth —macrosomia —respiratory distress syndrome —perinatal mortality	36
Cervical cerclage for history of previous 2nd trimester miscarriage	Reduced: —delivery before 33 weeks —miscarriage or perinatal death	40
External cephalic version at term for breech presentation	Reduced: —non-cephalic births —caesarean section	42
Antibiotics after prelabour rupture of membranes	Reduced: —puerperal infectious morbidity	43, 64
Effecting delivery when signs of infection after prelabour rupture of membranes	Reduced: —infectious morbidity	43, 64
Betamimetic tocolytics in preterm labour	Reduced: —delivery within 24 hours —delivery within 48 hours —delivery before 37 weeks	44
Indomethacin in preterm labour	Reduced: —delivery within 48 hours —delivery within 7–10 days —delivery before 37 weeks —birthweight below 2500 grams	44

Appendix 1 Forms of care that reduce negative outcomes of pregnancy and childbirth—*continued*

Intervention	Effects	Chapters
Oral betamimetics for maintenance after inhibition of preterm labour	Reduced: —recurrent preterm labour	44
Corticosteroids prior to preterm delivery	Reduced: —respiratory distress syndrome —periventricular haemorrhage —necrotizing enterocolitis —early neonatal death	43, 45
Social and psychological support during labour	Reduced: —augmentation of labour —caesarean section	49
Antacids before general anaesthesia	Reduced: —gastric acidity	52
Vaginal vs. rectal examinations to assess progress in labour	Reduced: —maternal discomfort from examination	53
Electronic fetal heart monitoring + scalp sampling vs. intermittent auscultation	Reduced: —early neonatal seizures	54
Intravenous preloading before epidural anaesthesia	Reduced: —maternal hypotension —fetal heart rate abnormalities	54
Upright vs. recumbent position during first stage of labour	Reduced: —use of narcotics/epidural	55
Systemic narcotics during labour	Reduced: —pain	52, 57
Epidural vs. systemic narcotics during labour	Reduced: —pain	57
Scheduled top-ups of epidural vs. top-ups at maternal request	Reduced: —episodes of severe pain	57
Epidural vs. placebo after 8 cm	Reduced: —pain in second stage	57
Methoxyflurane vs. nitrous oxide	Reduced: —nausea and vomiting	57
PGE_2 for cervical ripening	Reduced: —induction–delivery interval > 24 hours —operative delivery	61
$PGF_{2\alpha}$ for cervical ripening	Reduced: —induction–delivery interval > 24 hours —operative delivery	61
Oestrogens for cervical ripening	Reduced: —caesarean section	61
Amniotomy + early vs. + late oxytocin for induction	Reduced: —induction–delivery interval > 24 hours —operative delivery —postpartum haemorrhage	62
Oxytocin + amniotomy vs. oxytocin alone for induction	Reduced: —induction–delivery interval > 24 hours	62
Prostaglandins vs. placebo for induction	Reduced: —induction–delivery interval > 24 hours —caesarean section	62
Prostaglandins vs. oxytocin for induction	Reduced: —induction–delivery interval > 24 hours —operative delivery	63
Prostaglandins/analogues for induction after fetal death	Reduced: —failure to deliver vaginally	65
Low dose vs. high dose prostaglandin analogues for induction after fetal death	Reduced: —maternal morbidity	65

Appendix 1 Forms of care that reduce negative outcomes of pregnancy and childbirth—*continued*

Intervention	Effects	Chapters
Upright vs. recumbent position during second stage of labour	Reduced: —abnormal fetal heart rate patterns —severe pain —low umbilical artery pH (<7.25)	66
Lateral tilt vs. dorsal position during second stage of labour	Reduced: —low umbilical arterial pH	66
Exhalatory vs. sustained bearing down during second stage labour	Reduced: —abnormal fetal heart rate patterns —low Apgar scores	66
Late vs. early pushing with epidural during second stage of labour	Reduced: —use of rotational forceps	66
Restricted vs. liberal use of episiotomy at delivery	Reduced: —overall trauma —perineal trauma	66
Active management of third stage of labour	Reduced: —postpartum haemorrhage	67
Free bleeding from placental end of cord	Reduced: —feto–maternal transfusion	67
Early cord clamping	Reduced: —length of third stage	67
Prophylactic oxytocics in third stage	Reduced: —postpartum haemorrhage	67
Prostaglandins for otherwise uncontrollable postpartum haemorrhage due to uterine atony	Reduced: —emergency hysterectomy/internal iliac artery ligation	67
Continuous vs. interrupted sutures for perineal trauma	Reduced: —short-term perineal pain	68
Polyglycolic acid vs. catgut sutures	Reduced: —short-term perineal pain	68
Polyglycolic acid vs. silk or nylon sutures	Reduced: —short-term perineal pain	68
Policy of trial of labour after previous caesarean section	Reduced: —caesarean section —maternal morbidity	70
Vacuum extraction vs. forceps delivery (all indications)	Reduced: —maternal injury —use of major anaesthesia	71
Vacuum extraction vs. forceps for rotational deliveries	Reduced: —maternal injury —use of major anaesthesia	71
Cricoid pressure during induction of general anaesthesia	Reduced: —aspiration of gastric contents	72
Uterine exteriorization vs. intraperitoneal repair at caesarean, when exposure is difficult	Reduced: —serious infection	72
Prophylactic antibiotics with emergency caesarean section	Reduced: —endometritis —serious infection —wound infection —febrile morbidity	73
Prophylactic antibiotics with elective caesarean section	Reduced: —endometritis —serious infection —wound infection —febrile morbidity	73
Antibiotic vs. placebo irrigation with caesarean section	Reduced: —febrile morbidity	73
Ultrasound examination prior to preterm delivery	Reduced: —unnecessary caesarean sections for babies with lethal malformations	74

Appendix 1 Forms of care that reduce negative outcomes of pregnancy and childbirth—*continued*

Intervention	Effects	Chapters
Referral to institution with intensive care facilities for very preterm birth	Reduced: —neonatal mortality —neonatal morbidity	74
Neonatologist for immediate care of very preterm infant	Reduced: —neonatal morbidity	74, 75
Prevention of neonatal hypothermia in delivery room	Reduced: —acidosis	75
Prophylactic calf or human surfactant for preterm infants	Reduced: —moderate/severe respiratory distress syndrome —pneumothorax —periventricular haemorrhage —neonatal death	75
Prophylactic 'artificial lung expanding compound' for preterm infants	Reduced: —moderate/severe respiratory distress syndrome —neonatal death	75
Silver nitrate for prophylaxis against gonococcal conjunctivitis	Reduced: —gonococcal conjunctivitis	34, 75
Antibiotic prophylaxis against neonatal gonococcal conjunctivitis	Reduced: —gonococcal conjunctivitis	75
Erythromycin ointment vs. silver nitrate for prophylaxis against bacterial conjunctivitis	Reduced: —chemical conjunctivitis	34, 75
Unrestricted mother–infant contact following delivery	Reduced: —breastfeeding failure	77, 80
Prophylactic triple dye on umbilical cord	Reduced: —staphylococcal skin colonization	78
Prophylactic neomycin on umbilical cord	Reduced: —staphylococcal skin colonization	78
Local anaesthetic in aqueous form for perineal pain	Reduced: —perineal pain	79
Unrestricted breastfeeding	Reduced: —breastfeeding failure	80, 81
Social support and information for nursing mothers	Reduced: —breastfeeding failure	80, 81
Bromocriptine for non-breastfeeding mothers	Reduced: —breast pain during first week —continued lactation during first and second weeks —engorgement during first and second weeks	82
Synthetic oestrogens for non-breastfeeding mothers	Reduced: —breast pain during first week —continued lactation during first week —engorgement during first week	82
Oestrogen/testosterone combination for non-breastfeeding mothers	Reduced: —breast pain during first week —continued lactation during first week —engorgement during first week	82
Bromocriptine vs. breast binders for non-breastfeeding mothers	Reduced: —breast pain during first week —continued lactation during first week —engorgement during first week	82
Screening for phenylketonuria	Reduced: —symptomatic disease	84
Screening for congenital hypothyroidism	Reduced: —symptomatic disease	84
Enhanced care for bereaved parents	Reduced: —depression at 6 months postpartum —anxiety at 6 months postpartum	85

Appendix 2 Forms of care that appear promising, but require further evaluation

Intervention	Possible beneficial effects	Chapters
Folate supplements for malnourished/still growing pregnant women/girls	Possibly reduced: —low birthweight —stunted maternal growth	19
Antenatal classes	Possibly reduced: —low self-esteem —dissatisfaction in pregnancy and childbirth	20
Antenatal expression of colostrum	Possibly reduced: —breast engorgement —damaged nipples —breastfeeding failure	21
Anticipatory guidance for women wishing to breastfeed	Possibly reduced: —breastfeeding failure	21
Home monitoring of uterine contractions in women at increased risk of preterm labour	Possibly reduced: —preterm labour	22, 44
Routine ultrasound placentography in 3rd trimester	Possibly reduced: —low Apgar score —perinatal death	27
Dilute hydrochloric acid for heartburn	Possibly reduced: —heartburn	32
Prostigmine for heartburn	Possibly reduced: —heartburn	32
Sodium chloride for leg cramps	Possibly reduced: —leg cramps	32
Anti-platelet agents for increased risk of pre-eclampsia and fetal growth retardation	Possibly reduced: —proteinuria —severe pre-eclampsia —recurrent fetal growth retardation —perinatal death	33
Plasma volume expansion for severe pre-eclampsia	Possibly reduced: —oliguria —severe hypertension	33
Plasmapheresis in severe Rhesus disease	Possibly reduced: —perinatal morbidity and mortality	35
Hospitalization and bed rest for multiple pregnancy	Possibly reduced: —diastolic BP > 109 mm Hg	39
Abdominal decompression for compromised fetus	Possibly reduced: —proteinuria/pre-eclampsia —fetal distress in labour —birthweight less than 2500 grams —low Apgar score at 1 minute —perinatal death	41
Ultrasonography for surveillance after prelabour rupture of membranes preterm	Possibly reduced: —perinatal morbidity	43
Using prophylactic antibiotics with corticosteroids after prelabour rupture of membranes preterm	Possibly reduced: —maternal infectious morbidity —neonatal infectious morbidity	43
17-alpha hydroxyprogesterone caproate IM in women at increased risk of preterm delivery	Possibly reduced: —preterm delivery —low birthweight	44
Prophylactic progestagens for women at increased risk of preterm labour	Possibly reduced: —perinatal morbidity	44
Thyroid-releasing hormone in addition to corticosteroids prior to preterm delivery	Possibly reduced: —days on artificial ventilation —days in supplementary oxygen	45
Amnioinfusion for intrapartum 'fetal distress'	Possibly reduced: —persistent fetal heart rate abnormality	54
Intravenous betamimetics for intrapartum 'fetal distress'	Possibly reduced: —persistent fetal heart rate abnormality	54

Appendix 2 Forms of care that appear promising, but require further evaluation—*continued*

Intervention	Possible beneficial effects	Chapters
Piracetam for intrapartum 'fetal distress'	Possibly reduced: —caesarean section —neonatal morbidity	54
Self-administered vs. scheduled narcotics	Possibly reduced: —total dose of narcotics —pain	57
Amniotomy to augment spontaneous labour	Possibly reduced: —use of oxytocin —instrumental vaginal delivery	58
Prostaglandins when induction required after prelabour rupture of membranes	Possibly reduced: —operative delivery	64
Syntometrine vs. oxytocin for third stage of labour	Possibly reduced: —postpartum haemorrhage	67
Multiple vs. single doses of antibiotics with caesarean section	Possibly reduced: —febrile morbidity	73
Maternal phenobarbitone prior to preterm delivery	Possibly reduced: —intraventricular haemorrhage —perinatal death	74
Tracheal suction for depressed meconium-stained neonates	Possibly reduced: —severe meconium aspiration syndrome	75
Elective intubation for neonatal resuscitation	Possibly reduced: —asphyxial damage	75
Routine administration of Vitamin K to neonates	Possibly reduced: —haemorrhagic disease —intracranial haemorrhage	75
Antibiotic prophylaxis against neonatal chlamydial conjunctivitis	Possibly reduced: —chlamydial conjunctivitis	75
Oral proteolytic enzymes for perineal trauma	Possibly reduced: —short-term perineal pain —perineal oedema	79
Correct positioning of baby at breast	Possibly reduced: —breast engorgement —sore nipples —breastfeeding failure	80, 81
Oral proteolytic enzymes for breast engorgement	Possibly reduced: —breast engorgement	80, 81
Bromocriptine vs. stilboestrol for lactation suppression	Possibly reduced: —continued lactation during first week —breast pain during first week —engorgement during first week	82

Appendix 3 Forms of care with unknown effects, which require further evaluation

Intervention	Assessment of effects required in terms of:	Chapters
Modification of working patterns during pregnancy	—maternal and perinatal morbidity	6, 14
Periconceptional pre/proscriptions for women without overt problems	—maternal and perinatal morbidity	16
Periconceptional multivitamins and folate	—neural tube defects	16
Advice to abstain from coitus and alcohol during pregnancy	—perinatal morbidity	16
Nutritional advice and/or supplements	—pre-eclampsia —maternal and perinatal morbidity —childhood morbidity	17, 18
Routine iron and/or folate supplements	—maternal and perinatal morbidity	19
Different types of antenatal classes	—maternal and perinatal morbidity —paternal lack of involvement with child	20, 86
Woolwich shells for inverted nipples	—breastfeeding failure	21
Hoffman's exercises for inverted nipples	—breastfeeding failure	21
Frequency and timing of antenatal visits	—diagnosis of pre-eclampsia —antenatal hospital admission —maternal and perinatal morbidity	22–24
Formal risk scoring	—maternal anxiety —maternal and perinatal morbidity	22
Routine pelvic examination with antenatal visits	—preterm labour —perinatal morbidity	22
Chorion villus sampling vs. amniocentesis	—miscarriage —maternal and perinatal morbidity —childhood morbidity	23
Glucose tolerance testing	—maternal and perinatal morbidity —perinatal mortality	25
Serial fundal height/girth measurements	—perinatal morbidity	26
Routine ultrasound for fetal anthropometry and congenital malformations	—maternal and perinatal morbidity	27
Doppler ultrasound for fetal and uteroplacental blood flow	—maternal and perinatal morbidity	27
All biochemical tests of fetal wellbeing	—perinatal morbidity	29
All biophysical tests of fetal wellbeing	—perinatal morbidity	30
X-ray pelvimetry with breech presentation	—caesarean section —maternal and perinatal morbidity	31, 42
Calcium for leg cramps	—leg cramps	32
Vitamin D for leg cramps	—leg cramps	32
Quinine for leg cramps	—leg cramps	32
Routine screening for chlamydia	—neonatal infection	34
Routine screening for toxoplasmosis	—neonatal infection	34
Routine screening for HIV infection	—neonatal infection	34
Alternative treatment regimens for vaginitis	—symptomatic vaginitis	34
Treatment of mycoplasma colonization	—maternal and perinatal morbidity	34
Antiviral agents for active genital herpes	—persistent infection —herpes infection of newborn	34
Caesarean section for herpes with no clinical evidence of active disease	—herpes infection of newborn —maternal and perinatal morbidity	34
Repeated viral cultures for history of herpes	—herpes infection of newborn	34
Hospitalization for uncomplicated multiple pregnancy	—perinatal morbidity	39
Hospitalization for non-proteinuric hypertension	—development of proteinuria —severe hypertension —maternal and perinatal morbidity	39

Appendix 3 Forms of care with unknown effects, which require further evaluation—*continued*

Intervention	Assessment of effects required in terms of:	Chapters
Strict bed rest for proteinuric hypertension	—fulminating pre-eclampsia —maternal morbidity —perinatal morbidity and mortality	39
Cervical cerclage, other than for history of 2nd trimester miscarriage	—preterm delivery —admission to hospital —maternal and perinatal morbidity	40
Postural management for breech presentation	—non-cephalic birth —caesarean section —maternal and perinatal morbidity	42
Amniocentesis after prelabour rupture of membranes preterm	—maternal and perinatal morbidity	43
Routine digital or speculum examination after prelabour rupture of membranes	—maternal and perinatal morbidity	43, 64
Amnioinfusion during preterm labour after prelabour rupture of membranes	—caesarean section —perinatal morbidity	43
Betamimetics after prelabour rupture of membranes preterm	—maternal and perinatal morbidity	43, 44
Prophylactic oral betamimetics for twin pregnancy	—perinatal morbidity	44
Prophylactic oral betamimetics for other women at increased risk of preterm labour	—perinatal morbidity	44
Routine magnesium supplementation to prevent preterm delivery	—perinatal morbidity	44
Magnesium sulphate for inhibition of preterm labour	—maternal and perinatal morbidity	44
Diazoxide for inhibition of preterm labour	—maternal and perinatal morbidity	44
Oxytocin analogues for inhibition of preterm labour	—maternal and perinatal morbidity	44
Calcium antagonists to counteract side-effects of betamimetics	—maternal and perinatal morbidity	44
Beta blockers to counteract side-effects of betamimetics	—maternal and perinatal morbidity	44
Fetal weight estimations as a guide to care for preterm delivery	—caesarean section —perinatal morbidity	44
Elective induction of labour at 42 + weeks	—caesarean section —maternal and perinatal morbidity	47
Routine withholding of food and oral fluids during labour	—aspiration of gastric contents —maternal morbidity —operative delivery	52
Non-pharmacological methods of pain relief	—labour pain —use of pharmacological analgesia —maternal and perinatal morbidity	56
Epidural narcotics with or without local anaesthetic agents	—pain relief —maternal and perinatal morbidity	57
Early oxytocin to augment spontaneous labour	—use of analgesia —hyperstimulation —operative delivery —perinatal morbidity	58
Alternative oxytocic regimens for augmenting spontaneous labour	—use of analgesia —hyperstimulation —operative delivery —perinatal morbidity	58
Relaxin for cervical ripening	—caesarean section —perinatal morbidity	61
Sweeping (stripping) of membranes at term	—need for formal induction of labour —maternal morbidity —perinatal morbidity	62
Automatic oxytocin infusion apparatus for induction	—maternal discomfort and morbidity —perinatal morbidity	62

Appendix 3 Forms of care with unknown effects, which require further evaluation—*continued*

Intervention	Assessment of effects required in terms of:	Chapters
Prostaglandins vs. oxytocin for induction	—maternal discomfort and morbidity —perinatal morbidity	63
Induction of labour for prelabour rupture of membranes at term	—caesarean section —maternal and perinatal morbidity	64
Alternative regimens for prostaglandin analogues for induction after fetal death	—maternal morbidity	65
Perineal massage in labour	—perineal trauma —maternal discomfort	66
Midline vs. mediolateral episiotomy	—perineal pain —dyspareunia —longer-term maternal morbidity	66
Intraumbilical vein oxytocin for retained placenta	—manual removal of placenta —maternal morbidity	67
Non-absorbable synthetic suture vs. polyglycolic acid suture for subcuticular skin closure	—perineal pain —perineal irritation	68
Apposition vs. suturing of perineal skin for perineal trauma	—perineal pain —delayed wound healing	68
Vacuum extraction vs. forceps delivery	—short- and long-term effects on baby	71
Alternative designs of vacuum extractor	—instrument failure —maternal and fetal injury	71
Different antibiotic regimens for prophylaxis with caesarean section	—maternal morbidity —prevalence of commensal flora	73
Shorter vs. longer courses of antibiotics with caesarean section	—maternal morbidity	73
Routine vs. selective caesarean section for very preterm delivery	—maternal and perinatal morbidity	74
Routine vs. selective forceps for vaginal delivery preterm	—maternal and perinatal morbidity	74
Routine vs. selective episiotomy for vaginal delivery preterm	—maternal and perinatal morbidity	74
Routine pharyngeal suctioning of neonates at birth	—gas exchange —aspiration —colonization	75
Tracheal suction for non-depressed, meconium-stained neonates at birth	—meconium aspiration syndrome —pulmonary artery hypertension —infectious morbidity	75
Sodium bicarbonate administration to asphyxiated neonates	—intracranial haemorrhage —sequelae of asphyxia	75
Alcohol-based dressings for umbilical cord	—neonatal infection	78
Routine observations of maternal temperature, pulse, blood pressure, fundal height, lochia	—maternal morbidity	78
Ultrasound therapy for perineal pain	—perineal pain	79
Pulsed electromagnetic energy therapy for perineal pain	—perineal pain	79
Postnatal pelvic floor exercises	—perineal pain —urinary incontinence	79
Steroids added to local anaesthetics for perineal pain	—perineal pain —perineal wound infection	79
Dopamine antagonists for inadequate milk supply	—breastfeeding failure	80, 81
Nipple shields for nipple trauma	—nipple pain —nipple trauma —breastfeeding failure	81
Bromocriptine vs. breast binders and analgesics for non-breastfeeding mothers	—breast symptoms during first postpartum month	82
Routine paediatric examination of newborn	—infant morbidity	83

Appendix 4 Forms of care that should be abandoned in the light of the available evidence

Forms of care	Chapters
Failing to involve women in decisions about their care	7, 8, 15
Failing to provide continuity of care during pregnancy and childbirth	8–10, 49
Leaving women unattended during labour	8, 49, 58
Involving doctors in the care of all women during pregnancy	10–12
Involving obstetricians in the care of all women during pregnancy	10–13
Insisting on universal institutional confinement	11–13
Prescribing high-density protein supplements during pregnancy	17
Advising restriction of weight-gain during pregnancy	17, 18
Measuring maternal weight routinely throughout pregnancy	18, 26
Advising restriction of salt intake during pregnancy	18
Measuring haemoglobin at every antenatal visit	19
'Conditioning' nipples during pregnancy	21
Performing X-ray pelvimetry in cephalic presentations	31
Prescribing saline cathartics or lubricant oils for constipation	32
Prescribing stilboestrol during pregnancy	38
Using external cephalic version electively before term	42
Inducing labour for uncomplicated prelabour rupture of membranes preterm	43
Expanding plasma volume before using betamimetics in preterm labour	44
Prescribing ethanol for inhibition of preterm labour	44
Prescribing progesterone for inhibition of preterm labour	44
Prescribing aspirin for inhibition of preterm labour	44
Inducing labour routinely at less than 42 weeks' gestation	47
Shaving the perineum routinely prior to delivery	50, 51
Administering enemas or suppositories routinely during labour	50, 51
Limiting duration of second stage of labour arbitrarily	53, 66
Routine continuous monitoring of the fetal heart rate without fetal scalp blood sampling	54
Restricting maternal position during labour and delivery	55, 58, 66
Prescribing sedatives or tranquillizers routinely during labour	57
Using oxytocin for cervical ripening	61
Using mechanical methods for cervical ripening	61
Using breast stimulation for cervical ripening	61
Using oral prostaglandins for cervical ripening	61
Inducing labour with oral prostaglandin F_2 alpha	62
Inducing labour routinely after prelabour rupture of membranes at term	64
Inducing labour with oxytocin or oestrogens after fetal death preterm	65
Directing maternal pushing during second stage of labour	66
Performing episiotomy routinely	66
Using catgut, nylon, or silk sutures for skin closure of perineal trauma	68
Using glycerol-impregnated catgut sutures for repair of perineal trauma	68
Repeating caesarean section routinely after previous caesarean section	70
Selecting care for preterm delivery on the basis of estimated fetal weight	74
Failing to provide adequate warmth for newborn infants	74, 75
Performing gastric suctioning of newborn infants routinely	75
Separating healthy mothers and babies routinely	77, 78
Using prophylactic silver sulphadiazine on umbilical cord	78
Bathing newborn infants routinely in hexachlorophene	78
Prescribing routine use of gowns and masks in normal newborn nurseries	78
Prohibiting all sibling visiting postnatally	78
Restricting maternal access to non-prescription drugs postpartum	78
Administering laxatives routinely postpartum	78
Administering oral ergometrine routinely postpartum	80
Providing additional fluids to breastfed infants routinely	80
Scheduling the timing and duration of breastfeeds routinely	80, 81
Providing formula supplements to breastfed infants routinely	80
Test weighing term breastfed infants routinely	80
Giving free formula samples to breastfeeding mothers	80
Prescribing combined oral contraceptives for breastfeeding mothers	80
Prescribing increased fluid intake for breastfeeding mothers	80
Using topical applications for nipple trauma	80, 81
Scheduling duration of postnatal hospital stay inflexibly	78
Failing to take account of women's social circumstances postpartum	86

Index

bathing
  in labour 898, 899
  see also hydrotherapy
  newborn 1336
  for relief of perineal pain 1348,
    1349, 1350
bearing down 1129, 1130
  effect on duration of second
    stage 1130
  effect on instrumental vaginal
    delivery rate 1135
  effect on umbilical artery pH
    1130
bed rest in hospital 624–32
  economic evaluation 92
  hypertension 628–31
  multiple pregnancy 625–9
  threatened miscarriage 624, 625
  twin pregnancy 92
behaviour
  at birth, animal 798–801
  maternal 795, 796, 1323–7
    effect of restricting mother-
      infant contact 1323–7
    endocrine regulation of 796
    mammalian 798–801
behavioural modification, smoking
  246
Bendectin 503–6
  see also Debendox
benzodiazepines 923
  see also sedatives/tranquillizers
bereavement 106, 1423–32
  autopsy 1427
  care in community 1428
  care in hospital 1426
  communication 1427
  community care 1428
  counselling 1426–9
  counsellors 1429
  death registration 1427
  follow-up care 1428
  funeral arrangements 1427
  grief reactions 1423–377
  illness and impairment 1425,
    1426
  immediate care 1426, 1427
  perinatal death 1424, 1425, 1431
  self-help groups 1429
  specialist counsellors 1429
beta–1 blockers 712, 713
  use with betamimetics 712, 713
beta-blockers 521–4
  atenolol 522
  effect on perinatal death 522–4
  effect on proteinuria 522, 523
  effect on severe hypertension
    522, 523, 526
  labetalol 521, 522
  metoprolol 522
  oxyprenolol 522

versus methyldopa 523, 524
betamethasone for pulmonary
  maturity 747, 748
  versus ambroxol 761
  see also corticosteroids
betamimetics 696–715
  adverse effects 706–11
  cardiovascular effects 710, 711
  effect on preterm delivery 714
  effect on recurrence of preterm
    labour 714
  effect on respiratory distress
    syndrome 715
  for inhibition of active labour
    preterm 700–13
  intravenous for fetal distress in
    labour 855, 856
    effect on Apgar score 856
    effect on perinatal mortality
      856
    effect on persistent fetal heart
      rate abnormality 856
  for maintenance of tocolysis 713,
    714
    effect on perinatal death 714
  mechanisms of action 696, 697
  metabolic effects 711
  myocardial ischaemia 710
  prophylactic 697–700
    effect on low birthweight 698,
      700
    effect on perinatal death 698,
      699, 700
    effect on preterm delivery 698,
      699
    effect on respiratory distress
      syndrome 699, 701
    multiple pregnancy 697, 698
    in prelabour rupture of
      membranes preterm 674–
      7
  see also tocolytics, prophylactic
  pulmonary oedema 707–9
  range of drugs used 696, 697
  symptomatic effects 706
  use with other drugs 711–13
  versus ethanol in preterm labour
    723–695
    effect on delay in delivery 724
    effect on low birth weight 725
    effect on perinatal death 725
    effect on preterm delivery 724
    effect on respiratory distress
      syndrome 726
beta receptors 697
bias 15–20
  in allocation 15, 16
  in analysis 18–20
  in assessment of outcome 18
  citation 24
  in delivery of care 16, 17

in interpretation of diagnostic
  tests 75, 76
  publication 24–5
bilirubin, neonatal, effect of early
  cord clamping 1163
biochemical fetal monitoring in
  labour, continuous 876, 877
biochemical tests of fetal well-
  being 455–77
  see also alpha-fetoprotein;
    haemoglobin; human
    chorionic gonadotrophin;
    human placental lactogen;
    oestriol; oestrogens;
    placental proteins
biofeedback 324
biophysical tests of fetal well-being
  477–92
  see also individual tests
biparietal diameter, fetal 416
  in intrauterine growth
    retardation 416
  ultrasound assessment 421, 422
birth
  anthropology 99, 101, 105
  biology of 795–804
  ceremonies 99
  comparative 795–804
  medicalization 146
  rituals 106
birth centres 120, 121, 147, 149,
  152
birth companions 125, 222, 807–
  10, 816, 821, 822, 825
  at admission 821, 822, 825
  effect on intervention rate 808–
    10
  effect of social support 227
  fathers and husbands 807–9
  friends and relatives 104
  professionals (monitrice, doula)
    809–12
birth environment 806, 812
  effect on intervention rate 806,
    807, 812
  effect on stress 806, 812
  home 806
    see also home birth
  hospital 104, 107, 806, 807, 812
    see also hospital
  implications for support 806–7
birth experience 152
birth injury 407, 408
  gestational diabetes and 407, 408
  macrosomia and 407, 408
birth plans 175, 816, 821
birth rate 112, 113, 117
birth rooms 121, 137, 146, 812
  see also birth centres
birthweight
  assessment of 411–18

Down's syndrome 136
droperidol 923, 924
    see also sedatives/tranquillizers
Duchenne muscular dystrophy
    371, 1418, 1421
ductus arteriosus, effect of
    prostaglandin synthesis
    inhibitors 720, 721
duration of labour, effect of
    induction of labour for
    prelabour rupture of
    membranes at term 1115
dyslexia, ultrasound as possible
    aetiological factor 434, 435
dyspareunia 1348
    effect of absorbable versus non-
      absorbable sutures 1179
    effect of adding salt to bath
      water 1349
    effect of continuous versus
      interrupted suture 1172
    effect of glycerol-impregnated
      catgut 1176
    effect of polyglycolic acid versus
      catgut 1175
    gel for relief of 1348
dystocia 840–3
    amniotomy 954
    general measures 951, 952
    measures to increase uterine
      contractility 952–60
    measures to influence cervical
      resistance 960–2
    oxytocin 957
    treatment of 951–66
      see also augmentation of
        labour
      see also macrosomia, caesarean
        section for; shoulder
        dystocia

early discharge postpartum 121,
    1341–4
eclampsia 284, 382, 528, 529
    anticonvulsant agents 528, 529
economic evaluation of care 86–95
ectopic pregnancy, ultrasound
    diagnosis of 420
educational influentials 1192
educational strategies 1454–6
effacement of cervix 836
efficacy versus effectiveness 17, 27,
    28
efficiency of care 1458, 1462
elective delivery 981–7
    assessing place of 982, 983
    comparison of methods 983–6
    definition 981
    evaluation of 981–7

frequency 981, 982
outcomes used for assessment
    983–5
in post-term pregnancy 780–8
    clinical trials 781–3
    effect on Apgar scores 786
    effect on caesarean section rate
      788
    effect on epidural anaesthesia
      rate of use 787
    effect on fetal heart rate
      abnormalities 785
    effect on instrumental vaginal
      delivery 787, 788
    effect on meconium stained
      fluid 784
    effect on neonatal jaundice 786
    effects 780–8
    incidence 780, 781
    women's views 789
    preterm 1272, 1273
    trends 981, 982
    variations in practice 981, 982
electrocardiography, fetal 848
    see also fetal electrocardiography
electroencephalography, fetal 876
electronic fetal heart rate
    monitoring, continuous
    accuracy 850
    on admission 875, 876
      see also admission test
    equipment malfunction 853
    false positive interpretations 877
    interpretation 850–2
    methods 850
    observer variation 850–2
    predictive properties 852–4
    randomized trials 858–74
    women's views of 874
electronic fetal monitoring 41, 125,
    1319
    effect on cerebral palsies 1319
    liberal versus restrictive use
      effect on caesarean section rate
        865
      effect on instrumental vaginal
        delivery rate 866
      effect on neonatal seizures 873
      effect on perinatal mortality
        870
employment 206
    see also work
endometritis, effect of prophylactic
    antibiotics with
  caesarean section 1253, 1254
endorphins, intrathecal 942
enemas 107, 113, 117, 817, 823,
    824, 1341
    effect on faecal soiling 824
enflurane 921
    see also inhalation analgesia

Entonox 921
    see also inhalation analgesia
epidural 117, 169, 170, 321, 322,
    328, 461, 607, 926–42
    administration of top-ups by
      midwives 927
    availability of service 926
    for caesarean section 1238, 1239
    clinical trials 943–14
    complications of 929, 930
    continued administration after 8
      cm dilatation 927, 928
    continuous administration versus
      intermittent top-ups
      927, 928
    desire for 926
    effect on duration of first stage
      labour 927
    effect on instrumental delivery
      rate 927
    effect on instrumental vaginal
      delivery rate 1218
    effect on maternal pushing 1218
    effect on pain in labour 937
    frequency of use 924–6
    narcotics 934, 936
      clinical trials 936
      duration of analgesia 934, 936
      pruritis 934, 936
      respiratory depression 934
      urinary retention 934
    placenta praevia 607
    preloading with intravenous 855
    preterm delivery 1282, 1283
    with previous caesarean 1209
    rate of use 107
      effect of amniotomy with early
        versus late oxytocin
        for induction of labour 1062
      effect of antenatal classes on
        321, 324, 325
      effect of automated versus
        standard oxytocin for
        induction of labour 1065
      effect of continuous EFM
        versus intermittent
        auscultation 868
      effect of induction of labour
        for post-term pregnancy
        787
      effect of oestrogens for
        cervical ripening 1046
      effect of prostaglandins for
        cervical ripening 994,
        998, 1008
      effect of social support 231
      effect of sulprostone after fetal
        death 1123
      effect of TENS 904
    remuneration for 927
    safety 929, 930

oxytocin—*contd*
  intraumbilical vein 1146
  for postpartum haemorrhage
      1146
  prophylactic in third stage of
      labour 1147
  rate of use, effect of amniotomy
      954, 955
  for retained placenta 1146
  with second stage of labour 1217
  versus ergot alkaloids 1155–6
  versus syntometrine, effect on
      postpartum haemorrhage 53
oxytocin analogues for inhibition
    of preterm labour 736
oxytocinase (cystoaminopeptidase)
    469
  as test of fetal well-being 469
oxytocin challenge test (OCT) 479
oxytocin receptor blockers for
    inhibition of preterm labour
    736

paediatrician at preterm delivery
    1285
pain 104, 138, 597, 893–912
  adaptation 899
  attitudes towards 893, 894
  beliefs about 893, 894
  childbirth 99
  effect of forceps versus vacuum
      extraction 1227
  gate control theory 895
  labour 99, 885, 888
    effects of position during first
        stage of labour 885, 888
    see also labour pain
  modification of perception 895–
      905
  pathophysiology 894, 899
  perineal 1137, 1138, 1347–58
    effect of absorbable versus
        non-absorbable sutures
        1178
    effect of adding salt to bath
        water 1349
    effect of adding Savlon to bath
        water 1350
    effect of continuous versus
        interrupted suture 1172
    effect of episiotomy 1138
    effect of glycerol-impregnated
        catgut 1176
    effect of polyglycolic acid
        versus catgut 1174, 1175
    local anaesthetics 1351, 1352
    local antiseptics 1349
    non-pharmaceutical
        applications 1347–9
    oral analgesics 1355, 1356

pelvic floor exercises 1353
proteolytic enzymes 1353,
    1354, 1355
pulsed electromagnetic energy
    1352, 1353
relief of pressure 1352
therapeutic ultrasound 1352,
    1353
topical steroids 1351
placental abruption 597
postpartum 1340, 1341
stimuli 895
transmission of stimuli 894, 899
see also labour pain
paracervical block 117, 937–42
  clinical trials 939–41
  ease of administration 937
  effectiveness for pain relief 939–
      41
  effects on Apgar score 940, 941
  fetal bradycardia 940, 941
  fetal hazards 937, 938
  mechanism of effect 938
  side effects 938
  variations in use 937
  see also regional analgesia
paracetamol for perineal pain 1355
parity and post-term pregnancy
    770, 771
partogram 839, 840, 842, 843
  alert line 839, 840, 841
  transfer line 841
patent ductus arteriosus 1299,
    1301, 1302
payment for obstetrical services
    1452–4
pelvic floor exercises 1353
pelvic mass, ultrasound assessment
    of 424
pelvimetry
  clinical 493, 495
  X-ray 494–7
    computed tomographic 497
    see also X-ray pelvimetry
penicillin 540
  broad spectrum 537
    for bacteriuria 537
      effect on persistent bacteriuria
          537
    for pyelonephritis 537
  effect on febrile morbidity 1261
  prophylactic use with caesarean
      section 1247, 1248, 1249,
      1250, 1261, 1262
    versus cephalosporins 1261
  prophylaxis for ophthalmia
      neonatorum 540
pentazocine 918
  see also narcotics
pentobarbital 923
  see also sedatives/tranquillizers

perinatal death 628, 630, 1424,
    1425
  causes of in post-term pregnancy
      778
  effect of amnioinfusion in
      prelabour rupture of
      membranes 688
  effect of bed rest for
      hypertension 630
  effect of bed rest for twins 628
  effect of betamimetics
    in active preterm labour 707
    maintenance 714
    prophylactic 698, 700
      in prelabour rupture of
          membranes preterm 677
    versus ethanol for preterm
        labour 725
  effect of ethanol for inhibition of
      preterm labour 723
  effect of induction of labour in
      prelabour rupture of
      membranes preterm 681
  effect of oestrogens for cervical
      ripening 1036, 1047
  effect of progesterone 729
  effect of prophylactic antibiotics
      in prelabour rupture of
      membranes preterm 675
  effect of prostaglandins for
      cervical ripening 996, 1006
  endocervical 1028
  effect of prostaglandins for
      induction of labour
    intravenous, versus
        intravenous oxytocin 1102
    oral
      versus intravenous oxytocin
          1108
      versus oxytocin 1097
  effect of therapeutic tocolysis in
      prelabour rupture of
      membranes preterm 686
  see also mortality, perinatal;
      perinatal mortality
perinatal morbidity
  gestational diabetes and 406–10
  in post-term pregnancy 778,
      779, 781
perinatal mortality 207, 262, 263,
    265, 427, 457, 462, 578, 579,
    582, 584, 588, 589, 595, 596,
    649, 650, 657, 659, 855, 869
  diabetes 578, 579, 582, 584
  diabetic nephropathy 582
  effect of abdominal
      decompression 649
    for compromised fetus 651
  effect of antihypertensive
      therapy 527
  effect of antiplatelet therapy 520

size, fetal 411–18
  abdominal palpation 414
  fundal height 415
  ultrasound 415, 416
skin lesions of newborn 1406, 1407
smoking 242–7, 596
  behavioural modification 246
  congenital malformations 243
  counselling 245
  effect on birthweight 242, 246
  miscarriage and 243
  placental abruption 596
  pre-eclampsia 243
  as risk marker 348
  see also advice, smoking
social class 82, 132, 207–9
  caesarean section rate and 1189,
    1190
social policies 205, 207, 210
social sciences 81–6
sodium bicarbonate for
    resuscitation of newborn 1305,
    1306
sodium citrate 830
  to reduce gastric acidity 830
specialist counsellors 1429
  bereavement 1429
specificity of diagnostic test 70
speculum examination 605
  placenta praevia 605
  in prelabour rupture of
      membranes preterm 669–70
spina bifida, ultrasound diagnosis
    421
spinal anaesthesia 116, 117, 942
  for caesarean section 1239
  comparison with epidural 942
spiramycin 547
sprays, perineal 1347, 1348
station of fetal head 1217
  abdominal assessment 1217
  vaginal assessment 1217
statistical methods 47, 48, 62, 63
statistical significance 20, 21
steroids, topical, for perineal
    trauma 1351
stilboestrol
  for breast engorgement 1376
  effect on breast symptoms 1392–
    4
stillbirth 584
  diabetes 584
  effect of corticosteroids for
      pulmonary maturity 754
  effect of diethylstilboestrol 613
  effect of diuretics 516
  effect of folate supplementation
      314
  effect of progestagens 617
  preterm delivery 1272
stomach tube 829, 830
  to reduce gastric volume 829, 830

strategies to promote effective care
  local 1458–64
  national 1449–57
streptococcus, group B 551–5
  see also group B streptococcus
stress 250, 251
  biological effects of 801–2
  in labour 806, 812
    effect of environment 806
studies, research
  evaluation of quality 46, 47
  grouping 45
  heterogeneity 49–52
  identification 43, 44
  methodological quality 49–52
  unpublished 43, 44
study design 6–21
  see also controlled studies
Stutz pessary 643
  effect on delivery before 33
    weeks 643
  effect on pregnancy loss 643
  effect on preterm delivery 643
  versus cervical cerclage 642, 643
suckling, time of, effect on
    breastfeeding 1360, 1361
suction
  gastric, of newborn 1294
  nasopharyngeal, of newborn
    1294
    benefits 1294
    hazards 1294
    technique 1294
  tracheal, of newborn 1296
    with meconium 1296
  of very low birthweight infant
    1296, 1297
sulphonamide creams for perineal
    trauma 1350
sulphur and pre-eclampsia 291
sulpiride
  effect on breast milk production
    1381–5
  effect on prolactin levels 1381–5
sulprostone for induction of labour
    after fetal death 1122–4
  effect on diarrhoea 1123
  effect on epidural rate 1123
  effect on induction-delivery
      interval 1123
  effect on manual removal of
      placenta rate 1123
  effect on placental retention 1123
  effect on postpartum
      haemorrhage 1124
  effect on pyrexia 1123
  effect on vomiting 1123
supine position 884, 890
  effect on fetus 884
  effect on maternal
      haemodynamics 884
  effect on uterine contractions 884

see also position, maternal,
    during first stage of labour
supplementary feeding of breastfed
    babies 1366–8
  effect on duration of
      breastfeeding 1367
support
  for breastfeeding mothers 1370
  effect on breastfeeding 1370
  emotional 162
  financial 210
  in labour 321, 322, 805–14
    by companions 806
    by midwife 805, 809, 813
    definition 805
    effect on Apgar score 811
    effect on caesarean section rate
      811
    effect on instrumental delivery
      rate 811
    effect on intervention rate 806
    effect on labour augmentation
      rate 810
    effect on meconium stained
      liquor 811
    home 807
    hospital 806
    separation from other
        caregiving functions 805,
        806
  postpartum 1333, 1341
  psychological 221
  social 136, 145, 210, 221
surfactant
  effect on bronchopulmonary
      dysplasia 1298, 1299, 1300
  effect on intraventricular
      haemorrhage 1298, 1299,
      1301, 1302
  effect on necrotizing enterocolitis
      1299, 1300, 1301, 1302
  effect on periventricular
      haemorrhage 1298, 1299,
      1301, 1302
  effect on pneumothorax 1298,
      1299, 1301, 1302
  effect on respiratory distress
      syndrome 1298, 1300,
      1302
  for pulmonary immaturity 1297–
    303
suture, continuous versus
    interrupted 1172
  effect on dyspareunia 1172
  effect on perineal pain 1172
suture materials for repair of
    perineal trauma 1173–9
  absorbable versus non-
      absorbable 1177–9
  effect on dyspareunia 1175
  effect on perineal pain 1174,
      1175